Meyler's Side Effects of Drugs

The International Encyclopedia of Adverse Drug Reactions and Interactions

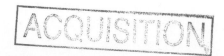

Complementary to this volume
Side Effects of Drugs Annuals 24–29 (1999–2006)
Edited by Jeffrey K. Aronson (Earlier annuals are no longer available in print)

Drugs During Pregnancy and Lactation, Second edition (2006)
Edited by Christof Schaefer et al.

The Law and Ethics of the Pharmaceutical Industry (2005)
By Graham Dukes

Introduction to Clinical Pharmacology, Fifth edition (2006)
By Marilyn Edmunds

Principles of Clinical Pharmacology, Second edition (2006)
Edited by Arthur Atkinson et al.

Writing Clinical Research Protocols (2006)
By E. De Renzo

A Pharmacology Primer (2003)
By Terry Kenakin

Publishing history of *Meyler's Side Effects of Drugs*

Volume*	Date of publication	Editors
First published in Dutch	1951	L Meyler
First published in English	1952	L Meyler
First updating volume	1957	L Meyler
Second volume	1958	L Meyler
Third volume	1960	L Meyler
Fourth volume	1964	L Meyler
Fifth volume	1966	L Meyler, C Dalderup, W Van Dijl, and HGG Bouma
Sixth volume	1968	L Meyler and A Herxheimer
Seventh volume	1972	L Meyler and A Herxheimer
Eighth volume	1975	MNG Dukes
Ninth edition	1980	MNG Dukes
Tenth edition	1984	MNG Dukes
Eleventh edition	1988	MNG Dukes
Twelfth edition	1992	MNG Dukes
Thirteenth edition	1996	MNG Dukes
Fourteenth edition	2000	MNG Dukes & JK Aronson
Fifteenth edition	2006	JK Aronson

*The first eight volumes were updates; the ninth edition was the first encyclopedic version and updating continued with the Side Effects of Drugs Annual (SEDA) series.

At various times, full or shortened editions of volumes in the Side Effects series have appeared in French, Russian, Dutch, German, and Japanese.
The website of *Meyler's Side Effects of Drugs* can be viewed at:
http://www.elsevier.com/locate/Meyler.

Meyler's Side Effects of Drugs

The International Encyclopedia of Adverse Drug Reactions and Interactions

Fifteenth edition

Editor

JK Aronson, MA, DPhil, MBChB, FRCP, FBPharmacol S
Oxford, United Kingdom

Honorary Editor

MNG Dukes, MA, DPhil, MB, FRCP
Oslo, Norway

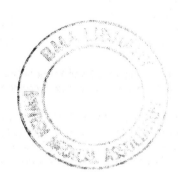

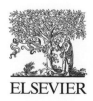

AMSTERDAM • BOSTON • HEIDELBERG • LONDON • NEW YORK • OXFORD
PARIS • SAN DIEGO • SAN FRANCISCO • SINGAPORE • SYDNEY • TOKYO

ELSEVIER

Elsevier
Radarweg 29, PO Box 211, 1000 AE Amsterdam, The Netherlands

Fifteenth edition 2006
Reprinted 2007

Notice
No responsibility is assumed by the publisher for any injury and/or damage to persons
or property as a matter of products liability, negligence or otherwise, or from any use
or operation of any methods, products, instructions or ideas contained in the material
herein. Because of rapid advances in the medical sciences, in particular, independent
verification of diagnoses and drug dosages should be made

British Library Cataloguing in Publication Data
A catalogue record for this book is available from the British Library

Library of Congress Cataloging-in-Publication Data
A catalog record for this book is available from the Library of Congress

ISBN: 978-0-444-50998-7 (Set)
ISBN: 978-0-444-52251-1 (Volume 1)
ISBN: 978-0-444-52252-8 (Volume 2)
ISBN: 978-0-444-52253-5 (Volume 3)
ISBN: 978-0-444-52254-2 (Volume 4)
ISBN: 978-0-444-52255-9 (Volume 5)
ISBN: 978-0-444-52256-6 (Volume 6)

For information on all Elsevier publications
visit our website at books.elsevier.com

Printed and bound in *Great Britain*

07 08 09 10 10 9 8 7 6 5 4 3 2

Working together to grow
libraries in developing countries

www.elsevier.com | www.bookaid.org | www.sabre.org

ELSEVIER   BOOK AID
             International   Sabre Foundation

Contents

Contributors

In this list the main contributors to the Encyclopedia are identified according to the original chapter material to which they made the most contribution. Most have contributed the relevant chapters in one or more editions of the *Side Effects of Drugs Annuals* 23-27 and/or the 14th edition of *Meyler's Side Effects of Drugs*. A few have contributed individual monographs to this edition.

M. Allwood
Derby, United Kingdom
Intravenous infusions—solutions and emulsions

M. Andersen
Odense, Denmark
Antihistamines

M. Andrejak
Amiens, France
Drugs affecting blood coagulation, fibrinolysis, and hemostasis

J.K. Aronson
Oxford, United Kingdom
Antiepileptic drugs
Antiviral drugs
Positive inotropic drugs and drugs used in dysrhythmias

S. Arroyo
Milwaukee, Wisconsin, USA
Antiepileptic drugs

I. Aursnes
Oslo, Norway
Drugs that affect lipid metabolism

H. Bagheri
Toulouse, France
Radiological contrast agents

A.M. Baldacchino
London, United Kingdom
Opioid analgesics and narcotic antagonists

D. Battino
Milan, Italy
Antiepileptic drugs

Z. Baudoin
Zagreb, Croatia
General anesthetics and therapeutic gases

A.G.C. Bauer
Rotterdam, The Netherlands
Antihelminthic drugs
Dermatological drugs, topical agents, and cosmetics

M. Behrend
Deggendorf, Germany
Drugs acting on the immune system

T. Bicanic
London, United Kingdom
Antiprotozoal drugs

L. Biscarini
Perugia, Italy
Anti-inflammatory and antipyretic analgesics and drugs used in gout

J. Blaser
Zurich, Switzerland
Various antibacterial drugs

C. Bokemeyer
Tübingen, Germany
Cytostatic drugs

S. Borg
Stockholm, Sweden
Antidepressant drugs

J. Bousquet
Montpellier, France
Antihistamines

P.J. Bown
Redhill, Surrey, United Kingdom
Opioid analgesics and narcotic antagonists

C.N. Bradfield
Auckland, New Zealand
General anesthetics and therapeutic gases

C.C.E. Brodie-Meijer
Amstelveen, The Netherlands
Metal antagonists

P.W.G. Brown
Sheffield, United Kingdom
Radiological contrast agents

A. Buitenhuis
Amsterdam, The Netherlands
Sex hormones and related compounds, including hormonal contraceptives

H. Cardwell
Auckland, New Zealand
Local anesthetics

A. Carvajal
Valladolid, Spain
Antipsychotic drugs

R. Cathomas
Zurich, Switzerland
Drugs acting on the respiratory tract

A. Cerny
Zurich, Switzerland
Various antibacterial drugs

G. Chevrel
Lyon, France
Drugs acting on the immune system

C.C. Chiou
Bethesda, Maryland, USA
Antifungal drugs

N.H. Choulis
Attika, Greece
Metals
Miscellaneous drugs and materials, medical devices, and techniques not dealt with in other chapters

L.G. Cleland
Adelaide, Australia
Corticotrophins, corticosteroids, and prostaglandins

P. Coates
Adelaide, Australia
Miscellaneous hormones

J. Costa
Badalona, Spain
Corticotrophins, corticosteroids, and prostaglandins

P. Cottagnoud
Bern, Switzerland
Various antibactcrial drugs

P.C. Cowen
Oxford, United Kingdom
Antidepressant drugs

S. Curran
Huddersfield, United Kingdom
Hypnosedatives and anxiolytics

H.C.S. Daly
Perth, Western Australia
Local anesthetics

A.C. De Groot
Hertogenbosch, The Netherlands
Dermatological drugs, topical agents, and cosmetics

M.D. De Jong
Amsterdam, The Netherlands
Antiviral drugs

A. Del Favero
Perugia, Italy
Anti-inflammatory and antipyretic analgesics and drugs used in gout

P. Demoly
Montpellier, France
Antihistamines

J. Descotes
Lyon, France
Drugs acting on the immune system

A.J. De Silva
Ragama, Sri Lanka
Snakebite antivenom

H.J. De Silva
Ragama, Sri Lanka
Gastrointestinal drugs

F.A. De Wolff
Leiden, The Netherlands
Metals

S. Dittmann
Berlin, Germany
Vaccines

M.N.G. Dukes
Oslo, Norway
Antiepileptic drugs
Antiviral drugs
Metals
Sex hormones and related compounds, including hormonal contraceptives

H.W. Eijkhout
Amsterdam, The Netherlands
Blood, blood components, plasma, and plasma products

E.H. Ellinwood
Durham, North Carolina, USA
Central nervous system stimulants and drugs that suppress appetite

C.J. Ellis
Birmingham, United Kingdom
Drugs used in tuberculosis and leprosy

P. Elsner
Jena, Germany
Dermatological drugs, topical agents, and cosmetics

T. Erikkson
Lund, Sweden
Thalidomide

E. Ernst
Exeter, United Kingdom
Treatments used in complementary and alternative medicine

M. Farré
Barcelona, Spain
Corticotrophins, corticosteroids, and prostaglandins

P.I. Folb
Cape Town, South Africa
Cytostatic drugs
Intravenous infusions—solutions and emulsions

J.A. Franklyn
Birmingham, United Kingdom
Thyroid hormones and antithyroid drugs

M.G. Franzosi
Milan, Italy
Beta-adrenoceptor antagonists and antianginal drugs

J. Fraser
Glasgow, Scotland
Cytostatic drugs

H.M.P. Freie
Maastricht, The Netherlands
Antipyretic analgesics

C. Fux
Bern, Switzerland
Various antibacterial drugs

P.J. Geerlings
Amsterdam, The Netherlands
Drugs of abuse

A.H. Ghodse
London, United Kingdom
Opioid analgesics and narcotic antagonists

P.L.F. Giangrande
Oxford, United Kingdom
Drugs affecting blood coagulation, fibrinolysis, and hemostasis

G. Gillespie
Perth, Australia
Local anaesthetics

G. Girish
Sheffield, United Kingdom
Radiological contrast agents

V. Gras-Champel
Amiens, France
Drugs affecting blood coagulation, fibrinolysis, and hemostasis

A.I. Green
Boston, Massachusetts, USA
Drugs of abuse

A.H. Groll
Münster, Germany
Antifungal drugs

H. Haak
Leiden, The Netherlands
Miscellaneous drugs and materials, medical devices, and techniques not dealt with in other chapters

F. Hackenberger
Bonn, Germany
Antiseptic drugs and disinfectants

J.T. Hartmann
Tübingen, Germany
Cytostatic drugs

K. Hartmann
Bern, Switzerland
Drugs acting on the respiratory tract

A. Havryk
Sydney, Australia
Drugs acting on the respiratory tract

E. Hedayati
Auckland, New Zealand
General anesthetics and therapeutic gases

E. Helsing
Oslo, Norway
Vitamins

R. Hoigné
Wabern, Switzerland
Various antibacterial drugs

A. Imhof
Seattle, Washington, USA
Various antibacterial drugs

L.L. Iversen
Oxford, United Kingdom
Cannbinoids

J. W. Jefferson
Madison, Wisconsin, USA
Lithium

D.J. Jeffries
London, United Kingdom
Antiviral drugs

M. Joerger
St Gallen, Switzerland
Drugs acting on the respiratory tract

G.D. Johnston
Belfast, Northern Ireland
Positive inotropic drugs and drugs used in dysrhythmias

P. Joubert
Pretoria, South Africa
Antihypertensive drugs

A.A.M. Kaddu
Entebbe, Uganda
Antihelminthic drugs

C. Koch
Copenhagen, Denmark
Blood, blood components, plasma, and plasma products

H. Kolve
Münster, Germany
Antifungal drugs

H.M.J. Krans
Hoogmade, The Netherlands
Insulin, glucagon, and oral hypoglycemic drugs

M. Krause
Scherzingen, Switzerland
Various antibacterial drugs

S. Krishna
London, United Kingdom
Antiprotozoal drugs

M. Kuhn
Chur, Switzerland
Drugs acting on the respiratory tract

R. Latini
Milan, Italy
Beta-adrenoceptor antagonists and antianginal drugs

T.H. Lee
Durham, North Carolina, USA
Central nervous system stimulants and drugs that
suppress appetite

P. Leuenberger
Lausanne, Switzerland
Drugs used in tuberculosis and leprosy

M. Leuwer
Liverpool, United Kingdom
Neuromuscular blocking agents and skeletal muscle
relaxants

G. Liceaga Cundin
Guipuzcoa, Spain
Drugs that affect autonomic functions or the
extrapyramidal system

P.O. Lim
Dundee, Scotland
Beta-adrenoceptor antagonists and antianginal drugs

H.-P. Lipp
Tübingen, Germany
Cytostatic drugs

C. Ludwig
Freiburg, Germany
Drugs acting on the immune system

T.M. MacDonald
Dundee, Scotland
Beta-adrenoceptor antagonists and antianginal drugs

G.T. McInnes
Glasgow, Scotland
Diuretics

I.R. McNicholl
San Francisco, California, USA
Antiviral drugs

P. Magee
Coventry, United Kingdom
Antiseptic drugs and disinfectants

A.P. Maggioni
Firenze, Italy
Beta-adrenoceptor antagonists and antianginal drugs

J.F. Martí Massó
Guipuzcoa, Spain
Drugs that affect autonomic functions or the
extrapyramidal system

L.H. Martín Arias
Valladolid, Spain
Antipsychotic drugs

M.M.H.M. Meinardi
Amsterdam, The Netherlands
Dermatological drugs, topical agents, and cosmetics

D.B. Menkes
Wrexham, United Kingdom
Hypnosedatives and anxiolytics

R.H.B. Meyboom
Utrecht, The Netherlands
Metal antagonists

T. Midtvedt
Stockholm, Sweden
Various antibacterial drugs

G. Mignot
Saint Paul, France
Gastrointestinal drugs

S.K. Morcos
Sheffield, United Kingdom
Radiological contrast agents

W.M.C. Mulder
Amsterdam, The Netherlands
Dermatological drugs, topical agents, and cosmetics

S. Musa
Wakefield, United Kingdom
Hypnosedatives and anxiolytics

K.A. Neftel
Bern, Switzerland
Various antibacterial drugs

A.N. Nicholson
Petersfield, United Kingdom
Antihistamines

L. Nicholson
Auckland, New Zealand
General anesthetics and therapeutic gases

I. Öhman
Stockholm, Sweden
Antidepressant drugs

H. Olsen
Oslo, Norway
Opioid analgesics and narcotic antagonists

I. Palmlund
London, United Kingdom
Diethylstilbestrol

J.N. Pande
New Delhi, India
Drugs used in tuberculosis and leprosy

J.K. Patel
Boston, Massachusetts, USA
Drugs of abuse

J.W. Paterson
Perth, Australia
Drugs acting on the respiratory tract

K. Peerlinck
Leuven, Belgium
Drugs affection blood coagulation, fibrinolysis, and
hemostasis

E. Perucca
Pavia, Italy
Antiepileptic drugs

E.H. Pi
Los Angeles, California, USA
Antipsychotic drugs

T. Planche
London, United Kingdom
Antiprotozoal drugs

B.C.P. Polak
Amsterdam, The Netherlands
Drugs used in ocular treatment

T.E. Ralston
Worcester, Massachusetts, USA
Drugs of abuse

P. Reiss
Amsterdam, The Netherlands
Antiviral drugs

H.D. Reuter
Köln, Germany
Vitamins

I. Ribeiro
London, United Kingdom
Antiprotozoal drugs

T.D. Robinson
Sydney, Australia
Drugs acting on the respiratory tract

Ch. Ruef
Zurich, Switzerland
Various antibacterial drugs

M. Schachter
London, United Kingdom
Drugs that affect autonomic functions or the
extrapyramidal system

A. Schaffner
Zurich, Switzerland
Various antibacterial drugs
Antifungal drugs

S. Schliemann-Willers
Jena, Germany
Dermatological drugs, topical agents, and cosmetics

M. Schneemann
Zürich, Switzerland
Antiprotozoal drugs

S.A. Schug
Perth, Australia
Local anesthetics

G. Screaton
Oxford, United Kingdom
Drugs acting on the immune system

J.P. Seale
Sydney, Australia
Drugs acting on the respiratory tract

R.P. Sequeira
Manama, Bahrain
Central nervous system stimulants and drugs that
suppress appetite

T.G. Short
Auckland, New Zealand
General anesthetics and therapeutic gases

D.A. Sica
Richmond, Virginia, USA
Diuretics

G.M. Simpson
Los Angeles, California, USA
Antipsychotic drugs

J.J. Sramek
Beverly Hills, California, USA
Antipsychotic drugs

A. Stanley
Birmingham, United Kingdom
Cytostatic drugs

K.J.D. Stannard
Perth, Australia
Local anesthetics

B. Sundaram
Sheffield, United Kingdom
Radiological contrast agents

J.A.M. Tafani
Toulouse, France
Radiological contrast agents

M.C. Thornton
Auckland, New Zealand
Local anesthetics

B.S. True
Campbelltown, South Australia
Corticotrophins, corticosteroids, and prostaglandins

C. Twelves
Glasgow, Scotland
Cytostatic drugs

W.G. Van Aken
Amsterdam, The Netherlands
Blood, blood components, plasma, and plasma products

C.J. Van Boxtel
Amsterdam, The Netherlands
Sex hormones and related compounds, including
hormonal contraceptives

G.B. Van der Voet
Leiden, The Netherlands
Metals

P.J.J. Van Genderen
Rotterdam, The Netherlands
Antihelminthic drugs

R. Verhaeghe
Leuven, Belgium
Drugs acting on the cerebral and peripheral circulations

J. Vermylen
Leuven, Belgium
Drugs affecting blood coagulation, fibrinolysis, and hemostasis

P. Vernazza
St Gallen, Switzerland
Antiviral drugs

T. Vial
Lyon, France
Drugs acting on the immune system

P. Vossebeld
Amsterdam, The Netherlands
Blood, blood components, plasma, and plasma products

G.M. Walsh
Aberdeen, United Kingdom
Antihistamines

T.J. Walsh
Bethesda, Maryland, USA
Antifungal drugs

R. Walter
Zurich, Switzerland
Antifungal drugs

D. Watson
Auckland, New Zealand
Local anesthetics

J. Weeke
Aarhus, Denmark
Thyroid hormones and antithyroid drugs

C.J.M. Whitty
London, United Kingdom
Antiprotozoal drugs

E.J. Wong
Boston, Massachusetts, USA
Drugs of abuse

C. Woodrow
London, United Kingdom
Antiprotozoal drugs

Y. Young
Auckland, New Zealand
General anesthetics and therapeutic gases

F. Zannad
Nancy, France
Antihypertensive drugs

J.-P. Zellweger
Lausanne, Switzerland
Drugs used in tuberculosis and leprosy

A. Zinkernagel
Zürich, Switzerland
Antiprotozoal drugs

M. Zoppi
Bern, Switzerland
Various antibacterial drugs

O. Zuzan
Hannover, Germany
Neuromuscular blocking agents and skeletal muscle relaxants

Foreword

My doctor is
A good doctor
He made me no
Iller than I was

Willem Hussem (The Netherlands) 1900–1974
Translation: Peter Raven

"*Primum non nocere*"—in the first place, do no harm—is often cited as one of the foundation stones of sound medical care, yet its origin is uncertain. Hippocrates? There are some who will tell you so;[1] but the phrase is not a part of the Hippocratic Oath, and the Father of Medicine wrote in any case in his native Greek.[2] It could be that the Latin phrase is from the Roman physician Galenius, while others attribute it to Scribonius Largus, physician to one of the later Caesars,[3] and there is a lot of reason to believe that it actually originated in 19th century England.[4] Hippocrates himself, in the first volume of his *Epidemics*, put it at all events better in context: "When dealing with diseases have two precepts in mind: to procure benefit and not to harm."[5] One must not become overly obsessed by the safety issue, but it is a necessary element in good medical care.

The ability to do good with the help of medicines has developed immensely within the last century, but with it has come the need to keep a watchful eye on the possibility of inflicting harm on the way. The challenge is to recognize at the earliest possible stage the adverse effects that a valuable drug may induce, and to find ways of containing them, so that risk never becomes disproportionate to benefit. The process of drug development will sometimes result in methods of treatment that are more specific to their purpose than were their predecessors and hence less likely to produce unwanted complications; yet the more novel a therapeutic advance the greater the possibility of its eliciting adverse effects of a type so unfamiliar that they are not specifically looked for and long remained unrecognized when they do occur. The entire process of keeping medicines safe today involves all those concerned with them, whether as researchers, manufacturers, regulators, prescribers, dispensers, or users, and it demands an effective and honest flow of information and thought between them.

For several decennia, concerned by its own errors in the past, the science of therapeutics put unbounded faith in the ability of well-planned clinical trials to arrive at the truth about the properties of medicines. Insofar as efficacy was concerned that was and remains a sound move, closing the door to charlatanism as well as to well-meant amateurism. Therapeutic trials with a new medicine were also able to delineate those adverse effects that occurred in a fair proportion of users. If serious, they would bar the drug from entry to the market altogether, while if transient and reasonably tolerable they would form the basis for warnings and precautions as well as the occasional contraindication. The problem lay with those adverse drug reactions that occurred rather less commonly or not at all in populations recruited for therapeutic trials, yet which could soon arise in the much broader spectrum of patients exposed to the drug once it was marketed across the world. The influence of race or climate might explain some of them; others might reflect interactions with foods, alcohol, or other drugs; yet others could only be explained, if at all, in terms of the particular susceptibility of certain individuals. Scattered across the globe, these effects might readily be overlooked, regarded as coincidental, or at worst dismissed contemptuously as "merely anecdotal".

The seriousness of the adverse effects issue became very apparent even as the reputation of controlled trials deservedly grew, and it touched on both newer and older drugs. The thalidomide calamity, involving several thousand cases of drug-induced phocomelia, was fortunately recognized by Widukind Lenz and others in the light of individual case reports within two years of the introduction of the product. On the other hand, generations elapsed between the patenting of aspirin in 1899 and the realization in 1965 that it might induce Reye's syndrome when used to treat fever in children. Such events, and many less spectacular, showed that, however vital well-controlled studies had become, there was good reason to remain alert for signals emerging from individual cases. Unanticipated events occurring during drug treatment might indeed reflect mere coincidence, but again they might not; and for many of the patients who suffered in consequence there was nothing in the least anecdotal about them.

Fortunately, the 1950s and 1960s of the 20th century saw the first positive reactions to the adverse reaction issue. Effective drug regulation emerged in one country after another. In 1952, Prof. Leo Meyler of The Netherlands produced his first "Side Effect of Drugs" to pull together data from the world literature. A number of national adverse reaction monitoring bureaux were established to gather data from the field and examine carefully reports of suspected side effects of medicines, creating the basis for the World Health Organization to establish its global reporting system. The pharmaceutical industry has increasingly realized its duty to collect and pass on the information that comes into its possession through its wide contacts with the health professions. Later years have seen the emergence, notably in Sweden and in Britain, of systems through which patients themselves can report possible adverse effects to the medicines they have taken. All these processes fit together in what the French language so appropriately terms "pharmacovigilance", with vigilance as the watchword for all concerned.

In this continuing development, the medical literature provides a resource with vast potential. The world is believed to have some 20 000 medical journals, of which a nuclear group of a thousand or so can be relied upon to publish reports and analyses of adverse effects—not only in the framework of formal investigations but also in letters, editorials, and reports of meetings large and small. Much of that information comprises not so much firm facts as emergent knowledge, based directly on experience in the field and calling urgently for attention. The book that Leo Meyler created has, in the course of fifteen editions and with the support of an ever-larger team of professionals, provided the means by which that attention can be mobilized. It has become the world's principal tool in bringing together, encyclopedically but critically, the evidence on the basis of which adverse drug effects and interactions can be recognized, discussed, and accommodated into medical practice. Together with its massive database and its complementary *Side Effects of Drugs Annuals*, it has evolved into a vital instrument in ensuring that drugs are used wisely and well and with due caution, in the light of all that is known about them.

There is nothing else like it, nor need there be; across the world, *Meyler* has become a pillar of responsible medical care.

M.N. Graham Dukes
Honorary Editor, *Meyler's Side Effects of Drugs*
Oslo, Norway

Notes

1. Lichtenhaeler C. Histoire de la Médicine, Fayard, Paris, 1978:117.
2. Smith CM. Origin and uses of *Primum non nocere*. J Clin Pharmacol 2005;45:371–7.
3. Albrecht H. Primum nil nocere. Die Zeit, 6 April, 2005.
4. Notably in a book by Inman T. *Foundation for a New Theory and Practice of Medicine*. London, 1860.
5. I am indebted to Jeffrey Aronson for his own translation of the Greek original from Hippocrates *Epidemics*, Book I, Section XI, which seems to convey the meaning of the original [ἀσκεῖν περὶ τὰ νοσημάτα δύο, ὠφελεῖν ἤ μὴ βλάπτειν] rather better than the published translations of his work.

Preface

This is a completely new edition of what has become the standard reference text in the field of adverse drug reactions and interactions since Leopold Meyler published his first review of the subject 55 years ago. Although we have retained the old title, *Meyler's Side Effects of Drugs*, the subtitle of this edition, *The Encyclopedia of Adverse Drug Reactions and Interactions*, reflects both modern terminology and the scope of the review. The structure of the book may have changed, but the *Encyclopedia* remains the most comprehensive reference source on adverse drug reactions and interactions and a major source of informed discussion about them.

Scope

The scope of the *Encyclopedia* remains wide. It covers not only the vast majority of prescription drugs, old and new, but also non-prescribed substances (such as anesthetics, antiseptics, lifestyle compounds, and drugs of abuse), herbal medicines, devices (such as blood glucose meters), and methods in alternative and complementary medicine. For this edition, entries on some substances that were regarded as obsolete, such as thalidomide and smallpox vaccine, have been rewritten and restored. Other compounds, such as diethylstilbestrol, although no longer in use, continue to cast their shadow and are included. Yet others, currently regarded as obsolete, have been retained, both for historical reasons and because one can never be sure when an old compound may once more become relevant or provide useful information in relation to another compound. Some drugs have been withdrawn from the market in some countries since the last edition of *Meyler* was published; rofecoxib, cisapride, phenylpropanolamine, and kava (see Piperaceae) are examples. Nevertheless, detailed monographs have been included on these substances because of the lessons that they can teach us and in some cases because of their relevance to other compounds in their classes that are still available; it is also not possible to predict whether these compounds will eventually reappear in some other form or for some new indication.

In the last 15 years there has been increasing emphasis on the use of high-quality evidence in therapeutic practice, principally as obtained from large, randomized clinical trials and from systematic reviews of the results of many such trials. However, while it has been possible to obtain useful information about the beneficial effects of interventions in this way, evidence about harms, including adverse drug reactions, has been more difficult to obtain. Even trials that yield good estimates of benefits are poor at providing evidence about harms for several reasons:

- benefits are usually single, whereas harms are usually multiple;
- the chance of any single form of harm is usually smaller than the chance of benefit and therefore more difficult to detect; however, multiple harms can accumulate and affect the benefit-to-harm balance;
- benefits are identifiable in advance, whereas harms are not or not always;
- the likely time-course of benefits can generally be predicted, while the time-course of harms often cannot and may be much delayed by comparison with the duration of a trial.

For all these reasons, larger and sometimes longer studies are needed to detect harms. In recent years attempts have been made to conduct systematic reviews of adverse reactions, but these have also been limited by several problems:

- harms are in general poorly collected in randomized trials and trials may not last long enough to detect them all;
- even when they are well collected, as is increasingly happening, they are often poorly reported;
- even when they are well reported in the body of a report, they may not be mentioned in titles and abstracts;
- even when they are well reported in the body of a report, they may be poorly indexed in large databases.

All this means that it is difficult to collect information on adverse drug reactions from randomized, controlled trials for systematic review. This can be seen from the evidence provided in Table 1, which shows the proportion of different types of information that have been used in the preparation of two volumes of the *Side Effects of Drugs Annual*, proportions that are likely be the same in this *Encyclopedia*.

Wherever possible, emphasis in this *Encyclopedia* has been placed on information that has come from systematic reviews and clinical trials of all kinds; this is reflected in new headings under which trial results are reported (observational studies, randomized studies, placebo-controlled studies). However, because many reports of adverse drug reactions (about 30%) are anecdotal, with evidence from one or just a few cases, many individual case studies (see below) have also been included. We need better methods to make use of the information that this large body of anecdotes provides.

Structure

The first major change that readers will notice is that the chapter structure of previous editions has given way to a monographic structure. That is because some of the information about individual drugs has previously been scattered over different chapters in the book; for example ciclosporin was previously covered in Chapter 37 and in scattered sections throughout Chapter 45; it is now dealt with in a single monograph. The monographs are arranged in alphabetical order, with cross-referencing as required. For example, if you turn to the monograph on cetirizine, you will be referred to the complementary general monograph on antihistamines, where much information that is relevant to cetirizine is given; the monograph on cetirizine itself contains information that is relevant only to cetirizine and not to other antihistamines. Within each monograph the material is arranged in the same way as in the *Side Effects of Drugs Annuals* (see "How to use this book").

Case Reports

A new feature, recognizable from the Annuals, but not incorporated into previous editions, is the inclusion of case reports of adverse effects. This feature reflects the fact that about 30% of all the literature that is reported and discussed in the Annuals derives from such reports (see Table 1). In some cases the only information about an adverse effect is contained in an anecdotal report; in other cases the report illustrates a variant form of the reaction. A case report also gives more immediacy to an adverse reaction, allowing the reader to appreciate more precisely the exact nature of the reported event.

Classification of Adverse Drug Reactions

Another new feature of this edition is the introduction of the DoTS method of classifying adverse drug reactions, based on the **Dose** at which they occur relative to the beneficial dose, the **Time-course** of the reaction, and individual **Susceptibility factors** (see "How to use this book"). This has been done for selected adverse effects, and I hope that as volumes of SEDA continue to be published and the *Encyclopedia's* electronic database is expanded, it will be possible to classify increasing numbers of adverse reactions in this way.

References

Because all the primary and secondary literature is thoroughly surveyed in the Annuals, the *Encyclopedia* has become increasingly compact relative to the amount of information available (even though it has increased in absolute size), with many unreferenced statements and cross-references to the Annuals, on the assumption that all the information would be readily available to the reader, although that may not always be the case. To restore all the reference material on which the *Encyclopedia* has been based as it has evolved over so many years would be a gargantuan task, but in this edition a major start has been made. Many references to original

material have been restored, and there is now hardly a statement that is not backed up by at least one reference to primary literature. In addition, almost all of the material that was published in Annuals 23 to 27 (SEDA-23 to SEDA-27) has been included, complete with citations. This has resulted in the inclusion of more than 40 000 references in this edition. Readers will still have to refer to earlier editions of the Annual (SEDA-1 to SEDA-22) and occasionally to earlier editions of *Meyler's Side Effects of Drugs* for more detailed descriptions, but now that the *Encyclopedia* is available electronically this will be repaired in future editions.

Methods and Contributors

I initially prepared the text of the *Encyclopedia* by combining text from the 14th edition of *Meyler's Side Effects of Drugs* and the five most recent annuals (SEDA-23 to SEDA-27). [Later literature is covered in SEDA-28 and the forthcoming SEDA-29.] I next restored missing references to the material and extended it where important information had not been included. The resulting monographs were then sent to experts for review, and their comments were incorporated into the finished monographs. I am grateful to all those, both authors of chapters in previous editions and Annuals and those who have reviewed the monographs for this edition, for their hard work and for making their expertise available.

Acknowledgements

This 15th edition of *Meyler's Side Effects of Drugs* was initiated and carefully planned with Joke Jaarsma at Elsevier, who has provided unstinting support during the production of several previous editions of *Meyler's Side Effects of Drugs* and the *Side Effects of Drugs Annuals*. Early discussions with Dieke van Wijnen at Elsevier about the structure of the text were invaluable. Professor Leufkens from the Faculty of Pharmacy at the University of Utrecht was instrumental in helping us to assemble the preliminary content for this edition; pharmacy students in his department entered the text

Table 1 Types of articles on adverse drug reactions published in 6576 papers in the world literature during 1999 and 2003 (as reviewed in SEDA-24 and SEDA-28)

Type of article	Number of descriptions* (%)
An anecdote or set of anecdotes (that is reported case histories)	2084 (29.9)
A major, randomized, controlled trial or observational study	1956 (28.1)
A minor, randomized, controlled trial or observational study or a non-randomized study (including case series)	1099 (15.8)
A major review, including non-systematic statistical analyses of published studies	951 (13.7)
A brief commentary (for example an editorial or a letter)	362 (5.19)
An experimental study (animal or in vitro)	263 (3.77)
A meta-analysis or other form of systematic review	172 (2.47)
Official statements (for example by Governmental organizations, the WHO, or manufacturers)	75 (1.07)
Total no. of descriptions*	6962
Total no. of articles	6576

* Some articles are described in more than one way

electronically into templates under the guidance of Joke Zwetsloot from Elsevier. Christine Ayorinde provided excellent assistance while I expanded and edited the material. The International Non-proprietary Names were checked by Renée Aronson. At Elsevier the references were then checked and collated by Liz Perill, who also copyedited the material, with Ed Stolting, and shepherded it through conversion to different electronic formats. Bill Todd created the indexes. Stephanie Diment oversaw the project and coordinated everyone's efforts.

The History of Meyler

The history of *Meyler's Side Effects of Drugs* goes back 55 years; a full account can be found at http://www.elsevier.com/locate/Meyler and the various volumes are listed before the title page of this set. When Leopold Meyler, a physician, experienced unwanted effects of drugs that were used to treat his tuberculosis, he discovered that there was no single text to which medical practitioners could turn for information about the adverse effects of drug therapy; Louis Lewin's text *Die Nebenwirkungen der Arzneimittel* ("The Untoward Effects of Drugs") of 1881 had long been out of print (SEDA-27, xxv–xxix). Meyler therefore surveyed the current literature, initially in Dutch as *Schadelijke Nevenwerkingen van Geneesmiddelen* (Van Gorcum, 1951), and then in English as *Side Effects of Drugs* (Elsevier, 1952). He followed up with what he called

surveys of unwanted effects of drugs. Each survey covered a period of two to four years and culminated in Volume VIII (1976), edited by Graham Dukes (SEDA-23, xxiii–xxvi), Meyler having died in 1973. By then the published literature was too extensive to be comfortably encompassed in a four-yearly cycle, and an annual cycle was started instead; the first *Side Effects of Drugs Annual* (SEDA-1) was published in 1977. The four-yearly review was replaced by a complementary critical encyclopaedic survey of the entire field; the first encyclopaedic edition of *Meyler's Side Effects of Drugs*, which appeared in 1980, was labeled the ninth edition.

Since then, *Meyler's Side Effects of Drugs* has been published every four years, providing an encyclopaedic survey of the entire field. Had the cycle been adhered to, the 15th edition would have been published in 2004, but over successive editions the quantity and nature of the information available in the text has changed. In the new millennium it was clear that for this edition a revolutionary approach was needed, and that has taken a little longer to achieve, with a great deal of effort from many different individuals.

We have come a long way since Meyler published his first account in a book of 192 pages. I think that he would have approved of this new *Encyclopedia*.

J. K. Aronson
Oxford, October 2005

How to use this book

In a departure from its previous structure, this edition of *Meyler's Side Effects of Drugs* is presented as individual drug monographs in alphabetical order. In many cases a general monograph (for example Antihistamines) is complemented by monographs about specific drugs (for example acrivastine, antazoline, etc.); in that case a cross-reference is given from the latter to the former.

Monograph Structure

Within each monograph the information is presented in sections as follows:

GENERAL INFORMATION

Includes, when necessary, notes on nomenclature, information about the results of observational studies, comparative studies, and placebo-controlled studies in relation to reports of adverse drug reactions, and a general summary of the major adverse effects.

ORGANS AND SYSTEMS

Cardiovascular (includes heart and blood vessels)
Respiratory
Ear, nose, throat
Nervous system (includes central and peripheral nervous systems)
Neuromuscular function
Sensory systems (includes eyes, ears, taste)
Psychological, psychiatric
Endocrine (includes hypothalamus, pituitary, thyroid, parathyroid, adrenal, pancreas, sex hormones)
Metabolism
Nutrition (includes effects on amino acids, essential fatty acids, vitamins, micronutrients)
Electrolyte balance (includes sodium, potassium)
Mineral balance (includes calcium, phosphate)
Metal metabolism (includes copper, iron, magnesium, zinc)
Acid–base balance
Fluid balance
Hematologic (includes blood, spleen, and lymphatics)
Mouth and teeth
Salivary glands
Gastrointestinal (includes esophagus, stomach, small bowel, large bowel)
Liver
Biliary tract
Pancreas
Urinary tract (includes kidneys, ureters, bladder, urethra)
Skin
Hair
Nails
Sweat glands
Serosae (includes pleura, pericardium, peritoneum)
Musculoskeletal (includes muscles, bones, joints)
Sexual function
Reproductive system (includes uterus, ovaries, breasts)
Immunologic (includes effects on the immune system and hypersensitivity reactions)
Autacoids

Infection risk
Body temperature
Multiorgan failure
Trauma
Death

LONG-TERM EFFECTS

Drug abuse
Drug misuse
Drug tolerance
Drug resistance
Drug dependence
Drug withdrawal
Genotoxicity
Mutagenicity
Tumorigenicity

SECOND-GENERATION EFFECTS

Fertility
Pregnancy
Teratogenicity
Fetotoxicity
Lactation

SUSCEPTIBILITY FACTORS (relates to features of the patient)

Genetic factors
Age
Sex
Physiological factors
Cardiac disease
Renal disease
Hepatic disease
Thyroid disease
Other features of the patient

DRUG ADMINISTRATION

Drug formulations
Drug additives
Drug contamination (includes infective agents)
Drug adulteration
Drug dosage regimens (includes frequency and duration of administration)
Drug administration route
Drug overdose

DRUG–DRUG INTERACTIONS
FOOD–DRUG INTERACTIONS
SMOKING
OTHER ENVIRONMENTAL INTERACTIONS
INTERFERENCE WITH DIAGNOSTIC TESTS
DIAGNOSIS OF ADVERSE DRUG REACTIONS
MANAGEMENT OF ADVERSE DRUG REACTIONS
MONITORING THERAPY

Classification of Adverse Drug Reactions

Selected major reactions are classified according to the DoTS system (BMJ 2003;327:1222–5). In this system adverse reactions are classified according to the **Dose** at which they usually occur relative to the beneficial dose, the **Time-course** over which they occur, and the **Susceptibility factors** that make them more likely, as follows:

1 Relation to dose
- *Toxic reactions* (reactions that occur at supratherapeutic doses)
- *Collateral reactions* (reactions that occur at standard therapeutic doses)
- *Hypersusceptibility reactions* (reactions that occur at subtherapeutic doses in susceptible patients)

2 Time-course
- *Time-independent reactions* (reactions that occur at any time during a course of therapy)
- *Time-dependent reactions*
  - Immediate reactions (reactions that occur only when a drug is administered too rapidly)
  - First-dose reactions (reactions that occur after the first dose of a course of treatment and not necessarily thereafter)
  - Early reactions (reactions that occur early in treatment then abate with continuing treatment)
  - Intermediate reactions (reactions that occur after some delay but with less risk during longer- term therapy, owing to the "healthy survivor" effect)
  - Late reactions (reactions the risk of which increases with continued or repeated exposure), including withdrawal reactions (reactions that occur when, after prolonged treatment, a drug is withdrawn or its effective dose is reduced)
  - Delayed reactions (reactions that occur some time after exposure, even if the drug is withdrawn before the reaction appears)

3 Susceptibility factors
- *Genetic*
- *Age*
- *Sex*
- *Physiological variation*
- *Exogenous factors* (for example drug–drug or food–drug interactions, smoking)
- *Diseases*

Drug Names And Spelling

Drugs are usually designated by their recommended or proposed International Non-proprietary Names (rINN or pINN); when these are not available, chemical names have been used. If a fixed combination has a generic combination name (for example co-trimoxazole for trimethoprim + sulfamethoxazole) that name has been used; in some cases brand names have been used.

Spelling

Where necessary, for indexing purposes, American spelling has been used, for example anemia rather than anaemia, estrogen rather than oestrogen.

Cross-references

The various editions of *Meyler's Side Effects of Drugs* are cited in the text as SED-l3, SED-14, etc.; the *Side Effects of Drugs Annuals* 1-22 are cited as SEDA-1, SEDA-2, etc. This edition includes most of the contents of SEDA-23 to SEDA-27. SEDA-28 and SEDA-29 are separate publications, which were prepared in parallel with the preparation of this edition.

Indexes

Index of drug names
An index of drug names provides a complete listing of all references to a drug for which adverse effects and/or drug interactions are described. The monograph on herbal medicines contains tabulated cross-indexes to the plants that are covered in separate monographs.

Index of adverse effects
This index is necessarily selective, since a particular adverse effect may be caused by very large numbers of compounds; the index is therefore mainly directed to adverse effects that are particularly serious or frequent, or are discussed in special detail; before assuming that a given drug does not have a particular adverse effect, consult the relevant monograph.

Alphabetical list of drug monographs

The number in parentheses after each heading is the number of the corresponding chapter in the Side Effects of Drug Annuals (SEDA-28 and later) in which the item is usually covered.

T

Tacrine

General Information

Tacrine (tetrahydroaminoacridine) was one of the first drugs to be widely marketed for the loss of memory and intellectual decline in Alzheimer's disease. However, its efficacy is controversial. A Cochrane review of the use of tacrine in Alzheimer's disease produced results that were compatible with improvement, no change, or even harm (1). For measures of overall clinical improvement, the intention-to-treat analyses did not detect any difference between tacrine and placebo (OR = 0.87; 95%CI = 0.61, 1.23). There was no effect on behavioral disturbance (SMD = 0.04; 95%CI = –0.52, 0.43) or cognitive function (SMD = 0.14; 95%CI = –0.02, 0.30). The odds ratio for withdrawal due to an adverse event was significantly different from 1, the control group experiencing fewer events (OR = 0.7; 95%CI = 4.1, 7.9). Raised serum liver enzymes caused the most withdrawals. Gastrointestinal adverse effects (diarrhea, anorexia, dyspepsia, and abdominal pain) were the other major adverse events and the odds ratio for withdrawal was also in favor of the control group (OR = 3.8; 95%CI = 2.8, 5.1). No deaths were reported in any of the studies, which lasted up to 6 months.

In a prospective randomized, double blind, parallel-group, multicenter comparison of idebenone 360 mg/day ($n = 104$) and tacrine up to 160 mg/day ($n = 99$) for 60 weeks in 203 patients with mild-to-moderate dementia of the Alzheimer's type, idebenone produced more benefit than tacrine (2). The benefit : harm balance was favorable for idebenone compared with tacrine. More patients taking tacrine (65%) reported adverse events than those taking idebenone (50%). The dropout rate in those taking tacrine was also higher. There were statistically significant differences between tacrine and idebenone for gastrointestinal adverse events (nausea, vomiting) and hepatobiliary toxicity (raised serum transaminase activity).

Organs and Systems

Nervous system

Myoclonus has been attributed to tacrine (3).

- A 68-year-old woman, who had had dementia of probable Alzheimer's type for 4 years, was given tacrine 40 mg/day and 24 hours later progressively developed generalized uncontrolled abnormal movements affecting all her limbs and her mouth, suggestive of myoclonus and controlled by clonazepam. The myoclonus disappeared 24 hours after tacrine was withdrawn. Causation was established a few months later by rechallenge: myoclonus occurred during the next 48 hours.

Liver

Hepatic failure associated with tacrine occurred outside the usual time of onset (within 9 months) and resulted in the death of a 75-year-old woman with Alzheimer's disease who had taken tacrine for 14 months (4). Thus, the potential for delayed, life-threatening hepatotoxicity with tacrine, although unusual, should not be overlooked.

The presence of the combined alleles M1 and T1, which mark deficiencies in glutathione-S-transferase genes, increases susceptibility to tacrine hepatotoxicity (5). It would be interesting to use this molecular epidemiological approach to identify the role of combinations of glutathione-S-transferase genotypes in other adverse drug reactions.

Tacrine-induced hepatotoxicity was reduced by ursodeoxycholic acid (13 mg/kg/day for 105 days) in a pilot study in 14 patients with Alzheimer's disease (6). Serum activity of alanine transaminase in 100 patients taking ursodeoxycholic acid was normal in 93% of cases, compared with 69% of patients who had taken tacrine alone.

Authors evaluating the adverse effects of tacrine in Alzheimer's disease recommend regular monitoring for hepatotoxicity (SEDA-15, 136).

References

1. Qizilbash N, Birks J, Lopez-Arrieta J, Lewington S, Szeto S. Tacrine for Alzheimer's disease. Cochrane Database Syst Rev 2000;(2):CD000202.
2. Gutzmann H, Kuhl KP, Hadler D, Rapp MA. Safety and efficacy of idebenone versus tacrine in patients with Alzheimer's disease: results of a randomized, double-blind, parallel-group multicenter study. Pharmacopsychiatry 2002;35(1):12–18.
3. Abillcira S, Viguera ML, Miquel F. Myoclonus induced by tacrine. J Neurol Neurosurg Psychiatry 1998;64(2):281.
4. Blackard WG Jr., Sood GK, Crowe DR, Fallon MB. Tacrine. A cause of fatal hepatotoxicity? J Clin Gastroenterol 1998;26(1):57–9.
5. Simon T, Becquemont L, Mary-Krause M, de Waziers I, Beaune P, Funck-Brentano C, Jaillon P. Combined glutathione-S-transferase M1 and T1 genetic polymorphism and tacrine hepatotoxicity. Clin Pharmacol Ther 2000;67(4):432–7.
6. Salmon L, Montet JC, Oddoze C, Montet AM, Portugal H, Michel BF. Acide ursodesoxycholique et prévention de l'hépatotoxicité de la tacrine: une étude pilote. [Ursodeoxycholic acid and prevention of tacrine-induced hepatotoxicity: a pilot study.] Therapie 2001;56(1):29–34.

Tacrolimus

General Information

Tacrolimus, a macrolide derivative, has similar immunosuppressive properties to ciclosporin and has effects on T lymphocytes by inhibiting interleukin-2 production. On a weight basis, tacrolimus is about 100 times more potent than ciclosporin. In view of the outcome of several multicenter trials, it has been used as an alternative to ciclosporin as a baseline regimen for the prophylaxis of renal and liver transplant rejection and in the treatment of acute rejection (SED-13, 1130) (SEDA-21, 390) (1). The clinical pharmacology, clinical use, and adverse effects profile of tacrolimus in organ transplantation have been extensively reviewed (2).

General adverse effects

The incidence of adverse effects (for example neurotoxicity, nephrotoxicity, and hyperglycemia), particularly those requiring drug withdrawal, was initially found to be higher in tacrolimus-treated liver transplant patients, but subsequently fell after the initial tacrolimus dose was reduced. This was in accordance with the results of very early trials, which showed that the initially proposed dose of tacrolimus was too high (3). In subsequent studies, tacrolimus and ciclosporin had a similar spectrum of adverse effects for nephrotoxicity, infectious complications, and lymphoproliferative disorders, and long-term adverse effects occurred at comparable rates, that is less than 2% (SED-13, 1130) (SEDA-21, 390).

Even though the glucocorticoid-sparing effect of tacrolimus is greater than that of ciclosporin, the initial hope that tacrolimus might prove less toxic than ciclosporin has not been realized. In trials in renal transplant patients, increased serum creatinine concentrations, tremor, paresthesia, gastrointestinal disorders, hyperglycemia, diabetes mellitus, pruritus, and angina pectoris occurred more often with tacrolimus, whereas there was a higher incidence of dysrhythmias, hyperkalemia, gingival hyperplasia, acne, alopecia, and hirsutism with ciclosporin (SEDA-21, 390). In the European Tacrolimus Multicenter Liver Trial, there was some evidence of possible advantages for tacrolimus over ciclosporin in terms of hypertension, cytomegalovirus infection, hirsutism, and gum hyperplasia (SEDA-21, 390). The safety profile of tacrolimus is very similar in children to that in adults, but in sharp contrast to ciclosporin, gingival hyperplasia, hirsutism, and coarsening of facial features have not been observed (4,5).

As the adverse effects of tacrolimus and ciclosporin are not strictly comparable, switching a patient from one to the other can sometimes be beneficial. Severe or persistent tacrolimus-related adverse effects, for example neurotoxicity, gastrointestinal disorders, or diabetes mellitus, can abate after replacement by ciclosporin (SEDA-20, 347) (6). Conversely, the change from ciclosporin to tacrolimus has been safely and successfully undertaken in patients with adverse effects from ciclosporin, such as nephrotoxicity, hemolytic–uremic syndrome, hypertension, neurological disorders, gingival hyperplasia, hypertrichosis, and dyslipidemia (SED-13, 1130) (SEDA-20, 347) (7,8). Replacing one drug by another is not always advantageous; in two patients switched to tacrolimus for ciclosporin-induced cortical blindness, visual abnormalities promptly resolved, but both patients rapidly developed thrombotic thrombocytopenic purpura and severe graft-versus-host disease, and finally died 33 days after bone marrow transplantation (9).

Long-term follow-up (mean of 93 months) of tacrolimus-based immunosuppression has been reported in 121 adult patients with liver transplants (10). Infections were the most common causes of deaths (17 patients out of 42), and half of them occurred during the first year after transplantation. Cardiovascular events (seven patients) or de novo malignancies (three patients) were also important causes of death. End-stage renal disease related to tacrolimus nephrotoxicity was noted in two patients who required renal transplantation. At 7 years, other important adverse effects included hyperkalemia (30%) or hypertension (31%) requiring treatment, and insulin-dependent diabetes mellitus (13%). Seven patients developed de novo malignancies and six had post-transplant lymphoproliferative disorders. The risks of tacrolimus in renal transplantation have been discussed (11).

Organs and Systems

Cardiovascular

The incidence of hypertension and the prevalence of anti-hypertensive drug use are lower with tacrolimus than with ciclosporin (5,12).

Severe recurrent, but usually reversible hypertrophic cardiomyopathy has been infrequently reported, both in adults and children (SEDA-19, 352) (SEDA-20, 346). Based on experimental data and one additional case report, the interaction of tacrolimus with calcium channel blockers in the cardiac muscle has been suggested as a possible mechanism (SEDA-21, 390). However, the role of tacrolimus in the development of cardiomyopathy is still hypothetical. Echocardiographic abnormalities were relatively common before and after liver transplantation in 12 adult patients, and there was no clear evidence that oral tacrolimus specifically alters cardiac function (13). Other investigators did not show differences in heart weight, ventricular thickness, or valve circumferences between 67 liver transplant recipients treated with tacrolimus and 72 non-transplanted patients who died from end-stage liver disease (14). In addition, more than 80% of patients in both groups had left ventricular hypertrophy.

Other isolated reports and preliminary studies have suggested a possible risk of life-threatening dysrhythmias, including sinus bradycardia or sinus arrest, asymptomatic but significant mean QT/QT_c interval prolongation in 33 patients (over 500 msec in seven patients), and recurrent episodes of ventricular tachycardia or torsade de pointes in two patients (SEDA-21, 391) (SEDA-22, 390) (15,16).

Several reports have previously focused on the possible occurrence of cardiomyopathy in tacrolimus-treated transplant patients, particularly children. In two further liver transplant children aged 2.5 and 14 years who died from multiorgan system failure due to sepsis and end-stage liver failure, pathological examination showed prominent concentric left ventricular hypertrophy (17). Although tacrolimus was regarded as a possible cause of asymptomatic hypertrophic cardiomyopathy in these patients, a direct causal relation was difficult to establish. The cause is probably multifactorial, and potential confounding factors (for example hypertension, glucocorticoids) are numerous in this population. In a retrospective review of 89 pediatric heart transplant patients who had survived for at least 6 months, repeated echocardiography showed signs of cardiac hypertrophy, particularly early after transplantation and in very young infants (18). However, there was no evidence of progressive hypertrophy on follow-up examinations, and no significant differences in the degree of cardiac hypertrophy between patients aged over 1 year at the time of transplantation who received ciclosporin ($n = 26$) or tacrolimus ($n = 41$).

In a retrospective study, the prevalence of hypertension 2 years after adult liver transplantation was significantly lower in patients treated with tacrolimus (64% of 28 patients) than in patients treated with ciclosporin (82% of 131 patients) (19). In addition, hypertension occurred later with tacrolimus. A similar benefit of tacrolimus over ciclosporin was found in a randomized, comparative trial in 85 heart transplant patients, and 41% of 39 tacrolimus-treated patients developed new-onset hypertension requiring treatment, compared with 71% of 46 ciclosporin-treated patients (20).

In 37 patients with liver transplants there was no difference between the pre- and post-transplant QT interval in the 25 taking oral ciclosporin and the 12 taking oral tacrolimus (21).

Cardiac symptoms manifesting as myocardial ischemia are uncommon, but can occur through tacrolimus toxicity (22).

- A 20-year-old woman with chest pain, dyspnea, and protracted electrocardiographic ST depression had very high blood tacrolimus concentrations (45 ng/ml). Subsequent coronary angiography ruled out any significant organic lesions, but showed vasospastic coronary arteries. She had no other cardiac symptoms when tacrolimus was restarted with careful surveillance of serum concentrations.

Nervous system

Tacrolimus mostly produces mild to moderate neurotoxic effects that are usually not treatment-limiting and rarely clinically relevant, at least in children (23). The occurrence of neurological symptoms, sometimes severe, is a well-known complication in the early post-transplant period, particularly in liver transplant recipients. It is therefore in most cases difficult to attribute these disorders to a particular immunosuppressive regimen.

When neurological symptoms occur in patients taking tacrolimus they are very similar to those seen in patients taking ciclosporin, with more frequent insomnia, tremor, and headaches, but a similar rate of severe neurological adverse effects, such as acute psychosis, peripheral neuropathy, seizures, encephalopathy, coma, and paralysis. Persistent speech disorders (dysarthria, apraxia, expressive aphasia, akinetic mutism), and visual blurring can also occur (SEDA-21, 391) (SEDA-22, 420) (24).

The higher incidence of moderate or severe late neurotoxicity from tacrolimus compared with ciclosporin was strongly associated with severe postoperative infections, multiple organ failure, and an increased bilirubin, creatinine, and transaminases (25).

It has been suggested that anxiety rather than akathisia can account for several symptoms caused by tacrolimus, such as restlessness (SEDA-21, 391).

Posterior leukoencephalopathy, with clinical, radiological, and neuropathological features resembling those previously described with ciclosporin has been reported in several patients (SEDA-22, 420) (26). Cortical blindness, generalized tonic-clonic seizures ($n = 2$), and diffuse MRI abnormalities were found in three of 50 patients taking tacrolimus after bone marrow transplantation (SEDA-20, 347); these findings have also been observed in patients taking ciclosporin. Acute neurotoxicity was fatal in one patient despite changing from tacrolimus to

ciclosporin, and autopsy showed multiple cerebral hemispheric infarcts due to cerebral vasculitis (SEDA-22, 420).

Six patients taking tacrolimus (including five children) developed signs of encephalopathy with generalized or focal seizures, reduced visual acuity or cortical blindness, altered mental status, and white matter lesions on MRI scan, particularly in the parieto-occipital regions (27–29). Three patients had tacrolimus blood concentrations above the target range before the neurological adverse event. Although there was complete resolution after tacrolimus withdrawal or reduction in dosage in four patients, two children still had persistent brain imaging abnormalities and recurrent episodes of seizures.

- A chronic inflammatory demyelinating polyneuropathy was considered to have been caused by tacrolimus in a 62-year-old patient (30).
- The presence of significant tacrolimus concentrations (5.2 and 1.3 ng/ml at 8 and 72 hours after the last dose) in the cerebrospinal fluid of a 64-year-old woman with a renal transplant, who developed an extremely severe form of encephalopathy after 21 months of treatment, suggested that tacrolimus can cross the blood–brain barrier (31).

Complete resolution of tacrolimus-induced neurotoxicity does not occur after tacrolimus withdrawal or dosage reduction (32).

- A 48-year-old man developed acute loss of speech and swallowing apraxia shortly after liver transplantation. Tacrolimus serum concentrations were very high. Although there was progressive improvement after tacrolimus withdrawal, residual speech deficits were still present 3 weeks later. A PET scan showed a marked reduction in metabolic rate in the temporal lobes and the adjacent parieto-occipital region bilaterally.

Other cases of severe neurotoxicity have been seen during tacrolimus treatment for graft-versus-host disease after allogeneic bone marrow transplantation.

- A 16-year-old girl had hypertension and generalized convulsions, which recurred after tacrolimus readministration; she subsequently died from cerebral hemorrhage and respiratory failure (33).

Based on this report and a review of previously published cases, concomitant hypertension and the use of high-dose methylprednisolone were discussed as precipitating factors of tacrolimus neurotoxicity. In two other patients aged 4 and 15 years who had prolonged leukoencephalopathy, the underlying chronic graft-versus-host disease was thought to be a risk factor (34).

In children one advantage of tacrolimus is that it can reduce the dose of glucocorticoids required for immunosuppression. This in turn improves growth. When in one center the immunosuppression protocol was changed to tacrolimus plus mycophenolate mofetil and prednisone, two patients developed transient encephalopathy associated with tacrolimus (35). In both cases, the encephalopathy was managed by treating the associated hypertension and fluid overload; tacrolimus was not withdrawn.

Both tacrolimus and ciclosporin are hydrophobic and can alter the properties of the cell membrane. They bind to an intracellular peptidylprolyl isomerase that regulates

T cell activation and can interfere with cytoskeletal components that prevent interleukin-2 synthesis and release. Cytotoxic edema caused by acute cerebral ischemia is associated with reduced diffusion, reflecting the failure of membrane sodium pumps. Altered electrolyte or fluid balance can precede the onset of encephalopathy. This can be shown by fluid-attenuated inversion recovery and diffusion-weighted MRI images (36).

A polymorphism of the ABCB1 gene may be associated with a risk of tacrolimus-induced neurotoxicity after liver transplantation. In six patients with neurotoxicity and 11 without neurotoxicity, high tacrolimus concentration, liver dysfunction, and a mutation in position 2677 in exon 21 were positive predictive factors for tacrolimus-induced neurotoxicity (37).

Sensory systems

Eyes

- Optic neuropathy has been reported in a 58-year-old liver transplant patient who had taken tacrolimus for 2 months (38). Further deterioration of vision occurred despite withdrawal.

Ears

Sudden hearing loss has been attributed to tacrolimus (39).

- A 38-year-old woman was switched from ciclosporin to tacrolimus 44 days after kidney and pancreas transplantation and 17 days later had sudden hearing loss with tinnitus. Her tacrolimus blood concentration 3 days later was 28 ng/ml and peaked at 35 ng/ml 8 days later. Audiograms showed bilateral hearing loss—80% for speech perception and mild to moderate sensorineural hearing loss. Her hearing improved on tacrolimus dosage reduction and after the tacrolimus blood concentration reached 15 ng/ml.

Although she was taking many other drugs, including muromonab, which was withdrawn 1 month before the hearing loss occurred, the role of tacrolimus was supported by its chemical similarity to erythromycin, which is ototoxic when given intravenously.

Endocrine

The risk of post-transplant diabetes mellitus is greater with tacrolimus than with ciclosporin, but this was mostly true in black patients and during the initial months after transplantation (40). In one study, insulin sensitivity, alpha and beta cell function, and beta cell reserve were studied in 14 hepatitis C-positive patients with liver transplants, who took tacrolimus or ciclosporin maintenance for 1 year (41). The patients were matched for low prednisolone dosage (1.1 mg/day versus 1.3 mg/day), body mass index, lean body mass, and sex, and compared with eight controls. Insulin sensitivity and insulin secretory reserve were significantly different from controls, but there was no significant difference between ciclosporin and tacrolimus.

The incidence, mechanism, and risk factors of tacrolimus-associated diabetes mellitus are still debated. In 58 patients investigated 1–3 years after liver transplantation there was a significantly higher incidence of diabetes mellitus with tacrolimus ($n = 32$) compared with ciclosporin ($n = 26$) (42). Newly-diagnosed diabetes occurred in nine of 28 tacrolimus-treated patients, of whom six required insulin, and in none of 25 ciclosporin-treated patients. Five patients taking tacrolimus also had islet cell-specific autoantibodies that correlated significantly with HLA risk haplotypes.

- A 32-year-old woman with previous autoimmune disorders and a susceptible HLA haplotype developed diabetes with newly positive glutamic acid decarboxylase antibody after taking tacrolimus for 5 months (43).

Together, these reports suggest that tacrolimus does not suppress the production of autoantibodies in patients genetically prone to develop autoimmune diabetes, with induction of an autoimmune phenomenon. This also suggests that tacrolimus treatment should be undertaken cautiously in predisposed patients.

Metabolism

Of 834 primary adult liver transplant recipients, of whom 499 were alive and taking tacrolimus, 70% were glucocorticoid-free after 1 year; this did not change over the next 5 years (44). However, glucocorticoid-associated adverse effects, such as hypertension, diabetes, and hyperlipidemia, were not statistically significantly less common in patients not taking glucocorticoids. This may have been because of the diabetogenic effect of tacrolimus.

Diabetes mellitus

Altered glucose metabolism and subsequent hyperglycemia or even insulin-dependent diabetes mellitus is an important issue in transplant patients, particularly in adults or patients taking high doses. In animals, high-dose tacrolimus causes glucose intolerance and reduced insulin release (45). This resolves after withdrawal. Diabetes mellitus after transplantation is a relatively common complication in pediatric thoracic organ recipients taking tacrolimus (46). Specific risk factors have not been identified. A switch from tacrolimus to ciclosporin for other reasons in two patients did not resolve the problem.

The incidence of hyperglycemia or diabetes mellitus requiring insulin at some point during treatment was 10–20% in adults (2% in children), an incidence about 2–3 times higher than with ciclosporin (SEDA-20, 347). However, more recent studies and case reports have shown that children could be also very sensitive to the diabetogenic effects of tacrolimus, with an incidence possibly higher than previously thought (47,48). While the diabetes mellitus tends to improve or abate after the dose of tacrolimus or glucocorticoid has been reduced, glucose intolerance was more frequent in the tacrolimus group after a median of 23 months (49). However, post-transplant diabetes mellitus requiring permanent insulin treatment was as frequent in patients with liver grafts taking ciclosporin or tacrolimus after 1 year (50). Finally, there was a possible correlation between impaired glucose tolerance or a diabetic pattern detected by a pretransplant 75 g oral glucose tolerance test and the later development of post-transplant diabetes mellitus (51).

In a pooled analysis of four randomized trials of tacrolimus versus ciclosporin after renal transplantation, the prevalence of post-transplant diabetes mellitus at 1 year (two studies, 532 patients) was five times higher with tacrolimus than with ciclosporin (OR = 5.0; 95% CI = 2.0, 12.4) (52). In the opinion of the US FDA, diabetes mellitus after transplantation was a significant hazard in tacrolimus-treated patients, even though about half of the patients were no longer taking insulin at 2 years after transplantation (53).

The exact mechanisms of tacrolimus-induced diabetes are unknown. In one renal transplant patient with genetic susceptibility, tacrolimus was associated with insulin-dependent diabetes mellitus and the simultaneous occurrence of anti-glutamic acid decarboxylase antibody (54). Within 2 months after conversion from tacrolimus to ciclosporin, the antibody was no longer detected and the patient's insulin requirements fell dramatically. Tacrolimus-induced direct beta cell toxicity, with subsequent development of beta cell autoimmunity, was therefore suggested as a possible mechanism in patients with genetic susceptibility for type I diabetes.

Hepatitis C virus infection has been associated with diabetes and is a significant risk in patients with renal transplants. In 427 patients with renal transplants and no previous diabetes mellitus, diabetes after transplantation occurred more often in hepatitis C virus-positive than hepatitis C virus-negative patients (39 versus 9.8%) (55). Diabetes mellitus after transplantation occurred more often in hepatitis C virus-positive patients taking tacrolimus than in those taking ciclosporin (58 versus 7.7%). In hepatitis C virus-negative patients, the rates of diabetes mellitus were similar. The authors concluded that hepatitis C is strongly associated with diabetes mellitus after renal transplantation because of the greater diabetogenicity of tacrolimus.

In 17 patients, in whom fasting blood samples were taken immediately before transplantation and at 1 and 3 months after transplantation for measurement of HbA, insulin, C-peptide, free fatty aids, lipids, urea, and creatinine, the incidence of diabetes mellitus was high (47%) (56). Diabetes was more common in black patients, but owing to the small number of patients the difference was not statistically significant. Insulin resistance seems to be the main pathogenic mechanism involved.

Lipid metabolism
In contrast to its effects on glucose metabolism, tacrolimus offers potential advantages over ciclosporin for lipid disorders (57). Compared with ciclosporin-based immunosuppressive regimens, total cholesterol and LDL cholesterol serum concentrations were lower in patients taking tacrolimus for 1 year (58). Both findings were considered to result from a significant glucocorticoid-sparing effect of tacrolimus.

Hematologic

Acute hemolysis occurred in eight of 1400 patients (59). Although multiple other causal factors could have been relevant, further hematological investigations suggested that tacrolimus can cause or promote hemolysis, particularly in patients with acquired anti-erythrocyte antibodies.

Pure red cell aplasia is an occasional complication of treatment (SED-13, 1131) (SEDA-20, 347) (60). In one case, tacrolimus was thought to have caused reversible pancytopenia with severely reduced granulopoiesis and megakaryocytopoiesis on bone marrow examination (SEDA-21, 391).

- The prothrombin time was prolonged to 36 seconds, with isolated factor V deficiency (5%), 2 weeks after a 46-year-old patient with a liver transplant was given tacrolimus and oxacillin (61). Factor V antigen was lower than 5%. In vitro investigations of the patient's plasma showed dose-dependent factor V inhibitory activity in the presence of tacrolimus. Factor V activity and the coagulation profile returned to normal after withdrawal.

The development of this transiently acquired inhibitor of coagulation factor V may have been due to either tacrolimus or oxacillin.

Microangiopathy and the resulting thrombotic thrombocytopenic purpura-like syndrome has been reported in three transplant patients taking tacrolimus, including one with a severe form (62). Microangiopathy was associated with high trough tacrolimus concentrations (over 24 ng/ml) and raised concentrations of endothelin and various cytokines, namely interleukin-8, interleukin-10, interleukin-12, tumor necrosis factor alfa, and interferon gamma.

Mouth and teeth

A brief case report has suggested that tacrolimus can cause gingival hyperplasia (63).

Gastrointestinal

Severe gastrointestinal toxicity with anorexia and weight loss is sometimes observed in patients taking tacrolimus (SEDA-19, 352).

Tacrolimus-associated *Clostridium difficile* diarrhea has been reported (64).

- A 29-year-old man was given mycophenolate and tacrolimus for an episode of renal transplant rejection that occurred 6.5 years after transplantation. Four weeks after tacrolimus was begun, he had diarrhea, nausea, and malaise. There was *C. difficile* toxin in the stools, and his symptoms abated with metronidazole. About 1 month later, he developed diarrhea, fever, and severe dehydration. *Clostridium difficile* toxin was again detected in the stools, and his symptoms completely resolved with oral vancomycin and withdrawal of tacrolimus.

Similar cases have been reported to the manufacturers. A possible relation between the macrolide molecular structure of tacrolimus and the development of *C. difficile* colitis remains to be established.

Liver

In children 0.1% tacrolimus ointment has been used daily without major adverse effects.

- In a 3-year-old African-American boy with moderate atopic dermatitis, tacrolimus caused raised transaminase and lactate dehydrogenase activities. Tacrolimus was withdrawn on day 29, but no further information was given about their liver function tests (65).

The finding of mild to moderate liver function test abnormalities that normalized on dosage reduction or withdrawal of tacrolimus has suggested possible dose-related hepatotoxicity (66). In liver transplant patients, liver biopsy showed a centrilobular hepatocellular dropout with sinusoidal dilatation and congestion, and no features of cellular rejection or acute hepatitis.

Pancreas

Acute pancreatitis has rarely been reported in clinical trials, but no detailed cases were available before the following report (67).

- A 28-year-old woman was switched from ciclosporin to tacrolimus for prophylaxis of graft-versus-host disease after allogeneic stem cell transplantation for chronic myelogenous leukemia. She also took methylprednisolone and inhaled pentamidine. After 2 weeks she developed acute abdominal pain, tachypnea, hypoxia, and oliguria. Amylase and lipase peaked at about four and five times the upper limits of the reference ranges, and urinary analysis was consistent with acute tubular necrosis. An abdominal CT scan showed an enlarged edematous pancreas with a peripancreatic inflammatory exudate. There was no biliary obstruction or dyslipidemia. Shortly after tacrolimus withdrawal, she became anuric and had an episode of acute respiratory distress, but then improved over the next few days.

Although treatment with methylprednisolone, pentamidine, and total parenteral nutrition could have contributed in this patient, they were either continued or readministered without ill effect.

Urinary tract

Tacrolimus nephrotoxicity has been reviewed (68) and is considered to be very similar to that described with ciclosporin. The clinical and histological characteristics of acute tacrolimus nephrotoxicity have been described from a retrospective analysis of 67 patients with renal transplants, of whom 27 developed acute nephrotoxicity, in seven of whom underlying moderate-to-severe renal arteriosclerosis might have predisposed to tacrolimus nephrotoxicity (69).

Tacrolimus-induced chronic nephrotoxicity has clinical and histopathological features very similar to those induced by ciclosporin, that is tubular lesions, hyaline arteriolopathy, and hemolytic–uremic syndrome-like changes in glomeruli and vessels (70). Isolated glomerular microthrombosis has also been described (71). Although tacrolimus was successfully used in several patients suffering from ciclosporin-induced hemolytic–uremic syndrome, thrombocytopenic purpura and hemolytic–uremic syndrome, including one fatal case, have also been reported in patients taking tacrolimus (SED-13, 1131) (SEDA-20, 347). In addition, ciclosporin and tacrolimus were significant risk factors for recurrence of hemolytic–uremic syndrome in patients who had undergone renal transplantation for end-stage renal disease (72). Late nephrotoxicity evaluated by the mean serum creatinine concentration and/or glomerular filtration rate at 1 year was similar in patients taking ciclosporin or tacrolimus (73,74). However, compared with ciclosporin, tacrolimus appears to be associated with more frequent and severe proximal or distal tubular acidosis 6 months after renal transplantation, although this conclusion is based on work with only a few patients in each group (SEDA-19, 352) (75). Overall, the reported incidence of tacrolimus-associated nephrotoxicity varies from 18 to 42% in liver transplant patients; among 128 patients who had early and late episodes of renal allograft dysfunction (1–156 weeks after transplantation) requiring biopsy, tacrolimus nephrotoxicity was estimated to account for only 17% of cases (76). There were higher than expected serum tacrolimus concentrations in most patients, and the highest concentrations were detected 1.6 days before the peak serum creatinine. However, renal histological lesions were independent of tacrolimus dosage or blood concentrations (77).

The nephrotoxic adverse effects of tacrolimus and ciclosporin are clinically indistinguishable. The pathological features of renal biopsies at 2 years of treatment in patients enrolled in a large multicenter comparison of tacrolimus and ciclosporin in renal transplantation have been reported (78). Of 412 patients initially randomized, renal biopsies were available from 79 taking tacrolimus and 65 taking ciclosporin. There were features of tacrolimus or ciclosporin nephrotoxicity (hyaline arteriolar change, tubular vacuolization) in 19 and 11 patients respectively. There were no differences in the rates of biopsy-proven acute rejection (8.9 versus 9.2%) or chronic allograft nephropathy (62 and 72%). In addition, the histological features of chronic allograft nephropathy were very similar. An older age of the donor, acute rejection, cytomegalovirus infection, and ciclosporin- and tacrolimus-associated nephrotoxicity during the first year of transplantation were the most significant factors associated with the occurrence of chronic nephropathy.

As with ciclosporin, tacrolimus used as a primary immunosuppressant has sometimes been associated with de novo thrombotic microangiopathy/hemolytic–uremic syndrome. Its role has been clearly confirmed in a 52-year-old heart transplant patient in whom hemolytic–uremic syndrome recurred 6 days after tacrolimus readministration (79). From a report of two additional cases and a review of 19 other reported cases, the incidence of tacrolimus-associated thrombotic microangiopathy has been suggested to be 1.0–4.7%; 15 cases were reported in renal transplant patients (80). The mean time to diagnosis was 9 months (4 days to 31 months), and the tacrolimus trough concentrations were usually within the target range. Most patients had the clinical features of hemolytic–uremic syndrome. Final outcomes were known in 18 patients: 10 had tacrolimus dosage reduction only (six recovered, three had an acute cellular rejection, one lost his renal graft); one stopped taking tacrolimus and recovered; seven had tacrolimus dosage reduction or withdrawal and underwent plasmapheresis, fresh-frozen plasma exchange, high-dose glucocorticoids, or anticoagulation (three died of sepsis and multiorgan failure, one lost her renal graft, and three recovered). Furthermore, and in contrast to previous reports (SEDA-19, 353), a change from ciclosporin to tacrolimus in patients with ciclosporin-associated hemolytic–uremic syndrome is not always successful.

- Two renal transplant patients developed resistant late acute rejection while taking ciclosporin (81). After a switch to tacrolimus, they had clinical and histological features of hemolytic–uremic syndrome, with biopsy-proven thrombotic microangiopathy within 2 and 12 days after conversion. Both finally required explantation of their renal allografts.

Skin

The long-term safety of topical tacrolimus ointment 0.1% for 6–12 months has been assessed in 316 patients with atopic dermatitis (82). The most common adverse effects clearly attributed to tacrolimus were a local burning sensation (47%), pruritus (24%), and erythema (12%); the incidences fell with time. The observed incidence of infections did not exceed the expected incidence in patients with atopic dermatitis, and there were no effects on circulating cell-mediated immunity.

In 631 adult patients with moderate to severe atopic dermatitis enrolled in a randomized, double-blind, multi-center comparison of tacrolimus (0.03% or 0.1%) with a vehicle applied twice-daily for 12 weeks, the most common adverse events were skin burning, erythema, and pruritus (83). Others were flu-like symptoms and headache. Withdrawal was required in 50 patients because of adverse events, twice as many as in the vehicle group. There was pruritus in 30 patients, skin burning in 19, skin erythema in 12, and skin infections in two. Skin burning and pruritus have consistently been observed with tacrolimus ointment, typically during the first days of treatment, reducing in incidence within the first week; they tend to be mild or moderate.

In 255 children with atopic dermatitis, tacrolimus 0.1% ointment caused transient skin burning and itching as the most common adverse events (65). Two patients required hospital admittance to control skin infections. A flu-like syndrome was the major non-topical adverse event.

- A diffuse, follicular, erythematous eruption has been reported in a 45-year-old patient with a previous history of allergies to multiple medications, including clarithromycin (84). It resolved after tacrolimus withdrawal.

The authors speculated on possible cross-sensitivity between tacrolimus and clarithromycin, which are both macrolides, but confirmatory skin-testing was not performed. In addition, the patient had taken many other drugs that might have been responsible.

Hair

In several studies, alopecia has been found more often with tacrolimus than ciclosporin, and severe alopecia has sometimes followed replacement of ciclosporin by tacrolimus. However, in the light of one detailed case report, and bearing in mind the minimal effect of tacrolimus on hair growth, it is not unlikely that alopecia has sometimes been mistakenly attributed to tacrolimus rather than to concomitant glucocorticoid-induced hair loss in the absence of the counteracting effects of ciclosporin (SEDA-21, 391).

Musculoskeletal

Severe acute rhabomyolysis with subsequent fatal acute renal insufficiency has been reported in an 18-month-old girl (SEDA-19, 353).

Like ciclosporin, tacrolimus has been thought to reduce bone mineral density, but this conclusion was based on a series of seven patients, all of whom had also taken azathioprine and glucocorticoids (85).

- Severe bone pain, previously reported in ciclosporin-treated patients (SED-14, 1291), also occurred as a possible consequence of tacrolimus treatment in a 50-year-old woman (86). Bilateral knee pain occurred within 2 months after renal transplantation and bone scintigraphy showed increased uptake in both knees. Calcitonin was ineffective, and she improved only after the dose of tacrolimus was reduced.

Sexual function

Priapism has been described in a patient with a liver transplant (87).

- One month after transplantation, a 19-year-old man who was taking tacrolimus, azathioprine, and prednisone, developed nausea and vomiting. He reported a 2-week history of painful spontaneous penile erections lasting 2–3 minutes and had had no previous episodes of priapism. An episode of spontaneous erection was confirmed during a medical examination that found no physical abnormalities. The tacrolimus blood concentration was 28 ng/ml. The digestive symptoms and priapism resolved after the tacrolimus concentration had fallen. Sickle cell disease was ruled out.

The authors discussed several mechanisms, including tacrolimus-induced vasodilatation, platelet aggregation, an increase in serotonin, or a fall in endothelin concentrations, based on in vitro data only.

Immunologic

Tacrolimus reduces IgE antibody synthesis, with a subsequent dramatic increase in IgE serum concentrations. This phenomenon has been reported in one asymptomatic patient but has also been advanced as an explanation for a case in which an infant girl treated with tacrolimus had milk hypersensitivity (SEDA-21, 391).

Fish allergy with increased IgE total concentrations and specific IgE antibodies against various fish products have been reported in two children with liver transplants (88). Even though both patients had a personal or familial history of allery, this again suggested a possible relation between tacrolimus and food allergy.

An increasing blood eosinophil count was associated with *Pneumocystis jiroveci* pneumonia in patients taking tacrolimus (89). The mean absolute eosinophil count was significantly higher and absolute eosinophilia (over 350×10^6/l) was more frequent in six patients who developed *P. jiroveci* pneumonia while taking tacrolimus compared with six patients with *P. jiroveci* pneumonia who were taking ciclosporin and eight patients without *P. jiroveci* pneumonia who were taking tacrolimus. A retrospective analysis also showed that the increase in eosinophil count preceded the diagnosis of *P. jiroveci* pneumonia.

Infection risk

Tacrolimus-based immunosuppression may be associated with a lower incidence of major infectious complications, namely CMV and pneumonia compared with other drugs (90). However, this hypothesis is based on a single paper, and other studies have been unable to find significant differences in the incidence of major infections between tacrolimus and ciclosporin (5,91). In addition, and as a direct consequence of excessive immunosuppression, a further retrospective study found an increased incidence of symptomatic Epstein–Barr virus infections and related lymphoproliferative disorders in children under 5 years of age who had taken tacrolimus rather than ciclosporin (92).

An unexplained change in the pattern of microbial causes of pneumonia has been noted in liver transplant patients taking tacrolimus, with an unexpectedly high incidence of *Legionella* and fungal pneumonia, the latter being involved in all deaths directly due to pneumonia (93).

In a randomized, double-blind, placebo-controlled study at 23 centers in the USA, children with moderate to severe atopic dermatitis applied the vehicle, tacrolimus ointment 0.03%, or tacrolimus ointment 0.1% for 12 weeks (94). Burning and pruritus were the main adverse effects. *Varicella* infection and vesiculobullous rashes on non-application areas occurred, but with a low incidence (below 5%). Since they occurred in those who used tacrolimus 0.03%, it is likely that they were random events rather than drug-related. Regardless of dose, there were some age-related differences in the incidence of individual adverse events. For example, otitis media was more common in younger children (2–6 years). Tacrolimus ointment had no age-selective effect that was not also observed with the vehicle. Each of the adverse events resolved without sequelae.

Long-Term Effects

Tumorigenicity

It has generally been considered that the incidence and pathological features of tacrolimus-induced cancers after transplantation are similar to those observed with other immunosuppressive agents, in particular ciclosporin (95). However, in a retrospective study in 392 children, who survived for more than 6 months after liver transplantation and were followed for a mean of 4.3 years, there was a five-fold higher rate of lymphoproliferative disease after transplantation in children who took tacrolimus ($n = 141$) than in those who took ciclosporin ($n = 251$) (96). As a result, the incidence density rate of lymphoproliferative disease was 4.8 per 100 person-years in tacrolimus-treated patients, with no difference among age groups. In addition, the mean time to lymphoproliferative disease (12.6 months) was five-fold shorter with tacrolimus than with ciclosporin. Most of the patients with lymphoproliferative disease had a primary Epstein–Barr virus infection after transplantation. The authors suggested that the 10-fold higher in vivo immunosuppressive effect of tacrolimus might have accounted for these findings.

Tacrolimus-induced post-transplant lymphoproliferative diseases are similar to those of the conditions induced by other immunosuppressants, particularly ciclosporin (SED-13, 1131). However, additional data from prolonged follow-up are still awaited. In children who are frequently Epstein–Barr virus-negative, the incidence of post-transplant lymphoproliferative disease varies from 6–11%

to 22% after liver transplantation (97). In 89 children, the incidence of post-transplant lymphoproliferative disease at 1 year was 20% (possibly related to Epstein–Barr virus in 89% of patients) (98). Excessive immunosuppression, for example as a result of prior muromonab or antithymocyte globulin administration and high tacrolimus blood concentrations during the period preceding Epstein–Barr virus infection are regarded as significant risk factors, emphasizing the need to secure low trough tacrolimus concentrations after the first post-transplant month. An increase in total gammaglobulin and the development of oligoclonal or polyclonal immunoglobulins were thought to be preliminary signs of this syndrome.

Second-Generation Effects

Pregnancy

Among 25 infants born after 27 pregnancies in tacrolimus-treated liver transplant patients there was an unexpectedly low incidence of hypertension, pre-eclampsia, and allograft function abnormalities, whereas preterm delivery, low birth weight, and transient mild renal impairment with hyperkalemia in neonates occurred at a similar rate (99).

It has been suggested that tacrolimus may be less likely than ciclosporin to cause maternal renal dysfunction or pre-eclampsia, but this hypothesis is based only on retrospective work in a small number of patients (100).

- Congestive heart failure with dilated cardiomyopathy occurred in twin boys born to a woman with a renal transplant who had taken tacrolimus throughout her pregnancy (101). One twin died from irreversible cardiac failure, and autopsy findings showed thrombogenic cardiomyopathy and degeneration of cardiac muscle. The other twin was more actively treated and had only mild tricuspid insufficiency on follow-up.

This report is in keeping with the possible and debated role of tacrolimus in the development of cardiomyopathy in children.

Teratogenicity

In the National Transplantation Pregnancy Registry, there was no evidence of an increased incidence of congenital malformations among 25 infants born after 27 pregnancies in tacrolimus-treated liver transplant patients (99).

Fetotoxicity

Among 25 infants born after 27 pregnancies in tacrolimus-treated liver transplant patients, there were two neonatal deaths whose conception had been close to the time of transplantation, and very high tacrolimus cord levels were found in one child who presented with neonatal anuria (99).

Drug Administration

Drug overdose

Acute tacrolimus overdosage usually produces only moderate toxicity or none at all. From the data available in 16 children or adults, overdosage up to 30 times the intended dose produced no symptoms in seven patients and reversible moderate increases in serum creatinine concentrations, or transaminase activities, nausea, and mild tremors in eight patients who underwent gastric decontamination and conservative measures only (102,103). An additional patient on maintenance treatment developed renal insufficiency, histoplasmosis, and sepsis within two days of overdosage. Continuous hemofiltration dramatically increased the rate of elimination of tacrolimus in two other patients who experienced acute renal and liver failure with high plasma tacrolimus blood concentrations (104).

Even large accidental overdosage of tacrolimus does not result in marked acute toxicity (105).

- The inadvertent administration of 25 times the intended dose in a 22-month-old infant produced minimal consequences, with only a five-fold reversible increase in serum amylase activity.

Drug–Drug Interactions

Antimicrobial agents

The hepatic metabolism of tacrolimus is primarily mediated by CYP3A, and experimental evidence suggests a theoretical potential for numerous interactions with drugs that induce or inhibit CYP3A. However, very few formal drug interaction studies have been carried out, and most of our current knowledge is based on case reports and small series of patients, or is derived from experience accumulated with ciclosporin. Among antimicrobial agents, erythromycin, chloramphenicol, clarithromycin, clotrimazole, danazol, oral (but not intravenous) fluconazole, itraconazole, and ketoconazole increase tacrolimus serum concentrations and can cause subsequent nephrotoxicity, whereas rifampicin reduces tacrolimus concentrations (SED-13, 1131) (SEDA-20, 348) (SEDA-22, 419) (106–109).

- A potential interaction with pristinamycin has been described in a 41-year-old renal transplant patient who had an approximate five-fold increase in tacrolimus trough concentrations within 4 days of pristinamycin treatment (110).
- A 10-fold increase in tacrolimus dosage was required in a 61-year-old patient with a renal transplant who took concomitant rifampicin (111).

The interaction of tacrolimus with rifampicin has been convincingly confirmed in six healthy volunteers who took a single oral or intravenous dose of tacrolimus (112). Rifampicin 600 mg/day for 18 days produced a significant 47% increase in tacrolimus clearance after intravenous administration and a 51% reduction in its oral systemic availability, consistent with induction by rifampicin of both hepatic and intestinal metabolism of tacrolimus.

Calcium channel blockers

A 3-day course of diltiazem 90 mg/day produced a four-fold increase in tacrolimus trough concentrations in a 68-year-old patient with a liver transplant (113).

In a non-randomized, pharmacokinetic study, four patients taking tacrolimus after kidney and liver transplantation were given diltiazem in seven incremental dosages of 0–180 mg at 2-week intervals (114). The mean tacrolimus-sparing effect was similar to the ciclosporin-sparing effect previously reported. This effect occurred at a lower dose of diltiazem in renal transplant patients than in liver transplant patients. Tacrolimus is metabolized by CYP3A4 and is also a substrate for P glycoprotein, and this interaction could have occurred by inhibition of these mechanisms.

A retrospective study has shown a significant improvement in kidney function and a 38% reduction in tacrolimus dosage requirements in patients taking both nifedipine and tacrolimus compared to patients not taking nifedipine (115).

Ibuprofen

Acute renal insufficiency in association with the use of ibuprofen and tacrolimus has been reported in two liver transplant recipients (116), and the relevance of this interaction is probably similar to that reported with ciclosporin.

Metronidazole

Metronidazole can produce a two-fold increase in blood concentrations of ciclosporin and tacrolimus, with a subsequent increase in serum creatinine in both cases (117).

Mibefradil

Mibefradil, a potent inhibitor of CYP3A, increased tacrolimus blood concentrations dramatically (118).

Nefazodone

Nefazodone may inhibit the metabolism of tacrolimus (119).

- A 16-year-old boy had a five-fold increase in tacrolimus blood concentrations and a two-fold increase in creatinine concentrations within 4 weeks of nefazodone treatment. Complete normalization occurred after replacement with paroxetine and a transient reduction in tacrolimus dosage.

Protease inhibitors

Various protease inhibitors are metabolic inhibitors and are predicted to have deleterious effects on tacrolimus metabolism.

- In a 52-year-old liver transplant patient with HIV infection, successive treatment with various antiretroviral combinations containing nelfinavir, ritonavir, or saquinavir increased tacrolimus blood concentrations and caused severe prolonged neurological symptoms suggestive of tacrolimus toxicity (120). The patient was finally stabilized with a regimen containing nelfinavir, stavudine, and lamivudine, and a more than 95% reduction in the dosage of tacrolimus.
- An acute drug interaction with nelfinavir has been described in a 49-year-old liver transplant man with HIV and hepatitis C infections (121). The patient had three consecutive episodes of increased blood tacrolimus concentrations during nelfinavir administration. Both drugs were finally continued, but the dose of tacrolimus was only one-seventieth of the usual dose.

Theophylline

An increase in tacrolimus trough blood concentrations has been attributed to concomitant theophylline therapy in a 33-year-old man with a renal transplant (122). A subsequent pharmacokinetic study showed that theophylline increased the AUC of oral tacrolimus six-fold.

Voriconazole

In a patient who took tacrolimus after liver transplant, co-administration of voriconazole resulted in raised trough tacrolimus concentrations (nearly 10-fold); there were no changes in another patient, who took a placebo (123). Voriconazole inhibits the metabolism of tacrolimus in liver microsomes by 50% in vitro.

Monitoring Therapy

In 14 patients with renal transplants, there was a closed relation between individual tacrolimus whole blood trough concentrations and the occurrence of adverse effects (124). The incidence of tacrolimus adverse effects was 76% with tacrolimus concentrations above 30 ng/ml and only 5.3% with concentrations below 10 ng/ml. This relation was found in all separate groups of adverse effects analysed, that is nephrotoxicity, neurotoxicity, infections, and others. In contrast, there was no relation between tacrolimus concentrations and rejection episodes. Accordingly, the authors stressed that tacrolimus whole blood trough concentrations should be strictly kept under 20 ng/ml.

There is no relation between tacrolimus blood concentrations and the occurrence of major neurotoxicity (125).

References

1. Spencer CM, Goa KL, Gillis JC. Tacrolimus. An update of its pharmacology and clinical efficacy in the management of organ transplantation. Drugs 1997;54(6):925–75.
2. Plosker GL, Foster RH. Tacrolimus: a further update of its pharmacology and therapeutic use in the management of organ transplantation. Drugs 2000;59(2):323–89.
3. Alessiani M, Cillo U, Fung JJ, Irish W, Abu-Elmagd K, Jain A, Takaya S, Van Thiel D, Starzl TE. Adverse effects of FK 506 overdosage after liver transplantation. Transplant Proc 1993;25(1 Pt 1):628–34.
4. Asante-Korang A, Boyle GJ, Webber SA, Miller SA, Fricker FJ. Experience of FK506 immune suppression in pediatric heart transplantation: a study of long-term adverse effects. J Heart Lung Transplant 1996;15(4):415–22.
5. Pham SM, Kormos RL, Hattler BG, Kawai A, Tsamandas AC, Demetris AJ, Murali S, Fricker FJ, Chang HC, Jain AB, Starzl TE, Hardesty RL, Griffith BP. A prospective trial of tacrolimus (FK 506) in clinical heart transplantation: intermediate-term results. J Thorac Cardiovasc Surg 1996;111(4):764–72.
6. Mor E, Sheiner PA, Schwartz ME, Emre S, Guy S, Miller CM. Reversal of severe FK506 side effects by conversion to cyclosporine-based immunosuppression. Transplantation 1994;58(3):380–2.
7. Pratschke J, Neuhaus R, Tullius SG, Haller GW, Jonas S, Steinmueller T, Bechstein WO, Neuhaus P. Treatment of cyclosporine-related adverse effects by conversion to tacrolimus after liver transplantation. Transplantation 1997;64(6):938–40.
8. Busque S, Demers P, St-Louis G, Boily JG, Tousignant J, Lemieux F, Smeesters C, Corman J, Daloze P. Conversion from Neoral (cyclosporine) to tacrolimus of kidney transplant recipients for gingival hyperplasia or hypertrichosis. Transplant Proc 1998;30(4):1247–8.
9. Tezcan H, Zimmer W, Fenstermaker R, Herzig GP, Schriber J. Severe cerebellar swelling and thrombotic thrombocytopenic purpura associated with FK506. Bone Marrow Transplant 1998;21(1):105–9.
10. Jain AB, Kashyap R, Rakela J, Starzl TE, Fung JJ. Primary adult liver transplantation under tacrolimus: more than 90 months actual follow-up survival and adverse events. Liver Transpl Surg 1999;5(2):144–50.
11. Kliem V, Brunkhorst R. Tacrolimus in kidney transplantation. A clinical review. Nephron 1998;79(1):8–20.
12. Hohage H, Bruckner D, Arlt M, Buchholz B, Zidek W, Spieker C. Influence of cyclosporine A and FK506 on 24 h blood pressure monitoring in kidney transplant recipients. Clin Nephrol 1996;45(5):342–4.
13. Dollinger MM, Plevris JN, Chauhan A, MacGilchrist AJ, Finlayson ND, Hayes PC. Tacrolimus and cardiotoxicity in adult liver transplant recipients. Lancet 1995;346(8973):507.
14. Jain AB, Fung JJ. Cyclosporin and tacrolimus in clinical transplantation. A comparative review. Clin Immunother 1996;5:351–73.
15. Johnson MC, So S, Marsh JW, Murphy AM. QT prolongation and torsades de pointes after administration of FK506. Transplantation 1992;53(4):929–30.
16. Sanoski CA, Vasquez EM, Bauman JL. QT interval prolongation associated with the use of tacrolimus in transplant recipients. Pharmacotherapy 1998;18:427.
17. Chang RK, Alzona M, Alejos J, Jue K, McDiarmid SV. Marked left ventricular hypertrophy in children on tacrolimus (FK506) after orthotopic liver transplantation. Am J Cardiol 1998;81(10):1277–80.
18. Scott JS, Boyle GJ, Daubeney PE, Miller SA, Law Y, Pigula F, Griffith BP, Webber SA. Tacrolimus: a cause of hypertrophic cardiomyopathy in pediatric heart transplant recipients? Transplant Proc 1999;31(1–2):82–3.
19. Canzanello VJ, Textor SC, Taler SJ, Schwartz LL, Porayko MK, Wiesner RH, Krom RA. Late hypertension after liver transplantation: a comparison of cyclosporine and tacrolimus (FK 506). Liver Transpl Surg 1998;4(4):328–34.
20. Taylor DO, Barr ML, Radovancevic B, Renlund DG, Mentzer RM Jr, Smart FW, Tolman DE, Frazier OH, Young JB, VanVeldhuisen P. A randomized, multicenter comparison of tacrolimus and cyclosporine immunosuppressive regimens in cardiac transplantation: decreased hyperlipidemia and hypertension with tacrolimus. J Heart Lung Transplant 1999;18(4):336–45.
21. Gonzalez MG, Hernandez-Madrid A, Sanroman AL, Monge G, De Vicente E, Barcena R. Comparison of post-liver transplantation electrocardiographic alterations between cyclosporine- and tacrolimus-treated patients. Transplant Proc 1999;31(6):2423–4.
22. Uchida N, Taniguchi S, Harada N, Shibuya T. Myocardial ischemia following allogeneic bone marrow transplantation: possible implication of tacrolimus overdose. Blood 2000;96(1):370–2.
23. Neu AM, Furth SL, Case BW, Wise B, Colombani PM, Fivush BA. Evaluation of neurotoxicity in pediatric renal transplant recipients treated with tacrolimus (FK506). Clin Transplant 1997;11(5 Pt 1):412–14.
24. Wijdicks EF, Wiesner RH, Dahlke LJ, Krom RA. FK506-induced neurotoxicity in liver transplantation. Ann Neurol 1994;35(4):498–501.
25. Mueller AR, Platz KP, Bechstein WO, Schattenfroh N, Stoltenburg-Didinger G, Blumhardt G, Christe W,

Neuhaus P. Neurotoxicity after orthotopic liver transplantation. A comparison between cyclosporine and FK506. Transplantation 1994;58(2):155–70.

26. Small SL, Fukui MB, Bramblett GT, Eidelman BH. Immunosuppression-induced leukoencephalopathy from tacrolimus (FK506). Ann Neurol 1996;40(4):575–80.

27. Steg RE, Kessinger A, Wszolek ZK. Cortical blindness and seizures in a patient receiving FK506 after bone marrow transplantation. Bone Marrow Transplant 1999; 23(9):959–62.

28. Tomura N, Kurosawa R, Kato K, Takahashi S, Watarai J, Takeda O, Watanabe A, Takada G. Transient neurotoxicity associated with FK506: MR findings. J Comput Assist Tomogr 1998;22(3):505–7.

29. Torocsik HV, Curless RG, Post J, Tzakis AG, Pearse L. FK506-induced leukoencephalopathy in children with organ transplants. Neurology 1999;52(7):1497–500.

30. Haviv YS, Friedlaender M, Dranitzki-Elhallel M. Chronic inflammatory demyelinating polyneuropathy possibly associated with tacrolimus. Clin Drug Invest 1999;18:169–72.

31. Grimbert P, Azema C, Pastural M, Dhamane D, Remy P, Salomon L, Schortgen F, Baron C, Lang P. Tacrolimus (FK506)-induced severe and late encephalopathy in a renal transplant recipient. Nephrol Dial Transplant 1999;14(10):2489–91.

32. Bronster DJ, Gurkan A, Buchsbaum MS, Emre S. Tacrolimus-associated mutism after orthotopic liver transplantation. Transplantation 2000;70(6):979–82.

33. Mori A, Tanaka J, Kobayashi S, Hashino S, Yamamoto Y, Ota S, Asaka M, Imamura M. Fatal cerebral hemorrhage associated with cyclosporin-A/FK506-related encephalopathy after allogeneic bone marrow transplantation. Ann Hematol 2000;79(10):588–92.

34. Misawa A, Takeuchi Y, Hibi S, Todo S, Imashuku S, Sawada T. FK506-induced intractable leukoencephalopathy following allogeneic bone marrow transplantation. Bone Marrow Transplant 2000;25(3):331–4.

35. Parvex P, Pinsk M, Bell LE, O'Gorman AM, Patenaude YG, Gupta IR. Reversible encephalopathy associated with tacrolimus in pediatric renal transplants. Pediatr Nephrol 2001;16(7):537–42.

36. Furukawa M, Terae S, Chu BC, Kaneko K, Kamada H, Miyasaka K. MRI in seven cases of tacrolimus (FK-506) encephalopathy: utility of FLAIR and diffusion-weighted imaging. Neuroradiology 2001;43(8):615–21.

37. Yamauchi A, Ieiri I, Kataoka Y, Tanabe M, Nishizaki T, Oishi R, Higuchi S, Otsubo K, Sugimachi K. Neurotoxicity induced by tacrolimus after liver transplantation: relation to genetic polymorphisms of the ABCB1 (MDR1) gene. Transplantation 2002;74(4):571–2.

38. Brazis PW, Spivey JR, Bolling JP, Steers JL. A case of bilateral optic neuropathy in a patient on tacrolimus (FK506) therapy after liver transplantation. Am J Ophthalmol 2000;129(4):536–8.

39. Min DI, Ku YM, Rayhill S, Corwin C, Wu YM, Hunsicker LG. Sudden hearing loss associated with tacrolimus in a kidney–pancreas allograft recipient. Pharmacotherapy 1999;19(7):891–3.

40. Weir MR, Fink JC. Risk for posttransplant diabetes mellitus with current immunosuppressive medications. Am J Kidney Dis 1999;34(1):1–13.

41. Fernandez LA, Lehmann R, Luzi L, Battezzati A, Angelico MC, Ricordi C, Tzakis A, Alejandro R. The effects of maintenance doses of FK506 versus cyclosporin A on glucose and lipid metabolism after orthotopic liver transplantation. Transplantation 1999;68(10):1532–41.

42. Lohmann T, List C, Lamesch P, Kohlhaw K, Wenzke M, Schwarz C, Richter O, Hauss J, Seissler J. Diabetes mellitus and islet cell specific autoimmunity as adverse effects of immunosuppressive therapy by FK506/tacrolimus. Exp Clin Endocrinol Diabetes 2000;108(5):347–52.

43. Kawai T, Shimada A, Kasuga A. FK506-induced autoimmune diabetes. Ann Intern Med 2000;132(6):511.

44. Jain A, Kashyap R, Marsh W, Rohal S, Khanna A, Fung JJ. Reasons for long-term use of steroid in primary adult liver transplantation under tacrolimus. Transplantation 2001;71(8):1102–6.

45. Tze WJ, Tai J, Murase N, Tzakis A, Starzl TE. Effect of FK 506 on glucose metabolism and insulin secretion in normal rats. Transplant Proc 1991;23(6):3158–60.

46. Paolillo JA, Boyle GJ, Law YM, Miller SA, Lawrence K, Wagner K, Pigula FA, Griffith BP, Webber SA. Posttransplant diabetes mellitus in pediatric thoracic organ recipients receiving tacrolimus-based immunosuppression. Transplantation 2001;71(2):252–6.

47. Furth S, Neu A, Colombani P, Plotnick L, Turner ME, Fivush B. Diabetes as a complication of tacrolimus (FK506) in pediatric renal transplant patients. Pediatr Nephrol 1996;10(1):64–6.

48. Moxey-Mims MM, Kay C, Light JA, Kher KK. Increased incidence of insulin-dependent diabetes mellitus in pediatric renal transplant patients receiving tacrolimus (FK506). Transplantation 1998;65(5):617–19.

49. Krentz AJ, Dmitrewski J, Mayer D, McMaster P, Buckels J, Dousset B, Cramb R, Smith JM, Nattrass M. Postoperative glucose metabolism in liver transplant recipients. A two-year prospective randomized study of cyclosporine versus FK506. Transplantation 1994;57(11):1666–9.

50. Jindal RM, Popescu I, Schwartz ME, Emre S, Boccagni P, Miller CM. Diabetogenicity of FK506 versus cyclosporine in liver transplant recipients. Transplantation 1994;58(3):370–2.

51. Tanabe K, Koga S, Takahashi K, Sonda K, Tokumoto T, Babazono T, Yagisawa T, Toma H, Kawai T, Fuchinoue S, Teraoka S, Ota K. Diabetes mellitus after renal transplantation under FK 506 (tacrolimus) as primary immunosuppression. Transplant Proc 1996;28(3):1304–5.

52. Knoll GA, Bell RC. Tacrolimus versus cyclosporin for immunosuppression in renal transplantation: meta-analysis of randomised trials. BMJ 1999;318(7191):1104–7.

53. Cavaille-Coll MW, Elashoff MR. Commentary on a comparison of tacrolimus and cyclosporine for immunosuppression after cadaveric renal transplantation. Transplantation 1998;65(1):142–5.

54. Yoshioka K, Sato T, Okada N, Ishii T, Imanishi M, Tanaka S, Kim T, Sugimoto T, Fujii S. Post-transplant diabetes with anti-glutamic acid decarboxylase antibody during tacrolimus therapy. Diabetes Res Clin Pract 1998;42(2):85–9.

55. Bloom RD, Rao V, Weng F, Grossman RA, Cohen D, Mange KC. Association of hepatitis C with posttransplant diabetes in renal transplant patients on tacrolimus. J Am Soc Nephrol 2002;13(5):1374–80.

56. Panz VR, Bonegio R, Raal FJ, Maher H, Hsu HC, Joffe BI. Diabetogenic effect of tacrolimus in South African patients undergoing kidney transplantation. Transplantation 2002;73(4):587–90.

57. Gomez E, Aguado S, Rodriguez M, Alvarez-Grande J. Kaposi's sarcoma after renal transplantation—disappearance after reduction of immunosuppression and reappearance 7 years later after start of mycophenolate mofetil treatment. Nephrol Dial Transplant 1998;13(12):3279–80.

58. Abouljoud MS, Levy MF, Klintmalm GB. Hyperlipidemia after liver transplantation: long-term results of the FK506/cyclosporine a US Multicenter trial. US Multicenter Study Group. Transplant Proc 1995;27(1):1121–3.

59. Abu-Elmagd KM, Bronsther O, Kobayashi M, Yagihashi A, Iwaki Y, Fung J, Alessiani M, Bontempo F,

Starzl T. Acute hemolytic anemia in liver and bone marrow transplant patients under FK 506 therapy. Transplant Proc 1991;23(6):3190–2.

60. Misra S, Moore TB, Ament ME, Busuttil RW, McDiarmid SV. Red cell aplasia in children on tacrolimus after liver transplantation. Transplantation 1998;65(4):575–7.

61. Leroy-Matheron C, Mallat A, Duvoux C, Metreau JM, Cherqui D, Dhumeaux D, Gouault-Heilmann M. Inhibitor against coagulation factor V after liver transplantation. Transplantation 1999;68(7):1054–6.

62. Burke GW, Ciancio G, Cirocco R, Markou M, Olson L, Contreras N, Roth D, Esquenazi V, Tzakis A, Miller J. Microangiopathy in kidney and simultaneous pancreas/kidney recipients treated with tacrolimus: evidence of endothelin and cytokine involvement. Transplantation 1999;68(9):1336–42.

63. Basile C, Marangi AL, Montanaro A, Giordano R, De Padova F, Ligorio VA, Santese D, Di Marco L, Semeraro A, Vernaglione L. Tacrolimus and gingival hyperplasia. Nephrol Dial Transplant 1998;13(11):2980–1.

64. Sharma AK, Holder FE. *Clostridium difficile* diarrhea after use of tacrolimus following renal transplantation. Clin Infect Dis 1998;27(6):1540–1.

65. Kang S, Lucky AW, Pariser D, Lawrence I, Hanifin JM. Long-term safety and efficacy of tacrolimus ointment for the treatment of atopic dermatitis in children. J Am Acad Dermatol 2001;44(Suppl 1):S58–64.

66. Fisher A, Mor E, Hytiroglou P, Emre S, Boccagni P, Chodoff L, Sheiner P, Schwartz M, Thung SN, Miller C. FK506 hepatotoxicity in liver allograft recipients. Transplantation 1995;59(11):1631–2.

67. Nieto Y, Russ P, Everson G, Bearman SI, Cagnoni PJ, Jones RB, Shpall EJ. Acute pancreatitis during immunosuppression with tacrolimus following an allogeneic umbilical cord blood transplantation. Bone Marrow Transplant 2000;26(1):109–11.

68. Finn WF. FK506 nephrotoxicity. Ren Fail 1999;21(3–4):319–29.

69. Shimizu T, Tanabe K, Tokumoto T, Ishikawa N, Shinmura H, Oshima T, Toma H, Yamaguchi Y. Clinical and histological analysis of acute tacrolimus (TAC) nephrotoxicity in renal allografts. Clin Transplant 1999;13(Suppl 1):48–53.

70. Ader JL, Rostaing L. Cyclosporin nephrotoxicity: pathophysiology and comparison with FK-506. Curr Opin Nephrol Hypertens 1998;7(5):539–45.

71. Antoine C, Thakur S, Daugas E, Fraoui R, Boudjeltia S, Julia P, Nochy D, Glotz D. Vascular microthrombosis in renal transplant recipients treated with tacrolimus. Transplant Proc 1998;30(6):2813–14.

72. Ducloux D, Rebibou JM, Semhoun-Ducloux S, Jamali M, Fournier V, Bresson-Vautrin C, Chalopin JM. Recurrence of hemolytic–uremic syndrome in renal transplant recipients: a meta-analysis. Transplantation 1998;65(10):1405–7.

73. Platz KP, Mueller AR, Blumhardt G, Bachmann S, Bechstein WO, Kahl A, Neuhaus P. Nephrotoxicity following orthotopic liver transplantation. A comparison between cyclosporine and FK506. Transplantation 1994;58(2):170–8.

74. Porayko MK, Gonwa TA, Klintmalm GB, Wiesner RH. Comparing nephrotoxicity of FK 506 and cyclosporine regimens after liver transplantation: preliminary results from US Multicenter trial. U.S. Multicenter Liver Study Group. Transplant Proc 1995;27(1):1114–16.

75. Heering P, Ivens K, Aker S, Grabensee B. Distal tubular acidosis induced by FK506. Clin Transplant 1998;12(5):465–71.

76. Katari SR, Magnone M, Shapiro R, Jordan M, Scantlebury V, Vivas C, Gritsch A, McCauley J, Starzl T,

Demetris AJ, Randhawa PS. Clinical features of acute reversible tacrolimus (FK 506) nephrotoxicity in kidney transplant recipients. Clin Transplant 1997;11(3):237–42.

77. Gaber LW, Moore LW, Reed L, Russell W, Alloway R, Hathaway D, Shokouh-Amiri MH, Gaber AO. Renal histology with varying FK506 blood levels. Transplant Proc 1997;29(1–2):186.

78. Solez K, Vincenti F, Filo RS. Histopathologic findings from 2-year protocol biopsies from a U.S. multicenter kidney transplant trial comparing tarolimus versus cyclosporine: a report of the FK506 Kidney Transplant Study Group. Transplantation 1998;66(12):1736–40.

79. Walder B, Ricou B, Suter PM. Tacrolimus (FK 506)-induced hemolytic uremic syndrome after heart transplantation. J Heart Lung Transplant 1998;17(10):1004–6.

80. Trimarchi HM, Truong LD, Brennan S, Gonzalez JM, Suki WN. FK506-associated thrombotic microangiopathy: report of two cases and review of the literature. Transplantation 1999;67(4):539–44.

81. Schmidt RH, Lenz T, Grone HJ, Geiger H, Scheuermann EH. Haemolytic–uraemic syndrome after tacrolimus rescue therapy for cortisone-resistant rejection. Nephrol Dial Transplant 1999;14(4):979–83.

82. Reitamo S, Wollenberg A, Schopf E, Perrot JL, Marks R, Ruzicka T, Christophers E, Kapp A, Lahfa M, Rubins A, Jablonska S, Rustin M. Safety and efficacy of 1 year of tacrolimus ointment monotherapy in adults with atopic dermatitis. The European Tacrolimus Ointment Study Group. Arch Dermatol 2000;136(8):999–1006.

83. Soter NA, Fleischer AB Jr., Webster GF, Monroe E, Lawrence I. Tacrolimus ointment for the treatment of atopic dermatitis in adult patients: part II, safety. J Am Acad Dermatol 2001;44(Suppl 1):S39–46.

84. Riley L, Mudd L, Baize T, Herzig R. Cross-sensitivity reaction between tacrolimus and macrolide antibiotics. Bone Marrow Transplant 2000;25(8):907–8.

85. Stempfle HU, Werner C, Echtler S, Assum T, Meiser B, Angermann CE, Theisen K, Gartner R. Rapid trabecular bone loss after cardiac transplantation using FK506 (tacrolimus)-based immunosuppression. Transplant Proc 1998;30(4):1132–3.

86. Villaverde V, Cantalejo M, Balsa A, Mola EM, Sanz A. Leg bone pain syndrome in a kidney transplant patient treated with tacrolimus (FK506). Ann Rheum Dis 1999;58(10):653–4.

87. Harmon JD, Ginsberg PC, Nachmann MM, Manzarbeita C, Harkaway RC. Stuttering priapism in a liver transplant patient with toxic levels of FK506. Urology 1999;54(2):366.

88. Inui A, Komatsu H, Fujisawa T, Matsumoto H, Miyagawa Y. Food allergy and tacrolimus. J Pediatr Gastroenterol Nutr 1999;28(3):355–6.

89. Dickenmann MJ, Tamm M, Tsinalis D, Binet I, Thiel G, Steiger J. Blood eosinophilia in tacrolimus-treated patients: an indicator of *Pneumocystis carinii* pneumonia Transplantation 1999;68(10):1606–8.

90. Hadley S, Samore MH, Lewis WD, Jenkins RL, Karchmer AW, Hammer SM. Major infectious complications after orthotopic liver transplantation and comparison of outcomes in patients receiving cyclosporine or FK506 as primary immunosuppression. Transplantation 1995;59(6):851–9.

91. Vincenti F, Laskow DA, Neylan JF, Mendez R, Matas AJ. One-year follow-up of an open-label trial of FK506 for primary kidney transplantation. A report of the U.S. Multicenter FK506 Kidney Transplant Group. Transplantation 1996;61(11):1576–81.

92. Cox KL, Lawrence-Miyasaki LS, Garcia-Kennedy R, Lennette ET, Martinez OM, Krams SM, Berquist WE, So SK, Esquivel CO. An increased incidence of Epstein–Barr virus infection and lymphoproliferative

disorder in young children on FK506 after liver transplantation. Transplantation 1995;59(4):524–9.

93. Singh N, Gayowski T, Wagener M, Marino IR, Yu VL. Pulmonary infections in liver transplant recipients receiving tacrolimus. Changing pattern of microbial etiologies. Transplantation 1996;61(3):396–401.

94. Paller A, Eichenfield LF, Leung DY, Stewart D, Appell M. A 12-week study of tacrolimus ointment for the treatment of atopic dermatitis in pediatric patients. J Am Acad Dermatol 2001;44(Suppl 1):S47–57.

95. Penn I. Post-transplant malignancy: the role of immunosuppression. Drug Saf 2000;23(2):101–13.

96. Younes BS, McDiarmid SV, Martin MG, Vargas JH, Goss JA, Busuttil RW, Ament ME. The effect of immunosuppression on posttransplant lymphoproliferative disease in pediatric liver transplant patients. Transplantation 2000;70(1):94–9.

97. McDiarmid SV. The use of tacrolimus in pediatric liver transplantation. J Pediatr Gastroenterol Nutr 1998;26(1):90–102.

98. Sokal EM, Antunes H, Beguin C, Bodeus M, Wallemacq P, de Ville de Goyet J, Reding R, Janssen M, Buts JP, Otte JB. Early signs and risk factors for the increased incidence of Epstein–Barr virus-related posttransplant lymphoproliferative diseases in pediatric liver transplant recipients treated with tacrolimus. Transplantation 1997;64(10):1438–42.

99. Jain A, Venkataramanan R, Fung JJ, Gartner JC, Lever J, Balan V, Warty V, Starzl TE. Pregnancy after liver transplantation under tacrolimus. Transplantation 1997;64(4):559–65.

100. Casele HL, Laifer SA. Association of pregnancy complications and choice of immunosuppressant in liver transplant patients. Transplantation 1998;65(4):581–3.

101. Vyas S, Kumar A, Piecuch S, Hidalgo G, Singh A, Anderson V, Markell MS, Baqi N. Outcome of twin pregnancy in a renal transplant recipient treated with tacrolimus. Transplantation 1999;67(3):490–2.

102. Curran CF, Blahunka PC, Lawrence ID. Acute overdoses of tacrolimus. Transplantation 1996;62(9):1376–7.

103. Mrvos R, Hodgman M, Krenzelok EP. Tacrolimus (FK 506) overdose: a report of five cases. J Toxicol Clin Toxicol 1997;35(4):395–9.

104. Hopp L, Lombardozzi S, Gilboa N, et al. Removal of FK 506 by continuous hemofiltration: report of two allograft recipients with renal and liver failures. Clin Transplant 1993;7:546–51.

105. Odoul F, Talbotec C, Boussa N, Le Guellec C, Furet Y, Maurage C, Breteau M. Massive ingestion of tacrolimus in a young liver transplant patient. Transplant Proc 1998;30(8):4327–9.

106. Mignat C. Clinically significant drug interactions with new immunosuppressive agents. Drug Saf 1997;16(4):267–78.

107. Capone D, Gentile A, Imperatore P, Palmiero G, Basile V. Effects of itraconazole on tacrolimus blood concentrations in a renal transplant recipient. Ann Pharmacother 1999;33(10):1124–5.

108. Gomez G, Alvarez ML, Errasti P, Lavilla FJ, Garcia N, Ballester B, Garcia I, Purroy A. Acute tacrolimus nephrotoxicity in renal transplant patients treated with clarithromycin. Transplant Proc 1999;31(6):2250–1.

109. Moreno M, Latorre A, Manzanares C, Morales E, Herrero JC, Dominguez-Gil B, Carreno A, Cubas A, Delgado M, Andres A, Morales JM. Clinical management of tacrolimus drug interactions in renal transplant patients. Transplant Proc 1999;31(6):2252–3.

110. Billaud EM, Chebassier C, Antoine C, Glotz D. Tacrolimus–pristinamycin drug interaction in renal transplant patient. Fundam Clin Pharmacol 1999;13:354.

111. Chenhsu RY, Loong CC, Chou MH, Lin MF, Yang WC. Renal allograft dysfunction associated with rifampin–tacrolimus interaction. Ann Pharmacother 2000;34(1):27–31.

112. Hebert MF, Fisher RM, Marsh CL, Dressler D, Bekersky I. Effects of rifampin on tacrolimus pharmacokinetics in healthy volunteers. J Clin Pharmacol 1999;39(1):91–6.

113. Hebert MF, Lam AY. Diltiazem increases tacrolimus concentrations. Ann Pharmacother 1999;33(6):680–2.

114. Jones TE, Morris RG. Pharmacokinetic interaction between tacrolimus and diltiazem: dose-response relationship in kidney and liver transplant recipients. Clin Pharmacokinet 2002;41(5):381–8.

115. Seifeldin RA, Marcos-Alvarez A, Gordon FD, Lewis WD, Jenkins RL. Nifedipine interaction with tacrolimus in liver transplant recipients. Ann Pharmacother 1997;31(5):571–5.

116. Sheiner PA, Mor E, Chodoff L, Glabman S, Emre S, Schwartz ME, Miller CM. Acute renal failure associated with the use of ibuprofen in two liver transplant recipients on FK506. Transplantation 1994;57(7):1132–3.

117. Herzig K, Johnson DW. Marked elevation of blood cyclosporin and tacrolimus levels due to concurrent metronidazole therapy. Nephrol Dial Transplant 1999;14(2):521–3.

118. Krahenbuhl S, Menafoglio A, Giostra E, Gallino A. Serious interaction between mibefradil and tacrolimus. Transplantation 1998;66(8):1113–15.

119. Campo JV, Smith C, Perel JM. Tacrolimus toxic reaction associated with the use of nefazodone: paroxetine as an alternative agent. Arch Gen Psychiatry 1998;55(11):1050–2.

120. Sheikh AM, Wolf DC, Lebovics E, Goldberg R, Horowitz HW. Concomitant human immunodeficiency virus protease inhibitor therapy markedly reduces tacrolimus metabolism and increases blood levels. Transplantation 1999;68(2):307–9.

121. Schvarcz R, Rudbeck G, Soderdahl G, Stahle L. Interaction between nelfinavir and tacrolimus after orthoptic liver transplantation in a patient coinfected with HIV and hepatitis C virus (HCV). Transplantation 2000;69(10):2194–5.

122. Boubenider S, Vincent I, Lambotte O, Roy S, Hiesse C, Taburet AM, Charpentier B. Interaction between theophylline and tacrolimus in a renal transplant patient. Nephrol Dial Transplant 2000;15(7):1066–8.

123. Venkataramanan R, Zang S, Gayowski T, Singh N. Voriconazole inhibition of the metabolism of tacrolimus in a liver transplant recipient and in human liver microsomes. Antimicrob Agents Chemother 2002;46(9):3091–3.

124. Bottiger Y, Brattstrom C, Tyden G, Sawe J, Groth CG. Tacrolimus whole blood concentrations correlate closely to side-effects in renal transplant recipients. Br J Clin Pharmacol 1999;48(3):445–8.

125. Burkhalter EL, Starzl TE, Van Thiel DH. Severe neurological complications following orthotopic liver transplantation in patients receiving FK 506 and prednisone. J Hepatol 1994;21(4):572–7.

Tafenoquine

General Information

Tafenoquine is an 8-aminoquinoline derivative that is more active than primaquine (SEDA-13, 811). It is active against all human forms of malaria. In animals, tafenoquine is several times more potent than primaquine and is effective against both blood and liver stages of the malaria parasite. It has a half-life of 14 days, which makes it a good candidate for prophylaxis, with the possibility of monthly dosing. It was effective and safe in early trials (1).

In a randomized, double-blind, placebo-controlled trial, in a single oral dose of 4–600 mg (base) in 48 men it was well tolerated, apart from minor gastrointestinal disturbances; the half-life was 14 days (2). However, although tafenoquine may well be safer than primaquine, patients were also excluded from this trial if they had glucose-6-phosphate dehydrogenase (G6PD) deficiency, so it remains to be seen whether tafenoquine can overcome the most important practical problem with primaquine. Further widespread use will be needed before rare adverse effects, if any, emerge (SEDA-14, 958) (SEDA-21, 296) (SEDA-22, 305) (SEDA-23, 306).

There has been a randomized placebo-controlled study of tafenoquine as chemoprophylaxis for malaria in 426 Gabonese schoolchildren aged 12–20 years (1). Children with G6PD deficiency were excluded. Radical cure of malaria was achieved with halofantrine followed by placebo or tafenoquine in the following daily doses: 250 mg, 125 mg, 62.5 mg, or 31.25 mg given for 3 days. Follow-up was for 77 days. Tafenoquine was highly effective in dosages over 62.5 mg/day. There were 180 adverse events thought to be related to the study drug. All were mild and self-limiting and none was considered to be serious. They included headache, fever, and abdominal pain. However, none was significantly more common with tafenoquine than with placebo. On day 28, but at no other time, there was a small (0.4 g/dl) but significant fall in hemoglobin concentration with tafenoquine 250 mg/day.

Susceptibility Factors

Age

In 104 healthy men (mean age 29 years, weight 60 kg) who took tafenoquine for malaria prophylaxis (loading dose 400 mg/day for 3 days followed by 400 mg/month in 5 consecutive months) age and weight affected the apparent volume of distribution, and subjects who contracted malaria had higher clearance rates (3). The population estimate of the first-order absorption half-life was 1.0 hour, clearance was 3.20 l/hour, volume of distribution was 1820 liters, and half-life was 16.4 days.

References

1. Lell B, Faucher JF, Missinou MA, Borrmann S, Dangelmaier O, Horton J, Kremsner PG. Malaria chemoprophylaxis with tafenoquine: a randomised study. Lancet 2000;355(9220):2041–5.
2. Brueckner RP, Lasseter KC, Lin ET, Schuster BG. First-time-in-humans safety and pharmacokinetics of WR 238605, a new antimalarial. Am J Trop Med Hyg 1998; 58(5):645–9.
3. Edstein MD, Kocisko DA, Brewer TG, Walsh DS, Eamsila C, Charles BG. Population pharmacokinetics of the new antimalarial agent tafenoquine in Thai soldiers. Br J Clin Pharmacol 2001;52(6):663–70.

Talc

General Information

Talc is a three-layered magnesium sheet with lubricant properties; it is rarely found as a pure entity in nature. The particle size varies considerably (1) depending on the manufacturing process, and may be an important factor in the development of adverse effects. Talc is principally used as inert filler material in medicinal tablets or as a drying ingredient in baby powders. The adverse effects of talc include empyema, dysrhythmias, and respiratory failure (2).

Use of talc in pleurodesis

Intrapleural therapy in humans was first reported by Bethune in 1935, when he described the dusting of pleural surfaces with talc before lobectomy to promote pleurodesis (3). Since this initial description, many different agents have been used intrapleurally to produce pleurodesis, both in patients with pleural effusion and in patients with pneumothorax. Some of these agents, talc in particular, have been associated with potentially serious adverse events. Over the last 25 years the role of intrapleural therapy has expanded and now includes the instillation of thrombolytic agents intrapleurally to hasten the resolution of complicated pleural space infections (empyema); both streptokinase and urokinase have been used for this purpose. Malignant pleural effusions represent 25–50% of all pleural effusions seen in a general hospital (4). Lung, breast, ovarian, genitourinary, and gastrointestinal tract malignancies are often associated with pleural effusions, and malignant effusion is often the first manifestation of malignancy (5,6).

The aim of pleurodesis is to produce fusion between the visceral and parietal pleural surfaces and so prevent the accumulation of air or fluid in the pleural space. In a chemical pleurodesis, this fusion is generally achieved by the instillation of agents that induce an inflammatory response on the pleural surfaces. These agents can be introduced into the pleural space through a chest tube at the bedside or during thoracoscopy/thoracotomy.

Mechanism of action

The mechanism of action of talc in pleurodesis has not been fully elucidated, although it is thought to stimulate a typical local inflammatory response, with reduced fibrinolytic activity, mesothelial cell injury, and fibroblast proliferation. Pneumonitis or respiratory failure can be secondary to downstream inflammatory mediators from more proximal talc injury (7). This acute-phase inflammatory response is dose-related (8,9) and is inhibited by glucocorticoids (10). Talc may also have an adhesion stimulating quality, since empyema alone stimulates a typical inflammatory response but does not lead to pleurodesis (11). In fact, talc stimulates intercellular adhesion molecule-1 in mesothelial cells (12). The mechanism of chronic fibrosis may involve continuous fibroblast activation by foreign body giant cell released mediators or macrophages.

Administration

Talc can be insufflated into the pleural space in a powder form, usually at thoracoscopy or thoracotomy (talc poudrage), or can be mixed with normal saline and instilled through a standard chest tube as talc slurry.

Comparative studies

The use of talc, one of the most common agents for chemical pleurodesis, has been documented in more than 3000 patients, largely in the form of case series (13). The intrapleural use of talc has been the subject of a number of recent comprehensive reviews (11,14,15).

Of 51 patients with malignant pleural effusions, 14 underwent slurry talc pleurodesis via a chest tube, 14 had talc poudrage during Video-Assisted Thoracoscopic exploration of the pleural cavity for suspected malignant effusion, and 24 underwent chemical pleurodesis with bleomycin via a chest tube (16). The most common adverse effects were chest pain and fever. The duration of adverse effects after talc pleurodesis was longer (2–3 days) than after bleomycin. There was chest pain in 15 of the 28 patients who received talc, with a duration of 18–52 (median 31) hours. There was fever in 22 of those who received talc, with a duration of 5–34 (median 12.5) hours. Complications were more common in those who received talc, such as thoracic empyema ($n = 1$), wound infection ($n = 2$), and respiratory distress ($n = 5$).

Adverse effects

Adverse events related to agents used in pleurodesis have been rare. However, almost any agent introduced into the pleural space can reach the circulation through inflamed pleural surfaces, with potential adverse effects (17). A case of fulminant pneumonitis following talc pleurodesis prompted a review of the existing experience (18). Of 78 patients with recurrent pleural effusions or pneumothorax treated by pleurodesis, five had bilateral pleural effusions, resulting in a total of 89 procedures. In 19 procedures talc was administered by poudrage and in 70 procedures it was given as a slurry with 50–500 ml of isotonic saline and 20–30 ml of 1% lidocaine. The dose was 5 g in 85 procedures, and 2.5 and 10 g each in two procedures. Of the patients who presented with malignant effusions, 18 had a primary carcinoma in the lung, 12 in the ovary, and 10 in the breast; there were six cases of lymphoma; 13 patients had less common primaries. Nine patients had benign or undiagnosed effusions and nine had spontaneous pneumothorax.

Of the procedures evaluated, 19 involved only minor complications, including fever over 38.1°C within 12 hours of pleurodesis in 13, asymptomatic hypoxemia in 19, dyspnea relieved by oxygen in six, and an increased need for narcotics in five. Subcutaneous emphysema, local infection, and asymptomatic hypotension each occurred after one procedure. There were major complications in 11 patients, including one patient with pulmonary embolism, three with unilateral pulmonary edema, eight who developed bilateral pulmonary edema, and one who died within 24 hours after bilateral talc administration. Patients developed respiratory complications after 24 of 28 talc pleurodesis procedures. The most significant respiratory complication was

adult respiratory distress syndrome, defined by bilateral diffuse infiltrates on chest X-ray and hypoxemia requiring mechanical ventilation, which occurred after eight procedures in seven patients. This figure includes one patient who died after simultaneous bilateral talc poudrage.

Minor adverse effects related to talc pleurodesis are common: chest pain occurs in about 7% of patients and fever in 16–69%. Fever characteristically starts within 4–12 hours of pleurodesis and rarely lasts more than 72 hours. Chest pain is usually only mild (11,13,14).

Respiratory complications

The most serious adverse effect of talc is a possible association between talc pleurodesis and the development of acute respiratory failure (usually in the form of ARDS); over 30 cases have been described (13) after intrapleural talc either as a slurry (8) or insufflated (18,19). The literature on acute respiratory failure after intrapleural talc has been reviewed, with recommendations on whether talc should continue to be used to produce pleurodesis (20). Some believe that intrapleural talc should not be used to produce a pleurodesis, since there are effective alternatives for producing pleurodesis (mechanical abrasion if thoracoscopy is performed, tetracycline derivatives or bleomycin if chest tubes are used).

Most cases of ARDS have occurred in patients with malignant pleural effusions, not all were clearly talc-related, and there is not enough information in some case reports to be certain of the role of talc. For example, in 1980, respiratory failure/pneumonia in seven of 197 patients who underwent talc poudrage for malignant pleural effusion was described in an abstract, but no further information regarding the clinical course of these patients is available (9). In 1983, Rinaldo et al. were the first to carefully document the development of ARDS after intrapleural talc instillation (8). They described three patients who developed progressive dyspnea and acute respiratory failure, characterized by bilateral diffuse pulmonary infiltrates, within 72 hours of the instillation of talc 10 g through a chest tube. All three had underlying malignancies and all required intubation and ventilation for respiratory failure. One patient died after 1 month of intensive care support. No other cause for ARDS was found in these patients and the authors were confident that talc had been responsible by unknown mechanisms. They recommended that other sclerosants be used for chemical pleurodesis. At around the same time, a patient who developed acute pneumonitis after chemical pleurodesis with talc 2 g was described (21). The clinical course of this patient was different to that described above: breathlessness occurred within 3 hours of pleurodesis, but the patient did not require intensive care support until 10 days later, when bilateral pulmonary infiltrates developed. At bronchoalveolar lavage 12 days after pleurodesis, talc particles were seen in the lavage fluid. No other cause for the pulmonary infiltrates was found and the patient recovered with oxygen and corticosteroid therapy alone. The authors suggested that systemic absorption of talc, with subsequent embolization to the lung, had produced this picture and they also suggested that pleural biopsies performed just before pleurodesis might have aided the systemic absorption of talc.

Three large case series were published after these reports. In two series (15,22) there were no episodes of respiratory distress after talc pleurodesis in 299 and 360 patients respectively. However, respiratory failure occurred in five of 58 patients treated with talc pleurodesis (23). Excess narcotic analgesia and infective pneumonia were considered causative in two patients, and two other patients recovered with oxygen and corticosteroids. No more information on these two patients was provided. The remaining patients developed bilateral pulmonary infiltrates and severe hypoxia consistent with ARDS, but recovered after intubation and ventilation for 5 days. This patient had undergone simultaneous bilateral talc pleurodesis and the authors thought that the higher dose of talc that this patient had received might have contributed to the development of ARDS. Again, the mechanism by which talc produced ARDS was unknown.

The possibility that talc can cause respiratory failure was explored further in 1997 (24). ARDS occurred in four of 338 patients treated with talc poudrage (2 g) via thoracoscopy. All four had malignant effusions and all developed bilateral pulmonary infiltrates, hypoxia, and hypotension within 24–48 hours of talc insufflation. All four required mechanical ventilation and three died. Bronchoalveolar lavage was performed in all four and talc crystals were recovered from lavage fluid in each case. Furthermore, at autopsy in one patient, talc crystals were found in almost every organ, showing that systemic distribution of talc did occur after pleurodesis. However, as the authors acknowledged, it was not possible to definitely attribute the symptoms in these patients to the talc pleurodesis. Studies in animals have shown systemic distribution of talc after pleurodesis (25). However, systemic dissemination may occur in all patients treated with pleurodesis and does not confirm that this is the cause of respiratory failure documented in a small number of patients.

The highest incidence of respiratory complications after talc pleurodesis was reported in 1999 in a retrospective review of 89 procedures in 78 patients (18). ARDS occurred in 9% (that is after eight procedures in seven patients). All seven patients had increased oxygen requirements, respiratory distress, and bilateral infiltrates on chest X-ray, and required a mean of 38 hours of mechanical ventilation. Six patients had malignant effusions. The other had AIDS, had undergone bilateral pleurodesis for pneumothoraces secondary to *Pneumocystis jiroveci* (*Pneumocystis carinii*) pneumonia, and died within 24 hours of the procedure. No more clinical information was given about the other six patients, particularly regarding the time-course of symptoms and investigations to exclude other diseases.

Since the literature on this topic largely comprises case reports and retrospective reviews, it is possible that complications may have been under-reported. In addition, there is marked variability in the reported incidence of respiratory complications from series to series, and there is the additional confounding factor that malignant pleural effusion, a condition with a poor short-term survival and significant associated morbidity, is often the indication for talc pleurodesis. Respiratory complications are common in these patients, and talc pleurodesis may be coincidental rather than causative. Other possible causes for respiratory distress in these patients include re-expansion pulmonary edema, sepsis related to the chest-tube, and bacterial contamination of talc. The presence of talc crystals in bronchoalveolar lavage fluid indicates systemic distribution but not necessarily causation of ARDS, and is likely to occur in all patients treated with talc. There is significant variability in the talc preparations available for pleurodesis, and it has been suggested that smaller particle size poses a higher risk for ARDS, although this is unproven. It has also been suggested that pleural biopsy before pleurodesis may increase the risk of ARDS (also unproven).

Organs and Systems

Respiratory

Intravenous injection of "solubilized" psychoactive pills containing talc can produce microemboli in small pulmonary vessels, leading to talc granulomatosis, a common finding in drug abusers. Medications intended for oral use can be injected or sniffed, together with talc particles. Pulmonary hypertension due to talc microemboli is a well-known cause of respiratory failure in heroin addicts.

- A heroin addicted patient, who had been followed up for 6 months for increasing dyspnea due to chronic cor pulmonale, was admitted to an intensive care unit. She died shortly after. Postmortem lung biopsies showed talc particles within alveolar walls and alveolar macrophages, as well as alterations in blood vessels (26).

Talc granulomatosis has been ascribed to sniffing cocaine (27).

Overzealous application of baby powder can cause severe pulmonary complications if the infant inhales the powder (28).

Formation of umbilical granulomas has been described as an adverse effect of talc in a newborn infant (29).

A group of patients underwent lung function testing 22–35 years after they were treated for idiopathic spontaneous pneumothorax either with talc poudrage or by simple drainage. The former caused mild restrictive impairment of lung function with a mean total lung capacity 89% of predicted, compared with a mean total lung capacity of 96% in subjects who had been treated by simple drainage. None of the subjects had developed a mesothelioma (30).

Although described in association with conglomerate masses and bullous disease in end-stage talc granulomatosis, spontaneous pneumothorax can also occur earlier in the course of talc-induced lung disease (31).

Gastrointestinal

An experimental animal study undertaken to determine whether cornstarch powder suspended in physiological saline causes intraperitoneal adhesions after laparotomy showed a significantly higher incidence of adhesions than in the control group two weeks after surgery. It was recommended that powder-free surgical gloves should be used to prevent adhesion formation after abdominal surgery (32).

Long-Term Effects

Tumorigenicity

Ovarian cancer has been increasing in frequency over the past 40 years, and a role for environmental factors in its etiology has been inferred from its higher incidence in industrialized countries. Cosmetic talc, deposited in the vagina after direct application to the perineum or to undergarments, sanitary napkins, or diaphragms, or through use of a talc-dusted condom during intercourse, may play an important role. In a case-control study of the use of talc in genital hygiene the risk of ovarian cancer was significantly increased in women who applied talc directly as a body powder, on a daily basis, for more than 10 years (33). The greatest risk of ovarian cancer was in the subgroup of women estimated to have made more than 10 000 talc applications during years when they were ovulating. However, this exposure was found in only 14% of women with ovarian cancer. The authors concluded that a life-time pattern of perineal talc use may increase the risk of epithelial ovarian cancer, but that it is unlikely to be the cause of most cases of epithelial ovarian cancers.

References

1. Ferrer J, Villarino MA, Tura JM, Traveria J, Light RW. Comparison of size and composition of nine different talcs: its relevance for pleurodesis. Am J Respir Crit Care Med 1998;157:A66.
2. Sahn SA. Is talc indicated for pleurodesis? Pro: Talc should be used for pleurodesis. J Branchol 2002;9:223–7.
3. Bethune N. A new technique for the deliberate production of pleural adhesions as a preliminary to lobectomy. J Thorac Surg 1935;4:251–61.
4. Deslauriers J, Beauchamp J, Desmeules M. Pleural neoplasms and malignant pleural effusion. In: Baue AE, Geha AS, Hammond GL, Laks H, Naunheim KS, editors. Glenn's Thoracic and Cardiovascular Surgery. 5th ed. Prentice-Hall International Inc, 1991;1:473–8.
5. Sahn SA. Malignant pleural effusions. In: Shields TW, LoCicero J, Ponn RB, editors. General Thoracic Surgery. 5th ed. Philadelphia: Lippincott Williams and Wilkins, 2000;1:795–803.
6. Rodriguez-Panadero F, Borderas Naranjo F, Lopez Mejias J. Pleural metastatic tumours and effusions. Frequency and pathogenic mechanisms in a post-mortem series. Eur Respir J 1989;2(4):366–9.
7. Kennedy L, Harley RA, Sahn SA, Strange C. Talc slurry pleurodesis. Pleural fluid and histologic analysis. Chest 1995;107(6):1707–12.
8. Rinaldo JE, Owens GR, Rogers RM. Adult respiratory distress syndrome following intrapleural instillation of talc. J Thorac Cardiovasc Surg 1983;85(4):523–6.
9. Todd TR, Delarue NC, Ilves R, Pearson FG, Cooper JD. Talc poudrage for malignant pleural effusion. Chest 1980;78:542–3.
10. Xie C, Teixeira LR, McGovern JP, Light RW. Systemic corticosteroids decrease the effectiveness of talc pleurodesis. Am J Respir Crit Care Med 1998;157(5 Pt 1):1441–4.
11. Kennedy L, Sahn SA. Talc pleurodesis for the treatment of pneumothorax and pleural effusion. Chest 1994;106(4):1215–22.
12. Nasreen N, Hartman DL, Mohammed KA, Antony VB. Talc-induced expression of C-C and C-X-C chemokines and intercellular adhesion molecule-1 in mesothelial cells. Am J Respir Crit Care Med 1998;158(3):971–8.
13. Sahn SA. Talc should be used for pleurodesis. Am J Respir Crit Care Med 2000;162(6):2023–4; discussion 2026.
14. Walker-Renard PB, Vaughan LM, Sahn SA. Chemical pleurodesis for malignant pleural effusions. Ann Intern Med 1994;120(1):56–64.
15. Rodriguez-Panadero F, Antony VB. Pleurodesis: state of the art. Eur Respir J 1997;10(7):1648–54.
16. Foroulis CN, Kotoulas C, Konstantinou M, Lioulias A. The management of malignant pleural effusions: talc pleurodesis versus bleomycin pleurodesis. J BUON 2001;6:397–400.
17. Wooten SA, Barbarash RA, Strange C, Sahn SA. Systemic absorption of tetracycline and lidocaine following intrapleural instillation. Chest 1988;94(5):960–3.
18. Rehse DH, Aye RW, Florence MG. Respiratory failure following talc pleurodesis. Am J Surg 1999;177(5):437–40.
19. Nandy P. Recurrent spontaneous pneumothorax: an effective method of talc poudrage. Chest 1980;77:493–5.
20. Light RW. Diseases of the pleura: the use of talc for pleurodesis. Curr Opin Pulm Med 2000;6(4):255–8.
21. Bouchama A, Chastre J, Gaudichet A, Soler P, Gibert C. Acute pneumonitis with bilateral pleural effusion after talc pleurodesis. Chest 1984;86(5):795–7.
22. Weissberg D, Ben-Zeev I. Talc pleurodesis. Experience with 360 patients. J Thorac Cardiovasc Surg 1993;106(4):689–95.
23. Kennedy L, Rusch VW, Strange C, Ginsberg RJ, Sahn SA. Pleurodesis using talc slurry. Chest 1994;106(2):342–6.
24. Campos JR, Werebe EC, Vargas FS, Jatene FB, Light RW. Respiratory failure due to insufflated talc. Lancet 1997;349(9047):251–2.
25. Werebe EC, Pazetti R, Milanez de Campos JR, Fernandez PP, Capelozzi VL, Jatene FB, Vargas FS. Systemic distribution of talc after intrapleural administration in rats. Chest 1999;115(1):190–3.
26. Magnan A, Ottomani A, Garbe L, Arnaud A, Manelli JC. Détresse respiratoire chez une héroïnomane séropositive pour le virus de l'immunodéficience humaine. [Respiratory failure in a HIV seropositive heroin addict female.] Ann Fr Anesth Reanim 1991;10(1):74–6.
27. Oubeid M, Bickel JT, Ingram EA, Scott GC. Pulmonary talc granulomatosis in a cocaine sniffer. Chest 1990;98(1):237–9.
28. Hollinger MA. Pulmonary toxicity of inhaled and intravenous talc. Toxicol Lett 1990;52(2):121–7.
29. Sparrow SA, Hallam LA. Talc granulomas. BMJ 1991;303(6793):58.
30. Lange P, Mortensen J, Groth S. Lung function 22–35 years after treatment of idiopathic spontaneous pneumothorax with talc poudrage or simple drainage. Thorax 1988;43(7):559–61.
31. Rhodes RE, Chiles C, Vick WW. Talc granulomatosis presenting as spontaneous pneumothorax. South Med J 1991;84(7):929–30.
32. Kamffer WJ, Jooste EV, Nel JT, de Wet JI. Surgical glove powder and intraperitoneal adhesion formation. An appeal for the use of powder-free surgical gloves. S Afr Med J 1992;81(3):158–9.
33. Harlow BL, Cramer DW, Bell DA, Welch WR. Perineal exposure to talc and ovarian cancer risk. Obstet Gynecol 1992;80(1):19–26.

Talipexole

General Information

Talipexole is a dopamine receptor agonist.

Long-term evaluations have indicated that no new adverse effects appear after the first 8 weeks of treatment and that overall adverse effects may abate with time.

Organs and Systems

Cardiovascular

Sinus bradycardia and hypotension have been attributed to talipexole (1).

- About 4 hours after a 65-year-old man with Parkinson's disease took talipexole hydrochloride 0.8 mg, he acutely developed sleepiness, delusion, akinesia, and faintness associated with hypotension and sinus bradycardia. A similar episode occurred when he took talipexole hydrochloride 1.2 mg/day in combination with co-careldopa (levodopa 200 mg/day plus carbidopa 20 mg/day). These symptoms persisted for 12 hours and abated gradually without any specific treatment.

The authors suggested that talipexole had caused bradycardia and hypotension by stimulating both D_2 dopamine receptors and alpha$_2$-adrenoceptors.

Nervous system

Frequent nervous system adverse effects of talipexole are drowsiness, dizziness, and fatigue (2); headache and confusion have also been reported. Talipexole can improve the negative symptoms of schizophrenia but exacerbate the positive symptoms (3).

Extrapyramidal reactions to talipexole are uncommon.

- A 60-year-old man with a 12-year history of Parkinson's disease was given talipexole for the wearing-off phenomenon 3 years after starting levodopa (4). His parkinsonism deteriorated and his serum creatine phosphokinase activity rose to 1875 IU/l. The talipexole was withdrawn after gradual dosage reduction and he gradually improved.

The authors suggested that talipexole had caused an incomplete form of the neuroleptic malignant syndrome.

References

1. Sakai T, Ii Y, Kuzuhara S. [Sinus bradycardia induced by talipexole hydrochloride in a patient with Parkinson disease.] Rinsho Shinkeigaku 1998;38(8):771–5.
2. Goetz CG, Stebbins GT, Thelen JA. Talipexole and adult Gilles de la Tourette's syndrome: double-blind, placebo-controlled clinical trial. Mov Disord 1994;9(3):315–17.
3. Benkert O, Muller-Siecheneder F, Wetzel H. Dopamine agonists in schizophrenia: a review. Eur Neuropsychopharmacol 1995;5(Suppl):43–53.
4. Osumi E, Imai T. [Increase in serum creatine phosphokinase following administration of talipexole hydrochloride.] Rinsho Shinkeigaku 2000;40(10):1041–3.

Talniflumate

See also Non-steroidal anti-inflammatory drugs

General Information

Talniflumate is an inhibitor of calcium-activated chloride channels, which has been developed to treat mucous hypersecretion (1). It is a phthalidyl ester of pyridine-carboxylic acid, related to niflumic acid.

Organs and Systems

Gastrointestinal

Gastrointestinal effects are the most frequent adverse effects of talniflumate (2).

References

1. Donnelly LE, Rogers DF. Therapy for chronic obstructive pulmonary disease in the 21st century. Drugs 2003;63(19):1973–98.
2. Torriani H. Talniflumate. Drugs Today 1983;19:97.

Tamoxifen

General Information

Tamoxifen is an estrogen receptor partial agonist with antiestrogenic properties in the breast and estrogenic effects in tissues such as bone and the cardiovascular system. In most cases there is endometrial thickening on ultrasonography, and additional tests, such as hydrosonography or hysteroscopy, are required to confirm the presence of an empty atrophic uterus, as seen in most asymptomatic women taking tamoxifen.

Tamoxifen is commonly used in the treatment of breast carcinoma (1); the overall rates published for adverse effects vary very greatly, between 1 and 60% (2,3). It has also been used as a form of HRT to reduce bone loss and the incidence of fractures in high-risk cases (4). A combination of tamoxifen with ovarian suppression is as effective as the use of cytostatic drugs, and has been claimed to be better tolerated (5–7).

The use of tamoxifen to prevent breast cancer has been reviewed (8). The merits of using tamoxifen to prevent mammary carcinoma in women who have never had the disease but are believed to be at high risk have been disputed (9), but it is clear that it would involve very long treatment and that one's view of the adverse effects might need to be revised for this class of users. The available data after 5, 10, and 15 years of follow up confirmed an increase in the incidence of endometrial cancer and of thromboembolic complications and suggested ocular toxicity, but these effects were not common and should be more than balanced by the reduced risk of coronary heart disease and osteoporosis (8).

Tamoxifen also has beneficial side effects: it protects the myocardium, reduces the incidence of ischemic heart disease, reduces the loss of bone mineral density, and has beneficial effects on lipids (10).

Observational studies

The effect of high-dose tamoxifen as an adjunct to post-operative brain irradiation has been studied for 40 weeks in 12 patients with glioblastoma multiforme, but without controls (11). Two weeks after surgery, the patients were given high-dose oral tamoxifen (120 mg/m^2 bd for 3 months) and 2 weeks later external beam radiotherapy (59.4 Gy, three daily fractions every 6.5 weeks). In one patient tamoxifen was associated with severe vomiting, necessitating dosage reduction and subsequent withdrawal; another patient had bilateral deep venous thrombosis after 51 weeks, but a causal relation was not firmly established. The authors concluded that adjuvant high-dose tamoxifen is relatively well tolerated, although in this series it did not appear to improve the prognosis.

Placebo-controlled studies

In the Breast Cancer Prevention Trial (P-1), initiated by the National Surgical Adjuvant Breast and Bowel Project (NSABP) in 1992, more than 13 000 eligible women were randomized to tamoxifen 20 mg/day or placebo for 5 years (12). During 69 months of follow-up tamoxifen reduced the risk of both invasive and non-invasive cancer and reduced fractures of the hip, radius, and spine; however, the rate of endometrial cancer increased (RR = 2.53; 95% CI = 1.35, 4.97), as did the frequency of vascular events.

General adverse effects

The adverse effects of tamoxifen are largely those that one would expect to be associated with a reduction in estrogenic activity, that is hot flushes (which can be severe), dry skin, mental or nervous system effects (such as mild depression, headache, fatigue, nervousness, and tremor), oligomenorrhea and amenorrhea, loss of libido, vaginal discharge, and rare events, such as pruritus, migraine, and edema (SED-12, 1034) (13). Nausea and vomiting are not uncommon. There are also reports of hirsutism, weight gain, rashes, thrombocytopenia, and leukopenia (SED-12, 1034); the hirsutism could reflect a relative dominance of endogenous androgen activity as the degree of estrogenic activity declines. The most specific and dangerous complication of tamoxifen is hypercalcemia, a direct consequence of the successful treatment of mammary carcinoma with bony metastases; the incidence varies greatly. Liver dysfunction and peliosis hepatis have been incidentally reported.

When tamoxifen is used in men (14), common adverse effects have included weight gain (25%), mood alterations (21%), hot flushes (21%), reduced libido (29%), and deep vein thrombosis (4%). The hot flushes respond well to oral clonidine 0.1 mg/day (15).

One expert in the USA (16) has publicly defended the safety of tamoxifen on the grounds that some of its supposed adverse effects may in fact have other causes. It is a difficult argument to follow, since she postulates that several of the unwanted effects referred to are in fact menopausal. However, these are largely likely to be inevitable consequences of the very changes that treatment with tamoxifen is intended to induce, that is suppression of estrogenic effects. Virtually the opposite belief can be derived from a Canadian study, which showed that 25 women taking tamoxifen were diffident about attributing adverse events to the drug, and therefore tended to under-report adverse effects (17). Menopause-like problems with these drugs are clearly likely to persist unless or until more selective SERMs become available, for example substances that act exclusively on the breast tumor.

Organs and Systems

Cardiovascular

Both deep vein thrombosis and pulmonary embolism have been described with tamoxifen.

- Cerebral sinus thrombosis, progressing to hemorrhagic cerebral infarction, occurred in a 52-year-old woman (18).

Although the authors pointed to the absence of risk factors other than the drug, it must be remembered that cerebral venous thrombosis is a recognized complication of various malignancies. In this case the breast tumor had been treated with various cytostatic drugs and stem cell transplantation, and tamoxifen had been given as an adjuvant, and it was believed that the tumor had been eliminated. Nevertheless, in this complex case one should perhaps be hesitant in attributing the complication solely to the drug.

In the light of three further cases of thrombosis, it has been suggested that there may be a particular predisposition to this complication in patients with high circulating concentrations of homocysteine, and that these should be checked for in advance of treatment (19).

In one case tamoxifen was associated with myocardial infarction (20).

Respiratory

An important synergistic reaction between radiation-related pulmonary fibrosis and tamoxifen has been described in 196 women followed for a minimum of 5 years, with a relative risk of 2.0 (21). However, others have shown that tamoxifen did not increase the pulmonary toxicity of agents such as carmustine and dacarbazine (22).

Nervous system

A short supplementary report on the US NSABP, originally published in 1999, later corrected the original data on adverse effects: among women who had used tamoxifen for an average of 29 months to complement irradiation after lumpectomy for intraductal carcinoma; there were five cases of stroke, compared with only one among the women who had not used tamoxifen (23). In a parallel study of breast cancer prevention there was also a slight but non-significant increase in the incidence of stroke in those taking tamoxifen. It may be wise to regard a history of stroke, transient ischemic attacks, uncontrolled hypertension, diabetes mellitus, or atrial fibrillation as relative contraindications to tamoxifen.

Sensory systems

There have been repeated reports of ophthalmic complications from tamoxifen, including irreversible retinopathy with seriously reduced visual acuity, refractile opacities, cystoid macular edema, retinal yellow-white dots, and keratopathy (SEDA-6, 356) (SEDA-7, 391) (SEDA-16, 466).

- Bilateral optic neuritis developed in a woman with breast cancer who was treated for 6 months with tamoxifen (24).

In a prospective study even in low doses (for example 10 mg/day or lower) tamoxifen caused ocular toxicity if given for a sufficiently long period; most of the changes were reversible but they justify very close monitoring (25). A related compound, MER-29 (triparanol), causes cataract and has various other adverse reactions in common with tamoxifen.

Metabolism

Steatosis and adipose tissue distribution has been evaluated using CT scanning in a cross-sectional study of 32 women taking tamoxifen for breast cancer and a similar control group (26). Tamoxifen users generally had more visceral adipose tissue and more liver fat than controls, and had a higher risk of diabetes. It is still unclear whether tamoxifen causes long-term metabolic abnormalities in obese patients, or whether patients with the metabolic syndrome X of obesity are at increased risk of the complications of tamoxifen. In view of this finding, and earlier results pointing in the same direction, it would be wise in future studies of tamoxifen to monitor metabolic changes in obese women with or without breast cancer.

Hematologic

Thrombosis and pulmonary embolism have been described with tamoxifen (27,28); the number of cases is small, but the association would not be unexpected in view of what is known about the effects of other sex hormones. The primary condition might be responsible, at least in part, for the occurrence of such complications. Tamoxifen does reduce antithrombin III but not to a degree at which a major risk would be expected, and other measurable effects on the coagulation process seem to be slight.

When tamoxifen 20 mg/day was compared with equieffective doses of anastrozole in 668 patients with advanced breast tumors that were hormone receptor-positive or of unknown receptor status, tamoxifen produced too high a rate of thromboembolism and vaginal bleeding to be considered the treatment of choice (29,30).

Liver

Liver dysfunction and peliosis hepatis are occasional complications of tamoxifen. There have also been reports of cirrhosis with fatty liver in women taking tamoxifen after surgery for breast cancer (31). The condition is reversible, and liver tests are advisable so that the tamoxifen can be promptly withdrawn if necessary.

- An elderly woman with a history of breast cancer developed multifocal steatohepatitis, but after tamoxifen was

withdrawn the CT features improved dramatically, and the hepatic transaminases normalized (32).

Skin

Tamoxifen has several adverse effects on the skin, including edema, flushing, rashes, hyperhidrosis, urticaria, alopecia, and hypertrichosis. Radiation recall dermatitis, a severe painful inflammatory skin reaction in sites that have previously been exposed to ionized radiation, can occur in patients taking tamoxifen (33). In one case the tamoxifen was withdrawn and the skin healed spontaneously in 7 weeks (34). Toremifene, a tamoxifen analogue, was well tolerated: during 18 months of continuous treatment no signs of radiation recall developed.

Hair

Effects of hormonal or antihormonal products on the hair are reported sporadically.

- A woman taking tamoxifen for metastatic cancer (presumably from the breast) developed alopecia; she began to lose her hair within 3 months and was entirely bald after 13 months of treatment (35).

The authors did not make it clear whether cytostatic drugs, which can cause alopecia, were also used, but it is striking that there have been several earlier reports of baldness with tamoxifen.

Musculoskeletal

In principle an anti-estrogen might precipitate osteoporosis, but tamoxifen has not been shown to do so; indeed, there is reason to believe that it protects the skeleton against steroid-induced bone loss (36), and in some studies of the state of the bones during treatment with tamoxifen there was actually a higher bone density than in controls.

Sexual function

Tamoxifen can cause loss of libido (37). In 57 patients sexual desire, arousal, and the ability to achieve orgasm were unaffected by tamoxifen (38). There was a 54% incidence of dyspareunia, but this seemed to be a consequence of co-administration of chemotherapy, which can cause vaginal dryness and loss of libido, rather than an effect of tamoxifen.

Reproductive system

Breasts

Tamoxifen can cause a sudden rapid increase in the growth rate of uterine leiomyomas (39).

- A leiomyoma of the breast occurred in a 50-year-old woman taking tamoxifen. It appeared as a discrete mass and had a microscopic pattern akin to leiomyomas at other sites (40).

Ovaries

In premenopausal women, tamoxifen has complex effects on ovarian function, compatible with accelerated development of multiple follicles, with ovarian enlargement and cyst formation (41,42); this might be expected in view of its similarity to clomiphene. Ovarian cysts have also been seen in postmenopausal patients with breast cancer during long-term adjuvant therapy with tamoxifen. Some premenopausal women with breast cancer had very marked increase in estrogen concentrations as a result of increased ovarian estrogen synthesis caused by tamoxifen. All premenopausal women with breast cancer taking tamoxifen should be under close gynecological and ultra-sonographic surveillance to detect such effects as soon as they occur.

Dutch workers concluded that patients who were still having a menstrual cycle had a high chance (81%) of developing ovarian cysts during tamoxifen treatment, but that postmenopausal women taking tamoxifen only developed ovarian cysts if their ovaries were able to respond to FSH stimulation, as shown by serum estradiol production (43). Differences in patient populations might explain why some workers (44) still find no association in their patients between tamoxifen and ovarian pathology.

Macroscopically visible cystic endosalpingiosis in the paraovarian region has been described in a woman who had been taking tamoxifen for breast cancer (45).

- A 2.5 cm multicystic lesion was seen on the external surface of the right ovary, and histological examination showed a mass of dilated glands lined by ciliated tubal-type epithelium and set in a fibrovascular stroma. Cystic endosalpingiosis resulting in a tumor-like mass is rarely described and is probably not well recognized by histo-pathologists.

Although unlikely to be mistaken for malignancy, this kind of lesion can result in diagnostic confusion. The role of tamoxifen in the development of the lesion in this case is not clear, but the estrogenic effects of tamoxifen may have contributed.

In one case, a complex cyst, thought to be due to ovarian hyperstimulation, resolved after monthly admin-istration of a depot gonadorelin (GnRH) receptor agonist without abandoning tamoxifen (46). One might expect some patients to react to tamoxifen with ovarian hyper-stimulation, since another non-steroidal antiestrogen (that is clomiphene) is used for ovarian stimulation and also on occasion produces cysts.

In one case reported from Japan, there was torsion of an ovarian cyst (47).

In a study of the mechanism and frequency of this complication, hormone concentrations in 20 premeno-pausal women taking tamoxifen (20 mg/day) were com-pared with those in untreated controls (48). Ovarian cysts were found in 80% of the treated patients but only in 8% of controls, and 17-beta-estradiol concentrations were significantly raised.

Uterus

Intermenstrual bleeding is a practical problem during tamoxifen therapy, particularly since it obliges the physi-cian to undertake repeated endometrial investigations to exclude malignancy. Monitoring the uterine cavity in women taking tamoxifen is mandatory, especially when there is postmenopausal bleeding.

Some preliminary but well-designed work has suggested that by inserting a levonorgestrel-releasing intrauterine

system it may be possible to limit considerably the pro-blems posed by unscheduled uterine bleeding (49).

Benign thickening of the endometrium is common dur-ing tamoxifen treatment, but appears to be fully reversi-ble within a few months of withdrawal (50,51).

Uterine polyps are not uncommon during postmeno-pausal treatment with tamoxifen (52), and up to 3% can show malignant changes. There has been an attempt to identify risk factors for the development of these polyps, by analysing the histories of 54 women in whom they occurred, as well as the histories of a larger control group without polyps (53). The women who developed polyps had a later menopause, had breast cancer for a longer period, and weighed more.

The pathology of tamoxifen-associated cases of myo-metrial adenomyosis has been compared with that in five cases of postmenopausal adenomyosis not associated with tamoxifen. The tumors were not identical: morphological features more often present in the tamoxifen-associated cases were cystic dilatation of glands (which sometimes resulted in grossly visible intramural cystic lesions), fibro-sis of the stroma, and various forms of epithelial metapla-sia. The proliferative activity in the adenomyosis, as determined by MIB1 staining, was higher in the tamox-ifen group (54), and this could be another mechanism of postmenopausal bleeding among tamoxifen users.

Tamoxifen can be associated with the formation of endometrial polyps and polypoid endometriosis; these polyps ("basilomas") can become malignant (55,56), per-haps because they lack progesterone receptors and are exposed to unopposed estrogen (57).

Whether one should routinely screen patients for endometrial changes is disputed; there seems to be no correlation between endometrial thickness and endome-trial pathology, and complications could be easily over-looked (58).

The gynecological consequences of antiestrogens (tamoxifen and toremifene) have been evaluated in 167 postmenopausal breast cancer patients in a 3-year pro-spective study. There was a proliferative endometrium more often in the tamoxifen group than in the toremifene group, but this did not translate into an increase in the rate of endometrial cancer. The authors did not recom-mend routine surveillance of the endometrium.

Immunologic

An acute inflammatory polyarthritis resembling rheuma-toid arthritis has been reported in three women tempo-rally related to the use of tamoxifen (59).

Long-Term Effects

Tumorigenicity

Several authors (60,61) have described a variety of cases, seven in all, of malignancies secondary to therapeutic dosages of tamoxifen given for 6 months to 10 years.

Uterine fibroids and endometrial polyps (sometimes with bleeding) have been reported in menopausal women who had taken tamoxifen for periods of months or years (SEDA-16, 466) (62,63). In view of this, the question of whether tamoxifen increases the risk of endometrial cancer has been widely discussed. The authors of a 1993 review of the outcome of six major trials tended strongly to the conclusion that tamoxifen can cause both endometrial hyperplasia and endometrial cancer proportional to the total dose (64); the figures pointed to an overall incidence of endometrial cancer of 0.5% in tamoxifen users and 0.1% in controls. Another major review up to 1992 concluded that in the world literature there were 70 cases of uterine malignancies with tamoxifen, including 61 cases of adenocarcinoma of the endometrium and four cases of uterine sarcoma (65).

Six cases of endometrial carcinoma were subsequently reported from France (66), and 36 cases in all had been reported up to that time (67). Although the effect can be caused by tamoxifen alone in women aged over 55, in younger women it is more likely to be an additive one, attributable to use of both tamoxifen and pelvic irradiation in the same subject.

Two distinct patterns of uterine cancer have been shown using magnetic resonance imaging of the tamoxifen-exposed uterus in 35 women (68). Patients with pattern 1 had homogeneous high signal intensity of the endometrium on T2-weighted images and enhancement of the endometrial–myometrial interface and a signal void in the lumen on gadolinium-enhanced images (18 patients). Patients with pattern 2 had heterogeneous endometrial signal intensity on T2-weighted images with enhancement of the endometrial–myometrial interface and lattice-like enhancement traversing the endometrial canal on gadolinium-enhanced images (17 patients).

Although the endometrial cancers associated with tamoxifen are usually pure adenocarcinomas, other types of rare tumors have also been reported. A pure uterine rhabdomyosarcoma has been reported (69), and a mesodermal mixed tumor of the endometrium occurred 5 years after 5 years of tamoxifen therapy (70). The tumor responded only to combined treatment with doxorubicin, cyclophosphamide, 5-fluorouracil, and carboplatin. It is possible that this type of tumor arises later than adenocarcinomas and should be looked for during long-term use of tamoxifen.

- Two well-documented cases of uterine carcinosarcoma have been reported in elderly women after 6 and 7 years of tamoxifen treatment (71). At laparotomy, a heterologous malignant mixed Mullerian tumor with peritoneal spread was found in each case and rapidly proved fatal; large uterine polyps with special histological features may represent an intermediate step in the formation of such tumors (72).

Ten similar cases have been described before.

When assessing the risk of endometrial malignancy in women with breast cancer taking tamoxifen, it is worth taking into account evidence that patients with breast cancer may at the outset have some endometrial pathology. In women with breast cancer scheduled for tamoxifen there were endometrial polyps in 9.3%, endometrial cysts in 16%, and synechiae in 12% at the outset. Tamoxifen significantly increased the incidence of these benign endometrial lesions, usually after less than 1 year of treatment. There were no cases of endometrial carcinoma in 34 patients who had taken tamoxifen for 12–24

months, and only one in 78 patients who had taken it for 5–72 months (73).

The risk that tamoxifen may cause endometrial cancer has been the subject of lively correspondence in the Lancet (74), fired by the paper published in 2000 by Bergman and her colleagues, who had concluded that the endometrial cancers seen with tamoxifen are unusually aggressive (75). Concern was expressed that such a conclusion could lead to even wider hesitation to use tamoxifen in breast cancer, despite the fact that it is already used very selectively, for example in women with positive estrogen receptors. A contradiction between Bergman's results and those of the NSABP P-1 were also highlighted, and doubts expressed whether Bergman's findings justify restricting the use of tamoxifen as a preventive agent. However, a Canadian group adduced its own work to support Bergman's findings, while French workers suggested that her unfavorable results, which were not seen in their own patients, could have been due to selection bias. It was also argued that a progestogen-releasing intrauterine contraceptive device might be used to counter the undesirable effects of tamoxifen on the endometrium. Clearly the issue raised by Bergman is still subject to debate, but it is obvious that physicians who use tamoxifen in advanced breast cancer or as a preventive agent should continue to do so selectively and that ways of protecting the endometrium during tamoxifen therapy need to be found.

The effects of norethisterone on endometrial abnormalities have been studied in 463 postmenopausal women taking tamoxifen or placebo (76). As in other studies, the results showed that any increased risk of endometrial cancer caused by tamoxifen is low and that transvaginal ultrasound screening is probably not justified for asymptomatic women taking tamoxifen. The authors found that 26% of women taking tamoxifen have endometrial thickening of 8 mm or more. It is possible to identify cysts in 7% of these women, polyps in 3%, and both cysts and polyps in 8%. These changes are characteristic of tamoxifen and unlike those seen with estrogen replacement therapy.

The usefulness of transvaginal ultrasound in detecting serious uterine changes in tamoxifen users has been disputed. According to one group it is a dependable diagnostic method (77), whereas others found it disappointing, with a high proportion of false positive results, even when the assessment criteria were chosen so as to exclude mild endometrial thickening (78). Setting these two papers beside one another it seems that one can detect marked endometrial changes but that ultrasound is not a dependable means of determining whether there is malignancy.

Second-Generation Effects

Teratogenicity

Since animal studies suggested the possibility of fetal and neonatal malformations it has for a long time been customary to exclude pregnancy before giving tamoxifen. However, there is currently reason to believe that the risk presented by tamoxifen to the human fetus is very slight or non-existent.

Susceptibility Factors

Genetic factors

Certain women have a genetic predisposition to develop an endometrial malignancy during tamoxifen treatment. There were significant amounts of tamoxifen-DNA adducts in the endometrium in eight of 16 women who took the drug but none at all in others, suggesting that a genotoxic mechanism may be responsible for tamoxifen-induced endometrial cancer (79). However, there is biochemical and histological evidence that tamoxifen-associated endometrial carcinoma is likely to be similar to type I and will therefore have a relatively favorable prognosis (80).

Drug–Drug Interactions

Cytotoxic drugs

An unusual case of rapidly fatal renal failure reported in 1993 could reflect an interaction between tamoxifen and one or more cytostatic agents, with mitomycin C a prime suspect; in a series of breast cancer patients some 10% of those treated both with tamoxifen and a cytostatic agent developed abnormal renal function, progressing towards various stages of hemolytic-uremic syndrome (81).

References

1. Jaiyesimi IA, Buzdar AU, Decker DA, Hortobagyi GN. Use of tamoxifen for breast cancer: twenty-eight years later. J Clin Oncol 1995;13(2):513–29.
2. Insler V, Lunenfeld B. Anovulation. Contrib Gynecol Obstet 1978;4:6–77.
3. De Muylder X, Neven P. Tamoxifen and potential adverse effects. Cancer J 1993;6:111.
4. Rosenfeld JA. Can the prophylactic use of raloxifene, a selective estrogen-receptor modulator, prevent bone mineral loss and fractures in women with diagnosed osteoporosis or vertebral fractures? West J Med 2000;173(3):186–8.
5. Boccardo F, Rubagotti A, Amoroso D, Mesiti M, Romeo D, Sismondi P, Giai M, Genta F, Pacini P, Distante V, Bolognesi A, Aldrighetti D, Farris A. Cyclophosphamide, methotrexate, and fluorouracil versus tamoxifen plus ovarian suppression as adjuvant treatment of estrogen receptor-positive pre-/perimenopausal breast cancer patients: results of the Italian Breast Cancer Adjuvant Study Group 02 randomized trial. J Clin Oncol 2000;18(14):2718–27.
6. Goldstein SR. Drugs for the gynecologist to prescribe in the prevention of breast cancer: current status and future trends. Am J Obstet Gynecol 2000;182(5):1121–6.
7. Reddy P, Chow MS. Safety and efficacy of antiestrogens for prevention of breast cancer. Am J Health Syst Pharm 2000;57(14):1315–25.
8. Bruzzi P. Tamoxifen for the prevention of breast cancer. Important questions remain unanswered, and existing trials should continue. BMJ 1998;316(7139):1181–2.
9. Kaufman CS, Bear HD. Another view of the tamoxifen trial. J Surg Oncol 1999;72(1):1–8.
10. Baum M. Tamoxifen—the treatment of choice. Why look for alternatives? Br J Cancer 1998;78(Suppl 4):1–4.
11. Muanza T, Shenouda G, Souhami L, Leblanc R, Mohr G, Corns R, Langleben A. High dose tamoxifen and radiotherapy in patients with glioblastoma multiforme: a phase IB study. Can J Neurol Sci 2000;27(4):302–6.
12. Dunn BK, Ford LG. Prevention of breast cancer. Sem Breast Dis 2000;3:90–9.
13. Sawka CA, Pritchard KI, Paterson AH, Sutherland DJ, Thomson DB, Shelley WE, Myers RE, Mobbs BG, Malkin A, Meakin JW. Role and mechanism of action of tamoxifen in premenopausal women with metastatic breast carcinoma. Cancer Res 1986;46(6):3152–6.
14. Anelli TF, Anelli A, Tran KN, Lebwohl DE, Borgen PI. Tamoxifen administration is associated with a high rate of treatment-limiting symptoms in male breast cancer patients. Cancer 1994;74(1):74–7.
15. Pandya KJ, Raubertas RF, Flynn PJ, Hynes HE, Rosenbluth RJ, Kirshner JJ, Pierce HI, Dragalin V, Morrow GR. Oral clonidine in postmenopausal patients with breast cancer experiencing tamoxifen-induced hot flashes: a University of Rochester Cancer Center Community Clinical Oncology Program study. Ann Intern Med 2000;132(10):788–93.
16. Jones J. Tamoxifen side effects may be attributable to other causes. J Natl Cancer Inst 2001;93(1):11–12.
17. Arnold BJ, Cumming CE, Lees AW, Handman MD, Cumming DC, Urion C. Tamoxifen in breast cancer: symptom reporting. Breast J 2001;7(2):97–100.
18. Finelli PF, Schauer PK. Cerebral sinus thrombosis with tamoxifen. Neurology 2001;56(8):1113–14.
19. Tisman G. Thromboses after estrogen hormone replacement, progesterone or tamoxifen therapy in patients with elevated blood levels of homocysteine. Am J Hematol 2001;68(2):135.
20. Ludwig M, Tolg R, Richardt G, Katus HA, Diedrich K. Myocardial infarction associated with ovarian hyperstimulation syndrome. JAMA 1999;282(7):632–3.
21. Bentzen SM, Skoczylas JZ, Overgaard M, Overgaard J. Radiotherapy-related lung fibrosis enhanced by tamoxifen. J Natl Cancer Inst 1996;88(13):918–22.
22. Rusthoven JJ, Quirt IC, Iscoe NA, McCulloch PB, James KW, Lohmann RC, Jensen J, Burdette-Radoux S, Bodurtha AJ, Silver HK, Verma S, Armitage GR, Zee B, Bennett K. Randomized, double-blind, placebo-controlled trial comparing the response rates of carmustine, dacarbazine, and cisplatin with and without tamoxifen in patients with metastatic melanoma. National Cancer Institute of Canada Clinical Trials Group. J Clin Oncol 1996;14(7):2083–90.
23. Dignam JJ, Fisher B. Occurrence of stroke with tamoxifen in NSABP B-24. Lancet 2000;355(9206):848–9.
24. Pugesgaard T, Von Eyben FE. Bilateral optic neuritis evolved during tamoxifen treatment. Cancer 1986;58(2):383–6.
25. Pavlidis NA, Petris C, Briassoulis E, Klouvas G, Psilas C, Rempapis J, Petroutsos G. Clear evidence that long-term, low-dose tamoxifen treatment can induce ocular toxicity. A prospective study of 63 patients. Cancer 1992;69(12):2961–4.
26. Nguyen MC, Stewart RB, Banerji MA, Gordon DH, Kral JG. Relationships between tamoxifen use, liver fat and body fat distribution in women with breast cancer. Int J Obes Relat Metab Disord 2001;25(2):296–8.
27. Ferrazzi E, Cartei G, De Besi P, Fornasiero A, Palu G, Paccagnella A, Sperandio P, Fosser V, Grigoletto E, Fiorentino M. Tamoxifen in disseminated breast cancer. Tumori 1977;63(5):463–8.
28. Millward MJ, Cantwell BM, Lien EA, Carmichael J, Harris AL. Intermittent high-dose tamoxifen as a potential modifier of multidrug resistance. Eur J Cancer 1992;28A(4–5):805–10.
29. Bonneterre J, Thurlimann B, Robertson JF, Krzakowski M, Mauriac L, Koralewski P, Vergote I, Webster A, Steinberg M, von Euler M. Anastrozole versus tamoxifen as first-line therapy for advanced breast cancer in 668

postmenopausal women: results of the Tamoxifen or Arimidex Randomized Group Efficacy and Tolerability study. J Clin Oncol 2000;18(22):3748–57.

30. Nabholtz JM, Buzdar A, Pollak M, Harwin W, Burton G, Mangalik A, Steinberg M, Webster A, von Euler M. Anastrozole is superior to tamoxifen as first-line therapy for advanced breast cancer in postmenopausal women: results of a North American multicenter randomized trial. Arimidex Study Group. J Clin Oncol 2000;18(22):3758–67.

31. Oien KA, Moffat D, Curry GW, Dickson J, Habeshaw T, Mills PR, MacSween RN. Cirrhosis with steatohepatitis after adjuvant tamoxifen. Lancet 1999;353(9146):36–7.

32. Cai Q, Bensen M, Greene R, Kirchner J. Tamoxifen-induced transient multifocal hepatic fatty infiltration. Am J Gastroenterol 2000;95(1):277–9.

33. Parry BR. Radiation recall induced by tamoxifen. Lancet 1992;340(8810):49.

34. Bostrom A, Sjolin-Forsberg G, Wilking N, Bergh J. Radiation recall—another call with tamoxifen. Acta Oncol 1999;38(7):955–9.

35. Puglisi F, Aprile G, Sobrero A. Tamoxifen-induced total alopecia. Ann Intern Med 2001;134(12):1154–5.

36. Fentiman IS, Fogelman I. Breast cancer and osteoporosis—a bridge at last. Eur J Cancer 1993;29A(4):485–6.

37. Malinovszky KM, Cameron D, Douglas S, Love C, Leonard T, Dixon JM, Hopwood P, Leonard RC. Breast cancer patients' experiences on endocrine therapy: monitoring with a checklist for patients on endocrine therapy (C-PET). Breast 2004;13(5):363–8.

38. Mortimer JE, Boucher L, Baty J, Knapp DL, Ryan E, Rowland JH. Effect of tamoxifen on sexual functioning in patients with breast cancer. J Clin Oncol 1999;17(5):1488–92.

39. Leo L, Lanza A, Re A, Tessarolo M, Bellino R, Lauricella A, Wierdis T. Leiomyomas in patients receiving tamoxifen. Clin Exp Obstet Gynecol 1994;21(2):94–8.

40. Son EJ, Oh KK, Kim EK, Son HJ, Jung WH, Lee HD. Leiomyoma of the breast in a 50-year-old woman receiving tamoxifen. Am J Roentgenol 1998;171(6):1684–6.

41. Sherman BM, Chapler FK, Crickard K, Wycoff D. Endocrine consequences of continuous antiestrogen therapy with tamoxifen in premenopausal women. J Clin Invest 1979;64(2):398–404.

42. Powles TJ, Jones AL, Ashley SE, O'Brien ME, Tidy VA, Treleavan J, Cosgrove D, Nash AG, Sacks N, Baum M, McKinna JA, Davey JB. The Royal Marsden Hospital pilot tamoxifen chemoprevention trial. Breast Cancer Res Treat 1994;31(1):73–82.

43. Mourits MJ, de Vries EG, Willemse PH, ten Hoor KA, Hollema H, Sluiter WJ, de Bruijn HW, van der Zee AG. Ovarian cysts in women receiving tamoxifen for breast cancer. Br J Cancer 1999;79(11–12):1761–4.

44. McGonigle KF, Vasilev SA, Odom-Maryon T, Simpson JF. Ovarian histopathology in breast cancer patients receiving tamoxifen. Gynecol Oncol 1999;73(3):402–6.

45. McCluggage WG, Weir PE. Paraovarian cystic endosalpingiosis in association with tamoxifen therapy. J Clin Pathol 2000;53(2):161–2.

46. Turan C, Unal O, Dansuk R, Guzelmeric K, Cengizoglu B, Esim E. Successful management of an ovarian enlargement resembling ovarian hyperstimulation in a premenopausal breast cancer patient receiving tamoxifen with cotreatment of GnRH-agonist. Eur J Obstet Gynecol Reprod Biol 2001;97(1):105–7.

47. Nasu K, Miyazaki T, Kiyonaga Y, Kawasaki F, Miyakawa I. Torsion of a functional ovarian cyst in a premenopausal patient receiving tamoxifen. Gynecol Obstet Invest 1999;48(3):200–2.

48. Cohen I, Figer A, Tepper R, Shapira J, Altaras MM, Yigael D, Beyth Y. Ovarian overstimulation and cystic

formation in premenopausal tamoxifen exposure: comparison between tamoxifen-treated and nontreated breast cancer patients. Gynecol Oncol 1999;72(2):202–7.

49. Gardner FJ, Konje JC, Abrams KR, Brown LJ, Khanna S, Al-Azzawi F, Bell SC, Taylor DJ. Endometrial protection from tamoxifen-stimulated changes by a levonorgestrel-releasing intrauterine system: a randomised controlled trial. Lancet 2000;356(9243):1711–17.

50. Love CD, Dixon JM. Thickened endometrium caused by tamoxifen returns to normal following tamoxifen cessation. Breast 2000;9(3):156–7.

51. Cohen I, Beyth Y, Azaria R, Flex D, Figer A, Tepper R. Ultrasonographic measurement of endometrial changes following discontinuation of tamoxifen treatment in postmenopausal breast cancer patients. BJOG 2000;107(9):1083–7.

52. Bakour SH, Khan KS, Newton JR. Evaluation of the endometrium in abnormal uterine bleeding associated with long-term tamoxifen use. Gynaecol Endosc 2000;9:19–22.

53. Cohen I, Azaria R, Bernheim J, Shapira J, Beyth Y. Risk factors of endometrial polyps resected from postmenopausal patients with breast carcinoma treated with tamoxifen. Cancer 2001;92(5):1151–5.

54. McCluggage WG, Desai V, Manek S. Tamoxifen-associated postmenopausal adenomyosis exhibits stromal fibrosis, glandular dilatation and epithelial metaplasias. Histopathology 2000;37(4):340–6.

55. Schlesinger C, Silverberg SG. Tamoxifen-associated polyps (basalomas) arising in multiple endometriotic foci: A case report and review of the literature. Gynecol Oncol 1999;73(2):305–11.

56. Cohen I, Bernheim J, Azaria R, Tepper R, Sharony R, Beyth Y. Malignant endometrial polyps in postmenopausal breast cancer tamoxifen-treated patients. Gynecol Oncol 1999;75(1):136–41.

57. Maia H Jr., Maltez A, Calmon LC, Moreira K, Coutinho EM. Endometrial carcinoma in postmenopausal patients using hormone replacement therapy: a report on four cases. Gynaecol Endosc 1999;8:235–41.

58. Seoud M, Shamseddine A, Khalil A, Salem Z, Saghir N, Bikhazi K, Bitar N, Azar G, Kaspar H. Tamoxifen and endometrial pathologies: a prospective study. Gynecol Oncol 1999;75(1):15–19.

59. Creamer P, Lim K, George E, Dieppe P. Acute inflammatory polyarthritis in association with tamoxifen. Br J Rheumatol 1994;33(6):583–5.

60. Clement PB, Oliva E, Young RH. Mullerian adenosarcoma of the uterine corpus associated with tamoxifen therapy: a report of six cases and a review of tamoxifen-associated endometrial lesions. Int J Gynecol Pathol 1996;15(3):222–9.

61. Orbo A, Lindal S, Mortensen E. Tamoxifen og endometriecancer. En kasuistikk. [Tamoxifen and endometrial cancer. A case report.] Tidsskr Nor Laegeforen 1996;116(16):1877–8.

62. Boudouris O, Ferrand S, Guillet JL, Madelenat P. Efféts paradoxaux du tamoxifène sur l'utérus de la femme. [Paradoxical effects of tamoxifen on the woman's uterus. Apropos of 7 cases of myoma that appeared while under anti-estrogen treatment.] J Gynecol Obstet Biol Reprod (Paris) 1989;18(3):372–8.

63. Nuovo MA, Nuovo GJ, McCaffrey RM, Levine RU, Barron B, Winkler B. Endometrial polyps in postmenopausal patients receiving tamoxifen. Int J Gynecol Pathol 1989;8(2):125–31.

64. Rutqvist LE, Mattsson A. Cardiac and thromboembolic morbidity among postmenopausal women with early-stage breast cancer in a randomized trial of adjuvant tamoxifen. The Stockholm Breast Cancer Study Group. J Natl Cancer Inst 1993;85(17):1398–406.

65. Seoud MA, Johnson J, Weed JC Jr. Gynecologic tumors in tamoxifen-treated women with breast cancer. Obstet Gynecol 1993;82(2):165–9.

66. Treilleux T, Mignotte H, Clement-Chassagne C, Guastalla P, Bailly C. Tamoxifen and malignant epithelial-nonepithelial tumours of the endometrium: report of six cases and review of the literature. Eur J Surg Oncol 1999;25(5):477–82.

67. Ramondetta LM, Sherwood JB, Dunton CJ, Palazzo JP. Endometrial cancer in polyps associated with tamoxifen use. Am J Obstet Gynecol 1999;180(2 Pt 1):340–1.

68. Ascher SM, Johnson JC, Barnes WA, Bae CJ, Patt RH, Zeman RK. MR imaging appearance of the uterus in postmenopausal women receiving tamoxifen therapy for breast cancer: histopathologic correlation. Radiology 1996;200(1):105–10.

69. Okada DH, Rowland JB, Petrovic LM. Uterine pleomorphic rhabdomyosarcoma in a patient receiving tamoxifen therapy. Gynecol Oncol 1999;75(3):509–13.

70. Dumortier J, Freyer G, Sasco AJ, Frappart L, Zenone T, Romestaing P, Trillet-Lenoir V. Endometrial mesodermal mixed tumor occurring after tamoxifen treatment: report on a new case and review of the literature. Ann Oncol 2000;11(3):355–8.

71. Jessop FA, Roberts PF. Mullerian adenosarcoma of the uterus in association with tamoxifen therapy. Histopathology 2000;36(1):91–2.

72. Fotiou S, Hatjieleftheriou G, Kyrousis G, Kokka F, Apostolikas N. Long-term tamoxifen treatment: a possible aetiological factor in the development of uterine carcinosarcoma: two case-reports and review of the literature. Anticancer Res 2000;20(3B):2015–20.

73. Andia D, Lafuente P, Matorras R, Usandizaga JM. Uterine side effects of treatment with tamoxifen. Eur J Obstet Gynecol Reprod Biol 2000;92(2):235–40.

74. Tempfer C, Kubista E, Atkins CD, Narod SA, Pal T, Graham T, Mitchell M, Fyles A, Lasset C, Bonadona V, Mignotte H, Bremond A, Van Leeuwen FE, Bergman L, Beelen MLR, Gallee MPW, Hollema H, Dickson MJ, Pandiarajan T, Kairies P, Marsh F, Mayfield M. Tamoxifen and risk of endometrial cancer. Lancet 2001;357(9249):65–8.

75. Bergman L, Beelen ML, Gallee MP, Hollema H, Benraadt J, van Leeuwen FE. Risk and prognosis of endometrial cancer after tamoxifen for breast cancer. Comprehensive Cancer Centres' ALERT Group. Assessment of Liver and Endometrial cancer Risk following Tamoxifen. Lancet 2000;356(9233):881–7.

76. Powles TJ, Bourne T, Athanasiou S, Chang J, Grubock K, Ashley S, Oakes L, Tidy A, Davey J, Viggers J, Humphries S, Collins W. The effects of norethisterone on endometrial abnormalities identified by transvaginal ultrasound screening of healthy post-menopausal women on tamoxifen or placebo. Br J Cancer 1998;78(2):272–5.

77. Strauss HG, Wolters M, Methfessel G, Buchmann J, Koelbl H. Significance of endovaginal ultrasonography in assessing tamoxifen-associated changes of the endometrium. A prospective study. Acta Obstet Gynecol Scand 2000;79(8):697–701.

78. Gerber B, Krause A, Muller H, Reimer T, Kulz T, Makovitzky J, Kundt G, Friese K. Effects of adjuvant tamoxifen on the endometrium in postmenopausal women with breast cancer: a prospective long-term study using transvaginal ultrasound. J Clin Oncol 2000;18(20):3464–70.

79. Shibutani S, Ravindernath A, Suzuki N, Terashima I, Sugarman SM, Grollman AP, Pearl ML. Identification of tamoxifen-DNA adducts in the endometrium of women treated with tamoxifen. Carcinogenesis 2000;21(8):1461–7.

80. Roy RN, Gerulath AH, Cecutti A, Bhavnani BR. Effect of tamoxifen treatment on the endometrial expression of human insulin-like growth factors and their receptor mRNAs. Mol Cell Endocrinol 2000;165(1–2):173–8.

81. Montes A, Powles TJ, O'Brien ME, Ashley SE, Luckit J, Treleaven J. A toxic interaction between mitomycin C and tamoxifen causing the haemolytic uraemic syndrome. Eur J Cancer 1993;29A(13):1854–7.

Tamsulosin

See also Alpha-adrenoceptor antagonists

General Information

Tamsulosin is an alpha$_1$-adrenoceptor antagonist that was specially designed for the treatment of benign prostatic hyperplasia, since it is highly selective for the urinary tract alpha$_{1A}$-adrenoceptors [1]. Indeed, it produces little or no cardiovascular effects, no first-dose effect, and much less dizziness. In clinical trials, adverse effects included dizziness, weakness, headache, and nasal congestion. Abnormal ejaculation was the most frequent adverse effect, in 8% of the patients at 0.4 mg/day, and in 18% at 0.8 mg/day [2,3].

References

1. Michel MC, de la Rosette JJ. Efficacy and safety of tamsulosin in the treatment of urological diseases. Expert Opin Pharmacother 2004;5(1):151–60.

2. Narayan P, Tewari A. Overview of alpha-blocker therapy for benign prostatic hyperplasia. Urology 1998;51(Suppl 4A):38–45.

3. de Mey C. Cardiovascular effects of alpha-blockers used for the treatment of symptomatic BPH: impact on safety and well-being. Eur Urol 1998;34(Suppl 2):18–28.

Taxaceae

See also Herbal medicines

General Information

The family of Taxaceae contains two genera:

1. *Taxus* (yew)
2. *Torreya* (torreya).

Taxus species

Taxus (yew) trees contain alkaloids called taxanes that have anticancer activity and are the basis of the semi-synthetic anticancer drugs paclitaxel and docetaxel (see separate monographs), which are based on taxol, from *Taxus brevifolia*.

Taxus baccata has been used as a means of suicide (1–3), successfully, because of cardiac dysrhythmias (4).

Taxoids from *Taxus cuspidata* (the Japanese yew) inhibit P glycoprotein and are candidates for reversing multidrug resistance in cancer cells (5).

Taxus celebica, which contains the flavonoid sciadopitysin, is traditionally used in China as an herbal treatment of diabetes mellitus.

Adverse effects
Hematologic
Thrombocytopenia has been attributed to the Chinese herbal mixture Jui, prepared from *T. cuspidata* (Japanese yew) (6).

- A 51-year-old Japanese woman developed gingival bleeding and petechiae. The only medication she had taken was Jui. She had thrombocytopenia and the causal relation was demonstrated by rechallenge. She recovered on withdrawal of the product.

Immunologic
Of 18 patients with seasonal allergic rhinitis, suffering mainly in April and May, five were sensitized to the pollen of *T. cuspidata* (7).

Drug overdose
In two cases the ingestion of a massive dose of *T. celebica* was followed by acute renal insufficiency; both patients initially presented with gastrointestinal upset and fever (8).

- A 40-year-old patient attempted suicide by drinking an extract made from 120 g of yew needles (*T. baccata*); recurrent episodes of ventricular tachycardia were successfully treated with high doses of lidocaine (9).
- Lethal intoxication with yew leaves (*T. baccata*) presented with dizziness 1 hour after ingestion, nausea, diffuse abdominal pain, unconsciousness, weak breathing, tachycardia, brief ventricular flutter followed by bradycardia, and finally death by respiratory arrest and cardiac standstill; the electrocardiogram showed atypical bundle branch block and absent P waves (10).
- A 14-year-old boy cut leaves from a yew tree (*T. baccata*), crushed them, and ingested them; he died soon afterwards (11). At autopsy pieces of partially crushed, partially preserved yew leaves were found in the stomach. The histological findings were non-specific.

Four prisoners drank a decoction of yew needles (*T. baccata*) (12). Two died in prison with cardiac arrest. One went into deep coma, and had several episodes of ventricular fibrillation, controlled by defibrillation; after return of consciousness his general condition deteriorated suddenly, he lost consciousness again, his circulation stopped, and he died on the fourth day. The other patient drank a much smaller amount of the decoction; he was conscious, had bradycardia requiring transient pacemaking, and had a mild ventricular dysrhythmia; he recovered after 10 days. In both cases there was excessive diuresis and severe hypokalemia and atropine was effective for a short time in the control of bradycardia.

Of 11 197 exposures to the berries of *Taxus* species children under 12 years of age were involved in 96% (under 6 years 93%; 6–12 years 3.7%) (13). When the final outcome of the exposure was documented ($n = 7269$), there were no adverse effects in 93% and minor effects in 7.0%. There were moderate (more pronounced, but not life-threatening) effects in 30 individuals and major (life-threatening) effects in four. There were no deaths. Decontamination therapy had no impact on outcome compared with no therapy. When symptoms occurred after exposure to *Taxus*, the most frequent were gastrointestinal (66%), followed by skin reactions (8.3%), nervous system effects (6.0%), and cardiovascular effects (6.0%).

References

1. Stebbing J, Simmons HL, Hepple J. Deliberate self-harm using yew leaves (*Taxus baccata*). Br J Clin Pract 1995;49(2):101.
2. Janssen J, Peltenburg H. Een klassieke wijze van zelfdoding: met *Taxus baccata*. [A classical method of committing suicide: with *Taxus baccata*.] Ned Tijdschr Geneeskd 1985;129(13):603–5.
3. Frohne D, Pribilla O. Todliche Vergiftung mit *Taxus baccata*. [Fatal poisoning with *Taxus baccata*.] Arch Toxikol 1965;21(3):150–62.
4. Willaert W, Claessens P, Vankelecom B, Vanderheyden M. Intoxication with *Taxus baccata*: cardiac arrhythmias following yew leaves ingestion. Pacing Clin Electrophysiol 2002;25(4 Pt 1):511–12.
5. Kobayashi J, Shigemori H, Hosoyama H, Chen Z, Akiyama S, Naito M, Tsuruo T. Multidrug resistance reversal activity of taxoids from *Taxus cuspidata* in KB-C2 and 2780AD cells. Jpn J Cancer Res 2000;91(6):638–42.
6. Azuno Y, Yaga K, Sasayama T, Kimoto K. Thrombocytopenia induced by Jui, a traditional Chinese herbal medicine. Lancet 1999;354(9175):304–5.
7. Maguchi S, Fukuda S. *Taxus cuspidata* (Japanese yew) pollen nasal allergy. Auris Nasus Larynx 2001;28 (Suppl):S43–7.
8. Lin JL, Ho YS. Flavonoid-induced acute nephropathy. Am J Kidney Dis 1994;23(3):433–40.
9. von Dach B, Streuli RA. Lidocainbehandlung einer Vergiftung mit Eibennadeln (*Taxus baccata* L.). [Lidocaine treatment of poisoning with yew needles (*Taxus baccata* L.).] Schweiz Med Wochenschr 1988;118(30):1113–16.
10. Schulte T. Todliche Vergiftung mit Eibennadeln (*Taxus baccata*). [Lethal intoxication with leaves of the yew tree (*Taxus baccata*).] Arch Toxicol 1975;34(2):153–8.
11. Wehner F, Gawatz O. Suizidale Eibenintoxikationen—von Casar bis heute—oder: Suizidanleitung im Internet. [Suicidal yew poisoning—from Caesar to today—or suicide instructions on the internet.] Arch Kriminol 2003;211 (1–2):19–26.
12. Feldman R, Chrobak J, Liberek Z, Szajewski J. Cztery przypadki zatrucia wywarem z igiel cisu (*Taxus baccata*). [4 cases of poisoning with the extract of yew (*Taxus baccata*) needles.] Pol Arch Med Wewn 1988;79(1):26–9.
13. Krenzelok EP, Jacobsen TD, Aronis J. Is the yew really poisonous to you? J Toxicol Clin Toxicol 1998;36(3):219–23.

Tea tree oil

General Information

Tea tree oil is extracted from *Melaleuca alternifolia*, a plant that is native to Australia. It is considered to have antibacterial properties, including an effect on methicillin-resistant *Staphylococcus aureus* (MRSA), while the commensal flora of the skin seem to be less susceptible (1). In addition, it is said to have antifungal, antiviral, anti-inflammatory, and analgesic properties, and has been increasingly incorporated into cosmetics for aromatherapy.

Organs and Systems

Nervous system

The systemic toxicity of tea tree oil is comparable to that of eucalyptus oil, and ingestion of 10–25 ml has resulted in ataxia, drowsiness, disorientation, or coma for 2 days, recovery was full without complications (2).

- A 4-year-old boy took a small quantity of tea tree oil and within 30 minutes became ataxic and shortly thereafter progressed to unresponsiveness; he was endotracheally intubated and his neurological status improved gradually over 10 hours (3).

Immunologic

Since the beginning of the 1990s, several case reports of allergic contact dermatitis to tea tree oil have been published (4,5). Most of these adverse effects emerged after the application of aged tea tree oil, and patients who are allergic to tea tree oil do not react to patch tests with freshly distilled tea tree oil (6). In a review of tea tree oil focussing on the allergic compounds in detail, the authors concluded that *d*-limonen, alpha-terpenes, and the aromadendrens are important allergens, whereas 1,8-cineole was not believed to be important, as has been previously stated (7). Tea tree oil undergoes photo-oxidation within a few days to several months, leading to degradation products, such as peroxides, epoxides, and endoperoxides, which are moderate to strong sensitizers. Experimental sensitization in guinea pigs was followed by patch tests with 15 constituents of oxidized tea tree oil in 11 patients with tea tree oil contact dermatitis (6). All the patients reacted to alpha-terpinene, terpinolene, and ascaridol, the latter being a deterioration product of alpha-terpinene.

Many people who are allergic to tea tree oil also react to turpentine, colophony, fragrances, balsam of Peru, and plant extracts of Compositae (8).

- A 46-year-old Chinese man developed an allergic contact dermatitis to tea tree oil, colophony, balsam of Peru, and abitol. He had used the tea tree oil under an occlusive dressing on a superficial abrasion on his left shin for 2 weeks, after which the treated area became red and itchy. During the next week, skin lesions appeared on his trunk and extremities, and were diagnosed as an erythema multiforme-like id reaction.

- A 38-year-old man developed an immediate hypersensitivity reaction, characterized by pruritus, throat constriction, and light-headedness, after topical application of tea tree oil (9). An intradermal test with tea tree oil gave a wheal and flare reaction. Specific IgG and IgE were not detected.

References

1. Carson CF, Riley TV, Cookson BD. Efficacy and safety of tea tree oil as a topical antimicrobial agent. J Hosp Infect 1998;40(3):175–8.
2. Seawright A. Comment: tea tree oil poisoning. Med J Aust 1993;(159):831.
3. Morris MC, Donoghue A, Markowitz JA, Osterhoudt KC. Ingestion of tea tree oil (*Melaleuca* oil) by a 4-year-old boy. Pediatr Emerg Care 2003;19(3):169–71.
4. Apted JH. Contact dermatitis associated with the use of tea-tree oil. Australas J Dermatol 1991;32(3):177.
5. Varma S, Blackford S, Statham BN, Blackwell A. Combined contact allergy to tea tree oil and lavender oil complicating chronic vulvovaginitis. Contact Dermatitis 2000;42(5):309–10.
6. Hausen BM, Reichling J, Harkenthal M. Degradation products of monoterpenes are the sensitizing agents in tea tree oil. Am J Contact Dermat 1999;10(2):68–77.
7. Beckmann B. Tea tree oil. Dermatosen 1998;46:120–4.
8. de Groot AC, Weyland JW. Systemic contact dermatitis from tea tree oil. Contact Dermatitis 1992;27(4):279–80.
9. Mozelsio NB, Harris KE, McGrath KG, Grammer LC. Immediate systemic hypersensitivity reaction associated with topical application of Australian tea tree oil. Allergy Asthma Proc 2003;24(1):73–5.

Teicoplanin

General Information

Teicoplanin has been used in the treatment of Gram-positive infections. Its pharmacological properties allow once-daily dosing. Its safety profile has been thoroughly investigated, and it is generally well tolerated. It diffuses well into bone tissue (1).

Teicoplanin is more effectively administered once daily than vancomycin and it can be given intramuscularly or intravenously; it is not absorbed after oral administration. It is 90% bound to plasma proteins and its elimination is primarily by renal excretion, allowing dosage adjustments to be made on the basis of the measured creatinine clearance. A dosing regimen of 12 mg/kg on day 1 followed by 6 mg/kg/day most often results in efficacious serum concentrations but premature neonates and children require higher dosages. However, doses of 10 mg/kg/day are required to achieve adequate bone concentrations, and there is little penetration into cerebrospinal fluid or aqueous or vitreous humors. In fat, concentrations can be subtherapeutic after a dose of 400 mg. Unlike vancomycin, routine drug monitoring is not required, although it may sometimes be useful for predicting the therapeutic effect of the drug.

Observational studies

In a study of the effects of teicoplanin (6–12 mg/day intravenously), 166 of 342 patients reported one or more adverse events, and in 119 they were thought to be associated with teicoplanin (2). Most had some form of hypersensitivity response (fever, rash, chills, or pruritus), and treatment was withdrawn in 59 patients. There was a clinically significant abnormality of liver function tests in 123 patients, but in only 33 was it judged to be possibly associated with teicoplanin. There was a rise in serum creatinine in 28 patients, in five of whom an association with teicoplanin was suggested.

Cell wall agents, such as glycopeptides, have concentration-independent bactericidal activity, and the time over which the antibiotic serum concentration persists over the minimal inhibitory concentration of the pathogen is a main pharmacodynamic determination of the outcome. In a two-way, randomized, open, two-period, crossover study in 10 healthy adults, teicoplanin given in two 200 mg doses intramuscularly produced steady-state trough concentrations even higher than those after once-daily intravenous administration of 400 mg (3). Conversion from intravenous to intramuscular administration may therefore allow better compliance with preserved efficacy. Intramuscular teicoplanin was well tolerated. Adverse effects reported were mild local pain for 2–3 hours, headache, and backache.

In 76 patients receiving long-term teicoplanin for chronic osteomyelitis due to oxacillin-resistant *Staphylococcus aureus*, teicoplanin had to be withdrawn in only one subject because of low-grade fever, muscular pain, and sleeplessness; these adverse effects abated after withdrawal (4).

Comparative studies

In a prospective study 56 patients with suspected or proven severe Gram-positive infections were randomized to receive vancomycin (1 g 12-hourly intravenously) or teicoplanin (200–400 mg/day intravenously or intramuscularly) (5). Clinical and bacteriological cure rates were similar, but vancomycin was associated with significantly greater toxicity (16 vancomycin, 7 teicoplanin), predominantly histamine-associated reactions (15, including two cases of red man syndrome) (SEDA-17, 312), and nephrotoxicity (five with vancomycin compared with one with teicoplanin). Four of the five vancomycin patients who developed nephrotoxicity were receiving netilmicin at the time, some with amphotericin as well.

The overall rate of adverse reactions in comparative trials was 19%, which is comparable with the rate observed with beta-lactams, but lower than the corresponding rate (39%) associated with vancomycin (6).

Only three of 422 patients treated with a single dose of teicoplanin for antimicrobial prophylaxis during hip or knee arthroplasty (400 mg by intravenous bolus at the time of anesthesia) reported adverse events compared with nine of 424 patients treated with five doses of cefazoline: one had nausea and two had erythema (7). Six patients given teicoplanin had surgical wound infections, and 57 had proven or suspected infections involving other body systems.

In another study, a single dose of teicoplanin (6 mg/kg intravenously) was compared with three doses of cefradine plus metronidazole as prophylaxis for vascular surgery. Efficacy was similar with the two regimens. Adverse events were reported by 40 of 136 patients treated with teicoplanin (versus 39 of 139 treated with cefradine plus metronidazole), and 19 (versus 15) were considered to be related to the study drug; however, none was considered definitely related (8).

In a prospective, randomized trial in 34 drug abusers a short course of a combination of a glycopeptide (vancomycin or teicoplanin) with gentamicin was significantly less effective in right-sided endocarditis caused by *S. aureus* than a combination of cloxacillin and gentamicin (9).

Pharmacoeconomics

In a randomized, prospective, cost-effectiveness study both teicoplanin and vancomycin were assessed as second-line therapy in 66 neutropenic patients after the failure of empirical treatment with a combination of piperacillin + tazobactam and amikacin (10). The primary success of second-line therapy was equivalent, and the direct total costs were similar. Acquisition costs per dose were in favor of vancomycin, but costs derived from administering vancomycin and serum concentration monitoring led to similar costs for both regimens. With the exception of the red man syndrome, which occurred in 10% of vancomycin-treated patients but none of the teicoplanin-treated patients, toxicity (renal, liver, and ear toxicity, diarrhea, phlebitis) was also similar.

In a retrospective cost analysis, the records of 527 patients with acute leukemia were studied (11). They had been treated in a multicenter, randomized trial for febrile neutropenia with ceftazidime and amikacin plus either teicoplanin (6 mg/kg in a single dose; $n = 275$) or vancomycin (30 mg/kg/day in 2 doses; $n = 252$). Clinical responses were equivalent. Again the higher acquisition costs for teicoplanin were counterbalanced by the lower incidence of adverse events and easier administration, resulting in overall similar costs for both regimens. A total of 8% of patients treated with vancomycin reported adverse events compared with 3.2% of patients treated with teicoplanin. Rashes occurred in 6.0 versus 1.4% respectively. Nephrotoxicity, ototoxicity, fever, and hypotension occurred in very few patients.

General adverse effects

The most common adverse events associated with teicoplanin are hypersensitivity, fever, rash, diarrhea, nephrotoxicity, and thrombocytopenia (12,13). Local reactions at the injection site include pain, redness, or discomfort after intramuscular injection, or phlebitis after intravenous injection. Erythroderma has occurred during infusion of teicoplanin with fever and hypotension. Allergic reactions have been reported with teicoplanin, with cross-reactivity between teicoplanin and vancomycin documented by in vitro studies showing IgE release by basophils in response to stimulation by both vancomycin and teicoplanin. However, known hypersensitivity to vancomycin is not a contraindication to teicoplanin. Tumor-inducing effects have not been reported.

Red man syndrome

The red man syndrome associated with rapid infusion of vancomycin, resulting in histamine release, is very rarely seen with teicoplanin. Teicoplanin can usually be safely administered to patients with a history of red man syndrome due to vancomycin, as has been confirmed in six children treated with teicoplanin for febrile neutropenia and Gram-positive bacteremia (14).

However, case reports have suggested that there can be cross-reactivity between vancomycin and teicoplanin in the induction of this syndrome, although the underlying mechanism remains elusive (15).

- A swinging pyrexia (peaking at 39–40°C during the day but settling overnight) developed after the fifth day of teicoplanin treatment in a 35-year-old man with infective endocarditis due to *Streptococcus mitis*. Two days after stopping the drug he became apyrexial. Therapy with vancomycin had previously had to be interrupted because of an extensive purpuric rash and erythema, which progressed to exfoliative dermatitis and was subsequently identified as red man syndrome secondary to vancomycin.

Organs and Systems

Cardiovascular

Hypotension has been observed as part of the manifestations of a hypersensitivity reaction to teicoplanin (16).

Respiratory

Bronchospasm required withdrawal of teicoplanin in two of 310 patients (17).

Sensory systems

Ototoxicity has been reported during treatment with teicoplanin (18). A fall in high-frequency auditory threshold was observed in one patient treated with teicoplanin for a serious Gram-positive infection (19). However, the causal relation between teicoplanin and alterations in auditory function has not been established in controlled clinical studies (20). Guinea pigs treated for 28 days with a maximum dose of 75 mg/kg/day remained without any evidence of functional, morphological, or histological changes indicative of ototoxicity (21). There were 11 cases of ototoxicity among 3377 patients treated with teicoplanin (20). It can be concluded that teicoplanin-associated ototoxicity is rare.

Hematologic

The overall rate of hematological adverse effects of teicoplanin was 2.2% in 1431 patients participating in a large non-comparative multicenter study (22).

Hemophagocytosis after vancomycin and teicoplanin occurred in a 45-year-old woman (23).

Leukocytes

The incidence of teicoplanin-induced leukopenia is low (0.33%) and the leukopenia is usually reversible.

- A 10-year-old Malay boy with G6PD deficiency received teicoplanin (300 mg/day) for an epidural abscess and 14 days later developed an erythematous, maculopapular, non-pruritic rash over his trunk and upper limbs and a mild fever with chills (24). He had a leukocyte count of 2×10^9/l. Teicoplanin was withdrawn and by 3 days the rash had almost completely subsided. After rechallenge with a single intravenous dose of teicoplanin 300 mg, he developed a fever (39.3°C), chills, and worsening of the rash on his arms. Teicoplanin was again withdrawn. His fever resolved after 4 days and his leukocyte count normalized by 7 days.
- Neutropenia developed in a patient after 20 days of treatment with teicoplanin (25).

In patients undergoing bone marrow transplantation receiving teicoplanin for the treatment of severe sepsis, the duration of neutropenia was not prolonged by teicoplanin (26).

Teicoplanin rarely causes eosinophilia (27).

Platelets

Thrombocytopenia was associated on two consecutive occasions with teicoplanin in a patient with acute myeloid leukemia (28). The exact mechanism for this adverse event is unknown. Teicoplanin does not alter platelet function or blood coagulation (29).

- Severe thrombocytopenia occurred in a 46-year-old white man treated with teicoplanin 6 mg/kg/day for methicillin-resistant *S. aureus* bacteremia (30). The platelet count fell to 25×10^9/l on day 8 (baseline 110). After drug withdrawal the platelet count improved within 4 days. The trough teicoplanin concentrations were 17 μg/ml on day 4 and 15.4 μg/ml on day 9.

Teicoplanin caused thrombocytopenia in one of 17 children (31).

In trials in the USA, thrombocytopenia occurred more commonly with teicoplanin than with vancomycin, but this was almost exclusively in patients who received much larger doses than are now recommended.

Gastrointestinal

Adverse events involving the gastrointestinal system are rare with teicoplanin. Diarrhea has been listed among non-specific events observed in 5.1% of patients (22).

Liver

In one study transient rises in liver enzymes occurred in 2.3% of patients taking teicoplanin (17). Other authors have reported abnormal liver enzymes (19,32–34).

Urinary tract

Teicoplanin can be nephrotoxic, but less often than vancomycin (6). However, concomitant aminoglycoside therapy in some patients makes the contribution of the glycopeptide antibiotic difficult to assess. Renal toxicity was observed more often in patients receiving the combination of netilmicin plus vancomycin than in patients treated with netilmicin plus teicoplanin (35). Similar differences in nephrotoxicity between vancomycin and teicoplanin were observed in febrile neutropenic patients receiving tobramycin plus piperacillin (36). There was significant deterioration of renal function when vancomycin and ciclosporin, but not teicoplanin and ciclosporin, were used together; the mechanism responsible for this interaction is unknown (36).

In two of 76 patients receiving long-term teicoplanin a reduction in dosage was required because of reduced renal function, which recovered within 30 days (4).

There was a fall in residual renal function during episodes of peritonitis in a prospective multicenter study in 152 children with peritoneal dialysis-associated peritonitis (37). The study evaluated the efficacy, safety, and clinical acceptance of combination treatment, including a glycopeptide (teicoplanin or vancomycin) and ceftazidime, each given either intermittently or continuously. Irreversible anuria developed in 19% of the patients with residual diuresis. In patients who retained residual renal function, there was a strong trend toward a decreased residual glomerular filtration rate (−11%). There was no difference with respect to the type of glycopeptide or the mode of use. Aminoglycosides were used concomitantly in only 12 patients and did not seem to affect the evolution of residual renal function. Underdosing/non-adherence or overdosing occurred in 8.2% of continuously treated versus 4.9% of intermittently treated patients. Intermittent and continuous intraperitoneal treatment with glycopeptides and ceftazidime were equally efficacious and safe when measured by objective clinical criteria.

In children with febrile neutropenia and Gram-positive bacteremia associated with antineoplastic drug therapy, teicoplanin was significantly less nephrotoxic than vancomycin (14).

The effect of co-administration of fosfomycin on glycopeptide antibiotic-induced nephrotoxicity for 3 days has been investigated in rats (38). Fosfomycin reduced glycopeptide antibiotic-induced nephrotoxicity, as shown by reduced urinary excretion of N-acetyl-beta-D-glucosaminidase and fewer histological signs of nephrotoxicity in those treated with a combination of glycopeptide and fosfomycin compared with a glycopeptide alone. In addition, the higher the dose of fosfomycin, the more it reduced urinary N-acetyl-beta-D-glucosaminidase activity, suggesting that the role of fosfomycin in alleviating nephrotoxicity is dose-dependent. There was significantly less accumulation of teicoplanin and vancomycin in the renal cortex of rats treated with glycopeptide antibiotics plus fosfomycin compared with the glycopeptide antibiotics alone.

Skin

A pustular skin eruption occurred in a 60-year-old woman who was given teicoplanin 400 mg as a loading dose followed by 200 mg/day (39). Following the sixth injection of teicoplanin she developed a pruritic eruption on her chest, which evolved into a widespread maculopapular eruption with tiny pustules and occasional vesicles on an erythematous base over the face, trunk, and limbs within 2 days. Teicoplanin was withdrawn and she was given prednisolone 60 mg/day. This resulted in improvement of the eruption and relieved the discomfort over the

next 7 days. In other cases teicoplanin caused an acute generalized rash and exanthematous pustulosis (24,40).

Vancomycin reportedly caused a severe delayed skin reaction with allergic cross-reactivity between vancomycin and teicoplanin requiring steroid therapy (41).

- A 68-year-old woman who was being treated with vancomycin for *Staphylococcus epidermidis* bacteremia developed pruritus and a generalized maculopapular skin rash after 2 weeks. After a short course of prednisolone, she was given teicoplanin and developed general malaise, fever, conjunctival injection, an extensive rash, and later blisters on the legs, again requiring treatment with steroids.

Musculoskeletal

Teicoplanin has been successfully used to treat bone and joint infections without any adverse reactions affecting bones or joints (42).

Immunologic

Allergic reactions have been reported with teicoplanin. Erythroderma during infusion of teicoplanin with fever and hypotension was described in a single patient. Re-exposure elicited the same reaction (16). Allergic cross-reactivity between teicoplanin and vancomycin has been reported (43,44). This cross-reactivity was documented by in vitro studies showing IgE release by basophils in response to stimulation by both vancomycin and teicoplanin in a further patient who had an allergic reaction to vancomycin (45). In other studies the second drug did not elicit allergic reactions in patients known to be allergic to one of the two compounds (46–48). Based on these small studies and individual case reports one can conclude that allergic reactions to teicoplanin can occur in patients with known allergic reactions to vancomycin, but the frequency of occurrence of this type of cross-reaction appears to be low. Therefore, known hypersensitivity to vancomycin is not a contraindication to the use of teicoplanin.

Local reactions at the injection site, including pain, redness, or discomfort after intramuscular injection, and phlebitis after intravenous injection, occur in about 3% of patients (6).

Long-Term Effects

Drug tolerance

In a study of antibiotic resistance in enterococci from raw meat, there was a high prevalence of glycopeptide-resistant strains (49). Resistance to vancomycin was significantly associated with resistance to teicoplanin, erythromycin, tetracycline, and chloramphenicol.

Susceptibility Factors

Renal disease

The administration of 5 and 10 mg/kg of teicoplanin to seven anuric patients immediately after the end of hemodialysis gave mean values of $C_{\max}$ of 63 and 122 µg/ml, mean AUCs of 526 and 1104 hours.µg/ml, mean half-lives of 109 and 107 hours, mean clearance rates of 13 and 12 ml/minute, mean apparent volumes of distribution of 1.68 and 1.68 l/kg, and mean volumes of distribution at steady state of 0.31 and 0.28 l/kg (50). Trough serum concentrations were above 10 µg/ml for 24 hours after the 5 mg/kg dose and for 48 hours after the 10 mg/kg dose. Teicoplanin was not detected in the dialysate. Its concentrations in the arterial and the venous lines of the fistulae were similar.

Drug Administration

Drug overdose

- A 10-day-old girl with a history of postasphyxia acute renal failure, which recovered within 7 days, was given teicoplanin for sepsis due to *Staphylococcus hominis* (51). The dosage used was erroneously high (20 mg/kg 12-hourly instead of an initial dose of 16 mg/kg followed by 6–8 mg/kg/day), and therapy was suspended after 5 days. She improved, and blood cultures were negative. Serum creatinine concentrations and cystatin C (as an early marker of glomerular damage) remained in the reference ranges. Urinary parameters for tubulotoxicity (*N*-acetyl-beta-D-glucosaminidase, beta$_1$-microglobulin) were higher than in the following days, but remained in the reference ranges. Urinary concentrations of epithelial growth factor were also higher during therapy than afterwards, probably indicating repair activity. Serum concentrations of teicoplanin were not determined.

Drug–Drug Interactions

Aminoglycosides

The risk of nephrotoxicity increases with the concomitant use of other nephrotoxic drugs, especially aminoglycosides (36).

Ciprofloxacin

Teicoplanin should be administered separately from ciprofloxacin, since precipitation has been provoked by concomitant parenteral administration (52).

Colestyramine

Since colestyramine binds teicoplanin in vitro and reduces its activity against *Clostridium difficile* almost completely, there is potential for a clinically important interaction (53).

Enalapril

A possible drug interaction with enalapril has been reported; a patient with diabetes receiving teicoplanin for osteomyelitis developed renal insufficiency requiring dialysis after the addition of enalapril (54).

Monitoring Therapy

There is evidence that predose concentrations of teicoplanin are related to clinical outcome; the evidence is less conclusive for vancomycin. Predose concentrations can be linked to some toxic effects (nephrotoxicity for vancomycin and thrombocytopenia to teicoplanin) (55,56). In severe infections monitoring serum teicoplanin concentrations is indicated to assure adequate trough concentrations (over 10 µg/ml) (57). For the treatment of *S. aureus* endocarditis trough concentrations should exceed 20 µg/ml (57). Inadequately low serum concentrations of teicoplanin may have been responsible for the high failure rate in intravenous drug users treated with teicoplanin for right-sided endocarditis (58). The fact that teicoplanin pharmacokinetics are unpredictably variable in intravenous drug users adds further weight to the importance of monitoring serum drug concentrations in this population during the treatment of severe infections such as endocarditis (59). Since the half-life of teicoplanin also varies greatly in patients with various degrees of renal insufficiency, monitoring serum concentrations can be helpful in guiding therapy in some patients with markedly reduced creatinine clearance (60).

References

1. Boselli E, Allaouchiche B. Diffusion osseuse des antibiotiques. [Diffusion in bone tissue of antibiotics.] Presse Méd 1999;28(40):2265–76.
2. LeFrock J, Ristuccia A. Teicoplanin Bone and Joint Cooperative Study Group A. Teicoplanin in the treatment of bone and joint infections: An open study. J Infect Chemother 1999;5(1):32–9.
3. Pea F, Furlanut M, Poz D, Baraldo M. Pharmacokinetic profile of two different administration schemes of teicoplanin. Single 400 mg intravenous dose vs double-refracted 200 mg intramuscular doses in healthy volunteers. Clin Drug Invest 1999;18:47–55.
4. Testore GP, Uccella I, Sarrecchia C, Mattei A, Impagliazzo A, Sordillo P, Andreoni M. Long-term intramuscular teicoplanin treatment of chronic osteomyelitis due to oxacillin-resistant *Staphylococcus aureus* in outpatients. J Chemother 2000;12(5):412–15.
5. Neville LO, Brumfitt W, Hamilton-Miller JMT, Harding I. Teicoplanin vs vancomycin for the treatment of serious infections: a randomised trial. Int J Antimicrob Agents 1995;5:187–93.
6. Campoli-Richards DM, Brogden RN, Faulds D. Teicoplanin. A review of its antibacterial activity, pharmacokinetic properties and therapeutic potential. Drugs 1990;40(3):449–86.
7. Periti P, Stringa G, Mini E. Comparative multicenter trial of teicoplanin versus cefazolin for antimicrobial prophylaxis in prosthetic joint implant surgery. Italian Study Group for Antimicrobial Prophylaxis in Orthopedic Surgery. Eur J Clin Microbiol Infect Dis 1999;18(2):113–19.
8. Kester RC, Antrum R, Thornton CA, Ramsden CH, Harding I. A comparison of teicoplanin versus cephradine plus metronidazole in the prophylaxis of post-operative infection in vascular surgery. J Hosp Infect 1999;41(3):233–43.
9. Fortun J, Navas E, Martinez-Beltran J, Perez-Molina J, Martin-Davila P, Guerrero A, Moreno S. Short-course therapy for right-side endocarditis due to *Staphylococcus aureus* in drug abusers: cloxacillin versus glycopeptides in combination with gentamicin. Clin Infect Dis 2001;33(1):120–5.

10. Vazquez L, Encinas MP, Morin LS, Vilches P, Gutierrez N, Garcia-Sanz R, Caballero D, Hurle AD. Randomized prospective study comparing cost-effectiveness of teicoplanin and vancomycin as second-line empiric therapy for infection in neutropenic patients. Haematologica 1999;84(3):231–6.

11. Bucaneve G, Menichetti F, Del Favero A. Cost analysis of 2 empiric antibacterial regimens containing glycopeptides for the treatment of febrile neutropenia in patients with acute leukaemia. Pharmacoeconomics 1999;15(1):85–95.

12. Harding I, Sorgel F. Comparative pharmacokinetics of teicoplanin and vancomycin. J Chemother 2000;12(Suppl 5):15–20.

13. Wilson AP. Clinical pharmacokinetics of teicoplanin. Clin Pharmacokinet 2000;39(3):167–83.

14. Sidi V, Roilides E, Bibashi E, Gompakis N, Tsakiri A, Koliouskas D. Comparison of efficacy and safety of teicoplanin and vancomycin in children with antineoplastic therapy-associated febrile neutropenia and Gram-positive bacteremia. J Chemother 2000;12(4):326–31.

15. Khurana C, de Belder MA. Red-man syndrome after vancomycin: potential cross-reactivity with teicoplanin. Postgrad Med J 1999;75(879):41–3.

16. Paul C, Janier M, Carlet J, Tamion F, Carlotti A, Fichelle JM, Daniel F. [Erythroderma induced by teicoplanin.] Ann Dermatol Venereol 1992;119(9):667–9.

17. Stille W, Sietzen W, Dieterich HA, Fell JJ. Clinical efficacy and safety of teicoplanin. J Antimicrob Chemother 1988;21(Suppl A):69–79.

18. Maher ER, Hollman A, Gruneberg RN. Teicoplanin-induced ototoxicity in Down's syndrome. Lancet 1986;1(8481):613.

19. Bibler MR, Frame PT, Hagler DN, Bode RB, Staneck JL, Thamlikitkul V, Harris JE, Haregewoin A, Bullock WE Jr. Clinical evaluation of efficacy, pharmacokinetics, and safety of teicoplanin for serious Gram-positive infections. Antimicrob Agents Chemother 1987;31(2):207–12.

20. Davey PG, Williams AH. A review of the safety profile of teicoplanin. J Antimicrob Chemother 1991;27(Suppl B):69–73.

21. Brummett RE, Fox KE, Warchol M, Himes D. Absence of ototoxicity of teichomycin A2 in guinea pigs. Antimicrob Agents Chemother 1987;31(4):612–13.

22. Lewis P, Garaud JJ, Parenti F. A multicentre open clinical trial of teicoplanin in infections caused by gram-positive bacteria. J Antimicrob Chemother 1988;21(Suppl A):61–7.

23. Lambotte O, Costedoat-Chalumeau N, Amoura Z, Piette JC, Cacoub P. Drug-induced hemophagocytosis. Am J Med 2002;112(7):592–3.

24. Wee IY, Oh HM. Teicoplanin-induced neutropenia in a paediatric patient with vertebral osteomyelitis. Scand J Infect Dis 2001;33(2):157–8.

25. Del Favero A, Patoia L, Bucaneve G, Biscarini L, Menichetti F. Leukopenia with neutropenia associated with teicoplanin therapy. DICP 1989;23(1):45–7.

26. Lang E, Schmid J, Fauser AA. A clinical trial on efficacy and safety of teicoplanin in combination with beta-lactams and aminoglycosides in the treatment of severe sepsis of patients undergoing allogeneic/autologous bone marrow transplantation. Br J Haematol 1990;76(Suppl 2):14–18.

27. Del Favero A, Menichetti F, Guerciolini R, Bucaneve G, Baldelli F, Aversa F, Terenzi A, Davis S, Pauluzzi S. Prospective randomized clinical trial of teicoplanin for empiric combined antibiotic therapy in febrile, granulocytopenic acute leukemia patients. Antimicrob Agents Chemother 1987;31(7):1126–9.

28. Terol MJ, Sierra J, Gatell JM, Rozman C. Thrombocytopenia due to use of teicoplanin. Clin Infect Dis 1993;17(5):927.

29. Agnelli G, Longetti M, Guerciolini R, Menichetti F, Grasselli S, Boldrini F, Bucaneve G, Nenci GG, Del Favero A. Effects of the new glycopeptide antibiotic teicoplanin on platelet function and blood coagulation. Antimicrob Agents Chemother 1987;31(10):1609–12.

30. Lambiotte F, Miczek S, Bierent S, Socolovsky C, Chagnon JL. Thrombopénie acquise sous teicoplanine. Med Mal Infect 2000;30:481–2.

31. Sunakawa K, Nonoyama M, Fujii R, Iwai N, Sakata H, Shirai M, Sato T, Kajino M, Toyonaga Y, Sano T, Naito A, Minagawa K, Niida Y, Oda T, Yokozawa M, Asanuma H, Shimura K, Fujimura M, Kitajima H, Fujinami K, Numazaki K, Fujikawa T, Kobayashi Y, Sato Y, Nishimura T, Iwata S, Tsuchihashi N, Oishi T, Matsumoto S, Motohiro T, Osawa M, Sunahara M, Shirakawa S, Nishida H, Takahashi N, Nakano R, Sai N, Iyoda K, Yoshimitsu K, Ogawa K, Okazaki T, Tsukimoto I, Motoyama O, Takada Y, Kawasaki M, Sunaoshi W, Nakamura S, Ueda Y, Kamata M, Kato T, Chiba M, Ouchi K, Sato S, Horiuchi T, Suzuki K, Shimoyama T, Masaki H, Aikyo M, Kawada M, Banba M, Furukawa S, Okada T, Yamaguchi S, Hirota O, Koizumi S, Wada H, Ohta K, Uehara T, Yukitake K, Mori T, Takakuwa S, Matsuyama K. [Pharmacokinetic and clinical studies on teicoplanin for sepsis by methicillin-cephem resistant *Staphylococcus aureus* in the pediatric and neonate field.] Jpn J Antibiot 2002;55(5):656–77.

32. Bochud-Gabellon I, Regamey C. Teicoplanin, a new antibiotic effective against Gram-positive bacterial infections of the skin and soft tissues. Dermatologica 1988;176(1):29–38.

33. Verhagen C, De Pauw BE. Teicoplanin for therapy of Gram-positive infections in neutropenic patients. Int J Clin Pharmacol Res 1987;7(6):491–8.

34. Webster A, Russell SJ, Souhami RL, Richards JD, Goldstone AH, Gruneberg RN. Use of teicoplanin for Hickman catheter associated staphylococcal infection in immunosuppressed patients. J Hosp Infect 1987;10(1):77–82.

35. Charbonneau P, Garaud J, Aubertin J, et al. Efficiency and safety of teicoplanin plus netilmicin compared to vancomycin plus netilmicin in the treatment of severe Gram-positive infections. 1987;110.

36. Kureishi A, Jewesson PJ, Rubinger M, Cole CD, Reece DE, Phillips GL, Smith JA, Chow AW. Double-blind comparison of teicoplanin versus vancomycin in febrile neutropenic patients receiving concomitant tobramycin and piperacillin: effect on cyclosporin A-associated nephrotoxicity. Antimicrob Agents Chemother 1991;35(11):2246–52.

37. Schaefer F, Klaus G, Muller-Wiefel DE, Mehls O. Intermittent versus continuous intraperitoneal glycopeptide/ceftazidime treatment in children with peritoneal dialysis-associated peritonitis. The Mid-European Pediatric Peritoneal Dialysis Study Group (MEPPS). J Am Soc Nephrol 1999;10(1):136–45.

38. Yoshiyama Y, Yazaki T, Wong PC, Beauchamp D, Kanke M. The effect of fosfomycin on glycopeptide antibiotic-induced nephrotoxicity in rats. J Infect Chemother 2001;7(4):243–6.

39. Unal S, Ikizoglu G, Demirkan F, Kaya TI. Teicoplanin-induced skin eruption. Int J Dermatol 2002;41(12):948–9.

40. Chu CY, Wu J, Jean SS, Sun CC. Acute generalized exanthematous pustulosis due to teicoplanin. Dermatology 2001;202(2):141–2.

41. Padial MA, Barranco P, Lopez-Serrano C. Erythema multiforme to vancomycin. Allergy 2000;55(12):1201.

42. Weinberg WG. Safety and efficacy of teicoplanin for bone and joint infections: results of a community-based trial. South Med J 1993;86(8):891–7.

43. McElrath MJ, Goldberg D, Neu HC. Allergic cross-reactivity of teicoplanin and vancomycin. Lancet 1986;1(8471):47.

44. Davenport A. Allergic cross-reactivity to teicoplanin and vancomycin. Nephron 1993;63(4):482.

45. Knudsen JD, Pedersen M. IgE-mediated reaction to vancomycin and teicoplanin after treatment with vancomycin. Scand J Infect Dis 1992;24(3):395–6.

46. Smith SR, Cheesbrough JS, Makris M, Davies JM. Teicoplanin administration in patients experiencing reactions to vancomycin. J Antimicrob Chemother 1989;23(5):810–12.

47. Wood G, Whitby M. Teicoplanin in patients who are allergic to vancomycin. Med J Aust 1989;150(11):668.

48. Schlemmer B, Falkman H, Boudjadja A, Jacob L, Le Gall JR. Teicoplanin for patients allergic to vancomycin. N Engl J Med 1988;318(17):1127–8.

49. Pavia M, Nobile CG, Salpietro L, Angelillo IF. Vancomycin resistance and antibiotic susceptibility of enterococci in raw meat. J Food Prot 2000;63(7):912–15.

50. Papaioannou MG, Marinaki S, Pappas M, Stamatiadis D, Giamarellos-Bourboulis EJ, Giamarellou H, Stathakis C. Pharmacokinetics of teicoplanin in patients undergoing chronic haemodialysis. Int J Antimicrob Agents 2002;19(3):233–6.

51. Fanos V, Mussap M, Khoory BJ, Vecchini S, Plebani M, Benini D. Renal tolerability of teicoplanin in a case of neonatal overdose. J Chemother 1998;10(5):381–4.

52. Jim LK. Physical and chemical compatibility of intravenous ciprofloxacin with other drugs. Ann Pharmacother 1993;27(6):704–7.

53. Pantosti A, Luzzi I, Cardines R, Gianfrilli P. Comparison of the in vitro activities of teicoplanin and vancomycin against Clostridium difficile and their interactions with cholestyramine. Antimicrob Agents Chemother 1985;28(6):847–8.

54. Frye R, Job M, Dretler R. Teicoplanin nephrotoxicity: first case report. Pharmacotherapy 1990;10:234.

55. Wilson AP. Comparative safety of teicoplanin and vancomycin. Int J Antimicrob Agents 1998;10(2):143–52.

56. MacGowan AP. Pharmacodynamics, pharmacokinetics, and therapeutic drug monitoring of glycopeptides. Ther Drug Monit 1998;20(5):473–7.

57. Brogden RN, Peters DH. Teicoplanin. A reappraisal of its antimicrobial activity, pharmacokinetic properties and therapeutic efficacy. Drugs 1994;47(5):823–54.

58. Fortun J, Perez-Molina JA, Anon MT, Martinez-Beltran J, Loza E, Guerrero A. Right-sided endocarditis caused by Staphylococcus aureus in drug abusers. Antimicrob Agents Chemother 1995;39(2):525–8.

59. Rybak MJ, Lerner SA, Levine DP, Albrecht LM, McNeil PL, Thompson GA, Kenny MT, Yuh L. Teicoplanin pharmacokinetics in intravenous drug abusers being treated for bacterial endocarditis. Antimicrob Agents Chemother 1991;35(4):696–700.

60. Lam YW, Kapusnik-Uner JE, Sachdeva M, Hackbarth C, Gambertoglio JG, Sande MA. The pharmacokinetics of teicoplanin in varying degrees of renal function. Clin Pharmacol Ther 1990;47(5):655–61.

Telenzepine

General Information

Telenzepine is a muscarinic M_1 receptor antagonist, like pirenzepine. On a weight-for-weight basis it is 25–50 times more potent than pirenzepine, but dose for dose it is, if anything, more likely to have undesired anticholinergic effects [1].

In 163 patients with endoscopically proven benign gastric ulcers randomly allocated to telenzepine 3 mg/day or ranitidine 300 mg/day for up to 8 weeks in a prospective, double-blind study, anticholinergic events occurred significantly more often in patients taking telenzepine, dry mouth being the most frequent adverse effect [2].

References

1. Levin SL. Pirenzepine, telenzepine, atropine and metacine as agonists for the muscarinic cholinoreceptors in the denervated human parotid gland. J Clin Pharm Ther 1990;15(6):455–62.

2. Simon B, Reinicke HG, Dammann HG, Müller P. 3 mg Telenzepin nocte in der Therapie der benignen Ulcusventriculi-Erkrankung: Eine doppelblinde Vergleichsstudie mit 300 mg Ranitidin nocte. [3 mg telenzepine nocte in the treatment of benign stomach ulcer disease: a double-blind comparative study with 300 mg ranitidine nocte.] Z Gastroenterol 1990;28(2):90–3.

Telmisartan

See also Angiotensin II receptor antagonists

General Information

Telmisartan is a highly selective antagonist at type 1 angiotensin II (AT_1) receptors.

Organs and Systems

Respiratory

The incidence of cough with telmisartan has been assessed in a multicenter, randomized, parallel-group, double-blind, placebo-controlled study, for 8 weeks using a visual analogue scale in 88 patients with hypertension who had previously had ACE inhibitor-related cough [1]. Cough was reported in 60% of the patients taking lisinopril 20 mg/day, 16% of those taking telmisartan 80 mg/day, and 9.7% with placebo.

Drug–Drug Interactions

Digoxin

Multiple-dose telmisartan 120 mg od administered with digoxin 0.25 mg od resulted in higher serum digoxin concentrations [2]. Digoxin AUC and C_{max} rose by 22% and 50% respectively; the rise in C_{min} (13%) was not significant. These results suggest that telmisartan reduces the clearance of digoxin. The magnitude of this effect is comparable to that observed with calcium channel blockers, carvedilol, captopril, amiodarone, quinidine, and propafenone. Monitoring serum digoxin concentrations should be considered when patients first receive telmisartan and in the event of any changes in the dosage of telmisartan.

Paracetamol or ibuprofen

The single-dose pharmacokinetics of telmisartan 120 mg were not affected by a concurrent single dose of paracetamol 1 g or ibuprofen 400 mg tds for 7 days (3).

References

1. Lacourciere Y. The incidence of cough: a comparison of lisinopril, placebo and telmisartan, a novel angiotensin II antagonist. Telmisartan Cough Study Group. Int J Clin Pract 1999;53(2):99–103.
2. Stangier J, Su CA, Hendriks MG, van Lier JJ, Sollie FA, Oosterhuis B, Jonkman JH. The effect of telmisartan on the steady-state pharmacokinetics of digoxin in healthy male volunteers. J Clin Pharmacol 2000;40(12 Pt 1):1373–9.
3. Stangier J, Su CA, Fraunhofer A, Tetzloff W. Pharmacokinetics of acetaminophen and ibuprofen when coadministered with telmisartan in healthy volunteers. J Clin Pharmacol 2000;40(12 Pt 1):1338–46.

Temazepam

See also Benzodiazepines

General Information

Temazepam is a benzodiazepine that was first discovered as a metabolite of diazepam. It is relatively short-acting, having a half-life of about 10 hours.

Temazepam has favorable kinetics for use as a hypnotic (1) and is widely prescribed for this purpose. Rather surprisingly, both 10 and 20 mg caused discernible and comparable psychomotor impairment the following morning (SEDA-20, 32), at a time when the subjective effects had virtually disappeared. This result emphasizes the often subtle but pervasive insight-impairing effects of benzodiazepines. Temazepam in soft capsules is more rapidly absorbed than from tablets. However, drug users have abused temazepam capsules by heating them to liquefaction and injecting the resultant fluid intravenously, often together with other substances; the resulting medical problems are varied and often serious.

Organs and Systems

Psychological, psychiatric

Temazepam produces a variety of adverse nervous system effects, including restlessness, agitation, irritability, aggression, rage, and psychosis. Perhaps because it is likely to be used recreationally, temazepam has also been used to facilitate crime, particularly in the UK (2).

The effects of oral temazepam 5, 10, and 30 mg on memory have been studied in healthy volunteers subjected to a battery of cognitive tests and analogue mood ratings (3). The lowest dose had no effect and 10 mg significantly increased only self-ratings of well-being. Temazepam 30 mg significantly improved recall of items learned before drug administration, but impaired recall and recognition of word lists acquired after drug administration. There was no impairment of retrieval, suggesting that automatic information processing was unaffected. Temazepam 30 mg significantly reduced self-ratings of anxiety and increased self-ratings of sedation. It also significantly impaired performance in symbol copying, digit-symbol substitution, and number cancellation tasks. It is striking that at a dose that was sedative and impaired many aspects of performance, temazepam nevertheless improved retrieval of items learned before drug administration. In a randomized, crossover study, psychomotor performance and memory were tested and mood assessed for 3 hours after single doses of placebo, temazepam 20 mg, or temazepam 30 mg in six healthy women aged 21–23 years (4). Psychomotor speed and explicit memory showed dose-dependent slowing and impairment, but there was no change in short-term memory.

Drug Administration

Drug dosage regimens

Benzodiazepine prescribing for sleep induction in an elderly medical inpatient population has been examined, to determine if hospital prescribing increases the use of benzodiazepines after discharge (5). The secondary objectives included monitoring for adverse effects and assessment of the quality of sleep in hospital compared with the quality of sleep at home. Inpatient and outpatient prescribing of benzodiazepines used for insomnia was recorded over 3 months. Benzodiazepines were prescribed for 20% of patients, and 94% of the prescriptions were for temazepam. Of the 57 patients who were given benzodiazepines during a hospital admission, 57% had not taken a benzodiazepine at home before admission. Benzodiazepines were effective in the short-term for inducing sleep in hospital, with little evidence of adverse effects.

Drug administration route

Inadvertent intra-arterial injection of temazepam can cause tissue damage.

- A 29-year-old unemployed man developed pain and swelling of the right hand following inadvertent intra-arterial injection of temazepam capsules (6). Over 10 days, necrotic areas involving the index, middle, and little fingers developed and the fingers had to be amputated. He reported episodes of intravenous drug use during the previous 3 days—a single heroin dose followed by temazepam four times (10 mg gel capsules dissolved in hot water). He had injected the drugs into a superficial blood vessel on the back of the right hand.

Drug overdose

In a retrospective analysis of 352 consecutive cases of fatal overdose, temazepam accounted for 65% of all deaths from benzodiazepine overdose (7). Acute rhabdomyolysis, usually associated with intravascular injection, has been seen after an oral overdose of temazepam (SEDA-17, 45).

- An 83-year-old woman developed coma, respiratory depression, hypotonia with generalized hyporeflexia, bilateral extensor plantar responses, and bullous eruptions containing serous fluid over the medial aspects of the knees after taking seven temazepam tablets (8).

Drug–Drug Interactions

Oral contraceptives

The clearance of temazepam was increased when oral contraceptives were co-administered (9). It is unlikely that this is an interaction of clinical importance.

References

1. Ashton H. Guidelines for the rational use of benzodiazepines. When and what to use. Drugs 1994;48(1):25–40.
2. Michel L, Lang JP. Benzodiazepine et passage à l'acte criminel. [Benzodiazepines and forensic aspects.] Encephale 2003;29(6):479–85.
3. File SE, Joyce EM, Fluck E, De Bruin E, Bazari F, Nandha H, Fitton L, Adhiya S. Limited memory impairment after temazepam. Hum Psychopharmacol 1998;13:127–33.
4. Wise MG, Griffies WS. A combined treatment approach to anxiety in the medically ill. J Clin Psychiatry 1995;56(Suppl 2):14–19.
5. Ramesh M, Roberts G. Use of night-time benzodiazepines in an elderly inpatient population. J Clin Pharm Ther 2002;27(2):93–7.
6. Feeney GF, Gibbs HH. Digit loss following misuse of temazepam. Med J Aust 2002;176(8):380.
7. Obafunwa JO, Busuttil A. Deaths from substance overdose in the Lothian and Borders region of Scotland (1983–91). Hum Exp Toxicol 1994;13(6):401–6.
8. Verghese J, Merino J. Temazepam overdose associated with bullous eruptions. Acad Emerg Med 1999;6(10):1071.
9. Patwardhan RV, Mitchell MC, Johnson RF, Schenker S. Differential effects of oral contraceptive steroids on the metabolism of benzodiazepines. Hepatology 1983;3(2):248–53.

Temocapril

See also Angiotensin converting enzyme inhibitors

General Information

Temocapril is an ACE inhibitor, a prodrug that is converted to the active metabolite temocaprilat after absorption.

Drug–Drug Interactions

Warfarin

Temocapril had no effect on the pharmacokinetics or pharmacodynamics of multiple-dose warfarin in 24 healthy subjects (1). There have been similar negative interaction studies with other ACE inhibitors and oral anticoagulants.

Reference

1. Lankhaar G, Eckenberger P, Ouwerkerk MJA, Dingemanse J. Pharmacokinetic–pharmacodynamic investigation of a possible interaction between steady-state temocapril and warfarin in healthy subjects. Clin Drug Invest 1999;17:399–405.

Tenidap sodium

See also Non-steroidal anti-inflammatory drugs

General Information

Tenidap sodium, an antirheumatic drug, combines the clinical and pharmacological properties of NSAIDs with those of a disease-modifying agent. Data from clinical studies have been reviewed (SEDA-19, 100).

Pfizer abandoned tenidap sodium for use in rheumatoid arthritis after a non-approval letter from the FDA was issued because of unresolved questions about its safety. The decision related only to the 120 mg dose. The FDA's Arthritis Drugs Advisory Committee also voted against approving tenidap sodium for osteoarthritis.

Organs and Systems

Nervous system

The adverse effects of tenidap sodium include headache (3.8%) (1).

Hematologic

Acute eosinophilic pneumonia has been described in a man with osteoarthritis taking tenidap sodium (2).

Gastrointestinal

As expected with a cyclo-oxygenase inhibitor, the adverse effects most frequently reported by patients taking tenidap sodium were gastrointestinal; serious gastrointestinal events occurred in 2.1% (1).

Liver

Increases in serum transaminases can occur, and severe abnormalities in liver function tests have been reported (1,3–5).

Urinary tract

Proteinuria, by an unknown mechanism, is a frequent adverse effect of tenidap sodium (13%), but is reversible and non-progressive in the long term, and with no evidence of deteriorating renal function (1,6).

Skin

The adverse effects of tenidap sodium include alopecia (3.2%) (1).

Drug–Drug Interactions

ACE inhibitors

Tenidap sodium reduces the antihypertensive effects of ACE inhibitors (7).

Diuretics

Tenidap sodium reduces the antihypertensive effects of diuretics (7).

Lithium

Tenidap sodium interacts with lithium, reducing its renal clearance and increasing steady-state lithium concentrations; the dosage of lithium should be reduced to avoid toxicity (7,8).

Phenytoin

Tenidap sodium displaces phenytoin from plasma albumin binding sites by about 25% (9).

Warfarin

Tenidap sodium interacts with warfarin by displacing it from plasma albumin, although there may be another mechanism; the dosage of warfarin may need to be reduced to avoid toxicity (7,10).

References

1. Breedveld F. Tenidap: a novel cytokine-modulating anti-rheumatic drug for the treatment of rheumatoid arthritis. Scand J Rheumatol Suppl 1994;100:31–44.
2. Martinez BM, Domingo P. Acute eosinophilic pneumonia associated with tenidap. BMJ 1997;314(7077):349.
3. Anonymous. Hepatic monitoring for tenidap. Scrip 1995;2073:21.
4. Blackburn WD Jr., Prupas HM, Silverfield JC, Poiley JE, Caldwell JR, Collins RL, Miller MJ, Sikes DH, Kaplan H, Fleischmann R, et al. Tenidap in rheumatoid arthritis. A 24-week double-blind comparison with hydroxychloro-quine-plus-piroxicam, and piroxicam alone. Arthritis Rheum 1995;38(10):1447–56.
5. Wylie G, Appelboom T, Bolten W, Breedveld FC, Feely J, Leeming MR, Le Loet X, Manthorpe R, Marcolongo R, Smolen J. A comparative study of teni-dap, a cytokine-modulating anti-rheumatic drug, and diclofenac in rheumatoid arthritis: a 24-week analysis of a 1-year clinical trial. Br J Rheumatol 1995;34(6):554–63.
6. Martel-Pelletier J, Quinissi H, Cloutier JM, Pellettier JP. Tenidap effectively reduces cytochine synthesis and expression by human rheumatoid arthritis synovium. Arth Rheum 1994;37.
7. Pullar T. The pharmacokinetics of tenidap sodium: introduction. Br J Clin Pharmacol 1995;39(Suppl 1):S1–2.
8. Apseloff G, Wilner KD, von Deutsch DA, Gerber N. Tenidap sodium decreases renal clearance and increases steady-state concentrations of lithium in healthy volunteers. Br J Clin Pharmacol 1995;39(Suppl 1):S25–8.
9. Blum RA, Schentag JJ, Gardner MJ, Wilner KD. The effect of tenidap sodium on the disposition and plasma protein binding of phenytoin in healthy male volunteers. Br J Clin Pharmacol 1995;39(Suppl 1):S35–8.
10. Apseloff G, Wilner KD, Gerber N. Effect of tenidap sodium on the pharmacodynamics and plasma protein binding of warfarin in healthy volunteers. Br J Clin Pharmacol 1995;39(Suppl 1):S29–33.

Tenofovir

See also Nucleoside analogue reverse transcriptase inhibitors (NRTIs)

General Information

Tenofovir is a nucleotide (nucleoside monophosphate) analogue reverse transcriptase inhibitor, given as a prodrug, tenofovir disoproxil fumarate. In contrast to the other members of this class, it only needs to be phosphorylated twice intracellularly before it is pharma-cologically active. Adverse effects have been reported as flatulence, raised transaminases, raised creatine kinase activity, and rarely a raised serum creatinine (1). Tenofovir does not currently appear to be nephrotoxic.

Reference

1. Barditch-Crovo P, Deeks SG, Collier A, Safrin S, Coakley DF, Miller M, Kearney BP, Coleman RL, Lamy PD, Kahn JO, McGowan I, Lietman PS. Phase I/II trial of the pharmacokinetics, safety, and antiretroviral activity of tenofovir disoproxil fumarate in human immuno-deficiency virus-infected adults. Antimicrob Agents Chemother 2001;45(10):2733–9.

Tenoxicam

See also Non-steroidal anti-inflammatory drugs

General Information

Tenoxicam is a piroxicam analogue with a half-life of 75 hours. Whether the differences in pharmacokinetics in elderly patients have any clinical significance is unknown (SEDA-12, 93).

The pattern of adverse effects is similar to that of piroxicam, but tenoxicam causes slightly fewer serious gastrointestinal effects (1). Fecal blood loss is lower than with aspirin (SEDA-8, 111). A large, multicenter, hospi-tal-based study confirmed that tenoxicam and piroxicam had similar tolerance ratings: 13% of patients had severe adverse effects, most often gastrointestinal (melena, hematemesis, rectal bleeding, exacerbation of ulcerative colitis) and serious rashes (SEDA-15, 103). Gastrointestinal adverse effects are more frequent with higher doses (2).

In an open, non-comparative study in 1267 patients, performed to test tenoxicam safety in general practice, the most common adverse reactions were gastrointestinal (11%), central and peripheral nervous system disorders (2.8%), and skin reactions (2.5%) (3). Patients who take long-term tenoxicam are at low risk of nephrotoxicity. The prevalence of urinary system adverse effects was 0.07% in trials that included 67 000 patients (4).

Other adverse effects include phototoxic dermatitis, thrombocytopenia, edema of the legs, pruritus, and hyper-salivation (SEDA-12, 93).

Organs and Systems

Respiratory

Tenoxicam can provoke severe bronchoconstriction and nasal obstruction in aspirin-sensitive asthmatic patients (SEDA-12, 93).

Liver

Mild chronic drug-induced hepatitis has been attributed to tenoxicam (SEDA-21, 108).

Skin

Three cases of toxic epidermal necrolysis (Lyell's syndrome) have been described in patients taking tenoxicam (SEDA-17, 114).

A fixed drug eruption with cross-sensitivity to droxicam and tenoxicam has been reported (SEDA-18, 107), but tenoxicam may not cross-react in patients with photosensitivity to piroxicam (SEDA-18, 107).

Drug Administration

Drug administration route

Tenoxicam can be given intravenously, but phlebitis and pain at the injection site occur, albeit rarely (SEDA-19, 99).

References

1. Bird HA. International experience with tenoxicam: a review. Scand J Rheumatol Suppl 1988;73:22–7.
2. Gonzalez JP, Todd PA. Tenoxicam. A preliminary review of its pharmacodynamic and pharmacokinetic properties, and therapeutic efficacy. Drugs 1987;34(3).289–310.
3. Caughey D, Waterworth RF. A study of the safety of tenoxicam in general practice. NZ Med J 1989; 102(879):582–3.
4. Heintz RC. Tenoxicam and renal function. Drug Saf 1995;12(2):110–19.

Terazosin

See also Alpha-adrenoceptor antagonists

General Information

The alpha$_1$-adrenoceptor antagonist terazosin has similar adverse effects to those of prazosin. The long-term efficacy and safety of terazosin have been reviewed, in both monotherapy and combination therapy in whites and blacks (1,2).

In order to investigate the mechanisms of adverse events associated with alpha$_1$-adrenoceptor antagonists, the Veterans Affairs Cooperative Study database was analysed with respect to the relation between adverse events and hypotension in 1229 men with benign prostate hyperplasia. Treatment with terazosin produced the following rates of adverse events: dizziness 19%, weakness 6%, postural hypotension 6%, and syncope 1%. Of these adverse events only postural hypotension was associated with orthostatic blood pressure changes. Weakness, dizziness, and postural hypotension occurred to the same extent in patients with falls in systolic blood pressure of 5 mmHg or more or less than 5 mmHg. Thus, dizziness and weakness do not seem to be associated with changes in blood pressure, suggesting that these adverse events associated with alpha-blockers are not related to vascular effects. Designing a subtype selective alpha$_1$-antagonist that has less effect on blood pressure may not result in marked improvement in tolerability over currently available alpha$_1$-antagonists (3).

Organs and Systems

Skin

Terazosin has reportedly caused a rash (4).

- A 59-year-old man developed a generalized rash 3 days after starting to take terazosin 2 mg/day for benign prostatic hyperplasia. He had mild fever, weakness, intense pruritus, and a widespread eruption of scaling erythematous plaques with a violaceous hue on the trunk and extremities. The clinical examination was otherwise unremarkable and laboratory and serological test were negative. A skin biopsy was suggestive of a drug reaction. Terazosin was stopped, and treatment with oral prednisolone and emollients resulted in complete recovery in 2 weeks.

Sexual function

Priapism is rare with alpha-blockers (5).

- A 20-year-old man with a cervical spinal cord injury and a neuropathic bladder was given terazosin 1 mg at night increasing 5 days later to 2 mg. He developed a full erection of his penis, which lasted 5 hours and subsided spontaneously. Terazosin was stopped and the patient experienced no further priapism.

References

1. Saunders E. The safety and efficacy of terazosin in the treatment of essential hypertension in blacks. Am Heart J 1991;122(3 Pt 2):936–42.
2. Cohen JD. Long-term efficacy and safety of terazosin alone and in combination with other antihypertensive agents. Am Heart J 1991;122(3 Pt 2):919–25.
3. Lepor H, Jones K, Williford W. The mechanism of adverse events associated with terazosin: an analysis of the Veterans Affairs Cooperative Study. J Urol 2000;163(4):1134–7.
4. Hernandez-Cano N, Herranz P, Lazaro TE, Mayor M, Casado M. Severe cutaneous reaction due to terazosin. Lancet 1998;352(9123):202–3.
5. Vaidyanathan S, Soni BM, Singh G, Sett P, Krishnan KR. Prolonged penile erection association with terazosin in a cervical spinal cord injury patient. Spinal Cord 1998;36(11):805.

Terbinafine

General Information

The allylamine derivative terbinafine can be used orally or topically. It is active against a broad range of fungi, including filamentous fungi and, to a lesser extent, yeast-like fungi. However, probably because of irreversible protein binding, its clinical usefulness is limited to the treatment of dermatophyte infections and perhaps lymphocutaneous sporotrichosis.

Terbinafine acts by inhibiting the synthesis of fungal ergosterol at the level of squalene oxidase, leading to depletion of ergosterol and accumulation of toxic squalenes in the fungal cell membrane.

Pharmacokinetics

Numerous reviews and studies of the pharmacokinetics of terbinafine have appeared (1–13). Independent of food, its oral availability is 70–80%. With a single dose of 250 mg, plasma concentrations reach around 0.97 μg/ml after two hours. Apparent steady-state plasma concentrations are reached after 10–14 days after only two-fold accumulation, although the half-life is up to 3 weeks and microbiologically active concentrations can be measured in plasma for weeks to months after the last dose, which is consistent with slow redistribution from the peripheral tissues and fat. Protein binding is over 99% and the apparent volume of distribution over 2000 liters, high concentrations reaching adipose tissues, the dermis, epidermis, and nails. Less than 0.2% reaches the breast milk. After several weeks, no further accumulation of the compound occurs (14,15). In renal or hepatic failure, elimination is slowed. Terbinafine undergoes extensive and complex hepatic biotransformation involving at least seven CYP450 enzymes (16); none of its metabolites is mycologically active. Urinary excretion accounts for more than 70% and fecal elimination for 10% of total excretion; the extent of enterohepatic recycling is unknown. Children have a shorter half-life, a lower mean AUC, and a higher volume of distribution, reflecting their higher proportion of lipophilic tissues (17,18).

Comparative studies

The safety and efficacy of terbinafine 250 mg/day and itraconazole 200 mg/day given for 12 weeks for toenail onychomycosis have been compared in a randomized, double-blind study in 372 patients (19). Adverse events were reported in 39% of the terbinafine-treated patients and in 35% of the itraconazole-treated patients. The mean values of biochemical parameters of liver and kidney function did not change significantly. Terbinafine produced higher rates of clinical cure (76 versus 58%) and mycological cure (73 versus 46%) than itraconazole.

In a randomized, double-blind comparison of terbinafine 250 mg/day ($n = 146$) with itraconazole 200 mg/day ($n = 146$), administered for 12 weeks for toenail onychomycosis, mycological cure rates at the 36-week follow-up end-point (67 versus 61%) and the proportion of patients with adverse effects (23 versus 22%) were similar in both study arms. However, more patients taking terbinafine

stopped treatment permanently because of treatment-related adverse events (8 versus 1%) (20).

In a double-blind, randomized, multicenter comparison of terbinafine (250 mg/day for 12 or 16 weeks) or itraconazole capsules (200 mg bd for 1 week every 4 weeks for 12 or 16 weeks), 236 patients reported at least one adverse event. All were within the known safety profile of both drugs, and there were no significant differences among the four treatment regimens. Continuous terbinafine was significantly more effective than intermittent itraconazole (mycological cure rates at week 72: 76, 81, 38, and 49%; significant for all comparisons between terbinafine and itraconazole) (21,22).

General adverse effects

Terbinafine is usually well tolerated. Gastrointestinal complaints (dyspepsia, nausea, diarrhea) were the most common reasons for withdrawal. Abdominal pain and loss of taste were reported, as well as mild nervous system symptoms (headache and dizziness) (23).

Organs and Systems

Sensory systems

Taste disturbance is a rare adverse effect of terbinafine. It is usually reversible, with a median time to recovery of 42 days. However, a 46-year-old woman had complete loss of taste after taking oral terbinafine, with persistent taste disturbances for 3 years after stopping the drug (24).

Hematologic

The projected rate of all blood dyscrasias associated with terbinafine has been estimated to be 32 per million patient-years (25). Pancytopenia has been reported (26).

Leukocytes

Neutropenia has been reported in patients taking terbinafine (25–28).

- A 55-year-old woman who was taking terbinafine and paroxetine presented with fever, diarrhea, and vomiting. A bone marrow biopsy showed overall reduced cellularity, and the aspirate showed a profound shift toward the production of immature myeloid cells, consistent with maturation arrest. Treatment consisted of withdrawal of all outpatient medications, hydration, intravenous fluids, broad-spectrum antibiotics, and G-CSF 5 μg/kg for 5 days. Mature granulocytes appeared in the peripheral blood on the fifth day in hospital, and she was discharged on the seventh hospital day with an absolute neutrophil count of 6.2×10^9/l. Paroxetine was resumed weeks after discharge from hospital without hematological toxicity over 6 months.
- A 60-year-old man presented with fever, oral mucositis, pedal cellulitis, and bacteremia after a 6-week course of terbinafine 250 mg. He was taking concurrent yohimbine for impotence. Bone marrow examination showed a hypocellular marrow with myeloid maturation arrest. Treatment consisted of withdrawal of outpatient medications, broad-spectrum antibiotics, hydration,

and G-CSF, and was ultimately successful. Yohimbine was resumed later without any adverse effects.

- A 42-year-old man presented with fever and granulocytopenia (absolute neutrophil count: $340 \times 10^6/l$; temperature: $39.5°C$) after a 30-day course of oral terbinafine 250 mg/day for presumed onychomycosis (27). The granulocyte count recovered promptly after withdrawal of the drug and administration of G-CSF for 2 days.
- Agranulocytosis occurred in a 15-year-old who took terbinafine 250 mg/day for toenail onychomycosis and tinea pedis (29). This effect was noted 4 weeks after starting terbinafine and resolved within 1 week after its withdrawal.

Platelets

Thrombocytopenia has been attributed to terbinafine (30), and the incidence has been estimated at 1 in 200 000 patients (25).

- A 25-year-old Yemeni woman with familial-ethnic leukopenia developed thrombocytopenia with epistaxis after taking terbinafine 250 mg for 4 weeks (30). The platelet count recovered from a nadir of $63 \times 10^9/l$ to $314 \times 10^9/l$ after drug withdrawal.
- A 53-year-old woman developed severe thrombocytopenia after a 6-week course of terbinafine (250 mg/day) for onychomycosis (31). A bone marrow aspirate showed a normocellular marrow. She received a platelet transfusion and recovered after a short course of prednisolone.

Mouth

- A 38-year-old man presented with acute right otitis media and unrelated painless bilateral enlargement of the parotid glands 15 days after taking oral terbinafine for tinea cruris (32). He stopped taking terbinafine and 12 days later the swelling had significantly abated and completely disappeared 4 weeks later.

Liver

Minor abnormalities in liver function tests have been reported in up to 4% of patients taking oral terbinafine (33), but have not generally been considered clinically important (SEDA-16, 297) (SEDA-18, 7) (SEDA-18, 25).

Terbinafine can cause hepatitis, with an estimated rate of about 1 in 50 000 (34). Idiosyncratic reactions can lead to liver cell necrosis as well as cholestasis. Prolonged cholestatic hepatitis and liver failure have been reported (35–39).

- In four patients with cholestatic hepatitis associated with terbinafine, all presented with jaundice and direct hyperbilirubinemia, various other clinical signs of hepatitis, and mild to moderate rises in alkaline phosphatase and hepatic transaminase activities (34,39). Biopsies in two patients showed cellular infiltrates in the portal tracts and hepatocellular and canalicular cholestasis ($n = 1$) and hepatocyte degeneration ($n = 1$). In the two cases with long-term follow-up, hepatitis was reversible after withdrawal of terbinafine and liver tests normalized within 6 months.

- A 41-year-old man developed severe hepatic dysfunction following a 3.5-week course of terbinafine (250 mg/day) (40). He had marked pruritus, jaundice, malaise, anorexia, and loin pain. His serum bilirubin rose to a peak of 718 μmol/l with alkaline phosphatase 569 U/l, alanine transaminase 90 U/l, aspartate transaminase 63 U/l, and a prolonged prothrombin time of 21 seconds, unresponsive to vitamin K. Liver biopsy showed canalicular cholestasis consistent with a drug reaction. His symptoms resolved 11 months after drug withdrawal, and his liver function tests normalized after 15 months.
- A previously healthy 46-year-old man developed acute fulminant hepatitis following treatment with rabeprazole, citalopram hydrobromide, terbinafine, and a multivitamin formulation (41). Liver biopsy showed submassive centrilobular necrosis and intrahepatic cholestasis with florid bile duct proliferation.

In the last case, because of the similarity of the clinical, laboratory, and histological effects of omeprazole and lansoprazole, as previously reported, the authors concluded that the reaction in the second patient might have been caused by the proton pump inhibitor rather than terbinafine.

- A 56-year-old woman developed chronic biliary ductopenia and portal fibrosis 2 years after a course of terbinafine (42). Terbinafine treatment at that time had resulted in jaundice and evidence of cholestasis. After withdrawal of terbinafine, she continued to have pruritus and persistently raised serum alkaline phosphatase activity. Investigations for various types of chronic liver disease were negative and so chronic bile duct loss and periportal fibrosis were attributed to terbinafine.

Because of the rare and unpredictable nature of hepatobiliary reactions to terbinafine, the mechanism of hepatotoxicity has been hypothesized to be either immunological or metabolically mediated. A potentially toxic reactive metabolite of terbinafine, 7,7-dimethylhept-2-ene-4-ynal (TBF-A), the N-dealkylation product of terbinafine, has been identified in vitro (43). The authors speculated that this allylic aldehyde metabolite, formed by liver enzymes and conjugated with glutathione, would be transported across the canalicular membrane of hepatocytes and concentrated in the bile. The reactive monoglutathione conjugate could bind to hepatobiliary proteins and cause direct toxicity. Alternatively, it could modify canalicular proteins and lead to an immune-mediated reaction, causing cholestatic dysfunction.

Skin

Cutaneous adverse effects reportedly occur in 1–3% of patients taking terbinafine. The overwhelming majority of these reactions consist of mild to moderate macular exanthemas.

The risk of serious skin disorders has been estimated in 61 858 users of oral antifungal drugs, aged 20–79 years, identified in the UK General Practice Research Database (44). They had received at least one prescription for oral fluconazole, griseofulvin, itraconazole, ketoconazole, or terbinafine. The background rate of serious cutaneous adverse reactions (corresponding to non-use of oral anti-fungal drugs) was 3.9 per 10 000 person-years (95% CI = 2.9, 5.2). Incidence rates for current use were 15 per 10 000 person-years (1.9, 56) for itraconazole, 11.1 (3.0, 29) for terbinafine, 10 (1.3, 38) for fluconazole, and 4.6 (0.1, 26) for griseofulvin. Cutaneous disorders associated with the use of oral antifungal drugs in this study were all mild.

Generalized rashes, fixed drug eruptions, toxic epidermolysis, and erythema exudativum multiforme have all been reported in association with terbinafine (45,46).

Pustular eruptions can occur occasionally (45–49).

- Acute generalized exanthematous pustulosis associated with terbinafine has been described in two patients (47,49). Both presented within 7–10 days after starting to take terbinafine with generalized pustular dermatosis and leukocytosis; fever was a presenting symptom in one patient. Treatment with systemic corticosteroids was successful in both cases.
- A 62-year-old diabetic man on stable oral medication with glibenclamide, metformin, Zestoretic (lisinopril + hydrochlorothiazide), gemfibrozil, and aspirin developed febrile generalized pustular eruptions after 44 days of therapy with oral terbinafine 250 mg/day (50). Withdrawal of terbinafine and symptomatic treatment with hydrotherapy and topical and systemic steroids resulted in complete resolution of fever and pustulosis within 4 days. The erythematous component responded more slowly, and mildly pruritic erythematous plaques persisted for more than 40 days.
- In another case of acute generalized exanthematous pustulosis attributed to terbinafine (250 mg/day), epicutaneous and intracutaneous skin tests were negative, and there was no evidence of viral infection (51).

Terbinafine can cause or exacerbate psoriatic lesions.

- Severe pustular psoriasis provoked de novo by oral terbinafine has been reported in a 65-year-old man 2 weeks after the start of therapy for onychomycosis (52). Treatment of psoriasis was complicated and ultimately required continuous systemic and topical antipsoriatic therapy.
- A 74-year-old woman developed inverse psoriasis after 14 days of therapy with terbinafine 250 mg/day for onychomycosis (53). The lesions resolved almost completely on withdrawal of terbinafine and topical therapy.

Probable psoriatic onychodystrophy, misdiagnosed as onychomycosis and treated with terbinafine, induced inverse psoriasis in the second case, underscoring the importance of mycological confirmation of onychomycosis before therapy.

Ten cases of severe skin reactions probably associated with terbinafine requiring drug withdrawal have been reported: erythema multiforme ($n = 5$), erythroderma ($n = 1$), severe urticaria ($n = 1$), pityriasis rosea ($n = 1$), and worsening of pre-existing psoriasis ($n = 2$) (54). All the patients made an uneventful recovery with appropriate therapy. The authors pointed out that patients should be counselled about discontinuing terbinafine at the onset of a skin eruption and about seeking medical advice about further management.

- Cutaneous lupus erythematosus attributed to terbinafine has been reported in two previously healthy women (55,56). In the first patient, the lesions improved but did not resolve completely; in the second the symptoms resolved completely with appropriate therapy and the patient remained disease-free after withdrawal of all medication.
- Another woman with a previous history suggestive of lupus erythematosus developed a widespread flare in her skin 1 week after starting oral terbinafine (57). The eruption ultimately responded to systemic treatment with corticosteroids.

Baboon syndrome has been attributed to terbinafine (58).

- A 26-year-old man developed a fixed drug eruption on his hands and inguinal and gluteal areas after oral treatment of onychomycosis with terbinafine 250 mg/day. The rash showed the characteristic distribution of the baboon syndrome. Although epicutaneous and intracutaneous tests were negative, the rash recurred 20 hours after oral rechallenge with terbinafine.

The underlying pathogenic mechanism for the baboon syndrome has been suggested to be a systemically induced allergic contact dermatitis.

Hair

Hair loss has been attributed to terbinafine (59).

- A 69-year-old woman took terbinafine 250 mg/day for 112 days for subungual hyperkeratosis and developed hair loss after 3 months. She was also taking hydrochlorothiazide, amiloride hydrochloride, and amlodipine besilate, all in the same dosage for more than 5 years. Clinical and laboratory investigations showed no other obvious causes, and hair loss completely reversed on withdrawal of terbinafine.

Musculoskeletal

Since its introduction, the Netherlands Pharmacovigilance Foundation Lareb has received eight reports of arthralgia in patients taking terbinafine (60). In four cases, skin reactions were also present and in two cases urticaria. Two patients who reported arthralgia also had a fever. Logistic regression modelling showed that both urticaria and arthralgia were statistically significantly associated with reports on terbinafine compared with all other reports in the database. These findings may point toward a clustering of these symptoms in patients using terbinafine, suggesting a shared immunological reaction.

Immunologic

Exacerbation of lupus erythematosus has been reported during terbinafine therapy (55–57,61). Of 21 consecutive patients with subacute cutaneous lupus erythematosus who attended an outpatient dermatology department in Germany during 1 year, 4 had terbinafine-associated disease (62). In addition to high titers of antinuclear antibodies with a homogeneous pattern, anti-Ro(SS-A) antibodies were present; in three of the four women, anti-La(SS-B) antibodies were also found. All the patients had antihistone antibodies, as in drug-induced lupus, and showed the characteristic genetic association with the HLA-B8,DR3 haplotype; moreover, in two cases HLA-DR2 was also present. After withdrawal of terbinafine, antinuclear antibody titers fell and antihistone antibodies became undetectable within 4.5 months in three patients.

- A 66-year-old man with giant cell arteritis and hypertension developed a hypersensitivity reaction 4.5 weeks after starting to take terbinafine, with a skin eruption, fever, lymphadenopathy, and hepatic dysfunction (63). Concomitant medications included prednisone, doxazosin, and aspirin. His symptoms and signs resolved within 6 weeks after withdrawal of terbinafine and continuation of all the other medications. The hypersensitivity syndrome reaction in this case was idiosyncratic, with no apparent predisposing factors.

Susceptibility Factors

Age

The pharmacokinetics of terbinafine and five known metabolites have been investigated in 12 children, (mean age 8 years; range 5–11 years), who took terbinafine 125 mg/day for 6–8 weeks for tinea capitis (15). The metabolism of terbinafine was similar to that observed in adults, and there were comparable steady-state plasma concentrations after administration of the same oral dose. Steady state was reached by day 21 with no further accumulation up to day 56. Terbinafine was effective in all patients and safe and well tolerated over 56 days.

In a randomized, double-blind comparison of terbinafine (n = 27) with itraconazole (n = 28) for 2 weeks for tinea capitis in Pakistani children (mean age 8 years), fever, body ache, and vertigo were seen with terbinafine in one patient each, and urticaria with itraconazole in two patients (64). There were no significant changes in hematological and biochemical profiles.

In an open assessment of the efficacy, safety, and tolerability of oral terbinafine 125–250 mg/day for 1, 2, and 4 weeks for tinea capitis in 132 Brazilian children aged 1–14 years, adverse events were reported in 10 patients (65). The drug was prematurely withdrawn in one patient. In the post-treatment evaluation, two patients had abnormal bilirubin concentrations and eight patients had abnormal alkaline phosphatase activities; none was considered clinically relevant.

In an open, non-comparative study of the use of terbinafine for 14 days to treat tinea capitis in 50 children and adolescents (mean age 7.6 years; range 24 months to 18 years), the clinical and mycological cure rates were 86%. The drug appeared to be well tolerated. Two children had reversible neutropenia, thought to be due to a preceding viral illness; other adverse effects were not observed (18).

In 14 children, aged 1–15 years, with *Microsporum canis* tinea capitis given oral terbinafine for 4 weeks, the recommended daily dose produced no response by week 4; the dose was doubled (to 250 mg/day) for a further 4–8 weeks in six patients and continued at the original dose in six patients (66). Two patients withdrew. Four patients were cured after 8–12 weeks of treatment, and all had taken the doubled dose of terbinafine, except for one who had taken the usual adult dose of 250 mg/day from the start. Oral terbinafine was well tolerated by all but one patient, who had gastrointestinal disturbance and slightly raised transaminase activities during the first 4 weeks of treatment.

In an open, prospective, uncontrolled study in 81 immunocompetent young children (aged 2–13 years) with tinea capitis due to *Microsporum canis*, oral terbinafine was given in dosages based on weight (62.5 mg for those weighing 10–20 kg and 125 mg for 20–40 kg), and applied topically to affected areas (1% cream bd) (67). Treatment lasted for 4 weeks, followed by an 8-week observation (treatment-free) period. All the subjects were assessed for efficacy and tolerability at 12 weeks. At 12 weeks: 32 had completely recovered, with no evidence of relapse during the observation period, and 21 had mycological cure but residual signs of infection. The effective cure rate was 65%. Terbinafine was well tolerated by these children: 75 had no adverse effects; the other six had abdominal pain (n = 2), vomiting (n = 1), generalized itching (n = 1), local itching (n = 1), and localized erythema (n = 1). Hematological and biochemical parameters remained normal during the study.

Drug–Drug Interactions

Rifamycins

Rifampicin 600 mg/day reduced terbinafine concentrations by about 50% by enzyme induction (68).

Theophylline

Theophylline is largely metabolized by CYP1A2 and terbinafine increases its half-life (69). In a randomized, crossover study in 12 healthy volunteers, terbinafine increased theophylline exposure by 16%, with a 14% reduction in clearance and a 24% increase in half-life (69). These pharmacokinetic changes may predispose individuals to accumulation of theophylline and unwanted toxicity. Caution should be taken in prescribing terbinafine for patients taking long-term theophylline.

Tricyclic antidepressants

Desipramine

Inhibition of CYP2D6 by terbinafine has been evaluated by assessing 48-hour concentration-time profiles of the tricyclic antidepressant desipramine in 12 healthy volunteers identified as extensive CYP2D6 metabolizers by genotyping and phenotyping (70). The pharmacokinetics were evaluated at baseline (50 mg oral desipramine given alone), steady state (after 250 mg oral terbinafine for 21 days), and 2 and 4 weeks after terbinafine withdrawal. The pharmacodynamics were evaluated before and 2 hours after each dose of desipramine, using Mini-Mental Status Examination and electroencephalography. Terbinafine inhibited CYP2D6 metabolism, as indicated by significant increases in desipramine C_{max} and AUC and reductions in the C_{max} and AUC of the CYP2D6-mediated metabolite, 2-hydroxydesipramine, both of which were still altered 4 weeks after terbinafine withdrawal. Caution should be exercised when co-prescribing terbinafine and drugs that are metabolized by CYP2D6, particularly those with a narrow therapeutic index.

Imipramine

- A 51-year-old patient developed imipramine toxicity and increased plasma concentrations associated with the introduction of terbinafine, possibly due to inhibition of CYP2D6 (71).

Nortriptyline

Metabolism by CYP2D6 is of major importance for the hydroxylation of nortriptyline, making it susceptible to competitive inhibition by terbinafine. Nortriptyline intoxication provoked by terbinafine has been reported (72).

- A 74-year-old man taking a stable dose of nortriptyline for depression developed signs of nortriptyline intoxication 14 days after he started to take terbinafine (72). Nortriptyline serum concentrations were several times higher than the usual target range and fell to baseline after withdrawal of terbinafine. Re-challenge led to the same clinical and laboratory findings.
- Nortriptyline intoxication secondary to terbinafine has been observed in a woman with a major depressive disorder (73). After rechallenge her serum nortriptyline concentration rose and the serum concentrations of its two hydroxylated metabolites fell. She had a normal genotype for CYP2D6, suggesting that this interaction can occur even in people without reduced CYP2D6 activity.

Warfarin

While terbinafine had no effect on warfarin in healthy volunteers, it can prolong the prothrombin time in some individuals (74–77), prompting intensification of laboratory control during terbinafine therapy.

- A 71-year-old woman taking a stable dose of warfarin and cimetidine was treated with terbinafine, and 32 days later developed profuse intestinal bleeding associated with a prothrombin time of 120 seconds, suggestive of an interaction between warfarin and terbinafine, either directly or through the mediation of cimetidine (which can reduce terbinafine clearance by 33%) (74).

However, a contrasting case has also been reported.

- A 68-year-old woman taking warfarin, glibenclamide, metformin, furosemide, and spironolactone was given terbinafine 250 mg/day and 4 weeks later required progressive increases in the warfarin dosage to maintain a therapeutic INR; after withdrawal of terbinafine, her warfarin requirements returned to baseline over 4 weeks, supporting enzyme induction with gradual onset and offset (75).

Since a pharmacokinetic study of a single dose of warfarin in 26 healthy volunteers treated with terbinafine showed no significant interaction, and since a large postmarketing study of terbinafine did not find any cases of interaction of warfarin with terbinafine, the manufacturers (78) and others (77) have cautioned about any generalization regarding an interaction between terbinafine and warfarin.

References

1. Shear NH, Villars VV, Marsolais C. Terbinafine: an oral and topical antifungal agent. Clin Dermatol 1991;9(4):487–95.
2. Balfour JA, Faulds D. Terbinafine. A review of its pharmacodynamic and pharmacokinetic properties, and therapeutic potential in superficial mycoses. Drugs 1992;43(2):259–84. Erratum in: Drugs 1992;43(5):699.
3. Finlay AY. Pharmacokinetics of terbinafine in the nail. Br J Dermatol 1992;126(Suppl 39):28–32.
4. Finlay AY. Global overview of Lamisil. Br J Dermatol 1994;130(Suppl 43):1–3.
5. Jones TC. Overview of the use of terbinafine (Lamisil) in children. Br J Dermatol 1995;132(5):683–9.
6. Gupta AK, Shear NH. Terbinafine: an update. J Am Acad Dermatol 1997;37(6):979–88.
7. Faergemann J, Zehender H, Jones T, Maibach I. Terbinafine levels in serum, stratum corneum, dermis–epidermis (without stratum corneum), hair, sebum and eccrine sweat. Acta Dermatol Venereol 1991;71(4):322–6.
8. Kovarik JM, Kirkesseli S, Humbert H, Grass P, Kutz K. Dose-proportional pharmacokinetics of terbinafine and its N-demethylated metabolite in healthy volunteers. Br J Dermatol 1992;126(Suppl 39):8–13.
9. Kovarik JM, Mueller EA, Zehender H, Denouel J, Caplain H, Millerioux L. Multiple-dose pharmacokinetics and distribution in tissue of terbinafine and metabolites. Antimicrob Agents Chemother 1995;39(12):2738–41.
10. Nedelman JR, Gibiansky E, Robbins BA, Cramer JA, Riefler JF, Lin T, Meligeni JA. Pharmacokinetics and pharmacodynamics of multiple-dose terbinafine. J Clin Pharmacol 1996;36(5):452–61.
11. Wildfeuer A, Faergemann J, Laufen H, Pfaff G, Zimmermann T, Seidl HP, Lach P. Bioavailability of fluconazole in the skin after oral medication. Mycoses 1994;37(3–4):127–30.
12. Faergemann J. Pharmacokinetics of fluconazole in skin and nails. J Am Acad Dermatol 1999;40(6 Pt 2):S14–20.
13. Humbert H, Cabiac MD, Denouel J, Kirkesseli S. Pharmacokinetics of terbinafine and of its five main metabolites in plasma and urine, following a single oral dose in healthy subjects. Biopharm Drug Dispos 1995;16(8):685–94.
14. Matsumoto T, Tanuma H, Kaneko S, Takasu H, Nishiyama S. Clinical and pharmacokinetic investigations of oral terbinafine in patients with tinea unguium. Mycoses 1995;38(3–4):135–44.
15. Humbert H, Denouel J, Cabiac MD, Lakhdar H, Sioufi A. Pharmacokinetics of terbinafine and five known metabolites in children, after oral administration. Biopharm Drug Dispos 1998;19(7):417–23.
16. Vickers AE, Sinclair JR, Zollinger M, Heitz F, Glanzel U, Johanson L, Fischer V. Multiple cytochrome P-450s involved in the metabolism of terbinafine suggest a limited potential for drug–drug interactions. Drug Metab Dispos 1999;27(9):1029–38.
17. Nejjam F, Zagula M, Cabiac MD, Guessous N, Humbert H, Lakhdar H. Pilot study of terbinafine in children suffering from tinea capitis: evaluation of efficacy, safety and pharmacokinetics. Br J Dermatol 1995;132(1):98–105.
18. Krafchik B, Pelletier J. An open study of tinea capitis in 50 children treated with a 2-week course of oral terbinafine. J Am Acad Dermatol 1999;41(1):60–3.
19. De Backer M, De Vroey C, Lesaffre E, Scheys I, De Keyser P. Twelve weeks of continuous oral therapy for toenail onychomycosis caused by dermatophytes: a double-blind comparative trial of terbinafine 250 mg/day versus itraconazole 200 mg/day. J Am Acad Dermatol 1998;38(5 Pt 3):S57–63.

20. Degreef H, del Palacio A, Mygind S, Ginter G, Pinto Soares A, Zuluaga de Cadena A. Randomized double-blind comparison of short-term itraconazole and terbinafine therapy for toenail onychomycosis. Acta Dermatol Venereol 1999;79(3):221–3.

21. Evans EG, Sigurgeirsson B. Double blind, randomised study of continuous terbinafine compared with intermittent itraconazole in treatment of toenail onychomycosis. The LION Study Group. BMJ 1999;318(7190):1031–5.

22. Sigurgeirsson B, Billstein S, Rantanen T, Ruzicka T, di Fonzo E, Vermeer BJ, Goodfield MJ, Evans EG. L.I.ON. Study: efficacy and tolerability of continuous terbinafine (Lamisil) compared to intermittent itraconazole in the treatment of toenail onychomycosis. Lamisil vs. Itraconazole in Onychomycosis. Br J Dermatol 1999;141(Suppl 56):5–14.

23. O'Sullivan DP, Needham CA, Bangs A, Atkin K, Kendall FD. Postmarketing surveillance of oral terbinafine in the UK: report of a large cohort study. Br J Clin Pharmacol 1996;42(5):559–65.

24. Bong JL, Lucke TW, Evans CD. Persistent impairment of taste resulting from terbinafine. Br J Dermatol 1998;139(4):747–8.

25. Gupta AK, Soori GS, Del Rosso JQ, Bartos PB, Shear NH. Severe neutropenia associated with oral terbinafine therapy. J Am Acad Dermatol 1998;38(5 Pt 1):765–7.

26. Kovacs MJ, Alshammari S, Guenther L, Bourcier M. Neutropenia and pancytopenia associated with oral terbinafine. J Am Acad Dermatol 1994;31(5 Pt 1):806.

27. Shapiro M, Li LJ, Miller J. Terbinafine-induced neutropenia. Br J Dermatol 1999;140(6):1196–997.

28. Ornstein DL, Ely P. Reversible agranulocytosis associated with oral terbinafine for onychomycosis. J Am Acad Dermatol 1998;39(6):1023–4.

29. Aguilar C, Mueller KK. Reversible agranulocytosis associated with oral terbinafine in a pediatric patient. J Am Acad Dermatol 2001;45(4):632–4.

30. Grunwald MH. Thrombocytopenia associated with oral terbinafine. Int J Dermatol 1998;37(8):634.

31. Tsai HH, Lee WR, Hu CH. Isolated thrombocytopenia associated with oral terbinafine. Br J Dermatol 2002;147(3):627–8.

32. Torrens JK, McWhinney PH. Parotid swelling and terbinafine. BMJ 1998;316(7129):440–1.

33. van der Schroeff JG, Cirkel PK, Crijns MB, Van Dijk TJ, Govaert FJ, Groeneweg DA, Tazelaar DJ, De Wit RF, Wuite J. A randomized treatment duration-finding study of terbinafine in onychomycosis. Br J Dermatol 1992;126(Suppl 39):36–9.

34. Gupta AK, del Rosso JQ, Lynde CW, Brown GH, Shear NH. Hepatitis associated with terbinafine therapy: three case reports and a review of the literature. Clin Exp Dermatol 1998;23(2):64–7.

35. van 't Wout JW, Herrmann WA, de Vries RA, Stricker BH. Terbinafine-associated hepatic injury. J Hepatol 1994;21(1):115–17.

36. Lazaros GA, Papatheodoridis GV, Delladetsima JK, Tassopoulos NC. Terbinafine-induced cholestatic liver disease. J Hepatol 1996;24(6):753–6.

37. Mallat A, Zafrani ES, Metreau JM, Dhumeaux D. Terbinafine-induced prolonged cholestasis with reduction of interlobular bile ducts. Dig Dis Sci 1997;42(7):1486–8.

38. Agarwal K, Manas DM, Hudson M. Terbinafine and fulminant hepatic failure. N Engl J Med 1999;340(16):1292–3.

39. Fernandes NF, Geller SA, Fong TL. Terbinafine hepatotoxicity: case report and review of the literature. Am J Gastroenterol 1998;93(3):459–60.

40. Chambers WM, Millar A, Jain S, Burroughs AK. Terbinafine-induced hepatic dysfunction. Eur J Gastroenterol Hepatol 2001;13(9):1115–18.

41. Johnstone D, Berger C, Fleckman P. Acute fulminant hepatitis after treatment with rabeprazole and terbinafine. Arch Intern Med 2001;161(13):1677–8.

42. Anania FA, Rabin L. Terbinafine hepatotoxicity resulting in chronic biliary ductopenia and portal fibrosis. Am J Med 2002;112(9):741–2.

43. Iverson SL, Uetrecht JP. Identification of a reactive metabolite of terbinafine: insights into terbinafine-induced hepatotoxicity. Chem Res Toxicol 2001;14(2):175–81.

44. Castellsague J, Garcia-Rodriguez LA, Duque A, Perez S. Risk of serious skin disorders among users of oral antifungals: a population-based study. BMC Dermatol 2002;2(1):14.

45. Carstens J, Wendelboe P, Sogaard H, Thestrup-Pedersen K. Toxic epidermal necrolysis and erythema multiforme following therapy with terbinafine. Acta Dermatol Venereol 1994;74(5):391–2.

46. Munn SE, Russell Jones R. Terbinafine and fixed drug eruption. Br J Dermatol 1995;133(5):815–16.

47. Condon CA, Downs AM, Archer CB. Terbinafine-induced acute generalized exanthematous pustulosis. Br J Dermatol 1998;138(4):709–10.

48. Kempinaire A, De Raeve L, Merckx M, De Coninck A, Bauwens M, Roseeuw D. Terbinafine-induced acute generalized exanthematous pustulosis confirmed by a positive patch-test result. J Am Acad Dermatol 1997;37(4):653–5.

49. Papa CA, Miller OF. Pustular psoriasiform eruption with leukocytosis associated with terbinafine. J Am Acad Dermatol 1998;39(1):115–17.

50. Bennett ML, Jorizzo JL, White WL. Generalized pustular eruptions associated with oral terbinafine. Int J Dermatol 1999;38(8):596–600.

51. Rogalski C, Hurlimann A, Burg G, Wuthrich B, Kempf W. Arzneimittelreaktion auf Terbinafin unter dem bild einer akuten generalisierten exanthematischen pustulose (AGEP). [Drug reaction to terbinafine simulating acute generalized exanthematous pustulosis.] Hautarzt 2001;52(5):444–8.

52. Wilson NJ, Evans S. Severe pustular psoriasis provoked by oral terbinafine. Br J Dermatol 1998;139(1):168.

53. Pauluzzi P, Boccucci N. Inverse psoriasis induced by terbinafine. Acta Derm Venereol 1999;79(5):389.

54. Gupta AK, Lynde CW, Lauzon GJ, Mehlmauer MA, Braddock SW, Miller CA, Del Rosso JQ, Shear NH. Cutaneous adverse effects associated with terbinafine therapy: 10 case reports and a review of the literature. Br J Dermatol 1998;138(3):529–32.

55. Brooke R, Coulson IH, al-Dawoud A. Terbinafine-induced subacute cutaneous lupus erythematosus. Br J Dermatol 1998;139(6):1132–3.

56. Murphy M, Barnes L. Terbinafine-induced lupus erythematosus. Br J Dermatol 1998;138(4):708–9.

57. Holmes S, Kemmett D. Exacerbation of systemic lupus erythematosus induced by terbinafine. Br J Dermatol 1998;139(6):1133.

58. Weiss JM, Mockenhaupt M, Schopf E, Simon JC. Fixes Arzneimittelexanthem auf Terbinafin mit charakteristischen Verteilungsmuster eines Baboon–Syndroms. [Reproducible drug exanthema to terbinafine with characteristic distribution of baboon syndrome.] Hautarzt 2001;52(12):1104–6.

59. Richert B, Uhoda I, De la Brassinne M. Hair loss after terbinafine treatment. Br J Dermatol 2001;145(5):842.

60. van Puijenbroek EP, Egberts AC, Meyboom RH, Leufkens HG. Association between terbinafine and arthralgia, fever and urticaria: symptoms or syndrome? Pharmacoepidemiol Drug Saf 2001;10(2):135–42.

61. Schilling MK, Eichenberger M, Maurer CA, Sigurdsson G, Buchler MW. Ketoconazole and pulmonary failure after esophagectomy: a prospective clinical trial. Dis Esophagus 2001;14(1):37–40.

62. Bonsmann G, Schiller M, Luger TA, Stander S. Terbinafine-induced subacute cutaneous lupus erythematosus. J Am Acad Dermatol 2001;44(6):925–31.

63. Gupta AK, Porges AJ. Hypersensitivity syndrome reaction to oral terbinafine. Australas J Dermatol 1998;39(3):171–2.

64. Jahangir M, Hussain I, Ul Hasan M, Haroon TS. A double-blind, randomized, comparative trial of itraconazole versus terbinafine for 2 weeks in tinea capitis. Br J Dermatol 1998;139(4):672–4.

65. Filho ST, Cuce LC, Foss NT, Marques SA, Santamaria JR. Efficacy, safety and tolerability of terbinafine for tinea capitis in children: Brazilian multicentric study with daily oral tablets for 1, 2 and 4 weeks. J Eur Acad Dermatol Venereol 1998;11(2):141–6.

66. Koumantaki E, Kakourou T, Rallis E, Riga P, Georgalla S. Doubled dose of oral terbinafine is required for *Microsporum canis* tinea capitis. Pediatr Dermatol 2001;18(4):339–42.

67. Silm H, Karelson M. Terbinafine: efficacy and tolerability in young children with tinea capitis due to *Microsporum canis*. J Eur Acad Dermatol Venereol 2002;16(3):228–30.

68. Jensen JC. Pharmacokinetics of Lamisil in humans. J Dermatol Treat 1990;1(Suppl 2):15.

69. Trepanier EF, Nafziger AN, Amsden GW. Effect of terbinafine on theophylline pharmacokinetics in healthy volunteers. Antimicrob Agents Chemother 1998;42(3):695–7.

70. Madani S, Barilla D, Cramer J, Wang Y, Paul C. Effect of terbinafine on the pharmacokinetics and pharmacodynamics of desipramine in healthy volunteers identified as cytochrome P450 2D6 (CYP2D6) extensive metabolizers. J Clin Pharmacol 2002;42(11):1211–18.

71. Teitelbaum ML, Pearson VE. Imipramine toxicity and terbinafine. Am J Psychiatry 2001;158(12):2086.

72. van der Kuy PH, Hooymans PM. Nortriptyline intoxication induced by terbinafine. BMJ 1998;316(7129):441.

73. Van Der Kuy PH, Van Den Heuvel HA, Kempen RW, Vanmolkot LM. Pharmacokinetic interaction between nortriptyline and terbinafine. Ann Pharmacother 2002;36(11):1712–14.

74. Gupta AK, Ross GS. Interaction between terbinafine and warfarin. Dermatology 1998;196(2):266–7.

75. Warwick JA, Corrall RJ. Serious interaction between warfarin and oral terbinafine. BMJ 1998;316(7129):440.

76. Guerret M, Francheteau P, Hubert M. Evaluation of effects of terbinafine on single oral dose pharmacokinetics and anticoagulant actions of warfarin in healthy volunteers. Pharmacotherapy 1997;17(4):767–73.

77. Clarke MF, Boardman HS. Interaction between warfarin and oral terbinafine. Systematic review of interaction profile of warfarin is needed. BMJ 1998;317(7152):205–6.

78. Gantmacher J, Mills-Bomford J, Williams T. Interaction between warfarin and oral terbinafine. Manufacturer does not agree that interaction was with terbinafine. BMJ 1998;317(7152):205.

Terbutaline

See also Beta$_2$-adrenoceptor agonists

General Information

Terbutaline is a selective beta$_2$-adrenoceptor agonist, with a similar profile to salbutamol, and its adverse effects profile is similar to that of salbutamol at equivalent doses (SEDA-21, 186) (SEDA-22, 193).

Nebulized terbutaline 5 mg has been compared with injected adrenaline (0.01 ml/kg of 1:1000 adrenaline to a maximum of 0.3 ml) in children with acute asthma. Those who received adrenaline had a significantly higher rate of adverse effects, 47 versus 11% (SEDA-21, 186).

Organs and Systems

Respiratory

The possibility of paradoxical bronchospasm due to terbutaline must be taken into consideration (SEDA-8, 145).

Nervous system

With terbutaline, somnolence has been reported in some studies, and may be characteristic of this drug, apparently occurring in some 25% of patients (SEDA-8, 145).

Acute paraparesis occurred after an injection of terbutaline sulfate for premature labor in a 26-year-old woman (1).

Metabolism

The effect of terbutaline on glucose metabolism has been studied in six healthy, pregnant women, with normal glucose tolerance, between the 30th and 34th weeks of pregnancy (2). The women took either oral terbutaline 5 mg every 6 hours for 24 hours or no medication. The study was repeated after 1 week and each subject acted as her own control. With terbutaline fasting blood glucose increased in each subject, the mean rising from 4.6 to 5.2 mmol/l (82 to 94 mg/dl). Basal serum insulin increased significantly, from 18 to 27 µU/ml. Glucagon fell from a mean of 166 to 144 pg/ml. There was a 12% rise in basal hepatic glucose production. The glucose infusion rate to maintain euglycemia fell by 33% while subjects were taking oral terbutaline. Indirect calorimetry showed that terbutaline caused a significant increase in energy expenditure. Oxygen consumption increased by 9% (270 to 294 ml/minute) and basal caloric expenditure increased by 14% (from 1.32 to 1.5 kcal/minute). Thus, oral terbutaline given for 24 hours is associated with a significant reduction in peripheral insulin sensitivity and an increase in energy expenditure. Increases in basal hepatic glucose metabolism and a reduced ability of insulin to suppress hepatic glucose output are consistent with an effect of terbutaline on maternal hepatic glucose metabolism.

Second-Generation Effects

Pregnancy

In pregnant women with a history of migraine or vascular headache the use of terbutaline (and its congeners) should be avoided because of the risk of cerebral ischemia (SEDA-8, 145). One pregnant woman with asthma suffered a hypotensive episode after treatment with subcutaneous terbutaline (SEDA-12, 123).

A severe and life-threatening hypotensive reaction in patients with quadriplegia after terbutaline medication warrants a warning against indiscriminate use of beta-adrenoceptor agonists in the absence of autonomic spinal function (SEDA-8, 145).

Drug–Drug Interactions

Phenylephrine

Sweating, tachycardia, and headache have been reported when terbutaline was added to phenylephrine (SEDA-18, 16).

Toloxatone

Sweating, tachycardia, and headache have been reported when terbutaline was added to toloxatone (SEDA-18, 16).

References

1. Herskowitz A, Herskowitz B. Acute paraparesis due to terbutaline sulfate. South Med J 2002;95(2):275–6.
2. Smigaj D, Roman-Drago NM, Amini SB, Caritis SN, Kalhan SC, Catalano PM. The effect of oral terbutaline on maternal glucose metabolism and energy expenditure in pregnancy. Am J Obstet Gynecol 1998;178(5):1041–7.

Terfenadine

See also Antihistamines

General Information

Launched as a peripherally acting antihistamine with little sedative activity, terfenadine largely fulfilled this promise, but proved to have cardiotoxic properties, which led to restrictions on its use (SEDA-17, 196) (SEDA-18, 182) (SEDA-18, 186) (SEDA-19, 176) (SEDA-20, 163) (SEDA-21, 177) (SEDA-22, 179).

Inhibitors of CYP3A4 can lead to accumulation of unchanged terfenadine, causing prolongation of the QT interval and ventricular dysrhythmias. However, little is known about the effects of terfenadine on the pharmacokinetics of other drugs, even though it is known that terfenadine itself inhibits CYP3A4 activity in human liver microsomes. In view of its mode of metabolism, interactions with many other drugs are likely.

Organs and Systems

Cardiovascular

Terfenadine can cause prolongation of the QT interval in overdose or during interactions with drugs that inhibit its metabolism, such as erythromycin (1), ketoconazole (2), and grapefruit juice (3). Torsade de pointes can result (4).

Nervous system

Terfenadine has been investigated in several thousands of patients and found to have a sedation rate comparable to placebo (5). It has not been shown to impair driving performance (6).

Liver

There have been reports of cholestatic hepatitis induced by terfenadine (SEDA-21, 177), but quantitative information has been lacking on the risk of acute liver disease among users of this drug. In a population-based cohort study using general practice data in the UK carried out by the Boston Collaborative Drug Surveillance Program, a causal connection to terfenadine could not be ruled out in only three cases of acute liver disease among 210 683 recipients (7). However, the three individuals were also taking other drugs known to cause liver toxicity.

Skin

Terfenadine has been reported to cause skin reactions, notably urticaria and rashes in a number of cases (SEDA-11, 148) (SEDA-13, 132). A photoallergic reaction to terfenadine has also been reported (SEDA-12, 143), and so have severe exacerbations of psoriasis (SEDA-14, 137).

Stevens–Johnson syndrome has been reported both with terfenadine (SEDA-21, 177).

Drug–Drug Interactions

Atorvastatin

Terfenadine is normally metabolized by CYP3A4 to fexofenadine, which has negligible cardiac effects. Atorvastatin is also a CYP3A4 substrate, and its effects on the pharmacokinetics of terfenadine have been studied in healthy volunteers who took atorvastatin 80 mg/day from 7 days before to 2 days after terfenadine 120 mg (8). Concentrations of terfenadine and fexofenadine were measured for 72 hours. There were no alterations in the pharmacokinetics of the parent compound or of its metabolite and there were no alterations in QT_c intervals after terfenadine alone or with atorvastatin.

Buspirone

Ten healthy volunteers took oral terfenadine 120 mg/day for 3 days and then took buspirone 10 mg; terfenadine had no significant effects on the pharmacokinetics of buspirone (9).

Erythromycin

Torsade de pointes has been reported in patients taking erythromycin and terfenadine (1).

Grapefruit juice

Grapefruit juice substantially increased the AUC and C_{max} of terfenadine (3).

Ketoconazole

Terfenadine can cause prolongation of the QT interval in overdose or during interactions with drugs that inhibit its metabolism, such as ketoconazole.

- Torsade de pointes occurred in a patient who was taking the recommended prescribed dose of terfenadine in addition to cefaclor, ketoconazole, and medroxyprogesterone (2). Measured serum concentrations of terfenadine and its main metabolite showed excessive levels of parent terfenadine and proportionately reduced concentrations of its metabolite, suggesting inhibition of terfenadine metabolism.

Nefazodone

Nefazodone is a phenylpiperazine antidepressant that is predominantly metabolized by CYP3A. In a randomized, double-blind, double-dummy, parallel-group, multiple-dose study in healthy men and women who were given terfenadine 60 mg every 12 hours or nefazodone 300 mg every 12 hours, the plasma concentrations of terfenadine were significantly increased by co-administration of nefazodone (10). The mean QT_c interval was unchanged by terfenadine alone, but was markedly prolonged with co-administration of nefazodone, and the extent of prolongation correlated with the plasma terfenadine concentration.

Norfluoxetine

A possible interaction with norfluoxetine, a metabolite of fluoxetine, has been reported (SEDA-20, 164).

Sertindole

Sertindole 30 mg/day had no effects on the pharmacokinetics of a single dose of terfenadine 120 mg or of its metabolite (11). The authors concluded that sertindole at this dose does not inhibit the metabolism of terfenadine.

Sparfloxacin

The effect of the concomitant administration of terfenadine and sparfloxacin on the QT_C interval has been studied in healthy men aged 18–49 years (12). Sparfloxacin was given in a dose of 400 mg on the first day and 200 mg/day thereafter for 3 days with terfenadine 60 mg bd. Terfenadine had no effect on the pharmacokinetics of sparfloxacin and there were no apparent effects on the QT_C interval.

Venlafaxine

Drugs used in the treatment of depression and psychosis can alter the metabolism of terfenadine. When the antidepressant venlafaxine was given to steady state (37.5 mg bd for 3 days and then 75 mg bd for 5 days), the pharmacokinetics of a single dose of terfenadine 120 mg were not altered and there were no changes in the electrocardiogram (13). The authors concluded that cardiotoxicity is unlikely to arise with co-administration of terfenadine and venlafaxine.

References

1. Paris DG, Parente TF, Bruschetta HR, Guzman E, Niarchos AP. Torsades de pointes induced by erythromycin and terfenadine. Am J Emerg Med 1994;12(6):636–8.
2. Monahan BP, Ferguson CL, Killeavy ES, Lloyd BK, Troy J, Cantilena LR Jr. Torsades de pointes occurring in association with terfenadine use. JAMA 1990;264(21):2788–90.
3. Clifford CP, Adams DA, Murray S, Taylor GW, Wilkins MR, Boobis AR, Davies DS. The cardiac effects of terfenadine after inhibition of its metabolism by grapefruit juice. Eur J Clin Pharmacol 1997;52(4):311–15.
4. Mathews DR, McNutt B, Okerholm R, Flicker M, McBride G. Torsades de pointes occurring in association with terfenadine use. JAMA 1991;266(17):2375–6.
5. McTavish D, Goa KL, Ferrill M. Terfenadine. An updated review of its pharmacological properties and therapeutic efficacy. Drugs 1990;39(4):552–74.
6. Nicholson AN. Antihistaminic activity and central effects of terfenadine. A review of European studies. Arzneimittelforschung 1982;32(9a):1191–3.
7. Myers MW, Jick H. Terfenadine and risk of acute liver disease. Br J Clin Pharmacol 1998;46(3):251–3.
8. Stern RH, Smithers JA, Olson SC. Atorvastatin does not produce a clinically significant effect on the pharmacokinetics of terfenadine. J Clin Pharmacol 1998;38(8):753–7.
9. Lamberg TS, Kivisto KT, Neuvonen PJ. Lack of effect of terfenadine on the pharmacokinetics of the CYP3A4 substrate buspirone. Pharmacol Toxicol 1999;84(4):165–9.
10. Abernethy DR, Barbey JT, Franc J, Brown KS, Feirrera I, Ford N, Salazar DE. Loratadine and terfenadine interaction with nefazodone: Both antihistamines are associated with QTc prolongation. Clin Pharmacol Ther 2001;69(3):96–103.
11. Wong SL, Cao G, Mack R, Granneman GR. Lack of CYP3A inhibition effects of sertindole on terfenadine in healthy volunteers. Int J Clin Pharmacol Ther 1998;36(3):146–51.
12. Morganroth J, Hunt T, Dorr MB, Magner D, Talbot GH. The effect of terfenadine on the cardiac pharmacodynamics of sparfloxacin. Clin Ther 1999;21(9):1514–24.
13. Amchin J, Zarycranski W, Taylor KP, Albano D, Klockowski PM. Effect of venlafaxine on the pharmacokinetics of terfenadine. Psychopharmacol Bull 1998;34(3):383–9.

Terguride

General Information

Terguride is an ergot derivative, a partial dopamine agonist with properties similar to those of bromocriptine. It has been used in the treatment of Parkinson's disease and hyperprolactinaemia.

In 21 patients with parkinsonism, terguride 0.25–0.5 mg caused improvement for periods of up to 6 hours, although eight of 21 subjects showed no improvement or deterioration with doses of 0.5–1.0 mg (1). In three patients the addition of terguride 0.75 mg/day for 5–10 days did not affect levodopa-induced psychosis. In three patients with levodopa-induced dyskinesias, the addition of terguride 0.75 mg/day for 14 days resulted in a slight increase in the severity of the involuntary movements. The adverse effects of terguride, nausea and hypotension, were similar to those of levodopa. Terguride caused prolonged inhibition of prolactin release, but unlike levodopa did not increase plasma growth hormone concentrations. Additionally, terguride caused considerable sedation. These results may have been due to the combined effects of terguride on both non-dopamine and dopamine neurotransmitter systems, rather than to partial or incomplete dopamine agonist effects.

In 32 women with ovarian dysfunction due to hyperprolactinemia treated with terguride for 2–33 months, increased prolactin concentrations were successfully normalized in 21 (2). Regular periods reappeared in 14, 13 became pregnant, 7 gave birth to healthy babies, and 2 aborted in the first trimester. Galactorrhea disappeared in 18 patients and was markedly inhibited in the others. There were adverse effects in 11 of the patients. They were mostly mild and included in most cases nausea, headache, and stomachache. The complaints were transient and abated after prolonged treatment.

References

1. Critchley P, Parkes D. Transdihydrolisuride in parkinsonism. Clin Neuropharmacol 1987;10(1):57–64.
2. Vetr M, Talas M, Pohanka J, Gazarek F, Fingerova H. Terguride in the treatment of hyperprolactinemia. Acta Univ Palacki Olomuc Fac Med 1990;125:155–60.

Terodiline

See also Anticholinergic drugs

General Information

Terodiline, an anticholinergic drug that was originally used for urinary incontinence (1), but was withdrawn in most countries in 1991 because of multiple reports of drug-related cardiac dysrhythmias (SEDA-17, 174).

Organs and Systems

Cardiovascular

A retrospective analysis of data from 19 patients has shown that the effect of terodiline on the QT interval is dose-related. The authors commented that terodiline has structural similarities to prenylamine, an antianginal drug that was previously shown to have prodysrhythmic properties, so that such problems should really not have been unexpected (SEDA-20, 147).

Reference

1. Langtry HD, McTavish D. Terodiline. A review of its pharmacological properties, and therapeutic use in the treatment of urinary incontinence. Drugs 1990;40(5):745–61.

Tetanus toxoid

See also Vaccines

General Information

Tetanus toxoid is prepared from *Clostridium tetani* and can be given either in a fluid form (plain) or an adsorbed form. The slight local reactions that tend to occur (induration, erythema, tenderness) are more common with the adsorbed type. Intramuscular injection of tetanus toxoid

is generally the route of choice, and the vaccine is best injected into a large muscle.

General adverse effects

Data on adverse events after tetanus immunization have been collected by Behringwerke, Germany (SED-12, 826) and in the framework of the US Monitoring System for Adverse Events Following Immunization (MSAEFI) (SEDA-13, 274). Some figures for particular types of complication are cited below.

Isolated reports of adverse effects have included: abscess formation (SEDA-11, 288); dermatomyositis, neuralgic amyotrophy, polyradiculoneuritis with paresis of the urinary bladder and bowel (SEDA-9, 283); asymmetrical polyneuropathy, demyelinating polyneuropathy, and Guillain–Barré syndrome (SEDA-14, 281); and subcutaneous nodules. Polyvinylpyrrolidone thesaurismosis, revealed by inflammatory manifestations after tetanus booster injection, has also been reported (SEDA-10, 288).

Combined diphtheria + tetanus + pertussis vaccination

An overview of clinical trials with a special diphtheria and tetanus toxoids and acellular pertussis (DTaP) vaccine has been published (1). The vaccine contains as pertussis components purified filamentous hemagglutinin, pertactin, and genetically engineered pertussis toxin. The vaccine induces high and long-lasting immunity and is at least as efficacious as most whole-cell pertussis vaccines and similar in efficacy to the most efficacious acellular pertussis vaccines that contain three pertussis antigens. The vaccine is better tolerated than whole cell vaccines and has a similar reactogenicity profile to other acellular vaccines.

A vaccine containing diphtheria and tetanus toxoids and acellular pertussis with reduced antigen content for diphtheria and pertussis (TdaP) has been compared with a licensed reduced adult-type diphtheria–tetanus (Td) vaccine and with an experimental candidate monovalent acellular pertussis vaccine with reduced antigen content (ap) (2). A total of 299 healthy adults (mean age 30 years) were randomized into three groups to receive one dose of the study vaccines. The antibody responses (anti-diphtheria, anti-tetanus, anti-pertussis toxin, anti-pertactin, anti-filamentous hemagglutinin) were similar in all groups. The most frequently reported local symptom was pain at the injection site (62–94%), but there were no reports of severe pain; redness and swelling with a diameter of 5 cm or more occurred in up to 13%. The incidence of local symptoms was similar after TdaP and Td immunization. The most frequently reported general symptoms were headache and fatigue (20–50%). The incidence of general symptoms was similar in the TdaP and Td groups. There were no reports of fever over 39°C. No serious adverse events were reported.

Data from the Third National Health and Nutrition Survey (1988–94) have been used to analyse the possible effects of DTP or tetanus immunization on allergies and allergy-related symptoms among 13 944 infants, children, and adolescents aged 2 months to 16 years in the USA (3). The authors concluded that DTP or tetanus immunization increases the risk of allergies and related respiratory symptoms in children and adolescents. However, the small number of non-immunized individuals and the study design limited their ability to make firm causal inferences about the true magnitude of effect.

Tetravalent, pentavalent, and hexavalent immunization

DTaP or DTwP vaccine can be combined with other antigens, such as *Haemophilus influenzae* type b (Hib), inactivated poliovirus (IPV), and hepatitis B vaccine. In children DTaP or DTwP vaccines are the basis for such combinations, while in adults it is mostly Td vaccine, Current safety concerns regarding combination vaccines have been defined and reviewed (4). The author concluded that there is no evidence that adding vaccines to combination products increases the burden on the immune system, which can respond to many millions of antigens. Combining antigens usually does not increase adverse effects, but it can lead to an overall reduction in adverse events. Before licensure, combination vaccines undergo extensive testing to assure that the new products are safe and effective.

The frequency, severity, and types of adverse reactions after DTP-Hib immunization in very preterm babies have been studied (5). Adverse reactions were noted in 17 of 45 babies: nine had major events (apnea, bradycardia, or desaturation) and eight had minor reactions (increased oxygen requirements, temperature instability, poor handling, and feeding intolerance). Babies who had major adverse reactions were significantly younger at the time of immunization than the babies who did not have major reactions. Of 27 babies immunized at 70 days or less, 9 developed major reactions compared with none of those who were immunized at over 70 days.

The Hexavalent Study Group has compared the immunogenicity and safety of a new liquid hexavalent vaccine against diphtheria, tetanus, pertussis, poliomyelitis, hepatitis B and *H. influenzae* type b (DTP + IPV + HB + Hib vaccine, manufactured by Aventis Pasteur MSD, Lyon, France) with two reference vaccines, the pentavalent DTP + IPV + Hib vaccine and the monovalent hepatitis B vaccine, administrated separately at the same visit (6). Infants were randomized to receive either the hexavalent vaccine ($n = 423$) or (administered at different local sites) the pentavalent and the HB vaccine ($n = 425$) at 2, 4, and 6 months of age. The hexavalent vaccine was well tolerated (for details see the monograph on Pertussis vaccines). At least one local reaction was reported in 20% of injections with hexavalent vaccine compared with 16% after the receipt of pentavalent vaccine or 3.8% after the receipt of hepatitis B vaccine. These reactions were generally mild and transient. At least one systemic reaction was reported in 46% of injections with hexavalent vaccine, whereas the respective rate for the recipients of pentavalent and HB vaccine was 42%. No vaccine-related serious adverse event occurred during the study. The hexavalent vaccine provided immune responses adequate for protection against the six diseases.

Organs and Systems

Cardiovascular

Myopericarditis has been attributed to Td-IPV vaccine (7).

- A 31-year-old man developed arthralgia and chest pain 2 days after Td-IPV immunization and had an acute myopericarditis. He recovered within a few days with high-dose aspirin.

The authors discussed two possible causal mechanisms, natural infection or an immune complex-mediated mechanism. Infection was excluded by negative bacterial and viral serology and a favorable outcome occurred within a few days without antimicrobial treatment.

Nervous system

Reports of neurological adverse effects after tetanus immunization have appeared (8). The most common reported complication is a polyneuropathy. In the majority of cases the onset occurred within 14 days of the last injection, and ranged in severity from a single nerve palsy to profound sensorimotor involvement of the nervous system, including cord and cortex. Recovery was usually complete (eight of 10 patients with onset at less than 14 days after injection) but three patients with onset at more than 14 days from injection had only partial recovery.

Mononeuritis and polyneuritis after tetanus immunization during 1970 and 1977 have been reviewed (9). The frequency of this adverse effect was 0.4 per one million distributed vaccine doses.

Sensory systems

Optic neuritis has been attributed to Td-IPV vaccine (10).

- Ten days after receiving Td-IPV vaccine a 56-year-old woman developed acute unilateral optic neuritis. Complete remission occurred within 6 weeks of prednisolone treatment. No other causes were found.

Skin

Bullous pemphigoid has been attributed to DTP-IPV vaccine (11).

- A previous healthy 3.5-month-old infant developed bullous pemphigoid 3 days after receiving a first dose of DTP-IPV vaccine. *Staphylococcus aureus* was isolated from purulent bullae. The lesions resolved rapidly after treatment with antibiotics and methylprednisolone.

The authors mentioned 12 other cases of bullous pemphigoid, reported during the last 5 years, that had possibly been triggered by vaccines (influenza, tetanus toxoid booster, and DTP-IPV vaccine).

- About 2 weeks after receiving a second dose of adsorbed tetanus toxoid a 50-year-old woman developed generalized morphea, a rare condition, in which multiple patches of skin sclerosis occur over much larger areas than in the localized variant. The patient denied taking any drugs. After prednisone therapy, a month later the lesions had dramatically improved (12).

The cause of this condition is unknown, but an autoimmune mechanism triggered by endogenous and exogenous factors has been suggested.

Immunologic

Allergic reactions to reinforcing doses of tetanus toxoid have been described by different investigators (SEDA-8, 300) (SEDA-11, 288). The association between high titers of antitoxin produced by active immunization and reactions is well established (13,14). Booster doses of tetanus toxoid are being given with unnecessary and indeed excessive frequency. Continuing to do this will produce a more highly toxoid-sensitive population without adding significantly to the already high protection that this immunized population has against tetanus. It is therefore recommended that routine boosters in individuals known to have had primary immunization including a reinforcing dose be given only at 10-year intervals, and that emergency boosters be given no less than 1 year apart (15). Allergic reactions may be due to an allergy to the toxoid or the proteins of *C. tetani* that co-purify with toxoid during the precipitation process used in its conventional preparation (16).

Susceptibility Factors

Age

In children aged 15–16 years receiving routine reinforcement tetanus immunization, adsorbed vaccine caused more intense and more frequent local reactions than did plain tetanus toxoid, and a higher incidence of pyrexia. The incidence of swelling and erythema at the inoculation site increased with serum antitoxin titre at the time of administration, whereas pain and tenderness were related to the presence of the aluminium hydroxide adjuvant (17). Based on similar experiences it has been widely recommended that plain and not adsorbed tetanus toxoid should be used when reinforcement of immunity to tetanus alone is desired.

Other features of the patient

The only contraindication to tetanus toxoid is a history of a severe allergic or neurological reaction after a previous dose. AIDS and HIV infections are not contraindications. Data on the immune response to tetanus in children with AIDS showed defective responses (18).

References

1. Matheson AJ, Goa KL. Diphtheria–tetanus–acellular pertussis vaccine adsorbed (Triacelluvax; DTaP3-CB): a review of its use in the prevention of Bordetella pertussis infection. Paediatr Drugs 2000;2(2):139–59.
2. Van der Wielen M, Van Damme P. Tetanus–diphtheria booster in non-responding tetanus–diphtheria vaccines. Vaccine 2000;19(9–10):1005–6.
3. Hurwitz EL, Morgenstern H. Effects of diphtheria–tetanus–pertussis or tetanus vaccination on allergies and allergy-related respiratory symptoms among children and adolescents in the United States. J Manipulative Physiol Ther 2000;23(2):81–90.
4. Halsey NA. Combination vaccines: defining and addressing current safety concerns. Clin Infect Dis 2001;33(Suppl 4):S312–18.
5. Sen S, Cloete Y, Hassan K, Buss P. Adverse events following vaccination in premature infants. Acta Paediatr 2001;90(8):916–20.
6. Mallet E, Fabre P, Pines E, Salomon H, Staub T, Schodel F, Mendelman P, Hessel L, Chryssomalis G, Vidor E, Hoffenbach A, Abeille A, Amar R, Arsene JP, Aurand JM, Azoulay L, Badescou E, Barrois S, Baudino N, Beal M, Beaude-Chervet V, Berlier P, Billard E, Billet L, Blanc B, Blanc JP, Bohu D, Bonardo C, Bossu C; Hexavalent Vaccine Trial Study Group. Immunogenicity and safety of a new liquid hexavalent combined vaccine compared with separate administration of reference licensed vaccines in infants. Pediatr Infect Dis J 2000;19(12):1119–27.
7. Boccara F, Benhaiem-Sigaux N, Cohen A. Acute myopericarditis after diphtheria, tetanus, and polio vaccination. Chest 2001;120(2):671–2.
8. Rutledge SL, Snead OC 3rd. Neurologic complications of immunizations. J Pediatr 1986;109(6):917–24.
9. Quast U, Hennessen W, Widmark RM. Mono- and polyneuritis after tetanus vaccination (1970–1977). Dev Biol Stand 1979;43:25–32.
10. Burkhard C, Choi M, Wilhelm H. Optikusneuritis als Komplikaton einer Tetanus–Diphtherie–Poliomyelitis–Schutzimpfung: ein Fallbericht. [Optic neuritis as a complication in preventive tetanus–diphtheria–poliomyelitis vaccination. a case report.] Klin Monatsbl Augenheilkd 2001;218(1):51–4.
11. Baykal C, Okan G, Sarica R. Childhood bullous pemphigoid developed after the first vaccination. J Am Acad Dermatol 2001;44(Suppl 2):348–50.
12. Drago F, Rampini P, Lugani C, Rebora A. Generalized morphoea after antitetanus vaccination. Clin Exp Dermatol 1998;23(3):142.
13. Levine L, Ipsen J Jr., McComb JA. Adult immunization. Preparation and evaluation of combined fluid tetanus and diphtheria toxoids for adult use. Am J Hyg 1961;73:20–35.
14. Relihan M. Reactions to tetanus toxoid. J Ir Med Assoc 1969;62(390):430–4.
15. Edsall G, Elliott MW, Peebles TC, Eldred MC. Excessive use of tetanus toxoid boosters. JAMA 1967;202(1):111–13.
16. Leen CL, Barclay GR, McClelland DB, Shepherd WM, Langford DT. Double-blind comparative trial of standard (commercial) and antibody-affinity-purified tetanus toxoid vaccines. J Infect 1987;14(2):119–24.
17. Collier LH, Polakoff S, Mortimer J. Reactions and antibody responses to reinforcing doses of adsorbed and plain tetanus vaccines. Lancet 1979;1(8131):1364–8.
18. Chen RT, Spira TJ. Tetanus prophylaxis in AIDS patients. JAMA 1986;255:1063.

Tetracaine

See also Local anesthetics

General Information

Tetracaine is a highly lipid-soluble, potent aminoester. It is primarily used as a constituent of many different topical formulations and for spinal anesthesia. It is four times as potent as lidocaine, and unless great caution is taken in dosage, serious systemic adverse effects can develop, owing to rapid absorption after topical use (for example in a 0.5% gargle) (1) or use in endoscopy. It is more effective than Emla in reducing the pain of venous cannulation in children.

Tetracaine can cause local reactions when applied to the skin, but because it is rapidly metabolized by plasma cholinesterase systemic reactions are unlikely (2).

Organs and Systems

Cardiovascular

- An 18-month-old child undergoing cardiac surgery developed discoloration of the hand, consistent with severe bruising, after application of 4% tetracaine gel, which was inadvertently left under an occlusive dressing for about 24 hours (3). There were no long-term sequelae and no treatment was required.

The authors blamed a combination of the vasodilatory properties of tetracaine and the fact that the child was heparinized for surgery, causing capillary leak at the area of application.

Hematologic

Adult cases of methemoglobinemia have been reported with Cetacaine (a proprietary mixture of 14% benzocaine, 2% tetracaine, and 2% butylaminobenzoate) (4–6).

Cetacaine spray used to anesthetize the oropharynx before endoscopy led to dyspnea, central cyanosis, and an oxygen saturation of 80%; methemoglobinemia was diagnosed, and the patient recovered rapidly with methylthioninium chloride 1 mg/kg over 5 minutes.

- A 77-year-old woman received two sprays of Cetacaine for an attempted emergency nasotracheal intubation. After intubation, she became cyanosed. The arterial blood was chocolate brown and the SaO_2 by CO oximetry was 54–58%, despite a high PaO_2. The methemoglobin concentration was 39% and she was treated with methylthioninium chloride. Three weeks later, Cetacaine again caused cyanosis with a drop in SpO_2 to 76% and a methemoglobin concentration of 24%, which resolved spontaneously.
- A 74-year-old man received Cetacaine spray to his oropharynx for transesophageal echocardiography. His SpO_2 fell to 85%, he became drowsy, then unresponsive, cyanotic, and apneic, and required intubation. His PaO_2 was 37 kPa (280 mmHg), SaO_2 40%, and methemoglobin concentration 60%. Intravenous methylthioninium chloride produced an immediate improvement in the cyanosis and the methemoglobin concentration fell to 0.6%.

Skin

Reported local adverse effects of tetracaine include itch and a high incidence of erythema as a consequence of vasodilatation, which may actually be an advantage. There was no evidence of dermatitis (SEDA-20, 127) (7).

In 272 children who required topical local anesthesia for venepuncture, there was no association between the duration of application of 4% tetracaine gel and the development of adverse skin reactions (8). However,

two reports discussed by the same authors highlighted rare adverse reactions.

- A 4-year-old child with no previous exposure complained of severe pain, erythema, and blistering 5 minutes after the application of 4% tetracaine gel.
- An anesthetist who was suspected of occupational exposure developed redness and blistering after applying a test dose of tetracaine.

The authors recommended minimizing occupational contact and quickly removing the cream in patients who report pain after application of tetracaine.

There may be a higher incidence of skin sensitization from tetracaine gel than Emla. At one hospital, in a 3-month period, there were seven site reactions to tetracaine (9). While the Summary of Product Characteristics says that significant skin reactions are rare, the authors estimated that seven reactions in their hospital represented a higher rate than 0.01–0.1% (usually regarded as the frequency of rare events). Indeed, the reported incidence of moderate to severe local skin reactions in clinical trials is 0.6–8.8%, compared with 0–1.7% with Emla. According to the Summary of Product Characteristics there is also a risk of sensitization with repeated exposure (four of the seven children who had reactions to tetracaine had had prior exposure to it), which is not known to happen with Emla.

Immunologic

Anaphylactic shock has been reported after spinal anesthesia (SED-12, 257) (10).

References

1. Patel D, Chopra S, Berman MD. Serious systemic toxicity resulting from use of tetracaine for pharyngeal anesthesia in upper endoscopic procedures. Dig Dis Sci 1989;34(6):882–4.
2. Geraint M. Check long contact with Ametop. Pharm Pract 1998;8:208
3. Hewitt T, Eadon H. Check long contact with Ametop. Pharm Pract 1998;8:47–8.
4. Maher P. Methemoglobinemia: an unusual complication of topical anesthesia. Gastroenterol Nurs 1998;21(4):173–5.
5. Khan NA, Kruse JA. Methemoglobinemia induced by topical anesthesia: a case report and review. Am J Med Sci 1999;318(6):415–18.
6. Stoiber TR. Toxic methemoglobinemia complicating transesophageal echocardiography. Echocardiography 1999;16(4):383–5.
7. Lawson RA, Smart NG, Gudgeon AC, Morton NS. Evaluation of an amethocaine gel preparation for percutaneous analgesia before venous cannulation in children. Br J Anaesth 1995;75(3):282–5.
8. Wongprasartsuk P, Main BJ. Adverse local reactions to amethocaine cream—audit and case reports. Anaesth Intensive Care 1998;26(3):312–14.
9. Clarkson A, Choonara I, O'Donnell K. Localized adverse skin reactions to topical anaesthetics. Paediatr Anaesth 1999;9(6):553–5.
10. Moriwaki K, Higaki A, Sasaki H, Murata K, Sumida T, Baba I. [A case report of anaphylactic shock induced by tetracaine used for spinal anesthesia.] Masui;35(8):1279–84.

Tetrachloroethylene

General Information

Tetrachloroethylene is a chlorinated derivative of a simple hydrocarbon, $H_2C{=}CH_2$, in which each of the four hydrogen atoms is replaced by chlorine, $Cl_2C{=}CCl_2$. It is a heavy liquid that has been used to treat hookworm infection. It is given orally in a dose of 0.1 ml/kg up to a maximum of 5 ml as a single dose on an empty stomach. Usually formulated as capsules or emulsion, it is unstable, especially if exposed to light. Concurrent *Ascaris* infection should be treated first to avoid migration of worms and the risk of peritonitis.

General adverse effects

The adverse effects of tetrachloroethylene are similar to those of carbon tetrachloride (CCl_4), but less severe. Tetrachloroethylene is hepatotoxic and neurotoxic, but gastrointestinal disturbance is the only common adverse effect when it is used carefully. There is some risk of addiction to the inhaled vapor: inhalation can result in vascular reactions, loss of consciousness, pulmonary edema, and fatal hepatic and renal damage. Alcohol and fatty foods increase absorption and hepatic toxicity. Exposure to tetrachloroethylene has been known to lead to vinyl chloride disease. Allergic reactions have not been reported.

It is highly unlikely that single-dose use of tetrachloroethylene could have a tumorigenic effect; however, animal studies conducted in connection with exposure to tetrachloroethylene in the course of industrial use showed an increased occurrence of liver tumors.

Organs and Systems

Cardiovascular

In cases of poisoning with tetrachloroethylene, hypotension can occur; sympathomimetic drugs should not be used to treat it, since ventricular fibrillation can be precipitated.

Respiratory

Hypersensitivity pneumonitis has been attributed to occupational exposure to tetrachloroethylene in a 42-year-old dry cleaner; the diagnosis was confirmed by lung biopsy (1).

Nervous system

Headache and vertigo are common with tetrachloroethylene (2,3). Patients should remain at rest for 3 hours after administration and take only water.

Inhalation of tetrachloroethylene vapor can cause stupor (4).

Psychological, psychiatric

Reversible neuropsychiatric symptoms, readily resembling alcoholic intoxication, have occurred after a single dose of 5 ml. Sleep apnea causing neuropsychiatric abnormalities has been attributed to exposure to high concentrations of tetrachloroethylene and *N*-butanol vapors; however, the patient was obese and the association with the solvents was not clear (5).

Gastrointestinal

Nausea, vomiting, colicky abdominal pain, and diarrhea are common with tetrachloroethylene (2).

Liver

Hepatotoxicity from tetrachloroethylene is similar to that caused by carbon tetrachloride and can occur after oral treatment or even inhalation of the vapor (6).

Urinary tract

Tetrachloroethylene can cause renal damage, especially after inhalation (7).

Skin

If tetrachloroethylene comes into contact with the skin, either directly or after vomiting, burn-like reactions can occur (8).

Erythema multiforme has followed oral administration of tetrachloroethylene (9).

Second-Generation Effects

Pregnancy

It is unwise to use tetrachloroethylene in pregnancy in view of its potential for hepatotoxicity, but there is no specific information on the risks to the fetus as a result of therapeutic use; however, work relating to industrial use (exposure of women in the dry-cleaning industry) suggests the need for caution (10).

Susceptibility Factors

Age

It is dangerous to use tetrachloroethylene in young children (11).

References

1. Tanios MA, El Gamal H, Rosenberg BJ, Hassoun PM. Can we still miss tetrachloroethylene-induced lung disease? The emperor returns in new clothes. Respiration 2004;71(6):642–5.
2. Ng TP, Tsin TW, O'Kelly FJ. An outbreak of illness after occupational exposure to ozone and acid chlorides. Br J Ind Med 1985;42(10):686–90.
3. Sorensen S, Melgaard B. Treatment of hookworm anemia. Scand J Infect Dis 1971;3(1):65–9.
4. Lackore LK, Perkins HM. Accidental narcosis. Contamination of compressed air system. JAMA 1970;211(11):1846.
5. Muttray A, Randerath W, Ruhle KH, Gajsar H, Gerhardt P, Greulich W, Konietzko J. Obstruktives Schlafapnoesyndrom durch eine berufliche Losungsmittelexposition. [Obstructive sleep apnea syndrome caused by occupational exposure to solvents.] Dtsch Med Wochenschr 1999;124(10):279–81.

6. Brautbar N, Williams J 2nd. Industrial solvents and liver toxicity: risk assessment, risk factors and mechanisms. Int J Hyg Environ Health 2002;205(6):479–91.

7. Salahudeen AK. Perchloroethylene-induced nephrotoxicity in dry-cleaning workers: is there a role for free radicals? Nephrol Dial Transplant 1998;13(5):1122–4.

8. Hake CL, Stewart RD. Human exposure to tetrachloroethylene: inhalation and skin contact. Environ Health Perspect 1977;21:231–8.

9. Hisanaga N, Jonai H, Yu X, Ogawa Y, Mori I, Kamijima M, Ichihara G, Shibata E, Takeuchi Y. [Stevens–Johnson syndrome accompanied by acute hepatitis in workers exposed to trichloroethylene or tetrachloroethylene.] Sangyo Eiseigaku Zasshi 2002;44(2):33–49.

10. Ahlborg G Jr. Pregnancy outcome among women working in laundries and dry-cleaning shops using tetrachloroethylene. Am J Ind Med 1990;17(5):567–75.

11. Balmer S, Howells G, Wharton B. The effects of tetrachlorethylene in children with kwashiorkor and hookworm infestation. J Trop Pediatr 1970;16(1):20–3.

Tetracyclines

See also Individual agents

General Information

The tetracyclines are a closely related group of antibiotics with comparable pharmacological properties but different pharmacokinetic characteristics. They have both the advantages and disadvantages of broad-spectrum antibiotics. Tetracyclines are effective not only against bacteria and spirochetes, but also against some forms of *Mycoplasma*, *Chlamydia*, and *Rickettsia*, as well as protozoa. They affect multiplying microorganisms by inhibiting ribosomal protein synthesis. Their effect is therefore primarily bacteriostatic rather than bactericidal, depending on the kind of microorganism.

Most of the adverse effects of the tetracyclines depend on the concentration of the antibiotic in the affected organ. The more lipophilic drugs are more potent with regard to their bacteriostatic efficacy and hence usually require daily doses below 1 g.

Use in non-infective conditions

Tetracyclines have many effects on non-infective inflammatory processes (SEDA-24, 278). They have been tried, and claimed to be of some value, in the treatment of rheumatoid arthritis, periodontal disease, myocardial infections, gastric disorders, and experimentally in the treatment of cancers. In all of these disorders, the proposed mechanisms for effects are on the host rather than the microbial side.

Tetracyclines have many effects on cells involved in inflammatory reactions, including inhibition of neutrophilic functions, such as migration, phagocytosis, degranulation, and the production of free oxygen radical (1). Most of these effects are supposed to be due to chelation of divalent ions and can be partly reversed by the addition of calcium ions or zinc ions. Their ability to inhibit synthesis

of mitochondrial proteins may be the background for their effects on lymphocytes, such as inhibition of lymphocyte proliferation in response to mitogens, inhibition of interferon gamma production, and inhibition of immunoglobulin production. Enzyme inactivation caused by tetracyclines has been studied in several models. Tetracyclines inhibited gingival collagenolytic activity in diabetic mice and in humans with periodontal disease (2). Subsequent studies showed that tetracyclines inactivated collagenases found in several places in the body (3,4). Most probably, the inhibitory effects of tetracyclines on collagenases are exerted through inactivation of metalloproteases, rather than serine proteases. Tetracycline also has radical-scavenging properties, which may be partly related to the ulcer-healing effect observed in a rat model of gastric mucosal injury (5).

As is to be expected, modified cycline molecules devoid of antibacterial effects are as effective as non-modified molecules. New derivatives with refined anti-inflammatory and enzyme inhibitory (and reduced antimicrobial) effects are being studied in experimental laboratories (6).

Tetracyclines and metalloproteinases

A major target for non-infective indications of the tetracyclines is inhibition of metalloproteinases. The following is a brief summary of what is known about tetracyclines and metalloproteinases, followed by some comments about possible adverse effects.

The matrix metalloproteinases (MMPs) are a family of calcium- and/or zinc-dependent endopeptidases involved in degradation of extracellular matrix and tissue remodelling (7). At least 21 mammalian MMPs have been described. They participate in various biological processes, such as embryonic development, ovulation, angiogenesis, apoptosis, wound healing, and nerve growth.

Under normal conditions, the activity of MMPs is very low and is strongly regulated by natural tissue inhibitors (TIMPs). The TIMPS are a family of four structurally related proteins (TIMP-1, 2, 3, and 4), exerting dual control of the MMPs by inhibiting both their active forms and their activation. In addition, the proteolytic activity of MMPs is inhibited by non-specific protease inhibitors, such as alpha$_2$-macroglobulin and alpha$_1$-antiprotease.

In the presence of specific stimuli, exemplified by cytokines and growth factors, MMPs can be up-regulated. Chronic activation of MMPs, due to an imbalance between the activity of MMPs and TIMPs, can result in excessive degradation of the extracellular matrix and is believed to contribute to the pathogenesis of several diseases, such as rheumatoid arthritis, osteoarthritis, periodontal disease, emphysema, atherosclerosis, skin ulceration, and cancer.

The physiological and pathophysiological roles of MMPs and TIMPs have been extensively studied in knockout mice (7). For most of the MMPs and TIMPs there seem to be significant overlaps in functions, and a deficiency of one enzyme can be compensated for by the presence of others (7,8). Each MMP is encoded by a distinct gene, and about half of the human MMP genes so far discovered are on chromosome 11 (7).

The mere fact that MMPs might be involved in the pathogenesis of several chronic disorders has made this field attractive to numerous pharmaceutical companies.

One major approach for controlling abnormal MMP activity has been the use of small molecular weight inhibitors, and several excellent reviews of the design of such inhibitors have been published (7).

Rheumatoid arthritis

In 1942, the Swedish doctor Nana Svartz introduced sulfasalazine into therapy and suggested that it might be useful in rheumatoid arthritis because of its antibacterial activity. Since then, many antimicrobial agents have been tried in the treatment of rheumatoid arthritis, based on the assumption that the disease may be due to an infectious agent. Interest has focused on tetracyclines for the treatment of rheumatoid arthritis (9), reactive arthritis (10), and osteoarthritis (11) and the state of the art has been reviewed (12). The theory that rheumatoid arthritis is due to an infectious agent has been refined to a statement that it may be a gene transfer disease in which some viruses act as vectors (13), thereby excluding a direct effect of antibacterial agents on the disease.

Two further perspectives on the use of tetracyclines in rheumatoid arthritis have been published (14,15). In addition to an effect on matrix metalloproteinases, the authors focused on a potential antiarthritic action of tetracyclines by their effects in the interaction between the generation of nitric oxide, matrix metalloproteinase release, and chondrocyte apoptosis. Both minocycline and doxycycline inhibit the production of nitric oxide from human cartilage and murine macrophages (16) in concentrations that are achieved in vivo. The authors suggested that tetracyclines may have several potential chondroprotective effects: direct inhibition of matrix metalloproteinase activity and, by inhibition of nitric oxide production, further reduction of matrix metalloproteinase activity, reversal of reduced matrix synthesis, and reduced chondrocyte apoptosis.

In double-blind, placebo-controlled studies, minocycline relieved clinical symptoms and reduced some laboratory measures of disease activity in patients with rheumatoid arthritis (17–19). However, the progression of radiographic damage was not significantly reduced and minocycline caused several adverse effects. This led to investigations of the therapeutic effects of doxycycline in patients with rheumatoid arthritis. In 13 patients with moderate rheumatoid arthritis, low-dose doxycycline 20 mg bd reduced the urinary excretion of pyridinoline (20). Pyridinolines are collagen cross-links that are released from joints during cartilage and bone resorption and correlate with the severity of joint destruction (21). In a later study, doxycycline produced a significant reduction in the number of tender joints and significant improvements in disability and behavior in 12 patients with rheumatoid arthritis (22).

However, these studies were not placebo-controlled, and it was possible that the observed effects were due to factors other than doxycycline. Two double-blind, placebo-controlled trials have since been reported (23,24).

In a crossover study, 66 patients took 50 mg doxycycline or placebo twice a day for 12, 24, or 36 weeks (23). Patients' assessments, swollen and tender joint counts, duration of morning stiffness, erythrocyte sedimentation rate, and the so-called modified disease activity score (25)

were used as measures of disease activity. Doxycycline had no significant effects on clinical and laboratory measures of disease activity, pyridinoline excretion, or progression of radiographic joint damage. Furthermore, there were adverse effects during treatment with doxycycline and not with placebo. The authors concluded that doxycycline 50 mg bd provided no therapeutic benefit in patients with rheumatoid arthritis.

In another study, a 16-week, randomized, double-blind, placebo-controlled trial, eligible subjects with active seropositive or erosive rheumatoid arthritis were randomly allocated to three treatment groups: doxycycline 200 mg intravenously, azithromycin 250 mg orally, or placebo (24). The primary end-points were changes between baseline and week 4 in the tender joint count, erythrocyte sedimentation rate, and urinary excretion of pyridinoline. The trial was stopped prematurely after 31 patients had been enrolled. Three subjects were withdrawn because of worsening arthritis. There were no significant differences across the groups in any of the three primary clinical end-points. The authors concluded that doxycycline did not reduce disease activity or collagen cross-link production.

Ten chemically modified tetracyclines (CMTs), minocycline, and doxycycline have been tested for their capacity to inhibit cartilage degradation in vitro (26). CMT-8 was the most active. The authors concluded that by carefully selecting a tetracycline-based MMP inhibitor and controlling dosages it should be possible to inhibit pathologically excessive MMP-8 and/or MMP-13 activity, especially that which causes bone erosion, without affecting the constitutive activity of MMP-1 needed for tissue remodelling and normal host function. They thought that of the CMTs, CMT-8 and to a lesser extent CMT-3 and CMT-7 were the most effective. However, the effects of these CMTs in a full-scale trial in rheumatoid arthritis have not been reported.

Reactive arthritis

It is well established that a number of microorganisms found in the gastrointestinal tract are associated with reactive arthritis and that most of these organisms might be susceptible to tetracyclines. Several investigations have shown clinical effects of tetracyclines in the treatment of reactive arthritis (12). In these cases, a more direct antibacterial effect of the triggering organism (if still present in the patient) might be the mechanism involved.

Osteoarthritis

Tetracyclines have been investigated in experimental osteoarthritis, because metalloproteases are involved in the breakdown of cartilage matrix seen in this condition. Doxycycline reduced the severity of knee osteoarthritis induced in dogs by ligamentous section (27) and also reduced the degradation of type XI collagen exposed to extract of human arthritic cartilage (28).

Periodontal disease

Periodontal disease is caused by microorganisms, but host responses are in large part responsible for destruction of the periodontal support structures. In these patients, pathological activity of host-derived matrix metalloproteinases occurs in response to the bacterial infection in the periodontal tissues, causing destruction of collagen, the primary structural component of periodontal matrix. This in turn leads to gingival recession, pocket formation, and increased tooth mobility. The final outcome is loss of the tooth.

Tetracyclines inhibit collagenolytic activity in gingival tissue (SEDA-23, 256) (29–31). Based on these findings, a large clinical development program was initiated to demonstrate the potential of a sub-antimicrobial dose of doxycycline to augment and maintain the beneficial effects afforded by conventional non-surgical periodontal therapy in adult periodontitis. A summary of these studies has been published (32). Several different dosage regimens and placebo were compared in patients who had had a variety of adjunctive non-surgical procedures. Of the various parameters studied, the following are worthy of mention: collagenase activity in gingival crevicular fluid and gingival specimens, so-called clinical attachment levels, probing pockets depths, bleeding on probing, and subtraction radiographic measurements of alveolar bone height.

Sub-antimicrobial doses of doxycycline reduced collagenase activity in both gingival crevicular fluid and gingival biopsies, augmented and maintained gains in clinical attachment levels and reductions in pockets depths, reduced bleeding on probing, and prevented loss of alveolar bone height. These clinical effects occurred in the absence of any significant effects on the subgingival microflora and without evidence of an increase in the incidence or severity of adverse reactions relative to the controls. The authors proposed that the main mechanism underlying these effects is inhibition of pathologically high matrix metalloproteinase activity in neutrophils (MMP-8) and bone cells (MMP-13).

Acne

Over the years, various tetracyclines have been used in the treatment of acne. Their mechanism of action is not clear, but appears to be not purely antimicrobial, since they reduce chemotaxis of polymorphonuclear leukocytes, modify complement pathways, and inhibit the polymorphonuclear leukocyte chemotactic factor and lipase production in *Propionibacterium acnes* (33). They may also have a direct effect on sebum secretion (34), for example by modification of free fatty acids (35).

Adult respiratory distress syndrome

Adult respiratory distress syndrome (ARDS) has many causes, is associated with severe lung damage, and is characterized by pulmonary edema and hypoxemia. It has a high mortality. The current method of treatment is supportive and there is no specific therapy. This was the background to a thorough review of the anti-inflammatory properties of tetracyclines in the prevention of acute lung injury (36). The authors ended with an optimistic forecast, that targeting the proteases that cause ARDS with chemically modified tetracyclines may be useful in prevention and treatment. They ended by suggesting that strategies to prevent ARDS should focus on targets downstream from the initial inflammatory signals that provoke the cascade of events.

Glaucoma

Tetracyclines, especially demeclocycline, are among the most effective ocular hypotensive agents, according to studies in rabbits and cats. The biochemical mechanism of this effect is unknown. The prolonged effect and apparent lack of adverse ocular adverse effects suggest their possible usefulness for treating glaucoma in man (SEDA-15, 260).

General adverse effects

Mild gastrointestinal disturbances are common. A common and nearly unique feature of all tetracyclines is the formation of drug–melanin complexes, resulting in pigment deposition at various sites. Except for enamel defects and presumable disturbances of osteogenesis these deposits do not give rise to abnormalities of organ function. In view of tooth discoloration and enamel hypoplasia, with a tendency to caries formation, tetracyclines should be avoided in children under 8 years of age and in women after the third month of pregnancy. The risk of photosensitivity reactions largely depends on the dose of the drug and the degree of exposure to sunlight. It may be increased in long-term treatment. Skin, nail, and other organ pigmentation often occur, even with low-dose long-term treatment. The syndrome of fatty liver degeneration is rarely encountered today, because risk factors such as pregnancy are respected, and formulations with lower doses are available. Adverse effects can occur with most tetracyclines if the dosage is not altered in patients with renal insufficiency.

Allergic reactions to tetracyclines are less than half as common as allergic reactions to penicillin. For this reason, tetracyclines are alternatives in patients with allergic reactions to other antibiotics. Exceptional observations of anaphylactic shock have been reported (37,38). In a few cases tetracyclines were assumed to be the cause of hypersensitivity myocarditis (39). Pneumonitis with eosinophilia has been described in association with tetracyclines (40). A serum sickness-like syndrome was probably associated with minocycline in a 19-year-old man treated for acne (41). Allergic and toxic reactions may in some cases have been caused by degraded formulations or additives (42). Tumor-inducing effects have not been reported.

Jarisch–Herxheimer reaction

The Jarisch–Herxheimer reaction is common in patients treated with tetracyclines for louse-borne relapsing fever (43). Two forms of reaction are described at the start of tetracycline therapy: (a) fever, rigor, increased respiratory and heart rates, and occasional delirium and coma (44); (b) fever and disseminated intravascular coagulation (45). At about the time the temperature reaches its peak, spirochetes disappear from the peripheral blood (44). Meptazinol, a partial opioid antagonist, reduces the Jarisch–Herxheimer reaction in relapsing fever (46).

Bleeding with thrombocytopenia and signs of intravascular coagulation in patients treated for louse-borne relapsing fever may be due to a Jarisch–Herxheimer reaction mediated by the release of endotoxins from disintegrating spirochetes (43).

Comparisons of individual tetracyclines

The spectra of bacterial effectiveness of the various tetracyclines are fairly similar. However, metabolism and excretion vary. In general, preference is currently given to drugs that can be given in relatively low doses (not above 1.0 g/day).

Tetracycline (chlortetracycline) and oxytetracycline

These tetracyclines are incompletely absorbed from the gastrointestinal tract. Plasma concentrations fall with half-lives of 6–12 hours. They are predominantly excreted by the kidney, extrarenal elimination amounting at most to 10–20%. They have a lower affinity for fat and membranes, which means that higher dosages to achieve therapeutic effectiveness. However, higher dosages can contribute to an increased risk of systemic toxic effects and, as absorption from oral administration is incomplete, also to an increased risk of gastrointestinal adverse reactions.

Demeclocycline (demethylchlortetracycline)

Demeclocycline produces a significantly higher rate of phototoxic skin reactions than other tetracyclines, presumably owing to its long half-life (about 16 hours), resulting in therapeutic plasma concentrations lasting 24–48 hours, and an even longer-lasting accumulation of the drug in membranes and fatty tissues. Demeclocycline is eliminated about 20–40% by glomerular filtration. In patients with liver cirrhosis, cardiac failure, or impaired renal function, it should be used cautiously, because of its pronounced effect on electrolyte and fluid balance (47).

Doxycycline and minocycline

Doxycycline and minocycline are more lipophilic tetracyclines. They are well absorbed after oral administration. Their half-lives are 16–18 hours. Their higher affinity for fatty tissues improves their effectiveness and changes their adverse effects profile. Local gastrointestinal irritation and disturbance of the intestinal bacterial flora occur less often than with the more hydrophilic drugs, which have to be given in higher oral doses for sufficient absorption.

Nevertheless, their toxic effects are similar to those of other tetracyclines and arise from accumulation in fatty tissues. Accumulation in a third compartment and the resulting long half-life may contribute to an increased incidence of various toxic adverse effects during long-term treatment, even if lower daily doses are used. This seems also to be the case for pigmentation disorders and possibly for neurological disturbances (48).

Minocycline and doxycycline are predominantly eliminated by the liver and biliary tract (70–90%). Therefore, no change in dose is needed in patients with impaired renal function. However, it should be considered that hepatic elimination of doxycycline or minocycline might be accelerated by co-administration of agents that induce hepatic enzymes.

Methacycline

Methacycline is rarely used. It has similar efficacy to ampicillin in acute exacerbations of chronic bronchitis.

Chemically modified tetracyclines

As early as the 1960s it was recognized that tetracyclines might inhibit bone growth, supposedly by interference with calcium metabolism. It was not until collagenase was discovered in 1983 (50) that intensive interest in the non-antimicrobial properties of tetracycline-based antibiotics developed. Most of the initial studies were done with doxycycline and minocycline, that is semi-synthetic tetracyclines with widespread medical and dental uses. However, in 1987, a non-antibacterial chemically modified tetracycline (CMT) that inhibited mammalian collagenase activity was described (51). At present, the CMTs (also known as COLs, from their having been introduced by CollaGenes Pharmaceuticals Inc, Newton, PA, USA) comprise a group of at least 10 analogues compounds (CMT-1 to CMT-10) that differ in their specificity and potency in inhibiting MMP. Comparative pharmacokinetic data, obtained from animals, have recently been published, as has a bibliography covering more than 75 papers and abstracts related to the basic biological properties of these compounds (52). Chemically modified tetracyclines are more active in interfering with mammalian processes than the classical tetracyclines, which is the main justification for their use in non-infective problems (52,53). From a qualitative point of view, it might be reasonable to assume similar host-related adverse effects as the classical tetracyclines, while from a quantitative point of view, dosages, duration of therapy, etc., will influence the number of adverse effects. However, the risks might be quite high.

Hematologic

Sideroblastic anemia is characterized by the accumulation of iron in the mitochondria of erythroblasts. In a Phase I study in 35 patients with refractory tumors, eight taking CMT-3 developed anemia without leukopenia or thrombocytopenia (54). Three of these patients underwent bone-marrow examination and each had ringed sideroblasts. The authors referred to several cases of aplastic anemia, megaloblastic anemia, and hemolytic anemia in which members of the tetracycline family have been implicated. However, they stated that there has been no previous reports of sideroblastic anemia associated with any tetracycline derivative and that the molecular mechanisms by which CMT-3 might cause sideroblastic anemia are unclear.

Immunologic

Based on the strategy that inhibition of angiogenesis is of importance in anticancer therapy, CMT-3 (COL-3) was used in a phase 1 study in 35 patients at the National Institutes of Health in the USA in patients with refractory metastatic cancer (55). The patients received a test dose of CMT-3, followed by pharmacokinetic testing during daily dosing for 7 days. After a few doses, three patients developed symptoms of drug-induced lupus, and the diagnoses were verified after a few days or weeks. CMT-3 was withdrawn and there was improvement.

Bacterial resistance

Prolonged treatment with the classical antibacterial tetracyclines results in bacterial resistance and/or opportunistic fungal infections. It has therefore been forecast, but not so far proven, that chemically modified tetracyclines without antibacterial activity may not cause microbial resistance. However, accepting that the major mechanism by which bacteria get rid of tetracyclines intracellularly is by increasing their efflux via P glycoprotein, the chemically modified tetracyclines might also trigger that mechanism, thereby causing reduced sensitivity of the exposed bacterial population to all types of tetracyclines. Before this possibility has been ruled out, the new chemically modified tetracyclines should be introduced with great care.

Organs and Systems

Cardiovascular

Cardiovascular reactions to tetracyclines have often been associated with other symptoms of hypersensitivity, such as urticaria, angioedema, bronchial obstruction, and arterial hypotension (37,56). Such reactions occurred in patients who had tolerated tetracyclines previously and were therefore considered as anaphylactic.

Respiratory

There have been a few cases of acute bronchial obstruction after the administration of a tetracycline (57).

Pneumonitis with eosinophilia has also been described (40,58).

When pleural tetracycline instillation is used to produce local inflammation for pleurodesis in spontaneous pneumothorax, there are no severe short-term or long-term adverse effects (59).

Nervous system

Tetracyclines rarely cause benign intracranial hypertension. This syndrome has primarily involved children (60,61), although it has also been observed in adults (48,62–69). Re-exposure can result in recurrence (59). As a rule, the symptoms develop within days or occasionally several months after the start of therapy, in one case only after 18 months of tetracycline therapy for acne (48). The syndrome includes headache, nausea and vomiting, dizziness, tinnitus, papilledema, and visual disturbances caused by scotoma or optic nerve damage. Intracranial pressure can be raised up to three-fold. Distinct intracerebral lesions are not visible on CT scan or angiography and the ventricular spaces are not enlarged (62). With the exception of raised intracranial pressure, all findings, including the cell count and protein concentration of the cerebrospinal fluid, are normal. After withdrawal, symptoms resolve over a period of hours to days or occasionally weeks. Increased use of long-term therapy with tetracyclines for acne may contribute to a higher prevalence of this syndrome (70).

Early studies showed that curare blockade was increased by tetracyclines (71–73). This effect can be antagonized by calcium ions (74). There was a short-term increase in muscular weakness in patients with myasthenia gravis after intravenous tetracycline. The mechanism may be a calcium-antagonizing effect of magnesium ions present in the tetracycline solvent, as the

symptoms could be provoked by similar amounts of magnesium alone. The formation of calcium complexes with non-protein-bound tetracycline, thus lowering the serum concentration of free calcium, may also be involved (75).

Sensory systems

Acute transitory myopia was described as an effect of tetracycline therapy, probably due to changes in refractive power (76).

Endocrine

Hormone production in patients with "black thyroid," who had taken a tetracycline for prolonged periods, was normal (77,78).

Metabolism

Tetracyclines can increase blood urea nitrogen or serum urea concentrations without a corresponding increase in serum creatinine (that is without accompanying renal damage). The mechanism is an excess nitrogen load of metabolic origin accompanied by negative nitrogen balance. This effect is termed "anti-anabolic" (79,80), but is in fact the result of inhibition of protein synthesis, which affects not only microorganisms but to some degree mammalian cells also. Sodium and water depletion, due to the diuretic effect of some tetracyclines, can further enhance uremia (80).

Tetracyclines have been associated with hypoglycemia (81). Insulin doses may have to be reduced (82).

Hematologic

Hematological changes with tetracyclines are extremely rare. However, in individual cases, hemolytic anemia (83), neutropenia or slight leukopenia, thrombocytopenia (84), and even aplastic anemia have all been described. In the light of the fact that such blood changes are often reported without a clear description of their cause, the relation to the drug often remains doubtful, especially if reactions are listed in tabular form and information on specific details or concomitant drug therapy is lacking.

Bleeding with thrombocytopenia and signs of intravascular coagulation in patients treated for louse-borne relapsing fever may be due to a Jarisch–Herxheimer reaction mediated by the release of endotoxins from disintegrating spirochetes (43).

Mouth and teeth

The long-term esthetic results of treating severely stained teeth due to tetracyclines by endodontics and internal bleaching have been assessed in 20 patients and found to be excellent (85). A therapeutic strategy may be bleaching after the preparation for porcelain laminate veneers or night-guard vital bleaching (86,87).

Stomatitis, other signs of irritation of the oropharynx, and a rash in and around the orifices have been described in patients taking tetracyclines. This may partly be considered as mucous membrane manifestations of allergic or toxic origin. Secondary infections by pathogenic organisms, such as *C. albicans*, viruses, or bacteria, should always be considered (88).

Gastrointestinal

Nausea, vomiting, and epigastric burning are the most common adverse effects of tetracyclines. This is also true for the lower-dose formulations. The symptoms are usually mild and seldom necessitate withdrawal. Nausea occurs in 8–15% of patients.

Esophageal damage

Esophageal ulcers have been described in association with oral doxycycline or tetracycline. Acute onset of substernal burning pain and dysphagia was noted within hours of taking the drug (89–93). Remaining parts of the ingested capsule were identified by esophagoscopy.

Thirty centers for pharmacovigilance in France have reported 81 cases of esophageal damage after treatment with tetracyclines collected between 1985 and 1992 (94). There were 64 ulcers, eight cases of dysphagia, and nine of esophagitis. Most (96%) of the cases were caused by doxycycline and 73% of the patients were female, mean age 29 years. Prescriptions were for dermatological (54%), urogenital (23%), and ENT diseases. In one patient, a 71-year-old man, an esophagobronchial fistulation required esophagectomy. In 92% the drugs were not taken correctly, that is at bedtime or without a sufficient quantity of fluid. Treatment with sucralfate 1 g tds did not change the outcome of tetracycline-induced esophageal ulcers (95).

In three studies of more than 600 children with chest pain, none had tetracycline-induced esophagitis as a cause of their pain (96–98).

Patients should not lie down immediately after taking a tetracycline capsule and the formulation should be swallowed with generous quantities of water (89,99).

Liver

A clinical syndrome, often with fatal outcome, has been recognized as a complication of high doses of tetracycline. It is characterized by nausea, vomiting, and spiking fever. Jaundice, acidosis, and uremia are also often present, while hematemesis and melena are only occasionally observed. Some patients die because of refractory hypotension. The histopathological findings are those of diffuse fatty liver degeneration (100–102). Although the syndrome was primarily described in pregnant women, it is not restricted to them. Impaired renal function, and thus reduced renal elimination of tetracyclines, as well as serious infections, increases the risk of this complication (100,103). Since the introduction of lower doses of tetracycline (under 1 g/day), the syndrome of fatty liver degeneration with severe hepatic insufficiency has become rare (101). However, a few reports have described liver reactions in previously healthy individuals with no pre-existing conditions and given usual oral doses of tetracyclines (104,105). Liver enzymes and renal function should be monitored, especially in patients at risk.

A personally experienced case of likely tetracycline-induced liver injury after low-dose tetracycline has been reported (106). The patient took oral doxycycline 200 mg/day for 8 days and had markedly altered liver function. The liver enzyme activities normalized only 109 days after withdrawal. The authors also reviewed all reports of liver damage to Swedish Adverse Drug Reactions Advisory Committee (SADRAC) in the period 1965–95. There were 23 liver reactions with a suspected causal relation to oral low-dose tetracycline derivatives. A causal relation was considered likely in three cases and possible in eight, giving an incidence of roughly one in 18 million defined daily doses. There were no deaths from these liver reactions, and liver enzyme activities normalized in all cases without any serious clinical consequences. The authors remarked that the frequency of liver reactions resulting from tetracyclines may be somewhat higher, as previous studies in Sweden suggest that only 20–50% of severe adverse reactions are reported to SADRAC (106).

Pancreas

Pancreatitis is a common feature of the clinical syndrome of fatty liver due to tetracyclines, although it has also been observed without overt liver disease in a patient after two separate exposures (107).

Urinary tract

Tetracyclines not uncommonly cause a raised serum urea concentration due to impaired protein synthesis rather than renal damage. However, renal insufficiency can occur, and patients with pre-existing renal insufficiency are particularly likely to develop raised blood urea nitrogen, serum phosphate, and serum sulfate concentrations during treatment with most tetracyclines. These changes may be associated with acidosis and even symptoms of uremia. Renal dysfunction can be missed if diuresis alone is monitored, since non-oliguric renal insufficiency has been reported (108). Interstitial nephritis is extremely rare (109–111).

Uremia, which may at least in part be due to a reduction in renal function, has been observed in patients with liver cirrhosis (112–114), cardiac failure, or interstitial nephritis (115), which is extremely rare (109–111).

Most observations suggest that a determining factor for the risk of renal insufficiency is a relative overdose of the drug in patients with pre-existing renal damage (113,114), particularly in those who are already dehydrated (for example due to diuretic therapy). The half-life of tetracyclines is prolonged several-fold in patients with renal dysfunction (116). With normal renal function, 20–70% of an intravenous dose of tetracycline is eliminated by glomerular filtration. Maintenance therapy must be adjusted to the degree of renal impairment.

Acquired Lignac–De Toni–Fanconi syndrome, with polyuria, polydipsia, glycosuria, aminoaciduria, hyperphosphaturia, and hypercalciuria, was described in a number of patients treated with outdated tetracycline formulations. The degeneration products responsible for the toxic action are probably epitetracycline, anhydro-4-epitetracycline, and anhydrotetracycline (117), as similar renal damage was produced in rats with anhydro-4-epitetracycline (118).

A few observations of a nephrogenic diabetes insipidus-like syndrome with demeclocycline (demethylchlortetracycline hydrochloride) and resistance to exogenous vasopressin suggested impairment of renal concentrating function by tubular damage (47). Demeclocycline has therefore been proposed for the treatment of inappropriate secretion of antidiuretic hormone (119–123).

Acute interstitial nephritis leading to acute renal insufficiency has been reported after a single repeated dose of tetracycline (124).

Skin

Pronounced responsiveness of the skin and nails to light is a complication of systemic therapy with tetracyclines. In general, the pathogenesis of skin reactions promoted by sunlight exposure is mediated by phototoxicity, as suggested by the high occurrence rate (up to 9 out of 10 patients), depending on sun exposure and drug dosage. Experimental studies identified a wavelength close to 320 nm within the ultraviolet spectrum as the most potent area for the induction of phototoxic reactions (125). It has been described with various tetracyclines and presumably occurs with all of them. The skin changes resemble those of minor to severe sunburn, with erythema, edema, papules, blisters, and urticaria (126,127). In some circumstances they resemble cutaneous porphyria and have therefore been described as "porphyria-like cutaneous changes" (128).

Pigmentation due to tetracyclines occurs, but the exact frequency is not known. It has been observed with newer and lower-dose formulations as well as with older drugs, and presumably occurs with all tetracyclines. In contrast to phototoxic reactions, pigmentation can appear without light exposure and without inflammation. Pigment deposits were observed in light-exposed and non-exposed skin, the conjunctivae, the oral mucosa, the tongue, and internal organs, such as the thyroid and heart valve endothelium (77,78,129,130). The pigment is presumed to be a drug–melanin–calcium complex and depends on the chelating properties of the tetracycline molecule. Although pigmentation usually tends to persist after withdrawal, it does not provoke any symptoms or organ dysfunction, except for cosmetic problems. A number of cases occurred in patients treated for acne, and may possibly have been due to more common use of long-term treatments (131), although there is no evidence that the risk is increased in these patients.

Allergic skin and mucous membrane reactions occur with a very low incidence of 0.3%, which is about 10-fold lower than the incidence of such reactions in patients treated with other antibiotics (132). A generalized rash can occur during tetracycline treatment. Various forms have been described, including generalized urticaria, maculopapular rash, erythema exudativum, multiforme-like eruptions, and rare cases of Stevens–Johnson syndrome (133–136). Even acute generalized exanthematous pustulosis has been described (137). Fixed drug eruptions due to systemic administration are rare (138–140), as is a serum sickness-like syndrome (41,141). Allergic contact dermatitis induced by local application of a tetracycline is an exception (133,142–144).

Antimicrobial drugs, especially co-trimoxazole, ampicillin, and tetracyclines, can cause fixed drug eruptions (145).

Nails

Pronounced photosensitivity of the skin and nails is a complication of systemic therapy with tetracyclines. Onycholysis is associated with nail discoloration.

Dystrophy is usually preceded by photosensitivity reactions of the skin (133). Depending on the degree and area of light exposure, onycholysis may also affect the toe nails (126). In contrast to idiopathic onycholysis, it not only affects women (146).

Musculoskeletal

Deposition of tetracyclines in bone tissue has been demonstrated in animals (147) and man (148). However, whereas osseous tissue in adult patients treated with tetracycline has shown deposits only in areas of repair or remodelling, children's bones contain extensive areas of deposition. Tetracycline deposition in bone has been reported to have an effect on longitudinal bone growth (149). In experimental tissue cultures, osteogenesis was impaired by tetracyclines in concentrations similar to serum concentrations that are associated with a therapeutic effect (that is 1 µg/ml) (150). The deposition of tetracyclines in human bone begins in utero as early as in the first trimester of pregnancy (148). With regular tissue turnover, the deposits disappear.

Infection risk

Monilial infections of the vulva and vagina in temporal association with tetracycline use can occur, even without other predisposing factors such as diabetes, pregnancy, immunodeficiency, and therapy with oral contraceptives and glucocorticoids. They also occur in patients treated with other antibiotics (151). *C. albicans* is not always the cause of vaginitis. The same is true for balanitis in men (152). If symptoms persist or change in patients with urethritis or adnexitis, this may be due to treatment failure, because of resistance of the causative pathogen (153).

Long-Term Effects

Drug resistance

Resistance to tetracyclines shows marked inter-regional variations and changes rapidly with time. The selection of resistant bacterial strains may be favored by widespread, often prophylactic, use in veterinary medicine and by long-term therapy for acne, periodontal disease, or symptomatic *Borrelia* infections. Many of the documented cases of resistance are of limited practical significance, since the tetracyclines are merely one of a number of therapeutic alternatives. The problem may be different when these drugs are the chemotherapeutic agents of first choice, that is in chronic *Borrelia* infections, especially arthritis due to Lyme disease and pulmonary or bubonic plague due to *Yersinia pestis* (154).

For infections with *Chlamydia* or *Mycoplasma*, effective alternative antibiotics are available. Increased rates of resistant strains of genital *Mycoplasma* may explain treatment failures (153,155).

A rather high resistance rate of 25–50% is reported for *Hemophilus* species (156), and this has to be taken into consideration if tetracyclines are given to patients with chronic pulmonary diseases or for the treatment of acute respiratory infections.

For infections with *Neisseria gonorrhoea*, tetracyclines are not indicated, owing to the higher prevalence of resistance, especially among penicillinase-producing strains (157). For these patients, better alternatives are usually available.

Second-Generation Effects

Teratogenicity

Teratogenic effects of tetracyclines have been demonstrated (158–160), as evidenced by increased rates of intrauterine death, congenital anomalies in general (161), and congenital cataracts (162) in fetuses exposed to tetracyclines. However, it is often impossible to distinguish between the drug and an underlying unidentified viral infection as a cause of the observed abnormalities.

Of 38 151 pregnant women who had babies without any defects (controls), 214 (0.6%) had taken oral oxytetracycline; in contrast, of 22 865 pregnant women who had offspring with congenital abnormalities, 216 (0.9%) had taken oxytetracycline (OR = 1.7; 95% CI = 1.4, 2.0) (163). More women whose babies had congenital abnormalities had taken oxytetracycline in the second month of pregnancy:

- neural-tube defects (OR = 9.7; CI = 2.0, 47);
- cleft palate (OR = 17; CI = 3.5, 84);
- multiple congenital abnormalities (particularly the combination of neural-tube defects and cardiovascular malformations) (OR = 13; CI = 3.8, 44).

The authors mentioned that their previous study had not shown a teratogenic potential of doxycycline (164), but concluded, far more prudently, that all tetracyclines are contraindicated during pregnancy.

Fetotoxicity

Discoloration of the first teeth is particularly likely if a tetracycline is given to the mother after the third month of pregnancy (165). Tetracyclines pass across the placenta and reach therapeutic concentrations in the fetal circulation (166,167).

Tooth discoloration is due to deposition of tetracyclines in the form of calcium complexes in the mineralizing zones of the teeth, and seems to be pathogenically related to the pigmentation of other organs. It occurs when tetracyclines are used during tooth formation. Tetracyclines pass through the placenta and are also found in high concentrations in the breast milk (168). As mineralization of the deciduous teeth takes place from the fourth month of intrauterine life until 1 year after birth and continues for the permanent teeth up to the age of 7–8 years (166), pregnant women after the third month of pregnancy, nursing women, and children under the age of 8 years should not be treated with tetracyclines. Discoloration of the teeth after intrauterine exposure to tetracyclines was observed in up to 50% of children at risk and was especially high when tetracyclines were used during the last trimester (166). Besides its merely cosmetic aspect, tooth discoloration in children is associated with enamel defects and hypoplasia in severe cases (169). Adult-onset tooth discoloration coincident with minocycline administration occurred in four of 72 patients (170).

Susceptibility Factors

Age

Pregnant women after the third month of pregnancy, nursing women, and children under the age of 8 years should not be treated with tetracyclines, because of the risk of discoloration of the teeth. Besides its merely cosmetic aspect, tooth discoloration in children is associated with enamel defects and hypoplasia in severe cases (169).

Renal disease

Tetracyclines are removed by hemodialysis, but significantly less than creatinine or urea (100,116). Severe adverse effects of tetracyclines occur almost exclusively with doses over 1.0 g/day (101) or in the treatment of pyelonephritis with concomitant renal insufficiency.

Drug Administration

Drug administration route

The intravenous formulation of tetracycline was instilled intrapleurally to produce chemical pleurodesis, with good effect, from the 1970s to the 1990s. The adverse effect most commonly seen with tetracycline was chest pain, which was often severe (171,172). In a comprehensive review of intrapleural therapy published in 1994 (173) the incidence of chest pain was estimated at 14%, and fever occurred in 10% of patients. However, the intravenous form of tetracycline has been withdrawn by the manufacturer and so this agent is no longer available for pleurodesis.

Drug–Drug Interactions

Antacids

Co-administration of tetracyclines with antacids or other drugs containing divalent or trivalent cations, such as calcium, magnesium, or iron, is contraindicated. Tetracyclines form complexes with such cations, which are very poorly or not at all absorbed (75,174,175).

To avoid this interaction, delay of 2–3 hours between the ingestion of tetracycline and the cation is recommended (175). Similarly, reduced systemic availability results from simultaneous intake of abundant quantities of milk or milk products.

Antidiarrheal drugs

Antidiarrheal drugs, such as kaolin-pectin and bismuth products (176,177), impair the absorption of tetracyclines by chelation (see the interaction with antacids in this monograph).

Coumarin anticoagulants

Although antibiotics can inhibit the production of vitamin K in the gut by intestinal bacteria, they do not thereby interfere with the actions of coumarin anticoagulation, since vitamin K that is produced by intestinal bacteria is of less importance than vitamin K that is obtained from dietary sources (178). Nevertheless, there have been sporadic reports that tetracyclines can enhance the effects of coumarin anticoagulants (179–182). The mechanism is not known, but evidence that tetracyclines can reduce the activity of prothrombin (183) suggests an additive pharmacodynamic interaction.

Diuretics

The combination of tetracyclines with diuretics is particularly detrimental to renal function (184). Tetracyclines accumulate in patients with pre-existing renal insufficiency (for example elderly people, even if the serum creatinine is in the reference range) and can cause nausea and vomiting, which causes dehydration and worsens renal function. This is exacerbated by the effects of diuretics.

Iron

See antacids above (174,175).

Methoxyflurane

In patients taking oral or parenteral tetracyclines who undergo methoxyflurane anesthesia, renal insufficiency and oxalate crystal formation in renal tissue was attributed to an interaction between these drugs (185–187). Tetracyclines are therefore not recommended preoperatively.

Risperidone and/or sertraline

An interaction of tetracycline with risperidone and/or sertraline has been described (188).

- A 15-year-old youth with Asperger's syndrome, Tourette's syndrome, and obsessive-compulsive disorder was stabilized on risperidone 1.5 mg bd and sertraline 100 mg od and had marked improvement in his social skills and tics, until he was given tetracycline 250 mg bd for acne. Within 2 weeks his tics were acutely exacerbated with pronounced neck jerking and guttural sounds. The sertraline was increased to 150 mg/day, but the tics did not resolve. The tetracycline was withdrawn after 1 month, and the tics improved within a few weeks.

The authors reviewed the major metabolic pathways of the three drugs used in this case. Tetracycline may have accelerated the hepatic metabolism of risperidone, but tetracycline has not been shown to induce CYP2D6, the major hepatic enzyme involved in the metabolism of risperidone. The authors claimed that it was more likely that tetracycline binds to risperidone or its active metabolite, making them inactive. They supported this suggestion by citing evidence that clozapine, which has similar pharmacology to risperidone, interacts with tetracycline in vitro (189). They also commented on the possibility that the effect could have come from increased concentrations of sertraline, which can increase tics (190). Tetracycline may inhibit the hepatic enzymes that metabolize sertraline; however, adequate evidence is lacking. Another possibility is a protein binding interaction, because all three drugs are highly protein bound. However, the observation that the tics were not worsened by an increase in sertraline dosage makes this possibility less likely. The mere fact that the withdrawal of tetracycline resulted in an improvement in the tics supports an interaction between tetracycline and risperidone.

References

1. Midtvedt T, Lingaas E, Melby K. The effect of 13 anti-microbial agents on the elimination phase of phagocytosis in human polymorphonuclear leukocytes. In: Eickenberg HU, Hahn A, Opferkuch W, editors. The Influence of Antibiotics on the Host-Parasite Relationship. Berlin: Springer Verlag; 1982:118–28.
2. Golub LM, Ramamurthy N, McNamara TF, Gomes B, Wolff M, Casino A, Kapoor A, Zambon J, Ciancio S, Schneir M, et al. Tetracyclines inhibit tissue collagenase activity. A new mechanism in the treatment of periodontal disease. J Periodontal Res 1984;19(6):651–5.
3. Greenwald RA, Golub LM, Lavietes B, Ramamurthy NS, Gruber B, Laskin RS, McNamara TF. Tetracyclines inhibit human synovial collagenase in vivo and in vitro. J Rheumatol 1987;14(1):28–32.
4. Lauhio A, Sorsa T, Lindy O, Suomalainen K, Saari H, Golub LM, Konttinen YT. The anticollagenolytic potential of lymecycline in the long-term treatment of reactive arthritis. Arthritis Rheum 1992;35(2):195–8.
5. Suzuki Y, Ishihara M, Segami T, Ito M. Anti-ulcer effects of antioxidants, quercetin, alpha-tocopherol, nifedipine and tetracycline in rats. Jpn J Pharmacol 1998;78(4):435–41.
6. Golub LM, Ramamurthy NS, Llavaneras A, Ryan ME, Lee HM, Liu Y, Bain S, Sorsa T. A chemically modified nonantimicrobial tetracycline (CMT-8) inhibits gingival matrix metalloproteinases, periodontal breakdown, and extra-oral bone loss in ovariectomized rats. Ann NY Acad Sci 1999;878:290–310.
7. Skiles JW, Gonnella NC, Jeng AY. The design, structure, and therapeutic application of matrix metalloproteinase inhibitors. Curr Med Chem 2001;8(4):425–74.
8. Hidalgo M, Eckhardt SG. Development of matrix metalloproteinase inhibitors in cancer therapy. J Natl Cancer Inst 2001;93(3):178–93.
9. Trentham DE, Dynesius-Trentham RA. Antibiotic therapy for rheumatoid arthritis. Scientific and anecdotal appraisals. Rheum Dis Clin North Am 1995;21(3):817–34.
10. Pott HG, Wittenborg A, Junge-Hulsing G. Long-term antibiotic treatment in reactive arthritis. Lancet 1988;1(8579):245–6.
11. Dejarnatt AC, Grant JA. Basic mechanisms of anaphylaxis and anaphylactoid reactions. Immunol Allergy Clin North Am 1992;12:33–46.
12. Toussirot E, Despaux J, Wendling D. Do minocycline and other tetracyclines have a place in rheumatology? Rev Rhum Engl Ed 1997;64(7–9):474–80.
13. Grubb R, Grubb A, Kjellen L, Lycke E, Aman P. Rheumatoid arthritis—a gene transfer disease. Exp Clin Immunogenet 1999;16(1):1–7.
14. Cooper SM. A perspective on the use of minocycline for rheumatoid arthritis. J Clin Rheumatol 1999;5:233–6.
15. Alarcon GS. Antibiotics for rheumatoid arthritis? Minocycline shows promise in some patients. Postgrad Med 1999;105(4):95–8.
16. Attur MG, Patel RN, Patel PD, Abramson SB, Amin AR. Tetracycline up-regulates COX-2 expression and prostaglandin E2 production independent of its effect on nitric oxide. J Immunol 1999;162(6):3160–7.
17. Kloppenburg M, Breedveld FC, Terwiel JP, Mallee C, Dijkmans BA. Minocycline in active rheumatoid arthritis. A double-blind, placebo-controlled trial. Arthritis Rheum 1994;37(5):629–36.
18. O'Dell JR, Haire CE, Palmer W, Drymalski W, Wees S, Blakely K, Churchill M, Eckhoff PJ, Weaver A, Doud D, Erikson N, Dietz F, Olson R, Maloley P, Klassen LW, Moore GF. Treatment of early rheumatoid arthritis with minocycline or placebo: results of a randomized,

double-blind, placebo-controlled trial. Arthritis Rheum 1997;40(5):842–8.

19. Tilley BC, Alarcon GS, Heyse SP, Trentham DE, Neuner R, Kaplan DA, Clegg DO, Leisen JC, Buckley L, Cooper SM, Duncan H, Pillemer SR, Tuttleman M, Fowler SE. Minocycline in rheumatoid arthritis. A 48-week, double-blind, placebo-controlled trial. MIRA Trial Group. Ann Intern Med 1995;122(2):81–9.

20. Greenwald RA, Moak SA, Golub LM. Low dose doxycycline inhibits pyridinoline excretion in selected patients with rheumatoid arthritis. Ann NY Acad Sci 1994;732:419–21.

21. Astbury C, Bird HA, McLaren AM, Robins SP. Urinary excretion of pyridinium crosslinks of collagen correlated with joint damage in arthritis. Br J Rheumatol 1994;33(1):11–15.

22. Nordstrom D, Lindy O, Lauhio A, Sorsa T, Santavirta S, Konttinen YT. Anti-collagenolytic mechanism of action of doxycycline treatment in rheumatoid arthritis. Rheumatol Int 1998;17(5):175–80.

23. van der Laan W, Molenaar E, Ronday K, Verheijen J, Breedveld F, Greenwald R, Dijkmans B, TeKoppele J. Lack of effect of doxycycline on disease activity and joint damage in patients with rheumatoid arthritis. A double blind, placebo controlled trial. J Rheumatol 2001;28(9):1967–74.

24. St Clair EW, Wilkinson WE, Pisetsky DS, Sexton DJ, Drew R, Kraus VB, Greenwald RA. The effects of intravenous doxycycline therapy for rheumatoid arthritis: a randomized, double-blind, placebo-controlled trial. Arthritis Rheum 2001;44(5):1043–7.

25. Prevoo ML, van't Hof MA, Kuper HH, van Leeuwen MA, van de Putte LB, van Riel PL. Modified disease activity scores that include twenty-eight-joint counts. Development and validation in a prospective longitudinal study of patients with rheumatoid arthritis. Arthritis Rheum 1995;38(1):44–8.

26. Greenwald RA, Golub LM, Ramamurthy NS, Chowdhury M, Moak SA, Sorsa T. In vitro sensitivity of the three mammalian collagenases to tetracycline inhibition: relationship to bone and cartilage degradation. Bone 1998;22(1):33–8.

27. Yu LP Jr., Smith GN Jr., Brandt KD, Myers SL, O'Connor BL, Brandt DA. Reduction of the severity of canine osteoarthritis by prophylactic treatment with oral doxycycline. Arthritis Rheum 1992;35(10):1150–9.

28. Yu LP Jr., Smith GN Jr., Hasty KA, Brandt KD. Doxycycline inhibits type XI collagenolytic activity of extracts from human osteoarthritic cartilage and of gelatinase. J Rheumatol 1991;18(10):1450–2.

29. Golub LM, Ryan ME, Williams RC. Modulation of the host response in the treatment of periodontitis. Dent Today 1998;17(10):102–6.

30. Sorsa T, Mantyla P, Ronka H, Kallio P, Kallis GB, Lundqvist C, Kinane DF, Salo T, Golub LM, Teronen O, Tikanoja S. Scientific basis of a matrix metalloproteinase-8 specific chair-side test for monitoring periodontal and peri-implant health and disease. Ann NY Acad Sci 1999;878:130–40.

31. Garrett S, Johnson L, Drisko CH, Adams DF, Bandt C, Beiswanger B, Bogle G, Donly K, Hallmon WW, Hancock EB, Hanes P, Hawley CE, Kiger R, Killoy W, Mellonig JT, Polson A, Raab FJ, Ryder M, Stoller NH, Wang HL, Wolinsky LE, Evans GH, Harrold CQ, Arnold RM, Southard GL, et al. Two multi-center studies evaluating locally delivered doxycycline hyclate, placebo control, oral hygiene, and scaling and root planing in the treatment of periodontitis. J Periodontol 1999;70(5): 490–503.

32. Ashley RA. Clinical trials of a matrix metalloproteinase inhibitor in human periodontal disease. SDD Clinical Research Team. Ann NY Acad Sci 1999;878:335–46.

33. Meynadier J, Alirezai M. Systemic antibiotics for acne. Dermatology 1998;196(1):135–9.

34. Del Rosso JQ. A status report on the use of subantimicrobial-dose doxycycline: a review of the biologic and antimicrobial effects of the tetracyclines. Cutis 2004;74(2):118–22.

35. Huber HP, Pflugshaupt C. Akne und freie Fettsäuren im Hauttalg, Beeinflussung durch Doxycyclin. [Acne and free fatty acids in sebum, modification by doxycycline.] Schweiz Rundsch Med Prax 1990;79(20):631–2.

36. Nieman GF, Zerler BR. A role for the anti-inflammatory properties of tetracyclines in the prevention of acute lung injury. Curr Med Chem 2001;8(3):317–25.

37. Sastre Dominguez J, Sastre Castillo A, Marin Nunez F. Anafilaxia sistémica a tetraciclinas. [Systemic anaphylaxis caused by tetracyclines.] Rev Clin Esp 1984;174(3–4):135–6.

38. Golbert TM, Patterson R, Pruzansky JJ. Systemic allergic reactions to ingested antigens. J Allergy 1969;44(2):96–107.

39. Fenoglio JJ Jr., McAllister HA Jr., Mullick FG. Drug related myocarditis. I. Hypersensitivity myocarditis. Hum Pathol 1981;12(10):900–7.

40. Guillon JM, Joly P, Autran B, Denis M, Akoun G, Debre P, Mayaud C. Minocycline-induced cell-mediated hypersensitivity pneumonitis. Ann Intern Med 1992;117(6):476–81.

41. Puyana J, Urena V, Quirce S, Fernandez-Rivas M, Cuevas M, Fraj J. Serum sickness-like syndrome associated with minocycline therapy. Allergy 1990;45(4):313–15.

42. Sulkowski SR, Haserick JR. Simulated systemic lupus erythematosus from degraded tetracycline. JAMA 1964;189:152–4.

43. Zein ZA. Louse borne relapsing fever (LBRF); mortality and frequency of Jarisch–Herxheimer reaction. J R Soc Health 1987;107(4):146–7.

44. Bryceson AD, Parry EH, Perine PL, Warrell DA, Vukotich D, Leithead CS. Louse-borne relapsing fever. Q J Med 1970;39(153):129–70.

45. Perine PL, Kidan TG, Warrell DA, Bryceson AD, Parry EH. Bleeding in louse-borne relapsing fever. II. Fibrinolysis following treatment. Trans R Soc Trop Med Hyg 1971;65(6):782–7.

46. Teklu B, Habte-Michael A, Warrell DA, White NJ, Wright DJ. Meptazinol diminishes the Jarisch–Herxheimer reaction of relapsing fever. Lancet 1983;1(8329):835–9.

47. Maxon HR 3rd, Rutsky EA. Vasopressin-resistant diabetes insipidus associated with short-term demethylchlortetracycline (declomycin) therapy. Mil Med 1973;138(8):500–1.

48. Lander CM. Minocycline-induced benign intracranial hypertension. Clin Exp Neurol 1989;26:161–7.

49. Chodosh S, Baigelman W, Medici TC. Methacycline compared with ampicillin in acute bacterial exacerbations of chronic bronchitis. A double-blind cross over study. Chest 1976;69(5):587–92.

50. Golub LM, Lee HM, Lehrer G, Nemiroff A, McNamara TF, Kaplan R, Ramamurthy NS. Minocycline reduces gingival collagenolytic activity during diabetes. Preliminary observations and a proposed new mechanism of action. J Periodontal Res 1983;18(5):516–26.

51. Golub LM, McNamara TF, D'Angelo G, Greenwald RA, Ramamurthy NS. A non-antibacterial chemically-modified tetracycline inhibits mammalian collagenase activity. J Dent Res 1987;66(8):1310–14.

52. Greenwald R, Golub L. Biologic properties of non-antibiotic, chemically modified tetracyclines (CMTs): a structured, annotated bibliography. Curr Med Chem 2001;8(3):237–42.

53. Liu Y, Ramamurthy N, Marecek J, Lee HM, Chen JL, Ryan ME, Rifkin BR, Golub LM. The lipophilicity, pharmacokinetics, and cellular uptake of different chemically-modified tetracyclines (CMTs). Curr Med Chem 2001;8(3):243–52.

54. Rudek MA, Horne M, Figg WD, Dahut W, Dyer V, Pluda JM, Reed E. Reversible sideroblastic anemia associated with the tetracycline analogue COL-3 Am J Hematol 2001;67(1):51–3.

55. Ghate JV, Turner ML, Rudek MA, Figg WD, Dahut W, Dyer V, Pluda JM, Reed E. Drug-induced lupus associated with COL-3: report of 3 cases. Arch Dermatol 2001;137(4):471–4.

56. Pollen RH. Anaphylactoid reaction to orally administered demethylchlortetracycline. N Engl J Med 1964;271:673.

57. Menon MP, Das AK. Tetracycline asthma—a case report. Clin Allergy 1977;7(3):285–90.

58. Sitbon O, Bidel N, Dussopt C, Azarian R, Braud ML, Lebargy F, Fourme T, de Blay F, Piard F, Camus P. Minocycline pneumonitis and eosinophilia. A report on eight patients. Arch Intern Med 1994;154(14):1633–40.

59. Almind M, Lange P, Viskum K. Spontaneous pneumothorax: comparison of simple drainage, talc pleurodesis, and tetracycline pleurodesis. Thorax 1989;44(8):627–30.

60. Fields JP. Bulging fontanel: a complication of tetracycline therapy in infants. J Pediatr 1961;58:74–6.

61. Maroon JC, Mealy J Jr. Benign intracranial hypertension. Sequel to tetracycline therapy in a child. JAMA 1971;216(9):1479–80.

62. Rush JA. Pseudotumor cerebri: clinical profile and visual outcome in 63 patients. Mayo Clin Proc 1980;55(9):541–6.

63. Bhowmick BK. Benign intracranial hypertension after antibiotic therapy. BMJ 1972;3(817):30.

64. Meacock DJ, Hewer RL. Tetracycline and benign intracranial hypertension. BMJ (Clin Res Ed) 1981;282(6271):1240.

65. Walters BN, Gubbay SS. Tetracycline and benign intracranial hypertension: report of five cases. BMJ (Clin Res Ed) 1981;282(6257):19–20.

66. Pearson MG, Littlewood SM, Bowden AN. Tetracycline and benign intracranial hypertension. BMJ (Clin Res Ed) 1981;282(6263):568–9.

67. Koch-Weser J, Gilmore EB. Benign intracranial hypertension in an adult after tetracycline therapy. JAMA 1967;200(4):345–7.

68. Lubetzki C, Sanson M, Cohen D, Schaison-Cusin M, Lhermitte F, Lyon-Caen O. Hypertension intracrénienne bénigne et minocycline. [Benign intracranial hypertension and minocycline.] Rev Neurol (Paris) 1988;144(3):218–20.

69. Haenggeli ChA, Laufer D. Pseudotumeur cérébrale chez un jeune homme traité aux tétracyclines pour une acne. Schweiz Med Wochenschr 1990;120(Suppl 34):25.

70. Askmark H, Lundberg PO, Olsson S. Drug-related headache. Headache 1989;29(7):441–4.

71. Bezzi G, Gessa GL. Rapporti tra antibiotici e curarismo (III). Tetracicline e curarismo. [Relation between antibiotics and curarism. III. Tetracycline and curarism.] Boll Soc Ital Biol Sper 1960;36:374–5.

72. Baisset A, Lareng L, Puig G. Incidence d'une thérapeutique antibiotique sur la curarisation. In: Comptes-Rendus, XII Congrès Français d'Anesthésiologie. Montpellier; 1962:813.

73. Snavely SR, Hodges GR. The neurotoxicity of antibacterial agents. Ann Intern Med 1984;101(1):92–104.

74. Kubikowski P, Szreniawski Z. The mechanism of the neuromuscular blockade by antibiotics. Arch Int Pharmacodyn Ther 1963;146:549–60.

75. Lambs L, Venturini M, Decock-Le Reverend B, Kozlowski H, Berthon G. Metal ion–tetracycline interactions in biological fluids. Part 8. Potentiometric and spectroscopic studies on the formation of Ca(II) and Mg(II) complexes with 4-dedimethylamino-tetracycline and 6-desoxy-6-demethyl-tetracycline. J Inorg Biochem 1988;33(3):193–210.

76. Edwards TS. Transient myopia due to tetracycline. JAMA 1963;186:69–70.

77. Billano RA, Ward WQ, Little WP. Minocycline and black thyroid. JAMA 1983;249(14):1887.

78. Reid JD. The black thyroid associated with minocycline therapy. A local manifestation of a drug-induced lysosome/substrate disorder. Am J Clin Pathol 1983;79(6):738–46.

79. Korkelia J. Antianabolic effect of tetracyclines. Lancet 1971;1(7706):974–5.

80. Morgan T, Ribush N. The effect of oxytetracycline and doxycycline on protein metabolism. Med J Aust 1972;1(2):55–8.

81. Seltzer HS. Drug-induced hypoglycemia. A review based on 473 cases. Diabetes 1972;21(9):955–66.

82. Garbitelli VP. Tetracycline reduces the need for insulin. NY State J Med 1987;87(10):576.

83. Simpson MB, Pryzbylik J, Innis B, Denham MA. Hemolytic anemia after tetracycline therapy. N Engl J Med 1985;312(13):840–2.

84. Kounis NG. Oxytetracycline-induced thrombocytopenic purpura. JAMA 1975;231(7):734–5.

85. Abou-Rass M. Long-term prognosis of intentional endodontics and internal bleaching of tetracycline-stained teeth. Compend Contin Educ Dent 1998;19(10):1034–8, 1040–2, 1044.

86. Leonard RH Jr. Efficacy, longevity, side effects, and patient perceptions of nightguard vital bleaching. Compend Contin Educ Dent 1998;19(8):766–70, 772, 774.

87. Sadan A, Lemon RR. Combining treatment modalities for tetracycline-discolored teeth. Int J Periodontics Restorative Dent 1998;18(6):564–71.

88. Topoll HH, Lange DE, Muller RF. Multiple periodontal abscesses after systemic antibiotic therapy. J Clin Periodontol 1990;17(4):268–72.

89. Baeriswyl G, Bengoa J, de Peyer R, Loizeau E. Importance des ulcérations médicamenteuses dans les lésions endoscopiques de l'oesophage. [Importance of drug-induced ulceration in endoscopic lesions of the esophagus.] Schweiz Med Wochenschr Suppl 1985;19:6–9.

90. Bonavina L, DeMeester TR, McChesney L, Schwizer W, Albertucci M, Bailey RT. Drug-induced esophageal strictures. Ann Surg 1987;206(2):173–83.

91. Zijnen-Suyker MP, Hazenberg BP. Oesophagusbeschadiging door doxycycline. [Esophageal lesions caused by doxycycline.] Ned Tijdschr Geneeskd 1981;125(35):1407–10.

92. Schneider R. Doxycycline esophageal ulcers. Am J Dig Dis 1977;22(9):805–7.

93. Crowson TD, Head LH, Ferrante WA. Esophageal ulcers associated with tetracycline therapy. JAMA 1976;235(25):2747–8.

94. Champel V, Jonville-Bera AP, Bera F, Autret E. Les tétracyclines peuvent être responsables d'ulcérations oesophagiennes si leur prise est incorrecte. Rev Prat Med Gen 1998;12:9–10.

95. Huizar JF, Podolsky I, Goldberg J. Ulceras esofagicas inducidas por doxiciclina. [Doxycycline-induced esophageal ulcers.] Rev Gastroenterol Mex 1998;63(2):101–5.

96. Pantell RH, Goodman BW Jr. Adolescent chest pain: a prospective study. Pediatrics 1983;71(6):881–7.

97. Selbst SM, Ruddy RM, Clark BJ, Henretig FM, Santulli T Jr. Pediatric chest pain: a prospective study. Pediatrics 1988;82(3):319–23.

98. Zavaras-Angelidou KA, Weinhouse E, Nelson DB. Review of 180 episodes of chest pain in 134 children. Pediatr Emerg Care 1992;8(4):189–93.

99. Kobler E, Nuesch HJ, Buhler H, Jenny S, Deyhle P. Medikamentös bedingte Oesophagusulzera. [Drug-induced esophageal ulcers.] Schweiz Med Wochenschr 1979;109(32):1180–2.

100. Dowling HF, Lepper MH. Hepatic reactions to tetracycline. JAMA 1964;188:307–9.

101. Peters RL, Edmondson HA, Mikkelsen WP, Tatter D. Tetracycline-induced fatty liver in nonpregnant patients. A report of six cases. Am J Surg 1967;113(5):622–32.

102. Burette A, Finet C, Prigogine T, De Roy G, Deltenre M. Acute hepatic injury associated with minocycline. Arch Intern Med 1984;144(7):1491–2.

103. Burette A, Finet C, Prigogine T, De Roy G, Deltenre M. Acute hepatic injury associated with minocycline. Arch Intern Med 1984;144(7):1491–2.

104. Hunt CM, Washington K. Tetracycline-induced bile duct paucity and prolonged cholestasis. Gastroenterology 1994;107(6):1844–7.

105. Schrumpf E, Nordgard K. Unusual cholestatic hepatotoxicity of doxycycline in a young male. Scand J Gastroenterol 1986;21(Suppl 120):68.

106. Bjornsson E, Lindberg J, Olsson R. Liver reactions to oral low-dose tetracyclines. Scand J Gastroenterol 1997;32(4):390–5.

107. Elmore MF, Rogge JD. Tetracycline-induced pancreatitis. Gastroenterology 1981;81(6):1134–6.

108. Gant NF Jr., Whalley PJ, Baxter CR. Nonoliguric renal failure. Report of a case. Obstet Gynecol 1969;34(5):675–9.

109. Walker RG, Thomson NM, Dowling JP, Ogg CS. Minocycline-induced acute interstitial nephritis. BMJ 1979;1(6162):524.

110. Wilkinson SP, Stewart WK, Spiers EM, Pears J. Protracted systemic illness and interstitial nephritis due to minocycline. Postgrad Med J 1989;65(759):53–6.

111. Murray KM, Keane WR. Review of drug-induced acute interstitial nephritis. Pharmacotherapy 1992;12(6):462–7.

112. Carrilho F, Bosch J, Arroyo V, Mas A, Viver J, Rodes J. Renal failure associated with demeclocycline in cirrhosis. Ann Intern Med 1977;87(2):195–7.

113. Miller PD, Linas SL, Schrier RW. Plasma demeclocycline levels and nephrotoxicity. Correlation in hyponatremic cirrhotic patients. JAMA 1980;243(24):2513–15.

114. Geheb M, Cox M. Renal effects of demeclocycline. JAMA 1980;243(24):2519–20.

115. Zegers de Beyl D, Naeije R, de Troyer A. Demeclocycline treatment of water retention in congestive heart failure. BMJ 1978;1(6115):760.

116. Kunin CM, Rees SB, Merrill JP, Finland M. Persistence of antibiotics in blood of patients with acute renal failure. I. Tetracycline and chlortetracycline. J Clin Invest 1959;38:1487–97.

117. Carey BW. Abnormal urinary findings and Achromycin V. Pediatrics 1963;31:697.

118. Lowe MB, Obst D, Tapp E. Renal damage caused by anhydro 4-EPI-tetracycline. Arch Pathol 1966;81(4):362–4.

119. Cherrill DA, Stote RM, Birge JR, Singer I. Demeclocycline treatment in the syndrome of inappropriate antidiuretic hormone secretion. Ann Intern Med 1975;83(5):654–6.

120. Forrest JN Jr., Cox M, Hong C, Morrison G, Bia M, Singer I. Superiority of demeclocycline over lithium in the treatment of chronic syndrome of inappropriate secretion of antidiuretic hormone. N Engl J Med 1978;298(4):173–7.

121. Singer I, Rotenberg D. Demeclocycline-induced nephrogenic diabetes insipidus. In-vivo and in-vitro studies. Ann Intern Med 1973;79(5):679–83.

122. De Troyer A, Pilloy W, Broeckaert I, Demanet JC. Correction of antidiuresis by demeclocycline. N Engl J Med 1975;293(18):915–18.

123. Troyer A, Pilloy W, Broeckaert I, Demanet JC. Letter: Demeclocycline treatment of water retention in cirrhosis. Ann Intern Med 1976;85(3):336–7.

124. Bihorac A, Ozener C, Akoglu E, Kullu S. Tetracycline-induced acute interstitial nephritis as a cause of acute renal failure. Nephron 1999;81(1):72–5.

125. Jones HE, Lewis CW, Reisner JE. Photosensitive lichenoid eruption associated with demeclocycline. Arch Dermatol 1972;106(1):58–63.

126. Frank SB, Cohen HJ, Minkin W. Photo-onycholysis due to tetracycline hydrochloride and doxycycline. Arch Dermatol 1971;103(5):520–1.

127. Frost P, Weinstein GD, Gomez EC. Phototoxic potential of minocycline and doxycycline. Arch Dermatol 1972;105(5):681–3.

128. Epstein JH, Tuffanelli DL, Seibert JS, Epstein WL. Porphyria-like cutaneous changes induced by tetracycline hydrochloride photosensitization. Arch Dermatol 1976;112(5):661–6.

129. Fenske NA, Millns JL, Greer KE. Minocycline-induced pigmentation at sites of cutaneous inflammation. JAMA 1980;244(10):1103–6.

130. Butler JM, Marks R, Sutherland R. Cutaneous and cardiac valvular pigmentation with minocycline. Clin Exp Dermatol 1985;10(5):432–7.

131. Shum DT, Smout MS, Pace WE, Headington JT. Unusual skin pigmentation from long-term methacycline and minocycline therapy. Arch Dermatol 1986;122(1):17–18.

132. Arndt KA, Jick H. Rates of cutaneous reactions to drugs. A report from the Boston Collaborative Drug Surveillance Program. JAMA 1976;235(9):918–23.

133. Shelley WB, Heaton CL. Minocycline sensitivity. JAMA 1973;224(1):125–6.

134. Fawcett IW, Pepys J. Allergy to a tetracycline preparation—a case report. Clin Allergy 1976;6(3):301–4.

135. Shoji A, Someda Y, Hamada T. Stevens–Johnson syndrome due to minocycline therapy. Arch Dermatol 1987;123(1):18–20.

136. Curley RK, Verbov JL. Stevens–Johnson syndrome due to tetracyclines—a case report (doxycycline) and review of the literature. Clin Exp Dermatol 1987;12(2):124–5.

137. Trueb RM, Burg G. Acute generalized exanthematous pustulosis due to doxycycline. Dermatology 1993;186(1):75–8.

138. Fiumara NJ, Yaqub M. Pigmented penile lesions (fixed drug eruptions) associated with tetracycline therapy for sexually transmitted diseases. Sex Transm Dis 1981;8(1):23–5.

139. Pasricha JS. Drugs causing fixed eruptions. Br J Dermatol 1979;100(2):183–5.

140. Kanwar AJ, Bharija SC, Singh M, Belhaj MS. Ninety-eight fixed drug eruptions with provocation tests. Dermatologica 1988;177(5):274–9.

141. Domz CA, McNamara DH, Holzapfel HF. Tetracycline provocation in lupus erythematosus. Ann Intern Med 1959;50(5):1217–26.

142. Bojs G, Moller H. Eczematous contact allergy to oxytetracycline with cross-sensitivity to other tetracyclines. Berufsdermatosen 1974;22(5):202–8.

143. Mahaur BS, Sharma VK, Kumar B, Kaur S. Prevalence of contact hypersensitivity to common antiseptics, antibacterials and antifungals in normal persons. Indian. J Dermatol Venerol Leprol 1987;53:269.

144. Burton J. A placebo-controlled study to evaluate the efficacy of topical tetracycline and oral tetracycline in the treatment of mild to moderate acne. Dermatology Research Group. J Int Med Res 1990;18(2):94–103.

145. Gaffoor PM, George WM. Fixed drug eruptions occurring on the male genitals. Cutis 1990;45(4):242–4.

146. Samman PD. The nails: onchylosis. In: Rook A, Wilkinson DS, Ebling FJG, editors. Textbook of

Dermatology. Oxford: Blackwell Scientific Publications; 1972;1647.

147. Rall DP, Loo TL, Lane M, Kelly MG. Appearance and persistence of fluorescent material in tumor tissue after tetracycline administration. J Natl Cancer Inst 1957;19(1):79–85.

148. Totterman LE, Saxen L. Incorporation of tetracycline into human foetal bones after maternal drug administration. Acta Obstet Gynecol Scand 1969;48(4):542–9.

149. Cohlan SQ, Bevelander G, Tiamsic T. Growth inhibition of prematures receiving tetracycline. Am J Dis Child 1963;105:453.

150. Kaitila I, Wartiovaara J, Laitinen O, Saxen L. The inhibitory effect of tetracycline on osteogenesis in organ culture. J Embryol Exp Morphol 1970;23(1):185–211.

151. Gilgor RS. Complications of tetracycline therapy for acne. N C Med J 1972;33(4):331–3.

152. Csonka GW, Rosedale N, Walkden L. Balanitis due to fixed drug eruption associated with tetracycline therapy. Br J Vener Dis 1971;47(1):42–4.

153. Elsner P, Hartmann AA, Burg G. Erfahrungen mit der Oxytetrazyklin-Therapie der nicht-gonorrhoischen Urethritis durch *Ureaplasma urealyticum*. [Experiences with oxytetracycline treatment of non-gonorrhea urethritis caused by *Ureaplasma urealyticum*.] Hautarzt 1990;41(2):94–7.

154. Crook LD, Tempest B. Plague. A clinical review of 27 cases. Arch Intern Med 1992;152(6):1253–6.

155. Jones RB, Van der Pol B, Martin DH, Shepard MK. Partial characterization of *Chlamydia trachomatis* isolates resistant to multiple antibiotics. J Infect Dis 1990;162(6):1309–15.

156. Ling JM, Khin-Thi-Oo H, Hui YW, French GL. Antimicrobial susceptibilities of *Haemophilus* species in Hong Kong. J Infect 1989;19(2):135–42.

157. Schlapfer G, Eichmann A. Penicillinaseproduzierende Stamme von N. gonorrhoeae (PPNG) im Raume Zurich, 1981–1988: Häufigkeit antibiotische Empfindlichkeit und Plasmidprofil (3. Mitteilung). [Penicillinase-producing strains of N. gonorrhoeae (PPNG) in the Zurich area, 1981–1988: incidence, antibiotic sensitivity and plasmid profile (3).] Schweiz Med Wochenschr 1990;120(4):92–7.

158. McColl JD, Globus M, Robinson S. Effect of some therapeutic agents on the developing rat fetus. Toxicol Appl Pharmacol 1965;11:409–17.

159. Krejci L, Brettschneider I. Congenital cataract due to tetracycline. Animal experiments and clinical observation. Ophthalmic Paediatr Genet 1983;3:59–60.

160. Mennie AT. Tetracycline and congenital limb abnormalities BMJ 1962;2:480.

161. Skosyreva AM. [Comparative evaluation of the embryotoxic effect of various antibiotics.] Antibiot Khimioter 1989;34(10):779–82.

162. Krejci L, Brettschneider I. Congenital cataract due to tetracycline. Ophthalmic Paediatr Genet 1983;3:59.

163. Czeizel AE, Rockenbauer M. A population-based case-control teratologic study of oral oxytetracycline treatment during pregnancy. Eur J Obstet Gynecol Reprod Biol 2000;88(1):27–33.

164. Czeizel AE, Rockenbauer M. Teratogenic study of doxycycline. Obstet Gynecol 1997;89(4):524–8.

165. Anthony JR. Effect on deciduous and permanent teeth of tetracycline deposition in utero. Postgrad Med 1970;48(4):165–8.

166. Seeliger HP, Ronde G. Die Wirkung von Tetracyclin-gaben auf das kindliche Gebiss bei Listeriosebehandlung von Schwangeren. [Effect of tetracycline administration on the child's dentition in the treatment of listeriosis in pregnant women.] Geburtshilfe Frauenheilkd 1968;28(3): 209–23.

167. Briggs GG, Freeman RK, Yaffe SJ. Drugs in Pregnancy and Lactation. 2nd ed. Baltimore, MD: Williams and Wilkins, 1986.

168. Charles D, Obst D. Placental transmission of antibiotics. J Obstet Gynaecol Br Emp 1954;61(6):750–7.

169. Witkop CJ Jr., Wolf RO. Hypoplasia and intrinsic staining of enamel following tetracycline therapy. JAMA 1963;185:1008–11.

170. Poliak SC, DiGiovanna JJ, Gross EG, Gantt G, Peck GL. Minocycline-associated tooth discoloration in young adults. JAMA 1985;254(20):2930–2.

171. Ruckdeschel JC, Moores D, Lee JY, Einhorn LH, Mandelbaum I, Koeller J, Weiss GR, Losada M, Keller JH. Intrapleural therapy for malignant pleural effusions. A randomized comparison of bleomycin and tetracycline. Chest 1991;100(6):1528–35.

172. Martinez-Moragon E, Aparicio J, Rogado MC, Sanchis J, Sanchis F, Gil-Suay V. Pleurodesis in malignant pleural effusions: a randomized study of tetracycline versus bleomycin. Eur Respir J 1997;10(10):2380–3.

173. Walker-Renard PB, Vaughan LM, Sahn SA. Chemical pleurodesis for malignant pleural effusions. Ann Intern Med 1994;120(1):56–64.

174. Neuvonen PJ, Gothoni G, Hackman R, Bjorksten K. Interference of iron with the absorption of tetracyclines in man. BMJ 1970;4(734):532–4.

175. Gothoni G, Neuvonen PJ, Mattila M, Hackman R. Iron–tetracycline interaction: effect of time interval between the drugs. Acta Med Scand 1972;191(5):409–11.

176. Albert KS, Welch RD, DeSante KA, DiSanto AR. Decreased tetracycline bioavailability caused by a bismuth subsalicylate antidiarrheal mixture. J Pharm Sci 1979;68(5):586–8.

177. Ericsson CD, Feldman S, Pickering LK, Cleary TG. Influence of subsalicylate bismuth on absorption of doxycycline. JAMA 1982;247(16):2266–7.

178. Koch-Weser J, Sellers EM. Drug interactions with coumarin anticoagulants. Part I. N Engl J Med 1971;285:487.

179. Westfall LK, Mintzer DL, Wiser TH. Potentiation of warfarin by tetracycline. Am J Hosp Pharm 1980;37(12):1620.

180. Danos EA. Apparent potentiation of warfarin activity by tetracycline. Clin Pharm 1992;11(9):806–8.

181. Caraco Y, Rubinow A. Enhanced anticoagulant effect of coumarin derivatives induced by doxycycline coadministration. Ann Pharmacother 1992;26(9):1084–6.

182. Chiavazza F, Merialdi A. Sulle interferenze fra dicumarolo ed antibiotici. [Interference between dicoumarol and antibiotics.] Minerva Ginecol 1973;25(11):630–1.

183. Searcy RL, Simms NM, Foreman JA, Bergquist LM. Evaluation of the blood-clotting mechanism in tetracycline-treated patients. Antimicrobial Agents Chemother 1964;10:179–83.

184. Boston Collaborative Drug Surveillance Program. Tetracycline and drug-attributed rises in blood urea nitrogen. JAMA 1972;220(3):377–9.

185. Albers DD, Leverett CL, Sandin JH. Renal failure following prostatovesiculectomy related to methoxyflurane anesthesia and tetracycline—complicated by *Candida infection*. J Urol 1971;106(3):348–50.

186. Kuzucu EY. Methoxyflurane, tetracycline, and renal failure. JAMA 1970;211(7):1162–4.

187. Proctor EA, Barton FL. Polyuric acute renal failure after methoxyflurane and tetracycline. BMJ 1971;4(788):661–2.

188. Steele M, Couturier J. A possible tetracycline–risperidone–sertraline interaction in an adolescent. Can J Clin Pharmacol 1999;6(1):15–17.

189. Csik V, Molnar J. Possible adverse interaction between clozapine and ampicillin in an adolescent with schizophrenia. J Child Adolesc Psychopharmacol 1994;4:123–8.

190. Hauser RA, Zesiewicz TA. Sertraline-induced exacerbation of tics in Tourette's syndrome. Mov Disord 1995;10(5):682–4.

Tetryzoline

General Information

Tetryzoline, an alpha-adrenoceptor agonist with vaso-constrictor and decongestant properties, is widely available without prescription for symptomatic relief of "pink eye" and is found in various products in a concentration of 0.05%.

Susceptibility Factors

Age

Tetryzoline eye-drops are considered to be safe when used appropriately. However, relatively small amounts can produce profound central nervous depression and can lead to serious toxicity, especially in children under 2 years of age. A Poison Center reported 64 cases of tetryzoline poisoning over a period of 3 years; ingestions accounted for 59 cases, but three were attributable to administration into the eye, ear, or nose (1).

Reference

1. Klein-Schwartz W, Gorman R, Oderda GM, Baig A. Central nervous system depression from ingestion of nonprescription eyedrops. Am J Emerg Med 1984;2(3):217–18.

Tezosentan

See also Endothelin receptor antagonists

General Information

Tezosentan is a dual endothelin-A and endothelin-B receptor antagonist. Its common adverse effects include headaches, nausea, and hypotension compared with placebo (1).

Organs and Systems

Nervous system

Tezosentan has been studied in single intravenous doses of 5, 20, 50, 100, 200, 400, and 600 mg for 1 hour in sequential groups of six men in a randomized, placebo-controlled, double-blind design (2). Headache was the most frequently reported adverse event and it was more common than with placebo at doses of 100 mg and over. There were no clinically important changes in vital signs, electrocardiography, or clinical laboratory tests. The volume of distribution at steady state, about 16 liters, and the clearance, 30 l/hour, were independent of dose. Endothelin-1 concentrations increased dose- and concentration-dependently and returned slowly to baseline after the end of the infusion.

During chronic double-blind, placebo-controlled infusion in healthy men, tezosentan 100 mg/hour for 6 hours in six subjects (total dose 600 mg) and 5 mg/hour for 72 hours in eight subjects (total dose 360 mg), headache was the most common adverse event (75–100% with tezosentan and 50% with placebo) (3).

References

1. Tovar JM, Gums JG. Tezosentan in the treatment of acute heart failure. Ann Pharmacother 2003;37(12):1877–83.
2. Dingemanse J, Clozel M, van Giersbergen PL. Entry-into-humans study with tezosentan, an intravenous dual endothelin receptor antagonist. J Cardiovasc Pharmacol 2002;39(6):795–802.
3. Dingemanse J, Clozel M, van Giersbergen PL. Pharmacokinetics and pharmacodynamics of tezosentan, an intravenous dual endothelin receptor antagonist, following chronic infusion in healthy subjects. Br J Clin Pharmacol 2002;53(4):355–62.

Thalidomide

General Information

Thalidomide was synthesized in 1953 by Wilhelm Kunz and Herbert Keller, working for Chemie Grünenthal. Kunz was preparing a series of peptides for antibiotic synthesis and in doing so isolated a non-peptide by-product, which Keller recognized as an analogue of the hypnotic glutethimide. They prepared a series of further analogues, one of which was thalidomide. It was introduced as a hypnotic in the late 1950s, as a supposedly safe sedative for children and pregnant women. Besides West Germany, Great Britain was the only country in which formulations containing thalidomide were sold on a large scale during the period 1959–60 inclusive. Following the discovery of its major teratogenic effects, thalidomide was withdrawn from the market in the early 1960s.

Modern uses

Since its withdrawal, thalidomide has been found to be effective in the treatment of erythema nodosum leprosum, and in 1997 it was marketed in the USA for this indication. The mechanism of action of thalidomide is still unclear (1,2), but it has many anti-inflammatory and immunomodulatory actions in vitro and in vivo (3,4).

In dermatological practice, thalidomide has also been used to treat patients with various diseases that are unresponsive to conventional therapy. Among these are aphthous stomatitis, Behçet's disease, discoid and systemic lupus erythematosus, uremic pruritus, actinic prurigo, prurigo nodularis, sarcoidosis, adult Langerhans cell histiocytosis, erosive lichen planus, and pyoderma gangrenosum (5). There has also been research on a possible antineoplastic action of thalidomide (6), which may be produced via antiangiogenic effects or direct effects on tumor cells, such as induction of apoptosis or G1 arrest of the cell cycle, inhibition of growth factor production, regulation of interactions between tumor and stromal cells, modulation of tumor immunity, modulation of adhesion molecules, and inhibition of cyclooxygenase type 2 (7,8). The malignancies in which thalidomide has been used include multiple myeloma, glioblastoma multiforme, renal cell carcinoma, and malignant melanoma.

The use of thalidomide in dermatology is based on its immunomodulatory properties. In vitro it inhibits leukocyte chemotaxis and reduces phagocytosis by monocytes and polymorphonuclear leukocytes, without signs of cytotoxicity (9,10). The production of TNF-alpha in human monocytes is selectively inhibited by enhanced degradation of TNF-alpha messenger RNA (11). In phytohemagglutinin-activated cultures of peripheral blood mononuclear cells the production of interleukin-4 and interleukin-5 (cytokines for type 2 T helper cells) is enhanced, while interferon-gamma production is inhibited by thalidomide (12). Its antiangiogenic activity is probably the cause of its teratogenic effects (13). There is evidence that angiogenesis is increased in multiple myeloma and that thalidomide is active in refractory myeloma (14). In organ bath experiments thalidomide antagonizes the actions of histamine, 5-hydroxytryptamine, acetylcholine, and prostaglandins; neither the mechanisms nor the clinical relevance of these effects is known (15).

Stereopharmacology of thalidomide

Thalidomide is given in a racemic mixture of its two enantiomers, R-thalidomide and S-thalidomide; the former is responsible for its hypnotic effects and the latter for its immunomodulatory and teratogenic effects (16).

Formulations

The full chemical name of thalidomide is α-(N-phthalimido)glutarimide or N-(2,6-dioxopiperid-3-yl)phthalimide. It has been marketed under a wide variety of brand names, including Contergan, Distaval, Glutanon, Hippuzon, Isomin, Kedavon, Kevadon, Neurosedine, Neurosedyn, Proban M, Sedalis, Softenon, Telagan, and Telargon. It has also been used in combination with various other drugs, for example in the proprietary combinations Tensival, Valgraine (with ergotamine tartrate), and Asmaval (with ephedrine).

The development of an intravenous formulation of rac-thalidomide is problematic, because of its poor solubility and rapid degradation in aqueous media (17). However, a chemically stable solution of the separate enantiomers of thalidomide for intravenous infusion has been described.

Pharmacokinetics

Thalidomide is slowly absorbed after oral administration; after an oral dose of 100 mg the t_{max} is 2–4 hours and the C_{max} is around 1 µg/ml (16). At larger doses its poor solubility in intestinal fluids reduces its rate of absorption even further. Co-administration with a high-fat meal causes small (<10%) changes in the AUC and C_{max} but prolongs the t_{max} markedly, to about 6 hours (18).

Thalidomide is slowly and variably absorbed after rectal administration (19). The mean availability of several formulations relative to oral administration was less than 40%.

The two enantiomers of thalidomide, R and S, undergo fast chiral interconversion at physiological pH (16). The apparent clearance rates in adults are 10 l/hour for R-thalidomide and 21 l/hour for S-thalidomide; however, each has a half-life of about 5 hours, implying different volumes of distribution (70 liters for the R-enantiomer and 150 liters for the S-enantiomer). Because of rapid interconversion, administration of R-thalidomide alone as a hypnotic would not avoid the teratogenic affects of S-thalidomide. Thalidomide does not induce its own metabolism. Its plasma protein binding is low.

The clearance of thalidomide is not altered in hepatic disease or in renal insufficiency, but hemodialysis increases it two-fold (20). Very small amounts of hydroxylated metabolites are detected in the blood and urine.

General adverse effects

Aside from teratogenicity, the main adverse effects of thalidomide include somnolence, dizziness, fatigue, tremor, rash, constipation, and edema. Although these adverse effects are generally mild and reversible, more severe adverse effects, such as peripheral neuropathy, deep vein thrombosis, and neutropenia, have occasionally been reported.

Organs and Systems

Cardiovascular

Bradycardia, hypotension, orthostatic hypotension, and dizziness have been reported with thalidomide; these effects may have been due to its central sedative effects or to vasovagal activation (21).

Of 96 patients taking thalidomide 52 had a heart rate below 60/minute at some time during follow-up and 10 developed symptomatic bradycardia; the symptoms abated with reduction of the dose in most cases (22).

Diabetic microvascular disease has been attributed to thalidomide (23).

- A 57-year-old man with type I diabetes mellitus started taking thalidomide after failed stem cell transplantation for multiple myeloma and after 10 months developed a sensory neuropathy with loss of pain sensation and ischemic changes in the legs.

The authors suggested that the antiangiogenic properties of thalidomide were implicated in the pathogenesis of diabetic foot disease in this patient.

Thromboembolic disease
DoTS classification (BMJ 2003;327:1222–5)
  Adverse effect: Deep venous thrombosis with thalidomide
  Dose-relation: collateral effect
  Time-course: intermediate
  Susceptibility factors: genetic; diseases (multiple myeloma, lupus erythematosus); drugs (chemotherapy, especially doxorubicin; darbepoetin)

Deep venous thrombosis is a common complication of thalidomide, especially when it is used in combination with chemotherapy and in patients with multiple myeloma (24–26).

Arterial thrombosis has also been reported. Of 23 patients with myeloma who took thalidomide 150 mg/day for 142 patient-months there were seven cases of thrombosis, five venous and two arterial; in a historical control group of 18 similar patients who did not take thalidomide there was only one case over 289 months (26,27).

Incidence

Of 50 patients with multiple myeloma, 14 developed a deep venous thrombosis after taking thalidomide 400 mg/day, compared with two of 50 patients who did not take it (24) All the episodes occurred during the first 3 cycles of therapy. One patient taking thalidomide had a pulmonary embolus. Most of the patients continued to take thalidomide with the addition of low molecular weight heparin followed by warfarin and there was no progression of deep venous thrombosis.

Of 23 men with advanced androgen-dependent prostatic cancer who received docetaxel alone, none developed a venous thrombosis, compared with nine of 47 men who received docetaxel + thalidomide (28).

Susceptibility factors

The risk of thrombosis from thalidomide may be increased in certain conditions, such as malignancies, cicatricial pemphigoid (29), and systemic lupus erythematosus. Four episodes of thrombosis (two arterial, two venous) occurred in three patients with systemic lupus erythematosus and one with severe atopic dermatitis within 10 weeks of starting treatment with thalidomide 50–100 mg/day (30). All four had at least one risk factor for thrombosis, but none had thrombosis before or after treatment with thalidomide.

The incidence of deep venous thrombosis is increased by the co-administration of doxorubicin, as suggested by a study in 232 patients with multiple myeloma who received a combination of thalidomide and chemotherapy in two protocols that differed only by the inclusion of doxorubicin in one: DT-PACE (dexamethasone + thalidomide + cisplatin + doxorubicin + cyclophosphamide + etoposide) and DCEP-T (dexamethasone + cyclophosphamide + etoposide + cisplatin + thalidomide) (25). There was an increased risk of deep venous thrombosis in those who received DT-PACE but not in those who received DCEP-T. Multivariate analysis confirmed that those who received thalidomide + doxorubicin had an increased risk of deep venous thrombosis. In two separate trials in patients taking thalidomide for multiple myeloma, deep venous thrombosis occurred in four of 15 patients who received concomitant treatment with doxorubicin + dexamethasone compared with three of 45 who received dexamethasone only (26).

Of 535 patients who received thalidomide with or without cytostatic chemotherapy, 82 developed a deep venous thrombosis (31). Multivariate analysis showed that the combination of thalidomide with chemotherapy that contained doxorubicin was associated with the highest odds ratio (OR = 4.3). Newly diagnosed disease (OR = 2.5) and chromosome 11 abnormalities (OR = 1.8) were also

independent predictors. After a median period of 2.9 years, survival was worse in those with chromosome 13 abnormalities, aged over 60 years, with a raised lactate dehydrogenase activity, and a raised serum creatinine concentration.

Three episodes of thrombosis occurred in patients who had taken thalidomide (25–100 mg/day) for up to 2 years (32). However, all had other risk factors (heterozygous protein C resistance in one and surgical intervention or trauma in the others), so a causal role of thalidomide was debatable.

In a trial of thalidomide in Behçet's disease there was superficial thrombophlebitis in 10 of 32 patients taking thalidomide 100 mg/day, two of 31 patients taking thalidomide 300 mg/day, and three of 32 patients taking placebo (33). The fact that this apparent increase in the incidence of thrombophlebitis in those taking 100 mg/day was not reproduced at the higher dosage suggests that the effect occurred by chance.

Management

Of 256 patients with myeloma randomized to thalidomide or not, 221 received no prophylactic anticoagulation and 35 received low-dose warfarin 1 mg/day (31). The incidence of deep venous thrombosis was higher in those who took thalidomide (hazard ratio 4.5). Warfarin did not reduce the risk, and prophylactic subcutaneous enoxaparin 40 mg/day was therefore introduced in 68 patients of a subsequent group of 130 patients who received thalidomide. This intervention eliminated the difference in the incidence of deep venous thrombosis between those who took thalidomide and those who did not.

Pulmonary hypertension

Pulmonary hypertension has been reported in one patient taking thalidomide (34).

- A 51-year-old man with multiple myeloma and a history of cardiovascular disease took thalidomide 100 mg/day and developed reversible pulmonary hypertension (pulmonary artery pressure 70 mmHg) with normal mitral valve and left ventricular function. After withdrawal of thalidomide for 2 months the pulmonary artery pressure fell to 47 mmHg. Rechallenge with a lower dose of thalidomide was again associated with a rise in pulmonary artery pressure.

Respiratory

In some early cases an increased incidence of asthmatic attacks was reported by asthmatic patients (35).

- A 65-year-old man with IgG multiple myeloma was given thalidomide and after 37 days developed acute cough, sweating, general malaise, and dyspnea at rest (36). There was an interstitial and alveolar pattern on the right side of a chest X-ray and arterial blood gases showed partial respiratory insufficiency (pH 7.40, PaCO$_2$ 40 mmHg, PaO$_2$ 47 mmHg). Microbiology was negative (sputum and blood cultures and urinary antigen detection for *Streptococcus pneumoniae* and *Legionella pneumophila*). He recovered when thalidomide was withdrawn and oxygen and intravenous glucocorticoids were given. A chest X-ray and arterial blood gases were normal 4 days later.

Nervous system

Somnolence is very common in patients taking thalidomide, and headache, dizziness, paresthesia, and peripheral neuropathy are common. Stupor, coma, and seizures have also been reported (21). The sedative effect possibly occurs through activation of the sleep center in the brainstem. However, even when it is taken in large doses, thalidomide is not associated with lack of coordination or respiratory depression (3).

In patients with leprosy, HIV infection, and multiple myeloma, the incidences of somnolence, fatigue, and weakness were 36–43%, 48%, and 6–22% respectively (21). Administration of thalidomide at bedtime minimizes appreciation of the drowsiness that it produces, and daytime drowsiness usually abates over several weeks.

Stupor has been reported in six patients with advanced refractory malignancies, complicated by severe weakness, anemia, nausea, vomiting, and dehydration, or tumor lysis syndrome with renal insufficiency; three developed fever, neutropenia, sepsis, and/or pneumonia, but the contribution of thalidomide was uncertain (21).

Seizures, including generalized tonic-clonic seizures, have been reported in patients taking thalidomide, 18 during the first 18 months of its availability in the USA; there was a past history of seizures or pre-existing nervous system disease in 11 (21).

Polyneuropathy
DoTS classification (BMJ 2003;327:1222–5)
Adverse effect: Polyneuropathy with thalidomide
Dose-relation: Collateral reaction
Time-course: Long-term
Susceptibility factors: sex (women more susceptible); age (elderly people more susceptible)

A chronic polyneuropathy was described soon after thalidomide was introduced. It is predominantly sensory, affecting distal nerves. Anatomically the lesion is a degeneration of the axis cylinder (37).

Mechanism
In six patients with multiple myeloma who developed a thalidomide-induced sensory polyneuropathy, spinal cord MRI showed high-signal intensity in the posterior columns in only one patient, with abnormal central conduction time at somatosensory-evoked potentials (38). These results suggest that thalidomide can induce either an axonal length-dependent neuropathy or, less often, a ganglionopathy.

Clinical features
The common symptoms are tingling of the hands, gradually increasing sensory disturbances, and finally motor disturbances, usually of the hands, although only after thalidomide has been taken over a lengthy period. A positive Babinsky reflex and disturbed vibration sense have also been reported (39). Unless the drug is discontinued promptly at the start of symptoms the polyneuropathy can be irreversible (40,41).

In 35 patients with polyneuropathy, mostly of the sensory type, which occurred after about 9 months of ingestion of thalidomide 100–200 mg/day, the principal symptoms were paresthesia and distal sensory disturbances in the feet. Withdrawal of the drug led to partial improvement, but complete resolution was not observed (42–45).

In 114 patients with thalidomide polyneuropathy other features included toxic psychosis, amnesic and aphasic symptoms, cerebellar syndromes, and autonomic dysfunction. An attempt was made to relate thalidomide toxicity to daily or total dose and duration of therapy but no association was found. The severity of the polyneuropathy was related to the age of the patient (46).

In 22 patients with thalidomide polyneuropathy, who were followed for 4–6 years after withdrawal, the symptoms and signs remained unchanged in 50% and improved in 25%; the rest recovered. Improvement was usually slow, and in some patients did not begin for 3 years (47).

- A 68-year-old woman took 20 tablets of thalidomide per month for 6 months and developed a severe peripheral neuropathy, which persisted for 3 years. Electromyography showed irreversible damage to several nerve trunks (48).

The distinguishing features of thalidomide polyneuropathy and of leprous polyneuropathy have been described. In thalidomide polyneuropathy the longest nerve fibers are affected first and the condition progressively involves fibers of decreasing length. Thus, the upper border of sensory loss in the limbs is roughly the same distance from the dorsal root ganglion cells; this can be estimated using a tape measure. Loss of tendon reflexes is also characteristic. In leprous polyneuropathy, the cells first affected are those in the coolest tissues, as *Mycobacterium leprae* is temperature-sensitive. This leads to the early involvement of the lobes of the ears, the nose, and the digits. Typically, deep reflexes are preserved (49).

Restlessness, agitation, queer sensations, difficulty in memorizing (40), and vertigo and convulsions (50) have also been reported. In nearly all cases there was a concomitant polyneuropathy. Muscle weakness or cramps, mild ataxia, carpal tunnel syndrome, and signs of pyramidal tract involvement have also been described (51).

Deterioration of the sensory nerve action potentials more than 40% from baseline may predict the development of neuropathy (51).

After withdrawal of thalidomide, symptoms are usually slow to recover, if they eventually do (3). The first symptoms of peripheral neuropathy can develop even after the withdrawal of thalidomide (33).

Incidence and susceptibility factors
The incidence of peripheral neuropathy, with symmetrical painful paresthesia of the hands and feet often accompanied by sensory loss in the legs, seems to vary with the condition that is being treated, and ranges from under 1% in patients with leprosy to over 70% in patients with prurigo nodularis (41,52). The symptoms do not correlate with either the duration of treatment or the dose. Women and elderly people seem to have an increased risk of neuropathy (53).

Incidences of 21–100% have been reported after treatment for up to 5 years (38,54–57).

Some have found no correlation between the occurrence of neuropathy and the cumulative dose (56); while others have found correlations with total dose (41,57) or daily dose. In 135 patients treated with thalidomide for various skin diseases, there were no cases in those who took daily doses of 25 mg/day or less, but the relative risk of neuropathy was 8.2 at a daily dose of 50–75 mg/day, and 20 at a daily dose of over 75 mg/day (54). It has been suggested that the risk increases at total doses over 20 g (58). Below this dose the risk of neuropathy is about 10% (57).

The incidence and susceptibility factors for thalidomide neuropathy have been studied in a prospective cohort study in 135 patients (54). Structured questionnaires were administered, standardized neurological and electrophysiological examinations were performed, and neuropathic signs and symptoms were classified by investigators who did not know the dose of thalidomide or the treatment duration. Definite thalidomide neuropathy occurred in 25% of patients, and another 30% developed atypical neuropathy, discordant clinical and electrophysiological features, or typical clinical signs without electrophysiological investigation. The only significant susceptibility factor was the daily dose: neuropathy did not develop at dosages below 25 mg/day.

Diagnosis and monitoring

Changes in nerve conductivity are frequent and predictable in thalidomide-induced neuropathy. Nerve conduction studies are required before and during therapy, irrespective of dose (55).

In 135 patients treated with thalidomide for various skin diseases who were prospectively monitored for 2 years there was clinical and electrophysiological evidence of a thalidomide-induced neuropathy in 25%; however, the neuropathy was subclinical in nearly a quarter of patients and when all potential cases were included, the rate was 56% (54). The incidence was maximal during the first year of treatment (20%).

Peripheral nerve function should be monitored by reviewing symptoms, regular neurological examination, and periodic screening of sensory nerve electrophysiology (58). If there is evidence of neuropathy, withdrawal of thalidomide should be considered; the decision should be made on an individual basis and should take into account the seriousness and severity of the underlying condition and the severity of the neuropathy.

Psychological, psychiatric

Mood changes are common with thalidomide (3). Three cases of paranoid reactions have been reported in patients with multiple myeloma taking thalidomide; however, causality was not proved (21).

- Reversible dementia occurred in a patient with multiple myeloma taking thalidomide 200 mg/day plus dexamethasone (59). Memory deficit and mania occurred about 2 months after the start of therapy and did not resolve on withdrawal of dexamethasone and administration of risperidone. The memory loss worsened and proceeded to disorientation, apraxia, and tremor 4 months after the start of therapy. The dementia

resolved completely within 48 hours after withdrawal of thalidomide.

Endocrine

Hypothyroidism has occasionally been reported in patients taking thalidomide (60,61).

- A 44-year-old man with an initial TSH concentration within the reference range took thalidomide 400 mg/day for multiple myeloma and within 4 weeks developed cold intolerance, fatigue, depression, dizziness, and bradycardia, and had a markedly raised TSH (62). He was given levothyroxine and the dose of thalidomide was reduced to 200 mg/day, after which he became euthyroid.

This case prompted further investigation of thyroid function in patients with multiple myeloma. TSH concentrations were measured in 174 patients who had been randomly assigned to chemotherapy plus thalidomide 400 mg/day ($n = 92$) or chemotherapy alone ($n = 82$). After 3–4 months 18 of the patients taking thalidomide had a serum TSH concentration over 5 IU/ml, including six with a concentration over 10 IU/ml (range 12–114 IU/ml), while seven receiving chemotherapy alone had a serum TSH concentration over 5 IU/ml and none had a concentration over 10 IU/ml. In 169 patients with relapsing multiple myeloma who took thalidomide 200–800 mg/day, of those with a serum TSH concentration in the reference range to begin with, 61 had increases after 2–6 months.

Metabolism

In a placebo-controlled study in six patients with type 2 diabetes mellitus thalidomide 150 mg/day for 3 weeks reduced insulin-stimulated glucose uptake by 31% and glycogen synthesis by 48% (63). However, it had no effect on rates of glycolysis, carbohydrate oxidation, non-oxidative glycolysis, lipolysis, free fatty acid oxidation, or re-esterification. The authors concluded that thalidomide increases insulin resistance in obese patients with type 2 diabetes.

This effect can have clinical consequences. For example, in patients with prostate cancer, reducing the dose of thalidomide improved hyperglycemia, suggesting that thalidomide may have exacerbated it in the first place (64).

- A 70-year-old man with no family history of diabetes or known diabetes took thalidomide 400 mg/day for refractory multiple myeloma. He developed hyperglycemia, which had to be treated with insulin and later with glipizide GITS 5 mg/day and which responded despite continuation of thalidomide (65).

Weight gain and edema have been reported in patients taking thalidomide (3). In 13 patients with minimally symptomatic HIV disease thalidomide for 14 days caused an increase in weight of 3.6% (66).

Electrolyte balance

Severe hyperkalemia occurred in six of eight patients with multiple myeloma and moderate to severe renal insufficiency who took thalidomide 100–200 mg/day for up to

12 days; three died and one recovered after withdrawal of thalidomide (67). Hyperkalemia occurred despite the fact that most of the patients also took dexamethasone.

Fluid balance

Thalidomide can cause painful edema of the legs, which is transitory and disappears as treatment continues (68). Peripheral edema was reported in 4.2% of patients with erythema nodosum leprosum, in patients with HIV infection (3.1% of those taking 100 mg/day and 8.3% of those taking 200 mg/day), and in up to 22% of patients with refractory multiple myeloma (21).

Hematologic

Thalidomide can cause leukopenia. In controlled trials in patients with HIV infection the incidences of neutropenia were 9%, 17%, and 25% in those who took placebo, thalidomide 100 mg/day, and thalidomide 200 mg/day respectively (21).

Neutropenia occurred in 14 of 80 patients treated with thalidomide for refractory chronic graft-versus-host disease (69). The median thalidomide dose at which neutropenia developed was 200 mg qds. Erythrocyte and platelet counts were not affected. After withdrawal of thalidomide the neutropenia resolved within a month (except in three patients, who died with refractory graft-versus-host disease). Six patients were rechallenged with thalidomide and again became neutropenic.

Of 44 patients who took thalidomide for refractory multiple myeloma, 10 developed grade 3 or 4 neutropenia, usually in the first or second week of treatment (70). There was concomitant progression of thrombocytopenia in five cases and bone marrow hypoplasia without a significant increase in myeloma cell numbers in five. Neutropenia was more common in patients with low neutrophil and platelet counts, anemia, or a high percentage of plasma cells in the bone marrow before thalidomide treatment.

Of 50 Taiwanese patients with relapsed and/or refractory multiple myeloma who took thalidomide on a dose-escalation schedule, 100–800 mg/day, 18 of 22 responders had reduced leukocyte counts before there was significant reduction in M proteins, compared with only four of the 28 non-responders (71). The median time from the start of thalidomide treatment to the minimum leukocyte count was 28 (range 7–150) days, with a mean cell count of 2.19 (range 0.96–3.35) $\times 10^9$/l. The leukopenia was generally transient, with rapid recovery despite continuation of thalidomide.

Myeloproliferative reactions have been reported in three patients with myelofibrosis taking thalidomide 200 mg/day (72). Thalidomide-associated leukemic transformation has also been reported in five patients with multiple myeloma (73).

Mouth and teeth

Xerostomia is common in patients taking thalidomide (2,3).

- An oral lichenoid eruption occurred in a 33-year-old woman after she had taken thalidomide 200 mg/day for

a few days for graft-versus-host disease after bone marrow transplantation for chronic myeloid leukemia (74).

Gastrointestinal

Constipation is common in patients taking thalidomide (2,3).

Liver

Severe hepatotoxicity has been attributed to thalidomide in multiple myeloma (75) and hepatic failure can occur (21,76,77).

Four post-marketing reports of hepatic failure have been reported; one patient with multiple myeloma developed severe jaundice, hepatic failure, and coma, and died 1 month after the start of thalidomide therapy; three other patients had pre-existing liver disease, and hepatic failure and death were probably not drug-related (21).

- A 50-year-old man with history of chronic hepatitis B had transient rises in serum transaminases after two successive episodes of autologous stem cell transplantation, with spontaneous resolution; at that time PCR for hepatitis B virus was negative (76). Later he was given thalidomide and after 5 months suddenly experienced dizziness and jaundice. The concentration of hepatitis B virus DNA was 1641 pg/ml and serological tests for other viruses were negative. Despite conventional supportive care, he died of septicemic shock caused by *Klebsiella* pneumonia. Other hepatotoxic agents were excluded.
- A 58-year-old woman, with a history of chronic stable hepatitis C infection, was given thalidomide 200 mg/day for end-stage plasma cell leukemia (77). Within 1 week she developed jaundice, light-coloured stools, and marked rises in serum transaminases, which had been stable before the introduction of thalidomide. The jaundice resolved promptly on withdrawal of all drugs; other drugs besides thalidomide that might have been implicated were reintroduced without ill effects.

Skin

Rash due to thalidomide is commonly described as erythematous, macular, and pruritic; it occurs over the back, trunk, and limbs and most commonly occurs 10–14 days after the start of treatment (21). In trials of thalidomide in patients with erythema nodosum leprosum the incidence of rash was 25%, in patients with HIV infection it was 42%, and in patients with myeloma it was up to 26%.

Other skin reactions to thalidomide include pustuloderma, exfoliative reactions, and hypersensitivity reactions, including toxic epidermal necrolysis (3). The frequency of erythema nodosum was increased compared with placebo during the first 8 weeks of thalidomide therapy for Behçet's syndrome, but not thereafter (33).

Redness of the palms was observed in four of 13 patients treated with thalidomide (43). Erythroderma and peripheral eosinophilia occurred in two patients with chronic renal insufficiency who were taking thalidomide for prurigo nodularis (78).

Three of forty patients taking thalidomide for leprosy developed dermatitis herpetiformis, which was thought to have been caused by the treatment (79).

In 87 patients with multiple myeloma in an open trial given thalidomide alone ($n = 50$) or thalidomide + dexamethasone ($n = 37$), there were minor to moderate skin eruptions in 23 patients taking thalidomide alone and in 16 of those taking thalidomide + dexamethasone (80). These included morbilliform, seborrheic, maculopapular, and non-specific dermatitis. Three patients taking thalidomide + dexamethasone had severe skin reactions (exfoliative erythroderma, erythema multiforme, and toxic epidermal necrolysis) that required hospitalization and withdrawal of thalidomide.

Worsening of psoriasis has been reported in a 46-year-old woman taking thalidomide for Behçet's disease (81).

Nails

Brittle nails occurred in three patients who took thalidomide (43), and in another case brittleness was accompanied by marked ridging of the nails (82). This last patient also had amenorrhea. She was taking 50–100 mg nightly at the time.

Sexual function

Erectile dysfunction and loss of libido have occasionally been attributed to thalidomide (83).

Reproductive system

Amenorrhea

In women taking thalidomide there have been occasional reports of amenorrhea (84–89).

Four of 13 women with cutaneous lupus erythematosus (either discoid or associated with systemic disease) treated with thalidomide 100–300 mg/day had amenorrhea during the first 4–5 months of treatment (85). They had high serum concentrations of pituitary gonadotrophins, normal prolactin concentrations, and low estradiol concentrations; antiovary antibodies were not detected. In one woman an ovarian biopsy showed severe ovarian atrophy and absence of ova or follicles. In all four women menstruation resumed 2–3 months after withdrawal of thalidomide. In two women thalidomide was reintroduced: one developed oligomenorrhea again after 5 months, with high concentrations of pituitary gonadotrophins; withdrawal of thalidomide resulted in remission. Other cases of ovarian failure in women taking thalidomide for aphthous ulcers have been described (87).

Among 21 women who took thalidomide, secondary amenorrhea occurred in four who took it for refractory cutaneous lupus erythematosus and in one who took it for aphthous ulcers (84). Menstruation resumed 2–3 months after withdrawal of thalidomide, and in one case amenorrhea recurred after reintroduction, in association with raised serum concentrations of pituitary gonadotrophins.

Four of thirteen women who took thalidomide for cutaneous lupus erythematosus developed amenorrhea (85). In one case a biopsy showed severe ovarian atrophy and absence of ova or follicles. In another case rechallenge with thalidomide 50 mg/day resulted in amenorrhea, which resolved on withdrawal.

Two young women with discoid lupus erythematosus developed amenorrhea after taking thalidomide 100–150 mg/day (86). In one patient the menstrual cycle returned to normal within 5 months after withdrawal of thalidomide; in another the dosage was reduced to 50 mg on alternate days but menstruation had not returned 6 months later.

Of seven women who took thalidomide for aphthous ulcers three developed amenorrhea (87).

- A 28-year-old woman took thalidomide 100 mg/day for Behçet's disease and after 3 months developed amenorrhea (89). She took an oral contraceptive for 8 months, but then had a deep vein thrombosis in association with a factor V Leiden mutation; the oral contraceptive was withdrawn and she was given warfarin. She remained amenorrheic. She had a raised serum concentration of follicle-stimulating hormone but all other laboratory tests were normal. Ultrasonography showed a normal uterus and an endometrial lining of 4 mm. The amenorrhea was attributed to thalidomide, which she decided to continue taking; she remained amenorrheic.

Thalidomide may destroy follicular cells by an action at follicle stimulating hormone receptors, either by directly inhibiting the binding of follicle stimulating hormone or by a post-receptor mechanism (87).

Gynecomastia

In men taking thalidomide there have been occasional reports of gynecomastia.

- A 69-year-old man developed right-sided gynecomastia after taking thalidomide 200 mg/day for 2 years (90). Mammography showed diffuse dense glandular right breast tissue in the retroareolar area with no discrete masses or microcalcification. He had taken no other drugs and had serum concentrations of prolactin, estradiol, and testosterone in the reference ranges. Thalidomide was withdrawn but the gynecomastia did not change during the following 3 months.
- A 55-year-old man developed unilateral gynecomastia after taking thalidomide 200 mg/day for 2 weeks (91). Mammography and ultrasonography showed an enlarged but otherwise normal mammary gland. He continued to take thalidomide for 4 months and the gynecomastia persisted.

Immunologic

Leukocytoclastic vasculitis has been reported in one of 260 patients (92).

Of 54 patients randomized to either placebo ($n = 26$) or thalidomide 200 mg/day ($n = 28$) starting 80 days after allogeneic bone marrow transplantation chronic graft-versus-host disease was significantly more common in those who took thalidomide; there was also a significant overall survival advantage in those who took placebo (93). These results suggest that while thalidomide is effective in treating chronic graft-versus-host disease, its use to prevent chronic graft-versus-host disease results in a paradoxical outcome.

Tumor lysis syndrome has been attributed to thalidomide in a 59-year-old woman with myeloma (94).

Infection risk

Disseminated infection with *Herpes simplex* virus and *Varicella zoster* virus occurred in a patient taking thalidomide for relapsed multiple myeloma (95).

Body temperature

Febrile reactions are common in patients taking thalidomide. In one study of 56 patients with HIV infection who took thalidomide for 14–21 days, 24 discontinued therapy owing to adverse reactions. Cutaneous and/or febrile reactions, which occurred in 20 patients, were the most frequent adverse effects (96).

Death

A randomized, placebo-controlled study of thalidomide in toxic epidermal necrolysis, undertaken because of the potent in vitro TNF-alpha-inhibitory properties of thalidomide, was stopped because of excess mortality in the thalidomide group (10 of 12 patients died compared with three of 10 in the placebo group) (97). There was an insignificant increase in plasma TNF-alpha in the thalidomide-treated patients on day 2.

Second-Generation Effects

Teratogenicity

Thalidomide should not be used during pregnancy because of its teratogenic effects (61,98–109). In 46 examined cases of malformations, 41 of the mothers had taken thalidomide, while in the other five cases the possibility could not be ruled out, while among 300 normal controls none of the mothers had taken thalidomide (110).

History

In the late 1950s and early 1960s thalidomide was used as a sedative in pregnant women in several countries in Europe and also distributed for trials in the USA, but was then identified as a cause of severe congenital limb malformations in many of the babies whose mothers had taken it while pregnant. The thalidomide disaster produced deep distrust in the way the public control of the effects of drugs was carried out. Suddenly, the edifices for the public control of drugs were in many countries perceived as gravely deficient and barely adapted to their purposes. People realized that drugs that were not safe could be produced by respected pharmaceutical companies, prescribed by trusted doctors, and sold by authorized pharmacies. It also became widely known that many marketed drugs were not providing their purported benefits and that claims of efficacy were barely checked by the drug regulatory authorities.

The outrage over thalidomide stimulated considerable reinforcement of the public control of drugs. In the USA, an amendment of the Food, Drug, and Cosmetic Act was approved by Congress in 1962 (111). Not only the safety but also the efficacy of drugs would henceforth be part of the criteria that the FDA used as benchmarks in decisions over whether drugs should be allowed on to the market. Since then pharmaceutical companies have had to show premarketing proof of both the safety and the efficacy of

any new drug they want to introduce. Moreover, manufacturers of drugs in the USA have since 1962 had a duty to report to the FDA any information on adverse effects of their products.

At that time, existing drugs on the US market also came under scrutiny, and a review of their efficacy conducted by the US National Academy of Sciences (112) led to the voluntary withdrawal by pharmaceutical manufacturers of about two-thirds of the approximately 7100 products that the FDA had previously approved (113).

Similar legislative changes were called for in other countries, with a strong emphasis on applying the principle of premarket testing of drugs, rather than relying on random, more or less voluntary, postmarket surveillance and monitoring.

In Britain the thalidomide tragedy led to calls for a revision of the existing drug safety regulations. However, the government's position was ambiguous. It expressed a belief in the value of premarket testing of all new drugs, but did not want to move against the interests of the pharmaceutical industry. The "goose which has laid so many golden therapeutic eggs" (114) was important for the economy. Instead of creating new legislation with far-reaching requirements on the testing of new drugs, a Committee on Safety of Drugs (CSD) was appointed in 1964, expecting voluntary cooperation from the pharmaceutical industry, and its chairman asserted that it was not going to impose unnecessary restraints on the industry. Moreover, a flexible approach was to be taken regarding the efficacy of medicines. The CSD would invite reports on the toxicological testing of drugs, consider whether clinical trials should be undertaken, and assess the results in terms of safety and efficacy. It pledged that information submitted to it by the manufacturers of new drugs would be kept confidential. In its first year the CSD received 600 submissions for new drugs from pharmaceutical manufacturers. Its reviews were rapid and it rejected only a small proportion of the submissions (115).

In 1967 the Association of the British Pharmaceutical Industry (ABPI) was facing radical political proposals to abolish brand names of drugs and introduce mandatory labeling with therapeutic classifications on all medicines. To avoid legislation with mandatory rules, the ABPI revised its Code of Practice to cover the inclusion in promotional material of information on adverse effects, precautions, and contraindications (116). When the Medicines Commission was established in 1969, under the 1968 Medicines Act, to regulate the quality, safety, efficacy, and promotion of drugs, the rules of confidentiality regarding data on the effects of drugs remained in place. The Medicines Commission saw its task as integrating consideration of the pharmaceutical industry's interests with the interest of public safety (115).

In Sweden, public outrage eased the acceptance of proposals for new legislation on drug control that were pending in the Riksdag (the Swedish Parliament). A new law in 1962 (115), and subsequent regulations issued in 1963 (117), stressed the importance of controlling drug safety and efficacy. Mandatory premarket testing, with results examined by the Swedish national drug control agency, was to be the main instrument in controlling the drug market.

The thalidomide disaster led to other initiatives in many countries to create mechanisms by which doctors

Wales the number of cases was calculated to be at least 800 (148).

The frequency in Bonn in 1962 was 3.56 per 1000 of all newborn children (200 times the frequency in 1960–61). In Liverpool, the frequency during 1960 and 1961 was lower (0.778 per 1000), but nevertheless considerably higher than in other countries. Cases have been reported from Australia, Scotland, and Sweden (149). The USA was relatively free from this adverse effect, since thalidomide (as Kevadon) failed to pass the Food and Drug Administration because of another adverse effect, namely polyneuropathy (119).

It was estimated that 10 000 deformed children were born in West Germany before thalidomide was withdrawn; of these, 4000 are believed to have survived. In Japan there were believed to be 1000 thalidomide children; in England 400; in the Scandinavian countries 280; in Canada 200; in Belgium 60; and 25 in the Netherlands. From 1958 to 1961, 223 kg of thalidomide were marketed in Austria; during this period 19 children were born showing abnormalities compatible with the dysmelia syndrome.

Dose relation

The actual dose of thalidomide taken is not as important as the fact of its ingestion (103,104,147). Neither the duration of administration of thalidomide nor the total dose was related to the teratogenic risk (77,119). Some cases have been observed after the ingestion of only 1, 2, or 3 tablets (150).

A baby with micromelia of all four limbs was born to a woman who had taken only a single dose of thalidomide 200 mg in the first weeks of pregnancy (151). In two other cases the total dose was less than 125 mg (152).

In one case the question arose as to whether ingestion of thalidomide by the father previous to or at the time of conception could have played a role (153).

- A baby was born with bilateral absence of radii and thumbs. The mother denied having taken thalidomide or any other drug. The father had been receiving thalidomide for some six months before the conception of the child.

However, the taking of a single sleeping tablet by the mother could easily have been forgotten in this case. Nevertheless, in one study in rabbits the effect on the offspring of the administration of thalidomide to the male parent was studied (154). It was concluded that in rabbits of a cross-bred colony of high fertility there was a deleterious effect on the progeny ascribable to paternal treatment with thalidomide.

Time course

During a 1-year period, 10 babies with major limb defects were born in Stirlingshire maternity units. At least eight of the mothers had had thalidomide prescribed in the early weeks of pregnancy (59,98–101).

The critical phase for teratogenic effects of thalidomide is from the 27th to the 40th day after conception or from the 37th to the 54th day after the first day of the last menstrual period (155). In 12 of 86 cases the date of conception was fairly well known and the narrowest

interval of time that spanned the taking of thalidomide was from the 27th to the 44th day after conception (150). In 205 cases, the mothers that were able to give precise accounts of the timing of administration of thalidomide had taken it from the 31st to 39th day from the first day of their last menstrual period, and in two cases they had taken only two tablets at 36–39 days (156).

In contrast, one woman gave birth to a baby with typical abnormalities after having taken thalidomide for 2 months before conception but only during the first 3 weeks of pregnancy (157).

Experimental data

Experimental work on thalidomide is complicated by the fact that different species respond in different ways to the drug (158). For example, oral thalidomide 25–200 mg/kg/day in rabbits produced a large number of fetal abnormalities, whereas very few occurred in rats. In contrast, after intravenous injection of thalidomide dissolved in propylene glycol or dimethylsulfoxide, abnormalities were produced in both species with doses as low as 2.5–10 mg/kg/day in rabbits, and 10 mg/kg/day in rats (159).

In vitro experiments

In leukocyte cultures, thalidomide is a potential antimitotic agent (160). There was a reduction in the percentage of lymphocytes transformed into the "blast" and "intermediate" types. The cells showed morphological abnormalities: pyknotic changes, chromatin clumping, and perinuclear pink halo of cytoplasm.

Mesanephric tissue from human embryos is normally capable of producing cartilage in vitro. However, when chondrogenic tissues from human embryos aged 5–8.5 weeks were exposed to thalidomide, it interfered with this process and the authors suggested that it may have a specific effect on similar tissues in vivo, accounting for the types of malformation of the fetus that have been observed (161).

Chickens

When chick eggs were injected with thalidomide, gross malformations were found only in the thalidomide-treated group after breeding; they affected 20% of the chickens and included encephalocele, anencephaly, microphthalmia, beak malformations, deformities of the jaw and legs (128).

In chick embryos, malformations were induced by introducing thalidomide into the amniotic cavity. However, other types of traumatic procedures similarly resulted in abnormalities (162).

Changes in the mitochondria of the endothelial cells of the axial limb bud artery occurred in chick embryos after treatment with thalidomide (163). However, there were no macroscopic abnormalities in chicks after thalidomide administration.

Thalidomide caused profound alterations in the morphogenesis of the encephalon in the developing chick embryo in vitro. Platyneuria occurred in 82% compared with 23% in the control group. Thalidomide has an inhibitory effect on growth, as measured by failure of closure of the neural plate, which can be reversed by the addition of ATP to the cultures (164).

The action of thalidomide on the production of limb abnormalities in the chick are similar to those produced by nitrogen mustard (165). Only mesodermal tissues are affected; differentiation is arrested and the mesodermal cells regroup beneath the ectodermal cap. The latter no longer induces development of the proximal portion of the limb, but only of its terminal part, which explains the occurrence of phocomelia.

Dogs
Of nine dogs treated with thalidomide 100 mg/kg/day in the first 3 weeks of pregnancy, three had no litters at all. Of a total of 30 pups, 19 appeared normal, two were stillborn and four died within 48 hours (of these six, two had malformations), and five survived for some days but had an abnormal tail bone (166).

Mice
In mice treated with thalidomide there was a marked reduction in litter size (167). The young had congenital anomalies, such as cleft lip, microphthalmia and malformation of the tail, in a frequency of 5–10%.

There was a high incidence (17.5%) of abnormal embryos in mice treated during the sixth to eighth days of pregnancy, whilst thalidomide-treated animals had a higher incidence of fetal resorption (168). Others, however, failed to find any malformations or other adverse effects when using doses ranging from 2 mg/kg up to 400 mg/kg (169).

In random-bred Charles River strain albino mice, thalidomide 1000 mg/kg/day given from the first day of mating failed to produce gross malformations of the offspring (170).

Monkeys
In seven pregnancies in monkeys, one normal fetus was obtained, four had deformities, and two had teratomas (171).

Rabbits
In rabbits treated with thalidomide there was a marked reduction in litter size (167). The frequency of malformations (encephalocele, anencephaly) was 30%. Experiments with thalidomide on pregnant rabbits showed that the young invariably showed deformities similar to those seen in humans (172).

In rabbits, malformations were found with doses of 5 mg/kg/day, 150 mg/kg/day, and 500 mg/day, given between the seventh and eleventh days of pregnancy. There were abnormalities of the extremities, skull, nose, and palate, as well as malformations of the kidneys. There seemed to be an increase in frequency with higher doses (173).

When 10 pregnant New Zealand white rabbits were fed thalidomide from the eighth to the eleventh days of pregnancy in doses of 150 mg/kg, 59 fetuses were produced, of which 56 were malformed. The 11 control rabbits gave birth to 94 normal fetuses (174).

In six male rabbits of proven fertility treated with 0.75–2.5 g of thalidomide for 10–21 days before mating, three of forty experimental matings did not result in pregnancies; six litters had five or fewer offspring; there

was gross abnormality of one male offspring in each of two different litters fathered by the same male; eight litters showed total loss of young and in another eight litters there was marked loss of young by day 14 of the postnatal period (154).

Rabbits have been found to be very sensitive to the action of thalidomide, but the types of abnormality produced vary with the strain of rabbit. In hybrid rabbits, in which the pregnant doe received thalidomide in a dose of 150 mg/kg on days 7–13, 13% of the young were deformed (175). Apart from the femur, only preaxial structures of both forelimbs and hind limbs were affected. Abnormalities were of both the supernumerary and reduction types. In contrast, only abnormalities of the forelimbs occurred in the New Zealand white strain of rabbits under the same dosage schedule (176). The pattern of these limb defects bore no resemblance to spontaneously occurring deformities, and it is suggested it is a characteristic pattern for the drug.

In Chinchilla and New Zealand white rabbits, thalidomide 150 mg/kg on days 6–15 of pregnancy caused increased incidences of conceptions undergoing resorption and of fetal malformations, and reductions in litter size and body weight of the 28-day fetuses; 22% of fetuses were deformed, with abnormalities affecting the locomotor, nervous, cutaneous, ocular, respiratory, and renal systems (177).

In liver-damaged rabbits, thalidomide 150 mg/kg on days 7–12 of pregnancy produced an 80% rate of fetal abnormalities. The teratogenic activity correlated with high blood and tissue concentrations of thalidomide (178). There was no correlation between the dose of thalidomide and blood thalidomide concentration in healthy rabbits (179).

Experimental work in six strains of rabbit showed that defective evolution of the spiral septum underlay many of the cardiac abnormalities. Incomplete evidence in the literature suggests the same effect may be present in human cardiac deformities (180).

A synthetic analogue of thalidomide, methyl-4-phthalimido-DL-glutamate, was teratogenic in rabbits (181).

Rats
In rats treated with thalidomide, congenital malformations were not seen, but the number of young per litter was reduced by 33% (167).

In rats thalidomide produced abnormalities of the ossification centers of the sternum and cervical vertebrae (182). These changes in ossification centers were more easily found after small doses than with large doses, since in the latter many of the young do not survive until birth.

In Wistar rats that received thalidomide 0.5–1% in the diet for periods from 9 days before mating up to the 20th day of pregnancy, 1% thalidomide produced the greatest number of fetal resorptions and extensive defects of ossification of thoracic centers, sternebrae, and pelvic girdles. Of 170 observed malformations, 150 (82%) occurred in rats treated with thalidomide before mating. The authors suggested that thalidomide may have a gonadal effect (183).

A histochemical study of the development of the sternum in thalidomide-treated rats showed increased storage of glycogen and reduced or absent alkaline phosphatase activity. These changes resulted in a delay in calcification of cartilage (184).

There were no macroscopic abnormalities in rats after thalidomide administration, although the number of resorption sites in the latter after 18 days gestation was increased (171).

Mechanisms

The mechanism by which thalidomide causes fetal abnormalities is not known. There is a high incidence of fetal resorption, but the cause of this is not known; it could be secondary to an abnormality of the fetus.

The more marked effect of thalidomide on some systems, for example the nervous system, the fetus, and erythrocytes, may be due to differing membrane permeabilities of different tissues to the drug (185). From a study of five head autopsies, and electroencephalographic and neurological findings in 17 individuals with the thalidomide embryopathy, it has been suggested that the action of thalidomide is not confined to mesoblastic tissue (186). This is especially true in children with an aural embryopathy. Cytogenic examination of mitotic cells in five children with ear deformities showed that the proportion of non-modal chromosomes was not greater than 10% and there were no structural changes in single chromosomes (187).

The abnormality of the ossification centers found in the rat could be connected with abnormal development of long bones. Radiographs of the limbs of 92 children with deformities due to thalidomide showed joint changes similar to those in neuropathic (Charcot's) joints in adults. The authors suggested that thalidomide causes joint changes by causing an embryonic sensory neuropathy. This hypothesis can be extended to explain other visceral and congenital malformations (188).

Thalidomide prolongs the survival time of skin homografts in the mouse, and the mechanism involved is thought to be immunosuppressive, because of the inhibition of the appearance of immunoblasts in the regional lymph nodes (189). The fetus is immunogenetically a homograft, and an early spontaneous abortion is homograft rejection. Thalidomide may therefore act by preventing spontaneous abortions, allowing damaged fetuses to reach term. If this were so, the abortion rate of those women who took thalidomide should be reduced (190). However, thalidomide has a direct toxic action on the pre-implantation blastocyst, especially the embryonic disc, and the immunological theory also cannot be reconciled with the fact that thalidomide produced teratogenic effects when given to the male rabbit before mating (191).

It has been suggested that thalidomide acts by a toxic action on the initial nerve impulses in the organogenetic phase of development due to accumulation of the drug in the nervous system of the embryo (192).

It has been suggested that in some way, thalidomide interferes with the action of certain of the B vitamins, that as a result of this antagonism fetal damage can occur, and that in the adult there may be a link between this effect and the polyneuropathy that thalidomide can cause (193). Thalidomide and its two isoglutamine derivatives caused an increase in sensitivity of intracellular hemoglobin to oxidation by nitrite ions in rats; simultaneous administration of pyridoxine and riboflavin prevented or corrected this change (185).

Prevention

Women of child-bearing age should take steps not to become pregnant while taking thalidomide, for example by using reliable contraception. If a woman taking thalidomide misses a menstrual period, thalidomide should be withdrawn for at least 9 weeks (120). Counseling about therapeutic abortion will be necessary.

Susceptibility Factors

The incidences of polyneuropathy and hypersensitivity reactions seem to be higher in HIV-infected patients (2,93).

Drug–Drug Interactions

Darbepoetin

In a study of the combination of thalidomide 100 mg/day with darbepoetin alfa 2.25 mg/kg/day in patients with myelodysplastic syndromes, there was an unexpectedly high incidence of thromboembolic events (194). Of the first seven patients enrolled, two developed deep vein thromboses and one died of a massive pulmonary embolus. The authors concluded that thalidomide may increase the thromboembolic risk associated with erythropoietic proteins in patients with myelodysplastic syndromes.

Dexamethasone

An interaction of thalidomide with dexamethasone has been postulated (195).

- A 64-year-old man with myeloma took dexamethasone and thalidomide 200 mg/day for 14 days and had no adverse effects. The dosage was increased to 400 mg/day and 10 days later a rash occurred; thalidomide was withdrawn. Within 3 days he developed toxic epidermal necrolysis.

Two other patients of eight who received thalidomide plus dexamethasone for multiple myeloma had unexpected severe skin rashes, including one who became seriously ill with erythroderma. Both recovered fully after thalidomide was withdrawn.

Docetaxel

The increased risk of venous thromboembolism in patients taking thalidomide and docetaxel is discussed in the cardiovascular section.

Sedative drugs

Thalidomide enhances the sedative actions of alcohol, barbiturates, chlorpromazine, and reserpine (118), perhaps by additive effects on their several pharmacodynamic actions (196), although other mechanisms have been described (197).

Sex steroids

Thalidomide does not interact with ethinylestradiol or norethindrone (198).

References

1. Calabrese L, Fleischer AB. Thalidomide: current and potential clinical applications. Am J Med 2000;108(6):487–95.

2. Gunzler V. Thalidomide in human immunodeficiency virus (HIV) patients. A review of safety considerations. Drug Saf 1992;7(2):116–34.

3. Tseng S, Pak G, Washenik K, Pomeranz MK, Shupack JL. Rediscovering thalidomide: a review of its mechanism of action, side effects, and potential uses. J Am Acad Dermatol 1996;35(6):969–79.

4. Koch HP. Thalidomide and congeners as anti-inflammatory agents. Prog Med Chem 1985;22:165–242.

5. Stirling DI. Thalidomide and its impact in dermatology. Semin Cutan Med Surg 1998;17(4):231–42.

6. Woodyatt B. Thalidomide. Lancet 1962;1:750.

7. Hattori Y, Iguchi T. Thalidomide for the treatment of multiple myeloma. Congenit Anom (Kyoto) 2004;44(3):125–36.

8. Fanelli M, Sarmiento R, Gattuso D, Carillio G, Capaccetti B, Vacca A, Roccaro AM, Gasparini G. Thalidomide: a new anticancer drug? Expert Opin Investig Drugs 2003;12(7):1211–25.

9. Faure M, Thivolet J, Gaucherand M. Inhibition of PMN leukocytes chemotaxis by thalidomide. Arch Dermatol Res 1980;269(3):275–80.

10. Barnhill RL, Doll NJ, Millikan LE, Hastings RC. Studies on the anti-inflammatory properties of thalidomide: effects on polymorphonuclear leukocytes and monocytes. J Am Acad Dermatol 1984;11(5 Pt 1):814–19.

11. Moreira AL, Sampaio EP, Zmuidzinas A, Frindt P, Smith KA, Kaplan G. Thalidomide exerts its inhibitory action on tumor necrosis factor alpha by enhancing mRNA degradation. J Exp Med 1993;177(6):1675–80.

12. McHugh SM, Rifkin IR, Deighton J, Wilson AB, Lachmann PJ, Lockwood CM, Ewan PW. The immunosuppressive drug thalidomide induces T helper cell type 2 (Th2) and concomitantly inhibits Th1 cytokine production in mitogen- and antigen-stimulated human peripheral blood mononuclear cell cultures. Clin Exp Immunol 1995;99(2):160–7.

13. D'Amato RJ, Loughnan MS, Flynn E, Folkman J. Thalidomide is an inhibitor of angiogenesis. Proc Natl Acad Sci USA 1994;91(9):4082–5.

14. Rajkumar SV, Witzig TE. A review of angiogenesis and antiangiogenic therapy with thalidomide in multiple myeloma. Cancer Treat Rev 2000;26(5):351–62.

15. Hastings RC, Morales MJ, Shannon EJ. Studies on the mechanism of action of thalidomide in leprosy. Pharmacologist 1976;18:218.

16. Eriksson T, Bjorkman S, Hoglund P. Clinical pharmacology of thalidomide. Eur J Clin Pharmacol 2001;57(5):365–76.

17. Eriksson T, Bjorkman S, Roth B, Hoglund P. Intravenous formulations of the enantiomers of thalidomide: pharmacokinetic and initial pharmacodynamic characterization in man. J Pharm Pharmacol 2000;52(7):807–17.

18. Teo SK, Scheffler MR, Kook KA, Tracewell WG, Colburn WA, Stirling DI, Thomas SD. Thalidomide dose proportionality assessment following single doses to healthy subjects. J Clin Pharmacol 2001;41(6):662–7.

19. Eriksson T, Wallin R, Hoglund P, Roth B, Qi Z, Ostraat O, Bjorkman S. Low bioavailability of rectally administered thalidomide. Am J Health Syst Pharm 2000;57(17):1607–10.

20. Eriksson T, Hoglund P, Turesson I, Waage A, Don BR, Vu J, Scheffler M, Kaysen GA. Pharmacokinetics of thalidomide in patients with impaired renal function and while on and off dialysis. J Pharm Pharmacol 2003;55(12):1701–6.

21. Clark TE, Edom N, Larson J, Lindsey LJ. Thalomid (thalidomide) capsules: a review of the first 18 months of spontaneous postmarketing adverse event surveillance, including off-label prescribing. Drug Saf 2001;24(2):87–117.

22. Fahdi IE, Gaddam V, Saucedo JF, Kishan CV, Vyas K, Deneke MG, Razek H, Thorn B, Bissett JK, Anaissie EJ, Barlogie B, Mehta JL. Bradycardia during therapy for multiple myeloma with thalidomide. Am J Cardiol 2004;93(8):1052–5.

23. Pitini V, Arrigo C, Aloi G, Azzarello D, La Gattuta G. Diabetic foot disease in a patient with multiple myeloma receiving thalidomide. Haematologica 2002;87(2):ELT07.

24. Zangari M, Anaissie E, Barlogie B, Badros A, Desikan R, Gopal AV, Morris C, Toor A, Siegel E, Fink L, Tricot G. Increased risk of deep-vein thrombosis in patients with multiple myeloma receiving thalidomide and chemotherapy. Blood 2001;98(5):1614–15.

25. Zangari M, Siegel E, Barlogie B, Anaissie E, Saghafifar F, Fassas A, Morris C, Fink L, Tricot G. Thrombogenic activity of doxorubicin in myeloma patients receiving thalidomide: implications for therapy. Blood 2002;100(4):1168–71.

26. Osman K, Comenzo R, Rajkumar SV. Deep venous thrombosis and thalidomide therapy for multiple myeloma. N Engl J Med 2001;344(25):1951–2.

27. Bowcock SJ, Rassam SM, Ward SM, Turner JT, Laffan M. Thromboembolism in patients on thalidomide for myeloma. Hematology 2002;7(1):51–3.

28. Horne MK 3rd, Figg WD, Arlen P, Gulley J, Parker C, Lakhani N, Parnes H, Dahut WL. Increased frequency of venous thromboembolism with the combination of docetaxel and thalidomide in patients with metastatic androgen-independent prostate cancer. Pharmacotherapy 2003;23(3):315–18.

29. Howell E, Johnson SM. Venous thrombosis occurring after initiation of thalidomide for the treatment of cicatricial pemphigoid. J Drugs Dermatol 2004;3(1):83–5.

30. Flageul B, Wallach D, Cavelier-Balloy B, Bachelez H, Carsuzaa F, Dubertret L. Thalidomide et thromboses. [Thalidomide and thrombosis.] Ann Dermatol Venereol 2000;127(2):171–4.

31. Zangari M, Barlogie B, Thertulien R, Jacobson J, Eddleman P, Fink L, Fassas A, Van Rhee F, Talamo G, Lee CK, Tricot G. Thalidomide and deep vein thrombosis in multiple myeloma: risk factors and effect on survival. Clin Lymphoma 2003;4(1):32–5.

32. Pouaha J, Martin S, Trechot P, Truchetet F, Barbaud A, Schmutz JL. Thalidomide et thromboses: trois observations. [Thalidomide and thrombosis: three observations.] Presse Méd 2001;30(20):1008–9.

33. Hamuryudan V, Mat C, Saip S, Ozyazgan Y, Siva A, Yurdakul S, Zwingenberger K, Yazici H. Thalidomide in the treatment of the mucocutaneous lesions of the Behçet syndrome. A randomized, double-blind, placebo-controlled trial. Ann Intern Med 1998;128(6):443–50.

34. Younis TH, Alam A, Paplham P, Spangenthal E, McCarthy P. Reversible pulmonary hypertension and thalidomide therapy for multiple myeloma. Br J Haematol 2003;121(1):191–2.

35. Mellin GW, Katzenstein M. The saga of thalidomide. Neuropathy to embryopathy, with case reports of congenital anomalies. N Engl J Med 1962;267:1184–92.

36. Carrion Valero F, Bertomeu Gonzalez V. Toxicidad pulmonar por talidomida. [Lung toxicity due to thalidomide.] Arch Bronconeumol 2002;38(10):492–4.

37. Seitelberger F. Thalidomid-poly-neuropathie. [Thalidomide polyneuropathy. Clinical biopsy studies.] Wien Klin Wochenschr 1968;80(3):41–3.

38. Isoardo G, Bergui M, Durelli L, Barbero P, Boccadoro M, Bertola A, Ciaramitaro P, Palumbo A, Bergamasco B, Cocito D. Thalidomide neuropathy: clinical, electrophysiological and neuroradiological features. Acta Neurol Scand 2004;109(3):188–93.

39. Broser F. [Polyneuritis and funicular myelosis after Contergan use.] Med Klin 1962;57:53–7.

40. Frenkel H. [Contergan—side effects. Central nervous system manifestations and polyneuritic symptoms in long-term medication with N-phthalyl glutamic acid imide.] Med Welt 1961;18:970–5.

41. Wulff CH, Hoyer H, Asboe-Hansen G, Brodthagen H. Development of polyneuropathy during thalidomide therapy. Br J Dermatol 1985;112(4):475–80.

42. Voss R. Nil nocere! Contergan–Polyneuritis. [Nil nocere. Contergan polyneuritis.] Münch Med Wochenschr 1961;103:1431–2.

43. Fullerton PM, Kremer M. Neuropathy after intake of thalidomide (Distaval). BMJ 1961;5256:855–8.

44. Hultsch EG, Hartmann J. Nil nocere! Die Thalidomid (Contergan) Polyneuritis. [Nil nocere. Thalidomide (Contergan) polyneuritis.] Münch Med Wochenschr 1961 Nov 3;103:2141–4.

45. Becker J. [Polyneuritis due to contergan.] Nervenarzt 1961;32:321–3.

46. Gibbels E. Toxische Schäden bei der Thalidomid-Medikation. [Toxic injuries in thalidomide medication.] Fortschr Neurol Psychiatr Grenzgeb 1967;35(8):393–411.

47. Fullerton PM, O'Sullivan DJ. Thalidomide neuropathy: a clinical electrophysiological, and histological follow-up study. J Neurol Neurosurg Psychiatry 1968;31(6):543–51.

48. Broser F, Hopf HC, Hohl J. Frage der Dauerschädigung bei der Contergan–Polyneuropathie und bei anderen Polyneuropathien bzw. Polyneuritiden. [Problems of permanent damage in Contergan polyneuropathy and other polyneuropathies or polyneuritides. Results of clinical and electromyographic follow ups.] Nervenarzt 1969;40(1):33–5.

49. Sabin TD. Thalidomine neuropathy and leprous neuritis. Lancet 1974;1(7849):165–6.

50. Schiefer I. [On clinical experiences with Contergan in tuberculous children.] Med Welt 1960;52–53:2765–8.

51. Gardner-Medwin JM, Smith NJ, Powell RJ. Clinical experience with thalidomide in the management of severe oral and genital ulceration in conditions such as Behçet's disease: use of neurophysiological studies to detect thalidomide neuropathy. Ann Rheum Dis 1994;53(12):828–32.

52. Clemmensen OJ, Olsen PZ, Andersen KE. Thalidomide neurotoxicity. Arch Dermatol 1984;120(3):338–41.

53. Ochonisky S, Verroust J, Bastuji-Garin S, Gherardi R, Revuz J. Thalidomide neuropathy: incidence and clinico-electrophysiologic findings in 42 patients. Arch Dermatol 1994;130(1):66–9.

54. Bastuji-Garin S, Ochonisky S, Bouche P, Gherardi RK, Duguet C, Djerradine Z, Poli F, Revuz J; Thalidomide Neuropathy Study Group. Incidence and risk factors for thalidomide neuropathy: a prospective study of 135 dermatologic patients. J Invest Dermatol 2002;119(5):1020–6.

55. Harland CC, Steventon GB, Marsden JR. Thalidomide-induced neuropathy and genetic differences in drug metabolism. Eur J Clin Pharmacol 1995;49(1–2):1–6.

56. Briani C, Zara G, Rondinone R, Della Libera S, Ermani M, Ruggero S, Ghirardello A, Zampieri S, Doria A. Thalidomide neurotoxicity: prospective study in patients with lupus erythematosus. Neurology 2004;62(12):2288–90.

57. Cavaletti G, Beronio A, Reni L, Ghiglione E, Schenone A, Briani C, Zara G, Cocito D, Isoardo G, Ciaramitaro P, Plasmati R, Pastorelli F, Frigo M, Piatti M, Carpo M. Thalidomide sensory neurotoxicity: a clinical and neurophysiologic study. Neurology 2004;62(12):2291–3.

58. Apfel SC, Zochodne DW. Thalidomide neuropathy: too much or too long? Neurology 2004;62(12):2158–9.

59. Morgan AE, Smith WK, Levenson JL. Reversible dementia due to thalidomide therapy for multiple myeloma. N Engl J Med 2003;348(18):1821–2.

60. Simpson JA. Myxoedema after thalidomide. BMJ 1962;1:55.

61. Lillicrap DA. Myxoedema after thalidomide (Distaval). BMJ 1962;1:477.

62. Badros AZ, Siegel E, Bodenner D, Zangari M, Zeldis J, Barlogie B, Tricot G. Hypothyroidism in patients with multiple myeloma following treatment with thalidomide. Am J Med 2002;112(5):412–13.

63. Iqbal N, Zayed M, Boden G. Thalidomide impairs insulin action on glucose uptake and glycogen synthesis in patients with type 2 diabetes. Diabetes Care 2000;23(8):1172–6.

64. Figg WD, Arlen P, Gulley J, Fernandez P, Noone M, Fedenko K, Hamilton M, Parker C, Kruger EA, Pluda J, Dahut WL. A randomized phase II trial of docetaxel (Taxotere) plus thalidomide in androgen-independent prostate cancer. Semin Oncol 2001;28(4 Suppl 15):62–6.

65. Pathak RD, Jayaraj K, Blonde L. Thalidomide-associated hyperglycemia and diabetes: case report and review of literature. Diabetes Care 2003;26(4):1322–3.

66. Haslett P, Hempstead M, Seidman C, Diakun J, Vasquez D, Freedman VH, Kaplan G. The metabolic and immunologic effects of short-term thalidomide treatment of patients infected with the human immunodeficiency virus. AIDS Res Hum Retroviruses 1997;13(12):1047–54.

67. Harris E, Behrens J, Samson D, Rahemtulla A, Russell NH, Byrne JL. Use of thalidomide in patients with myeloma and renal failure may be associated with unexplained hyperkalaemia. Br J Haematol 2003;122(1):160–1.

68. Jonquieres ED, Mosto SJ, Brusco CM. Talidomida y reacción leprosa lepromatosa. [Thalidomide and lepromatous leprosy reaction.] Arch Argent Dermatol 1967;17(3):279–86.

69. Parker PM, Chao N, Nademanee A, O'Donnell MR, Schmidt GM, Snyder DS, Stein AS, Smith EP, Molina A, Stepan DE, Kashyap A, Planas I, Spielberger R, Somlo G, Margolin K, Zwingenberger K, Wilsman K, Negrin RS, Long GD, Niland JC, Blume KG, Forman SJ. Thalidomide as salvage therapy for chronic graft-versus-host disease. Blood 1995;86(9):3604–9.

70. Hattori Y, Kakimoto T, Okamoto S, Sato N, Ikeda Y. Thalidomide-induced severe neutropenia during treatment of multiple myeloma. Int J Hematol 2004;79(3):283–8.

71. Huang SY, Tang JL, Yao M, Ko BS, Hong RL, Tsai W, Wang CH, Tien HF, Shen MC, Chen YC. Reduction of leukocyte count is associated with thalidomide response in treatment of multiple myeloma. Ann Hematol 2003;82(9):558–64.

72. Tefferi A, Elliot MA. Serious myeloproliferative reactions associated with the use of thalidomide in myelofibrosis with myeloid metaplasia. Blood 2000;96(12):4007.

73. Badros A, Morris C, Zangari M, Barlogie B, Tricot G. Thalidomide paradoxical effect on concomitant multiple myeloma and myelodysplasia. Leuk Lymphoma 2002;43(6):1267–71.

74. Bez C, Lodi G, Sardella A, Della Volpe A, Carrassi A. Oral lichenoid lesions after thalidomide treatment. Dermatology 1999;199(2):195.

75. Trojan A, Chasse E, Gay B, Pichert G, Taverna C. Severe hepatic toxicity due to thalidomide in relapsed multiple myeloma. Ann Oncol 2003;14(3):501–2.
76. Bang SM, Kim SS, Park SH, Ahn JY, Cho EK, Shin DB, Lee JH. Acute exacerbation of chronic hepatitis B during thalidomide therapy for multiple myeloma: a case report. Korean J Intern Med 2004;19(3):196–8.
77. Fowler R, Imrie K. Thalidomide-associated hepatitis: a case report. Am J Hematol 2001;66(4):300–2.
78. Bielsa I, Teixido J, Ribera M, Ferrandiz C. Erythroderma due to thalidomide: report of two cases. Dermatology 1994;189(2):179–81.
79. Sheskin J, Sagher F. Erupción tipo dermatitis herpetiforme en enfermos del mal de Hansen tratados con talidomida. [Dermatitis herpetiformis-like eruption in patients with Hansen disease treated with thalidomide.] Fontilles (Alicante) 1968;7:229.
80. Hall VC, El-Azhary RA, Bouwhuis S, Rajkumar SV. Dermatologic side effects of thalidomide in patients with multiple myeloma. J Am Acad Dermatol 2003;48(4):548–52.
81. Dobson CM, Parslew RA. Exacerbation of psoriasis by thalidomide in Behçet's syndrome. Br J Dermatol 2003;149(2):432–3.
82. Heathfield KW. Neuropathy after thalidomide ("Distaval"). BMJ 1961;2:1084.
83. Grosshans E, Illy G. Thalidomide therapy for inflammatory dermatoses. Int J Dermatol 1984;23(9):598–602.
84. Frances C, El Khoury S, Gompel A, Becherel PA, Chosidow O, Piette JC. Transient secondary amenorrhea in women treated by thalidomide. Eur J Dermatol 2002;12(1):63–5.
85. Ordi J, Cortes F, Martinez N, Mauri M, De Torres I, Vilardell M. Thalidomide induces amenorrhea in patients with lupus disease. Arthritis Rheum 1998;41(12):2273–5.
86. Passeron T, Lacour JP, Murr D, Ortonne JP. Thalidomide-induced amenorrhoea: two cases. Br J Dermatol 2001;144(6):1292–3.
87. Gompel A, Frances C, Piette JC, Blanc AS, Cordoliani F, Piette AM. Ovarian failure with thalidomide treatment in complex aphthosis: comment on the concise communication by Ordi, et al. Arthritis Rheum 1999;42(10):2259–60.
88. Gutierrez-Rodriguez O, Starusta-Bacal P, Gutierrez-Montes O. Treatment of refractory rheumatoid arthritis—the thalidomide experience. J Rheumatol 1989;16(2):158–63.
89. Dharia SP, Steinkampf MP, Cater C. Thalidomide-induced amenorrhea: case report and literature review. Fertil Steril 2004;82(2):460–2.
90. Mourad YA, Shamseddine A, Taher A. Thalidomide-associated gynecomasty in a patient with multiple myeloma. Hematol J 2003;4(5):372.
91. Pulik M, Genet P, Lionnet F, Touahri T. Thalidomide-associated gynecomasty in a patient with multiple myeloma. Am J Hematol 2002;70(3):265.
92. Witzens M, Moehler T, Neben K, Fruehauf S, Hartschuh W, Ho AD, Goldschmidt H. Development of leukocytoclastic vasculitis in a patient with multiple myeloma during treatment with thalidomide. Ann Hematol 2004;83(7):467–70.
93. Chao NJ, Parker PM, Niland JC, Wong RM, Dagis A, Long GD, Nademanee AP, Negrin RS, Snyder DS, Hu WW, Gould KA, Tierney DK, Zwingenberger K, Forman SJ, Blume KG. Paradoxical effect of thalidomide prophylaxis on chronic graft-vs.-host disease. Biol Blood Marrow Transplant 1996;2(2):86–92.
94. Cany L, Fitoussi O, Boiron JM, Marit G. Tumor lysis syndrome at the beginning of thalidomide therapy for multiple myeloma. J Clin Oncol 2002;20(8):2212.
95. Curley MJ, Hussein SA, Hassoun PM. Disseminated herpes simplex virus and varicella zoster virus coinfection in a patient taking thalidomide for relapsed multiple myeloma. J Clin Microbiol 2002;40(6):2302–4.
96. Haslett P, Tramontana J, Burroughs M, Hempstead M, Kaplan G. Adverse reactions to thalidomide in patients infected with human immunodeficiency virus. Clin Infect Dis 1997;24(6):1223–7.
97. Wolkenstein P, Latarjet J, Roujeau JC, Duguet C, Boudeau S, Vaillant L, Maignan M, Schuhmacher MH, Milpied B, Pilorget A, Bocquet H, Brun-Buisson C, Revuz J. Randomised comparison of thalidomide versus placebo in toxic epidermal necrolysis. Lancet 1998;352(9140):1586–9.
98. Kohler G, Fisher AM, Dunn PM. Thalidomide and congenital abnormalities. Lancet 1962;1:326.
99. Morgan BC. Thalidomide ("Distaval") and foetal abnormalities. BMJ 1962;1:792.
100. Ferguson AW, Rogerson G. Thalidomide and congenital abnormalities. Lancet 1962;1:691.
101. Speirs AL. Thalidomide and congenital abnormalities. Lancet 1962;1:303–5.
102. Pfeiffer RA, Kosenow W. Zur Frage einer exogenen Verursachung von schweren Extremitätenmißbildungen. [On the problem of exogenous causes of severe malformations of the extremities.] Munch Med Wochenschr 1962;104:68–74.
103. Burley DM, Lenz W. Thalidomide and congenital abnormalities. Lancet 1962;1:271.
104. Lenz W, Pfeiffer RA, Kosenow W, Hayman DJ. Thalidomide and congenital abnormalities. Lancet 1962;1:45–6.
105. Wiedemann HR. [Indications of a current increase of hypoplastic and aplastic deformities of the extremities.] Med Welt 1961;37:1863–6.
106. Yang TS, Shen Cheng CC, Wang CM. A survey of thalidomide embryopathy in Taiwan. Taiwan Yi Xue Hui Za Zhi 1977;76(7):546–62.
107. Edwards DH, Nichols PJ. The spinal abnormalities in thalidomide embryopathy. Acta Orthop Scand 1977;48(3):273–6.
108. Newman CG. Clinical observations on the thalidomide syndrome. Proc R Soc Med 1977;70(4):225–7.
109. McBride WG. Thalidomide embryopathy. Teratology 1977;16(1):79–82.
110. Lenz W. Kindliche Mißbildungen nach Medikament-Einnahme während der Gravidität? [Congenital abnormalities after drug use during pregnancy?] Dtsch Med Wochenschr 1961;86:2555–6.
111. USA, 76 Statute. 780, 87th Congress, 2nd session, October 10, 1962.
112. US National Academy of Sciences. Drug Efficacy Study. A Report to the Commissioner of Food and Drugs. Washington DC: National Academy of Sciences, 1969.
113. Bryan PA. "DESI Who?". FDA Consumer. DHEW Publication No 73-3031, 1972.
114. PSGB. Industry, Safety, Sainsbury and the Bill. Pharm J 1968;200:274–5.
115. Abraham J. In: Science, Politics and the Pharmaceutical Industry: Controversy and Bias in the Drug Regulation. New York: St Martin's Press, 1995:66–80.
116. PSGB. New ABPI code of practice. Pharm J 1967;198:692–3.
117. Riksdagen, Sweden. "Kungl Maj:ts läkemedelsförordning". Svensk Författningssamling 1962;701.
118. Beckman DA, Brent RL. Mechanisms of teratogenesis. Annu Rev Pharmacol Toxicol 1984;24:483–500.
119. Taussig HB. A study of the German outbreak of phocomelia. The thalidomide syndrome. JAMA 1962;180:1106–14.
120. Pliess G. Thalidomide and congenital abnormalities. Lancet 1962;1:1128.

121. Lenz W, Knapp K. Die Thalidomid–Embryopathie. [Thalidomide embryopathy.] Dtsch Med Wochenschr 1962;87:1232–42.

122. Franklin AW. Thalidomide babies. Memorandum from the British Paediatric Association. BMJ 1962;5303:522–4.

123. Ciciliani J, Tolks H. Ergebnisse systematischer Untersuchungen bei 96 Dysmeliekindern. [Results of systematic studies of 96 dysmelia children.] Med Welt 1966;43:2301–7.

124. Sakr R, el-Zawahry K, Khalifa AS, Aboul Hassan A, Khalil M. Hazards to the newlyborn infant from thalidomide-containing drugs administered to pregnant mothers. (Report on three cases). J Egypt Med Assoc 1966;49(1):78–87.

125. Brook CG, Jarvis SN, Newman CG. Linear growth of children with limb deformities following exposure to thalidomide in utero. Acta Paediatr Scand 1977;66(6):673–5.

126. Lecutier MA. Phocomelia and internal defects due to thalidomide. BMJ 1962;5317:1447–8.

127. Petersen CE. Thalidomidembryopathie mit seltener Symptomatik. Pädiatr Prax 1967;6:625.

128. Kemper F. Thalidomide and congenital abnormalities. Lancet 1962;2:836.

129. Rasore-Quartino A, Rovei S. Un caso di anotia talidomidica. [A case of thalidomide anotia.] Minerva Pediatr 1967;19(46):2056–60.

130. Archer J. Thalidomide and neurological damage revisited. JAMA 1978;239(16):1608–9.

131. Murphy R, Mohr P. Two congenital neurological abnormalities caused by thalidomide. BMJ 1977;2(6096):1191.

132. D Avignon M, Barr B. Ear abnormalities and cranial nerve palsies in thalidomide children. Arch Otolaryngol 1964;80:136–40.

133. Phelps PD. Congenital lesions of the inner ear, demonstrated by tomography. Arch Otolaryngol 1974;100(1):11–18.

134. Phelps PD, Roland PE. Thalidomide and cranial nerve abnormalities. BMJ 1977;2(6103):1672.

135. Zetterstrom B. Ocular malformations caused by thalidomide. Acta Ophthalmol (Copenh) 1966;44(3):391–5.

136. Rafuse EV, Arstikaitis M, Brent HP. Ocular findings in thalidomide children. Can J Ophthalmol 1967;2(3):222–5.

137. Canani MB, Raganati M, Tropodi V. Su di un caso di panmieloftsi con malformazioni multiple e probabile genesi talidomidica. [On a case of pan-myelophthisis with multiple malformations probably caused by thalidomide.] Pediatrica (Napoli) 1966;74(6):1009.

138. Axrup K, et al. Children with thalidomide embryopathy: odontologic observations and aspects. Dent Dig 1966;72(9):403.

139. Axrup K, et al. Children with thalidomide embryopathy: odontological observations and aspects. Acta Odontol Scand 1966;24(1):3.

140. Fogh-Andersen P. Thalidomide and congenital cleft deformities. Acta Chir Scand 1966;131(3):197–200.

141. Immeyer F. Lippen- Kiefer- Gaumen-spalten bei Thalidomid-geschädigten Kindern. [Cleft lip and palate in thalidomide-induced embryopathies.] Acta Genet Med Gemellol (Roma) 1967;16(3):244–74.

142. Bremner DN, Mooney G. Agenesis of appendix: a further thalidomide anomaly. Lancet 1978;1(8068):826.

143. Smithells RW. Thalidomide, absent appendix, and sweating. Lancet 1978;1(8072):1042.

144. Ives EJ. Thalidomide and anal abnormalities. Can Med Assoc J 1962;87:670–2.

145. McBride WG. Excessive sweating and reduction deformities. Lancet 1978;1(8068):826.

146. Stainsby GD, Quibell EP. Perthes-like changes in the hips of children with thalidomide deformities. Lancet 1967;2:242.

147. McBride WG. Thalidomide and congenital abnormalities. Lancet 1961;2:1358.

148. Smithells RW. Thalidomide and malformations in Liverpool. Lancet 1962;1:1270–3.

149. Weicker H, Hungerland H. Thalidomid–Embryopathie. [Thalidomide embryopathy. I. Incidence inside and outside Germany.] Dtsch Med Wochenschr 1962;87:992–8 passim.

150. Anonymous. Properties of thalidomide. BMJ 1962;2:785–6.

151. Tomsa DA, Hunter TAA, Ashley DJB, Woollam DHM, Applebey M. Thalidomide and congenital abnormalities. Lancet 1962;2:400.

152. Saunders H, Wright R, Hodgkin K. Thalidomide and congenital deformities. BMJ 1962;5307:796.

153. Jacobs J. Drugs and foetal abnormalities. BMJ 1962;2(5301):407.

154. Lutwak-Mann C. Observations on progeny of thalidomide-treated male rabbits. BMJ 1964;5390:1090–1.

155. Lenz W, Knapp K. Die Thalidomid–Embryopathie. [Thalidomide embryopathy.] Dtsch Med Wochenschr 1962;87:992.

156. Weicker H, Bachmann KD, Pfeiffer RA, Gleiss J. [Thalidomide embryopathy. II. Results of individual anamnestic findings in the areas of inquiry of the universities of Bonn, Cologne, Muenster and Duesseldorf pediatric clinics.] Dtsch Med Wochenschr 1962;87:1597–607.

157. Ward SP. Thalidomide and congenital abnormalities. BMJ 1962;5305:646–7.

158. Helm F. Tierexperimentelle Untersuchungen und Dysmeliesyndrom. [Studies in experiment animals and dysmelia syndrome.] Arzneimittelforschung 1966;16(9):1232–44.

159. Schumacher H, Blake DA, Gurian JM, Gillette JR. A comparison of the teratogenic activity of thalidomide in rabbits and rats. J Pharmacol Exp Ther 1968;160(1):189–200.

160. Roath S, Wales MB, Elves MW, Israels MCG. Effect of thalidomide on leucocyte cultures. Lancet 1962;2:812.

161. Lash JW, Saxen L. Human teratogenesis: invitro studies on thalidomide-inhibited chondrogenesis. Dev Biol 1972;28(1):61–70.

162. Williamson AP, Blattner RJ, Lutz HR. Abnormalities in chick embryos following thalidomide and other insoluble compounds in the amniotic cavity. Proc Soc Exp Biol Med 1963;112:1022–5.

163. Jurand A. Early changes in limb buds of chick embryos after thalidomide treatment. J Embryol Exp Morphol 1966;16(2):289–300.

164. Ruano Gil D. The influence of thalidomide on the development of chick embryos cultivated in vitro. Acta Anat (Basel) 1967;66(2):226–37.

165. Wolff E. La production des monstruosités par des substances chimiques et leur explication. [The induction of monstrosities by chemical substances and their explanation.] Ann Pharm Fr 1968;26(6):473–92.

166. Weidman WH, Young HH, Zollman PE. The effect of thalidomide on the unborn puppy. Mayo Clin Proc 1963;38:518–22.

167. Giroud A, Tuchmann-Duplessis H, Mercier-Parot L. Influence de la thalidomide sur le développement foetal. [Influence of thalidomide on fetal development.] Bull Acad Natl Med 1962;146:343–5.

168. DiPaolo JA, Buffalo PD. Congenital malformation in strain A mice. Its experimental production by thalidomide. JAMA 1963;183:139–41.

169. Mauss HJ, Stumpe K. Tierexperimentelle Untersuchungen zur Frage der Thalidomid–Embryopathie. [Animal experiments on the question of thalidomide embryopathy.] Klin Wschr 1963;41(1):21–5.

170. Szabo KT, Steelman RL. Effects of maternal thalidomide treatment on pregnancy, fetal development, and mortality of the offspring in random-bred mice. Am J Vet Res 1967;28(127):1823–8.

171. Delahunt CS, Lassen LJ, Rieser N. Some comparative teratogenic studies with thalidomide. Proc Eur Soc Study Drug Tox 1966;7:229.

172. Somers GF. Thalidomide and congenital abnormalities. Lancet 1962;1:912–3.

173. Ingalls TH, Curley FJ, Zappasodi P. Thalidomide embryopathy in hybrid rabbits. N Engl J Med 1964;271:441–4.

174. Dekker A, Mehrizi A. Use of thalidomide as a teratogenic agent in rabbits. Bull Johns Hopkins Hosp 1964;115(3):223–30.

175. Vickers TH. The thalidomide embryopathy in hybrid rabbits. Br J Exp Pathol 1967;48(1):107–17.

176. Pearn JH, Vickers TH. The rabbit thalidomide embryopathy. Br J Exp Pathol 1966;47(2):186–92.

177. Fabro S, Smith RL. The teratogenic activity of thalidomide in the rabbit. J Pathol Bacteriol 1966;91(2):511–19.

178. Heine W. Thalidomidembryopathie im Tierversuch. III. Teratologische Testung von Thalidomidabbauprodukten. [Thalidomide embryopathy in animal experiments. 3. Teratologic tests of thalidomide catabolic products.] Z Kinderheilkd 1966;96(2):141–6.

179. Heine W, Stuwe W. Thalidomidembryopathie im Tierversuch. II. Thalidomidblutspiegelwerte bei lebergesunden und lebergeschädigten Versuchstieren. [Thalidomide embryopathy in animal experiments. II. Thalidomide blood level in experimental animals with normal and damaged liver.] Z Kinderheilkd 1966;96(1):14–8.

180. Vickers TH. The cardiovascular malformations in the rabbit thalidomide embryopathy. Br J Exp Pathol 1968;49(2):179–96.

181. Wuest HM, Fox RR, Crary DD. Relationship between teratogeny and structure in the thalidomide field. Experientia 1968;24(10):993–4.

182. Klein Obbink HJ, Dalderup LM. Effects of thalidomide on the skeleton of the rat foetus. Experientia (Basel) 1964;20(5):283–4.

183. Cook MJ, Moore DF. The effect of thalidomide on the developing rat foetus. Br J Exp Pathol 1967;48(2):150–8.

184. Globus M, Gibson MA. A histological and histochemical study of the development of the sternum in thalidomide-treated rats. Teratology 1968;1(3):235–55.

185. Metcalf WK. The relation of vitamin-B complex to the effect of thalidomide on the sensitivity of intracellular haemoglobin to oxidation. Dev Med Child Neurol 1967;9(1):87–97.

186. Horstmann W. Hinweise auf zentral nervöse Schäden im Rahmen der Thalidomid–Embryopathie. [Reference to central nervous system damage within the context of thalidomide embryopathy. Pathological–anatomic, electroencephalographic and neurologic findings.] Z Kinderheilkd 1966;96(4):291–307.

187. Ahrens K. Cytogenische und klinische Untersuchungen bei thalidomidgeschädigten Kindern mit Ohrmissbildungen. [Cytogenetic and clinical studies in thalidomide damaged children with ear malformations.] Arch Klin Exp Ohren Nasen Kehlkopfheilkd 1966;186(3):264–78.

188. McCredie J. Thalidomide and congenital Charcot's joints. Lancet 1973;2(7837):1058–61.

189. Turk JL, Hellmann K, Duke DI. Effect of thalidomide on the immunological response in local lymph nodes after a skin homograft. Lancet 1966;1(7447):1134–6.

190. Hellmann K. Immunosuppression by thalidomide: implications for teratology. Lancet 1966;1(7447):1136–7.

191. Chard T. Immunosuppression by thalidomide. Lancet 1966;1:1373.

192. Gordon G. The mechanism of thalidomide deformities correlated with the pathogenic effects of prolonged dosage in adults. Dev Med Child Neurol 1966;8(6):761–7.

193. Evered DF, Randall HG. Thalidomide and B vitamins. BMJ 1963;1(5330):610.

194. Steurer M, Sudmeier I, Stauder R, Gastl G. Thromboembolic events in patients with myelodysplastic syndrome receiving thalidomide in combination with darbepoietin-alpha. Br J Haematol 2003;121(1):101–3.

195. Rajkumar SV, Gertz MA, Witzig TE. Life-threatening toxic epidermal necrolysis with thalidomide therapy for myeloma. N Engl J Med 2000;343(13):972–3.

196. Frederickson RC, Slater IH, Dusenberry WE, Hewes CR, Jones GT, Moore RA. A comparison of thalidomide and pentobarbital—new methods for identifying novel hypnotic drugs. J Pharmacol Exp Ther 1977;203(1):240–51.

197. Somers GF. Pharmacological properties of thalidomide (alpha-phthalimido glutarimide), a new sedative hypnotic drug. Br J Pharmacol Chemother 1960;15:111–16.

198. Trapnell CB, Donahue SR, Collins JM, Flockhart DA, Thacker D, Abernethy DR. Thalidomide does not alter the pharmacokinetics of ethinyl estradiol and norethindrone. Clin Pharmacol Ther 1998;64(6):597–602.

Theaceae

See also Herbal medicines

General Information

The genera in the family of Theaceae (Table 1) include camellia.

Table 1   The genera of Theaceae

Camellia (camellia)
Cleyera (cleyera)
Eurya (eurya)
Franklinia (Franklin tree)
Gordonia (gordonia)
Laplacea (laplacea)
Stewartia (stewartia)
Ternstroemia (ternstroemia)

Camellia sinensis

Camellia sinensis (green tea) contains caffeine and antioxidant polyphenols. It has been touted as being useful in a wide variety of conditions, including cancer prevention, mostly on relatively slim epidemiological evidence (1), cardiovascular disorders, and AIDS.

Adverse effects

The adverse effects of green tea are those of caffeine, with tremulousness and insomnia and withdrawal symptoms (headache, drowsiness, and fatigue).

Reference

1. Bushman JL. Green tea and cancer in humans: a review of the literature. Nutr Cancer 1998;31(3):151–9.

Theophylline

General Information

Owing to their ability to relax bronchial muscles, theophylline and related compounds are used chiefly in the maintenance treatment of asthma and chronic obstructive pulmonary disease. However, the availability of other therapeutic agents (for example beta-adrenoceptor agonists or steroid inhalers) with increased efficacy, fewer adverse effects, and greater ease of management has led to reduced use of these agents. Theophylline has also been used in the treatment of apnea associated with prematurity (1), congestive heart failure (2), and life-threatening Cheyne–Stokes respiration (3). In the emergency treatment of acute exacerbations of asthma (status asthmaticus), the controversy concerning the possible benefit of including theophylline or aminophylline has not been resolved (4,5) (and see the section under Drug–Drug Interactions in this monograph). A review has suggested that a combination of high doses of inhaled beta$_2$-adrenoceptor agonists, systemic corticosteroids, and oxygen is the treatment of choice; theophylline adds little to the bronchodilator effect of inhaled beta-agonists in most patients (6).

The bronchodilator effect of theophylline is related to serum concentrations, and begins at 5–8 µg/ml, with virtually no additional effects beyond 20 µg/ml. The relation of relatively minor adverse effects to serum concentration is idiosyncratic below 15 µg/ml; above that concentration, the relation becomes more consistent and more serious adverse effects also are increasingly likely, that is toxic effects; the latter are frequent at about 20 µg/ml. Therefore, the therapeutic range is usually considered to be 10–20 µg/ml; 10–15 µg/ml is optimal. However, there is still controversy. For example, the authors of one study found that the clinical response to theophylline correlated significantly with the log plasma theophylline concentration, while other authors have claimed that clinical aspects are more relevant for dose correction during therapy than the determination of serum concentrations (SEDA-12, 3). Various factors influence the metabolism of these compounds, including pronounced interindividual differences in metabolism, concurrent illnesses, and factors such as smoking, age, and weight. The use of these drugs requires extremely close attention, and many authors have stressed the importance of monitoring serum concentrations, the patient's clinical condition, and adverse effects.

An example of some of the complexity encountered is the initiation of chronic bronchodilator therapy with oral theophylline. Approximate initial daily doses are as follows: 6 mg/kg for adult nonsmokers; 10 mg/kg for adult smokers; 12 mg/kg for children under 12 years. Increases in dosage, if any, are made in small increments after about 3 days, depending on the clinical response and serum theophylline concentration. Proper dosing is complicated by two factors: variable systemic availability among the different products used and elimination kinetics in which saturable kinetics are probable but poorly defined.

Theophylline has been derivatized to produce aminophylline, choline theophyllinate, and other compounds.

Several modified-release formulations are available. Maximum serum concentrations occur at 1–3 hours with most of the standard formulations and at up to 6 hours with modified-release formulations. In aminophylline, the most widely used theophylline derivative, theophylline is combined with ethylenediamine to enhance its solubility. Since ethylenediamine is therapeutically inert, all the effects of aminophylline, except for allergic reactions, are considered to stem from the theophylline component.

Among the methylated xanthines, theophylline is the least active cerebral stimulant, its most pronounced features being stimulation of the medullary respiratory center, circulatory system, and smooth muscles of the bronchi. Therapeutic use and untoward responses will derive from these basic pharmacological features, which, apart from the desired actions, can produce untoward effects. Serious adverse reactions are rare with appropriate blood concentrations; however, it is difficult to control theophylline concentrations, especially when it is taken orally, absorption being erratic. When it is given intravenously, slow administration is advised. With both oral and parenteral administration, monitoring of serum theophylline concentrations with individual adjustment of dosage is necessary.

The adverse effects of other theophylline derivatives have been reviewed (SEDA-17, 1). Whether or not newer drugs have similar efficacy and/or better tolerability than the classic theophylline derivatives has not been carefully evaluated.

General adverse effects

Nausea, vomiting, headache, dizziness, tachycardia, dysrhythmias, vascular collapse, tremor, agitation, and convulsions have been described. Although 1% of children and 4% of adults cannot tolerate even low serum concentrations, the incidence of adverse effects during therapeutic use is generally related to the logarithm of the serum concentration. However, the relation between the severity of the symptoms of theophylline poisoning and serum–drug concentration is less clear and may well depend on the chronicity of the overdose (SEDA-9, 78) (see Drug overdose in this monograph).

True allergy to theophylline is rare. Hypersensitivity to aminophylline, when it occurs, is most likely due to the ethylenediamine component. Two immunogenic types of reactions have been described, one of urticaria and general pruritus and the other involving thrombocytopenia and a hemorrhagic diathesis (SED-8, 1). Also reported have been contact dermatitis, exfoliative erythroderma accompanied by bronchospasm and pruritus, generalized dermal reactions (SED-10, 4), severe generalized symptoms with a high fever (7), and aggressive behavior in a child (8).

The observation of excess mortality from cancer of the pancreas among US male veterans admitted to hospital for bronchial asthma and discharged on various bronchodilators has raised the question of a possible connection to the theophylline (see the monograph on Caffeine). Although not fully resolved, chronic use of theophylline does not appear to be associated with an increased risk of esophageal or gastric carcinoma (9).

Organs and Systems

Cardiovascular

The relation between toxicity and excessive serum theophylline concentrations has been confirmed, tachycardia being a frequent indication of toxic symptoms (SED-9, 3). It appears that the cardiac and metabolic effects of theophylline are at least partly related to catecholamine release (SEDA-13, 1). The importance of appropriate dosage has been stressed in several papers, all indicating the particular risk of ventricular fibrillation in subjects with respiratory distress (10). The authors have pointed to the potentially lethal effect of serum theophylline concentrations in excess of 20 µg/ml. In another study, half the patients with serum concentrations greater than 35 µg/ml had life-threatening dysrhythmias (SEDA-7, 7). In one study of the effect of oral aminophylline on cardiac dysrhythmias in 15 patients with chronic obstructive pulmonary disease, aminophylline had both dysrhythmogenic and chronotropic effects but did not change the grade of dysrhythmia (SEDA-7, 7). In another study of 16 patients there was a relation between the use of theophylline and multifocal atrial tachycardia (11). Whereas raised blood theophylline concentrations are likely in themselves to produce cardiovascular complications, patients with pre-existing cardiac disease are at greater risk.

Respiratory

Aminophylline sometimes aggravates bronchial asthma; sensitization to the ethylenediamine component is considered to be responsible (SEDA-6, 5).

Nervous system

In addition to the more common adverse effects of tremor, dizziness, anxiety, agitation, insomnia, visual disturbances, and seizures, depression, confusion (SEDA-6, 1), acute dyskinesias (SEDA-17, 1), and toxic psychosis (SED-10, 5) have also been reported.

Seizures with focal onset have been described during treatment of status asthmaticus in adult patients with no previous history of epilepsy (12). Although, serum theophylline concentrations are an unreliable predictor of seizures, seizures occur most commonly at serum concentrations over 40–50 µg/ml (13). Older patients are more likely to have seizures than younger ones at similar theophylline concentrations (14). Patients with pre-existing central nervous system abnormalities (15) or severe pulmonary disease may also be at increased risk (SEDA-17, 1). Theophylline-induced seizures have been reported in two neonates (SEDA-6, 2); the serum theophylline concentration during seizures was 51 µg/ml.

- A girl aged 3.5 months receiving theophylline had a seizure; in the next few months, she had a mixed seizure disorder and subsequently symptoms of moderately severe right brain damage (16).

Because toxic symptoms before seizures can be absent or undetected, such events underline the need for blood concentration monitoring during therapy.

Theophylline disturbs sleep more profoundly in caffeine-sensitive subjects (SEDA-15, 1). Exacerbation of spasticity has occurred when theophylline was used after a stroke (17).

Psychological, psychiatric

The concern that cognitive function may be impaired in children taking theophylline is still not resolved (SEDA-14, 1) (SEDA-15, 1); a review has suggested that detrimental effects of theophylline on various measures of cognitive function may be measure-specific (18).

Endocrine

The dangers of theophylline toxicity in hypothyroidism have been described (19).

Metabolism

The metabolic effects of intravenous infusions of aminophylline have been studied in a series of healthy young subjects with regard to serum glucose, insulin, glucagon, cortisol, and free fatty acid concentrations. Infusion of aminophylline, which produced theophylline concentrations in the usual target range (10–20 µg/ml) caused only small increases in plasma glucose concentrations but rapid, pronounced, and prolonged rises in free fatty acids. Increases in free fatty acid concentrations paralleled the rise in theophylline concentrations (SEDA-6, 6).

Gastrointestinal

The commonest gastrointestinal adverse effects of aminophylline in adults are nausea and gastrointestinal irritation, which are primarily a function of serum theophylline concentrations, although some additional local irritation may be produced by oral administration. Nausea was reported in six of 20 asthmatic patients with serum theophylline concentrations of 20 µg/ml (SED-9, 4). In a survey of 2766 theophylline-treated patients with cardiac or pulmonary diseases, 11% had adverse effects, most of which were gastrointestinal disturbances (7.8%) (SED-9, 4).

In two elderly patients hematemesis was thought to have been due to both a local irritant action of aminophylline and a susceptibility to systemic toxic effects at lower serum theophylline concentrations (SEDA-5, 5).

Esophageal ulceration can result from tablets that were taken with insufficient fluid and/or while lying down (20,21).

Non-allergic proctitis associated with an aminophylline suppository has been reported in a child (SEDA-17, 1).

Liver

Since about 90% of theophylline is eliminated by hepatic metabolism, liver function is related to toxic effects on other systems (see Susceptibility Factors in this monograph). Hepatitis has been reported in two patients (SEDA-15, 1).

Pancreas

An excess in mortality from pancreatic cancer has been noted among US male veterans admitted to hospital for bronchial asthma and discharged on various bronchodilators, suggesting a possible connection with theophylline

(SEDA-7, 8). A relation between coffee consumption and pancreatic cancer was reported in a case-control study (SEDA-7, 8), with an unexpected increase in pancreatic cancer associated with an increase in coffee drinking (relative risk in men, 2.6). The same workers studied changes in mortality from pancreatic cancer in different countries in relation to changes in coffee consumption and found a significant relation between increases in coffee consumption and increases in mortality from pancreatic cancer. However, the data on which the findings were based were crude.

Urinary tract

Methylxanthines, especially theophylline, in healthy subjects inhibit solute reabsorption in both the proximal nephron and the diluting segment without changing either glomerular filtration rate or renal blood flow appreciably. Accordingly, an apparent increase in creatinine clearance in a heavy tea drinker has been attributed to a discrepancy between GFR and creatinine clearance (22).

Skin

Three cases of skin eruptions have been reported in patients taking aminophylline who had probably been sensitized by the use of a multiantibiotic cream formulation also containing ethylenediamine (SEDA-12, 4). A case of Stevens–Johnson syndrome after modified-release theophylline has been reported (23).

Immunologic

Salivary IgA was significantly reduced in asthmatic children treated with theophylline compared with healthy controls or unmedicated patients with asthma (24). This finding is in harmony with earlier statements that theophylline reduces the bactericidal capacity of leukocytes and affects suppressor T cells (SEDA-11, 6). Theophylline also interferes with basophil and eosinophil responses; these immunomodulatory effects might participate in its therapeutic efficacy (25,26).

Long-Term Effects

Mutagenicity

Genetic effects of theophylline are not well known. Theophylline suppresses phosphodiesterase and cyclic AMP activity, and increases calcium transport in animals (SEDA-4, 25), suggesting a potential for teratogenicity. An increased rate of sister chromatid exchange rate, an indication of mutagenicity, has also been reported (SEDA-17, 1).

Second-Generation Effects

Pregnancy

Theophylline crosses the placenta, resulting in potentially dangerous serum theophylline concentrations in the neonate (SEDA-5, 3). This is of practical importance, since 1.3% of pregnant women have asthma. Fetal tachycardia has been observed when maternal blood concentration

exceeds 20 µg/ml (27). In one neonate the serum theophylline concentration of 14 µg/ml was 3 µg/ml higher than the cord or maternal serum concentrations. The authors concluded that neonates of mothers receiving theophylline products should be monitored for pharmacological effects of theophylline. In another study, women with asthma who used theophylline had a longer average duration of labor than did untreated women, since theophylline inhibited uterine contractions (SEDA-5, 3).

Fetotoxicity

Symptoms of irritability, vomiting, and jitteriness have been described in an infant, possibly related to ingestion of aminophylline during pregnancy by an asthmatic mother (28).

In pregnant women with bronchial asthma, bronchospasm can be exacerbated during labor, necessitating infusion of aminophylline. The placental transport of aminophylline and its effects on the fetus and the neonate are poorly understood. A recent report has highlighted the potential problems (29).

- A 26-year-old primigravida with bronchial asthma developed an acute exacerbation at 40 weeks gestation. She did not respond to salbutamol and was given hydrocortisone and aminophylline 250 mg intravenously, without improvement. She received two more doses of intravenous aminophylline, the last being 2 hours before delivery. At cesarean section she delivered a full-term female neonate weighing 3150 g with Apgar scores of 3 and 5 at 1 and 5 minutes respectively. Within 3 minutes of birth the neonate developed multifocal clonic convulsions, which failed to respond to intravenous glucose, calcium, phenobarbital, and phenytoin. She had a tachycardia, a normal blood pressure, and poor respiratory drive, and was comatose. The serum theophylline concentration was 8.6 µg/ml (47 µmol/l) at 1 hour of life. Despite ventilatory support and anticonvulsant therapy, she continued to have intermittent seizures and died 48 hours after birth. Postmortem showed normal brain structure and no evidence of hemorrhage or asphyxial brain injury.

The toxic concentrations for theophylline in neonates have not been well defined, and can vary from infant to infant. Other pharmacokinetic factors, such as low plasma protein binding and limited capacity for excretion could make neonates prone to aminophylline toxicity. Fetuses and neonates can develop theophylline toxicity even with plasma concentrations in the target range, since they can metabolize theophylline to caffeine, adding to the methylxanthine load.

Lactation

The kinetics of theophylline transfer into breast-milk have been studied in three lactating women given theophylline intravenously (SEDA-6, 2). The data suggested that theophylline accumulation to toxic concentrations should not occur in most breast-fed infants, but that serum theophylline concentrations in the mother should be kept as low as possible and transfer will be minimal if infants are nursed just before the mother takes the theophylline.

Susceptibility Factors

Age

Prematurity

Serious difficulties arise in giving theophylline to premature neonates. These are explained by peculiarities in biotransformation in prematurity. Transformation of theophylline to caffeine in premature neonates is explained by the lack of enzymes for desmethylation and *C*-hydroxylation and by predominant *N*-methylase activity. High serum caffeine concentrations have been found in two studies of premature newborns with respiratory disturbances who had received theophylline (SEDA-4, 3); caffeine and theophylline synergism was incriminated in the development of toxic reactions in these children. In another study, there was clinically significant hyperglycemia in 13% of preterm infants who received theophylline (30). Blood glucose concentrations should be monitored in preterm infants who receive theophylline. There is some evidence (SED-10, 5) that administration of 4.5 mg/kg of theophylline followed by a maintenance dose (1.2–1.52 mg/kg every 8–12 hours) is most likely to correct respiratory disturbances in premature neonates, while avoiding adverse effects. Because of simpler dosing regimens, some pediatricians prefer caffeine as the drug of choice in premature neonates (27,31).

Developmental differences in the balance between metabolic and renal elimination pathways determine the unique toxicokinetics of theophylline in neonates. Three premature neonates received inadvertent intravenous doses of theophylline for apnea of prematurity (32). All had sinus tachycardia and agitation. Maximum serum theophylline concentrations were 55–123 µg/ml; theophylline-derived caffeine concentrations plateaued at 8.4–13 µg/ml and did not fall during the sampling period. The half-life of theophylline was 28–37 hours and the clearance 0.02–0.05 l/kg/hour. This study shows that, in contrast to older children, theophylline elimination remains a first-order process during acute intoxication in premature infants, and that large overdoses of theophylline in neonates, while inducing symptoms and signs of overdose, do not uniformly result in life-threatening sequelae and do not necessarily require invasive treatment. Although the literature is rather scanty, the pharmacokinetics of theophylline in premature neonates do not seem to be different from those in full-term neonates. Furthermore, toxic concentrations in neonates have not been defined. It has been speculated that various factors in neonates, such as low plasma protein binding, metabolic interconversion to caffeine, and limited excretory capacity, make them susceptible to toxicity even at plasma concentrations within the usual adult therapeutic range (SEDA-23, 1)(SEDA-25, 1).

Term infants

Caution has been urged in using theophylline for wheezing in full-term infants under 3 months of age (SEDA-4, 3).

Cerebral blood flow velocity in infants treated with an intravenous bolus dose of aminophylline was reduced, perhaps because of a reduction in PCO_2, due to aminophylline (33).

Children

Convulsions have been attributed to theophylline given for bronchial asthma in the usual recommended dosage, with serum concentrations in the target range of 10–20 µg/ml (SEDA-5, 4). Young children may be more prone to excitement and dehydration due to diuresis and vomiting. Two afebrile children reported visual hallucinations during theophylline toxicity (SEDA-13, 2). Despite the recommendation for higher initial doses in young children, dosage management is more difficult, owing to the greater likelihood of toxicity, which is probably a reflection of more erratic pharmacodynamics.

Based on a retrospective investigation of theophylline-induced convulsions in epileptic children, it was concluded that infants under 1 year of age with epilepsy have a higher risk of theophylline-induced convulsions; theophylline should be avoided in this group (34).

Elderly patients

It is not entirely clear whether the risk of toxicity in the elderly is a function of an age-related reduction in the rate of metabolism, a tendency for systemic toxic effects to develop at relatively lower serum concentrations, or the greater likelihood of conditions that affect the pharmacokinetics of theophylline, for example cardiac failure, liver disease, or chronic obstructive pulmonary disease. In a review of 72 consecutive patients referred to a regional poisons center with chronic theophylline intoxication, stratification of data by chronological age showed a stepwise increase in the frequency of life-threatening events with advancing years; the authors suggested that elderly patients have a much greater risk of such events than younger patients (35).

In an investigation of 510 episodes of raised theophylline concentrations in 214 hospitalized patients, the authors concluded that life-threatening events can occur in critically ill patients or patients with past seizures or dysrhythmias with mildly raised theophylline concentrations (21–40 µg/ml) (36).

One study showed that in order to maintain plasma concentrations in the target range in elderly people, the maintenance dosage should be reduced by about 25% (SEDA-5, 1). Other reports have implicated chronic obstructive pulmonary disease and cardiac failure in elderly patients whose reduced theophylline clearances led to toxic reactions or potentially toxic plasma concentrations (SEDA-7, 6) (SEDA-8, 1). It was suggested that aminophylline dosages be reduced by 50% when there are clinical signs of cardiac failure, in order to avoid excessive drug accumulation.

Hepatic disease

In cirrhosis of the liver, drug clearance falls, the half-life of theophylline increases about threefold, and the incidence of adverse effects increases (SED-10, 6).

Drug Administration

Drug overdose

The effect of theophylline is cumulative, and there is a danger of overdosage if it is given repeatedly. However, intoxication has been described in young children after a single suppository (SED-9, 4).

The symptoms of overdosage are nausea, vomiting, headache, dizziness, tachycardia, dysrhythmias, vascular collapse, tremor, agitation, and convulsions. The highly variable interindividual differences in metabolism and disease-related alterations in metabolism of the various formulations can result in iatrogenically induced overdosage. The tendency of patients to increase the dose as their condition deteriorates is a second major source of overdosing.

The amount of drug administered, whether putative or known, is less likely to correlate with untoward reactions than the serum concentration is. Likewise, the serum concentration correlates poorly with relatively minor adverse effects. More reliable is the escalating correlation of serious toxic effects with serum concentrations rising above 15 µg/ml.

The relation between the severity of clinical manifestations of theophylline poisoning and serum drug concentrations is unclear. However, a start has been made in clarifying this, with the finding that patients with theophylline overdose caused by chronic repeated overmedication often develop seizures and dysrhythmias with serum concentrations of 40–70 µg/ml, while those with acute single ingestion are highly unlikely to suffer serious complications unless serum concentrations exceed 100 µg/ml. According to this study, patients who took a single overdose were easily recognized by the presence of hypotension, hypokalemia, and a low serum bicarbonate, features not present in patients with chronic overdose (SEDA-11, 5) (37). These findings could lead to better indicators for more aggressive treatment before the advent of major complications.

In healthy volunteers, theophylline reduced circulating pyridoxal phosphate (vitamin B6) concentrations, presumably by noncompetitive inhibition of pyridoxal kinase. Theophylline concentrations of approximately 10 µg/ml produced only partial inhibition, plasma pyridoxal kinase and pyridoxal concentrations being unaffected. The authors speculated that with theophylline overdose and greater inhibition, vitamin B6 deficiency might contribute to seizures (SEDA-14, 2).

Rhabdomyolysis is a rare complication of theophylline overdose (38).

- A 73-year-old man took an unknown number of theophylline modified-release tablets and furosemide 40 mg tablets. He developed a tachydysrhythmia, vomiting, and restlessness. His maximum theophylline concentration was 67 µg/ml and he had hypokalemia (2.8 mmol/l) and hyponatremia (123 mmol/l). The maximum creatine kinase activity was (32 mol/l [sic]) and the serum myoglobin concentration was 3789 µg/l. He was treated with oral activated charcoal, continuous venovenous hemodialysis, intravenous potassium and sodium chloride, forced diuresis, and continuous intravenous metoprolol, and survived without sequelae.

Management

The use of hemodialysis or hemoperfusion in the management of theophylline toxicity was initially controversial (SEDA-8, 11) (SEDA-9, 10) (SEDA-11, 5). In one study

(39) hemoperfusion provided a higher theophylline clearance rate than hemodialysis, but the latter appears to have comparable efficacy in reducing the morbidity of severe theophylline intoxication and is associated with a lower rate of procedural complications. The recommendation that these treatments be considered for patients who fail to respond to supportive care is complicated by findings that, once major complications have occurred, the benefits from these risky procedures are greatly reduced.

However, charcoal hemoperfusion is now regarded as the recommended method for rapid reduction of serum theophylline concentrations, if necessary, although access to this technique is limited in most hospitals. Venovenous hemofiltration, which is readily available in many hospitals, appears to be a realistic and practical alternative to charcoal hemoperfusion, in combination with oral activated charcoal, particularly in the hemodynamically unstable patient with severe theophylline toxicity without anticoagulation (40,41). A higher extraction ratio in neonates than in adults has also been described (41).

Drug–Drug Interactions

General

Both positive and negative drug interactions have been reported with theophylline. The usefulness of combination products has also been discussed (SEDA-6, 2) (SEDA-11, 7). The use of combinations complicates the evaluation of adverse effects, particularly those of theophylline and ephedrine. The likelihood of adverse effects of each component and synergistic effects between components must be evaluated in relation to the patient's clinical condition. A positive feature is the likelihood of greater compliance with an effective combination product.

Pharmacokinetic interactions

In one study, antacids increase the rate of theophylline absorption without a change in total systemic availability (42), although in an earlier study there was no interaction (43).

The concomitant use of drugs that reduce theophylline clearance can produce toxic serum concentrations with therapeutic doses of theophylline. Most of these drugs are believed to have this effect by inhibiting the hepatic microsomal P450-metabolizing enzymes that are responsible for the biotransformation of theophylline. Such drugs include the xanthine oxidase inhibitor allopurinol, some histamine H_2 receptor antagonists (cimetidine in particular), some antidepressants (fluvoxamine), and oral contraceptives. Also included are some antimicrobial drugs, for example tetracycline, the macrolides (erythromycin and troleandomycin), fluoroquinolones (ciprofloxacin, norfloxacin), possibly the cephalosporins, isoniazid, antihelminthic drugs (thiabendazole and possibly pyrantel), and antiviral drugs (influenza vaccine and vidarabine).

Other drugs that reduce theophylline clearance, but by unknown mechanisms, are cardiac medications: the beta-blocker propranolol, the calcium channel blockers nifedipine and verapamil, and mexiletine. Considering that increased theophylline concentrations can lead to an increased propensity for central and cardiac stimulation, it is prudent to avoid using a combination of theophylline and cardiac medications, especially antidysrhythmic drugs.

Lipophilic beta-adrenoceptor antagonists are metabolized to varying degrees by oxidation by liver microsomal cytochrome P450 (for example propranolol by CYP1A2 and CYP2D6 and metoprolol by CYP2D6). These agents can therefore reduce the clearance and increase the steady-state plasma concentrations of other drugs that undergo similar metabolism, potentiating their effects. Drugs that interact in this way include theophylline (44).

Conversely, drugs that induce P450 enzymes increase theophylline clearance and lower blood concentrations. These include the barbiturates, phenytoin, carbamazepine, and rifampicin. Increased clearance also occurs with a high-protein diet, marijuana, and tobacco. With phenytoin the interaction is two-sided: the plasma concentrations of both drugs fall. This can result in poor seizure and respiratory control and in drug toxicity.

Recommendations have been presented for correction of theophylline doses during concomitant medication with some of the above drugs (SEDA-8, 130) (45). Concomitant therapy with allopurinol, cimetidine, erythromycin, furosemide, isoprenaline, or propranolol requires a reduction in dose of about 20–30%; for oleandomycin the reduction should be about 50%.

Pharmacodynamic interactions
A debate was triggered by the suggestion some years ago of increased mortality because of greater use of theophylline, and additive toxicity between oral theophylline and inhaled beta-adrenoceptor agonists (SEDA-7, 1). Some authors concluded that a combination of theophylline and beta-adrenoceptor agonists in low doses will give equal and possibly superior results over full doses of either agent and may produce fewer adverse effects (SEDA-7, 2) (SEDA-8, 13). No one has yet documented any serious synergistic toxicity from a combination of theophylline and a beta-adrenoceptor agonist in appropriate doses (SEDA-15, 1), and it seems clear that the patient with severe asthma who is undertreated is much more at risk of dying than one who receives concomitant theophylline and adrenergic drug treatment in appropriate doses and sequence (SEDA-9, 10). At any rate, the most appropriate maintenance therapy continues to be debated. In recent years, it has been customary to use a combination of a beta-adrenoceptor agonist and a nontheophylline formulation, such as a steroid inhaler. However, it should be noted that the finding that theophylline has significant effects on basophils and eosinophils renewed an interest in theophylline.

Adverse reactions to theophylline are more common in patients who are concurrently taking a tetracycline (SED-9, 4).

Adenosine

Theophylline increases the dose of adenosine needed for conversion of supraventricular tachycardia, through competitive inhibition at purine receptors (46).

Caffeine

Caffeine can accumulate to toxic concentrations during treatment with theophylline (47). Likewise, concomitant administration of caffeine and theophylline can significantly increase plasma theophylline concentrations and reduce the clearance rates of theophylline and its metabolites (48).

Calcium channel blockers

Theophylline toxicity has been reported in several patients, apparently stabilized on theophylline, after the introduction of verapamil (49) or nifedipine (50).

Cephalosporins

The interaction between certain cephalosporins (including moxalactam) and the alcohol in theophylline elixir can cause a disulfiram-like reaction (51).

Citalopram

Both theophylline and citalopram are metabolized by CYP1A2. In an open, multiple-dose study in 13 healthy nonsmoking volunteers, steady-state citalopram therapy had no significant effect on theophylline metabolism. The authors suggested that dosage adjustment of theophylline may not be necessary in patients taking concurrent citalopram (52). The most frequent treatment-related adverse effects were fatigue and nausea.

Corticosteroids

In a single-dose study of the interaction of theophylline with prednisolone, the plasma concentrations of both drugs were slightly lower when they were given in combination than when given alone (53).

The kinetic behavior of theophylline given concomitantly with methylprednisolone and auranofin to six women suggested a possible interaction of theophylline with auranofin, although a role of the corticosteroid could not be ruled out. The observed concentrations of theophylline were lower than expected, suggesting the need to measure serum theophylline concentrations in patients who also take steroids and gold salts (54).

Digoxin

Despite the ability of theophylline to reduce blood concentrations of digitalis in digitalis intoxication (55), therapeutic doses of theophylline can cause dysrhythmias in the presence of concentrations of digoxin in the high part of the usual target range (56).

Fluvoxamine

Fluvoxamine is a potent inhibitor of cytochrome CYP1A2, which may lead to interactions with several tricyclic antidepressants and theophylline (57).

Furosemide

Intravenous furosemide reportedly increased steady-state theophylline concentrations by about 20% (SED-11, 428). However, this result has not been confirmed (58).

GABA receptor antagonists

Carbapenems (imipenem more than meropenem) are believed to increase central nervous system excitation by inhibition of GABA binding to receptors. Combinations with other GABA-inhibiting drugs, such as theophylline or quinolones, have been reported to provoke seizures (59,60).

Gold salts

The kinetic behavior of theophylline given concomitantly with methylprednisolone and auranofin to six women suggested a possible interaction of theophylline with auranofin, although a role of the corticosteroid could not be ruled out. The observed concentrations of theophylline were lower than expected, suggesting the need to measure serum theophylline concentrations in patients who also take steroids and gold salts (54).

Lithium

Theophylline increased the renal clearance of lithium, with resultant lowering of the serum lithium concentration (61).

Macrolides

The most frequently observed effects of macrolides on theophylline pharmacokinetics are increases in half-life and serum theophylline concentrations and reduced clearance (62). The interaction with theophylline is mainly seen with higher doses of macrolides and can result in theophylline toxicity (63).

Ciprofloxacin

Serious theophylline toxicity has been attributed to ciprofloxacin (64).

- A 79-year-old woman presented with a generalized seizure. She had long-standing asthma, and her admission medication included steroid and salbutamol inhalers, oral prednisolone, and oral modified-release aminophylline 450 mg bd. Plasma theophylline concentrations over the previous 3 years had been 8–12 µg/ml (44–66 µmol/l) without apparent toxicity. Seven days before presentation she had developed a fever and cough productive of green sputum, and had been given ciprofloxacin 500 mg bd. Despite adequate gas exchange, she developed repeated episodes of self-terminating supraventricular tachycardia, associated with hypokalemia (serum potassium 3.2 mmol/l), acidosis (pH 7.05), hypotension, and difficulty in breathing. The theophylline concentration was 33 µg/ml (183 µmol/l). Renal function was normal, and no other causes of fits or dysrhythmias were apparent. She was unable to tolerate oral activated charcoal and hemodialysis was started. After 2 hours of dialysis, the plasma theophylline had fallen to 15 µg/ml (177 µmol/l), she was in sinus rhythm, and her serum potassium was 3.8 mmol/l. She made an uneventful recovery.

Erythromycin

Erythromycin can increase the serum concentrations of theophylline by 20–25%. However, patients with an average serum concentration of theophylline under 15 µg/ml will probably have only a small increase in their serum theophylline concentration during erythromycin therapy, whereas patients with steady-state concentrations above 15 µg/ml deserve careful monitoring and close observation for symptoms of theophylline toxicity during treatment with erythromycin (65,66).

Fatal aminophylline toxicity has been described, precipitated by the concomitant administration of erythromycin (64).

- A 55-year-old man with a long history of bronchiectasis and severe obstructive pulmonary disease presented with a chest infection, having been taking oral modified-release aminophylline 450 mg bd for 4 years, with trough concentrations always in the range 6–12 µg/ml (33–66 µmol/l) and no apparent toxicity. Two days before admission, his general practitioner had prescribed trimethoprim 200 mg bd for a suspected urinary tract infection. On the day of admission, he was given cefotaxime 1 g intravenously bd and erythromycin 500 mg orally qds. Other medications included captopril 25 mg tds, furosemide 80 mg bd, ranitidine 150 mg bd, protriptyline 10 mg tds, and inhaled budesonide. He was anxious and had a fine tremor, but his gas exchange was satisfactory. He had chronic renal impairment of uncertain cause and hyperkalemia (5.5 mmol/l). The possibility of aminophylline toxicity was raised, but despite this, he received three doses of erythromycin. The plasma theophylline was 66 µg/ml (363 µmol/l). He had an episode of ventricular tachycardia and fibrillation, was successfully resuscitated, but had a second episode of ventricular tachycardia 30 minutes later, from which he could not be resuscitated. The plasma theophylline concentration at the time of his second cardiac arrest was 58 µg/ml (319 µmol/l).

These cases of interactions of aminophylline with macrolide antibiotics illustrate that serious, even fatal, adverse effects can occur when possible interactions are not considered. In both cases, experienced physicians prescribed appropriate antimicrobial drugs, but omitted to consider the possibility of interactions with aminophylline, and failed to reduce the dose of aminophylline or to measure theophylline concentrations. In the first case the development of tachycardia, hypokalemia, acidosis, vomiting, and convulsions can be explained on the basis of theophylline toxicity caused by ciprofloxacin, while in the second the anxiety, tremor, and cardiac arrests could all have resulted from an interaction of aminophylline and erythromycin. These cases add to an extensive literature that emphasizes the potential for interaction between aminophylline and drugs metabolized by CYP1A2.

Prulifloxacin

Prulifloxacin reduced the elimination of theophylline in healthy volunteers (67) presumably by inhibiting cytochrome CYP1A2.

Mexiletine

Mexiletine reduces the clearance of theophylline, and this combination has been reported to cause ventricular tachycardia (68). A similar interaction with caffeine has been reported (69).

Olanzapine

In healthy subjects, olanzapine did not affect theophylline pharmacokinetics (70). These results confirm the earlier reported *in vitro* findings that olanzapine is not a potent inhibitor of CYP1A2 (71).

Pancuronium

Antagonism to pancuronium has been found with theophylline concentrations in excess of the recommended target range (SEDA-5, 4).

Aminophylline appears to facilitate neuromuscular transmission, perhaps by increasing neurotransmitter release through raising cyclic AMP concentrations at the neuromuscular junction by phosphodiesterase inhibition (72). This would account for the antagonism of pancuronium-induced blockade that has been reported to occur in the presence of very high serum concentrations of theophylline (73). A similar effect should theoretically occur with other nondepolarizing relaxants.

Phenobarbital

Co-medication with phenobarbital may require an increase in the theophylline dose by about 30%; concurrent use with phenytoin may require an increase of as much as 75% (45).

Proton pump inhibitors

Co-administration of either lansoprazole or pantoprazole in healthy subjects did not affect the steady-state pharmacokinetics of theophylline in therapeutic doses (74).

Quinine

Quinine increased serum theophylline concentrations in an elderly patient (75).

Quinolones

Levofloxacin has been reported to interact with theophylline.

- A 59-year-old Japanese man taking theophylline for emphysema had stimulation, insomnia, and tachycardia owing to theophylline toxicity after he also took levofloxacin and clarithromycin (76). His theophylline clearance returned to normal and his symptoms resolved after withdrawal of levofloxacin, while clarithromycin was continued.

In a randomized, multiple-dose, period-balanced, three-way, crossover study in healthy nonsmoking male volunteers, moxifloxacin did not alter the pharmacokinetics of theophylline (77).

In seven healthy volunteers taking modified-release theophylline, intravenous pazufloxacin mesilate increased serum theophylline concentrations; analysis of the urinary excretion of theophylline and its metabolites suggested that CYP1A2 had been inhibited (78). Theophylline concentrations need to be monitored if pazufloxacin is co-administered.

Tacrolimus

An interaction of theophylline with tacrolimus has been described (79).

- A 33-year-old man with end-stage renal disease due to diabetic nephropathy received a cadaveric kidney graft. Immunosuppressive therapy after transplantation included tacrolimus (7 mg/day), azathioprine (75 mg/day), and prednisone (7.5 mg/day). He developed erythrocytosis 3 months later and was given drugs that reduce erythropoietin production, first enalapril, without success, and then theophylline (600 mg/day). After 1 month, his serum creatinine and tacrolimus concentrations were raised. The dosage of theophylline was therefore reduced to 300 mg/day four times a week. One month later, his serum creatinine and tacrolimus trough blood concentrations increased further. On withdrawal of theophylline, both renal function and tacrolimus trough blood concentration rapidly normalized. Theophylline was then reintroduced in a lower dose and increased the AUC of tacrolimus.

CYP3A4 is primarily responsible for tacrolimus biotransformation in the liver, but it has only a minor role in theophylline metabolism. It is therefore surprising that this tacrolimus–theophylline interaction occurred. The authors suggested that as long as renal function remains stable, low-dose theophylline can be used in transplant patients with erythrocytosis, provided that tacrolimus concentrations are closely monitored.

Tegaserod

The effect of tegaserod on the single-dose pharmacokinetics and safety profile of theophylline has been determined in a randomized, open, crossover study in 18 subjects (80). Tegaserod did not alter the pharmacokinetics of theophylline and the incidence of adverse events was similar after co-administration. However, since in vitro studies have shown that tegaserod inhibits CYP1A2 (81), more evidence is needed to claim that no dosage adjustment is required when theophylline is co-administered.

Terbinafine

In a randomized crossover study in 12 healthy volunteers, terbinafine increased the AUC of theophylline by 16%, with a 14% reduction in clearance and a 24% prolongation of half-life (82). The clinical impact of these results is difficult to define because of the small sample size in this study and because it is not known what effect terbinafine has on steady-state theophylline concentrations. An earlier study (83) showed that terbinafine reduced the clearance of caffeine, which is metabolized via similar pathways. Until more information is available, clinicians who prescribe terbinafine for patients taking chronic theophylline therapy should be cautious, and serum theophylline concentrations should be monitored.

Tocainide

Tocainide reduces the clearance of theophylline and increases its half-life, but to an extent that is probably clinically insignificant (84).

Trimethoprim

Two episodes of severe hyponatremia have been described in the same patient, one attributed to theophylline and the other to trimethoprim (85). The evidence to support an interaction is circumstantial, and the patient was taking multiple medications, making interpretations difficult.

Food-Drug Interactions

Food can affect both the absorption and the clearance of theophylline. One study showed that the absorption of a modified-release formulation of theophylline was very slow after an overnight fast, in contrast to absorption after a test meal (86). The effect may be dose-related. More specifically, dietary protein significantly affects theophylline clearance: a low-protein diet reduces theophylline clearance and a high-protein diet increases it. The implications for clinical practice have not been elaborated, but dietary extremes are contraindicated in patients taking theophylline (51).

References

1. Calhoun LK. Pharmacologic management of apnea of prematurity. J Perinat Neonatal Nurs 1996;9(4):56–62.
2. Hudgel DW, Thanakitcharu S. Pharmacologic treatment of sleep-disordered breathing. Am J Respir Crit Care Med 1998;15(3):691–9.
3. Pesek CA, Cooley R, Narkiewicz K, Dyken M, Weintraub NL, Somers VK. Theophylline therapy for near-fatal Cheyne–Stokes respiration: a case report. Ann Intern Med 1999;130(5):427–30.
4. Boyle CA, Berkowitz GS, LiVolsi VA, Ort S, Merino MJ, White C, Kelsey JL. Caffeine consumption and fibrocystic breast disease: a case-control epidemiologic study. J Natl Cancer Inst 1984;72(5):1015–19.
5. Weinmann S, Siscovick DS, Raghunathan TE, Arbogast P, Smith H, Bovbjerg VE, Cobb LA, Psaty BM. Caffeine intake in relation to the risk of primary cardiac arrest. Epidemiology 1997;8(5):505–8.
6. Levy BD, Kitch B, Fanta CH. Medical and ventilatory management of status asthmaticus. Intensive Care Med 1998;24(2):105–17.
7. Thompson PJ, Gibb WR, Cole P, Citron KM. Generalised allergic reactions to aminophylline. Thorax 1984;39(8):600–3.
8. Vaughan TL, Farrow DC, Hansten PD, Chow WH, Gammon MD, Risch HA, Stanford JL, Schoenberg JB, Mayne ST, Rotterdam H, Dubrow R, Ahsan H, West AB, Blot WJ, Fraumeni JF Jr. Risk of esophageal and gastric adenocarcinomas in relation to use of calcium channel blockers, asthma drugs, and other medications that promote gastroesophageal reflux. Cancer Epidemiol Biomarkers Prev 1998;7(9):749–56.
9. Niggemann B. Aggressives Verhalten als Nebenwirkung des Äthylendiamins (nicht aber des Theophyllins). [Aggressive behavior as a side effect of ethylenediamine (but not of theophylline).] Monatsschr Kinderheilkd 1985;133(7):487.
10. Chaithiraphan S. Fatal complication associated with intravenous use of aminophylline. J Med Assoc Thai 1976;59(11):507–9.
11. Levine JH, Michael JR, Guarnieri T. Multifocal atrial tachycardia: a toxic effect of theophylline. Lancet 1985;1(8419):12–14.
12. Schwartz MS, Scott DF. Aminophylline-induced seizures. Epilepsia 1974;15(4):501–5.
13. Burkle WS, Gwizdala CJ. Evaluation of "toxic" serum theophylline concentrations. Am J Hosp Pharm 1981;38(8):1164–6.
14. Aitken ML, Martin TR. Life-threatening theophylline toxicity is not predictable by serum levels. Chest 1987;91(1):10–14.
15. Covelli HD, Knodel AR, Heppner BT. Predisposing factors to apparent theophylline-induced seizures. Ann Allergy 1985;54(5):411–15.
16. Noetzel MJ. Theophylline neurotoxicity resulting in significant unilateral brain-damage. Dev Med Child Neurol 1985;27(2):242–5.
17. Clark JE, Devenport JK. Theophylline exacerbating spasticity. JAMA 1983;250(4):485.
18. International Coffee Organization. United States of America: coffee drinking study. London: International Coffee Organization; 1989.
19. Aderka D, Shavit G, Garfinkel D, Santo M, Gitter S, Pinkhas J. Life-threatening theophylline intoxication in a hypothyroid patient. Respiration 1983;44(1):77–80.
20. D'Arcy PF. Drug reactions and interactions. Pharm Int 1984;5:117.
21. Stoller JL. Oesophageal ulceration and theophylline. Lancet 1985;2(8450):328–9.
22. De Giorgi A, De Negri F, Fioriti R, Giannarelli C, Carmassi F. Creatinine clearance overestimated glomerular filtration rate in a heavy tea-drinker. Am J Kidney Dis 2001;37(4):877–8.
23. Brook U, Singer L, Fried D. Development of severe Stevens–Johnson syndrome after administration of slow-release theophylline. Pediatr Dermatol 1989;6(2):126–9.
24. Gozal D, Ben-Aryeh H, Szargel R, Colin A. Salivary composition in asthmatic children on theophylline. Isr J Med Sci 1985;21(5):460–1.
25. Ezeamuzie CI, Al-Hage M. Effects of some anti-asthma drugs on human eosinophil superoxide anions release and degranulation. Int Arch Allergy Immunol 1998;115(2):162–8.
26. Gibbs BF, Vollrath IB, Albrecht C, Amon U, Wolff HH. Inhibition of interleukin-4 and interleukin-13 release from immunologically activated human basophils due to the actions of anti-allergic drugs. Naunyn Schmiedebergs Arch Pharmacol 1998;357(5):573–8.
27. Serafin WE. Drugs used in the treatment of asthma. In: Hardman JG, Limbird LE, Molinoff PB, Ruddon RW, Gilman AG, editors. Goodman and Gilman's the pharmacological basis of therapeutics. 9th ed. New York: McGraw-Hill; 1996:659–82.
28. Khadem B. Aminophylline poisoning in children: report of two cases. Harper Hosp Bull 1962;20:179–84.
29. Agarwal HS, Nanavati RN, Bhagwat MS, Kabra NS, Udani RH. Transplancental aminophylline toxicity. Indian Pediatr 1998;35(5):467–70.
30. Srinivasan G, Singh J, Cattamanchi G, Yeh TF, Pildes RS. Plasma glucose changes in preterm infants during oral theophylline therapy. J Pediatr 1983;103(3):473–6.
31. LeGrady D, Dyer AR, Shekelle RB, Stamler J, Liu K, Paul O, Lepper M, Shryock AM. Coffee consumption and mortality in the Chicago Western Electric Company Study. Am J Epidemiol 1987;126(5):803–12.
32. Lowry JA, Jarrett RV, Wasserman G, Pettett G, Kauffman RE. Theophylline toxicokinetics in premature newborns. Arch Pediatr Adolesc Med 2001;155(8):934–9.
33. Rosenkrantz TS, Oh W. Aminophylline reduces cerebral blood flow velocity in low-birth-weight infants. Am J Dis Child 1984;138(5):489–91.
34. Miura T, Kimura K. Theophylline-induced convulsions in children with epilepsy. Pediatrics 2000;105(4 Part 1):920.
35. Shannon M, Lovejoy FH Jr. The influence of age vs peak serum concentration on life-threatening events after chronic

theophylline intoxication. Arch Intern Med 1990;150(10): 2045–8.

36. Emerman CL, Devlin C, Connors AF. Risk of toxicity in patients with elevated theophylline levels. Ann Emerg Med 1990;19(6):643–8.

37. Olson KR, Benowitz NL, Woo OF, Pond SM. Theophylline overdose: acute single ingestion versus chronic repeated overmedication. Am J Emerg Med 1985;3(5):386–94.

38. Teweleit S, Hippius M, Pfeifer R, Hoffmann A. Rhabdomyolyse als seltene Komplikation einer Theophyllinintoxikation. [Rhabdomyolysis as a rare complication of theophylline poisoning.] Med Klin (Munich) 2001;96(1):40–4.

39. Shannon MW. Comparative efficacy of hemodialysis and hemoperfusion in severe theophylline intoxication. Acad Emerg Med 1997;4(7):674–8.

40. Henderson JH, McKenzie CA, Hilton PJ, Leach RM. Continuous venovenous haemofiltration for the treatment of theophylline toxicity. Thorax 2001;56(3):242–3.

41. Gitomer JJ, Khan AM, Ferris ME. Treatment of severe theophylline toxicity with hemodialysis in a preterm neonate. Pediatr Nephrol 2001;16(10):784–6.

42. Gugler R, Allgayer H. Effects of antacids on the clinical pharmacokinetics of drugs: an update. Clin Pharmacokinet 1990;18(3):210–19.

43. Jonkman JH, Upton RA. Pharmacokinetic drug interactions with theophylline. Clin Pharmacokinet 1984;9(4):309–34.

44. Conrad KA, Nyman DW. Effects of metoprolol and propranolol on theophylline elimination. Clin Pharmacol Ther 1980;28(4):463–7.

45. Jonkman JHG, Koeter GH, Berg WC. Geneesmiddelen met een therapeutisch belangrijke invloed op de farmacokinetiek van theofylline. [Drugs with a therapeutically important influence on the pharmacokinetics of theophylline.] Pharm Weekbl 1983;118:185.

46. diMarco JP, Sellers TD, Lerman BB, Greenberg ML, Berne RM, Belardinelli L. Diagnostic and therapeutic use of adenosine in patients with supraventricular tachyarrhythmias. J Am Coll Cardiol 1985;6(2):417–25.

47. Iversen SA, Murphy PG, Leakey TE, Rydlewski A, Levy RD, Gertner D. Unsuspected caffeine toxicity complicating theophylline therapy. Hum Toxicol 1984;3(6):509–12.

48. Jonkman JH, Sollie FA, Sauter R, Steinijans VW. The influence of caffeine on the steady-state pharmacokinetics of theophylline. Clin Pharmacol Ther 1991;49(3):248–55.

49. Burnakis TG, Seldon M, Czaplicki AD. Increased serum theophylline concentrations secondary to oral verapamil. Clin Pharm 1983;2(5):458–61.

50. Parrillo SJ, Venditto M. Elevated theophylline blood levels from institution of nifedipine therapy. Ann Emerg Med 1984;13(3):216–17.

51. Brown KR, Guglielmo BJ, Pons VG, Jacobs RA. Theophylline elixir, moxalactam, and a disulfiram reaction. Ann Intern Med 1982;97(4):621–2.

52. Moller SE, Larsen F, Pitsiu M, Rolan PE. Effect of citalopram on plasma levels of oral theophylline. Clin Ther 2000;22(12):1494–501.

53. Anderson JL, Ayres JW, Hall CA. Potential pharmacokinetic interaction between theophylline and prednisone. Clin Pharm 1984;3(2):187–9.

54. Falcao AC, Rocha MJ, Almeida AM, Caramona MM. Theophylline pharmacokinetics with concomitant steroid and gold therapy. J Clin Pharm Ther 2000;25(3):191–5.

55. Tamburrini LR, Curri G, Mian G, et al. Digitaleteofillina: antagonismo della teofillina nella farmacocinetica della digossina in alcuni soggetti vecchi intossicati: implicazioni clinicobiometriche. Prog Med 1984;40:295.

56. Marchlinski FE, Miller JM. Atrial arrhythmias exacerbated by theophylline: response to verapamil and evidence for triggered activity in man. Chest 1985;88(6):931–4.

57. Barnes TR, Kidger T, Greenwood DT. Viloxazine and migraine. Lancet 1979;2(8156–8157):1368.

58. Janicke UA, Krudewagen B, Schulz A, Gundert-Remy U. Absence of a clinically significant interaction between theophylline and furosemide. Eur J Clin Pharmacol 1987;33(5):487–91.

59. De Sarro A, Ammendola D, De Sarro G. Effects of some quinolones on imipenem-induced seizures in DBA/2 mice. Gen Pharmacol 1994;25(2):369–79.

60. Semel JD, Allen N. Seizures in patients simultaneously receiving theophylline and imipenem or ciprofloxacin or metronidazole. South Med J 1991;84(4):465–8.

61. Cook BL, Smith RE, Perry PJ, Calloway RA. Theophylline–lithium interaction. J Clin Psychiatry 1985;46(7):278–9.

62. Watkins PB, Murray SA, Winkelman LG, Heuman DM, Wrighton SA, Guzelian PS. Erythromycin breath test as an assay of glucocorticoid-inducible liver cytochromes P-450: studies in rats and patients. J Clin Invest 1989;83(2):688–97.

63. Parish RA, Haulman NJ, Burns RM. Interaction of theophylline with erythromycin base in a patient with seizure activity. Pediatrics 1983;72(6):828–30.

64. Andrews PA. Interactions with ciprofloxacin and erythromycin leading to aminophylline toxicity. Nephrol Dial Transplant 1998;13(4):1006–8.

65. Zarowitz BJ, Szefler SJ, Lasezkay GM. Effect of erythromycin base on theophylline kinetics. Clin Pharmacol Ther 1981;29(5):601–5.

66. Paulsen O, Hoglund P, Nilsson LG, Bengtsson HI. The interaction of erythromycin with theophylline. Eur J Clin Pharmacol 1987;32(5):493–8.

67. Fattore C, Cipolla G, Gatti G, Bertoli A, Orticelli G, Picollo R, Millerioux L, Ciottoli GB, Perucca E. Pharmacokinetic interactions between theophylline and prulifloxacin in healthy volunteers. Clin Drug Invest 1998;16:387–92.

68. Kessler KM, Interian A Jr, Cox M, Topaz O, De Marchena EJ, Myerburg RJ. Proarrhythmia related to a kinetic and dynamic interaction of mexiletine and theophylline. Am Heart J 1989;117(4):964–6.

69. Joeres R, Richter E. Mexiletine and caffeine elimination. N Engl J Med 1987;317(2):117.

70. Macias WL, Bergstrom RF, Cerimele BJ, Kassahun K, Tatum DE, Callaghan JT. Lack of effect of olanzapine on the pharmacokinetics of a single aminophylline dose in healthy men. Pharmacotherapy 1998;18(6):1237–48.

71. Ring BJ, Catlow J, Lindsay TJ, Gillespie T, Roskos LK, Cerimele BJ, Swanson SP, Hamman MA, Wrighton SA. Identification of the human cytochrome P450 responsible for the in vitro formation of the major oxidative metabolites of the antipsychotic agent olanzapine J Pharmacol Exp Ther 1996;276(2):658–66.

72. Ono K, Nagano O, Ohta Y, Kosaka F. Neuromuscular effects of respiratory and metabolic acid-base changes in vitro with and without nondepolarizing muscle relaxants Anesthesiology 1990;73(4):710–16.

73. Doll DC, Rosenberg H. Antagonism of neuromuscular blockage by theophylline. Anesth Analg 1979;58(2):139–40.

74. Pan WJ, Goldwater DR, Zhang Y, Pilmer BL, Hunt RH. Lack of a pharmacokinetic interaction between lansoprazole or pantoprazole and theophylline. Aliment Pharmacol Ther 2000;14(3):345–52.

75. Shane R. Potential toxicity of theophylline in combination with Quinamm. Am J Hosp Pharm 1982;39(1):40.

76. Nakamura H, Ohtsuka T, Enomoto H, Hasegawa A, Kawana H, Kuriyama T, Ohmori S, Kitada M. Effect of levofloxacin on theophylline clearance during theophylline and clarithromycin combination therapy. Ann Pharmacother 2001;35(6):691–3.

77. Stass H, Kubitza D. Lack of pharmacokinetic interaction between moxifloxacin, a novel 8-methoxyfluoroquinolone, and theophylline. Clin Pharmacokinet 2001;40(Suppl 1):63–70.

78. Niki Y, Watanabe S, Yoshida K, Miyashita N, Nakajima M, Matsushima T. Effect of pazufloxacin mesilate on the serum concentration of theophylline. J Infect Chemother 2002;8(1):33–6.

79. Boubenider S, Vincent I, Lambotte O, Roy S, Hiesse C, Taburet AM, Charpentier B. Interaction between theophylline and tacrolimus in a renal transplant patient. Nephrol Dial Transplant 2000;15(7):1066–8.

80. Zhou H, Khalilieh S, Svendsen K, Pommier F, Osborne S, Appel-Dingemanse S, Lasseter K, McLeod JF. Tegaserod coadministration does not alter the pharmacokinetics of theophylline in healthy subjects. J Clin Pharmacol 2001;41(9):987–93.

81. Vickers AE, Zollinger M, Dannecker R, Tynes R, Heitz F, Fischer V. In vitro metabolism of tegaserod in human liver and intestine: assessment of drug interactions Drug Metab Dispos 2001;29(10):1269–76.

82. Trepanier EF, Nafziger AN, Amsden GW. Effect of terbinafine on theophylline pharmacokinetics in healthy volunteers. Antimicrob Agents Chemother 1998;42(3):695–7.

83. Wahllander A, Paumgartner G. Effect of ketoconazole and terbinafine on the pharmacokinetics of caffeine in healthy volunteers. Eur J Clin Pharmacol 1989;37(3):279–83.

84. Loi CM, Wei X, Parker BM, Korrapati MR, Vestal RE. The effect of tocainide on theophylline metabolism. Br J Clin Pharmacol 1993;35(4):437–40.

85. Dreiher J, Porath A. Severe hyponatremia induced by theophylline and trimethoprim. Arch Intern Med 2001;161(2):291–2.

86. D'Arcy PF. Theophylline toxicity from dose-dumping. Pharm Int 1985;6:289.

Thiacetazone

See also Antituberculosis drugs

General Information

Thiacetazone (thioacetazone, thiosemicarbazone) was greeted enthusiastically in 1946 as one of the first synthetic agents against tuberculosis. However, its use rapidly diminished with the increasing observation of untoward effects. It is currently rarely used and then only for economical reasons. Dosages should never exceed 200 mg/day.

Adverse effects of thiacetazone include bone marrow depression and hemolytic anemia. It can also cause serious skin rashes. Continuous laboratory and clinical observations are required (1).

Organs and Systems

Hematologic

Adverse effects of thiacetazone include bone marrow depression, with anemia, leukopenia, agranulocytosis, and thrombocytopenia (2–4). Hemolytic anemia has also been described (5).

Gastrointestinal

Anorexia, nausea, and vomiting are not uncommon with thiacetazone (1).

Urinary tract

Hepatotoxicity with jaundice is frequent with thiacetazone (1).

Skin

Adverse effects of thiacetazone on the skin are of various types, mainly erythematous and maculopapular rashes, angioedema, purpura (6), toxic epidermal necrolysis, Stevens–Johnson syndrome, and pigmentation (7).

Of 50 cases of cutaneous adverse effects of thiacetazone, there were 48 cases of erythema multiforme (25 cases of Stevens–Johnson syndrome and 23 of toxic epidermal necrolysis), one case of erythrodermia, and one case of lichenoid toxidermia; there were 20 deaths, 16 with toxic epidermal necrolysis and four with Stevens–Johnson syndrome (8).

In a retrospective study, 38 cases of toxic epidermal necrolysis were observed in Dakar, and were attributed to thiacetazone in 24 cases; 23 died, mainly because of hypovolemic shock during the first week and septic shock during the second (9). Those who died were generally aged over 50 years, had more than 50% skin involvement, and had evolving tuberculosis at the time of presentation or HIV infection. After-effects were vaginal synechia and two cases of blindness.

Immunologic

Cutaneous allergic reactions to thiacetazone are very common in HIV-positive patients, in the order of 20%. Ethambutol should therefore be used instead of thiacetazone in these patients (10).

Susceptibility Factors

Arguments have been advanced for the abandonment of thiacetazone as an antituberculosis drug (11,12), despite its cheapness, on the grounds that it often causes severe skin reactions, some rapidly fatal, in patients infected with HIV-1 (13). The WHO and IUATLD has recommended careful information and surveillance of possible adverse reactions, particularly cutaneous, in patients treated for tuberculosis in such countries and immediate replacement with ethambutol if there are any prodromal signs of toxicity.

Anergy to tuberculin and lymphopenia have been associated with an increased risk of adverse reactions to thiacetazone. In a randomized study of rifampicin- and thiacetazone-containing regimens in HIV-positive adults with pulmonary tuberculosis, eight of 13 patients who developed adverse reactions were tuberculin-anergic, compared with 12 of 77 patients who did not develop adverse reactions (13). An absolute lymphocyte count below 2.0×10^9/l was also associated with adverse reactions.

Drug–Drug Interactions

Isoniazid

Thiacetazone combined with isoniazid (and possibly thioacetazone alone) has been reported to damage chromosomes in cultured human lymphocytes (14).

References

1. Mandell GL, Sande MA. Antimicrobial agents: drugs used in the chemotherapy of tuberculosis and leprosy. In: Goodman Gilman A, Rall TW, Nies AS, Taylor P, editors. Goodman and Gilman's The Pharmacological Basis of Therapeutics. 8th ed. Chapter 49. New York: Pergamon Press, 1990:1146.

2. Chan SL. Chemotherapy of tuberculosis. In: Davies PDO, editor. Clinical Tuberculosis. London: Chapman and Hall, 1994:141.

3. Gupta SK, Bedi RS, Maini VK. Agranulocytosis due to thiacetazone. Indian J Tuberc 1983;30:146.

4. Jaliluddin, Mohsini AA. Fatal aplastic anaemia due to thiacetazone toxicity. J Indian Med Assoc 1981;77(11):176–7.

5. Anonymous. Antileprosy drugs. BMJ 1971;3(767):174–6.

6. Naraqi S, Temu P. Thiacetazone skin reaction in Papua New Guinea. Med J Aust 1980;1(10):480–1.

7. Short GM. Side-effect of thiacetazone. S Afr Med J 1980;58(1):5–6.

8. Dieng MT, Ndiaye B, Camara C. Toxidermies au thiacétazone (TB1) dans un service hospitalier à Dakar. [Skin toxicity of thiacetazone (TB1) at a hospital service in Dakar.] Dakar Med 2001;46(1):1–3.

9. Mame Thierno D, On S, Thierno Ndiaye S, Ndiaye B. Syndrome de Lyell au Senegal: responsabilité de la thiacétazone. [Lyell syndrome in Senegal: responsibility of thiacetazone.] Ann Dermatol Venereol 2001;128(12):1305–7.

10. Nunn P, Kibuga D, Gathua S, Brindle R, Imalingat A, Wasunna K, Lucas S, Gilks C, Omwega M, Were J, McAdam K. Cutaneous hypersensitivity reactions due to thiacetazone in HIV-1 seropositive patients treated for tuberculosis. Lancet 1991;337(8742):627–30.

11. Elliott AM, Foster SD. Thiacetazone: time to call a halt? Considerations on the use of thiacetazone in African populations with a high prevalence of human immunodeficiency virus infection. Tuber Lung Dis 1996;77(1):27–9.

12. Rieder HL, Enarson DA. Rebuttal: time to call a halt to emotions in the assessment of thioacetazone. Tuber Lung Dis 1996;77(2):109–11.

13. Okwera A, Johnson JL, Vjecha MJ, Wolski K, Whalen CC, Hom D, Huebner R, Mugerwa RD, Ellner JJ. Risk factors for adverse drug reactions during thiacetazone treatment of pulmonary tuberculosis in human immunodeficiency virus infected adults. Int J Tuberc Lung Dis 1997;1(5):441–5.

14. Ahuja YR, Jaju M, Jaju M. Chromosome-damaging action of isoniazid and thiacetazone on human lymphocyte cultures in vivo. Hum Genet 1981;57(3):321–2.

Thiamine

See also Vitamins

General Information

The requirement for thiamine depends on the utilization of energy-yielding substrates, and increases with energy expenditure; it is therefore expressed relative to energy intake (here given in mega-Joules, MJ, formerly often given per 1000 kilocalories (kcal) which is a better known but outdated terminology). The Average Requirement is 72 micrograms/MJ/day, the Population Reference Intake is 100 micrograms/MJ/day, and the Lowest Threshold Intake is 50 micrograms/MJ/day. Expressed for average energy expenditure, this would mean an Average Requirement of 0.8 mg/day for men and 0.6 for women, a Population Reference Intake of 1.1 and 0.9 mg/day, and a Lowest Threshold Intake of 0.6 and 0.4 mg/day (1).

Excess thiamine is normally readily cleared by the kidneys. Important adverse reactions are usually associated with parenteral feeding with doses much larger than the Population Reference Intake and over long periods of time. Most common are hypersensitivity reactions, which have been observed mainly after parenteral administration. The symptoms and signs are weakness, precordial pain, palpitation, dyspnea, epigastric pain, vomiting, itching, erythema, scaling of the facial skin, severe rash, tachycardia, hypotension, purpura, semicoma, and even fatal anaphylactic shock.

Despite its favorable safety profile, it cannot be assumed that thiamine is completely innocuous. Thiamine hydrochloride is routinely given to patients with Wernicke's encephalopathy or malnourished states (such as malabsorption, beri-beri, cancer, AIDS, and chronic alcohol abuse). Systemic reactions are rare but deaths can occur.

Organs and Systems

Respiratory

Respiratory failure has been reported after parenteral administration of high doses of thiamine, albeit on only a single occasion (2).

Skin

Thiamine hydrochloride, and possibly its intermediates such as thiothiamide, can cause allergic contact dermatitis (3,4). A prospective study of the toxicity of parenteral thiamine hydrochloride in a large group of patients showed adverse reactions in only 1.1% of the cases, mainly in the form of local irritation. Only one out of the 11 adverse reaction cases was serious (5).

Immunologic

Anaphylactic shock is a major adverse effect of thiamine, and can be life-threatening. It is IgE-mediated (6) and usually occurs after multiple parenteral dosages (6–10) but occasionally also after intramuscular injection. In some cases oral challenge did not produce any reaction (8,11,12).

- A 51-year-old woman with diabetes mellitus, chronic alcoholism, and anxiety disorder became acutely confused and was given 50% dextrose 25 g and thiamine hydrochloride 100 mg intravenously; 20 minutes later she became deeply cyanosed with shallow labored breathing at 28/minute, hypertensive, and tachycardic, with respiratory and metabolic acidosis and a blood alcohol concentration of 124 mg/dl (27 mmol/l) (13). The next morning she was communicative and oriented and her vital signs and blood gases were normal. She was given thiamine hydrochloride intravenously and within moments developed shortness of breath, warmth, and tightness of the throat. She had a tachycardia, hypotension, hypoxia, and central cyanosis. She recovered within 24 hours.

In 989 consecutive patients (1070 doses) there were 12 adverse reactions (1.1% of doses), comprising local irritation in 11 cases and a major skin reaction in the 12th. The authors concluded that thiamine hydrochloride can safely be given intravenously and that intradermal test doses before administration are not warranted unless patients have had previous allergic reactions (5).

Drug–Drug Interactions

Cancer chemotherapy

In a review it was suggested that thiamine when given to patients with cancer may interfere with chemotherapy in that thiamine may promote nucleic acid ribose synthesis and tumor cell proliferation via the transketolase pathway. The authors suggest that an oversupply of thiamine may actually do harm and may be responsible for the failure of therapeutic attempts to terminate cancer cell proliferation (14). Thiamine is directly involved in ribose synthesis in pancreatic adenocarcinoma cells through transketolase-catalysed non-oxidative pentose phosphate reactions. In addition, the chemically modified co-factor oxythiamine inhibited tumor cell proliferation in vitro and in vivo by 40% and 91% in two distinct tumor models (14). According to a review of thiamine supplementation in patients with cancer this raises serious suspicions that routine thiamine administration may not be warranted and could possibly be harmful (15). Thiamine deficiency in cancer patients is most often observed during or shortly after chemotherapy. Clinical and experimental data have shown increased thiamine utilization by human tumors and its interference with experimental chemotherapy. Current thiamine administration protocols oversupply thiamine by 200–20 000% of the RDA, because it is considered harmless and needed by cancer patients. However, since the thiamine-dependent transketolase pathway is the main reaction that supplies ribose phosphate for nucleic acids in tumors, excessive thiamine supplementation may be responsible for failed therapeutic attempts to terminate cancer cell proliferation. The authors therefore recommended that cancer management should include regular evaluation of thiamine status of the patient, especially during chemotherapy, and that dosages of thiamine should not exceed 1.2 mg/day unless necessary. Future studies should clarify whether oxythiamine as an inhibitor of transketolase is really safe and whether it is especially effective against cancer.

References

1. Scientific Committee for Food. Nutrient and energy intakes for the European Community. Directorate-General Industry, Commission of the European Communities. Luxembourg, 1993.
2. Fishman L, Goldstein M. Vitamins in dermatology. J Med Assoc Ga 1968;57(7):342–6.
3. Ingemann Larsen A, Riis Jepsen J, Thulin H. Allergic contact dermatitis from thiamine. Contact Dermatitis 1989;20(5):387–8.
4. Villas Martinez F, Joral A, Garmendia Goitia JF. Reaccion anafilactica por vitamina B1. [Anaphylactic reaction caused by vitamin B1.] Med Clin (Barc) 1993;100(8):316.
5. Wrenn KD, Murphy F, Slovis CM. A toxicity study of parenteral thiamine hydrochloride. Ann Emerg Med 1989;18(8):867–70.
6. Fernandez M, Barcelo M, Munoz C, Torrecillas M, Blanca M. Anaphylaxis to thiamine (vitamin B1). Allergy 1997;52(9):958–60.
7. Stephen JM, Grant R, Yeh CS. Anaphylaxis from administration of intravenous thiamine. Am J Emerg Med 1992;10(1):61–3.
8. Leung R, Puy R, Czarny D. Thiamine anaphylaxis. Med J Aust 1993;159(5):355.
9. Van Haecke P, Ramaekers D, Vanderwegen L, Boonen S. Thiamine-induced anaphylactic shock. Am J Emerg Med 1995;13(3):371–2.
10. Wrenn KD, Slovis CM. Is intravenous thiamine safe? Am J Emerg Med 1992;10(2):165.
11. Kolz R, Lonsdorf G, Burg G. Unverträglichkeitsreaktionen nach parenteraler Gabe von Vitamin B1. [Intolerance reactions following parenteral administration of vitamin B.] Hautarzt 1980;31(12):657–9.
12. Morinville V, Jeannet-Peter N, Hauser C. Anaphylaxis to parenteral thiamine (vitamin B1). Schweiz Med Wochenschr 1998;128(44):1743–4.
13. Johri S, Shetty S, Soni A, Kumar S. Anaphylaxis from intravenous thiamine—long forgotten? Am J Emerg Med 2000;18(5):642–3.
14. Boros LG, Brandes JL, Lee WN, Cascante M, Puigjaner J, Revesz E, Bray TM, Schirmer WJ, Melvin WS. Thiamine supplementation to cancer patients: a double edged sword. Anticancer Res 1998;18(1B):595–602.
15. Boros LG, Puigjaner J, Cascante M, Lee WN, Brandes JL, Bassilian S, Yusuf FI, Williams RD, Muscarella P, Melvin WS, Schirmer WJ. Oxythiamine and dehydroepiandrosterone inhibit the nonoxidative synthesis of ribose and tumor cell proliferation. Cancer Res 1997;57(19):4242–8.

Thiamphenicol

General Information

Thiamphenicol is a semisynthetic derivative of chloramphenicol, an amine derivative of hydrocarbylsulfonylpropandiol. It differs in that the NO_2 group in the para position is replaced by a methylsulfonyl group. The substitution in the para position of the molecule does not influence its effects on either protein or DNA synthesis in any recognizable way. The antibacterial spectrum is almost identical to that of chloramphenicol.

The two drugs are used in similar dosages, although there are large differences in their elimination. Glucuronidation is unimportant for thiamphenicol: over 90% of a therapeutic dose is excreted by the kidneys in unchanged form. The corresponding figure for chloramphenicol is only about 10%. Thus, in contrast to chloramphenicol, the half-life of thiamphenicol is prolonged in patients with reduced renal function in whom accumulation can occur.

Although the mechanism by which chloramphenicol causes aplastic anemia is not fully understood, all the available evidence suggests that the biochemical consequences of thiamphenicol administration and the risk of serious complications differ from those of chloramphenicol (1).

It does not seem unreasonable, therefore, to use thiamphenicol for wider indications than chloramphenicol, provided that the dosage is adjusted according to renal function. However, thiamphenicol has adverse effects on bone marrow, calling for a degree of caution. It is therefore generally recommended that thiamphenicol should not be given for more than 10–14 days.

The most important adverse effects are an immediate dose-related and reversible disturbance of erythropoiesis (2,3) and peripheral neuropathy. In contrast to chloramphenicol, aplastic anemia and the gray syndrome do not seem to occur with thiamphenicol.

Observational studies

Thiamphenicol has been used to treat 1171 patients with chancroid (4). Each patient was given granulated thiamphenicol 5.0 g orally in a single dose. Only 0.89% did not respond. A few patients had adverse effects, including epigastric pain, headache, nausea, and skin rashes; all were mild and of short duration.

Organs and Systems

Nervous system

Several cases of peripheral neuropathy after the administration of thiamphenicol for 3–5 months have been reported and were thought to be due to a vitamin deficiency. In most cases the sensory function of the nerves of the legs was primarily affected. When discovered early, the damage was reversible, but in other cases it tended to persist (5).

Hematologic

There is evidence that thiamphenicol is more potent than chloramphenicol in causing the early dose-related and therefore predictable type of bone marrow toxicity. Many studies have shown that thiamphenicol in a dose of 1.5 g, and to a much lesser extent 0.75 g/day, causes an immediate disturbance of erythropoiesis in almost every case (6). Alterations in the bone marrow become most evident in patients with renal disease and in elderly subjects (probably because of reduced renal function). Leukocytes and thrombocytes are only slightly affected (7).

Most reviewers have been impressed by the fact that the reported cases of peripheral cytopenia were never accompanied by bone marrow aplasia (8). There have been some doubtful case reports of marrow aplasia, in which factors such as advanced age (predisposing to antibiotic accumulation), neoplasia, concurrent treatment (myelotoxic drugs, anticoagulants), and major surgical interventions have to be mentioned. Even if these cases are to be ascribed to thiamphenicol, they fall within the normal spontaneous incidence of aplastic anemia (9–12).

The most severe hematological changes were reported after treatment of typhoid fever and sepsis with relatively high doses of thiamphenicol. These changes have always been reversible on withdrawal. The serum iron concentration returned to normal within a few days and was rapidly followed by reticulocytosis. Experimental results strongly suggest that the toxic effect of thiamphenicol is temporary and that recovery of the bone marrow after drug-induced suppression is complete, with no subsequent risk of myelodysplasia or leukemic transformation (13).

The occurrence of acute leukemia has been studied in relation to preceding use of drugs (before the 12 months preceding the diagnosis) in a case-control study of 202 patients aged over 15 years with a diagnosis of acute leukemia and age- and sex-matched controls (14). Among users of chloramphenicol or thiamphenicol the odds ratio for any use was 1.1 (0.6–2.2) whereas the odds ratio for high doses was 1.8 (0.6–5.3). Other systemic antibiotics showed no substantial relation with the occurrence of leukemia.

Gastrointestinal

Diarrhea, nausea, or constipation occur in under 10% of cases and are usually mild (15).

Skin

Alopecia has been reported in patients with renal insufficiency taking thiamphenicol, and can lead to complete baldness (6). After withdrawal, normal hair growth will recover. Other skin reactions are rare.

Immunologic

Thiamphenicol has immunosuppressive properties, which are ascribed to an effect on immunocompetent cells, rather than on immunoglobulin synthesis (16). In animals, thiamphenicol prolonged the survival of skin homografts (17).

Second-Generation Effects

Fetotoxicity

Although thiamphenicol penetrates the fetal circulation and is distributed evenly in fetal tissues, no fetal abnormalities have been related to thiamphenicol administration during pregnancy (18). Since mitochondrial protein synthesis in the fetal liver is inhibited by the drug concentrations normally attained, repeated administration of thiamphenicol to pregnant women is not recommended.

Susceptibility Factors

Renal disease

Impaired renal function is an important risk factor for toxic effects of thiamphenicol (19).

Other features of the patient

Pre-existing bone marrow dysfunction and prolonged treatment is an important risk factor for toxic effects of thiamphenicol (20).

References

1. Yunis AA. Chloramphenicol: relation of structure to activity and toxicity. Annu Rev Pharmacol Toxicol 1988;28:83–100.
2. International Symposium on Chloramphenicol, Thiamphenicol, Known and Unkown Aspects of Drug-Host Interactions, January 10–12, 1973. Sils-Maria, Switzerland, 1973.

3. Ferrari V. Salient features of thiamphenicol: review of clinical pharmacokinetics and toxicity. Sex Transm Dis 1984;11(Suppl 4):336–9.

4. Belda Junior W, Siqueira LF, Fagundes LJ. Thiamphenicol in the treatment of chancroid. A study of 1,128 cases. Rev Inst Med Trop Sao Paulo 2000;42(3):133–5.

5. Japanese Ministry of Health and Welfare. Information on adverse reactions to drugs. Peripheral nerve damage due to thiamphenicol. Jpn Med Gaz 1977;20:12.

6. Sotto JJ, Simon P, Subtil P, Rozenbaum A, Najean Y, Pecking A. Toxicité hématologique du thiophénicol. [Hematologic toxicity of thiophenicol.] Nouv Presse Méd 1976;5:2163.

7. Moeschlin S, Novotny Z, Koller F, Ruefli P. Zytostatische Nebenwirkungen des Thiamphenicols: Alopezie, reversible Zytopenien. [Cytostatic side effects of thiamphenicol: alopecia, reversible cytopenia.] Schweiz Med Wochenschr 1974;104(11):384–7.

8. Keiser G. Co-operative study of patients treated with thiamphenicol. Comparative study of patients treated with chloramphenicol and thiamphenicol. Postgrad Med J 1974;50(Suppl 5):143–5.

9. Najean Y, Guerin MN, Chomienne C. Etiology of acquired aplastic anemia. In: Najean Y, Tognoni G, Yunis AA, editors. Safety Problems Related to Chloramphenicol and Thiamphenicol Therapy. New York: Raven Press, 1981:61.

10. De Renzo A, Formisano S, Rotoli B. Bone marrow aplasia and thiamphenicol. Haematologica 1981;66(1):98–104.

11. Keiser G. Toxizitat von Choramphenicol und Thiamphenicol (CAP und TAP). In: Lohr GW, Arnold H, et al. editors. Probleme der Erythrozytopoese, Granulozytopoese und des malignen Melanoms. Berlin, Heidelberg: Springer Verlag, 1978:179.

12. Martinez-Dalmau A, Fernandez MN, Barbolla L. Haematological toxicity of thiamphenicol: analysis of a case with total irreversible bone marrow aplasia and general review of the problem. [Hematologic toxicity of thiamphenicol. Analysis of a case of irreversible total medullary aplasia and general review of the problem.] Sangre (Barc) 1972;17(1):59–66.

13. Yunis AA, Miller AM, Salem Z, Arimura GK. Chloramphenicol toxicity: pathogenetic mechanisms and the role of the p-NO$_2$ in aplastic anemia. Clin Toxicol 1980;17(3):359–73.

14. Traversa G, Menniti-Ippolito F, Da Cas R, Mele A, Pulsoni A, Mandelli F. Drug use and acute leukemia. Pharmacoepidemiol Drug Saf 1998;7(2):113–23.

15. Belda W. O tratamento da uretrite gonococica aguda masculina pelo tianfenicol: uma revisao. Rev Bras Clin Ter 1978;7:375–9.

16. Vindel JA, Khoury B. Inhibition by thiamphenicol of antibody production induced by different antigens. Postgrad Med J 1974;50(Suppl 5):108–10.

17. Ono K, Hattori T, Kusaba A, Inokuchi K. Prolongation of rat heart allograft survival by thiamphenicol. Surgery 1972;71(2):258–61.

18. Nau H, Welsch F, Ulbrich B, Bass R, Lange J. Thiamphenicol during the first trimester of human pregnancy: placental transfer in vivo, placental uptake in vitro, and inhibition of mitochondrial function. Toxicol Appl Pharmacol 1981;60(1):131–41.

19. Oldershausen HF, Menz HP, Hartmann I, Bezler HJ, Ilg R, Burck GC. Serum levels and elimination of thiamphenicol in patients with impaired liver function and with renal failure on dialysis. Postgrad Med J 1974;50(Suppl 5):44–6.

20. Franceschinis R. Drug utilization data for chloramphenicol and thiamphenicol in recent years. New York: Raven Press, 1981:81–9.

Thiamylal sodium

See also General anesthetics

General Information

Thiamylal sodium is a short-acting intravenous barbiturate anesthetic.

Organs and Systems

Electrolyte balance

Severe hypokalemia occurred in a 14-year-old boy undergoing emergency aortic arch replacement under deep hypothermic cardiopulmonary bypass (1). He was treated with thiamylal by infusion, total dose 30 mg/kg, for persistent convulsive waves on his electroencephalogram. This caused his serum potassium concentration to fall to 1.6 mmol/l. The hypokalemia was resistant to potassium chloride infusion 80 mmol/hour, but responded to replacing the thiamylal infusion with midazolam. It was noted that there have also been reports of severe hypokalemia in brain-injured patients undergoing thiopental coma therapy

Reference

1. Irita K, Kawasaki T, Uenotsuchi T, Sakaguchi Y, Takahashi S. Does barbiturate therapy cause severe hypokalemia? Anesth Analg 1998;86(1):214.

Thiazide diuretics

See also Diuretics

General Information

Although one thiazide diuretic may be 100 times more potent than another weight for weight, all these drugs have essentially the same properties. Their mechanism of action (inhibition of sodium and chloride reabsorption in the distal convoluted tubule of the kidney) is identical and they can therefore be dealt with as a group. Thiazide-like diuretics, structurally different from the thiazides, have similar actions. Thiazide and thiazide-like diuretics are listed in Table 1.

Like all diuretics, the thiazides can cause electrolyte abnormalities, such as hypokalemia and hyponatremia, and dehydration. These complications are uncommon in patients with uncomplicated hypertension, but are more common in patients with heart failure or decompensated hepatic cirrhosis with secondary hyperaldosteronism. Until a patient is accustomed to the effect of a diuretic, dizziness may be experienced. Serum lipid concentrations are slightly raised acutely and hyperglycemia can occur during long-term therapy. Rare effects are thrombocytopenia, rashes, drug fever, cholestatic jaundice, pancreatitis, and precipitation of hepatic

Table 1 Thiazide and thiazide-like diuretics (rINNs except where stated)

Thiazide diuretics	Thiazide-like diuretics
Althiazide	Chlortalidone
Bemetizide	Clopamide
Bendroflumethiazide	Clorexolone
Benzthiazide	Fenquizone (pINN)
Benzylhydrochlorothiazide	Indapamide
Butizide	Mefruside
Chlorothiazide	Metolazone
Cyclopenthiazide	Quinethazone
Cyclothiazide	Tripamide
Epithiazide	Xipamide
Hydrochlorothiazide	
Hydroflumethiazide	
Mebutizide	
Methylclothiazide	
Meticrane	
Paraflutizide	
Penflutizide	
Polythiazide	
Teclothiazide	
Trichlormethiazide	

encephalopathy in patients with hepatic cirrhosis. Generalized allergic vasculitis has been described occasionally. There is no evidence that the thiazides induce tumors. Second generation effects have not been reported.

Organs and Systems

Cardiovascular

Although dizziness is a fairly frequent complaint at the beginning of diuretic treatment (1), postural hypotension is rarely reported. Ischemic complaints (mesenteric infarction and transient cerebral ischemic attacks) have been observed in elderly patients, but it is not clear whether these resulted from diminished organ perfusion or from an effect of the drug itself. The former is more likely, since similar problems have arisen with any form of antihypertensive treatment in old people who have to some degree become dependent on their hypertension to ensure a blood supply through sclerotic vessels.

Criticism directed against the diuretics in recent years has among other things sought to show that they increase the risk of coronary events, including acute myocardial infarction. However, there is no real basis for such criticism. Properly used in hypertension the diuretics produce a beneficial effect out of all proportion to any incidental adverse cardiac effects.

- A 72-year-old woman had repeated episodes of sudden-onset pulmonary edema, each occurring immediately after she took a dose of hydrochlorothiazide 12.5 mg (2).

The close temporal relation between the ingestion of hydrochlorothiazide and the onset of symptoms, together with rapid and full clinical recovery after withdrawal of therapy, suggested drug-induced pulmonary edema and possible anaphylactoid hypotension.

Respiratory

In the older literature there were various reports of acute allergic interstitial pneumonitis caused by the thiazides, sometimes confirmed by rechallenge. Typically, it presents within an hour of taking the drug and causes chest pain, breathlessness, or both; the chest X-ray is characteristic (3,4). Recovery is rapid, but assisted ventilation may be needed. Most cases in the recent literature relate to hydrochlorothiazide, but that may simply reflect its wide use. A case involving chlorothiazide (5) suggests that this syndrome can arise with any thiazide, although it sometimes occurs after the first dose of hydrochlorothiazide when other thiazides have been well tolerated. The incidence is unknown, but recent work has confirmed that it is rare. No susceptibility factors have been identified. It can occur on initial exposure or subsequent rechallenge. The mechanism is obscure, but an immunological basis has been suggested.

The reason for concern about this adverse effect is that it may easily be mistaken for myocardial infarction or acute left ventricular failure, conditions that are not uncommon in patients requiring diuretics.

Diffuse interstitial pulmonary fibrosis has been reported after treatment with cyclopenthiazide and triamterene (6).

Sensory systems

Visual disturbances caused by dehydration of lens tissue or by retinal edema have been reported, particularly in the first few weeks of treatment. On the whole these effects are innocuous and transient (SED-9, 354). Presenile cataract has been attributed to long-term use of hydrochlorothiazide (7).

Electrolyte balance

Sodium balance
Hyponatremia is the most common electrolyte abnormality in the general hospital population and is associated with a wide range of diseases and a variety of drugs. Acute hyponatremic encephalopathy can develop rapidly with diuretics, particularly thiazides. Women, all patients with hypokalemia, and those with a low sodium and/or solute intake are particularly susceptible to diuretic-induced hyponatremia.

In a hospital-based survey of hypertensive patients with hyponatremia (serum sodium concentration below 135 mmol/l) the odds ratio for hyponatremia was three times higher in women. In those over 65 years there was a 10-fold higher risk. In many instances hyponatremia was insidious in its presentation and did not occur until several months after therapy had begun (8). However, hyponatremia can also develop rapidly.

- A 69-year-old woman with uncontrolled hypertension took two doses of hydrochlorothiazide 25 mg and her serum sodium fell to 115 mmol/l within 24 hours, with accompanying neurological symptoms (9). She recovered fully with the administration of 3% saline.

Potassium balance
The thiazides increase potassium excretion, but rarely to such an extent that total body potassium stores are appreciably affected. In most patients there is no reason to think

that long-term diuretic treatment will deplete body potassium at all. This is discussed in the monograph on Diuretics.

Mineral balance

Thiazides and related diuretics reduce the renal clearance of calcium by inhibiting the tubular secretion of calcium ions. This is discussed in the monograph on Diuretics.

Metal metabolism

Magnesium

Hypomagnesemia is common with both loop and thiazide diuretics. In 242 patients the frequency was 19% (10). It was corrected with potassium magnesium citrate, whereas potassium citrate or potassium chloride alone had little corrective effect.

Diuretic-induced hypomagnesemia is of particular relevance to patients with congestive heart failure (11). There is a reduced rate of sudden cardiac death in patients who take long-term diuretic therapy when potassium- and magnesium-sparing diuretics and/or magnesium supplements are also used. All potassium-sparing diuretics are also magnesium-sparing, and diuretic-induced hypokalemia is difficult to correct unless underlying magnesium deficiency is also addressed (12).

Zinc

Thiazide diuretics promote zinc loss in the urine and can reduce the zinc content of hair in the long term (13). It has sometimes been suggested that changes in zinc balance could be responsible for the effects of thiazides on sexual potency. There is evidence that diuretics deplete body zinc, which in turn interferes with testosterone production and causes erectile impotence (14).

Hematologic

Thrombocytopenia has been reported, but its incidence is low (SED-8, 484). Even rarer complications are autoimmune hemolytic anemia, granulocytopenia, and agranulocytosis (SED-9, 354).

Acute intravascular hemolysis has been described in a single case, and in this instance there were antibodies to hydrochlorothiazide; methyldopa, which had been given concurrently, might have facilitated antibody formation (15).

Gastrointestinal

Nausea and vomiting have often been reported, but if the incidence is compared to that in a control group taking placebo (1), it seems to be negligible, even in hospital (16), and such complaints rarely necessitate a change of therapy. The high incidence reported in the past (SED-9, 354) was probably related to the sheer size of the chlorothiazide tablets, and it has almost disappeared since the general change to more potent thiazides and related drugs.

Liver

Jaundice has very rarely been attributed to thiazide diuretics (SED-9, 354).

- Rash, lymphadenopathy, splenomegaly, periorbital edema, and hepatitis occurred in an 18-year-old

woman who was taking phenobarbital and hydrochlorothiazide (17). Tests for fluorescent antinuclear antibody and hepatitis-associated antigen and antibody were negative. Liver biopsy was not characteristic of viral hepatitis. She recovered within 2 weeks after withdrawal of the drugs and administration of methylprednisolone and diphenhydramine.

Biliary tract

Studies of the relation between diuretic use and cholecystitis have yielded conflicting results. A significant association of thiazide use with acute cholecystitis was reported in a case-control study (18). However, others examined the association between the use of thiazides and cholecystectomy and failed to show a relation between the use of thiazides and gallstone disease, except possibly in women who are not overweight (19).

Pancreas

Pancreatitis has been reported occasionally with thiazides (SED-9, 354) (SEDA-5, 228) (SEDA-17, 263).

Urinary tract

Toxic damage to the kidney has occasionally been reported (20), but is rare, and it is not clear whether nephrotoxicity was due to severe hypokalemia or the drug itself.

Thiazide diuretics cause hyperuricemia and can occasionally precipitate gout (21). They can also cause renal stones (22). Uric acid precipitation is not normally a problem, although it was with the uricosuric drug tienilic acid.

Renal vasculitis due to thiazides is rare (SEDA-18, 234).

Skin

Rashes due to thiazides are common but are only very occasionally severe and disabling (SEDA-11, 198). A state of chronic photosensitivity can persist for many years after drug withdrawal and is difficult to treat (23); it can mimic contact dermatitis, and there can be cross-reactivity with sulfonamides and phenothiazines. Patients who develop photosensitivity to thiazides should never take these drugs again.

Several cases of a reaction resembling systemic lupus erythematosus have been described (24–26). One patient taking hydrochlorothiazide developed unequivocal antinuclear antibody (ANA) positivity, with the homogeneous pattern most commonly found in drug-induced lupus (27). It is uncertain whether thiazides cause a lupus-like syndrome or activate latent disease in predisposed individuals.

Two of nine patients with drug-induced toxic epidermal necrolysis were taking hydrochlorothiazide, one with triamterene and allopurinol, the other with reserpine and hydralazine; both died (28).

In a patient who developed an allergic vasculitis affecting the skin during long-term treatment with hydrochlorothiazide the findings suggested that immediate (Type I) hypersensitivity may be involved in the induction of vasculitis (29).

- A 60-year-old man with a history of renal insufficiency and hypertension, taking hydrochlorothiazide, furosemide, and amiloride, developed pellagroid dermatitis involving light-exposed areas (30). The pigmentation disappeared slowly after withdrawal of hydrochlorothiazide and amiloride.

Hydrochlorothiazide, which is a well-known photoallergen, can also cause allergic photodermatitis (31).

- A 77-year-old man developed a florid photosensitive lichenoid eruption, histologically confirmed, while taking thiazide diuretics for heart failure (32). The eruption cleared on withdrawal of the drug. Although thiazide-induced photosensitivity is well documented, there have been no histologically proven cases of a lichenoid eruption in light exposed areas.

Immunologic

It has long been thought that loop and thiazide diuretics pose a theoretical risk of cross-sensitivity in patients with sulfonamide allergy because of their common structures. However, the available literature does not provide sufficient numbers of well-documented cases to support this impression (33). It seems that careful administration of diuretics is permissible in patients with documented sulfonamide allergy, but as always such a drug challenge should not be attempted without careful follow-up. A furosemide rechallenge protocol, based on a method that has been used to rechallenge with a sulfa-containing antimicrobial agent, safely allowed the long-term reinstitution of loop diuretic therapy with furosemide (34).

Second-Generation Effects

Pregnancy

In the past, thiazide diuretics have been considered as being contraindicated in pregnancy, because of risks to the mother and fetus. However, more recent evidence suggests that their use need not be contraindicated (35).

Susceptibility Factors

Age

The risks and benefits of distal tubular diuretics have been assessed in preterm infants under 3 weeks of age with or developing chronic lung disease (36). Acute and chronic administration of distal diuretics improved pulmonary mechanics; adverse effects were not reported. However, additional studies are needed to assess whether thiazide administration improves mortality, duration of oxygen dependency, ventilator dependency, length of hospital stay, and long-term outcome in patients exposed to corticosteroids and bronchodilators, and whether adding spironolactone to thiazides or adding metolazone to furosemide has any beneficial effect.

Other features of the patient

Thiazides should be used with caution in patients with a history of gout.

The use of thiazide diuretics in hepatic cirrhosis is associated with a high incidence of severe hypokalemia, asterixis, and precipitation of encephalopathy (9).

Thiazides should not be used in patients with advanced hepatic insufficiency.

Drug–Drug Interactions

ACE inhibitors

Even low dosages of angiotensin-converting enzyme (ACE) inhibitors, such as enalapril, can cause profound first-dose hypotension in hypertensive patients treated with a thiazide (37). This is rare if volume depletion and sodium depletion are avoided.

Angiotensin-converting enzyme inhibitors can cause renal insufficiency in patients with bilateral renal artery stenosis or stenosis of the artery supplying a single functioning kidney. Concomitant diuretic treatment may play a role in this adverse reaction (38).

Allopurinol

Adverse reactions to allopurinol, particularly toxic epidermal necrolysis and a hypersensitivity syndrome, are reputed to be more common in patients taking thiazides, but evidence to support this is hard to find (SEDA-11, 198) (SEDA-13, 188).

Angiotensin-II receptor antagonists

The value of low doses of thiazide diuretics in the management of hypertension is well attested, and low doses of diuretics have synergistic actions with other antihypertensive drug classes, including the angiotensin-II receptor antagonists (39–41). It is still unclear what represents the optimal dose of a thiazide diuretic in combination with either an ACE inhibitor or an angiotensin-II receptor antagonist. The addition of an angiotensin-II receptor antagonist to diuretic therapy seems to blunt the associated electrolyte disturbances. In particular, hydrochlorothiazide-induced hyperuricemia is specifically attenuated by losartan (42).

Beta-blockers

The combination of a thiazide and a beta-blocker can cause hyperglycemia (SEDA-10, 191) (SEDA-19, 192).

Calcium carbonate

Milk-alkali syndrome occurred in a patient who was taking chlorothiazide 500 mg/day for hypertension and calcium carbonate 7.5–10 g/day for heartburn (43).

Ciclosporin

Patients taking diuretics and ciclosporin may be at higher risk of hyperuricemia and gouty complications, perhaps because of tissue breakdown caused by ciclosporin (44).

Lithium

The thiazide diuretics inhibit the tubular excretion of lithium ions and can cause frank lithium intoxication (45). This is a potentially serious and well-documented interaction.

NSAIDs

Several non-steroidal anti-inflammatory drugs (NSAIDs) have been reported to interfere with the natriuretic effects of thiazides (SED-11, 423). A similar interaction is seen with tenidap, an antiarthritic cytokine modulating drug (46). The salt-retaining properties of the NSAIDs probably play the central role in this interaction.

Non-steroidal anti-inflammatory drugs (NSAIDs) are often reported to interfere with the blood pressure-lowering action of thiazide diuretics (SED-14, 667). In 17 women with arthritis and hypertension taking fosinopril and hydrochlorothiazide, ibuprofen, sulindac, and nabumetone, each for 1 month, had no effect on mean arterial pressure (47). These results suggest that the ACE inhibitor fosinopril may neutralize the tendency of NSAIDs to increase blood pressure in thiazide-treated hypertensive patients. However, the design of this study precluded such a conclusion, since no evidence was provided that any of the NSAIDs increased blood pressure in the absence of fosinopril. Furthermore, the numbers were small and the precision of the comparison is likely to have been low. Careful monitoring of blood pressure is necessary when NSAIDs are introduced in thiazide-treated hypertensive patients, even when ACE inhibitors are co-prescribed.

Oral hypoglycemic drugs and insulin

Thiazide drugs can oppose the blood glucose-lowering effects of oral hypoglycemic drugs and insulin (48) (although this effect is rarely serious).

Potassium-wasting drugs

Thiazide drugs have additive potassium-lowering effects with other drugs that reduce serum potassium, such as corticosteroids and carbenoxolone. Profound hypokalemia due to the latter combination has been reported to cause massive rhabdomyolysis and acute tubular necrosis (49).

References

1. Medical Research Council Working Party on Mild to Moderate Hypertension. Adverse reactions to bendrofluazide and propranolol for the treatment of mild hypertension. Lancet 1981;2(8246):539–43.
2. d'Aloia A, Fiorina C, Vizzardi E, Faggiano P, Dei Cas L. Episodi ricorrenti di edema polmonare acuto non cardiogeno indotti dall'assunzione di idroclorotiazide. [Recurrent episodes of acute non-cardiogenic pulmonary edema caused by ingesting hydrochlorothiazide.] Ital Heart J Suppl 2001;2(8):904–7.
3. Wagner AC. Interstitial pulmonary edema due to hydrochlorothiazide: case report. Va Med 1983;110(12):715–16.
4. Parfrey NA, Herlong HF. Pulmonary oedema after hydrochlorothiazide. BMJ (Clin Res Ed) 1984;288:1880.
5. Bowden FJ. Non-cardiogenic pulmonary edema after ingestion of chlorothiazide. BMJ 1989;298(6673):605.
6. Kheir A, Chabot F, Lesur O, Gerard H, Delorme N, Polu JM. [Fibrosing pneumopathy induced by cyclothiazide. Apropos of a case.] Rev Mal Respir 1992;9(2):208–12.
7. Kang JS, Kim TH, Park KB. Hydrochlorothiazide-induced phototoxic reaction. Korean J Dermatol 1992;30:529–34.
8. Sharabi Y, Illan R, Kamari Y, Cohen H, Nadler M, Messerli FH, Grossman E. Diuretic induced hyponatraemia in elderly hypertensive women. J Hum Hypertens 2002;16(9):631–5.
9. Al-Salman J, Pursell R. Hyponatremic encephalopathy induced by thiazides. West J Med 2001;175(2):87.
10. Pak CY. Correction of thiazide-induced hypomagnesemia by potassium-magnesium citrate from review of prior trials. Clin Nephrol 2000;54(4):271–5.
11. Seelig MS. Interrelationship of magnesium and congestive heart failure. Wien Med Wochenschr 2000;150(15–16):335–41.
12. Cohen N, Alon I, Almoznino-Sarafian D, Zaidenstein R, Weissgarten J, Gorelik O, Berman S, Modai D, Golik A. Metabolic and clinical effects of oral magnesium supplementation in furosemide-treated patients with severe congestive heart failure. Clin Cardiol 2000;23(6):433–6.
13. Mountokalakis T, Dourakis S, Karatzas N, Maravelias C, Koutselinis A. Zinc deficiency in mild hypertensive patients treated with diuretics. J Hypertens Suppl 1984;2(3):S571–2.
14. Geissler AH, Turnlund JR, Cohen RD. Effect of chlorthalidone on zinc levels, testosterone, and sexual function in man. Drug Nutr Interact 1986;4(3):275–83.
15. Beck ML, Cline JF, Hardman JT, Racela LS, Davis JW. Fatal intravascular immune hemolysis induced by hydrochlorothiazide. Am J Clin Pathol 1984;81(6):791–4.
16. Greenblatt DJ. Diuretics. In: Miller RR, Greenblatt DJ, editors. Drug Effects in Hospitalized Patients. New York: John Wiley and Sons, 1976:80.
17. Weisburst M, Self T, Peace R, Cooper J. Jaundice and rash associated with the use of phenobarbital and hydrochlorothiazide. South Med J 1976;69(1):126–7.
18. Van der Linden W, Ritter B, Edlund G. Acute cholecystitis and thiazides. BMJ (Clin Res Ed) 1984;289(6446):654–5.
19. Kakar F, Weiss NS, Strite SA. Thiazide use and the risk of cholecystectomy in women. Am J Epidemiol 1986;124(3):428–33.
20. Abry J, Cavusoglu M. Fatal tubular necrosis during chlorothiazide administration. NY State J Med 1960;60:1638–40.
21. Horwitz LR, Liebman JA, Cavolo DJ. Thiazide-induced hyperuricemia and gout. J Am Podiatry Assoc 1982;72(10):511–6.
22. Jorgensen FS, Brunner S. The long-term effect of bendroflumethiazide on renal calcium and magnesium excretion and stone formation in patients with recurring renal stones. Scand J Urol Nephrol 1974;8(2):128–31.
23. Robinson HN, Morison WL, Hood AF. Thiazide diuretic therapy and chronic photosensitivity. Arch Dermatol 1985;121(4):522–4.
24. Parodi A, Romagnoli M, Rebora A. Subacute cutaneous lupus erythematosus-like eruption caused by hydrochlorothiazide. Photodermatol 1989;6(2):100–2.
25. Reed BR, Huff JC, Jones SK, Orton PW, Lee LA, Norris DA. Subacute cutaneous lupus erythematosus associated with hydrochlorothiazide therapy. Ann Intern Med 1985;103(1):49–51.
26. Brown CW Jr., Deng JS. Thiazide diuretics induce cutaneous lupus-like adverse reaction. J Toxicol Clin Toxicol 1995;33(6):729–33.
27. Rich MW, Eckman JM. Can hydrochlorothiazide cause lupus? J Rheumatol 1995;22(5):1001.
28. Westly ED, Wechsler HL. Toxic epidermal necrolysis. Granulocytic leukopenia as a prognostic indicator. Arch Dermatol 1984;120(6):721–6.
29. Grunwald MH, Halevy S, Livni E. Allergic vasculitis induced by hydrochlorothiazide: confirmation by mast cell degranulation test. Isr J Med Sci 1989;25(10):572–4.
30. Stingeni L, Hansel K, Lisi P. Pellagroid allergic photodermatitis induced by hydrochlorothiazide. Ann Ital Dermatol Clin Sper 2000;54:36–8.
31. Wagner SN, Welke F, Goos M. Occupational UVA-induced allergic photodermatitis in a welder due to hydrochlorothiazide and ramipril. Contact Dermatitis 2000;43(4):245–6.

32. Johnston GA. Thiazide-induced lichenoid photosensitivity. Clin Exp Dermatol 2002;27(8):670–2.

33. Phipatanakul W, Adkinson NF Jr. Cross-reactivity between sulfonamides and loop or thiazide diuretics: a theoretical or actual risk? Allergy Clin Immunol Int 2000;12:26–8.

34. Earl G, Davenport J, Narula J. Furosemide challenge in patients with heart failure and adverse reactions to sulfa-containing diuretics. Ann Intern Med 2003;138(4):358–9.

35. Collins R, Yusuf S, Peto R. Overview of randomised trials of diuretics in pregnancy. BMJ (Clin Res Ed) 1985;290(6461):17–23.

36. Brion LP, Primhak RA, Ambrosio-Perez I. Diuretics acting on the distal renal tubule for preterm infants with (or developing) chronic lung disease (Cochrane Review). In: The Cochrane Library, Issue 4. Chichester, UK: John Wiley & Sons Ltd, 2003.

37. Webster J, Robb OJ, Witte K, Petrie JC. Single doses of enalapril and atenolol in hypertensive patients treated with bendrofluazide. J Hypertens 1987;5(4):457–60.

38. Watson ML, Bell GM, Muir AL, Buist TA, Kellett RJ, Padfield PL. Captopril/diuretic combinations in severe renovascular disease: a cautionary note. Lancet 1983;2(8346):404–5.

39. Ohma KP, Milon H, Valnes K. Efficacy and tolerability of a combination tablet of candesartan cilexetil and hydrochlorothiazide in insufficiently controlled primary hypertension—comparison with a combination of losartan and hydrochlorothiazide. Blood Press 2000;9(4):214–20.

40. Scholze J, Probst G, Bertsch K. Valsartan alone and in combination with hydrochlorothiazide in general practice. Clin Drug Invest 2000;20:1–7.

41. Koenig W. Comparison of the efficacy and tolerability of combination tablets containing candesartan cilexetil or losartan and hydrochlorothiazide in patients with moderate to severe hypertension. Results of the CARLOS-Study. Clin Drug Invest 2000;19:239–46.

42. Manolis AJ, Grossman E, Jelakovic B, Jacovides A, Bernhardi DC, Cabrera WJ, Watanabe LA, Barragan J, Matadamas N, Mendiola A, Woo KS, Zhu JR, Mejia AD, Bunt T, Dumortier T, Smith RD. Effects of losartan and candesartan monotherapy and losartan/hydrochlorothiazide combination therapy in patients with mild to moderate hypertension. Losartan Trial Investigators. Clin Ther 2000;22(10):1186–203.

43. Gora ML, Seth SK, Bay WH, Visconti JA. Milk–alkali syndrome associated with use of chlorothiazide and calcium carbonate. Clin Pharm 1989;8(3):227–9.

44. Tiller DJ, Hall BM, Horvarth JS, Duggin GG, Thompson JF, Sheil AG. Gout and hyperuricaemia in patients on cyclosporin and diuretics. Lancet 1985;1(8426):453.

45. Petersen V, Hvidt S, Thomsen K, Schou M. Effect of prolonged thiazide treatment on renal lithium clearance. BMJ 1974;3(924):143–5.

46. Rapeport WG, Grimwood VC, Korlipara K, Grillage MG, James I, Anderton JL, Selfridge DI. The effect of tenidap on the anti-hypertensive efficacy of thiazide diuretics in patients treated for mild to moderate hypertension. Br J Clin Pharmacol 1995;39(Suppl 1):S51–5.

47. Thakur V, Cook ME, Wallin JD. Antihypertensive effect of the combination of fosinopril and HCTZ is resistant to interference by nonsteroidal antiinflammatory drugs. Am J Hypertens 1999;12(9 Pt 1):925–8.

48. Kansal PC, Buse J, Buse MG. Thiazide diuretics and control of diabetes mellitus. South Med J 1969;62(11):1372–9.

49. Descamps C, Vandenbroucke JM, van Ypersele de Strihou C. Rhabdomyolysis and acute tubular necrosis associated with carbenoxolone and diuretic treatment. BMJ 1977;1(6056):272.

Thiazinamium metilsulfate

See also Antihistamines

General Information

Thiazinamium is a first-generation antihistamine (SED-13, 418).

Organs and Systems

Sensory systems

In long-term, double-blind study in 12 men with chronic bronchitis, three who took thiazinamium metilsulfate 900 mg/day had visual disturbances (1).

Gastrointestinal

Thiazinamium can cause attacks of sternal and epigastric pain, perhaps due to esophageal spasm. Esophageal ulceration has been reported (2).

References

1. Verheijen-Breemhaar L, Bogaard JM, Hilvering C. Comparison of the bronchodilatory action and side-effects of ipratropium bromide and thiazinamium methyl sulphate: a long-term, double-blind, crossover trial in patients with chronic bronchitis. Pharmatherapeutica 1982;3(3):180–7.

2. Pen J, Van Meerbeeck J, Pelckmans P, Van Maercke Y. Thiazinamium-induced oesophageal ulcerations. Acta Clin Belg 1986;41(4):278–83.

Thiazolidinediones

General Information

The thiazolidinediones include pioglitazone and rosiglitazone; darglitazone is in development; ciglitazone, englitazone, and troglitazone have been withdrawn owing to adverse effects on the liver (all names are rINNs).

The thiazolidinediones reduce insulin resistance and are sometimes designated as insulin sensitizers. They promote glucose utilization in peripheral tissues by stimulating non-oxidative glucose metabolism and suppressing gluconeogenesis. They activate the so-called Peroxisome Proliferator Activated Receptor Gamma (PPARγ), a nuclear hormone receptor that enhances a number of genes encoding enzymes involved in glucose and fat metabolism. PPARγ is essential for normal insulin sensitivity (1–3). They may also intervene directly in the fuel metabolism of skeletal muscle and liver, as suggested by in vitro experiments (4). They can reduce HbA_{1c}, the glucose AUC after a glucose tolerance test, and the glucose AUC after a meal in glucocorticoid-induced diabetes, as has been shown in seven patients taking troglitazone (5). They may ameliorate albuminuria in incipient diabetic nephropathy (6).

In some systems, troglitazone behaves as a partial agonist, but in fat cells it behaves as a full agonist. The transcriptional activities of troglitazone and rosiglitazone differ (7). The thiazolidinediones promote fat accumulation in subcutaneous tissue (8) rather than in the abdominal region, which plays such a bad role in the insulin resistance syndrome. Troglitazone lowers fasting glucose and postprandial glucose. Its effects persist for 2–3 weeks after withdrawal (9). It is also effective in insulin-resistant glucocorticoid-induced diabetes (10). It has a greater insulin-sparing effect than biguanides when given to patients on continuous subcutaneous insulin infusion (11).

The thiazolidinediones have been frequently reviewed (12–22). They can be prescribed as single drugs or in combination with other hypoglycemic drugs (23). In 12 healthy people, meals did not affect the absorption of rosiglitazone (24).

Comparative studies

In a parallel-group study in patients starting on hypoglycemic therapy with thiazolidinediones, 35 took troglitazone 600 mg/day, 36 took rosiglitazone 8 mg/day, and 30 took pioglitazone 45 mg/day (25). At 2 and 4 months, there was an equal effect on glucose lowering and greater weight gain with pioglitazone; pioglitazone had the largest beneficial effect on lipids and rosiglitazone the least.

In 203 patients, randomly assigned for 1 year to rosiglitazone 4 mg bd or glibenclamide to achieve optimal control, there was significant and sustained reduction in hyperglycemia and a significant reduction in diastolic blood pressure with rosiglitazone (26). There were no differences in adverse effects or in left ventricular mass index.

Placebo-controlled studies

Rosiglitazone monotherapy has been studied double-blind in 493 patients for 26 weeks (27). There was a dose-related fall in hemoglobin. Rosiglitazone caused more mild to moderate edema. One patient had a temporary rise in transaminases, which normalized spontaneously.

In a parallel-group, double-blind, placebo-controlled, dose-ranging study of rosiglitazone 4, 8, and 12 mg/day in 369 patients for 8 weeks after a run-in period, hematocrit and hemoglobin, C peptide, fasting blood glucose, and fructosamine all fell (28). Hepatotoxicity, significant cardiac events, or hypoglycemia were not different from placebo.

In 574 patients taking a sulfonylurea, twice-daily placebo ($n = 192$ patients) was compared with rosiglitazone 1 mg/day ($n = 199$ patients) or rosiglitazone 2 mg/day ($n = 183$ patients) for 26 weeks (29). Rosiglitazone improved HbA$_{1c}$. With the higher dose of rosiglitazone there were more cases of hypoglycemia and a small increase in mean body weight; some patients complained of headache and upper respiratory tract infections.

In a placebo-controlled study, 959 patients took placebo, rosiglitazone 4 mg od, 2 mg bd, 8 mg od, or 4 mg bd for 26 weeks (30). In the placebo group 38% withdrew and in the rosiglitazone groups 20%. Two patients (one in the placebo and one in the 4 mg bd group) had changes in alanine transaminase of more than three times the upper limit of the reference range. Other adverse events related to edema were seen in 1.6% of the placebo group and in 4.1% of those taking 2 mg bd and 6.6% in those taking 4 mg bd. There were small dose-dependent falls in hemoglobin and hematocrit.

In a multicenter, double-blind, placebo-controlled study, 408 patients took pioglitazone 7.5, 15, 30, or 45 mg/day (31). There was no hepatotoxicity and the overall adverse events profiles did not differ, except for edema in 12 of 329 patients who took pioglitazone. There was a significant fall in triglycerides and a small fall in LDL cholesterol. However, in another study in 150 patients, postprandial triglycerides were not reduced by pioglitazone (32).

In 561 patients with HbA$_{1c}$ concentrations of at least 8.0% on stable treatment with a sulfonylurea, pioglitazone was added for 16 weeks in a double-blind study (33). The incidence of edema increased from 2% in the placebo group to 7%. With pioglitazone there were more episodes of hypoglycemia, a dose-related increase in body weight, and a dose-related fall in hemoglobin. The frequency of adverse cardiovascular effects was the same.

Combinations of oral hypoglycemic drugs

The different mechanisms of action of the various classes of hypoglycemic drugs make combined therapy feasible: the sulfonylureas and meglitinides stimulate insulin production by different mechanisms, the biguanides reduce glucose production by the liver and excretion from the liver, acarbose reduces the absorption of glucose from the gut, and the thiazolidinediones reduce insulin resistance in fat. It is not necessary to wait until the maximal dose of one drug has been reached before starting another. However, sulfonylureas and meglitinides should no longer be used when endogenous insulin production is minimal. Combinations of insulin with sulfonylureas or meglitinides should only be used while the patient is changing to insulin, except when long-acting insulin is given at night in order to give the islets a rest and to stimulate daytime insulin secretion.

Large studies of the effects of lifestyle changes, the effects of drugs in preventing or postponing the complications of diabetes, or the usefulness of various combinations are regularly published. The different mechanisms of action of the various classes give different metabolic effects and different adverse effects profiles (34). Comparative costs of the various therapies in the USA have been presented (35).

This subject has been reviewed in relation to combined oral therapy. In a systematic review of 63 studies with a duration of at least 3 months and involving at least 10 patients at the end of the study, and in which HbA$_{1c}$ was reported, five different classes of oral drugs were almost equally effective in lowering blood glucose concentrations (36). HbA$_{1c}$ was reduced by about 1–2% in all cases. Combination therapy gave additive effects. However, long-term vascular risk reduction was demonstrated only with sulfonylureas and metformin.

The adverse effects of combined drug therapy are attributable to the adverse effects of the single drugs. Increased adverse effects or new adverse effects in patients taking combinations have not been reported.

Thiazolidinediones + biguanides

In a multicenter, randomized, double-blind study, 116 patients were treated for 26 weeks with metformin plus placebo, 119 with metformin plus rosiglitazone 4 mg/day, and 113 with metformin plus rosiglitazone 8 mg/day (37). In both rosiglitazone groups there were small but statistically significant falls in hemoglobin and hematocrit. Edema was rare but more common in the rosiglitazone groups (2.5% with 4 mg/day and 3.5% with 8 mg/day). Body weight fell by 1.2 kg from baseline with placebo but increased by 0.7 kg with rosiglitazone 4 mg/day and by 1.9 kg with 8 mg/day. No one taking rosiglitazone had an increase in alanine transaminase greater than three times the upper limit of the reference range.

In a placebo-controlled study in 116 patients who responded insufficiently to metformin 2.5 g/day, rosiglitazone 2 or 4 mg bd was added for 26 weeks (38). HbA_{1c} and fasting plasma glucose improved and hemoglobin fell. Edema was reported in 5.2% of the patients who took rosiglitazone and two patients withdrew because of headache.

Thiazolidinediones + meglitinides

In 585 patients in a double-blind, randomized, placebo-controlled, multicenter study lasting 16 weeks, nateglinide 40 mg tds alone, troglitazone 200 mg/day alone, and the combination were compared (39). The combination was most effective in lowering HbA_{1c}. The most frequent adverse effects were mild hypoglycemia, most often in the combination group. Three patients (two in the combination group and one in the troglitazone alone group) withdrew because of hypoglycemia. Most of the withdrawals were related to increased liver enzymes and weight gain, known adverse effects of troglitazone. Twelve patients withdrew because of predefined changes from baseline (transaminases more than 200% and alkaline phosphatase and bilirubin more than 100% over baseline); seven were taking troglitazone alone, four combined therapy, and one placebo.

In an open trial, 256 patients with type 2 diabetes with inadequate hypoglycemic control (HbA_{1c} over 7.0% during previous therapy) took repaglinide (0.5–4 mg at meals), troglitazone (200–600 mg/day), or a combination of the two for 22 weeks (40). Combination therapy was most effective. Repaglinide only was more effective than troglitazone only. Mean body weight increased in both groups. Serious adverse events were chest pain, cerebrovascular disorders, malignancies, dysrhythmias, electrocardiographic changes suggesting myocardial infarction, and increased aspartate transaminase activity (in one patient taking troglitazone). The serious adverse effects were similar in the different groups. Hypoglycemia occurred in 4% of the patients taking combined therapy, in 16% of those taking troglitazone only, and in 27% of those taking repaglinide only; none needed assistance. There were changes in liver function tests in three patients in the combined group and in one patient each in the two other groups; the drugs were withdrawn in the affected patients and liver function normalized. There were no differences in adverse effects in the different groups. Hypoglycemia occurred in 11 patients taking repaglinide, in seven taking combination therapy, and in one taking troglitazone. Anemia occurred

in four patients taking combined therapy and in two taking troglitazone only.

Thiazolidinediones + sulfonylureas

Troglitazone 100 or 200 mg/day or placebo was given for 16 weeks to 259 patients already taking sulfonylurea therapy (41). HbA_{1c} was 0.4 and 0.7% lower and blood glucose concentrations fell. The most common event was hypoglycemia, but this did not occur more often when troglitazone was added. Liver enzymes increased to the same extent in the three groups and never rose above normal. No patients withdrew because of drug-related effects.

Insulin + thiazolidinediones

Insulin plus metformin (27 patients, 2000 mg/day) or troglitazone (30 patients, 600 mg/day) in patients with type 2 diabetes using at least 30 U/day was compared with insulin alone (30 patients) for 4 months (42). Body weight increased in the insulin and the insulin plus troglitazone groups. In the insulin plus metformin group there were significantly more gastrointestinal adverse effects but less hypoglycemia than the other groups.

The addition of rosiglitazone to insulin for 26 weeks in a double-blind study in 315 patients with inadequately controlled type 2 diabetes improved glycemic control and was well tolerated (43). There was a significant fall in hemoglobin, and some patients in both the rosiglitazone and placebo groups developed edema.

General adverse effects

The adverse effects of the thiazolidinediones are comparable and include weight gain, upper respiratory tract infections, headache, and hypoglycemia (mostly in combination with other hypoglycemic drugs). Fluid retention sometimes occurs (19,21) and can lead to or exacerbate heart failure and pulmonary and general edema, which was reported in 1.5–12% of patients taking pioglitazone. Small clinically unimportant falls in hematocrit and hemoglobin occur because of hemodilution. Changes in liver enzymes and bilirubin have not been reported with rosiglitazone, and although there have been some reports of hepatic-related adverse effects, they have not been definitive (SEDA-25, 515). However, troglitazone causes liver complications, sometimes fatal, and this has led to its withdrawal from the market. There are no drug interactions with other hypoglycemic agents.

Organs and Systems

Cardiovascular

Reductions in VLDL cholesterol, LDL cholesterol, and chylomicrons may contribute to a reduction in cardiac complications. Pioglitazone reduced both lipoprotein(a) and the remnant particles (cholesterol-rich particles after the release of triglycerides from the chylomicrons), whereas troglitazone caused increases in lipoprotein(a) (44).

Respiratory

A single case of pleuropulmonary disease possibly induced by troglitazone has been reported (45).

Nervous system

Ataxia has been attributed to troglitazone in two patients aged about 80 years (a man and a woman) (46). The ataxia developed during treatment and disappeared in one case 2–3 days after withdrawal and in the other within 2 weeks. In one, the ataxia was accompanied by a dementia-like syndrome, which completely disappeared within 8 weeks. One of the patients was rechallenged and developed ataxia again.

Metabolism

The thiazolidinediones can cause hypoglycemia both when used alone or in combination with other hypoglycemic drugs (47).

The thiazolidinediones increase body weight. With troglitazone the increase in body weight is accompanied by changed fat distribution, but central fat, in part responsible for the cardiovascular changes seen in diabetes, remains the same; weight gain is accompanied by increased subcutaneous fat (48).

In one study, troglitazone increased body weight, adipocyte size, leptin concentrations, GLUT4 protein expression, basal and insulin-stimulated glucose transport, and insulin-stimulated whole-body glucose disposal rate (49).

In a 24-week study, in which 40 patients taking troglitazone and glibenclamide were compared with patients taking glibenclamide, serum fasting insulin, serum triglycerides, and insulin resistance were reduced when troglitazone was added. Fat deposition in the liver and the visceral fat area were reduced, but deposition in skeletal muscle was not (50).

When patients taking troglitazone were switched to equivalent amounts of rosiglitazone ($n = 60$) or pioglitazone ($n = 60$) there were no changes in HbA$_{1c}$ or other parameters, except that with pioglitazone there was a significant improvement in lipid profile, with an average fall in total cholesterol of 0.5 mmol/l (51).

However, in 23 patients who took pioglitazone for 16 weeks, in whom fasting and mean glucose concentrations and mean free fatty acid concentrations fell, weight gain of 3.6 kg was associated with an increase in peripheral fat without edema (52).

In 38 patients taking metformin 2550 mg/day and glimiperide 6 mg/day, rosiglitazone 4 or 8 mg/day was added for 20 weeks (53). HbA$_{1c}$ and fasting blood glucose fell significantly. There was hypoglycemia in 19% of those who took 4 mg/day and 28% of those who took 8 mg/day, and body weight increased by 4.2 and 4.6 kg respectively. There were no signs or symptoms of liver disease and no changes in liver function tests.

Fluid balance

Two cases of pulmonary and general edema have been reported with rosiglitazone (54).

- A 78-year-old man became short of breath. He had been taking rosiglitazone 8 mg/day for 6 months. He had renal insufficiency, atrial fibrillation, hypertension, and congestive heart failure, with pitting edema and bilateral pleural effusions. He was refractory to intravenous furosemide and metolazone. Withdrawal of rosiglitazone and administration of bumetanide

gave a net fluid output of 9.5 litres and the edema resolved.
- A 67-year-old man, who had taken troglitazone 600 mg/day for 4 months and who had renal insufficiency, stroke, and cardiomyopathy, developed pitting edema, hepatomegaly, ascites, and a pleural effusion. The edema was resistant to treatment until troglitazone was changed to glipizide 10 mg/day, when he had a diuresis of 18 litres in 6 days. Later he took rosiglitazone 4 mg bd for 3 weeks and had weight gain of 5 kg and pitting edema. Diuretic therapy failed until rosiglitazone was withdrawn, after which he reached his baseline weight in 4 days.

Pioglitazone also causes fluid retention, possibly because of increased production of vascular endothelial growth factor (55). The safety profile of monotherapy and combined therapy with pioglitazone has been evaluated in 3500 patients over 2500 patient-years, and some data from post-marketing surveillance were included; peripheral edema and hemodilution were common (56).

Hematologic

In 303 patients who took placebo or rosiglitazone for 8 weeks after a run-in period, rosiglitazone 4 mg bd had the same effect as 6 mg bd, but hemoglobin and hematocrit were lower with 6 mg bd (57). In another study troglitazone produced small reductions in hemoglobin, hematocrit, and erythrocyte counts and increases in lactate dehydrogenase and blood urea nitrogen (58).

Liver

The thiazolidinediones are hepatotoxic (59).

Troglitazone

Troglitazone causes liver damage more often than the other members of the family. Hepatotoxicity delayed and finally prevented the registration of troglitazone in Europe. In the US, a patient with diabetes who used troglitazone in a study, developed hepatic failure necessitating liver transplantation and died. Troglitazone was withdrawn from a major National Institutes of Health evaluation of various regimens for preventing type 2 diabetes. In Japan the government recommended in December 1997 that liver function tests should be assessed every month in patients taking troglitazone. In 1998 there were 21 fatal cases of liver failure and three liver transplantations in patients taking troglitazone (60). Monitoring of liver function was intensified and in 1998 troglitazone was withdrawn for monotherapy. In 1999 the FDA received 61 reports of fatal hepatic toxicity and seven cases requiring liver transplantation (61) and in spring 2000 troglitazone was withdrawn in America and in Japan.

- A 58-year-old man developed severe hepatitis after taking troglitazone 400 mg/day and glibenclamide 5 mg/day (62). Glibenclamide was stopped after 6 weeks as his HbA$_{1c}$ was 7.0%. About 2 weeks later he developed malaise and 1 week later jaundice. His bilirubin and transaminases were greatly raised and there was ascites. He had taken about 34 g of troglitazone. Drug-induced lymphocyte stimulation test was strongly positive for troglitazone and not for other drugs. Troglitazone was withdrawn and 3 days later the plasma concentration was below the limit of detection. Notwithstanding intensive therapy he died after 5 weeks. At autopsy, the liver showed yellow atrophy and massive hepatocellular coagulation necrosis with moderate neutrophil, monocyte, and eosinophil infiltration.

The positive lymphocyte stimulation test, the eosinophils, and the low blood concentrations 3 days after withdrawal suggest that hypersensitivity to troglitazone was the underlying cause. The authors reported that another patient with hepatitis after troglitazone had had a subacute course after withdrawal of the drug.

Late hepatic damage has also been reported.

- A 62-year-old woman with normal liver function tests took troglitazone 400 mg/day in combination with gliclazide 80 mg/day and pravastatin (63). After 9 months her transaminases were slightly above normal, but the HbA_{1c} was 7.0% and treatment was continued. Her liver enzymes were measured monthly and after 19 months rose abruptly. Troglitazone was withdrawn immediately and she received insulin. Her liver enzymes improved rapidly. A biopsy showed hepatic necrosis round the central vein and a mild inflammatory infiltrate and fibrosis in the portal area compatible with protracted acute hepatitis. A lymphocyte stimulation test and a skin test were negative for troglitazone.
- A 76-year-old man took troglitazone 400 mg in addition to glimepiride 4 mg/day, metformin 1 g/day, aspirin, and pravastatin (64). After 18 months his liver function deteriorated and improved after withdrawal of troglitazone.

There are no differences in outcome between these two patterns of hepatotoxicity, "rapid risers," in whom liver failure takes only a few days to develop, and "slower risers." The estimated death rate is one in 100 000, but the estimate of the FDA advisory committee was one in 15 154 at 8 months of treatment. It is unclear whether hepatotoxicity is a class effect of thiazolidinediones or whether the lipophilic alpha-tocopherol moiety of troglitazone is responsible for this effect. The basic quinone structure of alpha-tocopherol is common to other drugs that can form hepatotoxic free radicals by CYP2E1-mediated oxidation.

The relation of liver disease to oral hypoglycemic drugs has been investigated in 44 406 patients, of whom 605 had liver disease (65). When 185 patients with mild and transient disorders, 249 with a predisposing condition, and 113 with another cause were excluded, 57 cases with possibly drug-induced liver changes were left. Of these, 11 could be attributed to other drugs and eight were attributed to fatty liver disease caused by diabetes. In 51 patients, oral drugs were continued without worsening of the liver enzymes. In two cases (a 58-year-old woman, whose liver function improved after discontinuing metformin, and an 86-year-old woman, who developed jaundice and died shortly after metformin and glibenclamide were prescribed) a causal relation could not be excluded.

There has been a report of hepatic injury with troglitazone but not with rosiglitazone (66).

- A 38-year-old woman was given insulin when glibenclamide and acarbose failed. Troglitazone 400 mg/day

was added and increased to 800 mg/day 1 month later. After 2 months her liver function tests were normal, but she developed jaundice after 4 months. Total and direct bilirubin were 127 and 101 μmol/l and alanine transaminase was 34 μkat/l. After withdrawal of troglitazone her symptoms disappeared and her liver function tests normalized within several months. Metformin 1000 mg bd reduced her insulin requirement. Rosiglitazone 4 mg bd was added and her liver function tests remained normal for 10 months.

Pioglitazone

Hepatocellular damage has occasionally been attributed to pioglitazone.

- A 67-year-old man took pioglitazone 30 mg/day after having taken glibenclamide 2.5 mg/day for 10 years and voglibose 0.6 mg/day for 5 years (67). His liver function was normal before and during 6 months of pioglitazone therapy, but at 7 months he had abnormal liver function tests (total bilirubin 10 μmol/l, aspartate transaminase 1.95 μkat/l, alanine transaminase 5.65 μkat/l, alkaline phosphatase 17 μkat/l, gamma-glutamyl transferase 8 μkat/l). He was asymptomatic, with negative viral serology and normal liver ultrasonography. After withdrawal of pioglitazone his liver function normalized within a month.
- A 49-year-old man developed scleral icterus with raised bilirubin and transaminases after using pioglitazone 15-30 mg for 6 months and 45 mg for 1 week (68). No other cause for hepatitis was found. After withdrawal his liver function improved substantially within 14 days.
- A 49-year-old woman developed jaundice after taking pioglitazone 30 mg/day for 6 weeks, and after 3 weeks the alanine transaminase was 131 U/l and aspartate transaminase 79 U/l (69). Tests for viral hepatitis were negative. A liver biopsy showed marked portal edema, patchy chronic inflammation, a cellular infiltrate, and marked bile duct proliferation. There was no fibrosis. The laboratory results worsened after pioglitazone was withdrawn, and 1 month after withdrawal the bilirubin reached a peak of 585 μmol/l. Over the next 8 weeks the symptoms and laboratory tests improved, and after 6 months her condition was the same as when she had started to take pioglitazone.

Rosiglitazone

The frequency of liver damage with rosiglitazone is much lower than with troglitazone and the reported cases seem to have been less serious. No deaths have been reported.

- A 61-year-old man developed hepatotoxicity 8 days after starting to take rosiglitazone 4 mg/day, and it was withdrawn (70). The alanine transaminase was 28 μkat/l, aspartate transaminase 23 μkat/l, alkaline phosphatase 8.7 μkat/l, total bilirubin 14 μmol/l, and direct bilirubin 13 μmol/l. All the tests were normal 5 months later. He had taken troglitazone for 1 week 8 months before this incident but had stopped because of nausea and an upset stomach.
- A 69-year-old man taking rosiglitazone 4 mg/day and metformin 500 mg/day developed hepatic failure within

a week and both drugs were withdrawn (71). His alanine transaminase was 32 µkat/l, aspartate transaminase 47 µkat/l, total bilirubin 65 µmol/l, and direct bilirubin 41 µmol/l. He became comatose and the aspartate transaminase rose to 185 µkat/l. The enzyme activities were normal 7 weeks after withdrawal.

- A 58-year-old woman started to feel ill 2 weeks after starting to take rosiglitazone 4 mg/day (72). One week later her peak aspartate transaminase was 5.2 µkat/l, alanine transaminase 4.2 µkat/l, and bilirubin 41 µmol/l. Four weeks later all the values had returned to normal.

- In a 47-year-old woman, who took rosiglitazone 4 mg/day for a short, unspecified time, the alkaline phosphatase increased (11 µkat/l) and returned to normal 2 weeks after withdrawal (73).

- An obese 37-year-old man with type 2 diabetes, who used rosiglitazone for 15 months, at first 4 mg/day then 8 mg/day for 6 months, developed granulomatous hepatitis (74). His liver enzymes were normal at 6 and 8 months. After 14 months he developed fatigue, abdominal discomfort, and weight loss and 3 weeks later chills, nausea, vomiting, and diarrhea. No hepatic viruses were found. A liver biopsy showed a periportal mixed cellular infiltrate and granulomas within the portal triad and the parenchyma. There was no evidence of sarcoidosis. After withdrawal of rosiglitazone he improved and the liver enzymes became normal within 2 months.

- A 49-year-old man with pre-existing hepatic pathology took rosiglitazone 4 mg/day for 2 months and 8 mg/day for 5 months (75). He developed a "bull" face and then edema of the eyelids and neck. He had anorexia and nausea. His serum sodium was 110 mmol/l, potassium 3.3 mmol/l, chloride 81 mmol/l, cholesterol 21 mmol/l, triglycerides 33 mmol/l, and his liver enzymes were raised. Rosiglitazone was withdrawn and he was given saline and potassium, acarbose for his diabetes, spironolactone 200 mg/day for edema, and atorvastatin 10 mg/day for hyperlipidemia. He improved over 3 weeks.

Liver function was monitored in patients aged 30–80 years with type 2 diabetes taking rosiglitazone (76). When a patient had transaminase or alkaline phosphatase activities higher than 2.5 times the upper limit of the reference range, they were not included in the studies. In 5006 patients taking rosiglitazone as monotherapy or combined therapy there were no hepatotoxic effects. At entry to the studies, 5.6% of the patients had values between 1.0 and 2.5 times the upper limit. Of the placebo-treated patients, 39% had a fall to normal values and 39% had an increase, but not over three times the upper limit. In 66% of the patients treated with a hypoglycemic drug the values fell (often with a fall in HbA_{1c}); in 13% they increased to below three times the upper limit and in 2.0% to over three times (four patients).

Musculoskeletal

Rhabdomyolysis has been attributed to troglitazone in combination with alcohol (77).

- A 59-year-old man took troglitazone 400 mg/day for 6 months and alcohol about 40 g/day. He developed weakness and muscle pain. He had mild liver damage. His HbA_{1c} concentration was 9.0%. All his muscles were tender, his creatine kinase activity was 10 570 IU/ml, and his myoglobin, aldolase, and aspartate transaminase were raised. Troglitazone was withdrawn. He improved biochemically and clinically.

There was an increase in creatine phosphokinase activity to over 10 times the upper limit of the reference range in seven of 1510 patients taking pioglitazone in the USA; four normalized during treatment, two normalized after withdrawal, and one had fallen but not normalized at follow-up (21).

Immunologic

- Angioedema has been reported in an obese woman after she had taken pioglitazone 30 mg/day for 7 days (78). She developed a sore throat followed by dyspnea and swelling of the lips and tongue. There was no rash. After intravenous glucocorticoids her symptoms rapidly abated.

Susceptibility Factors

Renal disease

Dosage adjustment of rosiglitazone is not necessary when renal function is reduced (79).

Drug–Drug Interactions

Metformin

In 16 healthy men taking metformin 500 mg bd and/or rosiglitazone 2 mg bd for 4 days there were no significant effects on the steady-state pharmacokinetics of either drug (80).

Simvastatin

Troglitazone has been reported to reduce the effect of simvastatin, probably by induction of CYP3A4 (81).

References

1. Schwartz MW, Kahn SE. Insulin resistance and obesity. Nature 1999;402(6764):860–1.
2. Barroso I, Gurnell M, Crowley VE, Agostini M, Schwabe JW, Soos MA, Maslen GL, Williams TD, Lewis H, Schafer AJ, Chatterjee VK, O'Rahilly S. Dominant negative mutations in human PPARgamma associated with severe insulin resistance, diabetes mellitus and hypertension. Nature 1999;402(6764):880–3.
3. Auwerx J. PPARgamma, the ultimate thrifty gene. Diabetologia 1999;42(9):1033–49.
4. Furnsinn C, Waldhausl W. Thiazolidinediones: metabolic actions in vitro. Diabetologia 2002;45(9):1211–23.
5. Willi SM, Kennedy A, Brant BP, Wallace P, Rogers NL, Garvey WT. Effective use of thiazolidinediones for the treatment of glucocorticoid-induced diabetes. Diabetes Res Clin Pract 2002;58(2):87–96.
6. Imano E, Kanda T, Nakatani Y, Nishida T, Arai K, Motomura M, Kajimoto Y, Yamasaki Y, Hori M. Effect of troglitazone on microalbuminuria in patients with

incipient diabetic nephropathy. Diabetes Care 1998;21(12):2135–9.

7. Camp HS, Li O, Wise SC, Hong YH, Frankowski CL, Shen X, Vanbogelen R, Leff T. Differential activation of peroxisome proliferator-activated receptor-gamma by troglitazone and rosiglitazone. Diabetes 2000;49(4):539–47.

8. Mori Y, Murakawa Y, Okada K, Horikoshi H, Yokoyama J, Tajima N, Ikeda Y. Effect of troglitazone on body fat distribution in type 2 diabetic patients. Diabetes Care 1999;22(6):908–12.

9. Frias JP, Yu JG, Kruszynska YT, Olefsky JM. Metabolic effects of troglitazone therapy in type 2 diabetic, obese, and lean normal subjects. Diabetes Care 2000;23(1):64–9.

10. Fujibayashi K, Nagasaka S, Itabashi N, Kawakami A, Nakamura T, Kusaka I, Ishikawa S, Saito T. Troglitazone efficacy in a subject with glucocorticoid-induced diabetes. Diabetes Care 1999;22(12):2088–9.

11. Yu JG, Kruszynska YT, Mulford MI, Olefsky JM. A comparison of troglitazone and metformin on insulin requirements in euglycemic intensively insulin-treated type 2 diabetic patients. Diabetes 1999;48(12):2414–21.

12. Day C. Thiazolidinediones: a new class of antidiabetic drugs. Diabet Med 1999;16(3):179–92.

13. Scheen AJ, Lefebvre PJ. Troglitazone: antihyperglycemic activity and potential role in the treatment of type 2 diabetes. Diabetes Care 1999;22(9):1568–77.

14. Saleh YM, Mudaliar SR, Henry RR. Metabolic and vascular effects of the thiazolidinedione troglitazone. Diabetes Rev 1999;7:55–76.

15. Plosker GL, Faulds D. Troglitazone: a review of its use in the management of type 2 diabetes mellitus. Drugs 1999;57(3):409–38.

16. Balfour JA, Plosker GL. Rosiglitazone. Drugs 1999;57(6):921–30.

17. Caspi A. The promise of a new generation: rosiglitazone for the treatment of type 2 diabetes. P&T 1999;24:313–22.

18. Ducobu J, Sternon J. Les glitazones (thiazolidinediones). [Glitazones (thiazolidinediones).] Rev Med Brux 2000;21(5):441–6.

19. Scheen AJ, Charbonnel B. Effets antidiabétiques des thiazolidinediones. Med Ther 2001;7:672–9.

20. Werner AL, Travaglini MT. A review of rosiglitazone in type 2 diabetes mellitus. Pharmacotherapy 2001;21(9):1082–99.

21. Chilcott J, Tappenden P, Jones ML, Wight JP. A systematic review of the clinical effectiveness of pioglitazone in the treatment of type 2 diabetes mellitus. Clin Ther 2001;23(11):1792–823.

22. Wagstaff AJ, Goa KL. Rosiglitazone: a review of its use in the management of type 2 diabetes mellitus. Drugs 2002;62(12):1805–37.

23. Parulkar AA, Fonseca VA. Recent advances in pharmacological treatment of type 2 diabetes mellitus. Compr Ther 1999;25(8–10):418–26.

24. Freed MI, Allen A, Jorkasky DK, DiCicco RA. Systemic exposure to rosiglitazone is unaltered by food. Eur J Clin Pharmacol 1999;55(1):53–6.

25. King AB. A comparison in a clinical setting of the efficacy and side effects of three thiazolidinediones. Diabetes Care 2000;23(4):557.

26. St John Sutton M, Rendell M, Dandona P, Dole JF, Murphy K, Patwardhan R, Patel J, Freed M. A comparison of the effects of rosiglitazone and glyburide on cardiovascular function and glycemic control in patients with type 2 diabetes. Diabetes Care 2002;25(11):2058–64.

27. Lebovitz HE, Dole JF, Patwardhan R, Rappaport EB, Freed MI; Rosiglitazone Clinical Trials Study Group. Rosiglitazone monotherapy is effective in patients with type 2 diabetes. J Clin Endocrinol Metab 2001;86(1):280–8.

28. Nolan JJ, Jones NP, Patwardhan R, Deacon LF. Rosiglitazone taken once daily provides effective glycaemic control in patients with type 2 diabetes mellitus. Diabet Med 2000;17(4):287–94.

29. Wolffenbuttel BH, Gomis R, Squatrito S, Jones NP, Patwardhan RN. Addition of low-dose rosiglitazone to sulphonylurea therapy improves glycaemic control in Type 2 diabetic patients. Diabet Med 2000;17(1):40–7.

30. Phillips LS, Grunberger G, Miller E, Patwardhan R, Rappaport EB, Salzman A; Rosiglitazone Clinical Trials Study Group. Once- and twice-daily dosing with rosiglitazone improves glycemic control in patients with type 2 diabetes. Diabetes Care 2001;24(2):308–15.

31. Aronoff S, Rosenblatt S, Braithwaite S, Egan JW, Mathisen AL, Schneider RL. Pioglitazone hydrochloride monotherapy improves glycemic control in the treatment of patients with type 2 diabetes: a 6-month randomized placebo-controlled dose-response study. The Pioglitazone 001 Study Group. Diabetes Care 2000;23(11):1605–11.

32. Shimono D, Kuwamura N, Nakamura Y, Koshiyama H. Lack of effect of pioglitazone on postprandial triglyceride levels in type 2 diabetes. Diabetes Care 2001;24(5):971.

33. Kipnes MS, Krosnick A, Rendell MS, Egan JW, Mathisen AL, Schneider RL. Pioglitazone hydrochloride in combination with sulfonylurea therapy improves glycemic control in patients with type 2 diabetes mellitus: a randomized, placebo-controlled study. Am J Med 2001;111(1):10–7.

34. Inzucchi SE. Oral antihyperglycemic therapy for type 2 diabetes: scientific review. JAMA 2002;287(3):360–72.

35. Holmboe ES. Oral antihyperglycemic therapy for type 2 diabetes: clinical applications. JAMA 2002;287(3):373–6.

36. Van Gaal LF, De Leeuw IH. Rationale and options for combination therapy in the treatment of type 2 diabetes. Diabetologia 2003;46(Suppl 1):M44–50.

37. Fonseca V, Rosenstock J, Patwardhan R, Salzman A. Effect of metformin and rosiglitazone combination therapy in patients with type 2 diabetes mellitus: a randomized controlled trial. JAMA 2000;283(13):1695–702.

38. Gomez-Perez FJ, Fanghanel-Salmon G, Antonio Barbosa J, Montes-Villarreal J, Berry RA, Warsi G, Gould EM. Efficacy and safety of rosiglitazone plus metformin in Mexicans with type 2 diabetes. Diabetes Metab Res Rev 2002;18(2):127–34.

39. Rosenstock J, Shen SG, Gatlin MR, Foley JE. Combination therapy with nateglinide and a thiazolidinedione improves glycemic control in type 2 diabetes. Diabetes Care 2002;25(9):1529–33.

40. Raskin P, Jovanovic L, Berger S, Schwartz S, Woo V, Ratner R. Repaglinide/troglitazone combination therapy: improved glycemic control in type 2 diabetes. Diabetes Care 2000;23(7):979–83.

41. Buysschaert M, Bobbioni E, Starkie M, Frith L. Troglitazone in combination with sulphonylurea improves glycaemic control in Type 2 diabetic patients inadequately controlled by sulphonylurea therapy alone. Troglitazone Study Group. Diabet Med 1999;16(2):147–53.

42. Strowig SM, Aviles-Santa ML, Raskin P. Comparison of insulin monotherapy and combination therapy with insulin and metformin or insulin and troglitazone in type 2 diabetes. Diabetes Care 2002;25(10):1691–8.

43. Raskin P, Rendell M, Riddle MC, Dole JF, Freed MI, Rosenstock J; Rosiglitazone Clinical Trials Study Group. A randomized trial of rosiglitazone therapy in patients with inadequately controlled insulin-treated type 2 diabetes. Diabetes Care 2001;24(7):1226–32.

44. Nagai Y, Abe T, Nomura G. Does pioglitazone, like troglitazone, increase serum levels of lipoprotein(a) in diabetic patients? Diabetes Care 2001;24(2):408–9.

45. Koshida H, Shibata K, Kametani T. Pleuropulmonary disease in a man with diabetes who was treated with troglitazone. N Engl J Med 1998;339(19):1400–1.

46. Maher TD, Mirza SA. Ataxia and reversible dementia-like syndrome associated with troglitazone. Diabetes 1999;48(Suppl 1):A85.

47. Iwamoto Y, Kosaka K, Kuzuya T, Akanuma Y, Shigeta Y, Kaneko T. Effects of troglitazone: a new hypoglycemic agent in patients with NIDDM poorly controlled by diet therapy. Diabetes Care 1996;19(2):151–6.

48. Akazawa S, Sun F, Ito M, Kawasaki E, Eguchi K. Efficacy of troglitazone on body fat distribution in type 2 diabetes. Diabetes Care 2000;23(8):1067–71.

49. Ciaraldi TP, Kong AP, Chu NV, Kim DD, Baxi S, Loviscach M, Plodkowski R, Reitz R, Caulfield M, Mudaliar S, Henry RR. Regulation of glucose transport and insulin signaling by troglitazone or metformin in adipose tissue of type 2 diabetic subjects. Diabetes 2002;51(1):30–6.

50. Katoh S, Hata S, Matsushima M, Ikemoto S, Inoue Y, Yokoyama J, Tajima N. Troglitazone prevents the rise in visceral adiposity and improves fatty liver associated with sulfonylurea therapy—a randomized controlled trial. Metabolism 2001;50(4):414–17.

51. Khan MA, St Peter JV, Xue JL. A prospective, randomized comparison of the metabolic effects of pioglitazone or rosiglitazone in patients with type 2 diabetes who were previously treated with troglitazone. Diabetes Care 2002;25(4):708–11.

52. Miyazaki Y, Mahankali A, Matsuda M, Glass L, Mahankali S, Ferrannini E, Cusi K, Mandarino LJ, DeFronzo RA. Improved glycemic control and enhanced insulin sensitivity in type 2 diabetic subjects treated with pioglitazone. Diabetes Care 2001;24(4):710–19.

53. Kiayias JA, Vlachou ED, Theodosopoulou E, Lakka-Papadodima E. Rosiglitazone in combination with glimepiride plus metformin in type 2 diabetic patients. Diabetes Care 2002;25(7):1251–2.

54. Thomas ML, Lloyd SJ. Pulmonary edema associated with rosiglitazone and troglitazone. Ann Pharmacother 2001;35(1):123–4.

55. Baba T, Shimada K, Neugebauer S, Yamada D, Hashimoto S, Watanabe T. The oral insulin sensitizer, thiazolidinedione, increases plasma vascular endothelial growth factor in type 2 diabetic patients. Diabetes Care 2001;24(5):953–4.

56. Hanefeld M, Belcher G. Safety profile of pioglitazone. Int J Clin Pract Suppl 2001;(121):27–31.

57. Raskin P, Rappaport EB, Cole ST, Yan Y, Patwardhan R, Freed MI. Rosiglitazone short-term monotherapy lowers fasting and post-prandial glucose in patients with type II diabetes. Diabetologia 2000;43(3):278–84.

58. Kuzuya T, Iwamoto Y, Kosaka K, Takebe K, Yamanouchi T, Kasuga M, Kajinuma H, Akanuma Y, Yoshida S, Shigeta Y, et al. A pilot clinical trial of a new oral hypoglycemic agent, CS-045, in patients with non-insulin dependent diabetes mellitus. Diabetes Res Clin Pract 1991;11(3):147–53.

59. Tolman KG. Thiazolidinedione hepatotoxicity: a class effect? Int J Clin Pract Suppl 2000;(113):29–34.

60. Misbin RI. Troglitazone-associated hepatic failure. Ann Intern Med 1999;130(4 Pt 1):330.

61. Bailey CJ. The rise and fall of troglitazone. Diabet Med 2000;17(6):414–5.

62. Shibuya A, Watanabe M, Fujita Y, Saigenji K, Kuwao S, Takahashi H, Takeuchi H. An autopsy case of troglitazone-induced fulminant hepatitis. Diabetes Care 1998;21(12):2140–3.

63. Iwase M, Yamaguchi M, Yoshinari M, Okamura C, Hirahashi T, Tsuji H, Fujishima M. A Japanese case of liver dysfunction after 19 months of troglitazone treatment. Diabetes Care 1999;22(8):1382–4.

64. Bell DS, Ovalle F. Late-onset troglitazone-induced hepatic dysfunction. Diabetes Care 2000;23(1):128–9.

65. Jick SS, Stender M, Myers MW. Frequency of liver disease in type 2 diabetic patients treated with oral antidiabetic agents. Diabetes Care 1999;22(12):2067–71.

66. Lenhard MJ, Funk WB. Failure to develop hepatic injury from rosiglitazone in a patient with a history of troglitazone-induced hepatitis. Diabetes Care 2001;24(1):168–9.

67. Maeda K. Hepatocellular injury in a patient receiving pioglitazone. Ann Intern Med 2001;135(4):306.

68. May LD, Lefkowitch JH, Kram MT, Rubin DE. Mixed hepatocellular–cholestatic liver injury after pioglitazone therapy. Ann Intern Med 2002;136(6):449–52.

69. Pinto AG, Cummings OW, Chalasani N. Severe but reversible cholestatic liver injury after pioglitazone therapy. Ann Intern Med 2002;137(10):857.

70. Al-Salman J, Arjomand H, Kemp DG, Mittal M. Hepatocellular injury in a patient receiving rosiglitazone. A case report. Ann Intern Med 2000;132(2):121–4.

71. Forman LM, Simmons DA, Diamond RH. Hepatic failure in a patient taking rosiglitazone. Ann Intern Med 2000;132(2):118–21.

72. Ravinuthala RS, Nori U. Rosiglitazone toxicity. Ann Intern Med 2000;133(8):658.

73. Hachey DM, O'Neil MP, Force RW. Isolated elevation of alkaline phosphatase level associated with rosiglitazone. Ann Intern Med 2000;133(9):752.

74. Dhawan M, Agrawal R, Ravi J, Gulati S, Silverman J, Nathan G, Raab S, Brodmerkel G Jr. Rosiglitazone-induced granulomatous hepatitis. J Clin Gastroenterol 2002;34(5):582–4.

75. Kuschel U, Hesselbarth N, Hoffmann A, Hippius M, Hoffmann A. Schwere Elektrolytstörung und Ödeme unter Therapie mit Rosiglitazon. [Severe electrolyte imbalance and edema in therapy with rosiglitazone.] Med Klin (Munich) 2002;97(9):553–5.

76. Lebovitz HE, Kreider M, Freed MI. Evaluation of liver function in type 2 diabetic patients during clinical trials: evidence that rosiglitazone does not cause hepatic dysfunction. Diabetes Care 2002;25(5):815–21.

77. Yokoyama M, Izumiya Y, Yoshizawa M, Usuda R. Acute rhabdomyolysis associated with troglitazone. Diabetes Care 2000;23(3):421–2.

78. Shadid S, Jensen MD. Angioneurotic edema as a side effect of pioglitazone. Diabetes Care 2002;25(2):405.

79. Thompson-Culkin K, Zussman B, Miller AK, Freed MI. Pharmacokinetics of rosiglitazone in patients with end-stage renal disease. J Int Med Res 2002;30(4):391–9.

80. Di Cicco RA, Allen A, Carr A, Fowles S, Jorkasky DK, Freed MI. Rosiglitazone does not alter the pharmacokinetics of metformin. J Clin Pharmacol 2000;40(11):1280–5.

81. Lin JC, Ito MK. A drug interaction between troglitazone and simvastatin. Diabetes Care 1999;22(12):2104–6.

Thionamides

General Information

Several natural or synthetic substances interfere with the synthesis and/or secretion of the thyroid hormones. Two types of thionamides are used in the treatment of hyperthyroidism:

1. derivatives of thiouracil, especially propylthiouracil (rINN); methylthiouracil and iodothiouracil have

been used in the past, but are not currently used clinically;

2. derivatives of thioimidazole, especially thiamazole (rINN; methimazole) and its carbethoxy derivative carbimazole (rINN), which is converted in the body to thiamazole (1,2).

All of these drugs interfere with the thyroid peroxidase system and inhibit the synthesis of the thyroid hormones, reducing their overproduction in hyperthyroidism. However, if they are used in too high dosages, they can cause hypothyroidism and hypersecretion of thyrotrophin (TSH) which in turn will stimulate thyroid growth and the development of goiter. To avoid these problems, regular dosage adjustment or combination with synthetic thyroid hormones is necessary as soon as the euthyroid state is obtained.

Antithyroid drugs may also suppress lymphocytic infiltration into the thyroid and thereby directly modulate the basic disorder of autoimmune hyperthyroidism (SEDA-6, 364) (SEDA-9, 344). Propylthiouracil, but not the thioimidazoles, also inhibits the conversion of thyroxine to its more active derivative triiodothyronine. This effect is significant during high-dose treatment, and propylthiouracil may therefore be preferred if a more rapid onset of action is desired, for example thyrotoxic crisis, although clear experimental proof of the advantageous effect is still lacking (3).

The antithyroid drugs are well absorbed from the intestinal tract, but the half-life of propylthiouracil is much shorter (2 hours) than that of the thioimidazoles (6 hours). However, the in vivo half-life may be longer due to accumulation and retention of the drug in the thyroid gland (4).

General adverse effects

Both the thiouracils and the thioimidazoles can produce hypothyroidism and goiter. Most of their other adverse effects are allergic rather than toxic. The overall frequency of untoward reactions is 2–14%, but severe reactions occur in less than 1% of patients. Some data suggest that the thioimidazoles have a lower incidence of adverse effects than the thiouracils (5). An association between the dosage of thionamide and the development of untoward reactions has been found in several studies (6). It has therefore been proposed that the initial dose of carbimazole should not exceed 30 mg/day and that of propylthiouracil 300 mg/day (SEDA-17, 474). Allergic reactions include drug fever, lymphadenopathy, arthralgia, agranulocytosis, thrombocytopenia, leukopenia, and skin reactions (1,7). In view of the in vivo conversion of carbimazole to thiamazole, cross-allergy between the two compounds can be expected and has been observed. Cross-allergy between thiouracil and thioimidazoles is rare, but a few cases have been reported. Tumor-inducing effects have not been reported.

Organs and Systems

Nervous system

Neuritis has been described in patients taking thiamazole (8,9).

Sensory systems

Eyes

In contrast to ^{131}I, antithyroid drugs do not seem to increase the risk of new or worse exophthalmos in patients with Graves' disease (10,11).

Retrobulbar neuritis has been reported in a patient taking thiamazole (12).

Ears

Ototoxicity has rarely been attributed to antithyroid drugs (13). In one case progressive bilateral sensorineural hearing loss attributed to propylthiouracil was associated with myeloperoxidase-antineutrophil cytoplasmic antibodies (MPO-ANCA) (14).

Taste

Taste disturbance has been described in patients taking antithyroid drugs and has been attributed to zinc deficiency (SEDA-7, 398) (SEDA-11, 357).

Endocrine

Overtreatment with antithyroid drugs can cause hypothyroidism (15,16).

Metabolism

A specific form of hypoglycemia occurs in Hirata disease, a rare autoimmune syndrome in which large amounts of insulin can be released from autoantibodies. In a Japanese series of 197 cases, 43% of the patients had been taking medications before diagnosis: thiamazole for Graves' disease, alpha-mercaptopropionyl glycine for cataracts, liver disease, or rheumatoid arthritis, or glutathione for liver disease, all of which are sulfhydryl compounds. After these drugs were withdrawn, the hypoglycemic attacks subsided (17).

Hematologic

Neutropenia, agranulocytosis, aplastic anemia, and thrombocytopenia are the most important adverse effects of antithyroid drugs.

Neutropenia and agranulocytosis

There are two different types of neutropenia due to antithyroid drugs: a mild dose-related reduction in leukocyte count and a true allergic agranulocytosis (SEDA-10, 368) (18).

Allergic agranulocytosis
DoTS classification (BMJ 2003;327:1222–5)
  Dose-relation: hypersusceptibility effect
  Time-course: intermediate
  Susceptibility factors: genetic (HLA DRB1*08032 allele); age (over 40); sex (women)

Severe agranulocytosis (or more rarely pancytopenia) is usually only observed during the first few months of therapy. Since agranulocytosis can develop very rapidly, periodic leukocyte counts are usually considered to be of little help, but it has been suggested that weekly leukocyte counts during the first month of treatment can detect presymptomatic cases and allow more rapid intervention

(19). Patients should therefore be warned to seek immediate medical help if a fever or sore throat develops during antithyroid drug treatment. If the drug is withdrawn immediately recovery is the rule, but fatal cases have also been reported (20,21). In one case agranulocytosis unusually occurred after a second exposure to the drug, in this case propylthiouracil (22).

Frequency

The risk of agranulocytosis has been estimated during several surveys. A large European–Israeli study (23) showed a risk of about 3 per 10 000 users. However, the mortality in this survey was small (one in 45 cases) (SEDA-13, 376). In two hospital surveys of agranulocytosis (24,25) there was an increased risk in women aged over 40 years and when the dose of thiamazole (thiamazole) was more than 40 mg/day. In vitro lymphocyte testing can confirm the sensitization of the immune system to the antithyroid drugs and can occasionally indicate cross-sensitivity between thiamazole and propylthiouracil (SEDA-8, 372) (SEDA-9, 344). In a Japanese study, using an adverse drug reactions database, 24 of 91 cases of presumed drug-induced leukopenia were associated with thiamazole (26). The estimated overall risk was 3 per 10 000, largely in the first 3 months (RR = 182, 95% CI = 74, 449).

Mechanism

Laboratory studies have provided insights into the immune mechanisms underlying the hematological complications of antithyroid drugs (27). Sera from five patients taking thiamazole who presented with immune thrombocytopenia showed antibodies to the platelet cell adhesion molecule-1. Similar antibodies were present in the serum of a patient with carbimazole-associated neutropenia and mild thrombocytopenia, together with antibodies to the neutrophil-specific Fc gamma receptor IIIb (28). Antibodies against the rhesus component of erythrocyte proteins have also been described in patients with carbimazole-associated anemia, leading to the conclusion that carbimazole can induce cell lineage-specific drug-dependent antibodies that cause cytopenias.

In 24 patients with Graves' disease with thiamazole-induced agranulocytosis, 68 patients with Graves' disease without agranulocytosis, and 525 healthy controls, there was a strong positive association of the HLA DRB1*08032 allele with susceptibility to methimazole-induced agranulocytosis, suggesting that cellular autoimmunity may be involved in its development (29).

Time-course

In 18 cases of antithyroid drug-induced agranulocytosis in China, previous evidence that most cases occur early in treatment (2–12 weeks in 17 of 18 cases) and in those taking high doses was confirmed (30). This series also confirmed that agranulocytosis develops abruptly, arguing against routine monitoring of white cell count, and that fever and sore throat are the earliest symptoms.

Management

The treatment of this complication is controversial. There have been at least 15 reports of the use of granulocyte colony stimulating factor (G-CSF) in severe cases (granulocyte count under $100 \times 10^6/l$) of thionamide-induced agranulocytosis with the objective of shortening the period of neutropenia and hence the risk of infection (31). In another case the use of G-CSF in thionamide-induced agranulocytosis was associated with a number of iatrogenic complications (31). A review of treatment with G-CSF has shown that the average time to recovery from agranulocytosis is 8.2 days, not obviously different from the reported range of 7–14 days without the drug, leading the authors to argue against its routine use in afebrile patients, even in the face of a severe reduction in granulocyte count.

In 24 patients with Graves' disease who developed agranulocytosis during antithyroid drug therapy, randomized to receive G-CSF ($n = 14$) or an antibiotic only, recovery time (defined as the number of days required for neutrophil counts to exceed $0.5 \times 10^9/l$) did not differ between the treatments in patients with moderate or severe agranulocytosis, arguing against its routine use (32). These conclusions have been supported by retrospective data from a further 12 patients, four of whom received G-CSF (33). Again, there was no significant difference in terms of the speed of hematological recovery, the number of days of antibiotic treatment, or the duration of hospitalization.

In a retrospective cohort study of 90 cases of drug-induced agranulocytosis in Strasbourg, antithyroid drugs were implicated in 23% of cases, second only to antibiotics in terms of frequency of prescription in the affected cohort (34). The clinical presentation was often severe and included isolated fever (41% of cases), septicemia or septic shock (31%), and pneumonia (10%). The outcome was favorable in 98% of cases. All the patients were treated with broad-spectrum antibiotics and 42 received hemopoietic growth factors; in those given growth factors the mean durations for hematological recovery, antibiotic therapy, and hospitalization were significantly reduced. While patient selection may have contributed to these findings, they do suggest a useful role for such growth factors in supporting patients with this potentially life-threatening complication of thionamide therapy.

Aplastic anemia

Aplastic anemia due to antithyroid drugs is very rare and has been said to occur as an adverse effect of thionamide therapy with about one-tenth of the frequency of agranulocytosis.

- Aplastic anemia developed in a 58-year-old woman taking thiamazole for the third time; she responded well to drug withdrawal and treatment with human granulocyte colony stimulating factor (35).
- A 16-year-old girl who had taken thiamazole for 1 month (30 mg/day) developed a sore throat and dysphagia and had pancytopenia (36). Instead of the expected picture of hypoplasia, bone marrow aspiration showed replacement with plasma cells, a finding suggestive of myeloma and representing a picture not previously described in this context. Thiamazole was withdrawn and she was given antibiotics, dexamethasone, and granulocyte colony stimulating factor. Her

hematology and bone marrow findings normalized within days and she was well at follow-up at 24 months.

There have been anecdotal reports of the use of G-CSF in cases of thionamide-induced agranulocytosis (37). In a retrospective review (38) the outcomes in 10 severe cases treated with G-CSF and in 10 treated without were reviewed. The time to hematological recovery, the duration of antibiotic use, and the duration of hospitalization were all shorter in those treated with G-CSF, although there were no deaths in either group. These findings are in accord with the results of other non-randomized studies of the use of G-CSF in drug-induced agranulocytosis, but conflict with the results of one randomized study that showed no benefit (32). The latest findings must therefore be interpreted with caution, although it is notable that this study was confined to those with severe suppression of leukocyte counts and clinical evidence of infection.

Liver

Both carbimazole and propylthiouracil can cause liver damage, sometimes as part of a hypersensitivity reaction associated with pruritus, rash, fever, and arthralgia. Severe liver injury is believed to be rare, with only 20 reported cases up to 1993 (39). In contrast, subclinical hepatic dysfunction, characterized by a rise in hepatic enzymes, may be common and does not necessitate drug withdrawal in the absence of symptoms (39).

Of 14 cases of suspected drug-induced liver disease presenting to a gastroenterology department over a 3-year period, one was thought to be related to thiamazole, with a hepatitic pattern of liver function tests in a 39-year-old woman 6 days after the start of therapy; recovery was swift and complete (40). Delayed cholestatic hepatitis without antineutrophil cytoplasmic antibodies has been reported (41), and there have been fatal cases of hepatic necrosis (SEDA-21, 438) (7).

In a retrospective review of 497 patients taking propylthiouracil for hyperthyroidism, clinically overt hepatitis developed in six patients at 12–49 days after starting the drug (42). Jaundice and itching were present in five, fever in two, rash in two, and arthralgia in one. Serum bilirubin, alanine transaminase, and alkaline phosphatase were increased in five, four, and six patients respectively. The type of hepatic injury was cholestatic in three, hepatocellular in one, and mixed in two. There were no differences in age, sex, drug dose, or serum thyroid hormone concentrations at time of diagnosis in those with hepatic injury compared with those without. Liver function normalized in all patients at 16–145 days after withdrawal of propylthiouracil. In addition to these cases of overt liver injury, 14% of the cohort had mild asymptomatic liver enzyme rises at a mean of 75 days after the start of treatment.

The reported incidence of liver injury in this report is higher (at 1.2%) than in previous reports, perhaps reflecting patient selection or ethnic differences in study populations. An association with propylthiouracil in the six cases described was supported by the temporal association with the start of therapy and recovery after withdrawal. This complication is likely to be a hypersusceptibility reaction, given the lack of dose association within the therapeutic range, the unpredictable

occurrence, and an association with symptoms of hypersensitivity. The findings of this retrospective study do not indicate the need for regular monitoring of liver function tests in those taking propylthiouracil, but they do highlight the need to consider drug toxicity if overt hepatic injury develops, especially early in the course of propylthiouracil therapy.

Pancreas

Acute pancreatitis and parotitis without antineutrophil cytoplasmic antibodies has been attributed to thiamazole (43).

- A 33-year-old woman developed acute pancreatitis together with mild cholestatic hepatitis and erythema nodosum 1 month after starting carbimazole for Graves' disease; rechallenge with a single dose of carbimazole (10 mg) 7 days after initial recovery led to a further episode of acute pancreatitis, from which she recovered (44).

The temporal association with carbimazole therapy, the response to rechallenge, and the absence of other causes of acute pancreatitis suggested that the drug was causative in this case.

Urinary tract

Chronic tubulointerstitial nephritis with renal insufficiency without antineutrophil cytoplasmic antibodies has been attributed to propylthiouracil (45).

Skin

The most common reaction to antithyroid drugs is a benign skin rash or pruritus without rash. Although such a reaction is usually not serious and can even disappear during continuous treatment, it nevertheless indicates an allergic reaction and requires withdrawal of therapy. Thiouracil can then be replaced by thioimidazoles, but allergy to both products can occasionally occur.

Sexual function

Sexual precocity associated with hypothyroidism has been reported after long-term treatment of children with propylthiouracil, and may reflect relative overdosage (46).

Immunologic

Antineutrophil cytoplasmic antibody (ANCA)-positive vasculitis is a well-described complication, particularly with propylthiouracil and to a lesser extent with carbimazole, and has been most often described in patients with Graves' disease. The possible drug-induced causes of ANCA-positive vasculitis with high titers of antimyeloperoxidase antibodies in 30 new patients have been reviewed (47). The findings illustrated that this type of vasculitis is a predominantly drug-induced disorder. Only 12 of the 30 cases were not related to a drug. The most frequently implicated drug was hydralazine ($n = 10$); the remainder involved propylthiouracil ($n = 3$), penicillamine ($n = 2$), allopurinol ($n = 2$), and sulfasalazine ($n = 1$).

Cutaneous vasculitis is often a feature of such cases, although severe systemic manifestations often also occur.

Two patients with propylthiouracil hypersensitivity presented with skin manifestations but also had renal, rheumatological, and hematological features (48). A review of the literature showed that the symptoms and signs in patients with ANCA-associated thionamide-induced vasculitis are diverse. Acral purpuric skin lesions are typically seen; recognition of these classical clinical features may allow early diagnosis and limit associated morbidity and the requirement for other therapies, particularly immunosuppression. Several other reports have described cases of MPO-ANCA-positive cases of vasculitis presenting in a variety of ways in both adults and children treated with propylthiouracil (49–52).

There have been reports of propylthiouracil-induced ANCA-associated small vessel vasculitis (53,54), crescentic glomerulonephritis (55), and Wegener's granulomatosis (56). More common, however, may be a condition termed "antithyroid arthritis syndrome," which is a transient migratory polyarthritis occurring within 2 months of starting thionamides and resolving within 4 weeks of stopping therapy (57).

ANCA-positive vasculitis in a patient with multinodular goiter has been described, together with a review of the clinical features in a further 26 cases (58). Renal involvement, typically with crescentic or necrotizing glomerulonephritis on biopsy, and arthralgia were the most common manifestations. A few cases of diffuse proliferative lupus nephritis associated with ANCAs have been reported (SEDA-20, 394). Other cases of ANCA-associated disease in patients have been reported, including subjects presenting with neutrophilic dermatosis (59), pyoderma gangrenosum, secondary sterile pyoarthrosis (60), and purpura fulminans (61). Small vessel vasculitis leading to pulmonary alveolar hemorrhage and crescentic glomerulonephritis has also been described (61).

In 61 patients with Graves' hyperthyroidism, 32 of whom were taking propylthiouracil and 29 methimazole, there was a higher prevalence of antimyeloperoxidase ANCAs in those taking propylthiouracil than in those taking thiamazole (25 versus 3.4%) (62). There were no significant differences in age, duration of therapy, or drug dosage in those who developed antimyeloperoxidase ANCAs compared with those who did not. Two ANCA-positive patients in this study developed rheumatoid arthritis or membranous glomerulonephritis, but none developed classical ANCA-associated vasculitis.

There have been reports of antimyeloperoxidase ANCAs associated with diffuse pulmonary alveolar hemorrhage (63), IgA nephropathy (64), and drug-induced neutropenia (65) in patients who had Graves' hyperthyroidism taking propylthiouracil. Investigation using serum from the last of these patients implicated a complement-mediated mechanism. In another case ANCAs developed in two of three monozygotic triplets, both of whom had Graves' disease treated with propylthiouracil, supporting a genetic role in the development of this drug complication (66).

Long-term outcomes in a series of seven children who developed myeloperoxidase-specific ANCA-positive necrotizing crescentic glomerulonephritis associated with propylthiouracil were studied in Japan (67). Three had nephritis alone and four had extrarenal vasculitis. All had taken glucocorticoids, some with additional drugs, and all

had achieved remission. None had progressed to end-stage renal insufficiency or death during a mean period of follow-up of 58 months. This apparently benign course, albeit with a relatively short period of follow-up, is similar to that seen in adult patients with this drug complication and implies a better prognosis than in subjects with non-drug-induced ANCA-positive vasculitic disease.

The size of this problem has been addressed using serum samples from 117 patients with Graves' disease treated either with propylthiouracil or thiamazole, and from untreated patients (68). Myeloperoxidase ANCA and proteinase-3 antineutrophil cytoplasmic antibodies (PR3-ANCA) were tested by enzyme-linked immunosorbent assay. Myeloperoxidase ANCA was negative in all untreated patients and patients taking thiamazole, but positive in 21 of 56 patients taking propylthiouracil. In contrast, PR3-ANCA was not detected in any patient in the study. The proportion of patients who were positive for myeloperoxidase ANCA increased with the duration of propylthiouracil therapy. Of the 21 patients who were positive for myeloperoxidase ANCA, 12 had no symptoms, but nine complained of myalgia, arthralgia, or coryza-like symptoms after the appearance of the antibody; none had abnormal urinary findings. These findings suggest a specific association between propylthiouracil therapy and the development of myeloperoxidase ANCA in patients with Graves' disease.

ANCA positive microscopic polyangiitis has been associated with propylthiouracil, with a fatal outcome despite treatment with glucocorticoids and cyclophosphamide (69). Another patient presented atypically with acute pericarditis 10 months after starting to take propylthiouracil 100 mg tds (70). Another patient developed ANCA-negative leukocytoclastic vasculitis of the skin (71).

Several cases of "collagen-like" or "lupus-like" disease have been reported (joint pain, skin rash, and positive antinuclear antibodies) during treatment with either propylthiouracil or thiamazole (SEDA-8, 372) (SEDA-10, 368). Some cases of general vasculitis can be fatal, although high-dose glucocorticoid therapy can be helpful (72).

Other reports have described serious immunological complications of propylthiouracil in the absence of ANCA, including interstitial nephritis and fatal Stevens–Johnson syndrome in a 90-year-old woman treated for 5 weeks (73) and disseminated intravascular coagulation and vasculitis 2 weeks after the introduction of propylthiouracil in a 42-year-old woman (74). The latter was treated successfully by drug withdrawal and intravenous methylprednisolone.

Second-Generation Effects

Pregnancy

Both the thiouracils and thioimidazoles readily cross the placenta and can cause fetal hypothyroidism, resulting in a slight delay in neurological or bone maturation. Various degrees of goiter have also been observed, even to the extent of severe tracheal compression and death. Antithyroid drug dosage should therefore be reduced to the minimum required to maintain a euthyroid state without supplementation of levothyroxine (75).

Teratogenicity

Aplasia cutis congenita has been attributed to carbimazole, or its active metabolite thiamazole, given during early pregnancy (SEDA-14, 367) (76), and a review revealed 16 cases of solitary skin defects associated with intrauterine exposure to thiamazole (76). The defects can be restricted to a region of the body or can be widespread. Several causes have been documented, including chromosomal abnormalities (for example trisomy 13) and single gene mutations, such as Goltz syndrome. A few cases are believed to result from in utero exposure to teratogens, including thionamides. To date, 16 cases of solitary skin defects associated with intrauterine exposure to thiamazole have been reported. Additional cases of aplasia cutis congenita in thionamide-exposed infants associated with other congenital abnormalities, such as bilateral atresia of the nasal choana, esophageal atresia, imperforate anus, and cardiovascular defects have also been reported (76).

Additional cases of aplasia cutis congenita in thionamide-exposed infants associated with other congenital abnormalities, such as choanal atresia, esophageal atresia, imperforate anus, and cardiovascular defects, were also reviewed. This pattern of abnormalities has previously led to the term "methimazole [thiamazole] embryopathy" (77).

- A 3-year-old child, whose mother had been treated for Graves' hyperthyroidism with thiamazole throughout pregnancy, had two scalp lesions and other abnormalities of tissues of ectodermal origin, including dystrophic nails and syndactyly.

The authors suggested that a history of in utero exposure to thiamazole should be sought in all children with aplasia cutis congenita, as well as other ectodermal tissue abnormalities, to allow better definition of the "methimazole embryopathy." However, cautious interpretation of the literature is required, given the small number of thiamazole-associated cases of aplasia cutis congenita compared with the widespread prescription of this drug in pregnant women with hyperthyroidism. On the other hand, the absence of an apparent association with the use of the alternative thionamide, propylthiouracil, argues in favor of using the latter in pregnant patients.

In a prospective study in 241 women referred to a teratology service because of exposure to thiamazole during pregnancy, congenital abnormalities were compared with those found in offspring of 1089 controls referred because of exposure to non-teratogenic drugs or radiography (77). There were no statistically significant differences between the two groups in terms of major abnormalities, gestational age at delivery, neonatal weight, or head circumference, but among the thiamazole-exposed infants two had a major malformation consistent with "methimazole embryopathy." One had choanal atresia (exposed at 4–7 gestational weeks) and the other had esophageal atresia (exposed at 0–16 gestational weeks) (78). These are very rare malformations, and the number of cases in the cohort was insufficient to reach statistical significance, so the possibility of a chance association with thiamazole exposure cannot be excluded. These cases do, however, lend support to the view that thiamazole may be teratogenic, although thyrotoxicosis itself may be the associated factor. Until further data are available, treatment of thyrotoxicosis with propylthiouracil may be preferable in women who are planning a pregnancy.

- Scalp atresia has been described in an infant whose mother had taken carbimazole in a high dose (60 mg/day) during the first 12 weeks of pregnancy and propylthiouracil thereafter (79). The infant had other dysmorphic features (a flat face, low-set ears, upper lip retraction, and a low-set fifth finger) in addition to transient hypothyroidism.
- Choanal atresia has been described in an infant whose mother presented in early pregnancy with Graves' hyperthyroidism and who took carbimazole in doses up to 60 mg/day in the first trimester (80). She was also clinically and biochemically severely hyperthyroid at this time.

Propylthiouracil crosses the placenta as readily as the thioimidazoles, but the rare and probably real association between thioimidazoles and fetal anomalies makes the thioimidazoles less attractive first-line alternatives (81–83). When propylthiouracil is used cautiously in minimal amounts and with frequent dose adjustments, it is probably the safest form of treatment of hyperthyroidism during pregnancy (SEDA-8, 373) (SEDA-11, 357).

Fetotoxicity

Neonatal hypothyroidism has been reported after maternal use of antithyroid drugs (84,85). Transient neonatal hyperthyroidism in a female child born to a mother who had been treated with potassium iodide and carbimazole during pregnancy was followed by sexual precocity (86).

Lactation

The antithyroid drugs appear in human milk, and breast-feeding has therefore been considered contraindicated during such treatment. However, the amount of drug transferred in human milk is too small to affect thyroid function in the breastfed infant (87,88).

Susceptibility Factors

The antithyroid drugs should not be used in patients with a large intrathoracic goiter, which can further increase in size (89).

In severe hepatic disease, the dosages of antithyroid drugs should be very cautiously determined.

Drug Administration

Drug dosage regimens

There are two general patterns of use of antithyroid drugs: monotherapy with progressive reduction in dosage during recovery from hyperthyroidism and a higher dosage of antithyroid drugs complemented by thyroid replacement therapy to avoid hypothyroidism. There is no convincing evidence for a better short-term or long-term control of Graves' disease with either form of therapy, but combination therapy followed by monotherapy with levothyroxine increased the remission rate substantially. The administration of levothyroxine during antithyroid drug treatment reduces both the production of antibodies to TSH receptors and the frequency of recurrence of hyperthyroidism (90). During combination therapy with propylthiouracil and levothyroxine in normal therapeutic doses the inhibition of the conversion of T4 to T3 is of no importance. A single daily dose of antithyroid drugs cannot completely block iodine organification but can nevertheless control most cases of hyperthyroidism. Such therapy can therefore be used in some patients to improve compliance. The duration of therapy is also controversial, but a more prolonged duration of therapy is usually associated with a higher remission rate (SEDA-12, 354).

Drug overdose

Acute overdose of 13 g of propylthiouracil had no serious adverse effects, except for a temporary reduction in serum triiodothyronine (SEDA-5, 382).

Drug–Drug Interactions

Iodine

Since thionamides block the organification of iodine and incorporation of iodine into iodotyrosines, they inhibit the uptake of ^{131}I used therapeutically in hyperthyroidism. For this reason, thionamides are generally withdrawn for a period of up to a week before ^{131}I therapy is planned, and re-introduction is similarly delayed until several days after ^{131}I therapy. The effect of treatment with either thiamazole or propylthiouracil before ^{131}I has been studied retrospectively (91), the thionamide being withdrawn 5–55 days before ^{131}I administration. The findings confirmed the view that propylthiouracil, but not thiamazole, significantly reduced the cure rate after ^{131}I compared with that found in subjects not pretreated with propylthiouracil, and that discontinuation for 4 months was required for the cure rates to be similar. These findings highlight the fact that thionamides cause a relative "radio-resistance," and prolonged drug withdrawal or an increased dose of ^{131}I may be required to produce an acceptable cure rate.

References

1. Kampmann JP, Hansen JM. Clinical pharmacokinetics of antithyroid drugs. Clin Pharmacokinet 1981;6(6):401–28.
2. Langer P, Greer MA, editors. Antithyroid Substances and Naturally Occurring Goitrogens. Basel-Munchen-Paris-London-New York-Sidney: Karger, 1977:54.
3. Chopra IJ, Cody V. Triiodothyronines in health and disease. Gross F, editor. Monographs on Endocrinology. Berlin-Heidelberg-New York: Springer-Verlag, 1981;18:1.
4. Jansson R, Dahlberg PA, Johansson H, Lindstrom B. Intrathyroidal concentrations of methimazole in patients with Graves' disease. J Clin Endocrinol Metab 1983;57(1):129–32.
5. Marchant B, Lees JF, Alexander WD. Antithyroid drugs. Pharmacol Ther [B] 1978;3(3):305–48.
6. Reinwein D, Benker G, Lazarus JH, Alexander WD. A prospective randomized trial of antithyroid drug dose in Graves' disease therapy. European Multicenter Study

7. Group on Antithyroid Drug Treatment. J Clin Endocrinol Metab 1993;76(6):1516–21.
7. Cooper DS. Antithyroid drugs. N Engl J Med 1984;311(21):1353–62.
8. Stege R. Antithyroid drug therapy in hyperthyroidism. Recurrence, hypothyroidism and thyroid antibodies. Acta Chir Scand Suppl 1980;501:1–130.
9. Roldan EC, Nigrin G. Peripheral neuritis after methimazole therapy. NY State J Med 1972;72(23):2898–900.
10. Sridama V, DeGroot LJ. Treatment of Graves' disease and the course of ophthalmopathy. Am J Med 1989;87(1):70–3.
11. Tallstedt L, Lundell G, Torring O, Wallin G, Ljunggren JG, Blomgren H, Taube A. Occurrence of ophthalmopathy after treatment for Graves' hyperthyroidism. The Thyroid Study Group. N Engl J Med 1992;326(26):1733–8.
12. Sponzilli T, Tarroni P, D'Amico A, Vinciguerra V, Lupinacci L. Neurite ottica retrobulbare in corso di terapia con metimazolo (contributo clinico). [Retrobulbar optic neuritis in the course of methimazole therapy (a clinical case).] Riv Neurobiol 1979;25(2):233–8.
13. Smith KE, Spaulding JS. Ototoxic reaction to propylthiouracil. Arch Otolaryngol 1972;96(4):368–70.
14. Sano M, Kitahara N, Kunikata R. Progressive bilateral sensorineural hearing loss induced by an antithyroid drug. ORL J Otorhinolaryngol Relat Spec 2004;66(5):281–5.
15. Brewer C. Psychosis due to acute hypothyroidism during the administration of carbimazole. Br J Psychiatry 1969;115(527):1181–3.
16. Messina M, Manieri C, Spagnuolo F, Sardi E, Allegramente L, Monaco A, Ciccarelli E. A case of methimazole-induced hypothyroidism in a patient with endemic goiter: effects of endogenous TSH hyperstimulation after discontinuation of the drug. Thyroidology 1989;1(1):53–7.
17. Polychronakos C, Ligier S. Resuspension of intermediate-acting insulin as a source of error in insulin dosing. Diabetes Care 1994;17(10):1234–5.
18. Bartalena L, Bogazzi F, Martino E. Adverse effects of thyroid hormone preparations and antithyroid drugs. Drug Saf 1996;15(1):53–63.
19. Tajiri J, Noguchi S, Murakami T, Murakami N. Antithyroid drug-induced agranulocytosis. The usefulness of routine white blood cell count monitoring. Arch Intern Med 1990;150(3):621–4.
20. Beebe RT, Propp S, McClintock JC, Versaci A. Fatal agranulocytosis during treatment of toxic goiter with propylthiouracil. Ann Intern Med 1951;34(4):1035–40.
21. Tait GB. Fatal agranulocytosis during carbimazole therapy. Lancet 1957;272(6963):303.
22. Roeloffzen WW, Verhaegh JJ, van Poelgeest AE, Gansevoort RT. Fever or a soar throat after start of antithyroidal drugs? A medical emergency. Neth J Med 1998;53(3):113–17.
23. Retsagi G, Kelly JP, Kaufman DW. Risk of agranulocytosis and aplastic anaemia in relation to use of antithyroid drugs. International Agranulocytosis and Aplastic Anaemia Study. BMJ 1988;297(6643):262–5.
24. Cooper DS, Goldminz D, Levin AA, Ladenson PW, Daniels GH, Molitch ME, Ridgway EC. Agranulocytosis associated with antithyroid drugs. Effects of patient age and drug dose. Ann Intern Med 1983;98(1):26–9.
25. Kaaja R, Ebeling P, Lamberg BA. Tyreostaathioidon aiheuttama agranulosystoos. [Agranulocytosis induced by antithyroid drugs.] Duodecim 1986;102(13):872–8.
26. Ohtsu F, Yano R, Inagaki K, Sakakibara J. [Estimation of adverse drug reactions by the evaluation scores of subjective symptoms (complaints) and background of patients. III. Drug-induced leucopenia.] Yakugaku Zasshi 2000;120(4):397–407.

27. Kroll H, Sun QH, Santoso S. Platelet endothelial cell adhesion molecule-1 (PECAM-1) is a target glycoprotein in drug-induced thrombocytopenia. Blood 2000;96(4):1409–14.

28. Bux J, Ernst-Schlegel M, Rothe B, Panzer C. Neutropenia and anaemia due to carbimazole-dependent antibodies. Br J Haematol 2000;109(1):243–7.

29. Tamai H, Sudo T, Kimura A, Mukuta T, Matsubayashi S, Kuma K, Nagataki S, Sasazuki T. Association between the DRB1*08032 histocompatibility antigen and methimazole-induced agranulocytosis in Japanese patients with Graves disease. Ann Intern Med 1996;124(5):490–4.

30. Dai WX, Zhang JD, Zhan SW, Xu BZ, Jin H, Yao Y, Xin WC, Bai Y. Retrospective analysis of 18 cases of antithyroid drug (ATD)-induced agranulocytosis. Endocr J 2002;49(1):29–33.

31. Hirsch D, Luboshitz J, Blum I. Treatment of antithyroid drug-induced agranulocytosis by granulocyte colony-stimulating factor: a case of primum non nocere. Thyroid 1999;9(10):1033–5.

32. Fukata S, Kuma K, Sugawara M. Granulocyte colony-stimulating factor (G-CSF) does not improve recovery from antithyroid drug-induced agranulocytosis: a prospective study. Thyroid 1999;9(1):29–31.

33. Andres E, Maloisel F, Ruellan A. Use of colony-stimulating factors for the treatment of antithyroid drug-induced agranulocytosis: a retrospective study in twelve patients. Thyroid 2000;10(1):103.

34. Andres E, Maloisel F, Kurtz JE, Kaltenbach G, Alt M, Weber JC, Sibilia J, Schlienger JL, Blickle JF, Brogard JM, Dufour P. Modern management of non-chemotherapy drug-induced agranulocytosis: a monocentric cohort study of 90 cases and review of the literature. Eur J Intern Med 2002;13(5):324–8.

35. Mezquita P, Luna V, Munoz-Torres M, Torres-Vela E, Lopez-Rodriguez F, Callejas JL, Escobar-Jimenez F. Methimazole-induced aplastic anemia in third exposure: successful treatment with recombinant human granulocyte colony-stimulating factor. Thyroid 1998;8(9):791–4.

36. Breier DV, Rendo P, Gonzalez J, Shilton G, Stivel M, Goldztein S. Massive plasmocytosis due to methimazole-induced bone marrow toxicity. Am J Hematol 2001;67(4):259–61.

37. Calabro L, Alonci A, Bellomo G, D'Angelo A, Di Giacomo V, Musolino C. Methimazole-induced agranulocytosis and quick recovery with G-CSF: case report. Hepatology 2001;5:479–82.

38. Andres E, Kurtz JE, Perrin AE, Dufour P, Schlienger JL, Maloisel F. Haematopoietic growth factor in antithyroid-drug-induced agranulocytosis. QJM 2001;94(8):423–8.

39. Liaw YF, Huang MJ, Fan KD, Li KL, Wu SS, Chen TJ. Hepatic injury during propylthiouracil therapy in patients with hyperthyroidism. A cohort study. Ann Intern Med 1993;118(6):424–8.

40. Hartleb M, Biernat L, Kochel A. Drug-induced liver damage—a three-year study of patients from one gastroenterological department. Med Sci Monit 2002;8(4):CR292–6.

41. Hung YT, Yu WK, Chow E. Delayed cholestatic hepatitis due to methimazole. Hong Kong Med J 1999;5(2):200–1.

42. Kim HJ, Kim BH, Han YS, Yang I, Kim KJ, Dong SH, Kim HJ, Chang YW, Lee JI, Chang R. The incidence and clinical characteristics of symptomatic propylthiouracil-induced hepatic injury in patients with hyperthyroidism: a single-center retrospective study. Am J Gastroenterol 2001;96(1):165–9.

43. Taguchi M, Yokota M, Koyano H, Endo Y, Ozawa Y. Acute pancreatitis and parotitis induced by methimazole in a patient with Graves' disease. Clin Endocrinol (Oxf) 1999;51(5):667–70.

44. Marazuela M, Sanchez de Paco G, Jimenez I, Carraro R, Fernandez-Herrera J, Pajares JM, Gomez-Pan A. Acute pancreatitis, hepatic cholestasis, and erythema nodosum induced by carbimazole treatment for Graves' disease. Endocr J 2002;49(3):315–18.

45. Nakahama H, Nakamura H, Kitada O, Sugita M. Chronic drug-induced tubulointerstitial nephritis with renal failure associated with propylthiouracil therapy. Nephrol Dial Transplant 1999;14(5):1263–5.

46. Sadeghi-Nejad A, Senior B. Sexual precocity: an unusual complication of propylthiouracil therapy. J Pediatr 1971;79(5):833–7.

47. Choi HK, Merkel PA, Walker AM, Niles JL. Drug-associated antineutrophil cytoplasmic antibody-positive vasculitis: prevalence among patients with high titers of antimyeloperoxidase antibodies. Arthritis Rheum 2000;43(2):405–13.

48. Chastain MA, Russo GG, Boh EE, Chastain JB, Falabella A, Millikan LE. Propylthiouracil hypersensitivity: report of two patients with vasculitis and review of the literature. J Am Acad Dermatol 1999;41(5 Pt 1):757–64.

49. Morita S, Ueda Y, Eguchi K. Anti-thyroid drug-induced ANCA-associated vasculitis: a case report and review of the literature. Endocr J 2000;47(4):467–70.

50. Sera N, Yokoyama N, Abe Y, Ide A, Usa T, Tominaga T, Ejima E, Kawakami A, Ashizawa K, Eguchi K. Antineutrophil cytoplasmic antibody-associated vasculitis complicating Graves' disease: report of two adult cases. Acta Med Nagasaki 2000;45:33–6.

51. Otsuka S, Kinebuchi A, Tabata H, Yamakage A, Yamazaki S. Myeloperoxidase–antineutrophil cytoplasmic antibody-associated vasculitis following propylthiouracil therapy. Br J Dermatol 2000;142(4):828–30.

52. Matsubara K, Nigami H, Harigaya H, Osaki M, Baba K. Myeloperoxidase antineutrophil cytoplasmic antibody positive vasculitis during propylthiouracil treatment: successful management with oral corticosteroids. Pediatr Int 2000;42(2):170–3.

53. Harper L, Cockwell P, Savage CO. Case of propylthiouracil-induced ANCA associated small vessel vasculitis. Nephrol Dial Transplant 1998;13(2):455–8.

54. Miller RM, Savige J, Nassis L, Cominos BI. Antineutrophil cytoplasmic antibody (ANCA)-positive cutaneous leucocytoclastic vasculitis associated with antithyroid therapy in Graves' disease. Australas J Dermatol 1998;39(2):96–9.

55. Fujieda M, Nagata M, Akioka Y, Hattori M, Kawaguchi H, Ito K. Antineutrophil cytoplasmic antibody-positive crescentic glomerulonephritis associated with propylthiouracil therapy. Acta Paediatr Jpn 1998;40(3):286–9.

56. Pillinger M, Staud R. Wegener's granulomatosis in a patient receiving propylthiouracil for Graves' disease. Semin Arthritis Rheum 1998;28(2):124–9.

57. Bajaj S, Bell MJ, Shumak S, Briones-Urbina R. Antithyroid arthritis syndrome. J Rheumatol 1998;25(6):1235–9.

58. Gunton JE, Stiel J, Caterson RJ, McElduff A. Clinical case seminar: anti-thyroid drugs and antineutrophil cytoplasmic antibody positive vasculitis. A case report and review of the literature. J Clin Endocrinol Metab 1999;84(1):13–16.

59. Miller RM, Darben TA, Nedwich J, Savige J. Propylthiouracil-induced antineutrophil cytoplasmic antibodies in a patient with Graves' disease and a neutrophilic dermatosis. Br J Dermatol 1999;141(5):943–4.

60. Darben T, Savige J, Prentice R, Paspaliaris B, Chick J. Pyoderma gangrenosum with secondary pyarthrosis following propylthiouracil. Australas J Dermatol 1999;40(3):144–6.

61. Park KE, Chipps DR, Benson EM. Necrotizing vasculitis secondary to propylthiouracil presenting as purpura fulminans. Rheumatology (Oxford) 1999;38(8):790–2.

62. Wada N, Mukai M, Kohno M, Notoya A, Ito T, Yoshioka N. Prevalence of serum anti-myeloperoxidase antineutrophil cytoplasmic antibodies (MPO-ANCA) in patients with Graves' disease treated with propylthiouracil and thiamazole. Endocr J 2002;49(3):329–34.

63. Katayama K, Hata C, Kagawa K, Noda M, Nakamura K, Shimizu H, Fujimoto M. Diffuse alveolar hemorrhage associated with myeloperoxidase–antineutrophil cytoplasmic antibody induced by propylthiouracil therapy. Respiration 2002;69(5):473.

64. Winters MJ, Hurley RM, Lirenman DS. ANCA-positive glomerulonephritis and IgA nephropathy in a patient on propylthiouracil. Pediatr Nephrol 2002;17(4):257–60.

65. Akamizu T, Ozaki S, Hiratani H, Uesugi H, Sobajima J, Hataya Y, Kanamoto N, Saijo M, Hattori Y, Moriyama K, Ohmori K, Nakao K. Drug-induced neutropenia associated with anti-neutrophil cytoplasmic antibodies (ANCA): possible involvement of complement in granulocyte cytotoxicity. Clin Exp Immunol 2002;127(1):92–8.

66. Herlin T, Birkebaek NH, Wolthers OD, Heegaard NH, Wiik A. Anti-neutrophil cytoplasmic autoantibody (ANCA) profiles in propylthiouracil-induced lupus-like manifestations in monozygotic triplets with hyperthyroidism. Scand J Rheumatol 2002;31(1):46–9.

67. Fujieda M, Hattori M, Kurayama H, Koitabashi Y; Members and Coworkers of the Japanese Society for Pediatric Nephrology. Clinical features and outcomes in children with antineutrophil cytoplasmic autoantibody-positive glomerulonephritis associated with propylthiouracil treatment. J Am Soc Nephrol 2002;13(2):437–45.

68. Sera N, Ashizawa K, Ando T, Abe Y, Ide A, Usa T, Tominaga T, Ejima E, Yokoyama N, Eguchi K. Treatment with propylthiouracil is associated with appearance of anti-neutrophil cytoplasmic antibodies in some patients with Graves' disease. Thyroid 2000;10(7):595–9.

69. Seligman VA, Bolton PB, Sanchez IIC, Fye KII. Propylthiouracil-induced microscopic polyangiitis. J Clin Rheumatol 2001;7:170–4.

70. Colakovski H, Lorber DL. Propylthiouracil-induced perinuclear-staining antineutrophil cytoplasmic autoantibody-positive vasculitis in conjunction with pericarditis. Endocr Pract 2001;7(1):37–9.

71. Meister LH, Guerra IR, Carvalho GD. Images in thyroidology. Vasculitis secondary to treatment with propylthiouracil. Thyroid 2001;11(2):199–200.

72. Wing SS, Fantus IG. Adverse immunologic effects of antithyroid drugs. CMAJ 1987;136(2):121–7.

73. Dysseleer A, Buysschaert M, Fonck C, Van Ginder Deuren K, Jadoul M, Tennstedt D, Cosyns JP, Daumerie C. Acute interstitial nephritis and fatal Stevens–Johnson syndrome after propylthiouracil therapy. Thyroid 2000;10(8):713–16.

74. Khurshid I, Sher J. Disseminated intravascular coagulation and vasculitis during propylthiouracil therapy. Postgrad Med J 2000;76(893):185–6.

75. Hamburger JI. Diagnosis and management of Graves' disease in pregnancy. Thyroid 1992;2(3):219–24.

76. Martin-Denavit T, Edery P, Plauchu H, Attia-Sobol J, Raudrant D, Aurand JM, Thomas L. Ectodermal abnormalities associated with methimazole intrauterine exposure. Am J Med Genet 2000;94(4):338–40.

77. Clementi M, Di Gianantonio E, Pelo E, Mammi I, Basile RT, Tenconi R. Methimazole embryopathy: delineation of the phenotype. Am J Med Genet 1999;83(1):43–6.

78. Di Gianantonio E, Schaefer C, Mastroiacovo PP, Cournot MP, Benedicenti F, Reuvers M, Occupati B, Robert E, Bellemin B, Addis A, Arnon J, Clementi M. Adverse effects of prenatal methimazole exposure. Teratology 2001;64(5):262–6.

79. Bihan H, Vazquez MP, Krivitzky A, Cohen R. Aplasia cutis congenita and dysmorphic syndrome after antithyroid therapy during pregnancy. Endocrinologist 2002;12:87–91.

80. Barwell J, Fox GF, Round J, Berg J. Choanal atresia: the result of maternal thyrotoxicosis or fetal carbimazole? Am J Med Genet 2002;111(1):55–6.

81. Mandel SJ, Cooper DS. The use of antithyroid drugs in pregnancy and lactation. J Clin Endocrinol Metab 2001;86(6):2354–9.

82. Burrow GN. The management of thyrotoxicosis in pregnancy. N Engl J Med 1985;313(9):562–5.

83. Momotani N, Noh J, Oyanagi H, Ishikawa N, Ito K. Antithyroid drug therapy for Graves' disease during pregnancy. Optimal regimen for fetal thyroid status. N Engl J Med 1986;315(1):24–8.

84. Refetoff S, Ochi Y, Selenkow HA, Rosenfield RL. Neonatal hypothyroidism and goiter in one infant of each of two sets of twins due to maternal therapy with antithyroid drugs. J Pediatr 1974;85(2):240–4.

85. Low LC, Ratcliffe WA, Alexander WD. Intrauterine hypothyroidism due to antithyroid-drug therapy for thyrotoxicosis during pregnancy. Lancet 1978;2(8085):370–1.

86. Domenech E, Santisteban M, Moya M, Gonzalez C, Cortabarria C, Mendez A, Alvarez J, Rodriguez-Luis JC. Hipertiroidismo neonatal transitorio e hijo de madre hipertiroidea tratada. Posterior aparicion de precocidad sexual. [Transient neonatal hyperthyroidism in the child of a treated hyperthyroid mother. Subsequent appearance of sexual precocity.] An Esp Pediatr 1985;22(4):281–7.

87. Johansen K, Kampmann JP, Hansen JM, Andersen AN, Helweg J. Udskillelsen af antityreoide stoffer i modermaelk. [Excretion of antithyroid drugs in maternal milk.] Ugeskr Laeger 1982;144(22):1635–7.

88. Cooper DS, Bode HH, Nath B, Saxe V, Maloof F, Ridgway EC. Methimazole pharmacology in man: studies using a newly developed radioimmunoassay for methimazole. J Clin Endocrinol Metab 1984;58(3):473–9.

89. Hershey CO, McVeigh RC, Miller RP. Transient superior vena cava syndrome due to propylthiouracil therapy in intrathoracic goiter. Chest 1981;79(3):356–7.

90. Hashizume K, Ichikawa K, Sakurai A, Suzuki S, Takeda T, Kobayashi M, Miyamoto T, Arai M, Nagasawa T. Administration of thyroxine in treated Graves' disease. Effects on the level of antibodies to thyroid-stimulating hormone receptors and on the risk of recurrence of hyperthyroidism. N Engl J Med 1991;324(14):947–53.

91. Imseis RE, Vanmiddlesworth L, Massie JD, Bush AJ, Vanmiddlesworth NR. Pretreatment with propylthiouracil but not methimazole reduces the therapeutic efficacy of iodine-131 in hyperthyroidism. J Clin Endocrinol Metab 1998;83(2):685–7.

Thiopental sodium

See also General anesthetics

General Information

Thiopental sodium, a barbiturate and one of the oldest anesthetics, still remains the first-choice induction drug for cesarean section (1).

Organs and Systems

Cardiovascular

Cardiovascular depression is a well-documented complication of thiopental. However, the plasma concentrations necessary to produce loss of corneal reflex and trapezius muscle tone were only minimally depressant to the heart

(2). Problems can in any case be reduced or avoided by proper fluid administration before induction of anesthesia, as well as by cautious choice of dosage and administration in patients with uncompensated cardiac failure.

Surgery for cerebral artery aneurysms sometimes requires cardiopulmonary bypass and deep hypothermic circulatory arrest if they are to be operated on safely. During such bypass procedures patients with such aneurysms often receive large doses of thiopental, in the hope of providing additional cerebral protection. In 42 noncardiac patients thiopental loading to the point of suppressing electroencephalographic bursts caused only negligible cardiac impairment and did not impede withdrawal of cardiopulmonary bypass; however, there were no data on patients with cardiac disease (3).

Sensory systems

Patients sometimes notice a taste of onions or garlic before they lose consciousness; the incidence of this sensation was 42% in 113 adult patients (4).

Endocrine

Thiopental given for cerebral protection after cardiac arrest to patients in intensive care caused altered thyroid function (5). Five patients received 5 mg/kg as a bolus followed by 3 mg/kg/hour for 48–72 hours. Free T3 concentrations fell dramatically in three of them and remained near normal in the other two. In those in whom T3 concentrations fell they returned to near normal on withdrawal of thiopental. Reverse T3 concentrations increased in these patients. Although the study was not controlled, the authors speculated that thiopental causes conversion of T3 to reverse T3, and that this can intensify the sick euthyroid syndrome that can occur after cardiac arrest.

Electrolyte balance

Life-threatening hyperkalemia after therapeutic barbiturate coma with thiopental has been described in three patients; it was fatal in one (6). All the episodes occurred after the withdrawal of thiopental. Hypokalemia that is resistant to potassium replacement is common during thiopental coma and clinicians may choose to manage asymptomatic barbiturate-induced hypokalemia expectantly in an attempt to avoid rebound hyperkalemia.

Hematologic

- Immune hemolytic anemia with acute renal insufficiency has been reported in a 55-year-old patient after induction of anesthesia with thiopental 450 mg; a specific thiopental antibody was detected; the patient recovered fully (7).

Gastrointestinal

Vomiting is common during many types of anesthesia (8). By reducing upper esophageal sphincter pressure during induction, thiopental can contribute to this complication (9).

Skin

Fixed drug eruptions after thiopental administration have been reported (10).

Immunologic

Anaphylaxis has been repeatedly reported after thiopental (SED-10, 190) (SED-11, 211), but is rare, with an estimated incidence of one in 30 000.

- An extreme example reported in 1993 involved a 55-year-old obese man with no history of allergy to penicillin, who had on earlier occasions received sodium thiopental without reaction; on this occasion he stopped breathing and had severe bronchial constriction and vascular collapse requiring prolonged resuscitation and mechanical ventilation (11).

Second-Generation Effects

Fetotoxicity

A mother with eclampsia was unsuccessfully treated with diazepam, total dose 120 mg, and phenytoin 750 mg; she received thiopental and had an emergency cesarean section at 33 weeks gestation (12). The infant was unresponsive and floppy, requiring intubation and ventilation. At 10 hours after delivery a flumazenil infusion was begun; the baby responded with facial and limb movements within 30 seconds, resumed spontaneous ventilation, and was extubated 4 hours later. She was maintained on a slowly reducing flumazenil infusion over the next 4 days while the benzodiazepines were metabolized.

Susceptibility Factors

In one case, undetected congenital methemoglobinemia caused severe cyanosis during anesthesia with thiopental 500 mg and nitrous oxide 50% (13).

The use of thiopental or any other barbiturate is contraindicated in acute intermittent porphyria; a progressive neuropathy can occur and can be fatal.

Drug Administration

Drug administration route

Inadvertent injection into extravascular tissues causes pain, swelling, and possibly tissue necrosis. Pain on intravenous injection has been noted in 10% of patients (14). Intra-arterial injection causes vascular spasm and can cause gangrene of a distal extremity.

References

1. Celleno D, Capogna G, Emanuelli M, Varrassi G, Muratori F, Costantino P, Sebastiani M. Which induction drug for cesarean section? A comparison of thiopental sodium, propofol, and midazolam. J Clin Anesth 1993;5(4):284–8.
2. Becker KE Jr, Tonnesen AS. Cardiovascular effects of plasma levels of thiopental necessary for anesthesia. Anesthesiology 1978;49(3):197–200.
3. Stone JG, Young WL, Marans ZS, Khambatta HJ, Solomon RA, Smith CR, Ostapkovich N, Jamdar SC, Diaz J. Cardiac performance preserved despite thiopental loading. Anesthesiology 1993;79(1):36–41.

4. Nor NB, Fox MA, Metcalfe IR, Russell WJ. The taste of intravenous thiopentone. Anaesth Intensive Care 1996;24(4):483–5.

5. Kotake Y, Matsumoto M, Takeda J. Thiopental intensifies the euthyroid sick syndrome after cardiopulmonary resuscitation. J Anesth 2000;14(1):38–41.

6. Cairns CJ, Thomas B, Fletcher S, Parr MJ, Finfer SR. Life-threatening hyperkalaemia following therapeutic barbiturate coma. Intensive Care Med 2002;28(9):1357–60.

7. Habibi B, Basty R, Chodez S, Prunat A. Thiopental-related immune hemolytic anemia and renal failure. Specific involvement of red-cell antigen I. N Engl J Med 1985;312(6):353–5.

8. Vaughan GG, Grycko RJ, Montgomery MT. The prevention and treatment of aspiration of vomitus during pharmacosedation and general anesthesia. J Oral Maxillofac Surg 1992;50(8):874–9.

9. Vanner RG, Pryle BJ, O'Dwyer JP, Reynolds F. Upper oesophageal sphincter pressure and the intravenous induction of anaesthesia. Anaesthesia 1992;47(5):371–5.

10. Desmeules H. Nonpigmenting fixed drug eruption after anesthesia. Anesth Analg 1990;70(2):216–17.

11. Seymour DG. Anaphylactic reaction to thiopental. JAMA 1993;270:2503.

12. Dixon JC, Speidel BD, Dixon JJ. Neonatal flumazenil therapy reverses maternal diazepam. Acta Paediatr 1998;87(2):225–6.

13. Festimanni F, Orvieto A, Peduto VA. Metaemoglobinemia congenita come causi di cianosi durante l'anesthesia. Acta Anaesthesiol Ital 1980;31:601.

14. Kawar P, Dundee JW. Frequency of pain on injection and venous sequelae following the I.V. administration of certain anaesthetics and sedatives. Br J Anaesth 1982;54(9):935–9.

Thioridazine

See also Neuroleptic drugs

General Information

Thioridazine is a phenothiazine neuroleptic drug.

Organs and Systems

Cardiovascular

Cardiac dysrhythmias

Thioridazine has been associated with QT interval prolongation (1,2) and several cases of torsade de pointes have been reported (3,4).

Two types of T wave changes have also been described after treatment with thioridazine: type I (with rounded, flat, or notched T waves) and type II (with biphasic T waves) (5).

On July 7, 2000, doctors and pharmacists in the USA were notified about the addition of extensive new safety warnings, including a boxed warning to the professional product label for the neuroleptic drug thioridazine (Melleril, Novartis Pharmaceuticals). The text of the new boxed warning read: "Melleril (thioridazine) has been shown to prolong the QT_c interval in a dose-related manner, and drugs with this potential, including Melleril, have been associated with torsade de pointes-type arrhythmias and sudden death. Due to its potential for significant, possibly life-threatening, prodysrhythmic effects, Melleril should be reserved for use in the treatment of patients with schizophrenia who fail to show an acceptable response to adequate courses of treatment with other neuroleptic drugs, either because of insufficient effectiveness or the inability to achieve an effective dose due to intolerable adverse effects from those drugs."

The new labelling changes were based primarily on the FDA's review of three published studies. The first of these showed increased blood concentrations of thioridazine in patients with a genetic defect, resulting in the slow inactivation of debrisoquine (6). In this study, 19 healthy subjects (six poor and 13 extensive metabolizers of debrisoquine) took a single oral dose of thioridazine 25 mg. The poor metabolizers reached higher blood concentrations of thioridazine 2.4 times more quickly than the extensive metabolizers. There was a 4.5-fold increase in the systemic availability of the drug in the poor metabolizers, in whom thioridazine remained in the blood twice as long. The second study showed dose-related prolongation of the QT_c interval from 388 (range 370–406) to 411 (range 397–425) ms 4 hours after an oral dose of thioridazine 50 mg (7). The average maximal increase was 23 ms. This change was statistically greater than that for either placebo or thioridazine 10 mg. In the third study the effect of the selective serotonin re-uptake inhibitor (SSRI) fluvoxamine, 25 mg bd for 1 week, on thioridazine blood concentrations was evaluated in 10 hospitalized men with schizophrenia (8). The concentrations of thioridazine and its two active breakdown products, mesoridazine and sulforidazine, increased three-fold after the administration of fluvoxamine.

The possibility that some of the cardiac effects of thioridazine may be related to these metabolites as well as the parent compound has been explored (5,9) but needs further investigation.

Several regulatory measures (www.mca.gov.uk) (www.medsafe.govt.nz) (www.imb.ie) (www.hc-sc.gc.ca) (www.bpfk.org) (www.fda.gov) (www.who.int/medicines) have been adopted in different countries with regard to thioridazine.

The role of cardiac effects of neuroleptic drugs in sudden death is controversial (SEDA-18, 47) (SEDA-20, 26) (SEDA-20, 36). There may be multiple non-cardiac causes, including asphyxia, convulsions, or hyperpyrexia. However, some cases of sudden death in apparently young healthy individuals may be directly attributable to cardiac dysrhythmias after treatment with thioridazine or chlorpromazine (10), and from time to time, cases of sudden death are reported (SEDA-20, 36) (SEDA-22, 46), including four cases in which thioridazine in standard doses was implicated as the cause of death or as a contributing factor (11).

- A 68-year-old man with a 5-year history of Alzheimer's disease was treated with thioridazine 25 mg tds because of violent outbursts (12). His other drugs, temazepam 10–30 mg at night, carbamazepine 100 mg bd for neuropathic pain, and droperidol 5–10 mg as required, were unaltered. Five days later, he was found dead, having been in his usual condition 2 hours before. Post-mortem examination showed stenosis of the coronary arteries, but no coronary thrombosis, myocardial infarction, or other significant pathology. The certified cause of death was cardiac dysrhythmia due to ischemic heart disease. Thioridazine was considered as a possible contributing factor.

Hypotension

Hypotension is the most commonly observed cardiovascular adverse effect of neuroleptic drugs, particularly after administration of those that are also potent alpha-adrenoceptor antagonists, such as thioridazine. A central mechanism involving the vasomotor regulatory center may also contribute to the lowering of blood pressure.

Severe orthostatic hypotension has been observed in older volunteers ($n = 14$; aged 65–77 years) who participated in a randomized, double-blind, three-period, crossover study, in which they took single oral doses of thioridazine (25 mg), remoxipride (50 mg), or placebo (13). Compared with placebo, there were falls in supine and erect systolic and diastolic blood pressures after thioridazine, but not remoxipride. Standing systolic blood pressures fell by a maximum of 26 mmHg. There were similar falls in blood pressure in young volunteers.

Hypotension has been reported in two other elderly patients who were taking thioridazine (14). The patients, men aged 68 and 70 years, had traumatic brain injury and were taking oral thioridazine 25 mg/day for agitation. A few days later they developed mild hypotension (100/50 and 100/60 mmHg respectively).

Ear, nose, throat

Epistaxis has been reported in three patients with hypertension taking thioridazine (15).

Nervous system

In one study, there was no significant difference in serum concentrations of thioridazine, its metabolites, or radioreceptor activity between patients with and without tardive dyskinesia (16).

Sensory systems

Acute toxic effects of thioridazine on the eyes include nyctalopia, blurred vision, and dyschromatopsia, which typically become evident after 2–8 weeks of dosages over 800 mg/day.

Lens and corneal deposits

Deposits in the lens or cornea probably result from melanin-drug complex deposition and are best detected by slit-lamp examination. These deposits are probably dose- and time-related, since they generally occur only after years of treatment. Fortunately, they are in large part reversible, but if undetected they may progress to interfere with vision. They are most often reported with chlorpromazine or thioridazine and can occur in association with pigmentary changes in the skin.

Pigmentary retinopathy

Pigmentary retinopathy, which can seriously impair vision, is specifically associated with thioridazine, and has occurred more often with high and prolonged dosage

(for example 1200–1800 mg/day for weeks to months) (17), although in one case the daily dose was only 700 mg (18). Large-scale surveys have confirmed the relative safety of dosages up to 800 mg/day (19); at any dosage, however, any complaint of brownish discoloration of vision or impaired dark adaptation requires immediate evaluation.

- A 28-year-old woman with a long history of psychiatric problems was taking fluoxetine, diazepam, methylphenidate, and thioridazine 800 mg qds (17). Fluorescein angiography showed confluent areas of punctate hyperfluorescence, consistent with diffuse retinal pigment epithelial alteration secondary to acute thioridazine toxic effects.
- A 51-year-old woman with a long history of psychiatric problems and no family history of hereditary retinal degeneration had reduced vision in both eyes for several years while she was taking thioridazine 300 mg/day and chlorpromazine 600 mg/day (20). She had large patches of atrophy outside the arcades and within the macula, with sparing of foveal pigmentation; there were diffuse increases in hyperpigmentation in the peripheries of both eyes, and hypopigmented or unpigmented retinal epithelium.

The authors thought that the pigmentary changes were probably due to thioridazine, as adverse effects on the retina are rare with chlorpromazine.

Fluid balance

Water intoxication has been reported during treatment with thioridazine and may be due to its pronounced anticholinergic properties and/or direct stimulation of the hypothalamic thirst center (21).

Hematologic

The Committee on Safety of Medicines and the erstwhile Medicines Control Agency in the UK received 999 reports of hemopoietic disorders related to neuroleptic drugs between 1963 and 1996; there were 65 deaths (22). There were 182 reports of agranulocytosis; chlorpromazine and thioridazine were associated with the highest number of deaths—27 of 56 and nine of 24 respectively.

Sexual function

Thioridazine and other highly anticholinergic drugs can cause male sexual dysfunction, including impotence and retrograde ejaculation (23,24). A case of thioridazine-induced inhibition of female orgasm has also been reported (25).

Death

A retrospective case-control study conducted by the same group who first identified a relation effect of pimozide and thioridazine on the QT interval (SEDA-24, 55) has been published (26). The study was carried out in five large psychiatric hospitals in England and included all inpatients with sudden unexplained death over a period of 12 years (1984–1995) and two controls for each case from the same hospital matched for age, sex, and duration of inpatient stay, one of whom was also matched for primary psychiatric diagnosis. The patients were aged 18–74 years, and there were 69 cases and 132 controls (63 matched for diagnosis). Since the presence of an organic disorder was significantly associated with sudden unexpected death, this was adjusted for. Sudden death was associated with hypertension, ischemic heart disease, and thioridazine therapy (OR = 5.3; 95% CI = 1.7, 15). Among the limitations of this study was the incompleteness of the records, which often lacked information about important risk factors, including underlying cardiac disease, smoking, or the use of alcohol or illicit drugs; furthermore, the low rate of post-mortem examination raises the possibility that some of the deaths were from causes other than cardiac dysrhythmias, although other causes were found in only three of 30 cases when a post-mortem examination was done.

Long-Term Effects

Drug withdrawal

The consequences of restricting the indications for thioridazine in patients with learning disabilities have been a matter of reflection (27). Of 155 psychiatric patients, 18 were regularly taking thioridazine at the time of the directive; all stopped taking it and seven had moderate or severe difficulties during the following 3 months and one developed probable neuroleptic malignant syndrome 4 weeks after switching to an alternative drug. According to the authors, regulatory authorities should take account of the adverse consequences of drug changes when making judgements about the benefit-to-harm balance, especially in vulnerable patients, such as those with learning disabilities and psychiatric illnesses.

Other consequences of banning thioridazine have been reported in a rural general practice in Ireland, in which 29 of 40 GPs responded to a questionnaire and 17 reported management problems and adverse reactions (28). There was increased service demand, as 44% of the GPs described up to a 50% increase in referrals to the mental health service; although most of the GPs (67%) reported satisfaction with alternative agents, 37% described adverse effects associated with the alternative agents. It seems reasonable that directives should incorporate the flexibility required to accommodate the needs of patients who are already successfully stabilized on these drugs.

Susceptibility Factors

Genetic factors

The higher serum concentrations in poor CYP2D6 metabolizers are associated with an increased risk of thioridazine toxicity (11).

Age

Age increases the risk of thioridazine toxicity (11).

Sex

Female sex increases the risk of thioridazine toxicity (11).

Other features of the patient

Several factors increase the risk of thioridazine toxicity: pre-existing cardiac disease, hypokalemia, a glucose load, alcohol, exercise, and concomitant therapy with tricyclic antidepressants, erythromycin, co-trimoxazole, cisapride, risperidone, hydroxyzine, and drugs that inhibit CYP2D6 (some SSRIs, fluphenazine, and perphenazine) (11).

Drug–Drug Interactions

Beta-adrenoceptor antagonists

Lipophilic beta-adrenoceptor antagonists are metabolized to varying degrees by oxidation by liver microsomal cytochrome P450 (for example propranolol by CYP1A2 and CYP2D6 and metoprolol by CYP2D6). They can therefore reduce the clearance and increase the steady-state plasma concentrations of other drugs that undergo similar metabolism, potentiating their effects. Drugs that interact in this way include thioridazine (29).

The combination of propranolol or pindolol with thioridazine should be avoided if possible (30).

Diuretics

Diuretic-induced hypokalemia can potentiate thioridazine-induced cardiotoxicity (10).

Fluvoxamine

Fluvoxamine increased thioridazine concentrations threefold (8) in 10 patients with schizophrenia taking steady-state thioridazine who were given fluvoxamine (25 mg bd) for 1 week. Fluvoxamine interferes with the metabolism of thioridazine, probably via CYP2C19 and/or CYP1A2.

Lithium

Several cases of neurotoxicity in patients taking lithium and thioridazine have been reported. The cause of this interaction has not been resolved, but lithium seems compatible with all neuroleptic drugs, although patients should be carefully monitored (31–33).

Methylphenidate

Multiple involuntary movements, consisting of jaw grinding, oral dyskinesias, bilateral hand rolling, vermiform tongue movements, and bilateral choreiform movements of the digits, have been described in an 11-year-old boy taking thioridazine 150 mg/day and methylphenidate 10 mg bd (34). The methylphenidate was discontinued and within 4 weeks his movement disorder had completely disappeared.

Quinidine

Concurrent administration of quinidine with neuroleptic drugs, particularly thioridazine, can cause myocardial depression (10).

References

1. Warner JP, Barnes TR, Henry JA. Electrocardiographic changes in patients receiving neuroleptic medication. Acta Psychiatr Scand 1996;93(4):311–13.
2. Reilly JG, Ayis SA, Ferrier IN, Jones SJ, Thomas SH. QT_c-interval abnormalities and psychotropic drug therapy in psychiatric patients. Lancet 2000;355(9209):1048–52.
3. Kiriike N, Maeda Y, Nishiwaki S, Izumiya Y, Katahara S, Mui K, Kawakita Y, Nishikimi T, Takeuchi K, Takeda T. Iatrogenic torsade de pointes induced by thioridazine. Biol Psychiatry 1987;22(1):99–103.
4. Connolly MJ, Evemy KL, Snow MH. Torsade de pointes ventricular tachycardia in association with thioridazine therapy: report of two cases. New Trends Arrhythmias 1985;1:157.
5. Axelsson R, Aspenstrom G. Electrocardiographic changes and serum concentrations in thioridazine-treated patients. J Clin Psychiatry 1982;43(8):332–5.
6. von Bahr C, Movin G, Nordin C, Liden A, Hammarlund-Udenaes M, Hedberg A, Ring H, Sjoqvist F. Plasma levels of thioridazine and metabolites are influenced by the debrisoquin hydroxylation phenotype. Clin Pharmacol Ther 1991;49(3):234–40.
7. Hartigan-Go K, Bateman DN, Nyberg G, Martensson E, Thomas SH. Concentration-related pharmacodynamic effects of thioridazine and its metabolites in humans. Clin Pharmacol Ther 1996;60(5):543–53.
8. Carrillo JA, Ramos SI, Herraiz AG, Llerena A, Agundez JA, Berecz R, Duran M, Benitez J. Pharmacokinetic interaction of fluvoxamine and thioridazine in schizophrenic patients. J Clin Psychopharmacol 1999;19(6):494–9.
9. Dahl SG. Active metabolites of neuroleptic drugs: possible contribution to therapeutic and toxic effects. Ther Drug Monit 1982;4(1):33–40.
10. Risch SC, Groom GP, Janowsky DS. The effects of psychotropic drugs on the cardiovascular system. J Clin Psychiatry 1982;43(5 Pt 2):16–31.
11. Timell AM. Thioridazine: re-evaluating the risk/benefit equation. Ann Clin Psychiatry 2000;12(3):147–51.
12. Thomas SH, Cooper PN. Sudden death in a patient taking antipsychotic drugs. Postgrad Med J 1998;74(873):445–6.
13. Swift CG, Lee DR, Maskrey VL, Yisak W, Jackson SH, Tiplady B. Single dose pharmacodynamics of thioridazine and remoxipride in healthy younger and older volunteers. J Psychopharmacol 1999;13(2):159–65.
14. Rampello L, Raffaele R, Vecchio I, Pistone G, Brunetto MB, Malaguarnera M. Behavioural changes and hypotensive effects of thioridazine in two elderly patients with traumatic brain injury: post-traumatic syndrome and thioridazine. Gaz Med Ital Arch Sci Med 2000;159:121–3.
15. Idupuganti S. Epistaxis in hypertensive patients taking thioridazine. Am J Psychiatry 1982;139(8):1083–4.
16. Widerlov E, Haggstrom JE, Kilts CD, Andersson U, Breese GR, Mailman RB. Serum concentrations of thioridazine, its major metabolites and serum neuroleptic-like activities in schizophrenics with and without tardive dyskinesia. Acta Psychiatr Scand 1982;66(4):294–305.
17. Shah GK, Auerbach DB, Augsburger JJ, Savino PJ. Acute thioridazine retinopathy. Arch Ophthalmol 1998;116(6):826–7.
18. Meredith TA, Aaberg TM, Willerson WD. Progressive chorioretinopathy after receiving thioridazine. Arch Ophthalmol 1978;96(7):1172–6.
19. Simpson GM, Pi EH, Sramek JJ Jr. Adverse effects of antipsychotic agents. Drugs 1981;21(2):138–51.
20. Borodoker N, Del Priore LV, De A Carvalho C, Yannuzzi LA. Retinopathy as a result of long-term use of thioridazine. Arch Ophthalmol 2002;120(7):994–5.
21. Rao KJ, Miller M, Moses A. Water intoxication and thioridazine (Mellaril). Ann Intern Med 1975;82(1):61.
22. King DJ, Wager E. Haematological safety of antipsychotic drugs. J Psychopharmacol 1998;12(3):283–8.
23. Mitchell JE, Popkin MK. Antipsychotic drug therapy and sexual dysfunction in men. Am J Psychiatry 1982;139(5):633–7.
24. Siris SG, Siris ES, van Kammen DP, Docherty JP, Alexander PE, Bunney WE Jr. Effects of dopamine blockade on gonadotropins and testosterone in men. Am J Psychiatry 1980;137(2):211–14.
25. Shen WW, Park S. Thioridazine-induced inhibition of female orgasm. Psychiatr J Univ Ott 1982;7(4):249–51.
26. Reilly JG, Ayis SA, Ferrier IN, Jones SJ, Thomas SH. Thioridazine and sudden unexplained death in psychiatric in-patients. Br J Psychiatry 2002;180:515–22.
27. Davies SJ, Cooke LB, Moore AG, Potokar J. Discontinuation of thioridazine in patients with learning disabilities: balancing cardiovascular toxicity with adverse consequences of changing drugs. BMJ 2002;324(7352):1519–21.
28. Bailey P, Russell V. Restricting the use of thioridazine. Br J General Pract 2002;52(479):499–500.
29. Greendyke RM, Kanter DR. Plasma propranolol levels and their effect on plasma thioridazine and haloperidol concentrations. J Clin Psychopharmacol 1987;7(3):178–82.
30. Markowitz JS, Wells BG, Carson WH. Interactions between antipsychotic and antihypertensive drugs. Ann Pharmacother 1995;29(6):603–9.
31. Jefferson JW, Greist JH, Baudhuin M. Lithium: interactions with other drugs. J Clin Psychopharmacol 1981;1(3):124–34.
32. Waddington JL. Some pharmacological aspects relating to the issue of possible neurotoxic interactions during combined lithium-neuroleptic therapy. Hum Psychopharmacol 1990;5:293–7.
33. Batchelor DH, Lowe MR. Reported neurotoxicity with the lithium/haloperidol combination and other neuroleptics. A literature review. Hum Psychopharmacol 1990;5:275–80.
34. Connor DF. Stimulants and neuroleptic withdrawal dyskinesia. J Am Acad Child Adolesc Psychiatry 1998;37(3):247–8.

Thiurams

General Information

Thiurams are a group of chemicals that have been in commercial use since the 1920s. Their main uses are as accelerators and vulcanizing agents during rubber processing and as fungicides on seeds and plants.

Organs and Systems

Immunologic

Allergic contact dermatitis following exposure to thiuram compounds in rubber products, such as disposable rubber gloves, is well recognized (1).

- A 49-year-old man developed acute pruritic dermatitis of the hand, which settled quickly with oral glucocorticoids and antibiotics (2). Six months later he developed a similar eruption, which became more widespread, involving the trunk and limbs. He had no personal or family history of atopy, and had no known allergies or previous history of skin disease. He had a widespread dry eczematous eruption, most marked in exposed areas. The rash had developed soon after he had handled plants that had been sprayed with a fungicide. The safety data sheet for this product indicated that it contained 80% thiuram. Full blood count and serum electrolytes were normal, and autoantibodies and a porphyrin screen were negative. Biopsy of the lesion showed significantly sundamaged skin with a superficial perivascular chronic inflammatory infiltrate, confluent surface parakeratosis, and epidermal acanthosis with moderate spongiosis, consistent with a spongiotic dermatitis. He denied any previous contact with rubber gloves in both occupational and social settings, and had not had dermatitis before. He was treated with sun protection, topical and oral glucocorticoids, and a moisturizer. He had no further contact with the fungicide and the eruption resolved completely. He was advised to avoid all thiuram products, including rubber products and fungicides, in the future. Despite this, he subsequently developed one recurrence of hand dermatitis when he again used rubber gloves for protection at work.

Three Chinese national servicemen developed an itchy postauricular rash (3). None had a history of atopy and all three reported prior use of rubberized spectacle retainers as a curved pliable extension to the posterior ends of the earpieces of their spectacles, to stabilize them while undergoing rigorous military physical training. They were all patch-tested with the National Skin Center standard series and were positive to thiuram mix and the rubberized spectacle retainers. They were treated with topical corticosteroids and were advised to stop wearing their rubberized spectacle retainers.

References

1. von Hintzenstern J, Heese A, Koch HU, Peters KP, Hornstein OP. Frequency, spectrum and occupational relevance of type IV allergies to rubber chemicals. Contact Dermatitis 1991;24(4):244–52.
2. Saunders H, Watkins F. Allergic contact dermatitis due to thiuram exposure from a fungicide. Australas J Dermatol 2001;42(3):217–18.
3. Leow YH, Ng SK, Goh CL. An unusual cause of postauricular dermatitis. Contact Dermatitis 2000;42(5):308.

Thorotrast

General Information

Thorotrast (thorium dioxide), which has a radioactive half-life of about 400 years, was widely used in 1928–55 as an X-ray contrast medium.

By 1933 Thorotrast had been shown to induce malignancies in rats. It was prohibited in various countries from 1936 onwards, but continued to be used in some parts of the world for another three decades. Its late effects continue to be reported. Thorotrast deposits are predominantly localized in the liver and reticuloendothelial system; the major

late effects have been portal fibrosis, malignant liver tumors, and myeloproliferative disorders, but granulomatous, fibrotic, and malignant changes in many other organs have been described. Thorotrast is the most potent human leukemogen yet identified. The risk of a fatal blood dyscrasia after Thorotrast is very much greater than after external radiotherapy, and the latent period (20 years) is very much longer than after external irradiation (5–7 years).

In a 1993 follow-up study in Denmark of mortality among 999 patients who had received Thorotrast between 1935 and 1947 the excess mortality was explained in part by diseases known to be induced by Thorotrast, such as cirrhosis and cancer of the liver and leukemias and other hematological disorders; it was suggested that non-specific effects induced by the alpha particles emitted by Thorotrast may have contributed to this excess mortality (1).

Organs and Systems

Hematologic

The retention of Thorotrast in the bone marrow leads to the development of leukemia. Chromosome aberrations in bone marrow cells occurred at a high frequency in Japanese patients who had been given Thorotrast (2).

Liver

Various liver neoplasms due to chronic alpha-ray irradiation have been attributed to Thorotrast, most notably hepatocellular carcinoma, angiosarcoma, and cholangiocarcinoma. Multiple Thorotrast-induced primary tumors are rare but have been reported in a report from Japan (3).

- An 86-year-old man received intravenous Thorotrast to investigate a bullet wound to his shoulder in 1939. He presented in 1993 with jaundice, leading to liver failure and death. Autopsy showed four separate carcinomas: a cholangiocarcinoma in the left lobe of the liver, a well-differentiated tubular carcinoma of the antrum of the stomach, an invasive squamous carcinoma of the lung, and a well-differentiated adenocarcinoma of the ampulla of Vater. There were multiple mutations in the p53 tumor suppression gene caused by chronic alpha-ray irradiation.
- A 74-year-old developed nausea, night sweats, generalized fatigue, and weight loss (4). Thorotrast cerebral angiography had been performed 55 years before. Computed tomography of the abdomen showed areas of calcification within the liver, spleen, and peripancreatic lymph nodes, and there was a mass in the liver. Liver biopsy confirmed cholangiocarcinoma.

There has also been a report of nodular regenerative hyperplasia of the liver associated with previous Thorotrast administration (5).

Susceptibility Factors

Genetic factors

Several studies have shown that mutations of the TP53 gene (formerly known as p53) are important in the genesis of Thorotrast-induced tumors (6–8).

References

1. Andersson M, Juel K, Storm HH. Pattern of mortality among Danish Thorotrast patients. J Clin Epidemiol 1993;46(7):637–44.
2. Tanosaki S, Minamihisamatsu M, Ishihara T, Hachiya M, Kumatori T, Akashi M. Chromosome aberrations in bone marrow cells from Japanese patients with thorotrastosis. Radiat Res 1999;152(Suppl 6):S128–32.
3. Iwamoto KS, Mizuno T, Kurata A, Masuzawa M, Mori T, Seyama T. Multiple, unique, and common p53 mutations in a Thorotrast recipient with four primary cancers. Hum Pathol 1998;29(4):412–16.
4. Lipshutz GS, Brennan TV, Warren RS. Thorotrast-induced liver neoplasia: a collective review. J Am Coll Surg 2002;195(5):713–18.
5. Beer TW, Carr NJ, Buxton PJ. Thorotrast associated nodular regenerative hyperplasia of the liver. J Clin Pathol 1998;51(12):941–2.
6. Wada I, Horiuchi H, Mori M, Ishikawa Y, Fukumoto M, Mori T, Kato Y, Kitagawa T, Machinami R. High rate of small TP53 mutations and infrequent loss of heterozygosity in malignant liver tumors associated with Thorotrast: implications for alpha-particle carcinogenesis. Radiat Res 1999;152(Suppl 6):S125–7.
7. Kamikawa T, Amenomori M, Itoh T, Momoi H, Hiai H, Machinami R, Ishikawa Y, Mori T, Shimahara Y, Yamaoka Y, Fukumoto M. Analysis of genetic changes in intrahepatic cholangiocarcinoma induced by Thorotrast. Radiat Res 1999;152(Suppl 6):S118–24.
8. Iwamoto KS, Fujii S, Kurata A, Suzuki M, Hayashi T, Ohtsuki Y, Okada Y, Narita M, Takahashi M, Hosobe S, Doishita K, Manabe T, Hata S, Murakami I, Hata S, Itoyama S, Akatsuka S, Ohara N, Iwasaki K, Akabane H, Fujihara M, Seyama T, Mori T. p53 mutations in tumor and non-tumor tissues of Thorotrast recipients: a model for cellular selection during radiation carcinogenesis in the liver. Carcinogenesis 1999;20(7):1283–91.

Thrombolytic agents

General Information

The major thrombolytic agents are:

- streptokinase
- urokinase
- anistreplase (anisoylated plasminogen streptokinase activator complex or APSAC)
- pro-urokinase (single-chain urokinase-type plasminogen activator or scu-PA)
- alteplase (recombinant tissue plasminogen activator or rt-PA)
- reteplase (r-PA: a deletion mutant of rt-PA)
- tenecteplase (a triple combination mutant variant of alteplase).

Although their pharmacodynamic properties do not differ significantly, some characteristics, as a result of their origin or mode of action, explain specific differences in their adverse effects and pharmacokinetics.

General adverse effects

Hemorrhage is the major risk of thrombolytic drugs; there are some differences in risks between the various agents, and certain susceptibility factors can be identified. Transient hypotensive reactions have been described with all thrombolytic agents, but they are in principle reversible. Hypersensitivity reactions are most often seen in patients who have been treated with compounds derived from cultures of streptococci (streptokinase and anistreplase). Tumor-inducing effects have not been reported.

Organs and Systems

Cardiovascular

Transient hypotension can occur after thrombolysis, and the incidence after infusion of streptokinase in myocardial infarction is high. Hypotension has been related to plasminemia, which leads to bradykinin generation from kallikrein, activation of complement, and potentially endothelial prostacyclin release (1). During treatment of myocardial infarction, some other mechanisms may explain hypotension: vagal reflexes precipitated by posterior wall reperfusion (2) and left ventricular dysfunction associated with the infarct process. Hypotension occurs shortly after the start of infusion and can be accompanied by bradycardia, flushing, and anxiety. It is reversible if fluids are given and the infusion temporarily stopped (1); vasopressors may be needed. The magnitude of this hypotensive reaction is directly related to the rate of infusion of streptokinase. The incidence of such reactions does not seem to be affected by premedication with glucocorticoids. Like streptokinase, anistreplase can also cause transient hypotension (3). Alteplase seems to be associated with a lower risk of hypotension than streptokinase or anistreplase. In the ISIS-3 trial, the incidences of profound hypotension necessitating drug therapy were: 6.8% with streptokinase, 7.2% with anistreplase, and 4.3% with alteplase (4).

Embolic detachment of components of venous or mural thrombi can sometimes be involved in the development of thromboembolism or cholesterol embolization. There is a 10% incidence of pulmonary embolism during thrombolysis, lethal in 0–5% (5), pointing to the risk of detachment of white components of venous thrombi, especially if large veins, such as those in the pelvis, are involved (6). However, the risk has not been proven to exceed that reported in patients treated with heparin and/or oral anticoagulants.

Cholesterol embolization is thought to occur after removal of mural thrombi covering atherosclerotic plaques leading to direct exposure of the soft lipid-laden core of these plaques to the arterial circulation. The contents of the soft lipid core, including crystallized cholesterol, shower the downstream circulation. Cholesterol crystals are impervious to dissolution or lysis and they lodge in small arterioles, causing obstruction. Cholesterol embolization shortly after thrombolytic treatment is characterized by livedo reticularis or multiple necrotic lesions of the skin of both legs (7) but can also be associated with lower limb ischemia, gangrene, visceral ischemia, or pseudovasculitis (8). Cholesterol embolization is difficult to diagnose, and may therefore be more common than suspected. It can cause acute renal insufficiency (9), and renal biopsy shows acute tubular necrosis, in some instances with arteriolar clefts representing cholesterol crystals (10).

Reperfusion dysrhythmias can occur when thrombolytic drugs are used to treat myocardial infarction. The most common is transient ventricular tachycardia. However, controlled trials have failed to show an increase in serious ventricular dysrhythmias, the incidence of ventricular fibrillation being actually reduced by thrombolytic therapy in myocardial infarction (11).

- A coronary artery aneurysm occurred in a 49-year-old man 1 month after successful percutaneous transluminal coronary recanalization with streptokinase (12).

Phlebitis at the site of infusion of streptokinase has been reported.

Respiratory

Streptokinase can cause acute bronchospasm, sometimes fatal (13), or dyspnea.

Nervous system

Guillain–Barré syndrome has been reported in patients who were treated with streptokinase and anistreplase (14–18). As streptokinase and anistreplase are derived from streptococci, an immunological reaction is thought to have been responsible.

Sensory systems

Iritis and uveitis have been reported with streptokinase (19,20).

Hematologic

Hemorrhage is the major risk of the use of thrombolytic agents and can result from the lysis of thrombi at other sites where hemostasis is required. Hemostatic incompetence related to thrombolysis is also related to reductions in circulating fibrinogen and factors V and VIII and to the generation of fibrin and fibrinogen degradation products with anticoagulant properties. The most serious complication is intracranial hemorrhage, which has a high mortality (60% in the GUSTO-1 trial) and a high rate of severe disability (up to one-third of patients) (21).

In trials of intravenous streptokinase without angiography, hemorrhagic complications, apart from local venepuncture sites, were reported in about 4% of patients, with an absolute excess over controls of about 3% (11). Major bleeding, defined by transfusion requirements, occurred in only 0.5% of patients, and cerebral hemorrhage was seen in only 0.1%. In the AIMS trial, all hemorrhagic complications during hospitalization were 14% with anistreplase and 4.1% with placebo (22). Transfusion was required in 0.8% in each group. The absolute excess of cerebral hemorrhage rates was 0.3% with anistreplase compared with placebo. In the ASSET trial, the absolute excess risks of minor and major hemorrhagic complications with alteplase were respectively 6 and 0.9%. The excess risk of hemorrhagic strokes was 0.2% (23).

Several large clinical trials have compared alteplase and anistreplase with streptokinase. No clear-cut differences in severe or life-threatening bleeding were observed in these studies.

However, in interpreting these results, the role of adjunctive antithrombotic therapy must also be taken into account, since it can increase the risk of hemorrhage (24). In most of the trials, heparin-treated patients had significantly more major bleeding, and in the ISIS-3 trial, the incidence of cerebral hemorrhage was significantly increased by heparin (4). In the TIMI II B trial (25) in patients with unstable angina, the addition of a low dose of alteplase (0.8 mg/kg) to aspirin and heparin was associated with a 2.4% incidence of major hemorrhagic events (versus 0.6% with placebo) and a 0.55% incidence of intracranial hemorrhage (no such event occurring with placebo).

A study in general practice has suggested that intracranial hemorrhage during thrombolytic therapy for myocardial infarction may be more frequent than in clinical trials (10). The authors analysed the data accumulated in a US large registry called NRMI 2 (1484 hospitals, 71 073 patients having received alteplase in the initial treatment of acute myocardial infarction). The overall incidence of intracranial hemorrhage was 0.95%. This is a higher incidence than has been reported in clinical trials, and may have been due to the stringent enrolment criteria.

The susceptibility factors for intracranial hemorrhage have also been examined (10). The main factors were:

- advanced age; compared with patients under 65, the odds ratio was 2.71 (CI = 2.18, 3.37) for individuals aged 65–74 years and as high as 4.34 (3.45, 5.45) for patients aged 75 years or more
- female sex
- black ethnicity
- a history of stroke
- hypertension (an increased risk in patients with a systolic blood pressure of 140 mmHg or more and/or a diastolic of 100 mmHg or more)
- the dose of alteplase.

Because of the significant correlation with age and a previous history of stroke, it is now widely considered that in patients over 75 years with a history of stroke other therapies, such as primary coronary angioplasty, must be considered. As reported in the GUSTO-1 trial, patients with very high systolic blood pressures have an increased risk of death or disabling stroke (26), and the pulse pressure has been reported to be the clearest predictor of the blood pressure as regards the risk of intracranial hemorrhage (27).

The risk of major bleeding during thrombolytic therapy is undoubtedly a real problem, but it has to be considered against the background of the underlying mortality risk and the absolute benefit likely to be achieved in patients with acute myocardial infarction (28). This equation is fundamental in older patients, who have the highest mortality risk after myocardial infarction and thus the most to gain from thrombolysis (29).

Some reports of serious adverse consequences in patients with aortic dissection or pericarditis that mimic clinical or electrocardiographic myocardial infarction have emphasized the necessity for accurate diagnosis before thrombolysis is instituted in patients with chest pain or with atypical electrocardiographic changes (30).

The incidence of hemorrhagic complications is particularly high when high doses of streptokinase are used in the treatment of deep venous thrombosis (31). High-dose streptokinase thrombolysis for 2–3 days with an initial dose of 500 000 units followed by a maintenance dose of 3 600 000 U/day led to a 10% rate of major spontaneous bleeding complications, with a fatal outcome in four older subjects out of the total of 98 patients. The fatality rate of bleeding caused by streptokinase amounts to 7% in patients with peripheral arterial occlusion, but is much lower in younger patients with venous thromboembolism.

Secondary intraventricular hemorrhage has been described in two patients who received intraventricular tissue-type plasminogen activator to hasten the lysis of intraventricular hemorrhage (32).

Hemolysis after intravenous streptokinase is rare (33).

Transient lymphopenia, possibly related to immunological destruction of T-helper cells by streptokinase, has been described (34).

Platelet aggregation due to an antibody-mediated reaction has been suggested as a cause of streptokinase-enhanced coronary thrombosis in patients with a specific type of antistreptokinase antibodies (35).

Thrombocytopenia has been described after thrombolytic therapy but it is most probably multifactorial, since patients generally also received intravenous heparin (36).

Disseminated intravascular coagulation has been reported with urokinase (37).

Liver

There were no differences in the activities of serum transaminases, lactate dehydrogenase, or creatine kinase in patients with myocardial infarction who received an 18-hour infusion of urokinase compared with patients who received glucose alone (38), but subacute alterations of liver function tests have been described with streptokinase and anistreplase (39). Unexplained increases in transaminase activities have been reported in almost 25% of patients treated with streptokinase (40). In view of the greater prominence of liver dysfunction with streptokinase than with alteplase it could be wiser to choose alteplase rather than streptokinase in patients with previous impaired hepatic function (41).

A few cases of liver dysfunction with or without jaundice have been reported with streptokinase and urokinase (42–45). Jaundice with hepatic cytolysis can occur after allergic reactions to streptokinase (46).

Urinary tract

Hematuria and proteinuria can occur without alteration of immunohistochemical features, suggesting a non-immune cause, such as a direct effect on the glomeruli or a reflection of the hypocoagulable state.

- Acute interstitial nephritis associated with cholesterol embolization during streptokinase therapy has been reported (47). In this case, cholesterol clefts were found in the preglomerular and interlobular arterioles.

Cholesterol embolization can cause acute renal insufficiency (9), and renal biopsy shows acute tubular necrosis with, in some instances, arteriolar clefts representing cholesterol crystals (10).

Immunologic

Since streptokinase is a natural product of cultures of streptococci and therefore has similar antigenic properties, most of the population have anti-streptokinase antibodies. These antibodies may explain both the allergic reactions that can occur and resistance to the drug, which occurs in some cases. Within 3 or 4 days of streptokinase administration, the titer of neutralizing antibodies has become sufficient to inactivate the usual doses. Persistence of these antibodies is observed in up to 80% of patients 1 year after treatment and in about 50% of patients after 2–4 years (48,49). If streptokinase has to be re-administered within 8 months of previous exposure, the neutralizing effects of plasma should be taken into account and the dose of streptokinase should be adjusted to overcome these effects (50). However, the extent to which streptokinase antibodies decline after earlier exposure to streptokinase is controversial, and persistently raised titers are found in a large proportion of patients (51). For this reason, an alternative thrombolytic agent should be recommended in patients who have already received streptokinase. In addition, it appears that allergic reactions occur more often when streptokinase is reused (52).

Anistreplase, a compound consisting of streptokinase and anisoylated plasminogen, can also cause allergic reactions, but has a longer half-life, allowing intravenous administration in a relatively short interval of time.

Urokinase is extracted from human urine or prepared from cultures of fetal kidney cells and does not seem to cause allergic reactions.

Pro-urokinase, alteplase, reteplase, and tenecteplase, which are recombinant products, also appear to be free from allergic reactions. Pro-urokinase and alteplase have short half-lives (3–8 minutes) and require continuous infusion administration, which may in some cases be an advantage as it allows rapid surgical intervention when necessary (53). Reteplase and tenecteplase have substantially longer half-lives, allowing bolus administration.

The incidence of acute generalized allergic reactions in patients treated with streptokinase or anistreplase was originally reported to be high, but with the introduction of more highly purified forms of streptokinase the figure has fallen to 1–5%. The most common manifestations of non-anaphylactic reactions to streptokinase or anistreplase are skin rashes and pyrexia. However, anaphylactic shock with streptokinase is also well known, although rare; it occurred in 0.1% of the patients in the GISSI trial (54). Life-threatening angioedema has been described with streptokinase (55,56) and with alteplase (57–59). Skin rashes are seen especially with streptokinase, but rarely, if ever, with alteplase.

Several cases of low back pain associated with streptokinase or anistreplase injections for acute myocardial infarction have been described, with rapid resolution once the streptokinase was stopped (60,61). It is presumed that the mechanism is allergic, since no such report has been published with alteplase (62).

Streptokinase is regularly reported to have induced an immune complex syndrome, characterized by plasmacytosis, often severe, and accompanied by fever and the development of hemolytic anemia, occurring as early as the first week after the start of treatment; in some cases, temporary alterations in renal function also occur (63).

Vasculitis has been rarely described after streptokinase or anistreplase (64–67), but not after urokinase or alteplase. It is characterized by lymphocyte infiltration and deposition of immune complexes, fibrin, and complement in the skin microvasculature.

Other patients have the typical picture of serum sickness, sometimes associated with acute renal insufficiency (68–70) or of Henoch–Schönlein purpura (71) with a purpuric rash, joint and abdominal pains, and sometimes hematuria (72).

Adult respiratory distress syndromes and multisystem organ failure have been reported with streptokinase and anistreplase (73–76); the timing of the onset of symptoms and the antibody profile in one case suggested an immunological response (74).

The clinical efficacy of thrombolytic drugs such as streptokinase does not appear to be compromised by the occurrence of allergic reactions, according to data from GUSTO-1 (77).

There have been three reports of anaphylactoid reactions, mostly orolingual angioedema, after therapy of acute ischemic stroke with alteplase.

- In one patient there was marked edema of the lip about 45 minutes after a bolus dose of alteplase; it subsided within 2 hours without any intervention (78).

Of 105 consecutive patients treated with alteplase for acute ischemic stroke, 2 developed anaphylactoid reactions (79). The first had a rash and extensive bilateral swelling of the tongue, epiglottis, and uvula, requiring intubation. The second developed unilateral swelling of the tongue and lips without a rash or hypotension.

In 230 patients treated with alteplase for acute ischemic stroke, there were two cases of orolingual angioedema (80). Both presented with localized symptoms only, symmetrical in one and asymmetrical in the other.

IgE-associated anaphylactic reactions can also occur.

- A 70-year-old woman was treated with intravenous alteplase for thrombolysis in acute ischemic stroke and 30 minutes later had acute sinus tachycardia and hypotension, followed by cyanosis and loss of consciousness (81). Serum samples analysed by ELISA were positive for IgE antibodies to alteplase.

Such reactions are very rare; there have been four reported cases in over 1 million administrations.

Body temperature

Pyrexia can occur after the initial dose of streptokinase (82). Concurrent administration of glucocorticoids does not prevent it completely. A marked rise in body temperature with chills can be accompanied by hypotension, abdominal pain (particularly low back pain), and very occasionally mild psychotic reactions.

Second-Generation Effects

Pregnancy

Pregnancy is not considered to be incompatible with treatment with thrombolytic agents. No adverse effects on the fetus have been reported. Nevertheless, the possibility cannot be excluded that placental separation and uterine bleeding will occur. Only minimal amounts of streptokinase cross the placenta, and these are not sufficient to cause fibrinolysis in the fetus (83). Although the passage of streptokinase is blocked by the placenta, streptokinase antibodies do cross to the fetus (84). This passive sensitization would have clinical importance only if the neonate required streptokinase therapy. Septicemia during treatment with streptokinase has been also described (85). These different hazards may preclude the use of thrombolytic drugs during pregnancy but in acute life-threatening problems, efficacy has to be weighed up against the risk of adverse effects.

Drug Administration

Drug administration route

Pleural space infection is an important cause of sepsis, and traditional treatment comprises drainage of the pleural space, either through chest tubes or surgically, combined with antibiotics. Attempts at closed drainage with a chest tube often fail, owing to the development of loculations within the fluid and the high viscosity of the infected fluid. This problem has led to the use of intrapleural fibrinolytic drugs to improve drainage, hasten resolution of infection, and reduce the need for surgical intervention. At first, the use of intrapleural streptokinase and streptodornase was complicated by frequent allergic reactions, but with the availability of purified forms of streptokinase and urokinase these agents have been widely used for intrapleural fibrinolysis and this has been reviewed.

Streptokinase

Several reports, predominantly in the form of case series, have described the use of intrapleural streptokinase for complicated pleural effusions (86–92). The dose of streptokinase used varies, but is usually around 250 000 IU instilled once or twice daily, with tube clamping for 2–4 hours, repeated over several days. Local adverse effects are rare, but transient chest pain at the time of instillation occurs occasionally (93).

There are occasional reports of fever attributed to the intrapleural instillation of streptokinase (86,88), but the most important adverse event due to intrapleural streptokinase is systemic fibrinolysis. In many of the case series cited above, simple tests of clotting activity were performed before and after treatment and there were no significant changes. However, in 1984, a case report described major hemorrhage in one patient after the intrapleural use of streptokinase 500 000 IU, with tube clamping for 6 hours (94). Within 12 hours this patient developed a generalized coagulopathy, with features of disseminated intravascular coagulation. Following this report, in a carefully designed study, the systemic fibrinolytic effects of one dose (250 000 IU) and multiple doses of intrapleural streptokinase (250 000 IU bd for 3 days) were examined in healthy subjects (95). There were no physiological or statistical changes in any coagulation indices after intrapleural streptokinase. This suggests that the hemorrhage seen in the 1984 case report was probably not related to streptokinase, but was perhaps a complication of underlying sepsis.

Although intrapleural streptokinase does not cause systemic fibrinolytic effects, there can be local fibrinolytic effects. In a case series describing the use of intrapleural streptokinase or urokinase in 26 patients, one developed major "oozing" from rib fractures sustained 1 month before therapy (89). This local bleeding required two thoracotomies. It is not clear from the report if streptokinase or urokinase was used in this patient, but streptokinase was used in most of patients in this series. Furthermore, the dose used was also not clear, with streptokinase doses of 100 000–750 000 IU.

In 1998, major local hemorrhage after the use of intrapleural streptokinase was described in two patients (96). One patient had undergone mitral valve replacement 6 weeks before and collapsed after 2 days of standard intrapleural streptokinase, with hemorrhage into the chest. The second had undergone a mitral valve replacement 9 months before intrapleural streptokinase and collapsed with bleeding into the chest after 3 days. Both patients recovered, but the authors felt that recent cardiac surgery presented a contraindication to the use of intrapleural fibrinolytic drugs. It is not clear from this report if these two patients were taking oral anticoagulants, such as aspirin or warfarin, which may have confounded these findings. Another report of local hemorrhage has recently been published (97). The patient died after the instillation of intrapleural streptokinase for presumed empyema; autopsy showed an unsuspected abdominal aortic dissection with extension of blood clot into the thoracic cavity. These reports suggest that intrapleural streptokinase should be used with caution when there has been prior surgery or trauma involving the thorax.

Another potential adverse event associated with the use of intrapleural streptokinase is the development of antistreptokinase antibodies. These antibodies have been documented after intravenous streptokinase and can cause serious adverse events with re-exposure to streptokinase or can limit the efficacy of streptokinase in myocardial revascularization.

Urokinase

Urokinase has also been widely used intrapleurally for fibrinolysis, in doses of 40 000–250 000 IU and is as effective as streptokinase (98–101). Furthermore, urokinase is not antigenic and does not produce febrile reactions. As with streptokinase, transient chest pain at the time of instillation has occasionally been reported. These considerations have led some authors to prefer urokinase to streptokinase for intrapleural therapy, but urokinase is about twice as expensive and there is also more published experience with streptokinase.

Drug–Drug Interactions

Diltiazem

Clinical and experimental data suggested a possible increase of hemorrhage risk during thrombolytic therapy with alteplase in combination with diltiazem (102).

Heparin

The combination of thrombolytic agents with an anticoagulant and/or aspirin has been said to be life-threatening. An excess of major bleeding episodes with combined subcutaneous heparin and streptokinase or alteplase treatments (1.0% with heparin versus 0.5% without heparin) has been reported in the International Study Group Trial (103) in patients with suspected acute myocardial infarction.

Interference with Diagnostic Tests

Coagulation tests

Thrombolytic agents interfere with the measurement of plasma fibrinogen and other coagulation tests by promoting continuing fibrinolysis after the specimen is taken; thus, fibrinogen cannot be measured in a sample that is taken less than an hour after the administration of a thrombolytic agent.

References

1. Lew AS, Laramee P, Cercek B, Shah PK, Ganz W. The hypotensive effect of intravenous streptokinase in patients with acute myocardial infarction. Circulation 1985;72(6):1321–6.
2. Wei JY, Markis JE, Malagold M, Braunwald E. Cardiovascular reflexes stimulated by reperfusion of ischemic myocardium in acute myocardial infarction. Circulation 1983;67(4):796–801.
3. Been M, de Bono DP, Muir AL, Boulton FE, Fears R, Standring R, Ferres H. Clinical effects and kinetic properties of intravenous APSAC—anisoylated plasminogen-streptokinase activator complex (BRL 26921) in acute myocardial infarction. Int J Cardiol 1986;11(1):53–61.
4. ISIS-3 (Third International Study of Infarct Survival) Collaborative Group. ISIS-3: a randomised comparison of streptokinase vs tissue plasminogen activator vs anistreplase and of aspirin plus heparin vs aspirin alone among 41,299 cases of suspected acute myocardial infarction. Lancet 1992;339(8796):753–70.
5. Meissner AJ, Misiak A, Ziemski JM, Scharf R, Rudowski W, Huszcza S, Kucharski W, Wislawski S. Hazards of thrombolytic therapy in deep vein thrombosis. Br J Surg 1987;74(11):991–3.
6. Grimm W, Schwieder G, Wagner T. Todliche Lungenembolie bei Bein-Beckenvenenthrombose unter Lysetherapie. [Fatal pulmonary embolism in venous thrombosis of the leg and pelvis during lysis therapy.] Dtsch Med Wochenschr 1990;115(31–32):1183–7.
7. Queen M, Biem HJ, Moe GW, Sugar L. Development of cholesterol embolization syndrome after intravenous streptokinase for acute myocardial infarction. Am J Cardiol 1990;65(15):1042–3.
8. Blankenship JC. Cholesterol embolisation after thrombolytic therapy. Drug Saf 1996;14(2):78–84.
9. Gupta BK, Spinowitz BS, Charytan C, Wahl SJ. Cholesterol crystal embolization-associated renal failure after therapy with recombinant tissue-type plasminogen activator. Am J Kidney Dis 1993;21(6):659–62.
10. Gurwitz JH, Gore JM, Goldberg RJ, Barron HV, Breen T, Rundle AC, Sloan MA, French W, Rogers WJ. Risk for intracranial hemorrhage after tissue plasminogen activator treatment for acute myocardial infarction. Participants in

the National Registry of Myocardial Infarction 2. Ann Intern Med 1998;129(8):597–604.

11. Cairns JA, Kennedy JW, Fuster V. Coronary thrombolysis. Chest 1998;114(5 Suppl):S634–57.

12. Chen MF, Liau CS, Lee YT. Coronary arterial aneurysm after percutaneous transluminal coronary recanalization with streptokinase. Int J Cardiol 1990;28(1):117–19.

13. Shaw CE, Easthope RN. Fatal bronchospasm following streptokinase. NZ Med J 1993;106(956):207.

14. Ancillo P, Duarte J, Cortina JJ, Sempere AP, Claveria LE. Guillain–Barré syndrome after acute myocardial infarction treated with anistreplase. Chest 1994;105(4):1301–2.

15. Cicale MJ. Guillain–Barré syndrome after streptokinase therapy. South Med J 1987;80(8):1068.

16. Eden KV. Possible association of Guillain–Barré syndrome with thrombolytic therapy. JAMA 1983;249(15):2020–1.

17. Leaf DA, MacDonald I, Kliks B, Wilson R, Jones SR. Streptokinase and the Guillain–Barré syndrome. Ann Intern Med 1984;100(4):617.

18. Taylor BV, Mastaglia FL, Stell R. Guillain–Barré syndrome complicating treatment with streptokinase. Med J Aust 1995;162(4):214–15.

19. Gray MY, Lazarus JH. Iritis after treatment with streptokinase. BMJ 1994;309(6947):97.

20. Kinshuck D. Bilateral hypopyon and streptokinase. BMJ 1992;305(6865):1332.

21. Gore JM, Sloan M, Price TR, Randall AM, Bovill E, Collen D, Forman S, Knatterud GL, Sopko G, Terrin ML. Intracerebral hemorrhage, cerebral infarction, and subdural hematoma after acute myocardial infarction and thrombolytic therapy in the Thrombolysis in Myocardial Infarction Study. Thrombolysis in Myocardial Infarction, phase II, pilot and clinical trial. Circulation 1991;83(2):448–59.

22. AIMS Trial Study Group. Effect of intravenous APSAC on mortality after acute myocardial infarction: preliminary report of a placebo-controlled clinical trial. Lancet 1988;1(8585):545–9.

23. Wilcox RG, von der Lippe G, Olsson CG, Jensen G, Skene AM, Hampton JR. Trial of tissue plasminogen activator for mortality reduction in acute myocardial infarction. Anglo-Scandinavian Study of Early Thrombolysis (ASSET). Lancet 1988;2(8610):525–30.

24. Habib GB. Current status of thrombolysis in acute myocardial infarction. Part III. Optimalization of adjunctive therapy after thrombolytic therapy. Ches 1995;107(3):809–16.

25. Bovill EG, Tracy RP, Knatterud GL, Stone PH, Nasmith J, Gore JM, Thompson BW, Tofler GH, Kleiman NS, Cannon C, Braunwald E. Hemorrhagic events during therapy with recombinant tissue plasminogen activator, heparin, and aspirin for unstable angina (Thrombolysis in Myocardial Ischemia, phase IIIB trial). Am J Cardiol 1997;79(4):391–6.

26. Aylward PE, Wilcox RG, Horgan JH, White HD, Granger CB, Califf RM, Topol EJ. Relation of increased arterial blood pressure to mortality and stroke in the context of contemporary thrombolytic therapy for acute myocardial infarction. A randomized trial. GUSTO-I Investigators. Ann Intern Med 1996;125(11):891–900.

27. Selker HP, Beshansky JR, Schmid CH, Griffith JL, Longstreth WT Jr, O'Connor CM, Caplan LR, Massey EW, D'Agostino RB, Laks MM, et al. Presenting pulse pressure predicts thrombolytic therapy-related intracranial hemorrhage. Thrombolytic Predictive Instrument (TPI) Project results. Circulation 1994;90(4):1657–61.

28. Simoons ML, Maggioni AP, Knatterud G, Leimberger JD, de Jaegere P, van Domburg R, Boersma E, Franzosi MG, Califf R, Schroder R, et al. Individual risk assessment for intracranial haemorrhage during thrombolytic therapy. Lancet 1993;342(8886–8887):1523–8.

29. Woods KL, Ketley D. Utilisation of thrombolytic therapy in older patients with myocardial infarction. Drugs Aging 1998;13(6):435–41.

30. Blankenship JC, Almquist AK. Cardiovascular complications of thrombolytic therapy in patients with a mistaken diagnosis of acute myocardial infarction. J Am Coll Cardiol 1989;14(6):1579–82.

31. Conard J, Samama M, Milochevitch R, Horellou MH, Chabrun B, Prestat J. Complications hémorragiques au cours de 98 traitements par la stréptokinase. Place de la surveillance biologique. [Haemorrhagic complications using streptokinase during 98 treatments. Place of the biological surveillance.] Nouv Presse Méd 1979;8(16):1319–25.

32. Jenkins LA, Lau S, Crawford M, Keung YK. Delayed profound thrombocytopenia after c7E3 Fab (abciximab) therapy. Circulation 1998;97(12):1214–15.

33. Mathiesen O, Grunnet N. Haemolysis after intravenous streptokinase. Lancet 1989;1(8645):1016–17.

34. Blum A, Shohat B. CD-4 lymphopenia induced by streptokinase. Circulation 1995;91(6):1899.

35. Vaughan DE, Kirshenbaum JM, Loscalzo J. Streptokinase-induced, antibody-mediated platelet aggregation: a potential cause of clot propagation in vivo. J Am Coll Cardiol 1988;11(6):1343–8.

36. Harrington RA, Sane DC, Califf RM, Sigmon KN, Abbottsmith CW, Candela RJ, Lee KL, Topol EJ. Clinical importance of thrombocytopenia occurring in the hospital phase after administration of thrombolytic therapy for acute myocardial infarction. The Thrombolysis and Angioplasty in Myocardial Infarction Study Group. J Am Coll Cardiol 1994;23(4):891–8.

37. Oyama H, Iwakoshi T, Niwa M, Kida Y, Tanaka T, Kitamura R, Maezawa S, Kobayashi T. Coagulation and fibrinolysis study after local thrombolysis of a cerebral artery with urokinase. Neurol Med Chir (Tokyo) 1996;36(5):300–4.

38. A European Collaborative Study. Controlled trial of urokinase in myocardial infarction. Lancet 1975;2(7936):624–6.

39. Sallen MK, Efrusy ME, Kniaz JL, Wolfson PM. Streptokinase-induced hepatic dysfunction. Am J Gastroenterol 1983;78(8):523–4.

40. Maclennan AC, Ahmad N, Lawrence JR. Activities of aminotransferases after treatment with streptokinase for acute myocardial infarction. BMJ 1990;301(6747):321–2.

41. Freimark D, Leor R, Hod H, Elian D, Kaplinsky E, Rabinowitz B. Impaired hepatic function tests after thrombolysis for acute myocardial infarction. Am J Cardiol 1991;67(6):535–7.

42. Mager A, Birnbaum Y, Zlotikamien B, Strasberg B, Rechavia E, Sagie A, Sclarovsky S. Streptokinase-induced jaundice in patients with acute myocardial infarction. Am Heart J 1991;121(5):1543–4.

43. Phillips E, Woolfrey S, Cameron E. Streptokinase-induced jaundice. Postgrad Med J 1994;70(819):55.

44. Polkey MI, Oliver RM, Walker JM. Hepatic dysfunction induced by streptokinase. Am J Gastroenterol 1992;87(8):1062.

45. Pavlou H, Panagiotopoulos A, Graham A, Alexopoulos D. Urokinase-induced cyto-hepatolysis in a patient with acute myocardial infarction. Eur Heart J 1995;16(2):291–2.

46. Gilutz H, Cohn G, Battler A. Jaundice induced by streptokinase. Angiology 1996;47(3):281–4.

47. Adorati M, Pizzolitto S, Franzon R, Vallone C, Artero M, Moro A. Cholesterol embolism and acute interstitial nephritis: two adverse effects of streptokinase thrombolytic therapy in the same patient. Nephrol Dial Transplant 1998;13(5):1262–4.

48. Elliot JM, Cross DB, Cederholm-Williams S, et al. Streptokinase titers 1 to 4 years after intravenous streptokinase. Circulation 1991;84(Suppl 2):116.

49. Massel D, Turpie AGG, Oberhardt BJ, et al. Estimation of resistance to streptokinase: a preliminary report of a rapid bedside test. Can J Cardiol 1993;9:E134.

50. Jalihal S, Morris GK. Antistreptokinase titres after intravenous streptokinase. Lancet 1990;335(8683):184–5.

51. Cross DB. Should streptokinase be readministered? Insights from recent studies of antistreptokinase antibodies. Med J Aust 1994;161(2):100–1.

52. Cross DB, White HD. Allergic reactions to streptokinase: does antibody formation prevent reuse in a second myocardial infarction? Clin Immunother 1994;2:415.

53. Jolliet P, Magnin C, Unger PF. Pulmonary embolectomy after intravenous thrombolysis with alteplase. Lancet 1990;335(8684):290–1.

54. Gruppo Italiano per lo Studio della Streptocochinasi nell'Infarto miocardico (GSSI). Effectiveness of intravenous thrombolytic treatment in acute myocardial infarction. Lancet 1987;1:397.

55. Cooper JP, Quarry DP, Beale DJ, Chappell AG. Life-threatening, localized angio-oedema associated with streptokinase. Postgrad Med J 1994;70(826):592–3.

56. Stephens MB, Pepper PV. Streptokinase therapy. Recognizing and treating allergic reactions. Postgrad Med 1998;103(3):89–90.

57. Francis CW, Brenner B, Leddy JP, Marder VJ. Angioedema during therapy with recombinant tissue plasminogen activator. Br J Haematol 1991;77(4):562–3.

58. Purvis JA, Booth NA, Wilson CM, Adgey AA, McCluskey DR. Anaphylactoid reaction after injection of alteplase. Lancet 1993;341(8850):966–7.

59. Pancioli A, Brott T, Donaldson V, Miller R. Asymmetric angioneurotic edema associated with thrombolysis for acute stroke. Ann Emerg Med 1997;30(2):227–9.

60. Dickinson RJ, Rosser A. Low back pain associated with streptokinase. BMJ 1991;302(6768):111–12.

61. Hannaford P, Kay CR. Back pain and thrombolysis. BMJ 1992;304(6831):915.

62. Lear J, Rajapakse R, Pohl J. Low back pain associated with streptokinase. Lancet 1992;340(8823):851.

63. Chan NS, White H, Maslowski A, Cleland J. Plasmacytosis and renal failure after readministration of streptokinase for threatened myocardial reinfarction. BMJ 1988;297(6650):717–18.

64. Bucknall C, Darley C, Flax J, Vincent R, Chamberlain D. Vasculitis complicating treatment with intravenous anisoylated plasminogen streptokinase activator complex in acute myocardial infarction. Br Heart J 1988;59(1):9–11.

65. Gemmill JD, Sandler M, Hillis WS, Tillman J, Wakeel R. Vasculitis complicating treatment with intravenous anisoylated plasminogen streptokinase activator complex in acute myocardial infarction. Br Heart J 1988;60(4):361.

66. Ong AC, Handler CE, Walker JM. Hypersensitivity vasculitis complicating intravenous streptokinase therapy in acute myocardial infarction. Int J Cardiol 1988;21(1):71–3.

67. Sorber WA, Herbst V. Lymphocytic angiitis following streptokinase therapy. Cutis 1988;42(1):57–8.

68. Albert F, Dubourg O, Steg G, Delorme G, Bourdarias JP. Maladie sérique après fibrinoyse par streptokinase intraveineuse au cours d'un infarctus du myocarde. [Serum sickness after fibrinolysis using intravenous streptokinase in myocardial infarction.] Arch Mal Coeur Vaiss 1988;81(8):1013–15.

69. Davies KA, Mathieson P, Winearls CG, Rees AJ, Walport MJ. Serum sickness and acute renal failure after streptokinase therapy for myocardial infarction. Clin Exp Immunol 1990;80(1):83–8.

70. Noel J, Rosenbaum LH, Gangadharan V, Stewart J, Galens G. Serum sickness-like illness and leukocytoclastic vasculitis following intracoronary arterial streptokinase. Am Heart J 1987;113(2 Pt 1):395–7.

71. Verstraete M, Vermylen J, Donati MB. The effect of streptokinase infusion on chronic arterial occlusions and stenoses. Ann Intern Med 1971;74(3):377–82.

72. Argent N, Adam PC. Proteinuria and thrombolytic agents. Lancet 1990;335(8681):106–7.

73. Le SP, Chatterjee K, Wolfe CL. Adult respiratory distress syndrome following thrombolytic therapy with APSAC for acute myocardial infarction. Am Heart J 1992;123(5):1368–9.

74. Tio RA, Voorbij RH, Enthoven R. Adult respiratory distress syndrome after streptokinase. Am J Cardiol 1992;70(20):1632–3.

75. Montserrat I, Altimiras J, Dominguez M, Lamich R, Olle A, Fontcuberta J. Adverse reaction to streptokinase with multiple systemic manifestations. Pharm World Sci 1995;17(5):168–71.

76. Montgomery HE, McIntyre CW, Almond MK, Davies K, Pumphrey CW, Bennett D. Rhabdomyolysis and multiple system organ failure with streptokinase. BMJ 1995;311(7018):1472.

77. Tsang TS, Califf RM, Stebbins AL, Lee KL, Cho S, Ross AM, Armstrong PW. Incidence and impact on outcome of streptokinase allergy in the GUSTO-I trial. Global Utilization of Streptokinase and t-PA in Occluded Coronary Arteries. Am J Cardiol 1997;79(9):1232–5.

78. Papamitsakis NI, Kuyl J, Lutsep HL, Clark WM. Benign angioedema after thrombolysis for acute stroke. J Stroke Cerebrovasc Dis 2000;9:79–81.

79. Hill MD, Barber PA, Takahashi J, Demchuk AM, Feasby TE, Buchan AM. Anaphylactoid reactions and angioedema during alteplase treatment of acute ischemic stroke. CMAJ 2000;162(9):1281–4.

80. Rudolf J, Grond M, Schmulling S, Neveling M, Heiss W. Orolingual angioneurotic edema following therapy of acute ischemic stroke with alteplase. Neurology 2000;55(4):599–600.

81. Rudolf J, Grond M, Prince WS, Schmulling S, Heiss WD. Evidence of anaphylaxy after alteplase infusion. Stroke 1999;30(5):1142–3.

82. Marder VJ, Soulen RL, Atichartakarn V, Budzynski AZ, Parulekar S, Kim JR, Edward N, Zahavi J, Algazy KM. Quantitative venographic assessment of deep vein thrombosis in the evaluation of streptokinase and heparin therapy. J Lab Clin Med 1977;89(5):1018–29.

83. Pfeifer GW. Distribution and placental transfer of 131-I streptokinase. Australas Ann Med 1970;19(Suppl 1):17–18.

84. Ludwig H. Results of streptokinase therapy in deep venous thrombosis during pregnancy. Postgrad Med J 1973;49(Suppl 5).

85. Goring G. Kasuistischer Beitrag zur Streptokinase-behandlung in der Schwangerschaft. [Case report on streptokinase therapy during pregnancy.] Geburtshilfe Frauenheilkd 1971;31(4):348–53.

86. Robinson LA, Moulton AL, Fleming WH, Alonso A, Galbraith TA. Intrapleural fibrinolytic treatment of multiloculated thoracic empyemas. Ann Thorac Surg 1994;57(4):803–13; discussion 813–14.

87. Kennedy L, Rusch VW, Strange C, Ginsberg RJ, Sahn SA. Pleurodesis using talc slurry. Chest 1994;106(2):342–6.

88. Bouros D, Schiza S, Panagou P, Drositis J, Siafakas N. Role of streptokinase in the treatment of acute loculated parapneumonic pleural effusions and empyema. Thorax 1994;49(9):852–5.

89. Temes RT, Follis F, Kessler RM, Pett SB Jr, Wernly JA. Intrapleural fibrinolytics in management of empyema thoracis. Chest 1996;110(1):102–6.

90. Davies CW, Traill ZC, Gleeson FV, Davies RJ. Intrapleural streptokinase in the management of malignant multiloculated pleural effusions. Chest 1999;115(3):729–33.
91. Sasse SA. Parapneumonic effusions and empyema. Curr Opin Pulm Med 1996;2(4):320–6.
92. Sahn SA. Use of fibrinolytic agents in the management of complicated parapneumonic effusions and empyemas. Thorax 1998;53(Suppl 2):S65–72.
93. Taylor RF, Rubens MB, Pearson MC, Barnes NC. Intrapleural streptokinase in the management of empyema. Thorax 1994;49(9):856–9.
94. Godley PJ, Bell RC. Major hemorrhage following administration of intrapleural streptokinase. Chest 1984;86(3):486–7.
95. Davies CW, Lok S, Davies RJ. The systemic fibrinolytic activity of intrapleural streptokinase. Am J Respir Crit Care Med 1998;157(1):328–30.
96. Porter J, Banning AP. Intrapleural streptokinase. Thorax 1998;53(8):720.
97. Srivastava P, Godden DJ, Kerr KM, Legge JS. Fatal haemorrhage from aortic dissection following instillation of intrapleural streptokinase. Scott Med J 2000;45(3):86–7.
98. Moulton JS, Benkert RE, Weisiger KH, Chambers JA. Treatment of complicated pleural fluid collections with image-guided drainage and intracavitary urokinase. Chest 1995;108(5):1252–9
99. Bouros D, Schiza S, Tzanakis N, Drositis J, Siafakas N. Intrapleural urokinase in the treatment of complicated parapneumonic pleural effusions and empyema. Eur Respir J 1996;9(8):1656–9.
100. Bouros D, Schiza S, Patsourakis G, Chalkiadakis G, Panagou P, Siafakas NM. Intrapleural streptokinase versus urokinase in the treatment of complicated parapneumonic effusions: a prospective, double-blind study. Am J Respir Crit Care Med 1997;155(1):291–5.
101. Krishnan S, Amin N, Dozor AJ, Stringel G. Urokinase in the management of complicated parapneumonic effusions in children. Chest 1997;112(6):1579–83.
102. Becker RC, Caputo R, Ball S, Corrao JM, Baker S, Gore JM. Hemorrhagic potential of combined diltiazem and recombinant tissue-type plasminogen activator administration. Am Heart J 1993;126(1):11–14.
103. The International Study Group. In-hospital mortality and clinical course of 20,891 patients with suspected acute myocardial infarction randomised between alteplase and streptokinase with or without heparin. Lancet 1990;336(8707):71–5.

Thrombopoietin

General Information

Thrombopoietin is an endogenous colony-stimulating factor that increases the number of megakaryocyte colonies in bone marrow and also induces maturation of megakaryocytes [1]. Recombinant thrombopoietin is indicated for correction of thrombocytopenia, induced by chemotherapy or radiotherapy [1]. It has been tested in subcutaneous doses up to 5 micrograms/kg/day, resulting in increased numbers of platelets at 7 days, with a peak count at 17 days [1].

Organs and Systems

Hematologic

Thrombotic complications (deep venous thrombosis, pulmonary embolism, and superficial vein thrombosis) have been described in a few patients receiving thrombopoietin [2]. In none was thrombosis related to the platelet count, since none had more than 1000×10^9/l platelets. It could not be determined if the thrombosis was due to thrombopoietin or if an underlying malignancy predisposed these patients to thrombosis [2].

In in vitro studies thrombopoietin stimulates leukemic cell growth, but in clinical studies restimulation of leukemia has not been observed [2].

References

1. Ramsey G. Hematopoietic growth factors and transfusion medicine. Transfus Med Rev 1998;12(3):195–205.
2. Archimbaud E, Thomas X. Thrombopoietic factors potentially useful in the treatment of acute leukemia. Leuk Res 1998;22(12):1155–64.

Thyroid hormones

General Information

Nomenclature

In this monograph the following terms are used:

- thyroxine (T4): the endogenous hormone;
- triiodothyronine (T3): the endogenous hormone;
- levothyroxine (rINN) and dextrothyroxine (rINN): the stereoisomers of thyroxine, as used therapeutically;
- liothyronine (rINN): triiodothyronine, as used therapeutically.

Physiology

The normal adult thyroid gland secretes about 90 micrograms of thyroxine (T4) and less than 10 micrograms of liothyronine (triiodothyronine, T3) per day. Somewhat less than half of the T4 is converted to T3 by several tissues (especially the liver). Most of the daily production of T3 thus comes from peripheral 5′-deiodination of T4 and not by direct glandular secretion. The thyroid hormones are tightly bound (T4 even more than T3) to plasma transport proteins; this explains their prolonged half-lives (about 8 days for T4 and about 1 day for T3). Nuclear receptors for thyroid hormones bind T3 much more efficiently than T4, explaining the more rapid onset of action and greater biological potency of T3. The intestinal absorption and hepatic clearance of orally ingested thyroid hormones also differ. T3 has higher systematic availability than T4, only about 60% of which appears in the peripheral circulation after oral administration [1]. However, some formulations provide higher intestinal absorption of T4 (80%) [2]. These basic data form the background of optimal thyroid substitution.

Thyroid hormones are used either to replace the failing function of the thyroid gland (spontaneous or drug-induced) or to suppress the endocrine function of abnormal thyroid tissues (especially non-toxic struma or goiter or after thyroidectomy for thyroid neoplasms). Although there are abnormalities of the peripheral metabolism of thyroid hormones in some forms of undernutrition or overnutrition, thyroid drug therapy cannot be considered a safe way of treating obesity.

Treatment with thyroid hormones therefore poses only a few essential questions: which dosage should be used, which formulation should be chosen, and how can therapy best be monitored so as to avoid short-term and long-term risks.

Uses

Levothyroxine is used as replacement therapy in hypothyroidism and to suppress the production of thyrotrophin (thyroid-stimulating hormone) in patients with thyroid carcinoma.

Dextrothyroxine has been used as a lipid-lowering agent. It significantly lowers the serum cholesterol (3) as does levothyroxine; however, dextrothyroxine has a much smaller hormonal effect on body tissues than levothyroxine. The literature is confusing, since older formulations of dextrothyroxine contained considerable amounts of levothyroxine.

Liothyronine can be used for thyroid substitution, but it has the disadvantage of having a short-lived action and its intestinal absorption can give rise to unusually high post-absorption peaks, causing tachycardia. Moreover, the dosage necessary to obtain euthyroidism is more difficult to evaluate, owing to fluctuations in serum T3 concentrations; furthermore, in patients taking liothyronine, measurements of thyrotrophin are also probably less reliable, since its secretion by the pituitary gland depends more on the extracellular T4 concentration than on the T3 concentration. Therapeutic use of liothyronine is therefore generally only recommended when a more rapid onset of action is necessary, for example when thyroid therapy needs to be interrupted for the administration of ^{131}I in the treatment of thyroid cancer. In myxedematous coma it is controversial whether the therapeutic choice should be liothyronine, or levothyroxine, or a combination (4). Moreover, long-term therapy with liothyronine is more likely to cause secondary osteoporosis than T4.

The drug of choice for thyroid replacement therapy is therefore levothyroxine since it is the natural secretory product of the thyroid, has a long half-life, and is metabolized to T3 in the peripheral tissues.

Doses

The optimal dosage of levothyroxine should be based on repeated measurements of T3 and TSH serum concentrations. The daily recommended dose depends on the aim of the therapy. Thyroid replacement therapy for control of spontaneous or iatrogenic hypothyroidism should aim at a dosage of levothyroxine that maintains TSH concentrations within the low reference range. This will usually be associated with a free T4 concentration in the high reference range and a T3 concentration within the reference range. The mean requirement for such patients is

112 micrograms/day (2) or 1.57 micrograms/kg per day (5). This dose is lower than that recommended previously because of better knowledge of the real production rate of T4, the availability of better pharmaceutical formulations allowing better availability, and especially because of better methods for drug monitoring (SEDA-12, 353) (SEDA-15, 444) (6–8). Patients stabilized on one pharmaceutical formulation should not be switched to another without proper monitoring of thyroid hormones.

When thyroid therapy is used not only to replace deficiency but also to prevent the growth of remnants of a differentiated thyroid carcinoma, a suppressive dosage is used, aiming at T4 concentrations in the high reference range and an undetectable TSH concentration or at least one that is below the lower end of the reference range, as measured by two-sided assays. Such therapy is warranted because of its long-term safety, efficacy, and tolerance, but some additional therapy for osteoporosis prevention should be considered.

As with all forms of long-term therapy, adherence to the prescribed dosage of levothyroxine is not always optimal, and an unwarranted fear of thyroid-induced osteoporosis can add to this lack of adherence. Inadequacy of thyroxine replacement therapy is not always easily recognized. Several patients were reported with clearly inadequate or excessive consumption of levothyroxine despite a correct prescription. All patients had depression, which could be an additional susceptibility factor by promoting lack of adherence, and the resulting hypothyroidism or hyperthyroidism could further aggravate the depression (9).

When replacement therapy is with levothyroxine only, the T4/T3 ratio is increased compared with healthy subjects, suggesting that thyroid secretion of T3 is physiologically important. Animal studies have shown that euthyroidism is not restored in all tissues by levothyroxine alone (10). Mood and neuropsychological function improved in hypothyroid patients when 50 micrograms of thyroxine was replaced by 12.5 micrograms of liothyronine (11).

Several studies have failed to confirm the benefits of combined levothyroxine and liothyronine therapy. Liothyronine given once a day results in non-physiological peak serum concentrations of T3. Modified-release triiodothyronine plus thyroxine can normalize serum biochemistry, but it is not known whether this formulation is superior to levothyroxine alone (12).

In contrast to other protein-bound drugs for which a loading dose is given to achieve rapid steady-state concentrations, a slow and stepwise increase in thyroid hormone replacement therapy is advisable. This is preferred mainly to avoid sudden cardiac adverse effects, especially in older patients with long-standing myxedema. Moreover, since thyroid hormone substitution can change the metabolic clearance of this drug, steady-state concentrations are obtained only after several months (SEDA-6, 363).

General adverse effects

Ingestion of excessive amounts of thyroid hormones can cause symptoms and signs similar to those that result from endogenous overproduction. However, the symptoms and signs are generally relatively trivial in those who take standard doses of levothyroxine replacement therapy, although abnormalities have been evident in detailed studies of those who take levothyroxine in doses sufficient to suppress serum TSH (13). The adverse effects can therefore largely be avoided by adjusting the dosage according to the appropriately selected laboratory tests.

The adverse effects essentially comprise the symptoms of hyperthyroidism and include weight loss despite a normal or increased appetite, increased nervousness, tachycardia or dysrhythmias of various types, and increased general metabolism and its symptoms (hyperactivity, sweating, fever, etc.). Allergic reactions to pure thyroid formulations are rare and were first reported as late as 1986. Tumor-inducing effects have been investigated but not confirmed.

Organs and Systems

Cardiovascular

Overdosage of thyroid hormones causes tachycardia or palpitation but can also cause several types of dysrhythmia, for example atrial fibrillation. Evidence from the Framingham population that suppression of serum TSH is a susceptibility factor for atrial fibrillation has heightened concern that subclinical hyperthyroidism secondary to levothyroxine can also cause atrial fibrillation (14). Five women who reported frequent bouts of palpitation were investigated while taking levothyroxine and again after levothyroxine withdrawal (15). There was a clear increase in mean 24-hour heart rate during levothyroxine treatment, as well as an increase in atrial extra beats and the number of episodes of re-entrant atrioventricular nodal tachycardia. Four of these patients had evidence of abnormal conduction pathways, even when they were not taking levothyroxine, as evidenced by a short PR interval, but exacerbation of atrial dysrhythmias in these predisposed subjects is consistent with the view that thyroid hormones increase atrial excitability and may increase the risk of cardiac morbidity, especially if given in doses sufficient to suppress serum TSH.

Pre-existing cardiac disease, always to be suspected in elderly people or after long-standing hypothyroidism, can be severely aggravated by sudden thyroid substitution, resulting in severe angina pectoris, myocardial infarction, or sudden cardiac death (SEDA-13, 375). In such patients, the initial dosage should be low and the stepwise increase should be spaced out over a prolonged period and with careful clinical and cardiographic monitoring (16). In some circumstances, for example three-vessel disease, substitution should be postponed until after coronary bypass surgery (SEDA-6, 363). Cardiac decompensation can also result from the increased circulatory demand induced by thyroid hormone substitution or overtreatment. Long-term treatment with levothyroxine in doses that suppress thyrotrophin can have significant effects on cardiac function and structure, especially in patients with hyperthyroid symptoms (13,17), but large prospective studies are needed to assess cardiovascular risk in these patients.

In two cases of hypothyroidism myocardial infarction occurred at the start of thyroxine therapy in the absence of evidence of significant coronary artery disease (18).

- A 58-year-old man with a previous smoking history and a history of hypertension was severely biochemically hypothyroid (serum TSH 221 mU/l) and was given thyroxine, initially in a low dose (25 micrograms/day), increasing to 100 micrograms/day after 2 weeks. A month later he sustained a subendocardial myocardial infarction associated with only minor abnormalities on coronary angiography.
- A 61-year-old woman with severe hypothyroidism (serum TSH 115 mU/l) had an acute myocardial infarction (but no demonstrable abnormality on coronary angiography) 1 month after a thyroxine dosage increase from 50 to 100 micrograms/day.

Cautious introduction of thyroxine, especially in elderly people and those with severe or long-standing hypothyroidism, is prudent.

Myocardial infarction can also occur during long-term use of levothyroxine.

- A 71-year-old woman who had undergone total thyroidectomy with subsequent irradiation because of follicular carcinoma 3 years before (19). Since then, she had taken oral levothyroxine 0.15 mg and 0.2 mg on alternate days. When latent hypothyroidism became evident despite replacement therapy, the dose of levothyroxine was increased to 0.3 mg/day. Three weeks later, she had formed an acute posterior myocardial infarction, although she had no previous history of coronary artery disease. Subsequent coronary arteriograms revealed no evidence of disease of the major vessels. Myocardial scintigraphy 3 weeks after infarction still showed a persistent perfusion defect.

In the US Coronary Drug Project (20) a formulation of dextrothyroxine with a so-called low levothyroxine content was used. The study had to be terminated because of an excessive number of cardiac deaths and non-fatal infarcts.

Nervous system

Insomnia, psychic stimulation, general nervousness, and tremor are among the hyperthyroid symptoms that result from relative overdosage. Pseudotumor cerebri has incidentally been observed shortly after levothyroxine was given for juvenile hypothyroidism. The headache and bilateral papilledema without focal neurological defects subsequently disappeared even when levothyroxine was continued (21).

Psychological, psychiatric

Several cases of mania have been reported even after dosages of levothyroxine that are usually considered safe (22).

Musculoskeletal

A slipped capital femoral epiphysis has been described during the treatment of hypothyroidism (SEDA-3, 340). Since slipping occurs more often during the pubertal growth spurt, it is advisable to check for the occurrence of this complication during the pubertal period in children taking thyroid treatment.

Prolonged overtreatment with levothyroxine can result in osteopenia (23). Thyroid hormones have a direct effect on bone cells, thereby increasing both bone resorption and formation with subsequent mild adaptation of the systemic calciotrophic hormones (24). Increased bone turnover can result in a small deficit during each cycle and therefore finally result in mild osteoporosis. There are no good data regarding the incidence of fracture, but the bone mineral content of several areas known to be at risk of fracture (lumbar spine, forearm, femur) has been measured, mainly in cross-sectional studies, but also in a few prospective studies. During replacement therapy for hypothyroidism a small bone deficit was associated with a prior history of Graves' disease and/or later therapy with dosages of liothyronine or levothyroxine that suppress TSH concentrations (SEDA-16, 471). Since overt hyperthyroidism is associated with bone loss, it is possible that the reduction in bone density reported in some studies of levothyroxine treatment reflects an adverse effect of previous thyrotoxicosis rather than levothyroxine therapy itself (SEDA-17, 473).

In 50 women taking levothyroxine either for primary thyroid failure or for hypothyroidism secondary to radioiodine treatment for hyperthyroidism, there was no difference between the two groups in terms of bone density at the hip or spine and no difference from the reference population (25). In addition, there was no correlation between bone density and circulating thyroid hormone concentrations or duration of levothyroxine replacement. These findings are reassuring, although large studies of fracture risk are required, in view of previous evidence of an adverse effect of levothyroxine on bone mineral density, especially in post-menopausal women (26).

In a meta-analysis of cross-sectional studies suppressive levothyroxine was associated with mild but significant bone loss in postmenopausal women (SEDA-20, 394). The best measure of the effects of prolonged levothyroxine therapy can probably be obtained from bone mineral content in patients treated with suppressive doses of levothyroxine for thyroid carcinoma (Table 1).

Postmenopausal women with intact parathyroid glands on prolonged suppressive levothyroxine therapy may be more susceptible to osteoporosis and should have their bone mineral density measured and/or take preventive osteoporosis therapy. Cautious use of levothyroxine, avoiding overdosage and unnecessary use, is probably safe for bone.

Immunologic

Fever, liver dysfunction, and eosinophilia occurred during liothyronine or levothyroxine treatment of a hypothyroid patient and disappeared after withdrawal of therapy (31). In vitro lymphocyte testing confirmed sensitization for thyroid hormones.

Progressive re-institution of liothyronine subsequently proved possible in this patient without recurrence of hypersensitivity. Liothyronine was considered preferable because of the shorter biological half-life.

Long-Term Effects

Drug abuse

Abuse of thyroid hormones, causing factitious hyperthyroidism, can have adverse effects (32,33), including sudden death, attributed to ventricular fibrillation (34).

Partial empty sella syndrome (pituitary atrophy) has been described in an elite body builder who had abused various hormones, including testosterone, growth hormone, and triiodothyronine 25 micrograms qds for many years (35). He presented with infertility, and investigations showed suppression of serum TSH, a raised serum T3, and a partially empty pituitary sella.

It is likely that in this case long-standing suppression of pituitary function secondary to negative feedback from exogenous hormone ingestion (including liothyronine) resulted in pituitary atrophy.

Tumorigenicity

A possible link between breast cancer in women and thyroid hormone therapy was suggested on the basis of a retrospective study of patients with breast cancer (SEDA-3, 340). A subsequent statistical re-analysis of the original data failed, as did later studies, to confirm such a relation (SEDA-3, 340) (SEDA-4, 294) (36).

Second-Generation Effects

Pregnancy

The transplacental passage of maternal iodothyronines is quantitatively modest, although it might be sufficient to

---

Table 1 Summary of studies on the effects of thyroid hormones on bone mineralization

Reference	Number and sex (age in years)	Disease	Follow-up period (years)	Femur	Spine	Radius
(27)	7 F 1 M	Primary hypothyroidism; levothyroxine 125 micrograms/day	1	–	−9% per year	
(28)	6 F 4 M	Hypothyroidism (50 years); levothyroxine 135 micrograms/day	1	−7%	−5%	–
(29)	24 M (50)	Primary hypothyroidism (8 years) after [131]I	3	NS	NS	NS
(30)	18 F (60)	Hypothyroidism treated for 14 years	2			
		(a) low TSH (levothyroxine 170 micrograms/day)		−1.4% per year	−2.9% per year	−1.2% per year
		(b) normal TSH		−0.3% per year	−1.1% per year	−0.13% per year

ensure adequate fetal development. Maternal thyroid hormone secretion is markedly increased during pregnancy (by 25–50%); thyroid therapy should therefore be carefully adjusted during pregnancy (37).

Susceptibility Factors

Pre-existing cardiac disease and long-standing hypothyroidism carry serious risks.

Adrenal insufficiency can be associated with hypothyroidism (either by autoimmune destruction or due to hypophyseal disease) and carries the risk of acute Addisonian crisis if thyroid substitution precedes glucocorticoid therapy. The diagnostic problem presented by the fact that a few patients with central hypothyroidism have a moderately increased serum TSH should be kept in mind (38).

Some goitrous patients have autonomous thyroid hormone secretion, which is still within the reference range, but they become hyperthyroid even with relatively small amounts of exogenous thyroid hormones, since the latter accumulate with the endogenous autonomous thyroid secretion.

Rarely severe gastrointestinal disease can reduce the absorption of levothyroxine.

Since levothyroxine is occasionally used in supraphysiological doses to treat euthyroid people with refractory depression, adverse effects in healthy controls ($n = 13$) and patients with refractory depression also taking antidepressants ($n = 13$) have been studied in an 8-week, non-blind study (39). There was a higher rate of discontinuation of levothyroxine in the control subjects than in the patients, because of perceived adverse effects (38% versus 0%), together with a more marked rise in serum free T4 and free T3 in the controls. This suggests that the influence of supraphysiological doses of thyroxine is greater in healthy subjects than in those with psychiatric illness, perhaps reflecting the influence of the illness, or its therapy, on thyroid hormone metabolism in the latter.

Drug Administration

Drug overdose

Inadvertent excessive use of thyroid hormones (for example, by eating ground beef contaminated with thyroid hormones (40), the incorrect use of these drugs for the treatment of obesity (41), excessive thyroid substitution therapy, and factitious use of thyroid hormones for psychiatric reasons (42)) result in mild hyperthyroidism, but serious short-term adverse effects are rare.

Overdosage of levothyroxine causes increased metabolism resulting in increased heat production, with increased sweating and weight loss despite normal or even increased appetite. Accidental or suicidal injection of large amounts of thyroid hormones is exceptional (43). Clinical symptoms do not necessarily correlate well with plasma T4 concentrations and range from anxiety, confusion, or coma to tachycardia, atrial fibrillation, and angina. At least three lethal cases have been reported (SEDA-8, 371).

- A 34-year-old man took 900 tablets of veterinary levothyroxine, a total of 720 mg, and was given 60 g of activated charcoal (44). He became lethargic on days 2 and 3; on day 4 he had vomiting, sweating, and insomnia; on day 5 he became agitated and aggressive and stopped speaking intelligibly; and on day 6 he became combative and confused. He was sweating, mydriatic, hyper-reflexive, and tremulous, with clear lungs and active bowel sounds. He was given activated charcoal, haloperidol, diazepam, and phenobarbital, and had an endotracheal tube inserted. He was rehydrated and given propranolol and diazepam, but remained continuously tachycardic. On day 12 he became afebrile and his tachycardia resolved. Free T4 concentrations ranged from over 130 ng/l on day 6 to 12 ng/l on day 12. By discharge on day 15 he had lost 20 kg in weight, but was clinically euthyroid 2 weeks later.
- Self-induced thyrotoxicosis was associated with a marked rise in circulating free T4 and free T3 concentrations in a pregnant woman with an eating disorder who was abusing both levothyroxine and furosemide (45).

Treatment of thyroid overdosage is not standardized and can include gastric lavage, sedatives, beta-blockers, hydrocortisone, and specific antidysrhythmic drugs. Plasmapheresis (46) and exchange transfusion (47) have been used successfully to treat life-threatening cases. Iodine-containing organic radiographic agents (ipodate) can be effective, since they are potent inhibitors of the peripheral conversion of T4 to T3, but rebound effects can occur (43).

Drug–Drug Interactions

Antacids

Two patients with hypothyroidism taking a fixed dosage of levothyroxine took aluminium hydroxide and magnesium oxide (48). In both cases there was a marked increase in the serum concentration of TSH and low serum T4. After withdrawal of the antacids, TSH again fell. In vitro studies showed a dose-related adsorption of levothyroxine by a combination of aluminium hydroxide, magnesium hydroxide, and magnesium carbonate, but no effect of magnesium oxide alone.

Calcium carbonate

Calcium carbonate can reduce levothyroxine absorption (49).

- A 49-year-old woman, taking levothyroxine 150 micrograms/day and calcium carbonate (three tablets daily) for prevention of osteoporosis, developed symptoms of hypothyroidism and had a raised serum TSH concentration (22 mU/l). She was advised to continue taking the same dose of levothyroxine but to separate her medications. Repeat biochemical testing 8 months later showed a normal serum TSH (3.3 mU/l).
- A 61-year-old woman with hypothyroidism had celiac disease and a history of bowel resection for pancreatic cancer, was euthyroid taking thyroxine 175–188 micrograms/day (50). However, when she simultaneously took calcium carbonate (1250 mg/day) she had a raised serum thyrotropin (TSH) concentration of 41 mU/l. Delaying calcium carbonate ingestion by 4 hours returned her serum TSH concentration to high normal (5.7 mU/l) within a month.

Because of the possibility that calcium carbonate might impair levothyroxine absorption, another group carried out a prospective study in 20 patients taking stable long-term levothyroxine for hypothyroidism, who were given elemental calcium as calcium carbonate 1200 mg/day, taken with their levothyroxine for 3 months (51). Mean serum concentrations of free thyroxine and total thyroxine were significantly reduced during the calcium treatment period and rose after withdrawal. Mean concentrations of T3 did not change, but serum TSH rose during the calcium period, and 20% of the subjects had a serum TSH concentration above the reference range. The authors also reported the results of an in vitro study of thyroxine binding to calcium, which showed that there is adsorption of thyroxine to calcium at acidic pH. These findings show that calcium salts can have a modest put potentially clinically significant effect on levothyroxine treatment, probably by binding it and reducing its absorption; patients should be advised to separate their medications.

Colestyramine

Colestyramine can reduce thyroxine absorption (52).

Estrogens

Oral estrogens increase circulating concentrations of thyroxine-binding globulin, thereby increasing the bound fraction and reducing the free (bioactive) fraction of circulating thyroxine; this effect does not occur with transdermal estrogens (53). Thus, oral estrogens increase levothyroxine dosage requirements in women with primary hypothyroidism, at least during the first few months after the start of therapy.

Ferrous sulfate

Iron binds thyroxine in vitro (54) and ferrous sulfate can reduce thyroxine absorption (55). This can result in hypothyroidism (54,56). A similar interaction with ferrous fumarate has been described in a patient who took both medications simultaneously (57). Separation of thyroxine from iron may be prudent, since this interaction may reflect the formation of a non-absorbable complex in the gut (54).

Indinavir

Levothyroxine is metabolized in part through the action of glucuronyl transferase, which can be inhibited by some antiretroviral drugs, such as indinavir.

- Clinical and biochemical hyperthyroidism occurred in a 36-year-old woman, after previously stable levothyroxine replacement therapy, when antiretroviral drugs for HIV infection were introduced (58). She was reported to be taking a very large dose of levothyroxine (750 micrograms/day) after partial thyroidectomy for Graves' hyperthyroidism some 6 years before. One month after starting antiretroviral treatment she developed symptoms and signs suggestive of thyroid hormone excess and had markedly raised serum free T4 and free T3 concentrations, with suppression of TSH. The dose of levothyroxine was reduced progressively to 120 micrograms/day, and after about 2 months her thyroid function tests returned to normal.

While this pattern of biochemistry does not exclude transient relapse of Graves' hyperthyroidism (despite the finding of negative TSH receptor antibodies), or a transient thyroiditis, the authors speculated that indinavir (prescribed in this patient together with stavudine and lamivudine) had inhibited the glucuronidation of thyroxine and hence caused a rise in serum thyroid hormone concentrations.

Rifampicin

There was a modest rise in serum TSH concentration when rifampicin was given to a patient previously stabilized on thyroxine replacement (59). Rifampicin is believed to increase the metabolic clearance of both thyroxine and the inactive compound reverse triiodothyronine and in healthy volunteers it reduces circulating concentrations of total and free thyroxine, although in subjects without thyroid disease it has no effect on serum TSH (60).

Monitoring Therapy

Some diseases (liver disease, kidney disease, and malnutrition) interfere with the transport or metabolism of thyroid hormones and thereby alter thyroid function tests.

Several drugs (for example amiodarone, androgens, glucocorticoids, phenytoin, and salicylates) interfere with the transport or metabolism of thyroid hormones and thereby alter thyroid function tests. These have been reviewed (61). In patients taking levothyroxine serum TSH rises after treatment with sertraline (62) and antimalarial prophylaxis with chloroquine and proguanil (SEDA-22, 469).

References

1. Chopra IJ, Cody V. Triiodothyronines in health and disease. In: Gross F, editor. Monographs on Endocrinology. Berlin–Heidelberg–New York: Springer-Verlag, 1981;18:1.

2. Fish LH, Schwartz HL, Cavanaugh J, Steffes MW, Bantle JP, Oppenheimer JH. Replacement dose, metabolism, and bioavailability of levothyroxine in the treatment of hypothyroidism. Role of triiodothyronine in pituitary feedback in humans. N Engl J Med 1987;316(13):764–70.

3. Pristautz H, Leb G, Raber J, Goebel R, Steinberger R, Borkenstein J. Beeinflussung laborchemischer und nuklearmedizinischer Schilddrüsenparameter unter der Behandlung mit einem hochgereinigten D-Thyroxin-Präparat. [Influence of a highly purified D-thyroxine medication on thyroid iodine uptake and in vitro tests of thyroid function.] MMW Munch Med Wochenschr 1980;122(6):199–202.

4. Wartofsky L. Myxedema coma. In: Braverman LE, Utiger RD, editors. Werner and Ingbar's The Thyroid. 6th ed. Philadelphia: J.B. Lippincott, 1991:1089.

5. Carr D, McLeod DT, Parry G, Thornes HM. Fine adjustment of thyroxine replacement dosage: comparison of the thyrotrophin releasing hormone test using a sensitive thyrotrophin assay with measurement of free thyroid hormones and clinical assessment. Clin Endocrinol (Oxf) 1988;28(3):325–33.

6. Paul TL, Kerrigan J, Kelly AM, Braverman LE, Baran DT. Long-term L-thyroxine therapy is associated with decreased hip bone density in premenopausal women. JAMA 1988;259(21):3137–41.

7. Hiasa Y, Ishida T, Aihara T, Bando M, Nakai Y, Kataoka Y, Mori H. Acute myocardial infarction due to coronary spasm associated with L-thyroxine therapy. Clin Cardiol 1989;12(3):161–3.

8. Kologlu S, Baskal N, Kologlu LB, Laleli Y, Tuccar E. Hirsutism due to the treatment with L-thyroxine in patients with thyroid pathology. Endocrinologie 1988;26(3):179–85.

9. Exley A, O'Malley BP. Depression in primary hypothyroidism masquerading as inadequate or excessive L-thyroxine consumption. Q J Med 1989;72(269):867–70.

10. Escobar-Morreale HF, Obregon MJ, Escobar del Rey F, Morreale de Escobar G. Replacement therapy for hypothyroidism with thyroxine alone does not ensure euthyroidism in all tissues, as studied in thyroidectomized rats. J Clin Invest 1995;96(6):2828–38.

11. Bunevicius R, Kazanavicius G, Zalinkevicius R, Prange AJ Jr. Effects of thyroxine as compared with thyroxine plus triiodothyronine in patients with hypothyroidism. N Engl J Med 1999;340(6):424–9.

12. Hennemann G, Docter R, Visser TJ, Postema PT, Krenning EP. Thyroxine plus low-dose, slow-release triiodothyronine replacement in hypothyroidism: proof of principle. Thyroid 2004;14(4):271–5.

13. Biondi B, Fazio S, Cuocolo A, Sabatini D, Nicolai E, Lombardi G, Salvatore M, Sacca L. Impaired cardiac reserve and exercise capacity in patients receiving long-term thyrotropin suppressive therapy with levothyroxine. J Clin Endocrinol Metab 1996;81(12):4224–8.

14. Sawin CT, Geller A, Wolf PA, Belanger AJ, Baker E, Bacharach P, Wilson PW, Benjamin EJ, D'Agostino RB. Low serum thyrotropin concentrations as a risk factor for atrial fibrillation in older persons. N Engl J Med 1994;331(19):1249–52.

15. Biondi B, Fazio S, Coltorti F, Palmieri EA, Carella C, Lombardi G, Sacca L. Clinical case seminar. Reentrant atrioventricular nodal tachycardia induced by levothyroxine. J Clin Endocrinol Metab 1998;83(8):2643–5.

16. Toft AD, Boon NA. Thyroid disease and the heart. Heart 2000;84(4):455–60.

17. Ching GW, Franklyn JA, Stallard TJ, Daykin J, Sheppard MC, Gammage MD. Cardiac hypertrophy as a result of long-term thyroxine therapy and thyrotoxicosis. Heart 1996;75(4):363–8.

18. Kohno A, Hara Y. Severe myocardial ischemia following hormone replacement in two cases of hypothyroidism with normal coronary arteriogram. Endocr J 2001; 48(5):565–72.

19. Locker GJ, Kotzmann H, Frey B, Messina FC, Strez FR, Weissel M, Laggner AN. Factitious hyperthyroidism causing acute myocardial infarction. Thyroid 1995;5(6):465–7.

20. The Coronary Drug Project Research Group. The coronary drug project. Findings leading to further modifications of its protocol with respect to dextrothyroxine. JAMA 1972;220(7):996–1008.

21. Van Dop C, Conte FA, Koch TK, Clark SJ, Wilson-Davis SL, Grumbach MM. Pseudotumor cerebri associated with initiation of levothyroxine therapy for juvenile hypothyroidism. N Engl J Med 1983;308(18):1076–80.

22. Evans DL, Strawn SK, Haggerty JJ Jr, Garbutt JC, Burnett GB, Pedersen CA. Appearance of mania in drug-resistant bipolar depressed patients after treatment with L-triiodothyronine. J Clin Psychiatry 1986;47(10):521–2.

23. Medeiros-Neto GA. Osteopenia e tratamento com L-tiroxina. [Osteopenia and treatment with L-thyroxine.] Rev Assoc Med Bras 1995;41(1):34–6.

24. Auwerx J, Bouillon R. Mineral and bone metabolism in thyroid disease: a review. Q J Med 1986;60(232):737–52.

25. Hanna FW, Pettit RJ, Ammari F, Evans WD, Sandeman D, Lazarus JH. Effect of replacement doses of thyroxine on bone mineral density. Clin Endocrinol (Oxf) 1998;48(2):229–34.

26. Uzzan B, Campos J, Cucherat M, Nony P, Boissel JP, Perret GY. Effects on bone mass of long term treatment with thyroid hormones: a meta-analysis. J Clin Endocrinol Metab 1996;81(12):4278–89.

27. Krolner B, Jorgensen JV, Nielsen SP. Spinal bone mineral content in myxoedema and thyrotoxicosis. Effects of thyroid hormone(s) and antithyroid treatment. Clin Endocrinol (Oxf) 1983;18(5):439–46.

28. Ribot C, Tremollieres F, Pouilles JM, Louvet JP. Bone mineral density and thyroid hormone therapy. Clin Endocrinol (Oxf) 1990;33(2):143–53.

29. Toh SH, Brown PH. Bone mineral content in hypothyroid male patients with hormone replacement: a 3-year study. J Bone Miner Res 1990;5(5):463–7.

30. Stall GM, Harris S, Sokoll LJ, Dawson-Hughes B. Accelerated bone loss in hypothyroid patients overtreated with L-thyroxine. Ann Intern Med 1990;113(4):265–9.

31. Shibata H, Hayakawa H, Hirukawa M, Tadokoro K, Ogata E. Hypersensitivity caused by synthetic thyroid hormones in a hypothyroid patient with Hashimoto's thyroiditis. Arch Intern Med 1986;146(8):1624–5.

32. Keck FS, Loos U, Duntas L, Pfeiffer EF. Hyperthyreosis factitia acuta—Geringe klinische Symptome bei drei Fallen unter beta-Blocker-Behandlung. [Acute factitious hyperthyroidism—moderate clinical symptoms in 3 cases under beta-blocker treatment.] Klin Wochenschr 1986;64(7):319–26.

33. Galvan G. Hyperthyreosis factitia durch L-Thyroxinabusus: ein Fallbericht. [Factitious hyperthyroidism caused by L-thyroxin abuse. Case report.] Acta Med Austriaca 1983;10(2–3):79–81.

34. Bhasin S, Wallace W, Lawrence JB, Lesch M. Sudden death associated with thyroid hormone abuse. Am J Med 1981;71(5):887–90.

35. Dickerman RD, Jaikumar S. Secondary partial empty sella syndrome in an elite bodybuilder. Neurol Res 2001;23(4):336–8.

36. Gorman CA, Becker DV, Greenspan FS, Levy RP, Oppenheimer JH, Rivlin RS, Robbins J, Vanderlaan WP. Breast cancer and thyroid therapy. Statement by the American Thyroid Association. JAMA 1977;237(14):1459–60.

37. Glinoer D. Thyroid disease during pregnancy. In: Braverman LE, Utiger R, editors. Werner and Ingbar's The Thyroid. A Fundamental and Clinical Text. 8th ed. Philadelphia: J.B. Lippincott, 2000:1013–27.

38. Martino E, Bambini G, Bartalena L, Mammoli C, Aghini-Lombardi F, Baschieri L, Pinchera A. Human serum thyrotrophin measurement by ultrasensitive immunoradiometric assay as a first-line test in the evaluation of thyroid function. Clin Endocrinol (Oxf) 1986;24(2):141–8.

39. Bauer M, Baur H, Berghofer A, Strohle A, Hellweg R, Muller-Oerlinghausen B, Baumgartner A. Effects of supraphysiological thyroxine administration in healthy controls and patients with depressive disorders. J Affect Disord 2002;68(2–3):285–94.

40. Hedberg CW, Fishbein DB, Janssen RS, Meyers B, McMillen JM, MacDonald KL, White KE, Huss LJ, Hurwitz ES, Farhie JR, et al. An outbreak of thyrotoxicosis caused by the consumption of bovine thyroid gland in ground beef. N Engl J Med 1987;316(16):993–8.

41. Krotkiewski M. Thyroid hormones in the pathogenesis and treatment of obesity. Eur J Pharmacol 2002;440(2–3):85–98.

42. Fuessl HS. Verwirrende Schilddruse. Hyperthyreosis factitia. [The confusing thyroid gland. Factitious hyperthyroidism.] MMW Fortschr Med 1999;141(36):53–4.

43. Cohen JH 3rd, Ingbar SH, Braverman LE. Thyrotoxicosis due to ingestion of excess thyroid hormone. Endocr Rev 1989;10(2):113–24.

44. Hack JB, Leviss JA, Nelson LS, Hoffman RS. Severe symptoms following a massive intentional L-thyroxine ingestion. Vet Hum Toxicol 1999;41(5):323–6.

45. Wark H, Wallace EM, Wigg S, Tippett C. Thyroxine abuse: an unusual case of thyrotoxicosis in pregnancy. Aust NZ J Obstet Gynaecol 1998;38(2):221–3.

46. May ME, Mintz PD, Lowry P, Geller R, Curnow RT. Plasmapheresis in thyroxine overdose: a case report. J Toxicol Clin Toxicol 1983;20(5):517–20.

47. Gerard P, Malvaux P, De Visscher M. Accidental poisoning with thyroid extract treated by exchange transfusion. Arch Dis Child 1972;47(256):981–2.

48. Mersebach H, Rasmussen AK, Kirkegaard L, Feldt-Rasmussen U. Intestinal adsorption of levothyroxine by antacids and laxatives: case stories and in vitro experiments. Pharmacol Toxicol 1999;84(3):107–9.

49. Butner LE, Fulco PP, Feldman G. Calcium carbonate-induced hypothyroidism. Ann Intern Med 2000;132(7):595.

50. Csako G, McGriff NJ, Rotman-Pikielny P, Sarlis NJ, Pucino F. Exaggerated levothyroxine malabsorption due to calcium carbonate supplementation in gastrointestinal disorders. Ann Pharmacother 2001;35(12):1578–83.

51. Singh N, Singh PN, Hershman JM. Effect of calcium carbonate on the absorption of levothyroxine. JAMA 2000;283(21):2822–5.

52. Farmer JA, Gotto AM Jr. Antihyperlipidaemic agents. Drug interactions of clinical significance. Drug Saf 1994;11(5):301–9.

53. Mazer NA. Interaction of estrogen therapy and thyroid hormone replacement in postmenopausal women. Thyroid 2004;14(Suppl 1):S27–34.

54. Campbell NR, Hasinoff BB, Stalts H, Rao B, Wong NC. Ferrous sulfate reduces thyroxine efficacy in patients with hypothyroidism. Ann Intern Med 1992;117(12):1010–13.

55. Schlienger JL. Accroissement des besoins en thyroxine par le sulfate de fer. [Increased need for thyroxine induced by iron sulfate.] Presse Méd 1994;23(10):492.

56. Shakir KM, Chute JP, Aprill BS, Lazarus AA. Ferrous sulfate-induced increase in requirement for thyroxine in a patient with primary hypothyroidism. South Med J 1997;90(6):637–9.

57. Leger CS, Chye T. Ferrous fumarate-induced malabsorption of thyroxine. Endocrinologist 1999;9:493–5.

58. Lanzafame M, Trevenzoli M, Faggian F, Marcati P, Gatti F, Carolo G, Concia E. Interaction between levothyroxine and indinavir in a patient with HIV infection. Infection 2002;30(1):54–5.

59. Nolan SR, Self TH, Norwood JM. Interaction between rifampin and levothyroxine. South Med J 1999;92(5):529–31.

60. Ohnhaus EE, Studer H. A link between liver microsomal enzyme activity and thyroid hormone metabolism in man. Br J Clin Pharmacol 1983;15(1):71–6.

61. Davies PH, Franklyn JA. The effects of drugs on tests of thyroid function. Eur J Clin Pharmacol 1991;40(5):439–51.

62. McCowen KC, Garber JR, Spark R. Elevated serum thyrotropin in thyroxine-treated patients with hypothyroidism given sertraline. N Engl J Med 1997;337(14):1010–11.

Thyrotrophin and thyrotropin

General Information

Thyrotrophin is native thyroid-stimulating hormone. Recombinant human thyrotrophin is called thyrotropin.

Thyrotropin stimulates iodine uptake, and this facilitates the diagnosis and treatment of recurrent disease or metastases in the follow-up of differentiated thyroid cancer. It is used as an alternative to thyroid hormone withdrawal, to avoid symptomatic hypothyroidism (1). Headache and nausea occur in 6–40% of patients after intramuscular administration, but are usually mild and transient (2,3).

The adverse effects of thyrotropin have been reviewed (4).

Organs and Systems

Immunologic

Many years ago bovine thyrotrophin was used for diagnostic purposes and to increase ^{131}I uptake. However, for diagnostic purposes it has been replaced by sensitive TSH assays, and because of antibody development and hypersensitivity reactions it is not used therapeutically. There is no evidence that thyrotropin causes allergic reactions, even after multiple injections (4).

Rapid tumor expansion has been occasionally reported after thyrotropin, including four of 55 patients with central nervous system metastases enrolled in a compassionate use protocol (5). Two patients with locally recurrent papillary carcinoma had tumor growth 12–48 hours after their second injection of recombinant thyrotropin (rTSH); rapid improvement in neck pain, stridor, and dysphonia after glucocorticoids suggested an inflammatory etiology (5). There were no features to suggest an allergic reaction; only one such case has been reported and there are no reports of antibody formation even after repeated dosing (1).

References

1. McDougall IR, Weigel RJ. Recombinant human thyrotropin in the management of thyroid cancer. Curr Opin Oncol 2001;13(1):39–43.

2. Haugen BR, Pacini F, Reiners C, Schlumberger M, Ladenson PW, Sherman SI, Cooper DS, Graham KE, Braverman LE, Skarulis MC, Davies TF, DeGroot LJ, Mazzaferri EL, Daniels GH, Ross DS, Luster M, Samuels MH, Becker DV, Maxon HR 3rd, Cavalieri RR, Spencer CA, McEllin K, Weintraub BD, Ridgway EC. A comparison of recombinant human thyrotropin and thyroid hormone withdrawal for the detection of thyroid remnant or cancer. J Clin Endocrinol Metab 1999;84(11):3877–85.

3. Durski JM, Weigel RJ, McDougall IR. Recombinant human thyrotropin (rhTSH) in the management of differentiated thyroid cancer. Nucl Med Commun 2000;21(6):521–8.

4. Robbins RJ, Robbins AK. Clinical review 156: Recombinant human thyrotropin and thyroid cancer management. J Clin Endocrinol Metab 2003;88(5):1933–8.

5. Braga M, Ringel MD, Cooper DS. Sudden enlargement of local recurrent thyroid tumor after recombinant human TSH administration. J Clin Endocrinol Metab 2001;86(11):5148–51.

Tiabendazole

See also Benzimidazoles

General Information

Tiabendazole is a non-carbamate benzimidazole which inhibits cellular enzyme systems specific to some species of helminths. It is active against *Giardia lamblia*, but less effective than albendazole and mebendazole. It was at one time the drug of choice against *Strongyloides stercoralis*, both the enteric and tissue forms, but has been superseded by more modern drugs. It is also effective against *Enterobius*, hookworms, and *Trichuris trichiura*. Normally given orally, it is rapidly absorbed, with peak serum concentrations 1–2 hours after ingestion. It is rapidly metabolized and excreted; 40% of the drug and its metabolites are excreted during the first 4 hours and 80% during the first 24 hours. Its main metabolite, 5-hydroxythiabendazole, is inactive.

General adverse effects

Common toxic effects of tiabendazole include nausea, vomiting, and dizziness. Malaise and drowsiness are also common. Liver disorders can occur and are the most serious complications. Most systems can on occasion be affected. Allergic reactions are essentially due to parasite destruction rather than a direct effect of the drug itself. Chills, fever, lymphadenopathy, angioedema, and pruritic rashes all can occur; and treatment should in that case be stopped, since otherwise more serious reactions (for example Stevens–Johnson syndrome) can follow. Tumor-inducing effects have not been reported.

Organs and Systems

Cardiovascular

Bradycardia, hypotension, and syncope can occur with tiabendazole, even to the point of collapse (1).

Nervous system

Somnolence has been described with high doses of tiabendazole rectally or orally, and drowsiness, headache, malaise, and fatigue are common (1). Patients should be warned not to drive or carry out other potentially hazardous pursuits during treatment.

More severe symptoms of neurotoxicity are not unusual and include disorientation, confusional states, feelings of detachment, overt psychosis (2), and possibly epileptiform convulsions (3), although the latter have been observed only in a case of Down syndrome.

Sensory systems

Effects of tiabendazole on vision are not uncommon: abnormal sensations in the eyes, xanthopsia (a yellow tinge to objects), blurred vision, drying of mucous membranes, and sicca syndrome all have been described (4).

Allergic reactions to tiabendazole can cause keratoconjunctivitis sicca as part of Sjögren's syndrome (5).

Tinnitus has been attributed to tiabendazole (6).

Metabolism

Instances of both hypoglycemia and hyperglycemia have been recorded in patients taking tiabendazole.

Hematologic

Marked peripheral eosinophilia has also been described after rectal thiabendazole (7).

Gastrointestinal

Nausea, anorexia, vomiting, abdominal pain, and diarrhea are common and occur in a high proportion of patients taking tiabendazole (8).

Liver

Parenchymal liver damage can occur in patients taking tiabendazole and abnormal liver function tests have been documented (9). There have been well-studied cases of bile duct injury, which can lead to micronodular cirrhosis (10), and a case in which these various forms of liver disorder co-existed and liver transplantation proved necessary (11).

Persistent cholestasis can occur in patients taking tiabendazole (12).

- A 27-year-old patient from Surinam with beta-thalassemia took tiabendazole 1250 mg bd for 2 days for strongyloidiasis (13). One week later she became icteric, with raised total and conjugated bilirubin, alkaline phosphatase, gamma-glutamyltransferase, and transaminases. Tests for antinuclear antibodies, parietal cells antibodies, smooth muscle antibodies, mitochondrial antibodies, hepatitis A, B, C, cytomegalovirus, Epstein–Barr virus, mumps, and measles were negative. Ultrasonography showed normal intrahepatic and extrahepatic bile ducts. Liver biopsy showed intrahepatic cholestasis and a slightly increased infiltrate in the portal areas. One week later she developed a generalized urticarial rash. She had mildly abnormal liver tests for the next 7 years, at which time a liver biopsy showed a slight lymphatic infiltrate in the portal fields, without signs of cirrhosis, chronic hepatitis, or primary biliary cirrhosis.

- A 42-year-old woman, also from Surinam, with beta-thalassemia and non-insulin dependant diabetes mellitus took tiabendazole 1250 mg bd for 2 days for strongyloidiasis (13). Five weeks later she developed general malaise, anorexia, weight loss, icterus, and a tender liver. She had raised total and direct bilirubin, gamma-glutamyltransferase, and alkaline phosphatase, but only marginally raised transaminases. Tests for Hepatitis A, B, and C, cytomegalovirus, and schistosomiasis were negative. Tests for antinuclear antibodies and antibodies against liver cell membranes, smooth muscle, and mitochondria were negative, but there were parietal cell antibodies. Ultrasonography and ERCP showed normal intrahepatic and extrahepatic bile ducts. Liver biopsy showed severe centrally localized cholestasis. A year later all clinical and laboratory abnormalities had disappeared.

In view of these and previous cases of severe cholestasis after tiabendazole and the availability of less toxic equally effective drugs (albendazole or preferably ivermectin), tiabendazole must be considered obsolete in the treatment of strongyloidiasis.

Urinary tract

Crystalluria has been noted in patients taking tiabendazole, sometimes with hematuria (1).

Tiabendazole can give the urine an asparagus-like smell because of the presence of a mercaptan metabolite of tiabendazole (14).

Skin

Pruritus and skin rashes can occur (15). Much more rarely, toxic epidermal necrolysis has occurred after a total dose of 1800 mg, and Stevens–Johnson syndrome and erythema multiforme have also been reported (16).

Very occasionally a topical form of tiabendazole is used, for example to treat rosacea, and in one such case contact dermatitis aggravated by sunlight occurred as a complication, with positive tests for tiabendazole sensitivity (17).

Musculoskeletal

Tiabendazole can cause severe muscle pain on exercise (18).

Second-Generation Effects

Teratogenicity

There is no firm information on adverse reactions during pregnancy, but animal evidence points to teratogenicity and there have been official warnings against use by pregnant women (19).

Susceptibility Factors

Renal disease

Tiabendazole is metabolized almost completely by the liver, and its active metabolites are substantially excreted by the kidney; the risk of toxicity may therefore be greater in patients with impaired renal function (20).

Hepatic disease

Because tiabendazole is metabolized almost completely by the liver (20), it should be used with caution in hepatic impairment.

Drug–Drug Interactions

Theophylline

Tiabendazole can markedly increase serum concentrations of theophylline, with a prolonged half-life and a reduced clearance rate; concomitant administration of theophylline and thiabendazole resulted in severe nausea and vomiting (21).

References

1. Bagheri H, Simiand E, Montastruc JL, Magnaval JF. Adverse drug reactions to anthelmintics. Ann Pharmacother 2004;38(3):383–8.
2. Schantz PM, Van den Bossche H, Eckert J. Chemotherapy for larval echinococcosis in animals and humans: report of a workshop. Z Parasitenkd 1982;67(1):5–26.
3. Tchao P, Templeton T. Thiabendazole-associated grand mal seizures in a patient with Down syndrome. J Pediatr 1983;102(2):317–18.
4. Medwatch. Summary of safety-related drug labeling changes approved by FDA Center for Drug Evaluation and Research (CDER). Mintezole (Thiabendazole). 01/06/2001.
5. Fink AI, MacKay CJ, Cutler SS. Sicca complex and cholangiostatic jaundice in two members of a family probably caused by thiabendazole. Ophthalmology 1979;86(10):1892–6.
6. Council on Drugs. Evaluation of a broad-spectrum anthelmintic thiabendazole (Mintezol). JAMA 1968;205(3):172–3.
7. Boken DJ, Leoni PA, Preheim LC. Treatment of *Strongyloides stercoralis* hyperinfection syndrome with thiabendazole administered per rectum. Clin Infect Dis 1993;16(1):123–6.
8. Igual-Adell R, Oltra-Alcaraz C, Soler-Company E, Sanchez-Sanchez P, Matogo-Oyana J, Rodriguez-Calabuig D. Efficacy and safety of ivermectin and thiabendazole in the treatment of strongyloidiasis. Expert Opin Pharmacother 2004;5(12):2615–19.
9. Hennekeuser HH, Pabst K, Poeplau W, Gerok W. Thiabendazole for the treatment of trichinosis in humans. Tex Rep Biol Med 1969;27(Suppl 2):581.
10. Manivel JC, Bloomer JR, Snover DC. Progressive bile duct injury after thiabendazole administration. Gastroenterology 1987;93(2):245–9.
11. Skandrani K, Richardet JP, Duvoux C, Cherqui D, Zafrani ES, Dhumeaux D. Transplantation hépatique pour ductopénie sévère associée la prise de thiabendazole. [Hepatic transplantation for severe ductopenia related to ingestion of thiabendazole.] Gastroenterol Clin Biol 1997;21(8–9):623–5.
12. Ishizaki T, Kamo E, Boehme K. Double-blind studies of tolerance to praziquantel in Japanese patients with *Schistosoma japonicum* infections. Bull World Health Organ 1979;57(5):787–91.
13. Eland IA, Kerkhof SC, Overbosch D, Wismans PJ, Stricker BH. Cholestatische hepatitis toegeschreven aan her gebruik van tiabendazole. [Cholestatic hepatitis ascribed to the use of thiabendazole.] Ned Tijdschr Geneeskd 1998;142(23):1331–4.
14. Morgan M. Practice management of helminth infections. Practitioner 2000;11(10).
15. Sanchez del Rio J, Ramos Polo E, Nosti Martinez D, Rozado Fernandez S, Ribas Barcelo A. Exantema fijo generalizado por thiabendazol. [Fixed, generalized exanthema caused by thiabendazole.] Actas Dermosifiliogr 1982;73(3–4):125–8.
16. Humphreys F, Cox NH. Thiabendazole-induced erythema multiforme with lesions around melanocytic naevi. Br J Dermatol 1988;118(6):855–6.
17. Izu R, Aguirre A, Goicoechea A, Gardeazabal J, Diaz Perez JL. Photoaggravated allergic contact dermatitis due to topical thiabendazole. Contact Dermatitis 1993;28(4):243–4.
18. Parasitic infections. In: Merck Manual. 17th ed. Section 13, Chapter 161.
19. Anonymous. Communication from the Department of Health and Social Security. London, 22-02-1988.
20. Letter from the US Department of Health and Human Services to Merck Inc, 2000.
21. Schneider D, Gannon R, Sweeney K, Shore E. Theophylline and antiparasitic drug interactions. A case report and study of the influence of thiabendazole and mebendazole on theophylline pharmacokinetics in adults. Chest 1990;97(1):84–7.

Tiagabine

See also Antiepileptic drugs

General Information

Tiagabine is a nipecotic acid derivative which inhibits GABA re-uptake. It is highly bound to plasma proteins (96%) and is mainly eliminated by CYP3A-mediated oxidation, with a half-life of about 7 hours (1). It is used in add-on treatment of refractory partial seizures. Its adverse effects are mostly on the central nervous system.

In a review of safety data from nearly 3100 patients included in 53 clinical trials, tiagabine had no significant effect on hepatic metabolic processes, serum concentrations of concomitant anticonvulsants, and blood chemistry and hematology tests (2). Allergic reactions, such as skin rashes, were less common with tiagabine than with most other anticonvulsants. Adverse effects were generally mild and affected mainly the central nervous system, the most common being dizziness, weakness, nervousness, tremor, difficulty with concentration and attention, speech disorders, depression, and abdominal pain. About 1% of patients given tiagabine experienced weakness severe enough to cause falls or inability to walk, and some form of weakness occurred in about 9% of patients, especially at high dosages or after stopping a single concomitant enzyme-inducing antiepileptic drug.

The safety of long-term tiagabine has been studied retrospectively in 42 patients with refractory partial epilepsy who took tiagabine for longer than 6 months (3). The most common adverse events were tiredness (56%), headache (46%), dizziness (44%), visual symptoms (blurring, difficulty in focusing, and diplopia; 39%), altered thinking (32%), and tremor (31%). The adverse events profile was comparable among those who had taken tiagabine for 6–12 months, 12–24 months, and more than 24 months.

The use of tiagabine 4–16 mg/day in preventing migraine has been studied in 41 patients who had failed treatment with divalproex sodium because of adverse effects or lack of efficacy (4). There was at least a 50% reduction in the frequency of migraine headaches in 33 patients. There were adverse events in 12 patients, most commonly tiredness; a few patients had weight gain or confusion.

The effects of tiagabine have been studied in a 4-month, single-blind study in 52 children over the age of 2 years with different syndromes of refractory epilepsy (5). Adverse events, mostly mild to moderate, were reported by 39% of the children during the single-blind placebo period and by 83% of the children during tiagabine treatment. The events predominantly affected the nervous system; weakness (19%), nervousness (19%), dizziness (17%), and somnolence (17%) were the most common. One child had hallucinations that responded to dosage reduction. Only three children withdrew because of adverse events.

The efficacy and safety of tiagabine have been assessed in a study with an open screening phase (in which patients were titrated to the optimal tiagabine dose), followed by a double-blind, placebo-controlled, crossover phase (6).

Of the 88 patients who entered the double-blind phase, seizure frequency was significantly reduced in 44, and there was an over 50% reduction of partial seizures in 33%. There were adverse events in 77% of the patients during the screening phase and 22% during the double-blind phase. The most frequent adverse events were dizziness (32%), somnolence (30%), and weakness (19%). Two patients taking tiagabine withdrew during the double-blind phase because of adverse events.

Organs and Systems

Nervous system

In add-on trials, adverse events significantly more common with tiagabine than with placebo were dizziness (30 versus 13%), weakness (24 versus 12%), nervousness (12 versus 3%), tremor (9 versus 3%), depressed mood (5 versus 1%), and emotional lability (4 versus 1%) (SEDA-19, 73) (SEDA-20, 65) (SEDA-22, 91) (7). Somnolence, amnesia, confusion, difficulty in concentrating, paresthesia, headache, and ataxia can also occur.

In a randomized, double-blind, add-on trial of tiagabine (16, 32, or 56 mg/day) in 297 patients with refractory partial seizures, adverse events significantly more common with tiagabine were dizziness in the 32 mg group (33 versus 15% with placebo), tremor in the 32 and 56 mg groups (15 and 21 versus 3%), mental lethargy or difficulty in concentrating in the 56 mg group (14 versus 3%), and depressed mood in the 16 and 56 mg groups (7% in both groups versus 0%) (8). In a similar study with a dosage of 10 mg tds, the most common adverse events were dizziness, weakness, headache, and somnolence (9), but only dizziness was significantly more common than with placebo (29 versus 10%).

A few more cases of non-convulsive status epilepticus associated with tiagabine have been reported (10–12).

Exacerbation of seizures

Tiagabine can reportedly exacerbate seizures and non-convulsive status epilepticus (SEDA-21, 74). Two of nine patients with partial epilepsy in a trial of tiagabine 30 mg/day developed non-convulsive status and features consistent with atypical absence seizures, although neither had had such seizure types before; drug withdrawal was followed by sustained remission (13). GABAergic drugs aggravate absence seizures, but the de novo occurrence of absences in patients with partial epilepsy is unusual. Tiagabine is only recommended for partial seizures (with or without secondary generalization).

- After an increase in tiagabine dose to 32 mg/day, a 28-year-old woman with partial epilepsy developed a prolonged and disoriented state associated with generalized spike-and-wave discharges on the electroencephalogram. Tiagabine was withdrawn and the status did not recur.
- Two similar episodes occurred in a 28-year-old man taking 24 and 32 mg/day (14).
- Both patients were taking a non-enzyme-inducing agent (valproate and lamotrigine respectively), which probably resulted in higher serum tiagabine concentrations than those seen in enzyme-induced patients.

Although the manufacturer's database suggested that non-convulsive status is rare during tiagabine therapy (2), the possibility of status needs to be considered in patients who develop episodes of confusion or atypical behavior while taking tiagabine, especially high dosages. A critical analysis of the available literature suggests that misdiagnosis can occur and that some reported cases of putative non-convulsive status epilepticus might in fact have been due to drug-induced encephalopathy (2,15). Overall, the risk of tiagabine-induced generalized non-convulsive status is likely to be greater in patients with a history of absence or generalized epileptic discharges, which are known to be aggravated by GABAergic agents, but patients without such a history can be also affected.

Generalized non-convulsive status needs to be differentiated not only from non-epileptic encephalopathy, but also from partial non-convulsive status, which can also be occasionally precipitated by tiagabine (2,15).

There have been cases of generalized non-convulsive status epilepticus in patients with chronic partial epilepsy treated with tiagabine, on one occasion specifically associated with frontal lobe discharges (15).

- A 12-year-old boy with familial bilateral perisylvian polymicrogyria, mental retardation, and refractory partial seizures was given tiagabine in addition to sodium valproate, and the dosage was increased to 10 mg tds (1 mg/kg/day). This produced complete seizure control. After 1 week he developed hypoactivity, reduced reactivity, and affective detachment. Electroencephalography showed subcontinuous sharp-wave discharges, with irregular runs of atypical spike-wave complexes over the anterior regions of both hemispheres, consistent with a diagnosis of frontal non-convulsive status epilepticus. The dosage of tiagabine was reduced to 15 mg/day and there was complete regression of the behavioral and affective changes and normalization of the electroencephalogram.
- A 21-year-old woman with partial epilepsy had seizure aggravation and complex partial status epilepticus after stepwise increase of tiagabine to 60 mg/day in addition to carbamazepine and vigabatrin (16). The electroencephalogram showed bilateral rhythmic slow activity, which disappeared, together with clinical signs, when intravenous clonazepam (2 mg) was given.

Tiagabine 0.45–40.57 mg/kg/day was associated with long-standing non-convulsive status epilepticus in three girls, two aged 12 years and one aged 17 years, with refractory localization-related epilepsy (17). Resolution followed withdrawal of tiagabine or a reduction in dosage.

Dystonias

Three patients had transient dystonic reactions while taking tiagabine 20–30 mg/day in addition to carbamazepine (18). The dystonic reactions occurred during the first few weeks of treatment. The patients each had a different type of dystonia: focal limb dystonia, oromandibular dystonia, and writer's cramp. In each case the dystonia resolved spontaneously without withdrawal of tiagabine and without any other treatment. Although paroxysmal dystonic movements have been well described with

carbamazepine, these patients had been taking carbamazepine for years without this adverse effect.

In placebo-controlled trials, the overall incidence of non-convulsive status epilepticus was no higher with tiagabine than with placebo. However, there have been isolated reports of tiagabine-related non-convulsive status epilepticus (19).

The frequency of status during tiagabine trials has been compared with the occurrence of status epilepticus in four large epidemiological cohorts from Rochester (Minnesota), Turku (Finland), New York, and New Haven (Connecticut) (20). A review of 13 cases with non-convulsive status showed that most of them had had generalized discharges on prior electroencephalography. Only three had encephalographic evidence of status during tiagabine treatment. In the placebo-controlled trials, there was no difference in the frequency of status or complex partial status between patients taking tiagabine or placebo (0.8–1.0 versus 1.5%). In long-term safety studies, which included 2248 patients, there was a 5% frequency of status and a 3% frequency of complex partial status in the tiagabine-treated patients, which was similar to the rates of occurrence in the four external cohorts. Thus, tiagabine does not appear to increase the risk of status or non-convulsive status.

Sensory systems

Following reports of concentric visual field defects associated with vigabatrin (SEDA-21, 78), there has been concern that other drugs that enhance GABAergic inhibition might cause a similar disorder. Although visual field defects were detected in six of 12 patients treated with tiagabine in Australia, no details were given, and this report seems to have remained isolated (21). In a controlled study, none of 15 patients who took tiagabine monotherapy for 1.5–3.5 years (mean daily dose 22 mg) had evidence of a concentric visual field defect (22).

The effect of tiagabine on visual function has been studied in 15 patients with chronic partial epilepsy treated for 23–55 months with tiagabine monotherapy after failure with standard antiepileptic drug monotherapy (23). Three patients had localized field losses (two quadrantanopic and one hemianopic) from earlier brain lesions. Tiagabine had no effect on visual fields but acquired color vision defects were found in seven of 14 patients; contrast sensitivity was unaffected.

Psychological, psychiatric

Although psychosis has been described occasionally (24), in three double-blind trials the incidence of psychotic symptoms was comparable to placebo (SEDA-21, 74). However, patients with a past history of psychiatric disturbances are often excluded from trials, and caution is recommended when using tiagabine in these patients.

Metabolism

Changes in body weight have been evaluated in 349 patients taking carbamazepine, phenytoin, or tiagabine. Carbamazepine add-on therapy caused a significant mean weight gain of 1.5% (25). However, tiagabine add-on therapy to either phenytoin or carbamazepine caused no significant weight change.

Hematologic

- A 42-year-old woman developed thrombocytopenia (platelet count $4 \times 10^9/l$), ecchymoses, and petechiae after taking tiagabine 50 mg/day for about 1 month (26). Bone-marrow biopsy showed a moderate increase in megakaryocytes without signs of disturbed maturation. Withdrawal of tiagabine led to gradual recovery.

However, the authors failed to mention that ecchymoses have been reported before in patients taking tiagabine, as discussed in the manufacturer's prescribing information (7).

Gastrointestinal

Nausea, vomiting, diarrhea, abdominal pain, and ecchymoses can occur, but they are not common (SEDA-22, 91) (7).

Susceptibility Factors

Hepatic disease

Hepatic dysfunction is associated with impaired tiagabine elimination and can result in greater susceptibility to adverse effects (SEDA-21, 75). Tiagabine should only be used cautiously and in reduced dosages in these patients.

Other features of the patient

Caution is also required in patients with a history of depression or behavioral disorders (24).

Drug Administration

Drug dosage regimens

Two different dosage regimens (twice or three times a day) of add-on tiagabine have been compared in a multicenter, open, randomized, parallel-group study in 347 patients (27). The tiagabine dosage was titrated over 12 weeks to a target of 40 mg/day. The patients were followed for a further 12 weeks. Significantly more patients in the thrice-daily group completed the titration period (81 versus 73%). The proportion of responders during the last 8 weeks of the flexible phase was similar in the two groups (42% for twice-daily and 47% for thrice-daily administration). Thus, although both regimens appeared to offer similar efficacy, significantly more patients completed the study in the thrice-daily group, probably because tolerability is less when high doses are given undivided.

In a large comparison of 16 mg bd with 8 mg qds, the twice-daily schedule tended to be associated with more adverse events (SEDA-22, 91).

Drug overdose

In four adults who took 300–800 mg, the most common symptoms were agitation, hostility, and myoclonus. Supportive care, including in some cases gastric lavage and activated charcoal, was effective. One patient developed status epilepticus, which was managed with phenobarbital (SEDA-21, 74).

Tiagabine overdose (1 g) was associated with convulsive status epilepticus in a 39-year-old man, previously well controlled (28). The tiagabine plasma concentration was 2620 ng/ml, over 10 times higher than the concentrations found in trials.

Drug–Drug Interactions

Contraceptive steroids

Tiagabine, unlike carbamazepine and oxcarbazepine, felbamate, phenobarbital, phenytoin, and topiramate, does not affect the metabolism of oral contraceptive steroids (29).

Enzyme-inducing anticonvulsants

The most important interactions of tiagabine involve induction of its metabolism by enzyme-inducing anticonvulsants (30). This results in larger tiagabine dosage requirements compared with patients taking monotherapy or valproic acid co-medication.

References

1. Perucca E, Bialer M. The clinical pharmacokinetics of the newer antiepileptic drugs. Focus on topiramate, zonisamide and tiagabine. Clin Pharmacokinet 1996;31(1):29–46.
2. Leppik IE, Gram L, Deaton R, Sommerville KW. Safety of tiagabine: summary of 53 trials. Epilepsy Res 1999;33(2–3):235–46.
3. Fakhoury T, Uthman B, Abou-Khalil B. Safety of long-term treatment with tiagabine. Seizure 2000;9(6):431–5.
4. Freitag FG, Diamond S, Diamond ML, Urban GJ, Pepper BJ. An open use trial of tiagabine in migraine. Headache Q 2000;11:133–4.
5. Uldall P, Bulteau C, Pedersen SA, Dulac O, Lyby K. Tiagabine adjunctive therapy in children with refractory epilepsy: a single-blind dose escalating study. Epilepsy Res 2000;42(2–3):159–68.
6. Crawford P, Meinardi H, Brown S, Rentmeester TW, Pedersen B, Pedersen PC, Lassen LC. Tiagabine: efficacy and safety in adjunctive treatment of partial seizures. Epilepsia 2001;42(4):531–8.
7. Adkins JC, Noble S. Tiagabine. A review of its pharmacodynamic and pharmacokinetic properties and therapeutic potential in the management of epilepsy. Drugs 1998;55(3):437–60.
8. Uthman BM, Rowan AJ, Ahmann PA, Leppik IE, Schachter SC, Sommerville KW, Shu V. Tiagabine for complex partial seizures: a randomized, add-on, dose-response trial. Arch Neurol 1998;55(1):56–62.
9. Kalviainen R, Brodie MJ, Duncan J, Chadwick D, Edwards D, Lyby K. A double-blind, placebo-controlled trial of tiagabine given three-times daily as add-on therapy for refractory partial seizures. Northern European Tiagabine Study Group. Epilepsy Res 1998;30(1):31–40.
10. Zhu Y, Vaughn BV. Non-convulsive status epilepticus induced by tiagabine in a patient with pseudoseizure. Seizure 2002;11(1):57–9.
11. Kellinghaus C, Dziewas R, Ludemann P. Tiagabine-related non-convulsive status epilepticus in partial epilepsy: three case reports and a review of the literature. Seizure 2002;11(4):243–9.

12. Brouns R, Van Paesschen W. Recurrent complex partial status epilepticus associated with tiagabine rechallenge. Acta Neurol Belg 2002;102(1):19–20.

13. Eckardt KM, Steinhoff BJ. Nonconvulsive status epilepticus in two patients receiving tiagabine treatment. Epilepsia 1998;39(6):671–4.

14. Ettinger AB, Bernal OG, Andriola MR, Bagchi S, Flores P, Just C, Pitocco C, Rooney T, Tuominen J, Devinsky O. Two cases of nonconvulsive status epilepticus in association with tiagabine therapy. Epilepsia 1999; 40(8):1159–62.

15. Piccinelli P, Borgatti R, Perucca E, Tofani A, Donati G, Balottin U. Frontal nonconvulsive status epilepticus associated with high-dose tiagabine therapy in a child with familial bilateral perisylvian polymicrogyria. Epilepsia 2000;41(11):1485–8.

16. Trinka E, Moroder T, Nagler M, Staffen W, Loscher W, Ladurner G. Clinical and EEG findings in complex partial status epilepticus with tiagabine. Seizure 1999;8(1):41–4.

17. Balslev T, Uldall P, Buchholt J. Provocation of non-convulsive status epilepticus by tiagabine in three adolescent patients. Eur J Paediatr Neurol 2000;4(4):169–70.

18. Wolanczyk T, Grabowska-Grzyb A. Transient dystonias in three patients treated with tiagabine. Epilepsia 2001;42(7):944–6.

19. Fitzek S, Hegemann S, Sauner D, Bonsch D, Fitzek C. Drug-induced nonconvulsive status epilepticus with low dose of tiagabine. Epileptic Disord 2001;3(3):147–50.

20. Shinnar S, Berg AT, Treiman DM, Hauser WA, Hesdorffer DC, Sackellares JC, Leppik I, Sillanpaa M, Sommerville KW. Status epilepticus and tiagabine therapy: review of safety data and epidemiologic comparisons. Epilepsia 2001;42(3):372–9.

21. Beran RG, Hung A, Plunkett M, Currie J, Sachinwalla R. Predictability of visual field defects in patients exposed to GABAergic agents, vigabatrin, or tiagabine. Neurology 1999;52(Suppl 2):A249.

22. Kalviainen R, Nousiainen I, Mantyjarvi M, Riekkinen PJ. Absence of concentric visual field defects in patients with long-term tiagabine monotherapy. Neurology 1999;52(Suppl 2):A236.

23. Nousiainen I, Mantyjarvi M, Kalviainen R. Visual function in patients treated with the GABAergic anticonvulsant drug tiagabine. Clin Drug Invest 2000;20:393–400.

24. Trimble MR, O'Donoghue M, Sander L, Duncan J. Psychosis with tiagabine. Epilepsia 1997;38(Suppl 3):40.

25. Hogan RE, Bertrand ME, Deaton RL, Sommerville KW. Total percentage body weight changes during add-on therapy with tiagabine, carbamazepine and phenytoin. Epilepsy Res 2000;41(1):23–8.

26. Willert C, Englisch S, Schlesinger S, Runge U. Possible drug-induced thrombocytopenia secondary to tiagabine. Neurology 1999;52(4):888.

27. Biraben A, Beaussart M, Josien E, Pestre M, Savet JF, Schaff JL, Tourniaire D, Sevestre M, Renault-Djouadi J. Comparison of twice- and three times daily tiagabine for the adjunctive treatment of partial seizures in refractory patients with epilepsy: an open label, randomised, parallel-group study. Epileptic Disord 2001;3(2):91–100.

28. Ostrovskiy D, Spanaki MV, Morris GL 3rd. Tiagabine overdose can induce convulsive status epilepticus. Epilepsia 2002;43(7):773–4.

29. Crawford P. Interactions between antiepileptic drugs and hormonal contraception. CNS Drugs 2002;16(4):263–72.

30. So EL, Wolff D, Graves NM, Leppik IE, Cascino GD, Pixton GC, Gustavson LE. Pharmacokinetics of tiagabine as add-on therapy in patients taking enzyme-inducing antiepilepsy drugs. Epilepsy Res 1995;22(3):221–6.

Tiapride

See also Neuroleptic drugs

General Information

Tiapride is a substituted benzamide related to sulpiride, a selective dopamine D_2 and D_3 receptor antagonist with little propensity for causing catalepsy and sedation. It has antidyskinetic activity, reflecting its antidopaminergic action, and also anxiolytic activity mediated by mechanisms that are poorly understood. Unlike the benzodiazepines, tiapride does not affect vigilance and has a low potential for interaction with ethanol, and possibly for abuse. From a clinical point of view, it can be considered as an atypical neuroleptic drug. It has reported efficacy in neuroleptic-drug induced tardive dyskinesia, levodopa-induced dyskinesias, psychomotor agitation in elderly patients, and chorea (1).

Tiapride appears to be useful in alcohol withdrawal as an alternative to the benzodiazepines (2). It facilitates the management of ethanol withdrawal, but its use in patients at risk of severe reactions in acute withdrawal should be accompanied by adjunctive therapy for hallucinosis and seizures. Since it may prove difficult to identify such patients and since there is also a small risk of the neuroleptic malignant syndrome (particularly with parenteral administration), the usefulness of tiapride in this setting is likely to be limited. The potential risk of tardive dyskinesia at the dosage used in alcoholic patients following detoxification (300 mg/day) requires evaluation and necessitates medical supervision. It is unlikely to produce problems of dependence or abuse.

Tiapride has been assessed for the treatment of agitation and aggressiveness in elderly patients with cognitive impairment in a multicenter, double-blind study, in which patients were randomly allocated to tiapride 100 mg/day ($n = 102$), haloperidol 2 mg/day ($n = 101$), or placebo ($n = 103$) (3). The percentage of responders after 21 days, according to the Multidimensional Observation Scale for Elderly Subjects (MOSES) irritability/aggressiveness subscale, was significantly greater in both of the active treatment groups (haloperidol 63%, tiapride 69%) than in the placebo group (49%). There were 10 dropouts in the tiapride group, 21 in the haloperidol group, and 16 in the placebo group. The number of patients with at least one extrapyramidal symptom was significantly smaller with tiapride (16%) than with haloperidol (34%) and identical to that with placebo (17%); there was no significant difference across the groups in the numbers of patients with endocrinological adverse events. Four deaths were reported: one with placebo (stroke), one with tiapride (pneumonia), and two with haloperidol (stroke and heart failure).

Organs and Systems

Cardiovascular

Torsade de pointes has been attributed to tiapride.

- A 76-year-old man developed torsade de pointes while taking tiapride 300 mg/day; the QT_c interval 1 day after starting treatment was 600 ms; the dysrhythmia resolved when tiapride was withdrawn (4).

References

1. Dose M, Lange HW. The benzamide tiapride: treatment of extrapyramidal motor and other clinical syndromes. Pharmacopsychiatry 2000;33(1):19–27.
2. Peters DH, Faulds D. Tiapride. A review of its pharmacology and therapeutic potential in the management of alcohol dependence syndrome. Drugs 1994;47(6):1010–32.
3. Allain H, Dautzenberg PH, Maurer K, Schuck S, Bonhomme D, Gerard D. Double blind study of tiapride versus haloperidol and placebo in agitation and aggressiveness in elderly patients with cognitive impairment. Psychopharmacology (Berl) 2000;148(4):361–6.
4. Iglesias E, Esteban E, Zabala S, Gascon A. Tiapride-induced torsade de pointes. Am J Med 2000;109(6):509.

Tiaprofenic acid

See also Non-steroidal anti-inflammatory drugs

General Information

Data are available on the incidence of adverse effects of this drug (1–3). A review of published studies showed that about 13–15% of patients have adverse effects. The withdrawal rate because of unwanted reactions was 3.2–12% in short-term studies and 4% in one long-term trial. Adverse effects involved the gastrointestinal tract in 8–12% of patients, the central nervous system in 1–10% and the skin (rash, sweating, and itching) in 1–4%. Cutaneous photosensitivity and edema have also been reported.

The adverse effects profile does not differ from that of other propionic acid derivatives and includes the whole spectrum of gastrointestinal adverse reactions usually found with NSAIDs (SED-10, 166) (SEDA-10, 84) (4). The claim of good tolerance and gastric protection, based on animal data, which the company extrapolated to humans, has not been confirmed by appropriate clinical studies (SEDA-12, 89).

Organs and Systems

Urinary tract

Although many NSAIDs have rarely been reported to be responsible for increased urinary frequency and dysuria, and never for severe cystitis, tiaprofenic acid causes severe cystitis (SEDA-18, 106) (SEDA-20, 94) (SEDA-21, 107) (5,6).

If this complication occurs, the drug should be withdrawn immediately (7). A report has given some data on the frequency with which tiaprofenic acid cystitis-related disorders were reported to the UK's Committee on Safety of Medicines. Between 1981 and 1996, 770 adverse drug reactions involving 221 patients were reported. A peak in the reporting of cystitis was noted in 1994, when tiaprofenic acid product information was changed and advice

was sent to UK doctors warning about cystitis-related disorders. This peak was followed by a fall in the number of reports, but it is not clear if this was due to reduced drug usage or also to a fall in the reporting rate of such adverse reactions (8).

References

1. Anonymous. The side effects of tiaprofenic acid. Reactions 1985;118:11.
2. Rave O, Penth B. Arzneimittelsicherheit bei Antirheumatika: Ergebnisse einer Breitenprufung mit Tiaprofensaure an 20,947 Patienten. Med Welt 1984;35:1587.
3. Poletto B. Tiaprofenic acid. Clin Rheum Dis 1984;10(2):333–51.
4. Anonymous. Tiaprofenic acid (Surgam) — a major claim is dropped. Drug Ther Bull 1983;21(13):49–50.
5. Crew JP, Donat R, Roskell D, Fellows GJ. Bilateral ureteric obstruction secondary to the prolonged use of tiaprofenic acid. Br J Clin Pract 1997;51(1):59–60.
6. Crawford ML, Waller PC, Wood SM. Severe cystitis associated with tiaprofenic acid. Br J Urol 1997;79(4):578–84.
7. Drake MJ, Nixon PM, Crew JP. Drug-induced bladder and urinary disorders. Incidence, prevention and management. Drug Saf 1998;19(1):45–55.
8. Brown EG, Waller PC, Sallie BA. Tiaprofenic acid and severe cystitis. Postgrad Med J 1998;74(873):443–4.

Tick-borne meningoencephalitis vaccine

See also Vaccines

General Information

Tick-borne meningoencephalitis vaccine is an adsorbed formalin-inactivated virus vaccine prepared on chicken embryo tissue. Mild local reactions (soreness, redness, swelling) have been reported in 10–25% of vaccinees; systemic reactions occur at similar rates. Fever over 39°C is rare.

Positive merthiolate tests were found in eight of 30 patients with suspected adverse reactions to tetanus or tick-borne encephalitis vaccine (local inflammatory reactions at the injection site, fever, lymphadenopathy, urticarial or lichenoid exanthemas) (1).

An improved tick-borne encephalitis vaccine for children, produced by Baxter, has been licensed and is being used without safety concerns in many countries.

Organs and Systems

Nervous system

In 1989, 172 reports on adverse effects after tick-borne meningoencephalitis immunization were collected in the Federal Republic of Germany, among them 72 reports of suspect neurological complications. Among the 72 reports, there were only three cases of peripheral neuropathy that suggested a causal link with immunization (2). Three cases of mild meningitis, encephalitis, and convulsions were, because of incomplete diagnosis, difficult to evaluate.

The database of the Swiss Drug Monitoring Center included 20 spontaneous reports (1987 to July 1992) of adverse events after the administration of tick-borne meningoencephalitis vaccine, among them 11 reports of cases with neurological symptoms (for example meningism, polyradiculitis, ataxia, vestibulopathy, facialis paresis). Most recovered completely within a few days. The incompleteness of the data did not allow conclusions regarding the causality of immunization (3).

Individual reports of neuropathy (SEDA-13, 290), multifocal cerebral vasculitis and infarction (4), cervical myelitis (5), myelopolyradiculitis (5), and suspected encephalitis (SEDA-17, 363) have appeared.

During the period 1987–2000, the Swiss Center for Adverse Events Drug Monitoring (Schweizerische Arzneimittel-Nebenwirkungszentrale) received 33 reports, including 39 neurological adverse events, following the receipt of tick-borne encephalitis vaccine: headache (36% of reports), neuropathy (18%), and meningeal signs (13%); 12 of 33 patients were hospitalized and all recovered (6).

Immunologic

A case of facial edema and pain and swelling of the left knee following the receipt of tick-borne meningoencephalitis vaccine was suspected to be caused by thiomersal allergy (7).

Body temperature

Following the use of tick-borne encephalitis vaccine ("Ticovac," produced by Baxter) in German children, there was a sudden increase in the number of cases of high fever, and 20–30% of vaccinees, primarily those 3 years of age and younger, reacted with a high fever (39°C or more) after the first dose (8). The increased number of cases of high fever was observed after changes in the production of tick-borne encephalitis vaccine were made: the vaccine no longer contains thiomersal and human albumin. Currently, according to the German licensing authority, the Paul Ehrlich institute, the vaccine is no longer recommended for children under 3 years; children aged 3–15 years should only receive half a dose of Ticovac, and the vaccine should only be used when strongly indicated. The reason for the changed reactogenicity is still unclear.

References

1. Lindemayr H, Drobil M, Ebner H. Impfreaktionen nach Tetanus- und Frühsommer-meningoenzephalitisschutzimpfung durch Merthiolat (Thiomersal). [Reactions to vaccinations against tetanus and tick-borne encephalitis caused by merthiolate (thiomersal).] Hautarzt 1984;35(4):192–6.
2. Kappos L. Mogliche neurologische Nebenwirkungen nach FSME-Impfung. Fachpressegedprach, Frankfurt Press Club. 20 February 1990.
3. Bohus M, Glocker FX, Jost S, Deuschl G, Lucking CH. Myelitis after immunisation against tick-borne encephalitis. Lancet 1993;342(8865):239–40.
4. Schabet M, Wiethoelter H, Grodd W, Vallbracht A, Dichgans J, Becker W, Berg PA. Neurological complications after simultaneous immunisation against tick-borne encephalitis and tetanus. Lancet 1989;1(8644):959–60.
5. Goerre S, Kesselring J, Hartmann K, Kuhn M, Reinhart WH. Neurologische Nebenwirkungen nach Impfung gegen die Fruhsommer–Mening–Enzephalitis. Fahlbericht und Erfahrungen der Schweizerischen Arzneimittel–Nebenwirkungs–Zentrale (SANZ). [Neurological side effects following vaccination of early-summer meningoencephalitis. Case report and experiences of the Swiss Center for Adverse Drug Effects.] Schweiz Med Wochenschr 1993;123(14):654–7.
6. Doser AK, Hartmann K, Fleisch F, Kuhn M. Vermutete neurologische Nebenwirkungen der FSME–Impfung: Erfahrung Schweizerischen Arzneimittel–Nebenwirkungs–Zentrale (SANZ). [Suspected neurological side-effects of tick-borne meningoencephalitis vaccination: experiences of the Swiss Adverse Drug Reaction Reporting Center.] Schweiz Rundsch Med Prax 2002;91(5):159–62.
7. Ackermann R. Allergische Reaktion nach FSME-Auffrischimpfung (Anfrage und Antwort). Dtsch Med Wochenschr 1990;115:1213.
8. Statement of Paul Ehrlich Institute. Use of Ticovac TBE vaccine. Langen: Germany. http://www.pei.de/ticova_info.htm, 4/11/2000.

Ticlopidine

General Information

Ticlopidine is a thienopyridine derivative with potent antiplatelet activity associated with inhibition of ADP-induced platelet aggregation. It was first used in Europe in 1978 in the secondary prevention of stroke and coronary events, the treatment of peripheral vascular disease, and after vascular stent placement. However, the use of ticlopidine has been progressively restricted in some countries because of its serious adverse effects. It has largely been superseded by clopidogrel.

General adverse effects

There is a risk of hemorrhage from drugs that inhibit platelet aggregation. The adverse effects most commonly reported with ticlopidine are skin rashes and gastrointestinal effects, including nausea, dyspepsia, vomiting, anorexia, epigastric pain, and diarrhea. Hypersensitivity reactions underly some of the hematological complications of ticlopidine, such as thrombotic thrombocytopenic purpura.

Organs and Systems

Respiratory

Bronchiolitis obliterans organizing pneumonia has been attributed to ticlopidine (1).

- A 76-year-old non-smoking woman with giant-cell arteritis who had a normal chest X-ray was taking prednisone 45 mg/day and ticlopidine 250 mg bd for persistence of cloudy vision. After 1 month of ticlopidine therapy, she developed increasing dyspnea and a pruritic rash. Chest radiography showed diffuse interstitial infiltrates, predominantly affecting the peripheries of both lungs. Transbronchial biopsy showed widening of the alveolar fields, with a mixed inflammatory infiltrate. Ticlopidine was withdrawn and prednisone was continued in the same dosage. Her symptoms completely resolved within 3 months and her chest X-ray normalized within 5 months.

Sensory systems

Two patients developed retinal vasculitis 3 and 4 weeks after starting to take ticlopidine (2). The symptoms and signs of retinitis resolved within 4–6 weeks after withdrawal of ticlopidine, with no reactivation within the next 2 or 3 years.

Hematologic

Ticlopidine can prolong bleeding time by up to 30 minutes. In well-controlled studies the incidence of minor bleeding was 10% (menorrhagia, bruises, and epistaxis) (3). Since the effect on platelet function is irreversible, the bleeding time does not return to normal sooner than 5–10 days after withdrawal, although it can be corrected immediately by platelet transfusion. In a retrospective comparison of the hemorrhagic risk in patients who had received platelet antiaggregants preoperatively for coronary surgery revascularization, there was a significant increase in postoperative hemorrhage and a higher incidence of reoperations in the patients who received ticlopidine compared with other antiaggregants (4).

Various other hematological complications have been observed during ticlopidine treatment (5). They include neutropenia, agranulocytosis, thrombocytopenia, aplastic anemia, pancytopenia, and thrombotic thrombocytopenic purpura (6). These reactions are potentially severe and some are fatal. Major bleeding is rare. Among 188 cases of hematological complications associated with ticlopidine and reported to the US Food and Drug Administration, 36 (19%) resulted in death (7).

Neutropenia

Neutropenia was the most common hematological complication in some of the major trials with ticlopidine. Severe neutropenia occurs in about 1% of patients. Neutropenia typically occurs in the first few months after the start of therapy, but is seen infrequently in the first 2–3 weeks. The mechanism has been reported to be inhibition of myeloid colony growth. On the basis of major randomized, controlled studies with ticlopidine, there is a 2.4% overall incidence of neutropenia and a 0.85% incidence of severe neutropenia and agranulocytosis (6). The neutropenia generally occurs at 2–5 weeks after the start of treatment (8). In some cases, neutropenia is delayed (9) or can develop after drug withdrawal. It has therefore been recommended that one should perform a complete blood count at baseline and every 2 weeks for the first 3 months of treatment, and that ticlopidine should be withdrawn if the neutrophil count falls below 1.2×10^9/l. In some cases, granulocyte colony-stimulating factors have been used, but their efficacy needs to be evaluated further (10). Although some fatal cases have been reported, neutropenia induced by ticlopidine is usually reversible.

Thrombocytopenia

Isolated thrombocytopenia has been reported at anything from 4 weeks to 5 years after the start of drug therapy (11,12). In these cases, platelet antibodies were also detected.

Thrombotic thrombocytopenic purpura has been repeatedly reported (6). The incidence has been estimated at 1 in 1600 (based on the observation of 5 cases out of a total of 7842 patients studied after coronary stent placements) (13). This rare adverse reaction is generally observed after a short exposure period of about 3–8 weeks. The clinical features are generally indistinguishable from those of idiopathic thrombotic thrombocytopenic purpura (14). The pathogenesis is unknown. Platelet antibodies were found in one patient, suggesting an immunologic mechanism (6). The outcome appears to be favorable in comparison to that of idiopathic thrombotic thrombocytopenic purpura, but several authors have reported cases in which death resulted (15,16). Early diagnosis and the rapid institution of plasmapheresis provide the best hope of complete recovery.

Sixty cases of thrombotic thrombocytopenic purpura have been reviewed (17). Ticlopidine had been prescribed for under 1 month in 80% of the patients, and platelet counts were normal within 2 weeks of the onset of thrombotic thrombocytopenic purpura in most patients. Mortality rates were higher among patients who were not treated with plasmapheresis than among those who underwent plasmapheresis (50% compared with 24%). The authors concluded that the onset of ticlopidine-associated thrombotic thrombocytopenic purpura is difficult to predict, despite close monitoring of platelet counts.

In 43 322 patients treated with coronary stents and ticlopidine for 1 year there were 9 cases of thrombotic thrombocytopenic purpura (0.02%) (18). The risk of thrombotic thrombocytopenic purpura during the use of ticlopidine after coronary stenting was 50-fold higher than in the general population. Ten other cases of thrombotic thrombocytopenic purpura related to ticlopidine were identified from the participating centers. Four of the 19 patients died, and all four deaths occurred in patients who were not treated with plasmapheresis. The authors stressed that early recognition and treatment is crucial for minimizing mortality.

Deficiency of, or auto-antibodies to, a von Willebrand-cleaving metalloproteinase are pathogenic in idiopathic thrombotic thrombocytopenic purpura (19). Seven consecutive patients, who developed thrombotic thrombocytopenic purpura 2–7 weeks after starting to take ticlopidine, had markedly reduced concentrations of von Willebrand factor metalloproteinase. In six cases initial samples were available and were positive for immunoglobulin G inhibitors to von Willebrand factor metalloproteinase.

Aplastic anemia

Rare cases of aplastic anemia have been reported (20). Some authors have suggested that the incidence of this complication may have been underestimated (21). The reaction is characterized by pancytopenia and the bone marrow shows profound hypocellularity, absence of precursor cells, and fatty replacement. Some studies have suggested a direct toxic effect of ticlopidine on bone marrow cells, particularly the myeloid line. In some cases, agranulocytosis or thrombocytopenia have been reported to precede the development of aplastic anemia. One should be alert to the fact that this reaction may still occur after the recommended 3 months of hematological monitoring have elapsed (6).

Gastrointestinal

Diarrhea is among the most common adverse effects of ticlopidine. It can occur in up to 20% of those who take it, in contrast to an incidence of 10% among placebo- and aspirin-treated patients (22) and usually occurs early in the course of treatment. It can be prevented by taking ticlopidine with food or by reducing the dosage. In rare cases, severe chronic diarrhea with marked body weight loss and anorexia can occur, sometimes long after the start of therapy (23).

In a few reports, lymphocytic colitis has been attributed to ticlopidine; in some cases the pathological features in the colon biopsy resolved after withdrawal of the drug (24–26).

Liver

Several cases of ticlopidine-induced hepatotoxicity have been reported (27). Between 10 days and 12 weeks after the start of treatment, patients develop jaundice, usually without fever, eosinophilia, or pain. Laboratory tests show a cholestatic or mixed cholestatic-hepatocellular pattern of injury. There is usually clinical and biochemical recovery within 1–11 months. Frank ticlopidine-associated liver injury is uncommon, but in one study, 44% of patients had abnormal liver function tests and about one-half of them had to stop taking the drug (22).

Skin

In a 1-year prospective study of 136 patients taking ticlopidine to prevent thrombosis after coronary stenting, 16 had adverse skin reactions (28). The most common were urticaria, pruritus, and maculopapular eruptions. Three patients had previously unreported reactions: a fixed drug eruption, an erythromelalgia-like eruption, and an erythema multiforme-like eruption.

Immunologic

A lupus-like illness (fever, rash, arthritis, renal involvement, and positive antinuclear and antihistone antibodies) developed in three patients 2–8 weeks after they started to take ticlopidine (29). After withdrawal, there was slow but complete resolution in all patients.

Susceptibility Factors

If it is considered necessary to withdraw ticlopidine before elective surgery, it should be done 1 week in advance (30). In emergencies, desmopressin or fresh platelet concentrates reduce the risk of bleeding.

Drug–Drug Interactions

Carbamazepine

In one patient taking ticlopidine and carbamazepine, serum carbamazepine concentrations rose in association with nervous system toxicity (31).

Omeprazole

In six Japanese CYP2C19 extensive metabolizers, ticlopidine 300 mg/day for 6 days significantly increased the C_{max} of a single oral dose of omeprazole 40 mg and reduced its oral clearance of omeprazole (32). The authors concluded that ticlopidine inhibits CYP2C19 but not, or to a lesser extent, CYP3A4, and that the magnitude of inhibition by ticlopidine is related to the in vivo activity of CYP2C19 before inhibition.

Phenytoin

Several reports have described ticlopidine-induced phenytoin toxicity with increased serum phenytoin concentrations (33–36). Data obtained in vitro using hepatic microsomal preparations have shown that ticlopidine inhibits the activity of CYP2C19 (37).

References

1. Alonso-Martinez JL, Elejalde-Guerra JI, Larrinaga-Linero D. Bronchiolitis obliterans–organizing pneumonia caused by ticlopidine. Ann Intern Med 1998;129(1):71–2.
2. Barak A, Morse LS, Schwab IR. Atypical reginal vasculitis associated with ticlopidine hydrochloridine use. Am J Ophthalmol 2000;129(5):684–5.
3. Editorial. Ticlopidine. Lancet 1991;23:459.
4. Criado A, Juffe A, Carmona J, Otero C, Avello F. Ticlopidine as a hemorrhagic risk factor in coronary surgery. Drug Intell Clin Pharm 1985;19(9):673–6.
5. Sharis PJ, Cannon CP, Loscalzo J. The antiplatelet effects of ticlopidine and clopidogrel. Ann Intern Med 1998;129(5):394–405.
6. Love BB, Biller J, Gent M. Adverse haematological effects of ticlopidine. Prevention, recognition and management. Drug Saf 1998;19(2):89–98.
7. Wysowski DK, Bacsanyi J. Blood dyscrasias and hematologic reactions in ticlopidine users. JAMA 1996;276:952.
8. Haushofer A, Halbmayer WM, Prachar H. Neutropenia with ticlopidine plus aspirin. Lancet 1997;349(9050):474–5.
9. Farver DK, Hansen LA. Delayed neutropenia with ticlopidine. Ann Pharmacother 1994;28(12):1344–6.
10. Gur H, Wartenfeld R, Tanne D, Solomon F, Sidi Y. Ticlopidine-induced severe neutropenia. Postgrad Med J 1998;74(868):126–7.
11. Claas FH, de Fraiture WH, Meyboom RH. Thrombopénie causée par des anticorps induits par la ticlopidine. [Thrombocytopenia due to antibodies induced by ticlopidine.] Nouv Rev Fr Hematol 1984;26(5):323–4.
12. Takishita S, Kawazoe N, Yoshida T, Fukiyama K. Ticlopidine and thrombocytopenia. N Engl J Med 1990;323(21):1487–8.
13. Bennett CL, Kiss JE, Weinberg PD, Pinevich AJ, Green D, Kwaan HC, Feldman MD. Thrombotic thrombocytopenic purpura after stenting and ticlopidine. Lancet 1998;352(9133):1036–7.
14. Muszkat M, Shapira MY, Sviri S, Linton DM, Caraco Y. Ticlopidine-induced thrombotic thrombocytopenic purpura. Pharmacotherapy 1998;18(6):1352–5.

15. Ellie E, Durrieu C, Besse P, Julien J, Gbipki-Benissan G. Thrombotic thrombocytopenic purpura associated with ticlopidine. Stroke 1992;23(6):922–3.

16. Kupfer Y, Tessler S. Ticlopidine and thrombotic thrombocytopenic purpura. N Engl J Med 1997;337(17):1245.

17. Bennett CL, Weinberg PD, Rozenberg-Ben-Dror K, Yarnold PR, Kwaan HC, Green D. Thrombotic thrombocytopenic purpura associated with ticlopidine. A review of 60 cases. Ann Intern Med 1998;128(7):541–4.

18. Steinhubl SR, Tan WA, Foody JM, Topol EJ. Incidence and clinical course of thrombotic thrombocytopenic purpura due to ticlopidine following coronary stenting. EPISTENT Investigators. Evaluation of Platelet IIb/IIIa Inhibitor for Stenting. JAMA 1999;281(9):806–10.

19. Tsai HM, Rice L, Sarode R, Chow TW, Moake JL. Antibody inhibitors to von Willebrand factor metalloproteinase and increased binding of von Willebrand factor to platelets in ticlopidine-associated thrombotic thrombocytopenic purpura. Ann Intern Med 2000;132(10):794–9.

20. Elias M, Reichman N, Flatau E. Bone marrow aplasia associated with ticlopidine therapy. Am J Hematol 1993;44(4):289–90.

21. Lesesve JF, Callat MP, Lenormand B, Monconduit M, Noblet C, Moore N, Caron F, Humbert G, Stamatoullas A, Tilly H. Hematological toxicity of ticlopidine. Am J Hematol 1994;47(2):149–50.

22. Gent M, Blakely JA, Easton JD, Ellis DJ, Hachinski VC, Harbison JW, Panak E, Roberts RS, Sicurella J, Turpie AG. The Canadian American Ticlopidine Study (CATS) in thromboembolic stroke. Lancet 1989;1(8649):1215–20.

23. Mansoor GA, Aziz K. Delayed chronic diarrhea and weight loss possibly due to ticlopidine therapy. Ann Pharmacother 1997;31(7–8):870–2.

24. Martinez Aviles P, Gisbert Moya C, Berbegal Serra J, Lopez Benito I. Colitis linfocitaria inducida por ticlopidina. [Ticlopidine-induced lymphocytic colitis.] Med Clin (Barc) 1996;106(8):317.

25. Swine C, Cornette P, Van Pee D, Delos M, Melange M. Ticlopidine, diarrhée et colite lymphocytaire. [Ticlopidine, diarrhea and lymphocytic colitis.] Gastroenterol Clin Biol 1998;22(4):475–6.

26. Brigot C, Courillon-Mallet A, Roucayrol AM, Cattan D. Colite lymphocytaire et ticlopidine. [Lymphocytic colitis and ticlopidine.] Gastroenterol Clin Biol 1998;22(3):361–2.

27. Martinez Perez-Balsa A, De Arce A, Castiella A, Lopez P, Ruibal M, Ruiz-Martinez J, Lopez De Munain A, Marti Masso JF. Hepatotoxicity due to ticlopidine. Ann Pharmacother 1998;32(11):1250–1.

28. Yosipovitch G, Rechavia E, Feinmesser M, David M. Adverse cutaneous reactions to ticlopidine in patients with coronary stents. J Am Acad Dermatol 1999;41(3 Pt 1):473–6.

29. Braun-Moscovici Y, Schapira D, Balbir-Gurman A, Sevilia R, Menachem Nahir A. Ticlopidine-induced lupus. J Clin Rheumatol 2001;7:102–5.

30. Harder S, Klinkhardt U, Alvarez JM. Avoidance of bleeding during surgery in patients receiving anticoagulant and/or antiplatelet therapy: pharmacokinetic and pharmacodynamic considerations. Clin Pharmacokinet 2004;43(14):963–81.

31. Brown RI, Cooper TG. Ticlopidine–carbamazepine interaction in a coronary stent patient. Can J Cardiol 1997;13(9):853–4.

32. Tateishi T, Kumai T, Watanabe M, Nakura H, Tanaka M, Kobayashi S. Ticlopidine decreases the in vivo activity of CYP2C19 as measured by omeprazole metabolism. Br J Clin Pharmacol 1999;47(4):454–7.

33. Riva R, Cerullo A, Albani F, Baruzzi A. Ticlopidine impairs phenytoin clearance: a case report. Neurology 1996;46(4):1172–3.

34. Privitera M, Welty TE. Acute phenytoin toxicity followed by seizure breakthrough from a ticlopidine–phenytoin interaction. Arch Neurol 1996;53(11):1191–2.

35. Rindone JP, Bryan G 2nd. Phenytoin toxicity associated with ticlopidine administration. Arch Intern Med 1996;156(10):1113.

36. Klaassen SL. Ticlopidine-induced phenytoin toxicity. Ann Pharmacother 1998;32(12):1295–8.

37. Donahue SR, Flockhart DA, Abernethy DR, Ko JW. Ticlopidine inhibition of phenytoin metabolism mediated by potent inhibition of CYP2C19. Clin Pharmacol Ther 1997;62(5):572–7.

Tienilic acid

See also Diuretics

General Information

Tienilic acid, a uricosuric diuretic (1), had to be withdrawn soon after its release in 1980, after it had caused several hundreds of cases of severe liver damage, many of them fatal (SEDA-5, 229). In France almost 500 reports of liver injury were received. Tienilic acid had no advantage over other diuretics; it certainly had the worst benefit:harm balance (SEDA-17, 269). For a time it was considered that the hepatic complication might be geographically limited (for example because of differences in manufacturing in different countries), but there is now no doubt that the drug itself was responsible. The hepatic complication was thoroughly studied in retrospect (SED-11, 424). Other adverse effects, including acute renal insufficiency, urate stones, and interactions with other drugs, such as oral anticoagulants and phenytoin, helped tienilic acid to its early demise.

Reference

1. Maass AR, Snow B, Beg M, Stote RM. Pharmacokinetics and mode of action of tienilic acid. Clin Exp Hypertens A 1982;4(1–2):139–60.

Timegadine

See also Non-steroidal anti-inflammatory drugs

General Information

Timegadine, a guanidine derivative, inhibits cyclo-oxygenase, lipoxygenase, and phospholipase activity. Reported adverse effects are skin rashes, oral lesions, epigastric pain, nausea, dysuria, dizziness, vertigo, and sleep disturbances. Liver enzyme changes and pneumonitis have also been described (1–4).

References

1. Egsmose C, Lund B, Andersen RB. Timegadine: more than a non-steroidal for the treatment of rheumatoid arthritis. A controlled, double-blind study. Scand J Rheumatol 1988;17(2):103–11.
2. Mbuyi-Muamba JM, Dequeker J. A comparative trial of timegadine and D-penicillamine in rheumatoid arthritis. Clin Rheumatol 1983;2(4):369–74.
3. Caruso I, Fumagalli M, Montrone F, Greco M, Boccassini L. Timegadine: long-term open study in rheumatoid arthritis. Clin Rheumatol 1983;2(4):363–7.
4. Berry H, Bloom B, Fernandes L, Morris M. Comparison of timegadine and naproxen in rheumatoid arthritis. A placebo controlled trial. Clin Rheumatol 1983;2(4):357–61.

Timolol

See also Beta-adrenoceptor antagonists

General Information

Timolol is a hydrophilic, non-selective beta-blocker with little partial agonist and membrane-stabilizing activity.

Organs and Systems

Cardiovascular

Of 153 consecutive patients treated with timolol eye-drops, three complained of unexplained falls and two of them had dizziness and blackouts (1). Two had a cardioinhibitory carotid sinus syndrome (a period of asystole greater than 3 seconds after carotid sinus massage) and the third a vasodepressor carotid sinus syndrome (a reduction in systolic blood pressure higher than 50 mmHg after carotid sinus massage). In all three cases, timolol eye-drops were withdrawn. Follow-up carotid sinus massage in the two patients with a cardioinhibitory carotid sinus syndrome was negative, and all reported complete remission of symptoms.

Significant cardiovascular adverse effects have been reported after topical administration of timolol maleate. Bradycardia with frank syncope can occur, especially in elderly patients (2). After topical administration its action begins in 20 minutes, peaks in 4 hours, and lasts 24 hours. Episodes of dizziness and occasional falls can occur 1–2 hours after instillation of timolol, as has been described in an otherwise healthy elderly patient (3).

- An 80-year-old woman with gastrointestinal bleeding had a sinus bradycardia (52/minute) despite acute blood loss. The only drug she had used that was an AV nodal depressant was timolol maleate 0.5%, one drop to both eyes every day. Continuous electrocardiography showed transient complete AV block without ventricular escape for nearly 6 seconds about 1 hour after instillation of timolol eye drops. She also reported having previously had episodes of dizziness and occasional falls 1–2 hours after instillation of her eye drops.

Timolol was withheld and a temporary pacemaker was inserted. Rechallenge with timolol was associated with recurrence of third-degree AV block. She subsequently had a permanent dual chamber pacemaker implanted.

Psychological, psychiatric

Depressive symptoms were reported in 17 of 165 patients after the administration of timolol over two decades (4). Depression accounted for 17% of 369 central nervous system reactions to timolol reported to a National Registry of Drug-induced Ocular Side Effects during 7 years: of these, 20 cases were of acute suicidal depression.

Long-Term Effects

Tumorigenicity

The development of liver tumors in mice and an increased incidence of mammary fibroadenomata in female rats at one time caused concern in the USA, although animal studies elsewhere and clinical studies have shown no evidence of tumor-forming potential.

Drug–Drug Interactions

Brimonidine

The effects of topical brimonidine and timolol have been compared in two trials in 926 subjects with glaucoma or ocular hypertension already using systemic beta-blockers (5). Concurrent systemic beta-blocker therapy had no deleterious effects on ocular hypotensive efficacy and no impact on safety with topical brimonidine, but the combination of timolol and brimonidine significantly reduced systolic and diastolic blood pressures and heart rate compared with brimonidine alone. This observation suggests that ocular hypotensive agents other than beta-blockers, such as brimonidine, may be appropriate as a first-choice therapy for glaucoma in patients concurrently taking systemic beta-blockers.

References

1. Mulcahy R, Allcock L, O'Shea D. Timolol, carotid sinus hypersensitivity, and elderly patients. Lancet 1998;352(9134):1147–8.
2. Frishman WH, Kowalski M, Nagnur S, Warshafsky S, Sica D. Cardiovascular considerations in using topical, oral, and intravenous drugs for the treatment of glaucoma and ocular hypertension: focus on beta-adrenergic blockade. Heart Dis 2001;3(6):386–97.
3. Sharifi M, Koch JM, Steele RJ, Adler D, Pompili VJ, Sopko J. Third degree AV block due to ophthalmic timilol solution. Int J Cardiol 2001;80(2–3):257–9.
4. Schweitzer I, Maguire K, Tuckwell V. Antiglaucoma medication and clinical depression. Aust NZ J Psychiatry 2001;35(5):569–71.
5. Schuman JS. Effects of systemic beta-blocker therapy on the efficacy and safety of topical brimonidine and timolol. Brimonidine Study Groups 1 and 2. Ophthalmology 2000;107(6):1171–17.

Tinidazole

General Information

The adverse effects of tinidazole resemble those of metronidazole. It can be given intravenously and is well tolerated, although thrombophlebitis has been reported. In one healthy volunteer, fainting with low blood pressure and nausea and tiredness for several hours was reported (SEDA-11, 597) (1).

Organs and Systems

Gastrointestinal

Drug-induced esophagitis is rare, accounting for about 1% of all cases of esophagitis. An incidence of 3.9 in 100 000 has been reported. After the first description, there have been more than 250 observations, with more than 50 different drugs. Among those, the principal antibiotics included tetracyclines (doxycycline, metacycline, minocycline, oxytetracycline, and tetracycline), penicillins (amoxicillin, cloxacillin, penicillin V, and pivmecillinam), clindamycin, co-trimoxazole, erythromycin, lincomycin, spiramycin, and tinidazole. Doxycycline alone was involved in one-third of all cases. Risk factors included prolonged esophageal passage, due to motility disorders, stenosis, cardiomegaly, the formulation, supine position during drug ingestion, and failure to use liquid to wash down the tablet. Direct toxic effects of the drug (pH, accumulation in epithelial cells, non-uniform dispersion) also seem to contribute to the development of drug-induced esophagitis (2).

Skin

Skin reactions can occasionally occur in patients taking tinidazole.

- A fixed eruption with pruritus was observed in a 27-year-old man treated for *Entamoeba histolytica* with tinidazole 500 mg, four tablets in a single dose for 3 days.
- An erythematous patch with a sensation of burning appeared over the left buttock in a 32-year-old man while he was taking tinidazole for giardiasis; the allergic lesion was provoked by a challenge dose.

Both of these patients reacted with the same skin reaction on rechallenge with metronidazole (SEDA-16, 310).

In a patient with a fixed drug eruption to metronidazole, a provocation test showed cross-reactivity with tinidazole but not with secnidazole (3).

References

1. Aase S, Olsen AK, Roland M, Fagerhol MK, Liavag I, Bergan T, Leinebo O. Severe toxic reaction to tinidazole. Eur J Clin Pharmacol 1983;24(3):425–7.
2. Zerbib F. Les oesophagites médicamenteuses. Hepato-Gastro 1998;5:115–20.

3. Thami GP, Kanwar AJ. Fixed drug eruption due to metronidazole and tinidazole without cross-sensitivity to secnidazole. Dermatology 1998;196(3):368.

Tioguanine

See also Cytostatic and immunosuppressant drugs

General Information

Tioguanine is an analogue of the physiological purines, guanine and hypoxanthine, and is a purine antimetabolite. It is incorporated into DNA and RNA, resulting in a variety of cytotoxic effects. It has been used to treat hematological malignancies, psoriasis, and more recently, inflammatory bowel disease, such as Crohn's disease. Its main adverse effects are liver damage and hemotoxicity.

Among 111 patients taking tioguanine for inflammatory bowel disease, 29 had laboratory abnormalities, most commonly rises in liver enzymes and reduced platelet counts (1). Of the patients who underwent liver biopsy, there was nodular regenerative hyperplasia in 76% of those with laboratory abnormalities and 33% of those without.

Organs and Systems

Hematologic

Tioguanine can cause blood dyscrasias, in particular thrombocytopenia (2).

In 23 children taking tioguanine and a matched group taking mercaptopurine, there was no difference in the pattern of anemia or neutropenia between the two groups, but dose-limiting thrombocytopenia was more common in those taking tioguanine, four of whom had a fall in platelet count to below 20×10^9/l compared with only one taking mercaptopurine (3).

Liver

Nodular regenerative hyperplasia of the liver has been reported in three patients with inflammatory bowel disease who had taken tioguanine for more than a year and who had raised serum liver enzymes; all three had histological foci of nodular regenerative hyperplasia, which was best seen with reticulin silver impregnation (4).

The United Kingdom Medical Research Council Chronic Myeloid Leukemia Group reported 18 cases of tioguanine-induced non-cirrhotic portal hypertension, commonly associated with deterioration in liver function (5).

A patient developed acute sinusoidal obstruction syndrome after taking tioguanine for 14 months for Crohn's disease (6).

- A patient with acute myeloblastic leukemia, who took tioguanine for 2 months, developed severe peliosis hepatis associated with mild lesions of the centrilobular veins; withdrawal was followed by progressive improvement of liver dysfunction (7).

Several cases of hepatic veno-occlusive disease have been reported (8–11).

- A 23-year-old man with acute lymphocytic leukemia took tioguanine for 10 months and developed intense sinusoidal engorgement which resolved on withdrawal with some residual subintimal fibrosis around the terminal hepatic veins (12).

Of 12 patients aged 3–10 years, who had taken tioguanine 25–77 mg/m^2/day for acute lymphoblastic leukemia, one had persistent pancytopenia and intermittent splenomegaly. MRI/MRA scans showed a dilated splenic vein and collaterals, consistent with portal hypertension; esophagoscopy showed esophageal varices (13). A liver biopsy showed periportal fibrosis and marked dilatation of veins and venules. Of the other 12 patients, nine had abnormal MRI/MRA scans with evidence of varices in four. Liver biopsies in two cases showed periportal fibrosis, dilatation of venules and sinusoids, and minimal focal fatty changes.

References

1. Dubinsky MC, Vasiliauskas EA, Singh H, Abreu MT, Papadakis KA, Tran T, Martin P, Vierling JM, Geller SA, Targan SR, Poordad FF. 6-thioguanine can cause serious liver injury in inflammatory bowel disease patients. Gastroenterology 2003;125(2):298–303.
2. Wenzl HH, Hogenauer C, Fickert P, Petritsch W. Thioguanine-induced symptomatic thrombocytopenia. Am J Gastroenterol 2004;99(6):1195.
3. Lancaster DL, Lennard L, Rowland K, Vora AJ, Lilleyman JS. Thioguanine versus mercaptopurine for therapy of childhood lymphoblastic leukaemia: a comparison of haematological toxicity and drug metabolite concentrations. Br J Haematol 1998;102(2):439–43.
4. Shastri S, Dubinsky MC, Fred Poordad F, Vasiliauskas EA, Geller SA. Early nodular hyperplasia of the liver occurring with inflammatory bowel diseases in association with thioguanine therapy. Arch Pathol Lab Med 2004;128(1):49–53.
5. Shepherd PC, Fooks J, Gray R, Allan NC. Thioguanine used in maintenance therapy of chronic myeloid leukaemia causes non-cirrhotic portal hypertension. Results from MRC CML. II. Trial comparing busulphan with busulphan and thioguanine. Br J Haematol 1991;79(2):185–92.
6. Kane S, Cohen SM, Hart J. Acute sinusoidal obstruction syndrome after 6-thioguanine therapy for Crohn's disease. Inflamm Bowel Dis 2004;10(5):652–4.
7. Larrey D, Freneaux E, Berson A, Babany G, Degott C, Valla D, Pessayre D, Benhamou JP. Peliosis hepatis induced by 6-thioguanine administration. Gut 1988;29(9):1265–9.
8. Krivoy N, Raz R, Carter A, Alroy G. Reversible hepatic veno-occlusive disease and 6-thioguanine. Ann Intern Med 1982;96(6 Pt 1):788.
9. Satti MB, Weinbren K, Gordon-Smith EC. 6-thioguanine as a cause of toxic veno-occlusive disease of the liver. J Clin Pathol 1982;35(10):1086–91.
10. Kao NL, Rosenblate HJ. 6-Thioguanine therapy for psoriasis causing toxic hepatic venoocclusive disease. J Am Acad Dermatol 1993;28(6):1017–18.
11. Romagosa R, Kerdel F, Shah N. Treatment of psoriasis with 6-thioguanine and hepatic venoocclusive disease. J Am Acad Dermatol 2002;47(6):970–2.
12. Gill RA, Onstad GR, Cardamone JM, Maneval DC, Sumner HW. Hepatic veno-occlusive disease caused by 6-thioguanine. Ann Intern Med 1982;96(1):58–60.
13. Broxson EH, Dole M, Wong R, Laya BF, Stork L. Portal hypertension develops in a subset of children with standard-risk acute lymphoblastic leukemia treated with oral 6-thioguanine during maintenance therapy. Pediatr Blood Cancer 2005;44(3):226–31.

Tiopronin

General Information

Tiopronin has been extensively used as an antirheumatic drug in France and Japan. Adverse effects occur in about 45% of patients and led to withdrawal in about one-fifth.

Observational studies

In 140 patients with classic or definite rheumatoid polyarthritis treated with tiopronin 1 g/day over a mean duration of 1 year and retrospectively studied, adverse effects occurred in 55% and required withdrawal in 40% (1). These effects occurred during the first 6 months of treatment in 75% of cases. They mainly affected the skin and mucosae: in 46 cases (33%) treatment was withdrawn because of stomatitis, pruritus, various types of erythema, and pemphigus (1 case). There was renal insufficiency in 14 patients (10%) requiring withdrawal in eight cases (5.7%) because of nephrotic syndrome ($n = 3$) or proteinuria ($n = 5$). There were hematological disorders in 13 (9.2%), justifying withdrawal in 10 cases (7.1%) because of thrombocytopenia or leukopenia. The other adverse effects included digestive disorders ($n = 15$), requiring withdrawal in three, and ageusia ($n = 6$), requiring withdrawal in one case.

Comparative studies

In 69 patients with rheumatoid arthritis, tiopronin 1500 mg/day was as effective as penicillamine (2). The adverse effects of the two drugs were similar. Tiopronin was associated with obstructive bronchiolitis in one case. There was little cross-intolerance: the same unwanted effect was only observed in four cases; one of pemphigus, one of toxic dermatitis, and two instances of proteinuria.

In 66 patients with cystinuria, adverse reactions to tiopronin (mean dose 1193 mg/day) were common, and occurred in 76% of the patients with a history of D-penicillamine treatment and 65% of those without a history of D-penicillamine treatment, compared with 84% who had adverse effects with D-penicillamine (3). Serious adverse reactions requiring drug withdrawal were less common with tiopronin. Among the patients who took both drugs 31% had to stop taking tiopronin, whereas 69% could not tolerate D-penicillamine.

General adverse effects

Tiopronin has a roughly similar pattern of adverse effects to that of penicillamine (1–6), including rashes, toxic dermatitis, ageusia, and proteinuria; these effects resolve on withdrawal (6). If a patient has an adverse reaction to D-penicillamine, the risk of that adverse reaction to tiopronin is only slightly increased.

Organs and Systems

Sensory systems

Tiopronin can cause impaired taste and ageusia (6).

Endocrine

Autoimmune hypoglycemia with anti-insulin antibodies, a complication of penicillamine and pyritinol, has also been reported with tiopronin (7).

- Autoimmune hypoglycemia occurred in a 49-year-old woman with regular menstrual periods accompanied by marked enlargement of the breasts, and was probably induced by tiopronin (8). Her breasts were red and painful; histological examination showed extensive lymphocytic inflammation and edema in the connective tissue. She recovered after stopping tiopronin and taking danazol.

Hematologic

Hematological reactions, such as thrombocytopenia and leukopenia, occur in about 6–9% of patients using tiopronin (1,5).

- Aplastic anemia with fever and pancytopenia developed in a 29-year-old woman, probably as a reaction to tiopronin (500 mg/day), which she had taken for 71 days for seronegative rheumatoid arthritis (9). A bone marrow examination confirmed acute marrow aplasia. She recovered within 5 weeks after withdrawal.

Another detailed case report described profound granulocytopenia, probably caused by tiopronin (10).

Gastrointestinal

Gastrointestinal adverse effects of tiopronin include nausea, vomiting, oral ulcers, and stomatitis (1–3,5,6).

Liver

Of 140 patients taking tiopronin, three had cholestasis (1). A detailed report described liver injury, with steatosis, intrahepatic cholestasis, and centrilobular inflammation, in association with tiopronin (11). In another patient cholestatic hepatitis plus toxic epidermal necrolysis developed in suspected association with tiopronin (12).

Urinary tract

Some degree of renal damage occurs in about 10% of patients taking tiopronin (1–3,5,6). As with penicillamine, proteinuria can progress to nephrotic syndrome (13,14). Biopsy may show minimal change membranous glomerulonephritis and granular depositions of IgG and C3 (13,15).

In a comparison of tiopronin and penicillamine in the treatment of cystinuria in 15 children, nephrotic syndrome developed in one of the patients taking tiopronin; no further details were given (16).

Skin

Cutaneous or mucous reactions occur in about 15–30% of patients using tiopronin. Alopecia, erythema, eczema, cutaneous vasculitis, lichenoid eruptions, skin wrinkling, or a perforating elastoma can develop (1–3,5,6).

There have been several cases of tiopronin-induced pemphigus, characterized by intra-epidermal bullae with acantholysis and epidermal intercellular deposition of IgG and C3 (17,18). The eruption can present as multiple red crusted macules. One patient first had pemphigus in association with penicillamine and later had a relapse while taking tiopronin (19). In skin explant cultures, tiopronin can cause acantholysis with intra-epidermal splits and bulla formation (20).

In a patient with a tiopronin-associated lichenoid skin eruption, the rash was associated with alopecia (21). In another report of a lichenoid eruption, positive rechallenge confirmed the role of tiopronin (22).

In four patients with pluriform skin eruptions in association with tiopronin, the pathological findings were characteristic of a graft-versus-host reaction (23).

In one patient, cholestatic hepatitis plus toxic epidermal necrolysis developed in suspected association with tiopronin (12).

Musculoskeletal

There have been a few cases of myasthenia gravis in association with tiopronin (24,25).

Immunologic

Tiopronin can cause fever, with or without a rash (3). In a patient with a prior hypersensitivity reaction to penicillamine, there was no cross-hypersensitivity to tiopronin (26).

Tiopronin has occasionally been described as a cause of polymyositis (27,28).

- A 62-year-old woman with rheumatoid arthritis, hypothyroidism, and hypertension, treated for 6 years with tiopronin (dosage not specified), developed severe polymyositis. She had dysphagia and muscle weakness and pain in all limbs; there were no skin abnormalities. Her creatine kinase activity was 12 000 U/l (reference range 25–160) and her LDH 23 000 U/l (240–480). Her C-reactive protein was 58 µg/ml and the erythrocyte sedimentation rate 42 mm/hour (both raised). Electromyography of her proximal and distal muscles showed pseudomyotonic fibrillations. A biopsy of the deltoid muscle showed necrosis of muscle fibers and interstitial mononuclear infiltrates. There was no evidence of a paraneoplastic syndrome. Tests for toxoplasmosis, trichinosis, picornavirus, HIV, and hepatitis A, B, and C were negative, and there were no autoantibodies (anti-Jo, anti-KU, anti-PM/SCL, anti-DNA, anti-SSA, anti-SSB, anti-ECT, antithyroid, rheumatoid factor, or cryoglobulins), although ANF was positive on one occasion (1/100). Tiopronin was withdrawn, she was given glucocorticoids and methotrexate, and made a good recovery.

References

1. Sany J, Combe B, Verdie-Petibon D, Tagemouati A, Daures JP. Etude de la tolérance á long terme de la thiopronine (Acadione) A propos de 140 cas personnels. dans le traitement de la polyarthrite rhumatoïde. [Long-term tolerability of tiopronin (Acadione) in the treatment of rheumatoid arthritis. Apropos of 140 personal cases.] Rev Rhum Mal Osteoartic 1990;57(2):105–11.

2. Sigaud M, Maugars Y, Maisonneuve H, Prost A. Tiopronine dans 69 cas de polyarthrite rhumatoïde traités antérieurement par la D-pénicillamine. [Tiopronin in 69 cases of rheumatoid polyarthritis treated earlier with D-penicillamine.] Rev Rhum Mal Osteoartic 1988;55(6):467–71.

3. Pak CY, Fuller C, Sakhaee K, Zerwekh JE, Adams BV. Management of cystine nephrolithiasis with alpha-mercaptopropionylglycine. J Urol 1986;136(5):1003–8.

4. Jaffe IA. Adverse effects profile of sulfhydryl compounds in man. Am J Med 1986;80(3):471–6.

5. Ehrhart A, Chicault P, Fauquert P, Le Goff P. Effets secondaires dus au traitement par la tiopronine de 74 polyarthrites rhumatoïdes. [Side-effects of treatment of 74 rheumatoid polyarthritis with tiopronin.] Rev Rhum Mal Osteoartic 1991;58(3):193–7.

6. Amor B, Mery C, de Gery A. L'acadione, un nouveau traitement de fond de la polyarthrite rhumatoïde. [Acadione, a new long-term treatment of rheumatoid polyarthritis.] Rev Rhum Mal Osteoartic 1988;55(6):462–6.

7. Faguer de Moustier B, Burgard M, Boitard C, Desplanque N, Fanjoux J, Tchobroutsky G. Syndrome hypoglycémique auto-immune induit par le pyritinol. [Auto-immune hypoglycemic syndrome induced by pyritinol.] Diabete Metab 1988;14(4):423–9.

8. Gregoir C, Hilliquin P, Acar F, Lessana-Leibowitch M, Renoux M, Menkes CJ. Mastite aiguë au cours d'une polyarthrite rhumatoïde avec syndrome de Gougerot–Sjögren traitée par tiopronine (acadione). [Acute mastitis in rheumatoid polyarthritis with Gougerot–Sjögren syndrome treated with tiopronin (Acadione).] Rev Rhum Mal Osteoartic 1991;58(3):203–6.

9. Taillan B, Nectoux F, Vinti H, Fuzibet JG, Verdier JM, Dujardin P, Chichmanian RM, Vitetta A. Aplasie médullaire au cours d'une polyarthrite rhumatoïde traitée par tiopronine. [Bone marrow aplasia in rheumatoid polyarthritis treated with tiopronin.] Rev Rhum Mal Osteoartic 1990;57(5):443–4.

10. Corda C, Tavernier C, Oriol P, Sgro C, Escousse A, Strauss J. Tiopronin-induced agranulocytosis. Therapie 1990;45(2):161.

11. Mori T, Ohta M, Nakagawa Y, Hayashi K, Sobajima J, Okuda M, Mochi T, Shimamoto K, Kagawa K, Okanoue T, Kashima K. A case report of non-alcoholic steatohepatitis associated with tiopronin-induced liver injury. Acta Hepatol Jpn 1990;31:449–53.

12. Matsueda K, Matsuoka Y, Mizuno M, et al. A case of drug-induced toxic epidermal necrolysis complicated with severe liver injury. Acta Hepatol Jpn 1988;29:949–55.

13. Lindell A, Denneberg T, Enestrom S, Fich C, Skogh T. Membranous glomerulonephritis induced by 2-mercaptopropionylglycine (2-MPG). Clin Nephrol 1990;34(3):108–15.

14. Shibasaki T, Murai S, Kodama K, Nakano H, Ishimoto F, Sakai O. A case of nephrotic syndrome due to alpha-mercaptopropionyl glycine in a patient with familial cystinuria. Nippon Jinzo Gakkai Shi 1990;32(8):933–7.

15. Azar R, Mercier D, Codaccioni MX. Néphropathie a lésions glomérulaires minimes secondaire a un traitement par la triopronine. Semin Hop 1992;68:209–10.

16. Asanuma H, Nakai H, Takeda M, Shishido S, Kawamura T, Nagakura K, Yamafuji M. [Clinical study on cystinuria in children—the stone management and the prevention of calculi recurrence.] Nippon Hinyokika Gakkai Zasshi 1998;89(9):758–65.

17. Ohno S, Fujita M, Miyachi Y. Tiopronine-induced pemphigus-like lesions. 532–7.

18. Meunier L, Combes B, Marck Y, Barneon G, Sany J, Meynadier J. Pemphigus induit par l'alpha-mercaptopropionylglycine (Acadione). [Pemphigus induced by alphamercaptopropionylglycine (Acadione).] Ann Dermatol Venereol 1990;117(12):959–61.

19. Meunier L, Krause E, Guillot B, Barneon G, Sany J, Meynadier J. Pemphigus induit par l'alpha-mercaptopropionylglycine. [Pemphigus induced by alpha-mercaptopropionylglycine.] Presse Méd 1988;17(13):647.

20. Ruocco V, de Angelis E, Lombardi ML, Pisani M. In vitro acantholysis by captopril and thiopronine. Dermatologica 1988;176(3):115–23.

21. Kawabe Y, Mizuno N, Yoshikawa K, Matsumoto Y. Lichenoid eruption due to mercaptopropionylglycine. J Dermatol 1988;15(5):434–9.

22. Kurumaji Y, Miyazaki K. Tiopronin-induced lichenoid eruption in a patient with liver disease and positive patch test reaction to drugs with sulfhydryl group. J Dermatol 1990;17(3):176–81.

23. Kitamura K, Aihara M, Osawa J, Naito S, Ikezawa Z. Sulfhydryl drug-induced eruption: a clinical and histological study. J Dermatol 1990;17(1):44–51.

24. Menkes CJ, Job-Deslandre C, Bauer-Vinassac D, Rouillon A, Rousseau R. Myasthénie induite par la tiopronine au cours du traitement de la polyarthrite rhumatoïde. [Myasthenia caused by tiopronin during treatment of rheumatoid polyarthritis.] Presse Méd 1988;17(22):1156–7.

25. Arfi S, Caplanne D, Jean-Baptiste G, Habault Ch, Panelatti G, Vernant JC. Myasthénie induite par la tiopronine au cours du traitement d'une polyarthrite rhumatoïde. Bull SMNFI 1991;12:489.

26. Matsukawa Y, Saito N, Nishinarita S, Horie T, Ryu J. Therapeutic effect of tiopronin following D-penicillamine toxicity in a patient with rheumatoid arthritis. Clin Rheumatol 1998;17(1):73–4.

27. Koeger AC, Rozenberg S, Chaibi P, Camus JP, Bourgeois P. Polymyosite induite par la tiopronine, confirmée par l'histologie. [Tiopronin-induced polymyositis confirmed by histology.] Rev Rhum Ed Fr 1993;60(1):78–9.

28. Cacoub P, Sbai A, Azizi P, Gatfosse M, Godeau P, Piette JC. Polymyosite induite par la tiopronine. [Polymyositis induced by tiopronine.] Presse Méd 1999;28(17):911–12.

Tiotixene

See also Neuroleptic drugs

General Information

Tiotixene is a thioxanthene neuroleptic drug.

Organs and Systems

Nervous system

Neuroleptic malignant syndrome has been reported as a severe complication of tiotixene (SEDA-21, 49).

- A 42-year-old man with a history of paranoid schizophrenia developed confusion and emesis. His medications included buspirone and tiotixene. He also had a generalized seizure that resolved spontaneously. His serum sodium concentration was 114 mmol/l, which was thought to be secondary to psychogenic polydipsia and which was corrected. The next day his temperature rose to 40°C and the day after that he became lethargic and non-verbal and developed generalized muscle rigidity. A diagnosis of probable neuroleptic malignant syndrome was made, and he was given dantrolene sodium 1 mg/kg intravenously; neuroleptic drugs were withdrawn. The serum creatine kinase activity was over 234 500 U/l. Urinalysis showed more than 3 g/l of protein, a trace of ketones, and hemoglobin and leukocytes. By the following day, his muscle rigidity and fever had resolved and his mental status was markedly improved.

Skin

Cutaneous lesions consisting of telangiectatic macules have been reported with tiotixene (1).

Reference

1. Matsuoka LY. Thiothixene drug sensitivity. J Am Acad Dermatol 1982;7(3):405.

Tiotropium bromide

See also Anticholinergic drugs

General Information

Tiotropium bromide is a long-acting anticholinergic bronchodilator that binds with similar affinity to the three muscarinic receptor subtypes (SEDA-20, 190) (1). However, it dissociates more slowly from M_1 and M_3 receptors in bronchial smooth muscle than from M_2 receptors (1). This results in a long half-life of the bound complex, allowing once-daily administration.

Tiotropium is inhaled from the HandiHaler, a dry-powder, breath-activated inhaler system that delivers particles to the lung over a wide range of airflow limitations in patients with chronic obstructive pulmonary disease (COPD); it can be effectively delivered at inspiratory flow rates as low as 20 l/minute (2). Pharmacodynamic steady-state studies have shown that most of the bronchodilator activity is achieved with one to two doses within 48 hours, although a carryover effect on forced vital capacity was observed beyond 48 hours (3).

The efficacy and safety of tiotropium have been studied in vitro and in early clinical trials, and dose-ranging studies have shown that tiotropium dry powder 18 micrograms/day is safe and efficacious (1,4,5). Since the quaternary structure of tiotropium limits its absorption through the mucous membrane of the respiratory and gastrointestinal tract, systemic adverse effects are in general minimal.

Therapeutic studies

Placebo-controlled studies

In repeated dose studies of 4.5, 9, 18, and 36 micrograms od for 28 days, in 169 patients with COPD, each dose was significantly more effective than placebo, as shown by increased effects with increasing dose on FEV_1 and peak expiratory flow. At doses of 9 micrograms and above there were detectable concentrations of the drug at peak (5 minutes after inhalation), but a trough plasma concentration was only measurable with the 36 micrograms dose. At the highest dose, three of 34 patients reported a dry mouth compared with none of 35 patients taking placebo. This preliminary study suggests that the anticholinergic activity of tiotropium will cause some systemic adverse effects at high doses.

In a randomized, double-blind study, 470 patients with stable COPD (mean FEV_1 38.6% predicted) received tiotropium 18 micrograms or placebo as a once-daily medication via a lactose-based dry-powder inhaler device (6). Spirometry was measured on days 1 and 8 and at regular intervals for 3 months. Tiotropium produced significant improvements in trough FEV_1 and FVC (measured immediately before the next dose), averaging 12% greater than baseline on day 8. The bronchodilatation resulting from tiotropium did not diminish over the 3 months of the study. Upper respiratory tract infections were reported in 15% of the patients in each of the treatment groups and exacerbations of COPD were reported in 22% of patients taking placebo and 16% of patients taking tiotropium. Dry mouth was significantly more common with tiotropium (9.3 versus 1.6%). There was a 6.8% incidence of serious adverse events or events leading to withdrawal (2.5% with tiotropium and 5.8% with placebo). A patient with a long history of cardiovascular disease, who was randomized to receive tiotropium, was found dead and was suspected to have died of a cardiac dysrhythmia. There were no differences in electrocardiograms between the treatment groups or changes in laboratory values.

In a multicenter, double-blind, placebo-controlled trial in patients with stable COPD, tiotropium 18 micrograms/day for 1 year ($n = 550$) significantly improved lung function (mean trough FEV_1, FVC, PEFR) and reduced dyspnea compared with placebo ($n = 371$) (7). Moreover, tiotropium recipients had better health status scores, fewer exacerbations of COPD, and fewer hospitalizations. There was no evidence of tachyphylaxis over one year.

Comparative studies

In a randomized, double-blind trial tiotropium 18 micrograms/day for 1 year ($n = 356$) was compared with ipratropium 160 micrograms/day ($n = 179$) in patients with COPD (8). Tiotropium maintained superior efficacy (FEV_1 and FVC) throughout the study, improved dyspnea, and reduced the number of exacerbations by 24%.

In a placebo-controlled, double-blind study, tiotropium 18 micrograms/day for 6 months ($n = 209$) was compared with salmeterol 50 micrograms bd ($n = 213$) and placebo ($n = 201$) in 623 patients with moderate to severe COPD

(8). Tiotropium improved dyspnea and trough FEV_1 and FVC significantly more than salmeterol. The patients who used tiotropium had better quality-of-life scores than those who used salmeterol, but the difference was not statistically significant.

Organs and Systems

Mouth and teeth

In placebo-controlled studies adverse events were comparable to those with placebo, except for dry mouth, which was reported in 10–16% of patients (1,7,8).

References

1. Disse B, Speck GA, Rominger KL, Witek TJ Jr, Hammer R. Tiotropium (Spiriva): mechanistical considerations and clinical profile in obstructive lung disease. Life Sci 1999;64(6–7):457–64.
2. van Noord JA, Smeets JJ, Custers FL, Korducki L, Cornelissen PJ. Pharmacodynamic steady state of tiotropium in patients with chronic obstructive pulmonary disease. Eur Respir J 2002;19(4):639–44.
3. Casaburi R, Mahler DA, Jones PW, Wanner A, San PG, ZuWallack RL, Menjoge SS, Serby CW, Witek T Jr. A long-term evaluation of once-daily inhaled tiotropium in chronic obstructive pulmonary disease. Eur Respir J 2002;19(2):217–24.
4. Beeh KM, Welte T, Buhl R. Anticholinergics in the treatment of chronic obstructive pulmonary disease. Respiration 2002;69(4):372–9.
5. Chodosh S, Flanders JS, Kesten S, Serby CW, Hochrainer D, Witek TJ Jr. Effective delivery of particles with the HandiHaler dry powder inhalation system over a range of chronic obstructive pulmonary disease severity. J Aerosol Med 2001;14(3):309–15.
6. Casaburi R, Briggs DD Jr, Donohue JF, Serby CW, Menjoge SS, Witek TJ Jr. The spirometric efficacy of once-daily dosing with tiotropium in stable COPD: a 13-week multicenter trial. The US Tiotropium Study Group. Chest 2000;118(5):1294–302.
7. Vincken W, van Noord JA, Greefhorst AP, Bantje TA, Kesten S, Korducki L, Cornelissen PJ, Van de Bosch JMM, Bunnik MCM, Creemers JPHM, Dalinghaus WH, Eland ME, Evers WBM, Gans SJM, Gooszen Hch, Van Harreveld AJ, Van Kasteren JHLM, Kuipers AF, Nossent GD, Pannekoek BJM, Pasma HR, Peters A, Pieters WR, Postmus PE, Schreurs AJM, Sinninghe Damste HEJ, Sips AP, Van Spiegel PI, Westbroek J, Aumann JL, Janssens E, Pauwels R, Radermecker M, Slabbynck H, Stappaerts I, Verhaert J, Vermeire P; Dutch/Belgian Tiotropium Study Group. Improved health outcomes in patients with COPD during 1 yr's treatment with tiotropium. Eur Respir J 2002;19(2):209–16.
8. Donohue JF, van Noord JA, Bateman ED, Langley SJ, Lee A, Witek TJ Jr, Kesten S, Towse L. A 6-month, placebo-controlled study comparing lung function and health status changes in COPD patients treated with tiotropium or salmeterol. Chest 2002;122(1):47–55.

Titanium

General Information

Titanium is a strong, light, metallic element (symbol Ti; atomic no. 22) that is mostly found as oxides in minerals such as anatase, brookite, ilmenite, rutile, and sphene, and also as the antimonate in lewisite.

Titanium is used in medicine mainly for its mechanical benefits in surgical and dental materials in a host of orthopedic and orthodontic appliances, with or without other metals (for example nickel, cobalt, chromium), and generally without serious adverse effects. Titanium and its alloys are in use as implants in bone surgery (1,2) and in dental materials (3,4). Research on the biocompatibility of metal and tissue continues (5).

Titanium is also a constituent of some anticancer compounds (6). Titanium dioxide is used in sunscreens. Non-therapeutic exposure to the metal also occurs.

Titanium in metal implants and prostheses

Titanium is very biocompatible (7). Complications from the use of metal implants and prostheses can arise because of biochemical and histological reactions to some of the materials used (SEDA-22, 250). These include titanium, stainless steel (10–14% nickel, 17–20% chromium), and cobalt chrome alloys (27–30% chromium, 57–68% cobalt, and up to 2.5% nickel). All of these metals can produce sensitization or elicit toxic reactions when they are solubilized and come into contact with tissues; it can be difficult or even impossible to differentiate between hypersensitivity and toxic reactions.

Metals from prostheses can continue to be released into the system for many years. The development of hypersensitivity takes time, and allergic reactions are usually delayed for weeks, months, or 1–2 years. The symptoms can assume a variety of forms. Local reactions can cause loosening of the device or local pain. Dermatological reactions include eczema, bullous pemphigoid, urticaria, and "muscle tumors."

Attempts continue to predict metal sensitivity in the individual patient so that the choice of material can be made accordingly. In vitro tests for metal allergies have been developed on the basis of lymphokine (MIF) release from sensitized T lymphocytes exposed to metal-protein complexes (8). About 6% of patients without a previous metal implant had positive reactions to nickel, chromium, or cobalt. However, it is still not clear whether such a positive reaction is a reliable predictor of clinical problems. In practice few patients have either local or systemic reactions; when symptoms occur and other causes are ruled out, the implant should be removed. Some workers recommend removal of an implant whenever there is both a positive MIF test and a positive skin test, even in the current absence of a serious reaction. Allergic dermatitis will clear up as soon as the metal has begun to be cleared from the tissue. The type of metal and the amount released into the tissue will affect the time taken for the disappearance of toxic dermatological phenomena.

Of 120 consecutive patients (66 women, 54 men; mean age 66 years) with 126 prostheses inserted between March and December 1989, who were followed prospectively both clinically and radiologically for a mean of 9.1 years (9), 40 (41 hips) died, 9 (9 hips) were interviewed by telephone, and 71 (76 hips) were available for follow-up. Four hips had been revised, two of them because of aseptic loosening of the femoral component, one because of a late infection—all after 9 years—and one because of a periprosthetic fracture after 6 years. The 9-year survival was 97% and for aseptic loosening of the stem 98%. None of the cups had to be revised for aseptic loosening. The result was excellent or good in 88%, moderate in 8%, and poor in 4%. Radiological analysis showed no osteolysis or radiolucent lines in 59 prostheses (78%). Nine stems (12%) showed a radiolucent line. Focal osteolysis was detected in eight cases (10%) in one or more Gruen zones. The distribution of the osteolytic areas showed that zones II, V, VI, and VII were predominantly affected in increasing frequency. There was no osteolysis on the acetabular side. These results do not confirm the high rate of osteolysis and revisions with the Muller titanium alloy Straight Stem used in some other institutions.

Organs and Systems

Skin

Titanium tetrachloride ($TiCl_4$) is an intermediate compound in the production of white pigment, which can cause severe chemical burns (10). In two reported cases titanium tetrachloride caused 18–20% total body surface area burns, as a combined consequence of hydrochloric acid and the heat that was generated in areas in which this otherwise stable compound was mixed with sweat. Titanium tetrachloride combined with water is extremely dangerous, and its immediate treatment (towel drying before irrigation) makes it unique among chemicals. The experience of the authors suggested that in most cases grafting will be required. These chemical burns were self-limiting and had no notable systemic sequelae. Wound biopsy specimens were taken on days 3 and 6 and the burns were subjected to immunostaining, which showed that titanium tetrachloride did not retard wound healing. The exposure time to titanium tetrachloride vapor will determine the pulmonary and ophthalmological effects in each case. Clinical awareness of the propensity of titanium tetrachloride to react with water—even in the form of sweat—is vital, because prompt management can limit the extent of injury.

Exacerbation of atopic dermatitis has been attributed to titanium clips (11).

- A 28-year-old woman with breast cancer underwent breast conservation, and three titanium clips were placed at the margin of the excision cavity, followed 2 months later by rapid exacerbation of her atopic dermatitis. The skin lesions developed progressively and involved the whole body. Patch tests and lymphocyte stimulation tests could not be performed, owing to the severity of the skin lesions. Various drugs were suspected, but the results of a bidigital O-ring test suggested an allergic reaction to titanium clips. She underwent a second operation to remove the titanium clips under local anesthesia. By 12 months after surgery, the atopic dermatitis had not completely resolved.

A contact allergic reaction has been reported in three individuals of a group of 23 volunteers who participated in a study with topically applied ammonium titanium lactate 10% (12).

Immunologic

Allergic reactions to titanium can occur (13). Inflammatory reactions and contact sensitivity have been reported after insertion of titanium implants. Osseointegration of the implant tends to occur, but around the area there can be an intense inflammatory reaction and persistent irritation of soft tissues (SEDA-22, 250) (14,15).

Occasionally, reactions to titanium can occur at a distance from a hip implant, probably because small particles of titanium become detached and enter the system.

- Distant granulomatous reactions occurred in an elderly man, who developed symptomless lymph node histiocytosis, which was discovered incidentally.
- Another man had a visceral granulomatosis reaction (liver, spleen, and lymph node) associated with hepatic and splenic enlargement; in affected tissue specimens particles from the hip arthroplasty were detected, and titanium was found in the spleen (16).

Despite its widespread use, titanium is only rarely linked with contact allergic reactions. A hypersensitivity reaction has been attributed to titanium in a pacemaker (17).

- An 86-year-old Japanese man received a pacemaker for atrioventricular block, and 2 months later developed a scaly erythema over the implantation site and later widespread nummular eczema. Histologically, the lesions showed slight spongiosis, intracellular edema, moderate acanthosis in the epidermis, and perivascular infiltration with thickened capillary walls in the dermis. The pacemaker contained titanium and a variety of other metals, but patch tests were all negative. However, titanium sensitivity was demonstrated by intracutaneous and lymphocyte stimulation tests.

Titanium is so widely used that the risk of contact sensitivity to it must be very small. If a patient shows contact sensitivity to titanium, a replacement pacemaker should be completely encased in patch-tested non-allergenic material.

Long-Term Effects

Tumorigenicity

A rhabdomyosarcoma has been reported near the site of a pacemaker (18).

- An 85-year-old man developed a voluminous, rapidly evolving tumor beneath the right clavicle where a titanium pacemaker had been implanted 5 years before. Immunohistochemistry showed that it was a rhabdomyosarcoma.

The role of the pacemaker and especially of titanium in the development of this tumor was not clear.

References

1. Disegi JA. Titanium alloys for fracture fixation implants. Injury 2000;31(Suppl 4):14–17.
2. Pohler OE. Unalloyed titanium for implants in bone surgery. Injury 2000;31(Suppl 4):7–13.
3. Thompson SA. An overview of nickel–titanium alloys used in dentistry. Int Endod J 2000;33(4):297–310.
4. Kononen M, Kivilahti J. Fusing of dental ceramics to titanium. J Dent Res 2001;80(3):848–54.
5. Parma-Benfenati S, Tinti C, Albrektsson T, Johansson C. Histologic evaluation of guided vertical ridge augmentation around implants in humans. Int J Periodontics Restorative Dent 1999;19(5):424–37.
6. Melendez E. Titanium complexes in cancer treatment. Crit Rev Oncol Hematol 2002;42(3):309–15.
7. Schlegel KA, Eppeneder S, Wiltfang J. Soft tissue findings above submerged titanium implants—a histological and spectroscopic study. Biomaterials 2002;23(14):2939–44.
8. Hierholzer S, Hierholzer G. Untersuchungen zur Metalallergie nach Osteosynthesen. [Allergy to metal following osteosynthesis.] Unfallchirurgie 1982;8(6):347–52.
9. Acklin YP, Berli BJ, Frick W, Elke R, Morscher EW. Nine-year results of Muller cemented titanium Straight Stems in total hip replacement. Arch Orthop Trauma Surg 2001;121(7):391–8.
10. Paulsen SM, Nanney LB, Lynch JB. Titanium tetrachloride: an unusual agent with the potential to create severe burns. J Burn Care Rehabil 1998;19(5):377–81.
11. Tamai K, Mitsumori M, Fujishiro S, Kokubo M, Ooya N, Nagata Y, Sasai K, Hiraoka M, Inamoto T. A case of allergic reaction to surgical metal clips inserted for postoperative boost irradiation in a patient undergoing breast-conserving therapy. Breast Cancer 2001;8(1):90–2.
12. Basketter DA, Whittle E, Monk B. Possible allergy to complex titanium salt. Contact Dermatitis 2000;42(5):310–11.
13. Farronato G, Tirafili C, Alicino C, Santoro F. Titanium appliances for allergic patients. J Clin Orthod 2002;36(12):676–9.
14. Holgers KM, Thomsen P, Tjellstrom A. Persistent irritation of the soft tissue around an osseointegrated titanium implant. Case report. Scand J Plast Reconstr Surg Hand Surg 1994;28(3):225–30.
15. Piattelli A, Scarano A, Piattelli M, Bertolai R, Panzoni E. Histologic aspects of the bone and soft tissues surrounding three titanium non-submerged plasma-sprayed implants retrieved at autopsy: a case report. J Periodontol 1997;68(7):694–700.
16. Peoc'h M, Pasquier D, Ducros V, Moulin C, Bost F, Faure C, Pasquier B. Réactions granulomateuses systémiques et prothèse de hance. Deux observations anatomocliniques. [Systemic granulomatous reaction in hip prosthesis. Apropos of 2 anatomoclinical cases.] Rev Chir Orthop Reparatrice Appar Mot 1996;82(6):564–7.
17. Yamauchi R, Morita A, Tsuji T. Pacemaker dermatitis from titanium. Contact Dermatitis 2000;42(1):52–3.
18. Carpentier O, Dubost-Brama A, Martin De Lassalle E, Piette F, Delaporte E. Rhabdomyosarcome sur site d'implantation d'un stimulateur cardiaque. [Rhabdomyosarcoma at site of pacemaker implantation.] Ann Dermatol Venereol 2000;127 (10):837–40.

Tizanidine

General Information

Tizanidine is a centrally acting benzothiadiazol derivative with myotonolytic activity. Although its mechanism of action has not been fully clarified, facilitation of glycine-mediated transmission in the spinal cord may play an important role (1). A total daily dose of 15 mg (5 mg 3 times) is reported to be effective and well tolerated by most patients (2).

The documentation of adverse effects is still fragmentary. Tizanidine seems to be a relatively well tolerated and useful antispastic agent. The most frequently reported adverse effects include drowsiness, dry mouth, and muscle weakness (3). Occasionally, hypotension can occur; it is usually mild (4,5) but can be more severe in patients taking antihypertensive drugs (6–8), in whom tizanidine should be used with great caution. A small fall in heart rate has also been reported (9).

In an open study of tizanidine for neuropathic pain, several adverse effects were noted, such as dizziness, drowsiness, fatigue/weakness, dry mouth, gastrointestinal upset, and sleep difficulty (10).

Organs and Systems

Liver

In an open study of tizanidine for neuropathic pain, one patient developed abnormal liver function tests accompanied by nausea and vomiting, fatigue, confusion, weakness, and muscle aches (10). Within three weeks after withdrawal of tizanidine, the liver function tests returned to baseline and the symptoms resolved. Two other patients had transient asymptomatic rises in liver function tests, which returned to normal despite continuation of tizanidine. Transiently raised liver function tests during tizanidine treatment have occasionally been reported before (11–13).

References

1. Sayers AC, Burki HR, Eichenberger E. The pharmacology of 5-chloro-4-(2-imidazolin-2-yl-amino)-2,1, 3-benzothiadiazole (DS 103-282), a novel myotonolytic agent. Arzneimittelforschung 1980;30(5):793–803.
2. Rinne UK. Tizanidine treatment of spasticity in multiple sclerosis and chronic myelopathy. Curr Ther Res 1980;28:827.
3. Hutchinson DR. Modified release tizanidine: a review. J Int Med Res 1989;17(6):565–73.
4. Fryda-Kaurimsky Z, Muller-Fassbender H. Tizanidine (DS 103-282) in the treatment of acute paravertebral muscle spasm: a controlled trial comparing tizanidine and diazepam. J Int Med Res 1981;9(6):501–5.
5. Goei HS, Whitehouse IJ. Acomparative trial of tizanidine and diazepam in the treatment of acute cervical muscle spasm. Clin Trials J 1982;19:20.
6. Hennies OL. A new skeletal muscle relaxant (DS 103-282) compared to diazepam in the treatment of muscle spasm of local origin. J Int Med Res 1981;9(1):62–8.

7. Hassan N, McLellan DL. Double-blind comparison of single doses of DS103-282, baclofen and placebo for suppression of spasticity. J Neurol Neurosurg Psychiatry 1980;43(12):1132–6.

8. Stien R, Nordal HJ, Oftedal SI, Slettebo M. The treatment of spasticity in multiple sclerosis: a double-blind clinical trial of a new anti-spastic drug tizanidine compared with baclofen. Acta Neurol Scand 1987;75(3):190–4.

9. Mathias CJ, Luckitt J, Desai P, Baker H, el Masri W, Frankel HL. Pharmacodynamics and pharmacokinetics of the oral antispastic agent tizanidine in patients with spinal cord injury. J Rehabil Res Dev 1989;26(4):9–16.

10. Semenchuk MR, Sherman S. Effectiveness of tizanidine in neuropathic pain: an open-label study. J Pain 2000; 1(4):285–92.

11. de Graaf EM, Oosterveld M, Tjabbes T, Stricker BH. A case of tizanidine-induced hepatic injury. J Hepatol 1996;25(5):772–3.

12. Saper JR, Winner PK, Lake AE 3rd. An open-label dose-titration study of the efficacy and tolerability of tizanidine hydrochloride tablets in the prophylaxis of chronic daily headache. Headache 2001;41(4):357–68.

13. Lapierre Y, Bouchard S, Tansey C, Gendron D, Barkas WJ, Francis GS. Treatment of spasticity with tizanidine in multiple sclerosis. Can J Neurol Sci 1987; 14(Suppl 3):S13–17.

Tobramycin

See also Aminoglycoside antibiotics

General Information

Tobramycin closely resembles gentamicin in its microbiological and toxicological properties. The two drugs have similar half-lives, peak serum concentrations, lack of protein binding, volumes of distribution, and predominantly renal excretion by glomerular filtration. The main advantage of tobramycin may be its greater intrinsic activity against *Pseudomonas aeruginosa*. Not all bacterial strains resistant to gentamicin are invariably also resistant to tobramycin. Because of its inherent potential for ototoxicity and nephrotoxicity, renal function and eighth nerve function should be closely monitored (1,2).

Comparative studies

In a randomized comparison of nebulized tobramycin and nebulized colistin in patients with cystic fibrosis, 26 of 53 patients treated with tobramycin had at least one respiratory adverse event, most commonly pharyngitis (3). In 520 patients, inhaled tobramycin (300 mg bd for three 28-day cycles, each cycle being separated by a 28-day period of no treatment) was compared with placebo. Respiratory function was significantly improved as early as the second week and remained so for the rest of the study, even during periods without aerosol treatment. There was also a parallel reduction in the relative risk of hospitalization, the number of days of hospitalization, and the number of days of intravenous antibiotic treatment (4).

Organs and Systems

Respiratory

Nebulized antipseudomonal antibiotic treatment improves lung function and reduces the frequency of exacerbations of infection in patients with cystic fibrosis and Wegener's granulomatosis (5–7), but the significance of development of antibiotic-resistant organisms remains to be determined (8). In 10 healthy adults, the inhalation of tobramycin 80 mg resulted in the deposition of 11.8 mg in the lungs (9). In a double-blind, randomized, placebo-controlled study, inhaled tobramycin significantly reduced sputum density of *P. aeruginosa*. More patients in the treatment group reported increased cough, dyspnea, wheezing, and non-cardiac chest pain, but the symptoms did not limit therapy (10).

Inhalation of the intravenous formulation of tobramycin can cause bronchoconstriction, as has been confirmed in 26 children with mild to moderate cystic fibrosis (11). Nevertheless, while bronchoconstriction did occur, many patients did not have bronchoconstriction in response to the standard intravenous formulation. The risk of bronchoconstriction may further be reduced by pretreatment with salbutamol.

In a comparison of different dosage regimens, inhaled tobramycin caused bronchial obstruction (12). However, after 10 minutes of inhalation, lung function returned to baseline; the effect was independent of dose.

In two placebo-controlled, randomized studies, inhaled tobramycin significantly reduced sputum density of *P. aeruginosa*; however, more patients in the treatment group reported increased dyspnea and wheezing, although the symptoms did not limit therapy (13,14).

Neuromuscular function

The aminoglycosides have a curare-like action, which can be antagonized by calcium ions and prostigmine. In cases requiring general anesthesia, the effect of muscle relaxants such as D-tubocurarine can be potentiated by aminoglycosides.

Aminoglycoside-induced neuromuscular blockade can be clinically relevant in patients with respiratory acidosis, in myasthenia gravis, and in other neuromuscular diseases. Severe illness, the simultaneous use of anesthetics, for example in the immediate postoperative phase, and the application of the antibiotic to serosal surfaces are predisposing factors to be considered (15). Severe clinical manifestations are rare in patients treated with aminoglycosides that are administered in low doses, such as tobramycin.

Sensory systems

Eyes

Subconjunctival injection of tobramycin has caused macular infarction (SEDA-20, 238). This potentially devastating consequence suggests that care must be exercised when contemplating instillation of aminoglycosides directly into the eye.

Allergic contact dermatitis causing conjunctivitis and blepharitis has been reported with topical ophthalmic tobramycin (16).

Ears

Tobramycin affects the cochlear and vestibular systems to a similar extent as gentamicin. A survey of 24 trials showed the following mean frequencies of ototoxicity: gentamicin 7.7%, tobramycin 9.7%, amikacin 13.8%, netilmicin 2.3% (17). There was also a lower incidence of netilmicin-induced inner-ear damage compared with tobramycin in two studies (18,19).

Of 60 adult patients with cystic fibrosis randomized to tobramycin, either 10 mg/kg/day or 3.3 mg/kg tds, two patients (one in each group) had bilateral impairment in pure tone audiography after treatment (20).

Histological examination of the temporal bones from two individuals with ototoxicity due to tobramycin showed reductions in the numbers of both ganglion cells and hair cells (21). Spiral ganglion cell loss was not necessarily subadjacent to areas of hair cell loss in cases of aminoglycoside ototoxicity. Instead, there may be a reduction in the number of ganglion cells in segments of the cochlea with normal-appearing hair cells.

Psychological, psychiatric

As with gentamicin, toxic psychoses can occur with tobramycin (22).

Metal metabolism

Repeated courses of intravenous tobramycin can cause hypomagnesemic tetany (23).

Liver

Certain aminoglycosides affect liver function tests. Increases in alkaline phosphatase after tobramycin have been described (24).

Urinary tract

The following order of relative nephrotoxicity was found in animal experiments: neomycin > gentamicin > tobramycin > amikacin > netilmicin (25,26). However, in humans, conclusive data regarding the relative toxicity of the various aminoglycosides are still lacking. An analysis of 24 controlled trials showed the following average rates for nephrotoxicity: gentamicin, 11%; tobramycin, 11.5%; amikacin, 8.5%; and netilmicin, 2.8% (17). In contrast to this survey, direct comparison in similar patient groups showed no significant differences between the various agents in most trials (27–33). One prospective trial showed a significant advantage of tobramycin over gentamicin (34). However, these findings could not subsequently be confirmed (35). Nephrotoxicity remains a serious risk with all the currently available aminoglycoside antibiotics, and no drug in this series can be regarded as safe.

- Nephrotoxicity due to inhaled tobramycin has recently been described in a 20-year-old patient with cystic fibrosis who developed acute non-oliguric renal insufficiency after taking inhaled tobramycin 300 mg bd for 1 week; the clinical and renal biopsy findings were consistent with aminoglycoside-induced changes (36).

Skin

Ultraviolet recall has been reported after piperacillin, tobramycin, and ciprofloxacin, with a reaction pattern different from that of chemotherapy-induced reactions.

- A 31-year-old woman with a *Pseudomonas* pneumonia was given intravenous ciprofloxacin 400 mg 12-hourly, tobramycin 400 mg/day, and piperacillin 4 g 6-hourly (37). Three days after the initial administration of the intravenous antibiotics, she developed a morbilliform eruption on the sun-exposed areas of her chest, back, and arms, corresponding to sites of intense sunburn that had occurred a month before.

Immunologic

- Hypersensitivity to inhaled tobramycin has been reported in a 9-year-old boy who developed a rash after a course of gentamicin (38). The rash resolved after withdrawal, but returned all over his body when inhaled tobramycin was restarted. He was desensitized using escalating doses of inhaled tobramycin, tolerated the procedure well, and was still using once-a-day tobramycin 9 months after desensitization.

Long-Term Effects

Drug tolerance

Intermittent administration of inhaled tobramycin has been recommended in patients with cystic fibrosis, as it improves pulmonary function, reduces the density of *P. aeruginosa* in sputum, and reduces the risk of hospitalization. The proportion of patients with isolates of *P. aeruginosa* with higher minimal inhibitory concentrations of tobramycin may increase (39). Treatment with inhaled tobramycin does not increase isolation of *Burkholderia cepacia*, *Stenotrophomonas maltophilia*, or *Alcaligenes xylosoxidans*; however, isolation of *Candida albicans* and *Aspergillus* species may increase (40).

With nebulized tobramycin the introduction or selection of resistant bacteria is relatively rare but is a matter of concern (41).

Second-Generation Effects

Teratogenicity

During pregnancy the aminoglycosides cross the placenta and they might theoretically be expected to cause otological and perhaps nephrological damage to the fetus. However, no proven cases of intrauterine damage by tobramycin have been recorded.

Susceptibility Factors

Renal disease

Reduced tobramycin clearance can be associated with a normal creatinine clearance in serum concentration-adjusted dosage of once-daily tobramycin therapy in critically ill patients (42).

Other features of the patient

The pharmacokinetics of tobramycin in patients with cystic fibrosis is significantly altered after lung transplantation, and early and close drug monitoring is recommended (43).

Hydrophilic contact lenses may increase the penetration of tobramycin into the aqueous humor (44).

Drug Administration

Drug dosage regimens

The addition of tobramycin reduced the amount of cefuroxime-induced endotoxin released per killed *Escherichia coli* to a level that was even lower than that of tobramycin alone, despite an increased killing rate (45). Increasing concentrations of tobramycin led to a reduction in endotoxin release, pointing to a possible benefit of once-daily dosing regimens.

In an analysis of sera from 60 adults with cystic fibrosis, it was suggested that the potential benefit of achieving a greater peak/MIC with once-daily aminoglycoside administration may be offset by the significantly greater time that the concentration was below the MIC, compared with that achieved with multiple daily dosing regimens (46)

Based on a study of 10 patients with automated peritoneal dialysis, it was recommended that for empirical treatment of dialysis-related peritonitis, the dosage of intermittent intraperitoneal tobramycin must be 1.5 mg/kg for one exchange during the first day and then 0.5 mg/kg thereafter, to reduce the risk of adverse effects (47).

Drug administration route

With combined inhalational and intravenous tobramycin, toxic serum drug concentrations can occur (48).

Wound irrigation

Although the efficacy of peroperative wound irrigation with aminoglycosides has yet to be firmly established in prospective comparative trials, they are often used during intra-abdominal and thoracic surgery. Depending on the amount of drug used and the nature of the operation, it is likely that significant amounts of tobramycin are absorbed (SEDA-20, 237).

Inhalation

Tobramycin has been used extensively in cystic fibrosis because of its effect on *Pseudomonas* organisms. Used as an adjunct to intravenous antibiotics in acute infections, it can lower sputum colony counts. Aerosolized antibiotics over prolonged periods can improve lung function and reduce hospital admissions, but they carry the potential risk of drug toxicity and resistance. In a review of clinical studies it was concluded that there was no evidence of nephrotoxicity or ototoxicity (49), although long-term toxicity studies at higher dosages are awaited.

The efficacy of nebulized tobramycin 300 mg bd for 4 weeks has been studied in a randomized, double-blind, placebo-controlled trial in 74 patients with bronchiectasis and *Pseudomonas* infection, without cystic fibrosis (31).

After 4 weeks there was a significant fall in the density of *Pseudomonas* infection in the sputum of the treated group. This correlated with an improvement in general medical condition, as assessed subjectively 2 weeks later. There was no difference in lung function. Tobramycin resistance (MIC over 16 µg/ml) developed in 4 patients in the treated group and 1 patient in the placebo group. Adverse events were reported by 31 of the 37 patients in each arm. There were significantly increased incidences of dyspnea (32%), chest pain (19%), and wheezing (16%) in the treated group compared with placebo (8%, 0%, 0% respectively). Cough increased in 15 patients (41%) in the treated group and 9 (24%) in the placebo group. The investigators felt that the majority of these respiratory adverse events had been related to the drug. They commented that these adverse events did not generally result in withdrawal of the patients from the trial. No more details were given but the apparent adverse effects profile of nebulized tobramycin in this group is of concern.

Topical administration into the ear

The primary target for the topical effects of aminoglycosides in the ear is controversial. It has been generally believed that outer hair cells are primarily affected, followed by loss of inner hair cells; that degeneration starts basally and proceeds towards the apex; and that neural fibers and ganglion cells would degenerate secondarily to loss of hair cells. However, the possibility that spiral ganglion cells may be a primary target has been raised. In a postmortem study of 10 temporal bones from 6 patients (aged 11–40 years) with cystic fibrosis, whose pulmonary infections had been treated with systemic aminoglycosides (mainly tobramycin), in most cases combined with nebulized tobramycin, cytocochleograms were analysed for each bone (50). Four bones showed typical manifestations of aminoglycoside-induced ototoxicity, with loss of hair cells in the lower turns and degeneration of ganglion cells. Six bones showed no loss or scattered loss of hair cells, but there was degeneration of the spiral ganglion cells. This study supports the hypothesis that degeneration of spiral ganglion cells may occur as a primary manifestation in some cases of aminoglycoside-induced ototoxicity.

Drug overdose

Multiple-dose activated charcoal does not increase the elimination of tobramycin and is therefore not recommended for treatment of poisoning (SEDA24.26.74) (51).

Monitoring Therapy

During multiple daily dosing peak serum concentrations of tobramycin over 5–7 µg/ml are associated with improved survival in patients with septicemia and pneumonia caused by Gram-negative bacteria (52,53). On the other hand, excessive peak concentrations (over 10–12 µg/ml) and trough concentrations (over 2 µg/ml) of tobramycin increase the risk of ototoxicity and nephrotoxicity (54).

References

1. Bendush CL, Weber R. Tobramycin sulfate: a summary of worldwide experience from clinical trials. J Infect Dis 1976;134(Suppl):S219–34.

2. Neu HC. Tobramycin: an overview. J Infect Dis 1976;134(Suppl):S3–19.

3. Hodson ME, Gallagher CG, Govan JR. A randomised clinical trial of nebulised tobramycin or colistin in cystic fibrosis. Eur Respir J 2002;20(3):658–64.

4. Geller DE, Pitlick WH, Nardella PA, Tracewell WG, Ramsey BW. Pharmacokinetics and bioavailability of aerosolized tobramycin in cystic fibrosis. Chest 2002;122(1):219–26.

5. Niedzielska G, Katska E. Rodzinne wystepowanie niedosluchu odbiorczego zwiazanego z leczeniem streptomycyna. [Familial occurrence of hearing loss following streptomycin (SM) treatment.] Otolaryngol Pol 2001;55(3):313–15.

6. Bothamley G. Drug treatment for tuberculosis during pregnancy: safety considerations. Drug Saf 2001;24(7):553–65.

7. Govan J. TOBI: reducing the impact of pseudomonal infection. Hosp Med 2002;63(7):421–5.

8. Ryan G, Mukhopadhyay S, Singh M. Nebulised antipseudomonal antibiotics for cystic fibrosis (Cochrane Review). Oxford: Update Software, 2000.

9. Coates AL, Dinh L, MacNeish CF, Rollin T, Gagnon S, Ho SL, Lands LC. Accounting for radioactivity before and after nebulization of tobramycin to insure accuracy of quantification of lung deposition. J Aerosol Med 2000;13(3):169–78.

10. Barker AF, Couch L, Fiel SB, Gotfried MH, Ilowite J, Meyer KC, O'Donnell A, Sahn SA, Smith LJ, Stewart JO, Abuan T, Tully H, Van Dalfsen J, Wells CD, Quan J. Tobramycin solution for inhalation reduces sputum *Pseudomonas aeruginosa* density in bronchiectasis Am J Respir Crit Care Med 2000;162(2 Pt 1):481–5.

11. Ramagopal M, Lands LC. Inhaled tobramycin and bronchial hyperactivity in cystic fibrosis. Pediatr Pulmonol 2000;29(5):366–70.

12. Nikolaizik WH, Trociewicz K, Ratjen F. Bronchial reactions to the inhalation of high-dose tobramycin in cystic fibrosis. Eur Respir J 2002;20(1):122–6.

13. Hinojosa R, Nelson EG, Lerner SA, Redleaf MI, Schramm DR. Aminoglycoside ototoxicity: a human temporal bone study. Laryngoscope 2001;111(10):1797–805.

14. Moss RB. Administration of aerosolized antibiotics in cystic fibrosis patients. Chest 2001;120(Suppl 3):S107–13.

15. Holtzman JL. Letter: Gentamicin and neuromuscular blockade. Ann Intern Med 1976;84(1):55.

16. Caraffini S, Assalve D, Stingeni L, Lisi P. Allergic contact conjunctivitis and blepharitis from tobramycin. Contact Dermatitis 1995;32(3):186–7.

17. Cone LA. A survey of prospective, controlled clinical trials of gentamicin, tobramycin, amikacin, and netilmicin. Clin Ther 1982;5(2):155–62.

18. Lerner AM, Reyes MP, Cone LA, Blair DC, Jansen W, Wright GE, Lorber RR. Randomised, controlled trial of the comparative efficacy, auditory toxicity, and nephrotoxicity of tobramycin and netilmicin. Lancet 1983;1(8334):1123–6.

19. Gatell JM, SanMiguel JG, Araujo V, Zamora L, Mana J, Ferrer M, Bonet M, Bohe M, Jimenez de Anta MT. Prospective randomized double-blind comparison of nephrotoxicity and auditory toxicity of tobramycin and netilmicin. Antimicrob Agents Chemother 1984;26(5):766–9.

20. Whitehead A, Conway SP, Etherington C, Caldwell NA, Setchfield N, Bogle S. Once-daily tobramycin in the treatment of adult patients with cystic fibrosis. Eur Respir J 2002;19(2):303–9.

21. Gardner TB, Hill DR. Treatment of giardiasis. Clin Microbiol Rev 2001;14(1):114–28.

22. McCartney CF, Hatley LH, Kessler JM. Possible tobramycin delirium. JAMA 1982;247(9):1319.

23. Adams JP, Conway SP, Wilson C. Hypomagnesaemic tetany associated with repeated courses of intravenous tobramycin in a patient with cystic fibrosis. Respir Med 1998;92(3):602–4.

24. Martines G, Butturini L, Menozzi I, Restori G, Boiardi L, Bernardi S, Baldassarri P. Amikacin-induced liver toxicity: correlations between biochemical indexes and ultrastructural features in an experimental model. Rev Med Univ Navarra 1988;32(1):41–5.

25. Luft FC, Yum MN, Kleit SA. Comparative nephrotoxicities of netilmicin and gentamicin in rats. Antimicrob Agents Chemother 1976;10(5):845–9.

26. Hottendorf GH, Gordon LL. Comparative low-dose nephrotoxicities of gentamicin, tobramycin, and amikacin. Antimicrob Agents Chemother 1980;18(1):176–81.

27. Smith CR, Baughman KL, Edwards CQ, Rogers JF, Lietman PS. Controlled comparison of amikacin and gentamicin. N Engl J Med 1977;296(7):349–53.

28. Feld R, Valdivieso M, Bodey GP, Rodriguez V. Comparison of amikacin and tobramycin in the treatment of infection in patients with cancer. J Infect Dis 1977;135(1):61–6.

29. Love LJ, Schimpff SC, Hahn DM, Young VM, Standiford HC, Bender JF, Fortner CL, Wiernik PH. Randomized trial of empiric antibiotic therapy with ticarcillin in combination with gentamicin, amikacin or netilmicin in febrile patients with granulocytopenia and cancer. Am J Med 1979;66(4):603–10.

30. Lau WK, Young LS, Black RE, Winston DJ, Linne SR, Weinstein RJ, Hewitt WL. Comparative efficacy and toxicity of amikacin/carbenicillin versus gentamicin/carbenicillin in leukopenic patients: a randomized prospective trail. Am J Med 1977;62(6):959–66.

31. Fong IW, Fenton RS, Bird R. Comparative toxicity of gentamicin versus tobramycin: a randomized prospective study. J Antimicrob Chemother 1981;7(1):81–8.

32. Bock BV, Edelstein PH, Meyer RD. Prospective comparative study of efficacy and toxicity of netilmicin and amikacin. Antimicrob Agents Chemother 1980;17(2):217–25.

33. Barza M, Lauermann MW, Tally FP, Gorbach SL. Prospective, randomized trial of netilmicin and amikacin, with emphasis on eighth-nerve toxicity. Antimicrob Agents Chemother 1980;17(4):707–14.

34. Smith CR, Lipsky JJ, Laskin OL, Hellmann DB, Mellits ED, Longstreth J, Lietman PS. Double-blind comparison of the nephrotoxicity and auditory toxicity of gentamicin and tobramycin. N Engl J Med 1980;302(20):1106–9.

35. Matzke GR, Lucarotti RL, Shapiro HS. Controlled comparison of gentamicin and tobramycin nephrotoxicity. Am J Nephrol 1983;3(1):11–17.

36. Hoffmann IM, Rubin BK, Iskandar SS, Schechter MS, Nagaraj SK, Bitzan MM. Acute renal failure in cystic fibrosis: association with inhaled tobramycin therapy. Pediatr Pulmonol 2002;34(5):375–7.

37. Terzano C, Taurino AE, Peona V. Nebulized tobramycin in patients with chronic respiratory infections during clinical evolution of Wegener's granulomatosis. Eur Rev Med Pharmacol Sci 2001;5(4):131–8.

38. Spigarelli MG, Hurwitz ME, Nasr SZ. Hypersensitivity to inhaled TOBI following reaction to gentamicin. Pediatr Pulmonol 2002;33(4):311–14.

39. Ramsey BW, Pepe MS, Quan JM, Otto KL, Montgomery AB, Williams-Warren J, Vasiljev-K M, Borowitz D, Bowman CM, Marshall BC, Marshall S,

Smith AL. Intermittent administration of inhaled tobramycin in patients with cystic fibrosis. Cystic Fibrosis Inhaled Tobramycin Study Group. N Engl J Med 1999;340(1):23–30.

40. Burns JL, Van Dalfsen JM, Shawar RM, Otto KL, Garber RL, Quan JM, Montgomery AB, Albers GM, Ramsey BW, Smith AL. Effect of chronic intermittent administration of inhaled tobramycin on respiratory microbial flora in patients with cystic fibrosis. J Infect Dis 1999;179(5):1190–6.

41. Sermet-Gaudelus I, Le Cocguic Y, Ferroni A, Clairicia M, Barthe J, Delaunay JP, Brousse V, Lenoir G. Nebulized antibiotics in cystic fibrosis. Paediatr Drugs 2002;4(7):455–67.

42. Reimann IR, Meier-Hellmann A, Pfeifer R, Traut T, Schilling A, Stein G, Reinhart K, Hoffmann A. Serumspiegelorientierte Dosierung der einmal täglichen Aminoglykosidtherapie beim kritisch Kranken: Ergebnisse einer prospektiven Untersuchung. [Serum level-adjusted dosage of once-daily aminoglycoside therapy in critical illness: results of a prospective study.] Anasthesiol Intensivmed Notfallmed Schmerzther 1999;34(5):288–95.

43. Moore RA, DeShazer D, Reckseidler S, Weissman A, Woods DE. Efflux-mediated aminoglycoside and macrolide resistance in *Burkholderia pseudomallei*. Antimicrob Agents Chemother 1999;43(3):465–70.

44. Hehl EM, Beck R, Luthard K, Guthoff R, Drewelow B. Improved penetration of aminoglycosides and fluoroquinolones into the aqueous humour of patients by means of Acuvue contact lenses. Eur J Clin Pharmacol 1999;55(4):317–23.

45. Sjolin J, Goscinski G, Lundholm M, Bring J, Odenholt I. Endotoxin release from *Escherichia coli* after exposure to tobramycin: dose-dependency and reduction in cefuroxime-induced endotoxin release Clin Microbiol Infect 2000;6(2):74–81.

46. Beringer PM, Vinks AA, Jelliffe RW, Shapiro BJ. Pharmacokinetics of tobramycin in adults with cystic fibrosis: implications for once-daily administration. Antimicrob Agents Chemother 2000;44(4):809–13.

47. Manley HJ, Bailie GR, Frye R, Hess LD, McGoldrick MD. Pharmacokinetics of intermittent intravenous cefazolin and tobramycin in patients treated with automated peritoneal dialysis. J Am Soc Nephrol 2000;11(7):1310–16.

48. Elidemir O, Maciejewski SR, Oermann CM. Falsely elevated serum tobramycin concentrations in cystic fibrosis patients treated with concurrent intravenous and inhaled tobramycin. Pediatr Pulmonol 2000;29(1):43–5.

49. Touw DJ, Brimicombe RW, Hodson ME, Heijerman HG, Bakker W. Inhalation of antibiotics in cystic fibrosis. Eur Respir J 1995;8(9):1594–604.

50. Sone M, Schachern PA, Paparella MM. Loss of spiral ganglion cells as primary manifestation of aminoglycoside ototoxicity. Hear Res 1998;115(1–2):217–23.

51. American Academy of Clinical Toxicology; European Association of Poisons Centres and Clinical Toxicologists. Position statement and practice guidelines on the use of multi-dose activated charcoal in the treatment of acute poisoning. J Toxicol Clin Toxicol. 1999;37(6):731–51.

52. Moore RD, Smith CR, Lietman PS. The association of aminoglycoside plasma levels with mortality in patients with Gram-negative bacteremia. J Infect Dis 1984;149(3):443–8.

53. Moore RD, Smith CR, Lietman PS. Association of aminoglycoside plasma levels with therapeutic outcome in Gram-negative pneumonia. Am J Med 1984;77(4):657–62.

54. Wenk M, Vozeh S, Follath F. Serum level monitoring of antibacterial drugs. A review. Clin Pharmacokinet 1984;9(6):475–92.

Tocainide

See also Antidysrhythmic drugs

General Information

The clinical pharmacology, uses, efficacy, and adverse effects of tocainide have been extensively reviewed (1–9).

The adverse effects of tocainide occur with increasing frequency above plasma concentrations of 10 µg/ml. They are mostly related to the nervous system. In two large series withdrawal of tocainide was required in 11–16% of patients because of adverse effects (10,11). The high incidence of blood dyscrasias severely limits the use of tocainide.

Organs and Systems

Cardiovascular

Adverse cardiovascular effects have been reported in 6–55% of cases. After a single dose of tocainide the most common effect is hypotension with bradycardia (12). Angina pectoris has also been reported (13).

During repeated administration cardiovascular adverse effects are relatively uncommon. Increasing heart failure (14,15), worsening dysrhythmias (15,16), pericarditis (15,17,18), and sinus arrest with sinoatrial block (19) have all been reported. Tocainide can worsen ventricular tachycardia (20).

Respiratory

There have been several reports of interstitial pneumonitis attributable to tocainide (21,22), and it may also cause severe pulmonary fibrosis (23,24).

Nervous system

A wide variety of central nervous system symptoms has been reported in almost every study, varying in incidence from 10 to 100%. Common reactions include dizziness, tremor and tremulousness, dysesthesia and paresthesia, light-headedness, and blurred vision. Various mental changes have been described, including paranoid psychosis (25–27). Nausea is common and probably central in origin, since it occurs after intravenous as well as oral administration. These adverse effects can be reduced in frequency during oral administration by taking the tablets with food.

Sensory systems

There have been not infrequent reports of odd taste sensations (peppermint and menthol) and of coolness of the throat, hands, and feet.

Hematologic

Tocainide can cause blood dyscrasias (neutropenia, thrombocytopenia, pancytopenia, and aplastic anemia) in one in 300 patients (28–31). There have been isolated reports of eosinophilia with an allergic rash and anemia with pericarditis (17,32).

Gastrointestinal

Nausea is very common, particularly during the initial stages of treatment, after which it tends to disappear (14). There have been occasional reports of constipation (17) and of anorexia and vomiting (14).

Liver

Tocainide can increase the activities of serum transaminases (33) and can cause fatty change (33) and granulomatous hepatitis (34).

Urinary tract

Non-membranous glomerulonephritis has been reported (35).

Skin

There have been a few reports of skin rashes attributed to tocainide (17,36).

Hair, nails, sweat glands

Night sweats have been reported in three patients taking tocainide (17).

Immunologic

Arthralgia has been reported in two cases with positive antinuclear antibody titers, suggesting the possibility of a lupus-like syndrome (37). In another case tocainide treatment was associated with both a lupus-like syndrome and neutropenia (38). Cross-reactivity of tocainide with lidocaine has been reported (39).

Drug Administration

Drug overdose

Convulsions, complete heart block, and asystole developed in a case of fatal self-poisoning with 400 mg of tocainide (40).

Drug–Drug Interactions

Theophylline

Tocainide reduces the clearance of theophylline and increases its half-life, but to an extent that is probably clinically insignificant (41).

References

1. Nattel S, Zipes DP. Clinical pharmacology of old and new antiarrhythmic drugs. Cardiovasc Clin 1980;11(1):221–48.
2. Danilo P Jr. Tocainide. Am Heart J 1979;97(2):259–62.
3. Holmes B, Brogden RN, Heel RC, Speight TM, Avery GS. Tocainide. A review of its pharmacological properties and therapeutic efficacy. Drugs 1983;26(2):93–123.
4. ADIS Editors and Consultants. Tocainide (Tonocard): a review of its pharmacological properties and therapeutic efficacy. Curr Ther 1984;July:17.
5. Schweyen DH. Tocainide: a new antiarrhythmic. Hosp Pharm 1984;19:558–65.
6. Keefe DL, Somberg JC. New therapy focus: tocainide. Cardiovasc Rev Rep 1984;5:1023–30.
7. Lynch JJ, Lucchesi BR. New antiarrhythmic agents. IV. The pharmacology and clinical use of tocainide. Pract Cardiol 1985;2:108.
8. Hasegawa GR. Tocainide: a new oral antiarrhythmic. Drug Intell Clin Pharm 1985;19(7–8):514–17.
9. Kutalek SP, Morganroth J, Horowitz LN. Tocainide: a new oral antiarrhythmic agent. Ann Intern Med 1985; 103(3):387–91.
10. Horn HR, Hadidian Z, Johnson JL, Vassallo HG, Williams JH, Young MD. Safety evaluation of tocainide in the American Emergency Use Program. Am Heart J 1980;100(6 Pt 2):1037–40.
11. Young MD, Hadidian Z, Horn HR, Johnson JL, Vassallo HG. Treatment of ventricular arrhythmias with oral tocainide. Am Heart J 1980;100(6 Pt 2):1041–5.
12. Greenspon AJ, Mohiuddin S, Saksena S, Lengerich R, Snapinn S, Holmes G, Irvin J, Sappington E, et al. Comparison of intravenous tocainide with intravenous lidocaine for treating ventricular arrhythmias. Cardiovasc Rev Rep 1989;10:55–9.
13. Winkle RA, Anderson JL, Peters F, Meffin PJ, Fowles RE, Harrison DC. The hemodynamic effects of intravenous tocainide in patients with heart disease. Circulation 1978;57(4):787–92.
14. Maloney JD, Nissen RG, McColgan JM. Open clinical studies at a referral center: chronic maintenance tocainide therapy in patients with recurrent sustained ventricular tachycardia refractory to conventional antiarrhythmic agents. Am Heart J 1980;100(6 Pt 2):1023–30.
15. Cheesman M, Ward DE. Exacerbation of ventricular tachycardia by tocainide. Clin Cardiol 1985;8(1):47–50.
16. Winkle RA, Meffin PJ, Harrison DC. Long-term tocainide therapy for ventricular arrhythmias. Circulation 1978; 57(5):1008–16.
17. Roden DM, Reele SB, Higgins SB, Carr RK, Smith RF, Oates JA, Woosley RL, Tocainide therapy for refractory ventricular arrhythmias. Am Heart J 1980;100(1):15–22.
18. Gould LA, Betzu R, Vacek T, Muller R, Pradeep V, Downs L. Sinoatrial block due to tocainide. Am Heart J 1989;118(4):851–3.
19. Van Natta B, Lazarus M, Li C. Irreversible interstitial pneumonitis associated with tocainide therapy. West J Med 1988;149(1):91–2.
20. Perlow GM, Jain BP, Pauker SG, Zarren HS, Wistran DC, Epstein RL. Tocainide-associated interstitial pneumonitis. Ann Intern Med 1981;94(4 Pt 1):489–90.
21. Braude AC, Downar E, Chamberlain DW, Rebuck AS. Tocainide-associated interstitial pneumonitis. Thorax 1982;37(4):309–10.
22. Anonymous. Tocainide hydrochloride pulmonary fibrosis. Swed Adv Drug React Adv Comm Bull 1988;54.
23. Feinberg L, Travis WD, Ferrans V, Sato N, Bernton HF. Pulmonary fibrosis associated with tocainide: report of a case with literature review. Am Rev Respir Dis 1990; 141(2):505–8.
24. Currie P, Ramsdale DR. Paranoid psychosis induced by tocainide. BMJ (Clin Res Ed) 1984;288(6417):606–7.
25. Harrison DJ, Wathen CG. Paranoid psychoses induced by tocainide. BMJ (Clin Res Ed) 1984;288(6422):1010–11.
26. Clarke CW, el-Mahdi EO. Confusion and paranoia associated with oral tocainide. Postgrad Med J 1985; 61(711):79–81.
27. Woosley RL, McDevitt DG, Nies AS, Smith RF, Wilkinson GR, Oates JA. Suppression of ventricular ectopic depolarizations by tocainide. Circulation 1977;56(6):980–4.
28. Anonymous. Tocainide and blood disorders. Aust Adv Drug React Bull 1986;April.

29. Drost RA. Voorzorgen bij gebruik van Tonocard (tocainide). Meded Coll Beoord Geneesmidd 1986;121:167.
30. Soff GA, Kadin ME. Tocainide-induced reversible agranulocytosis and anemia. Arch Intern Med 1987;147(3):598–9.
31. Morrill GB, Gibson SM. Tocainide-induced aplastic anemia. DICP 1989;23(1):90–1.
32. Engler R, Ryan W, LeWinter M, Bluestein H, Karliner JS. Assessment of long-term antiarrhythmic therapy: studies on the long-term efficacy and toxicity of tocainide. Am J Cardiol 1979;43(3):612–18.
33. Farquhar DL, Davidson NM. Possible hepatoxicity of tocainide. Scott Med J 1984;29(4):238.
34. Tucker LE. Tocainide-induced granulomatous hepatitis. JAMA 1986;255(24):3362.
35. Winkle RA, Mason JW, Harrison DC. Tocainide for drug-resistant ventricular arrhythmias: efficacy, side effects, and lidocaine responsiveness for predicting tocainide success. Am Heart J 1980;100(6 Pt 2):1031–6.
36. Nyquist O, Forssell G, Nordlander R, Schenck-Gustafsson K. Hemodynamic and antiarrhythmic effects of tocainide in patients with acute myocardial infarction. Am Heart J 1980;100(6 Pt 2):1000–5.
37. Mohiuddin SM, Esterbrooks D, Mooss AN, Dahl JM, Hilleman DE. Efficacy and tolerance of tocainide during long-term treatment of malignant ventricular arrhythmias. Clin Cardiol 1987;10(8):457–62.
38. Oliphant LD, Goddard M. Tocainide-associated neutropenia and lupus-like syndrome. Chest 1988;94(2):427–8.
39. Duff HJ, Roden DM, Marney S, Colley DG, Maffucci R, Primm RK, Oates JA, Woosley RL. Molecular basis for the antigenicity of lidocaine analogues: tocainide and mexiletine Am Heart J 1984;107(3):585–9.
40. Barnfield C, Kemmenoe AV. A sudden death due to tocainide overdose. Hum Toxicol 1986;5(5):337–40.
41. Loi CM, Wei X, Parker BM, Korrapati MR, Vestal RE. The effect of tocainide on theophylline metabolism. Br J Clin Pharmacol 1993;35(4):437–40.

Tolazoline

General Information

Tolazoline is an alpha$_2$-adrenoceptor antagonist that increases skin blood flow in healthy subjects and has been used to relieve acute vasospasm. However, convincing evidence of its therapeutic value in patients with chronic conditions, such as claudication or cerebrovascular impairment, is not available. It has a pulmonary vasodilator action and seems to be a useful adjunct in the management of neonates with persistent fetal circulation.

Tolazoline has a histamine-like action. Its most common adverse effects are palpitation, tachycardia, flushing, sweating, headache, and paresthesia of the skin with piloerection. Unwanted gastrointestinal effects include nausea, vomiting, and diarrhea. Postural hypotension and failure to ejaculate have also been reported.

Organs and Systems

Gastrointestinal

An infant with persistent fetal circulation treated with tolazoline developed gastric ulceration and perforation (1). The first symptoms occurred 14 hours after the start of therapy, and there was free air in the abdomen 34 hours later. Duodenal perforation also occurred in a 31-hour-old infant with meconium aspiration treated with tolazoline for 6 hours; the defect required surgical correction (2).

Drug–Drug Interactions

Clonidine

Tolazoline can antagonize the effects of intravenous clonidine and prevent the brief hypertensive reaction that it often causes (SEDA-2, 192) (SEDA-3, 180).

References

1. von Muhlendahl KE. Perforating gastric ulceration during tolazoline therapy for persistent foetal circulation. Z Kinderchir 1988;43(1):48–9.
2. Matsuo M, Aida M, Yamada T, Takemine H, Tsugawa C, Kimura K, Matsumoto Y. Duodenal perforation with tolazoline therapy. J Pediatr 1982;100(6):1005–6.

Tolcapone

General Information

Tolcapone is an inhibitor of catchol-O-methyltransferase, which catalyses a relatively minor pathway of dopamine metabolism. It therefore enhances the action of dopamine.

The introduction of tolcapone had a major impact on the management of Parkinson's disease, and within months tens of thousands of patients throughout the world were treated with it. Tolcapone was considered to be useful in prolonging the half-life of levodopa, thereby allowing dosage reduction and possibly smoother therapeutic responses.

In early studies the most frequent adverse effects of tolcapone were dyskinesias, nausea, sleep disorders, dystonia, orthostatic hypotension, diarrhea, dizziness, and hallucinations (1). However, very soon tolcapone was withdrawn in most countries, because of reports of severe hepatotoxicity. The background to these events has been briefly reviewed (2).

Organs and Systems

Gastrointestinal

Raised liver enzymes due to tolcapone were often associated with diarrhea and occurred within 6 weeks to 6 months of the start of tolcapone therapy. Diarrhea developed in 16–18% of patients taking tolcapone and was severe in 3–4% of the cases.

Liver

A number of cases of severe hepatotoxicity (3) led the health authorities to withdraw tolcapone from most European countries following an EMEA ruling in November 1998. Increases of more than three times the upper limit of the reference range for alanine aminotransferase and aspartate aminotransferase occurred in respectively 1% and 3% of patients taking tolcapone 100 mg tds and 200 mg tds. Increases of more than eight times the upper limit of normal alanine aminotransferase and aspartate aminotransferase occurred in respectively 0.3% and 1.7% of patients taking tolcapone 100 mg tds and 200 mg tds. Subsequently there were three deaths from acute liver failure in patients taking tolcapone during a total exposure of 40 000 patient-years, leading to the complete withdrawal of the drug. An earlier review, predating the withdrawal of tolcapone, had suggested that it could be safely used provided liver function was closely monitored in the first 6 months of therapy (4), and some neurologists believe that this course of action may still be reasonable because of what they regard as the superior efficacy of this drug.

Skin

- Progressive vitiligo occurred in a 50-year-old Caucasian who took tolcapone 300 mg/day in combination with co-careldopa (5). The first depigmented lesions appeared a week after starting the drug.

The authors speculated that the increased concentrations of dopamine may have interfered with melanin synthesis.

References

1. Micek ST, Ernst ME. Tolcapone: a novel approach to Parkinson's disease. Am J Health Syst Pharm 1999;56(21):2195–205.
2. Colosimo C. The rise and fall of tolcapone. J Neurol 1999;246(10):880–2.
3. Watkins P. COMT inhibitors and liver toxicity. Neurology 2000;55(11 Suppl 4):S51–2.
4. Olanow CW. Tolcapone and hepatotoxic effects. Tasmar Advisory Panel. Arch Neurol 2000;57(2):263–7.
5. Sabate M, Bosch A, Pedros C, Figueras A. Vitiligo associated with tolcapone and levodopa in a patient with Parkinson's disease. Ann Pharmacother 1999;33(11):1228–9.

Tolfenamic acid

See also Non-steroidal anti-inflammatory drugs

General Information

The main adverse effects of tolfenamic acid (particularly nephrotoxicity) are similar to those of the other anthranilic acid derivatives. However, dysuria has been reported more often and confirmed by rechallenge (SEDA-4, 68).

Skin disorders are frequent (40% of all reported effects), and fixed drug eruption has occurred (SEDA-18, 107). Diarrhea (10%) and upper gastrointestinal symptoms (including dyspepsia, nausea, vomiting, gastric pain, and ulcer) (6%) are common (SEDA-19, 98). Hepatitis has been described with positive rechallenge. Six patients with pulmonary infiltrates, possibly caused by tolfenamic acid, were reported to the Finnish National Centre for Adverse Drug Reaction Monitoring over a 12-year period. In some patients with hemolytic anemia, a positive Coombs' test and antinuclear antibodies suggested an immunological mechanism (SEDA-13, 83).

Organs and Systems

Electrolyte balance

Hyperkalemia has been attributed to tolfenamic acid (1).

- A hemodialysis patient with nephritic syndrome and diabetic end-stage renal disease developed severe hyperkalemia with muscle paresis after taking tolfenamic acid 300 mg/day for chronic headache. Five days after starting treatment he reported pain and tenderness affecting the muscles of his back and lower extremities. He had hyponatremia and severe hyperkalemia. During the following days he developed increasing weakness and became unable to move his head and limbs. Tolfenamic acid was withdrawn and aggressive treatment and repeated hemodialysis started, leading to complete recovery in a few days.

In this case, end-stage renal disease with nephrotic syndrome and insulin-dependent diabetes mellitus were predisposing factors to the development of hyperkalemia, but a possible role of accumulated tolfenamic acid metabolites could not be excluded. Patients with severe renal insufficiency should not receive NSAIDs.

Reference

1. Nielsen EH. Hyperkalaemic muscle paresis—side-effect of prostaglandin inhibition in a haemodialysis patient. Nephrol Dial Transplant 1999;14(2):480–2.

Tolmetin

See also Non-steroidal anti-inflammatory drugs

General Information

In 32 207 patients taking part in a short (1–4 weeks) postmarketing study of tolmetin, adverse effects occurred in 12%, and led to withdrawal in 3.6% (1). Tolerability was similar to that of naproxen, indometacin (SEDA-7, 114), and ibuprofen (SED-9, 152) (2). In another retrospective study in patients treated for 1 year or more with tolmetin, 64% reported generally mild transitory adverse effects. In controlled studies, about 10% of patients withdrew owing to adverse effects (3). In another study of

25 000 prescription records (4), tolmetin caused adverse reactions severe enough to merit hospitalization in only two cases (drug fever and membranous glomerulopathy).

Organs and Systems

Cardiovascular

Increased blood pressure can occur after long-term treatment with tolmetin (5).

Nervous system

The usual adverse reactions of NSAIDs on the nervous system have been attributed to tolmetin (SEDA-6, 98). One woman developed aseptic meningitis, similar to that seen with ibuprofen (6).

Sensory systems

Hearing loss has been documented (SED-9, 152) (7).

Hematologic

Acute reversible thrombocytopenic purpura and tolmetin-related antibodies have been reported in a patient with a history of multiple allergies; rechallenge was positive (8). Peripheral blood eosinophilia has also been found (SEDA-6, 98).

Gastrointestinal

Gastrointestinal adverse effects occurred in 31% of patients taking tolmetin and peptic ulceration in 2% (3). In older patients, the percentage of peptic ulceration and gastrointestinal bleeding was somewhat higher (9).

Urinary tract

Reversible renal insufficiency and acute interstitial nephritis have been reported. Nephrotic syndrome was attributed to tolmetin, but a firm causal relation was not established (10). Nephrotic syndrome has also been described in a 16-year-old girl after she had taken tolmetin for 6 months (SEDA-16, 122).

Immunologic

From early on, the high incidence of hypersensitivity reactions with tolmetin was striking, for example in spontaneous adverse reaction reports. However, the high incidence was not confirmed in a retrospective comparative review (SEDA-6, 98) (SEDA-7, 134) (11). Several factors can explain the discrepancy. For example, patients covered by the review may have persisted with treatment, since they did not experience such reactions.

Multiorgan failure

Fatal multisystem toxicity including both renal and hepatic failure, with microvesicular fatty change in the liver, has been reported with tolmetin in a young woman (12).

Drug–Drug Interactions

Warfarin

Tolmetin combined with warfarin can markedly prolong the prothrombin time and cause bleeding (SEDA-13, 82).

References

1. Sarchi C, Cioffi T, Bertelletti D, Guslandi M. Tolmetin sodium in clinical practice: a survey of 32,207 treated patients. J Int Med Res 1981;9(6):482–9.
2. Brogden RN, Heel RC, Speight TM, Avery GS. Tolmetin: a review of its pharmacological properties and therapeutic efficacy in rheumatic diseases. Drugs 1978;15(6):429–50.
3. Reid RT, Levin J, Ricca LR, et al. Tolmetin sodium in the treatment of osteoarthrtis: an analysis of 725 patients with a year or more of therapy. Curr Ther Res 1982;28:173.
4. Jick H, Jick SS, Hunter JR, Walker AM. Follow-up study of tolmetin users. Pharmacotherapy 1989;9(2):91–4.
5. Maibach E. European experiences with tolmetin in the treatment of rheumatic diseases. Curr Ther Res Clin Exp 1976;19(3):350–62.
6. Ruppert GB, Barth WF. Tolmetin-induced aseptic meningitis. JAMA 1981;245(1):67–8.
7. Brown JH, Hull J, Biundo JJ. Results of a one-year trial of tolmetin in patients with rheumatoid arthritis. J Clin Pharmacol 1975;15(5–6):455–63.
8. Stefanini M, Nassif RI. Acute thrombocytopenic purpura traced to tolmetin-related antibody. Va Med 1982;109(3):171–5.
9. O'Brien WM. Long-term efficacy and safety of tolmetin sodium in treatment of geriatric patients with rheumatoid arthritis and osteoarthritis: a retrospective study. J Clin Pharmacol 1983;23(7):309–23.
10. Chatterjee GP. Nephrotic syndrome induced by tolmetin. JAMA 1981;246(14):1589.
11. Strom BL, Carson JL, Schinnar R, Sim E, Morse ML. The effect of indication on the risk of hypersensitivity reactions associated with tolmetin sodium vs other nonsteroidal anti-inflammatory drugs. J Rheumatol 1988;15(4):695–9.
12. Shaw GR, Anderson WR. Multisystem failure and hepatic microvesicular fatty metamorphosis associated with tolmetin ingestion. Arch Pathol Lab Med 1991;115(8):818–21.

Toloxatone

See also Monoamine oxidase inhibitors

General Information

Like moclobemide, toloxatone, a selective and reversible inhibitor of monoamine oxidase type A, is thought to be relatively safe in combination with sympathomimetics (SEDA-18, 16). However, sweating, tachycardia, and headache have been reported when terbutaline was added to toloxatone and phenylephrine (SEDA-18, 16). In healthy volunteers, doses up to 600 mg/day did not produce hypertensive reactions on challenge with oral tyramine (SEDA-17, 17). Two fatal cases of fulminant hepatitis have been reported (SEDA-16, 7).

Interactions with toloxatone are similar to those with moclobemide (1).

Reference

1. Livingston MG, Livingston HM. Monoamine oxidase inhibitors. An update on drug interaction. Drug Saf 1996; 14(4):219–27.

Tolterodine

See also Anticholinergic drugs

General Information

Tolterodine is an anticholinergic drug that is used to treat bladder detrusor instability. It has antimuscarinic actions that are relatively bladder-selective. Its efficacy and tolerability have been reviewed (1,2). The general conclusion is that tolterodine is better tolerated than the previous standard medication oxybutinin, particularly with regard to the frequency and severity of dry mouth, but also comparing other autonomic adverse effects, although this is not universally agreed (SEDA-22, 157). The rate of adverse effects-related withdrawals was 2–3 times higher with oxybutinin than tolterodine.

The adverse effects of tolterodine and other antimuscarinic anticholinergic drugs have been reviewed in patients with incontinence and bladder overactivity (3–6).

The findings are not unexpected: dry mouth is by far the most commonly reported adverse effect, with a frequency of about 40% in patients taking 2 mg of the immediate-release formulation bd. The next most common effects are consistently headache, constipation, and abdominal discomfort. Hallucinations and tachycardia have also been reported. It is agreed that higher doses should not be used because of the risk of urinary retention. About 5% of patients stopped taking tolterodine because of adverse effects and in about 10% the dosage was reduced. In one comparison of tolterodine 2 mg twice-daily with 4 mg once-daily in a modified-release formulation the latter produced about a 23% lower incidence of dry mouth, with increased efficacy (7).

Comparative studies

Tolterodine and oxybutynin have been compared (8). The authors concluded that the efficacy of tolterodine 2 mg bd is equivalent to that of oxybutynin 5 mg bd, but that tolterodine causes fewer autonomic adverse effects, less need for dosage reduction, and fewer dropouts because of adverse effects.

Organs and Systems

Mouth

In over 300 patients modified-release oxybutynin once-daily produced less dry mouth (28 versus 33%) than immediate-release tolterodine 2 mg bd (9).

Immunologic

Anticholinergic drugs can rarely cause immunological reactions.

- An 81-year-old Swiss woman took immediate-release tolterodine 2 mg bd and 18 days later had fever, malaise, and nausea with vomiting (10). Liver function tests showed a mixed hepatitic and cholestatic pattern and she also had leukocytosis and eosinophilia.

The authors suggested that this was a hypersensitivity reaction; if so it is the first of its kind to be reported with tolterodine.

References

1. Drutz HP, Appell RA, Gleason D, Klimberg I, Radomski S. Clinical efficacy and safety of tolterodine compared to oxybutynin and placebo in patients with overactive bladder. Int Urogynecol J Pelvic Floor Dysfunct 1999;10(5):283–9.
2. Anonymous. Tolterodine offers new hope for those with overactive bladder. Drugs Ther Perspect 1999;13:1–4.
3. Clemett D, Jarvis B. Tolterodine: a review of its use in the treatment of overactive bladder. Drugs Aging 2001;18(4):277–304.
4. Abrams P, Malone-Lee J, Jacquetin B, Wyndaele JJ, Tammela T, Jonas U, Wein A. Twelve-month treatment of overactive bladder: efficacy and tolerability of tolterodine. Drugs Aging 2001;18(7):551–60.
5. Crandall C. Tolterodine: a clinical review. J Womens Health Gend Based Med 2001;10(8):735–43.
6. Layton D, Pearce GL, Shakir SA. Safety profile of tolterodine as used in general practice in England: results of prescription-event monitoring. Drug Saf 2001;24(9):703–13.
7. Van Kerrebroeck P, Kreder K, Jonas U, Zinner N, Wein A; Tolterodine Study Group. Tolterodine once-daily: superior efficacy and tolerability in the treatment of the overactive bladder. Urology 2001;57(3):414–21.
8. Malone-Lee JG. The efficacy, tolerability and safety profile of tolterodine in the treatment of overactive/unstable bladder. Rev Contemp Pharmacother 2000;11:(29–42).
9. Appell RA, Sand P, Dmochowski R, Anderson R, Zinner N, Lama D, Roach M, Miklos J, Saltzstein D, Boone T, Staskin DR, Albrecht D. Overactive Bladder: Judging Effective Control and Treatment Study Group. Prospective randomized controlled trial of extended-release oxybutynin chloride and tolterodine tartrate in the treatment of overactive bladder: results of the OBJECT Study. Mayo Clin Proc 2001;76(4):358–63.
10. Schlienger RG, Keller MJ, Krahenbuhl S. Tolterodine-associated acute mixed liver injury. Ann Pharmacother 2002;36(5):817–19.

Tonazocine

General Information

Tonazocine is a partial opioid receptor agonist that has not been reported to have adverse effects on the cardiovascular system or to cause clinically significant respiratory depression. When single doses of tonazocine 2, 4, and 8 mg were compared in 150 adults postoperatively, drowsiness was the most frequent adverse effect and visual hallucinations occurred in two patients (1).

Reference

1. Lippmann M, Mok MS, Farinacci JV, Lee JC. Tonazocine mesylate in postoperative pain patients: a double-blind placebo controlled analgesic study. J Clin Pharmacol 1989;29(4):373–8.

Topiramate

See also Antiepileptic drugs

General Information

Topiramate is used in the adjunctive therapy of partial seizures and some types of generalized seizure. Most of its adverse effects relate to the central nervous system.

Observational studies

In an open study of the effects of topiramate 100–1600 mg/day in 292 adults (mean age 33 years) with partial and/or generalized seizures previously resistant to antiepileptic drug therapy over 50% of the patients achieved at least a 50% reduction in seizures (1). The most commonly reported adverse events were related to the central nervous system, including headache, difficulty in concentrating, somnolence, anorexia, fatigue, dizziness, nervousness, nausea, confusion, and paresthesia; 32% discontinued because of adverse events.

Topiramate had a beneficial effect on benign essential tremor in an open study in nine patients (2). Six patients complained of fatigue and two discontinued therapy; four complained of paresthesia.

The effectiveness and tolerability of topiramate has been studied in an open study in 56 patients with bipolar disorder (3). The most common adverse effects were neurological and gastrointestinal, including reduced appetite ($n = 11$), cognitive impairment ($n = 10$), fatigue ($n = 5$), and sedation ($n = 5$). Six patients dropped out during acute treatment and four during maintenance therapy because of adverse effects (cognitive impairment, poor appetite and weight loss, sedation, paresthesia, psychosis, anxiety, tremor, nausea, altered taste, and rash).

In a 3-year retrospective review of the use of topiramate in 51 children aged 3–16 years with partial and generalized epilepsy, 15 children had a greater than 50% reduction in their seizure frequency and four became seizure free (4). Adverse effects were reported in 29 patients; most were related to behavioral and cognitive difficulties; less common effects included anorexia, weight loss, and headache. Topiramate was withdrawn in 25 patients; in 20 cases because of adverse effects.

In 18 patients with severe myoclonic epilepsy in infancy topiramate caused reduced seizure frequency in most (5). There were adverse effects in nine patients, eight with a weekly titration schedule and one with a fortnightly schedule. They were usually minor and transient nervous system effects, except for weight loss, which lasted longer and occurred in four patients.

Among the adverse effects of topiramate are reduced appetite and weight loss, and this has been put to use in the treatment of binge eating in an open study in 13 patients (6). Nine patients had a moderate or better response, two had moderate or marked responses that subsequently diminished, and two had a mild response or none. Neurological adverse effects were the most common. Three patients discontinued topiramate because of adverse effects, and two resumed at a later date without significant recurrence.

The efficacy and tolerability of topiramate have been studied in 170 patients with refractory epilepsy (7). The most common adverse effects resulting in withdrawal were fatigue, weight loss, irritability, paresthesia, depression, and headache. Three patients developed renal calculi but continued therapy.

The effect of topiramate for 6–18 months in 34 children with drug-resistant epilepsy has been studied (8). Adverse effects were reported in nine patients, appetite suppression in five, behavioral disturbances in three, somnolence in two, and poor concentration in one.

In a long-term open extension to a double-blind, placebo-controlled trial of topiramate in 83 children with partial-onset seizures, with or without secondary generalization, seizure frequency over the last 3 months of therapy was reduced by at least 50% in 47 children (9). Anorexia was common during long-term therapy. Five children withdrew because of adverse events.

Topiramate has been used for the treatment of psychiatric disorders, especially bipolar disease. The adverse events profile is similar to that in patients with epilepsy. In a retrospective assessment of 76 patients taking topiramate for bipolar spectrum disorders there was mild improvement in 47% and moderate-to-marked improvement in 13% (10). Responders took a significantly higher mean dose (180 mg/day) than non-responders (83 mg/day). There was weight loss (mean 6.4 kg) in 50% of the patients; the dose was significantly higher in patients who lost weight. Other adverse events were reported by 82% of patients: cognitive effects, sedation, paresthesia, nausea, insomnia, headache, and dizziness. Adverse effects led to withdrawal in 36% of the total patient population. Similar anecdotal experiences in the treatment of bipolar disorders have been reported by others (11,12).

Placebo-controlled studies

In a double-blind, placebo-controlled, add-on trial of topiramate (300 mg/day) in 177 Korean patients with epilepsy, adverse events that were significantly more common in the active treatment group were anorexia (21 versus 6% on placebo), abdominal pain or discomfort (21 versus 2%), speech disturbances (10 versus 1%), psychomotor slowing (9 versus 1%), and weight loss (9 versus 0%) (13). The relatively high incidence of gastrointestinal disturbances was not seen in Western trials, suggesting that Koreans may be more sensitive to this type of adverse effect. Of seven patients who withdrew because of adverse events, four did so because of abdominal symptoms, nausea, and/or vomiting.

The results of six double-blind, placebo-controlled trials with topiramate in adults with treatment-resistant partial-onset seizures with or without secondary generalization have been analysed (14). Seizures were reduced by at least 50% in 43% of topiramate-treated patients and in 12% of placebo-treated patients. The most common treatment-related adverse events were dizziness, somnolence, fatigue, psychomotor slowing, nervousness, paresthesia, ataxia, memory difficulty, and speech problems. These effects were generally mild to moderate, usually occurred early in treatment, often during titration, and resolved with continued treatment. Other adverse effects were weight loss and, in a few patients, renal calculi.

The efficacy and safety of topiramate has been studied in 46 adult Chinese patients with refractory partial epilepsy in a randomized, double-blind, placebo-controlled study (15). Adverse events were mostly mild and transient, with no significant differences between treatment groups. Two patients taking topiramate had weight loss.

Organs and Systems

Cardiovascular

It is unclear whether topiramate played any role in rare cardiovascular events. These included symptoms of Raynaud's phenomenon in three patients, and third-degree atrioventricular block requiring emergency cardiac pacemaker implantation in one patient with pre-existing right bundle branch block (SEDA-21, 76).

Respiratory

Topiramate inhibits carbonic anhydrase isozymes II and IV, which are present in the central nervous system. Respiratory alkalosis in a 15-year-old girl, who presented with hyperpnea, was not therefore surprising (16). The problem resolved within 24 hours of withdrawal.

Nervous system

In controlled trials, adverse effects with a minimum incidence of 20% in any dosage group included dizziness, fatigue, diplopia, nystagmus, somnolence, confusion, mental slowing, ataxia, anorexia, impaired concentration, and headache (17). The most common complaint was dizziness (40 versus 13% on placebo) in those assigned to the highest dosage (1000 mg/day). Taking events that were probably or definitely drug-related, those with a frequency of 5% or greater were ataxia, impaired concentration, confusion, dizziness, fatigue, paresthesia, somnolence, and mental slowing. All the events were usually mild or moderate and tended to be more frequent at dosages above 600 mg/day, although some, such as dizziness and somnolence, showed no clear dose-dependency. These studies may have overestimated the adverse potential of the drug, because excessively fast dosage escalations were used and maintenance dosages in many groups were larger than those that were later found to be optimal. However, signs of cognitive dysfunction, including word-finding difficulties and impaired memory, have occurred in an appreciable proportion of patients in many studies (SEDA-20, 66).

In monotherapy studies, the incidence of adverse effects was lower than in add-on studies, except for paresthesia which tended to occur more often.

Ataxia was twice as common in patients taking two concomitant anticonvulsants compared with those taking only one other drug (17).

In the comparison of four anticonvulsants mentioned above, the commonest adverse effect of topiramate in 28 patients was irritability, which occurred in seven of ten patients who discontinued therapy because of adverse effects (18).

The response to topiramate has been evaluated in 97 patients with Lennox–Gastaut syndrome in a long-term, open-label extension to a double-blind, placebo-controlled trial (19). The most common adverse events, apart from childhood illnesses, were somnolence and anorexia.

There have been a few reports of hemiparesis in patients taking topiramate.

- Hemiparesis developed in a 41-year-old man and a 59-year-old woman during the first few weeks on topiramate at dosages up to 250 and 200 mg/day respectively (20). The condition resolved gradually after drug withdrawal.

Both patients had pre-existing cerebral damage (contralateral cerebral palsy and temporal lobe infarction respectively), which might have facilitated this hitherto unreported possible adverse effect.

Reversible hemiparesis occurred in a boy taking topiramate (21).

- A 5.5-year-old boy with partial motor seizures secondary to heterotopic gray matter in the atrium of the left lateral ventricle and postictal Todd's paresis was given topiramate in addition to baseline valproate and carbamazepine, and became seizure-free for 6 months. However, he then started to have a new type of seizure, characterized as complex partial. The dosage of topiramate was increased and carbamazepine was withdrawn. He then had a change in behavior, clumsiness, and persistent right hemiparesis. Electroencephalography showed continuous independent left and right centrotemporal epileptiform discharges. There were no changes on an MRI scan. Topiramate was withdrawn and ethosuximide was added. He became seizure-free and his hemiparesis resolved after 1 month. The electroencephalogram improved remarkably.

It is very difficult to find a causal relation between topiramate and this patient's hemiparesis. An alternative interpretation is that he had complex partial status (as suggested by his electroencephalogram) when carbamazepine was withdrawn, associated with reversible hemiparesis.

Sensory systems

On 26 September 2001 OrthoMacneil/Jansen-Cilag issued a "Dear Doctor" letter about an ocular syndrome in patients taking topiramate. The syndrome is characterized by acute myopia and secondary angle-closure glaucoma. Several case reports have been published (22–24).

As of 17 August 2001 there were 23 reported cases (22 adults and 1 child) out of 825 000 patients. Symptoms typically occur within the first month of therapy, and the patients report acutely reduced visual acuity and/or ocular pain. There is myopia, redness, swelling of the anterior chamber, and raised ocular pressure, with or without pupil dilatation. Supraciliary effusion can displace the lens and iris anteriorly, secondarily causing angle-closure glaucoma. The symptoms are reversible if topiramate is withdrawn. Acute myopia has been described as a rare idiosyncratic reaction to other sulfonamides. It has been postulated that the pathogenic mechanism is related to partial inhibition of carbonic anhydrase and to ciliary body swelling.

Psychological, psychiatric

Psychiatric

Depression and psychosis have been observed in respectively 15 and 3% of patients taking topiramate (SEDA-22, 91) (17). Three patients taking topiramate for bipolar disorder developed substantial depression (25). The symptoms began or increased within 1 week of topiramate treatment (25 mg/day) or with an increase in dosage to 50 mg/day. All had significant relief from depression 1–2 weeks after withdrawal of topiramate. The close associa tion with the onset of the most severe depression these patients had ever experienced suggests an adverse effect of topiramate. However, all these patients had bipolar disorder, so the onset of depression could have been coincidental. Moreover, their depression might also have been due to a synergistic interaction between topiramate and their other medications.

Two adult patients with refractory partial seizures without a previous history of psychosis had an acute psychotic episode with hallucinations and psychomotor agitation after taking topiramate 200–300 mg/day (26).

A single case report of new-onset panic attacks has been described.

- A 24-year-old woman with a history of bipolar disorder and binge eating had a history of "isolated" panic attacks 8 years before and the attacks subsided 14 days after topiramate withdrawal (27).

Because she had a history of psychiatric diseases and panic attacks, the relation of these symptoms to topiramate was doubtful.

Cognitive effects

All anticonvulsants have been associated with adverse cognitive events, and many, sometimes contradictory, studies of classical anticonvulsants have been published (28). Cognitive adverse effects are large for phenobarbital, and possibly larger for phenytoin than for carbamazepine or valproic acid (28). Most often cognitive adverse events result in mild general psychomotor slowing. Although the severity of cognitive adverse effects is considered mild to moderate for most anticonvulsants, their impact may be substantial in some patients, especially in those with pre-existing impaired cognitive function. There is relatively little reliable information on cognitive adverse events of new anticonvulsants. Most of the published studies are on

polytherapy and there is little information about healthy volunteers (29).

Topiramate can cause cognitive adverse effects in some patients. Those affected often have impaired verbal learning and fluency. Slow titration reduces the likelihood of cognitive adverse events. Two patients had neuropsychological deficits during topiramate treatment and cognitive improvement after withdrawal (30). One patient was assessed during and after topiramate withdrawal and the other before, during, and after.

The cognitive adverse effects of gabapentin, lamotrigine, and topiramate in healthy volunteers have been compared in a randomized, single-blind, parallel-group study (29). Neurobehavioral testing was conducted at baseline, during the acute oral dosing period 3 hours after medication administration, and at 2 and 4 weeks during chronic dosing. Acutely, those who took topiramate (2.8 mg/kg) performed significantly worse than those who took gabapentin (17 mg/kg) or lamotrigine (3.5 mg/kg) on tasks of letter and category word fluency and visual attention; cognitive effects were not different between those who took gabapentin or lamotrigine. The doses were then increased to topiramate 5.7 mg/kg/day, lamotrigine 7.1 mg/kg/day, and gabapentin 35 mg/kg/day. At 2 and 4 weeks, those taking topiramate had significant verbal memory deficit and slow psychomotor speed compared with baseline; those taking gabapentin and lamotrigine did not. However, the clinical impact of the trial was limited, owing to the small sample size (17 patients) and the very rapid topiramate titration, much faster than is currently recommended (31).

There has been a retrospective analysis of neuropsychological scores before and after the use of topiramate 125–600 mg/day for at least 3 months in 18 patients (32). Topiramate was associated with significant deterioration in verbal IQ, learning, and fluency. Withdrawal or dosage reduction was associated with significant improvement. There was no correlation between individual topiramate dose and the change in test score. This study was retrospective and the patients were selected because they had cognitive problems; the resultant bias makes it difficult to generalize these results to wider populations.

A group of 14 US epilepsy centers has published the results of a post-marketing surveillance study of 701 patients taking topiramate (33). Although 41% of the patients reported cognitive adverse events at any time during treatment, only 5.8% of them discontinued for that reason. Cognitive effects were the most frequent reason for withdrawal because of adverse events (41/170 or 24% of those who discontinued). The central nervous system-related adverse effects profile in these patients included psychomotor slowing, fatigue, slurred speech, irritability, behavioral changes, confusion, inappropriate laughter, and hallucinations. Only 2.4% of the patients were taking monotherapy, and the mean dose of topiramate at 6 months was 385 mg/day, with a mean weekly dose during titration of 36 mg/day. Risk factors for discontinuation were evaluated. A slow titration rate (slower than 25 mg/week), but not the total dose at discontinuation, was significantly associated with a lower discontinuation rate. There was no specific population, dose titration, or concomitant antiepileptic drug that increased the risk of treatment discontinuation because of cognitive complaints. Psychomotor slowing was the most common complaint, but most patients elected to continue treatment because of improved seizure control.

In a retrospective survey, behavioral changes occurred in nine of 69 children (median age 12 years) taking topiramate (34). Dosages in the affected children were 2.4–8.5 mg/kg, and three children were taking monotherapy. Manifestations included school difficulties (4), mood swings (2), and aggression, irritability, and hallucinations (one case each). There was no apparent relation to dosage or titration rate.

The cognitive effects of topiramate and valproate as adjunctive therapy to carbamazepine have been compared in 53 patients (35). Topiramate was given in an initial dose of 25 mg and increased weekly by 25 mg/day increments to a minimum of 200 mg/day. Cognition was significantly worsened by topiramate and improved by valproate. Gradual introduction of topiramate reduced the extent of cognitive impairment.

The effects of topiramate and valproate, when added to carbamazepine, on cognitive status in adults have been compared in a randomized, observer-blinded, parallel-group study (35). Topiramate was introduced slowly at a starting dose of 25 mg/day and increased weekly by 25 mg/day increments over 8 weeks to a minimum dosage of 200 mg/day. The target dosages were 200–400 mg/day for topiramate and 1800 mg/day for valproate. There were significant differences between topiramate and valproate in short-term verbal memory—worsening with topiramate and improvement with valproate—but the differences were small. There were no effects on mood disorders, psychiatric symptoms, or motor and mental speed and language tests. These results suggest that if the dose of topiramate is slowly titrated cognitive adverse events can be minimized. However, although most patients tolerated topiramate if properly titrated and dosed, a subset of patients had clinically significant deficits, possibly as an idiosyncratic reaction. In another multicenter, parallel-group, randomized study similar results were obtained when topiramate or valproate was added to carbamazepine (36,37).

The effects of topiramate on tests of intellect and other cognitive processes have been studied in 18 patients (32). Repeat assessments in those taking topiramate were associated with a significant deterioration in many domains, which were not seen in controls. The greatest changes were for verbal IQ, verbal fluency, and verbal learning. There were improvements in verbal fluency, verbal learning, and digit span in patients who had topiramate withdrawn or reduced.

The factors associated with behavioral and cognitive abnormalities in children taking topiramate have been studied retrospectively (38). There were behavioral or cognitive abnormalities in 11 of 75 children at 2–4 months after the start of therapy. The mean dosage (4.6 mg/kg/day) at which these abnormalities were observed was similar to the mean final dose (5.8 mg/kg/day) in children without abnormalities. Five of the eleven children with behavioral or cognitive abnormalities had a previous history of behavioral or cognitive abnormalities, but only nine of the 64 children without abnormalities had a previous history of behavioral or cognitive abnormalities.

Angelman's syndrome, a genetic disorder that involves a defect in the DNA coding for subunits of the GABA-A receptor, is often associated with intractable epilepsy. Topiramate was effective in five children with Angelman's syndrome and epilepsy (39). One patient had transient insomnia and one had akathisia and insomnia that persisted until topiramate was withdrawn.

Slowed mental function is a relatively common adverse effect of topiramate, especially at high dosages, and has been confirmed in a randomized single-blind, parallel-group study in healthy volunteers. After single doses, topiramate (2.8 mg/kg) reduced performance in attention and word fluency tests, whereas lamotrigine (3.5 mg/kg) and gabapentin (17 mg/kg) had no effects (29). After 4 weeks of multiple dosing, topiramate (5.7 mg/kg) was still associated with impairment in verbal memory and psychomotor speed, while there was no impairment with lamotrigine (7.1 mg/kg) or gabapentin (35 mg/kg). While these data suggests that topiramate can cause greater cognitive dysfunction in the short-term than lamotrigine and gabapentin, these findings should be interpreted cautiously. First, the design was less than ideal: the use of a double-blind, crossover design and inclusion of placebo would have been preferable. Secondly, the speed of topiramate titration was much faster than currently recommended, and it is known that neurotoxicity can be reduced by slow dose escalation. Finally, the dosage of topiramate was very high, in view of the fact that no enzyme-inducing co-medication was present.

Word-finding difficulties are a known adverse effect of topiramate. Language disturbances (anomia or impaired verbal expression) without other complaints suggestive of impaired cognition were reported by four of 51 patients; five others had language problems associated with cognitive dysfunction (40). One severely retarded patient with a limited vocabulary became mute, although otherwise alert. Anomia or dysnomia were also seen in two of eight patients treated with zonisamide, which shares with topiramate a sulfa structure and carbonic anhydrase inhibitory properties. Psychotic symptoms are a significant adverse effect in occasional patients. In a retrospective survey, five of 80 patients developed psychosis 2–46 days after starting to take topiramate; manifestations included paranoid delusions in four and auditory hallucinations in three (41). The dosage at the time of onset of symptoms was 50–500 mg/day, and recovery occurred rapidly after drug withdrawal (three patients), dosage reduction (one patient), or neuroleptic drug treatment (one patient). Three of the patients had no significant psychiatric history.

Metabolism

Topiramate causes a fall in body weight, ranging from a mean of 1.1 kg at 200 mg/day to 5.9 kg at 800–1000 mg/day (17). Loss of weight may be linked to anorexia. Women tend to lose more weight than men, and weight loss is greatest in patients with the highest weight at baseline.

Weight loss with topiramate can occasionally be extensive (42).

- A 37-year-old obese white woman with affective instability and obesity taking topiramate (up to

275 mg/day) lost 10 kg over 10 weeks, although she remained obese (BMI 52 kg/m^2). She also improved mentally.

In this case the weight loss was a beneficial collateral effect of topiramate.

In a retrospective chart review, weight loss was assessed in 214 patients with psychiatric disorders taking topiramate (43). Patients taking either lithium or valproate gained a mean (SD) of 6.3 (9.0) kg and 6.4 (9.0) kg respectively, whereas patients taking topiramate lost 1.2 (6.3) kg. Similar statistically significant results were found in the bone mass index.

Acid–base balance

Topiramate lowers serum bicarbonate by inhibiting carbonic anhydrase. In 20 of 29 children there was a greater than 10% fall in serum bicarbonate after starting topiramate (mean absolute reduction 4.7 mmol/l), but none had significant symptoms of metabolic acidosis, except possibly for anorexia in one (44). In another report, mild to moderate metabolic acidosis (bicarbonate concentrations, 16–21 mmol/l) developed in three topiramate-treated patients aged 25–51 years; the condition was not considered clinically significant, but it led to diagnostic tests to exclude other causes (45).

While the fall in serum bicarbonate is asymptomatic in most cases, special caution is required in patients already at risk of metabolic acidosis, such as those with respiratory acidosis, renal disease, frequent severe infections and sepsis, gastrointestinal disorders with recurrent dehydration, inborn errors of metabolism, or treatment with a ketogenic diet (44).

Mental changes and metabolic acidosis can occur with topiramate, through inhibition of carbonic anhydrase.

- A 20-year-old man taking topiramate, valproate, and phenytoin had acute mental changes with hyperchloremic metabolic acidosis (46). He had been receiving a modest dose of topiramate for 9 months. His mental status returned to normal within 48 hours of withdrawal.

Two children developed symptomatic metabolic acidosis while taking topiramate (47).

- An 11-year-old boy with refractory partial epilepsy who had been taking topiramate 300 mg/day for 13 months developed hyperventilation. He had a hyperchloremic metabolic acidosis with partial respiratory compensation. The hyperventilation and acidosis resolved after the administration of sodium bicarbonate and reduction of the dose of topiramate.
- A 16-month-old girl developed increasing irritability associated with topiramate; it resolved promptly on withdrawal. Venous blood showed a metabolic acidosis.

The authors postulated that the mechanism of topiramate-induced acidosis is inhibition of carbonic anhydrase in the proximal renal tubule, resulting in impaired proximal bicarbonate reabsorption. Blood gases should be obtained in patients taking topiramate who develop hyperventilation and changes in mental status.

Metabolic acidosis developed in eight of nine infants and toddlers aged 5 months to 2.3 years, weights 8.2–26 (median 11) kg, taking topiramate (48). Five patients were taking other antiepileptic drugs. The metabolic acidosis developed early in treatment (after 8–26 days). Four of the nine children had hyperventilation. This study suggests that metabolic acidosis may not be rare in young children taking topiramate, although it is often asymptomatic. However, the very rapid titration and high doses used make it difficult to generalize the data.

Gastrointestinal

Nausea, abdominal pain, and severe constipation occur rarely, although nausea and abdominal symptoms have been seen commonly in Korean patients (13).

Liver

Hepatitis, reversible on topiramate withdrawal, occurred in one child, but no details were given (49).

- Fulminant liver failure developed in a 39-year-old woman after she had taken topiramate for about 4 months, in addition to carbamazepine. The condition occurred after she increased the dosage of topiramate to 300 mg/day, and was preceded for a few days by tiredness and somnolence (50). She made an uncomplicated recovery after liver transplantation. Histological examination showed centrilobular necrosis, compatible with drug-induced fulminant liver failure.

A causative role of the drug could not be determined with certainty in this case.

Urinary tract

By inhibiting carbonic anhydrase, topiramate reduces the urinary excretion of citrate and increases urinary pH, leading to higher calcium phosphate saturation and a risk of nephrolithiasis. During 1074 patient-years of topiramate exposure in 1183 patients, 18 (1.5%) had 21 episodes of renal calculi, suggesting an incidence of nephrolithiasis comparable to that reported for acetazolamide (SEDA-20, 66).

Body temperature

Reduced sweating, heat and exercise intolerance, and fever have been associated with topiramate. Three patients (aged 17 months, 9 years, and 16 years) developed hyperthermia because of reduced sweating capacity during the summer and/or during exercise 2–3 months after reaching the target dose of topiramate (51). A reduction in the dosage of topiramate did not correct the symptoms, which disappeared on topiramate withdrawal. This adverse effect may be related to carbonic anhydrase inhibition by topiramate, as it has been described with zonisamide (another carbonic anhydrase inhibitor).

- A 9-year-old boy with partial epilepsy taking topiramate 4 mg/kg/day developed hyperthermia, reduced sweating, and tiredness after exercise 4 months after the start of treatment (51). Sudomotor function showed 180 sweat glands/cm^2 (normal 286, fifth percentile 221). After topiramate withdrawal he became asymptomatic and 5 weeks later he had 392 sweat glands/cm^2.

Long-Term Effects

Drug withdrawal

Two patients with hemiparesis reversible after topiramate withdrawal have been reported (20).

Second-Generation Effects

Lactation

The concentrations of topiramate have been measured in plasma and breast milk in five women with epilepsy during pregnancy and lactation (52). The umbilical cord plasma/maternal plasma ratios were close to unity, suggesting extensive transplacental transfer of topiramate. The mean milk/maternal plasma concentration ratio was 0.86 (range 0.67–1.1) at 2–3 weeks after delivery. The milk/maternal plasma concentration ratios at sampling 1 and 3 months after delivery were similar. Two of the breast-fed infants had detectable (>0.9 µmol/l) concentrations of topiramate 2–3 weeks after delivery, although they were below the limit of quantification (2.8 µmol/l), and one had an undetectable concentration. Thus, breast-fed infants had very low topiramate concentrations. No adverse effects were observed in the infants.

Drug Administration

Drug dosage regimens

Slow dosage titration of topiramate has been advocated by clinicians for improving tolerability. In a multicenter, double-blind trial in adults with refractory partial epilepsy 188 patients were randomized to add-on topiramate by either "slow" titration (initial dose 50 mg/day increased weekly by 50 mg/day) or "fast" titration (initial dose 100 mg/day increased weekly by 100–200 mg/day) (31). The maximum dosage of 400 mg/day in both groups was achieved by 3 or 8 weeks. Efficacy was comparable, but slow titration was significantly associated with a lower frequency of adverse events or withdrawals because of adverse events.

Drug–Drug Interactions

Digoxin

Topiramate slightly impairs digoxin clearance (53), but the interaction is probably not clinically significant.

Enzyme-inducing anticonvulsants

Enzyme-inducing anticonvulsants reduce serum topiramate concentrations to an important extent (SEDA-20, 67).

Oral contraceptives

Topiramate reduces plasma estrogen concentrations in women taking oral contraceptives, by an unknown mechanism (53), potentially reducing the efficacy of the oral contraceptive. In one study topiramate dose-dependently reduced the plasma concentrations of ethinylestradiol by 18–30% (SEDA-20, 67) (54).

Phenytoin

An increase in serum phenytoin concentration has occasionally been observed in patients taking topiramate, possibly in relation to inhibition of CYP2C19 (SEDA-20, 67), but it is usually of little significance.

In 12 patients taking phenytoin monotherapy, topiramate 400–800 mg/day was added progressively; after stabilization phenytoin was tapered and withdrawn (55). Although there were no changes in phenytoin serum concentrations in nine patients, in three of them the peak phenytoin plasma concentrations increased (from 60 to 84 µmol/l, from 112 to 144 µmol/l, and from 108 to 164 µmol/l). Human liver microsomal studies showed that topiramate partially inhibits CYP2C19 at very high concentrations (about 5–15 times higher than the recommended dose). Topiramate clearance was about two-fold higher during co-administration of phenytoin.

Valproic acid

Topiramate can reduce serum valproic acid concentrations to a minor extent (SEDA-20, 67). Conversely, the metabolism of topiramate can be inhibited by valproate (53).

Three children taking valproate developed hyperammonemia after topiramate was added (56). Ammonia was normalized after topiramate was reduced or withdrawn. Thus, topiramate could potentially enhance the risk of hyperammonemia in patients taking valproate. The authors did not discuss the mechanism of this purported interaction.

References

1. Abou-Khalil B. Topiramate in the long-term management of refractory epilepsy. Topiramate YOL Study Group. Epilepsia 2000;41(Suppl 1):S72–6.
2. Galvez-Jimenez N, Hargreave M. Topiramate and essential tremor. Ann Neurol 2000;47(6):837–8.
3. McElroy SL, Suppes T, Keck PE, Frye MA, Denicoff KD, Altshuler LL, Brown ES, Nolen WA, Kupka RW, Rochussen J, Leverich GS, Post RM. Open-label adjunctive topiramate in the treatment of bipolar disorders. Biol Psychiatry 2000;47(12):1025–33.
4. Mohamed K, Appleton R, Rosenbloom L. Efficacy and tolerability of topiramate in childhood and adolescent epilepsy: a clinical experience. Seizure 2000;9(2):137–41.
5. Nieto-Barrera M, Candau R, Nieto-Jimenez M, Correa A, del Portal LR. Topiramate in the treatment of severe myoclonic epilepsy in infancy. Seizure 2000;9(8):590–4.
6. Shapira NA, Goldsmith TD, McElroy SL. Treatment of binge-eating disorder with topiramate: a clinical case series. J Clin Psychiatry 2000;61(5):368–72.
7. Stephen LJ, Sills GJ, Brodie MJ. Topiramate in refractory epilepsy: a prospective observational study. Epilepsia 2000;41(8):977–80.
8. Yeung S, Ferrie CD, Murdoch-Eaton DG, Livingston JH. Topiramate for drug-resistant epilepsies. Eur J Paediatr Neurol 2000;4(1):31–3.
9. Ritter F, Glauser TA, Elterman RD, Wyllie E. Effectiveness, tolerability, and safety of topiramate in

children with partial-onset seizures. Topiramate YP Study Group. Epilepsia 2000;41(Suppl 1):S82–5.

10. Ghaemi SN, Manwani SG, Katzow JJ, Ko JY, Goodwin FK. Topiramate treatment of bipolar spectrum disorders: a retrospective chart review. Ann Clin Psychiatry 2001;13(4):185–9.

11. Davanzo P, Cantwell E, Kleiner J, Baltaxe C, Najera B, Crecelius G, McCracken J. Cognitive changes during topiramate therapy. J Am Acad Child Adolesc Psychiatry 2001;40(3):262–3.

12. Chengappa KN, Gershon S, Levine J. The evolving role of topiramate among other mood stabilizers in the management of bipolar disorder. Bipolar Disord 2001;3(5):215–32.

13. Lee BI, Kim WJ, Kim DK; Korean Topiramate Study Group. Topiramate in medically intractable partial epilepsies: double-blind placebo-controlled randomized parallel group trial. Epilepsia 1999;40(12):1767–74.

14. Reife R, Pledger G, Wu SC. Topiramate as add-on therapy: pooled analysis of randomized controlled trials in adults. Epilepsia 2000;41(Suppl 1):S66–71.

15. Yen DJ, Yu HY, Guo YC, Chen C, Yiu CH, Su MS. A double-blind, placebo-controlled study of topiramate in adult patients with refractory partial epilepsy. Epilepsia 2000;41(9):1162–6.

16. Laskey AL, Korn DE, Moorjani BI, Patel NC, Tobias JD. Central hyperventilation related to administration of topiramate. Pediatr Neurol 2000;22(4):305–8.

17. Shorvon SD. Safety of topiramate: adverse events and relationships to dosing. Epilepsia 1996;37(Suppl 2):S18–22.

18. Collins TL, Petroff OA, Mattson RH. A comparison of four new antiepileptic medications. Seizure 2000;9(4):291–3.

19. Glauser TA, Levisohn PM, Ritter F, Sachdeo RC. Topiramate in Lennox-Gastaut syndrome: open-label treatment of patients completing a randomized controlled trial. Topiramate YL Study Group. Epilepsia 2000;41(Suppl 1):S86–90.

20. Stephen LJ, Maxwell JE, Brodie MJ. Transient hemiparesis with topiramate. BMJ 1999;318(7187):845.

21. Patel H, Asconape JJ, Garg BP. Reversible hemiparesis associated with the use of topiramate. Seizure 2002;11(7):460–3.

22. Sankar PS, Pasquale LR, Grosskreutz CL. Uveal effusion and secondary angle-closure glaucoma associated with topiramate use. Arch Ophthalmol 2001;119(8):1210–11.

23. Rhee DJ, Goldberg MJ, Parrish RK. Bilateral angle-closure glaucoma and ciliary body swelling from topiramate. Arch Ophthalmol 2001;119(11):1721–3.

24. Banta JT, Hoffman K, Budenz DL, Ceballos E, Greenfield DS. Presumed topiramate-induced bilateral acute angle-closure glaucoma. Am J Ophthalmol 2001;132(1):112–14.

25. Klufas A, Thompson D. Topiramate-induced depression. Am J Psychiatry 2001;158(10):1736.

26. Stella F, Caetano D, Cendes F, Guerreiro CA. Acute psychotic disorders induced by topiramate: report of two cases. Arq Neuropsiquiatr 2002;60(2-A):285–7.

27. Goldberg JF. Panic attacks associated with the use of topiramate. J Clin Psychopharmacol 2001;21(4):461–2.

28. Aldenkamp AP. Effects of antiepileptic drugs on cognition. Epilepsia 2001;42(Suppl 1):46–9.

29. Martin R, Kuzniecky R, Ho S, Hetherington H, Pan J, Sinclair K, Gilliam F, Faught E. Cognitive effects of topiramate, gabapentin, and lamotrigine in healthy young adults. Neurology 1999;52(2):321–7.

30. Rorsman I, Kallen K. Recovery of cognitive and emotional functioning following withdrawal of topiramate maintenance therapy. Seizure 2001;10(8):592–5.

31. Biton V, Edwards KR, Montouris GD, Sackellares JC, Harden CL, Kamin, M; Topiramate TPS-TR Study Group.

Topiramate titration and tolerability. Ann Pharmacother 2001;35(2):173–9.

32. Thompson PJ, Baxendale SA, Duncan JS, Sander JW. Effects of topiramate on cognitive function. J Neurol Neurosurg Psychiatry 2000;69(5):636–41.

33. Tatum WO IV, French JA, Faught E, Morris GL III, Liporace J, Kanner A, Goff SL, Winters L, Fix APADS Investigators. Post-marketing antiepileptic drug survey. Postmarketing experience with topiramate and cognition. Epilepsia 2001;42(9):1134–40.

34. Hamiwka LD, Gerber PE, Connolly MB, Farrell K. Topiramate-associated behavioural changes in children. Epilepsia 1999;40(Suppl 7):116.

35. Aldenkamp AP, Baker G, Mulder OG, Chadwick D, Cooper P, Doelman J, Duncan R, Gassmann-Mayer C, de Haan GJ, Hughson C, Hulsman J, Overweg J, Pledger G, Rentmeester TW, Riaz H, Wroe S. A multicenter, randomized clinical study to evaluate the effect on cognitive function of topiramate compared with valproate as add-on therapy to carbamazepine in patients with partial-onset seizures. Epilepsia 2000;41(9):1167–78.

36. Meador KJ, Hulihan JF, Karim R. Cognitive function in adults with epilepsy; effect of topiramate and valproate added to carbamazepine. Epilepsia 2001;42(Suppl 2):75.

37. Meador KJ. Effects of topiramate on cognition. J Neurol Neurosurg Psychiatry 2001;71(1):134–5.

38. Gerber PE, Hamiwka L, Connolly MB, Farrell K. Factors associated with behavioral and cognitive abnormalities in children receiving topiramate. Pediatr Neurol 2000;22(3):200–3.

39. Franz DN, Glauser TA, Tudor C, Williams S. Topiramate therapy of epilepsy associated with Angelman's syndrome. Neurology 2000;54(5):1185–8.

40. Ojemann LM, Crawford CA, Dodrill CB, Holmes MD, Kutsy R, Wilensky AJ. Language disturbances as a side effect of topiramate and zonisamide therapy. Epilepsia 1999;40(Suppl 7):66.

41. Khan A, Faught E, Gilliam F, Kuzniecky R. Acute psychotic symptoms induced by topiramate. Seizure 1999;8(4):235–7.

42. Teter CJ, Early JJ, Gibbs CM. Treatment of affective disorder and obesity with topiramate. Ann Pharmacother 2000;34(11):1262–5.

43. Chengappa KN, Chalasani L, Brar JS, Parepally H, Houck P, Levine J. Changes in body weight and body mass index among psychiatric patients receiving lithium, valproate, or topiramate: an open-label, nonrandomized chart review. Clin Ther 2002;24(10):1576–84.

44. Takeoka M, Holmes GR, Thiele E, Bourgeois B, Helmers SL, Duffy FH, Riviello JJ Jr. Topiramate and metabolic acidosis in pediatric epilepsy. Epilepsia 1999;40(Suppl 7):126.

45. Sethi PP, Tulyapronchote R, Faught E, Gilliam F. Topiramate-induced metabolic acidosis. Epilepsia 1999;40(Suppl 7):148.

46. Stowe CD, Bollinger T, James LP, Haley TM, Griebel ML, Farrar HC 3rd. Acute mental status changes and hyperchloremic metabolic acidosis with long-term topiramate therapy. Pharmacotherapy 2000;20(1):105–9.

47. Ko CH, Kong CK. Topiramate-induced metabolic acidosis: report of two cases. Dev Med Child Neurol 2001;43(10):701–4.

48. Philippi H, Boor R, Reitter B. Topiramate and metabolic acidosis in infants and toddlers. Epilepsia 2002;43(7):744–7.

49. Kugler S, Mandelbaum D, Traeger E, Meulener M, Taft T, Sachdeo R. Broad spectrum efficacy of topiramate in children. Epilepsia 1998;39(Suppl 6):1640–51.

50. Bjoro K, Gjerstad L, Bentdal O, Osnes S, Schrumpf E. Topiramate and fulminant liver failure. Lancet 1998;352(9134):1119.

51. Arcas J, Ferrer T, Roche MC, Martinez-Bermejo A, Lopez-Martin V. Hypohidrosis related to the administration of topiramate to children. Epilepsia 2001;42(10):1363–5.

52. Ohman I, Vitols S, Luef G, Soderfeldt B, Tomson T. Topiramate kinetics during delivery, lactation, and in the neonate: preliminary observations. Epilepsia 2002;43(10):1157–60.

53. Garnett WR. Clinical pharmacology of topiramate: a review. Epilepsia 2000;41(Suppl 1):S61–5.

54. Rosenfeld WE, Doose DR, Walker SA, Nayak RK. Effect of topiramate on the pharmacokinetics of an oral contraceptive containing norethindrone and ethinyl estradiol in patients with epilepsy. Epilepsia 1997;38(3):317–23.

55. Sachdeo RC, Sachdeo SK, Levy RH, Streeter AJ, Bishop FE, Kunze KL, Mather GG, Roskos LK, Shen DD, Thummel KE, Trager WF, Curtin CR, Doose DR, Gisclon LG, Bialer M. Topiramate and phenytoin pharmacokinetics during repetitive monotherapy and combination therapy to epileptic patients. Epilepsia 2002;43(7):691–6.

56. Longin E, Teich M, Koelfen W, Konig S. Topiramate enhances the risk of valproate-associated side effects in three children. Epilepsia 2002;43(4):451–4.

Topoisomerase inhibitors

See also Cytostatic and immunosuppressant drugs

General Information

Inhibitors of topoisomerase I and topoisomerase II are the most commonly used anticancer drugs. The camptothecins—topotecan and irinotecan (CPT-11)—interact with the enzyme topoisomerase I; the podophyllotoxins—etoposide and teniposide—target topoisomerase II. They cause various forms of single- and double-strand breaks in DNA (1–7). Other drugs inhibit both enzymes simultaneously (8) (see below).

The anthracyclines and related compounds, such as mitoxantrone and amsacrine (9), also exert their cytotoxic effects via inhibition of topoisomerase II. However, they differ from the camptothecins and podophyllotoxins in respect to DNA intercalation and have a different pattern of cardiac toxicity.

Inhibitors of topoisomerase I

Camptothecins were originally isolated from the wood, bark, and fruit of the oriental tree *Camptotheca acuminata* ("tree of joy"). Why the tree produces these highly toxic alkaloids is not known, but the most likely reason is that the toxins are part of a survival strategy in combating herbivores. Among a lot of isolated plant constituents, the naturally occurring alkaloid camptothecin (CAM, NSC94600) was identified as a highly potent inhibitor of topoisomerase I, which is overexpressed in many cancers. The water-soluble salt CAM-sodium, which was introduced in early preclinical trials in the 1960s, was highly toxic in animals. Hemorrhagic cystitis, leukopenia, and thrombocytopenia were its dose-limiting toxic effects. In addition, sterile hemorrhagic cystitis, myelosuppression, and gastrointestinal toxic effects were common in patients during phase I studies. Clinical testing of CAM-sodium was therefore discontinued in the 1970s. However, the semisynthetic derivatives irinotecan and topotecan are highly active in several malignancies and do not cause hemorrhagic cystitis, because of their greater physicochemical stability and solubility at lower pH values. However, the drugs differ from each other in approved therapeutic uses, recommended doses, toxicity profiles, and pharmacokinetics (1–5).

Several camptothecin analogues are currently being investigated. The water-soluble derivatives lurtotecan (GI147211) and exatecan (DX-8951-f) and the poorly water-soluble analogues 9-aminocamptothecin and 9-nitrocamptothecin, which can be given orally, are in various stages of development (3,10–13).

Exatecan is a novel synthetic camptothecin derivative with a unique hexacyclic structure. It does not require metabolic activation, whereas irinotecan does. In vitro experiments in various cell lines have suggested that exatecan may be 6 and 28 times more active than SN-38 (7-ethyl-10-hydroxycamptothecin, the active metabolite of irinotecan) and topotecan respectively. Furthermore, it has a 2–10 times higher therapeutic index than irinotecan and topotecan. In addition, exatecan may even be active in P-glycoprotein-mediated multidrug-resistant tumor cells. Its dose-limiting adverse effects are neutropenia and liver dysfunction. The recommended dosages of exatecan for phase II trials are 0.5 mg/m^2/day or 0.3 mg/m^2/day as a 30-minute infusion on 5 consecutive days for minimally pretreated and heavily pretreated patients respectively (14,15).

Current clinical investigations with topoisomerase I inhibitors include the feasibility of oral administration of topotecan and irinotecan, the use of a liposomal lurtotecan formulation (NX211), and the use of a pegylated derivative of the naturally occurring camptothecin, which is soluble in aqueous solutions even at low pH values (3,10).

Inhibitors of topoisomerase II

Etoposide and teniposide are semisynthetic derivatives of podophyllin, which was originally isolated from the root of the Indian podophyllum plant. After extensive isolation procedures, the most effective "antileukemic" factor was identified as 4'-demethylepipodophyllin benzylidiene glucoside (DEPBG). Etoposide, its water-soluble derivative etoposide phosphate, and teniposide are semisynthetic analogues of DEPBG with increased antineoplastic activity. Etoposide is active in testicular tumors, non-Hodgkin's lymphoma, Hodgkin's disease, other lymphomas, ovarian carcinoma, gastric carcinoma, breast cancer, small-cell and non-small-cell lung cancers, and cancers of unknown origin. The major indications for teniposide include lymphoma, bladder cancer, acute lymphoblastic leukemia, and glioblastoma (6,7).

Dual inhibitors of topoisomerases I and II

Intoplicin is one of the first congeners of the so-called dual inhibitors of topoisomerases I and II (16). These new antitumor drugs interact with both topoisomerase I and II simultaneously. This mechanism of action appears to be advantageous, because selective inhibition of topoisomerase I has been reported to increase topoisomerase II enzyme activity and vice versa, which may be important for the development of drug resistance (17–20). Intoplicin may overcome this limitation. In phase I trials, intoplicin has been reported to cause dose-limiting liver toxicity; other adverse effects were sporadic and mild (16).

Another dual inhibitor of topoisomerase I and topoisomerase II is XR 5000 (N-2-[(dimethylamino)ethyl]acriacridine-4-carboxamine). Its cytotoxicity was not affected by the presence of P-glycoprotein, and it seems to be a promising candidate, even in highly resistant tumor cells. However, neither complete nor partial remission was observed during a phase II trial in 20 patients with advanced or metastatic colorectal cancer (21).

A novel pentafluorinated epipodophylloid characterized by marked antitumor activity in vivo is F11872. It is a dual inhibitor of the catalytic activity of both topoisomerases I and II, with markedly superior activity in vivo compared with other dual inhibitors, such as intoplicin, TAS-103, and others (22).

Mechanisms of action

Topoisomerase I is the target enzyme for the inhibitory effects of camptothecins. It modulates the topological structure of DNA by inducing transient DNA breaks. Single-strand breaks help to remove excessive positive and negative DNA supercoils, which arise during DNA replication and transcription. The interaction between the camptothecins and the enzyme results in the formation of a topoisomerase-I-DNA complex (23).

Etoposide and teniposide interact with topoisomerase II within the tumor cell. This nuclear enzyme catalyses the passage of DNA across adjacent strands during cell division and is most active during the late S and G2 phases of the cell cycle. If the tumor cell is exposed to etoposide during this stage, stabilization of the enzyme-DNA complex results in double- and single-strand breaks in DNA as well as cell-cycle arrest. Several studies have shown that the activity of etoposide is schedule dependent, which means that its antiproliferative effect on tumor cells is greater when it is given over several consecutive days rather than on a single day. At higher dosages, podophyllotoxins may also act as spindle poisons (24).

In contrast to topoisomerase II, cellular concentrations of topoisomerase I are relatively independent of the cell-cycle phase in normal tissues. Thus, topoisomerase I activity is only slightly increased in cells and tissues under conditions of proliferation. However, higher constitutive activities of this enzyme can be detected in several tumor tissues (for example adenocarcinoma of the colon and rectum) compared with healthy tissues (25).

Pharmacokinetics

Camptothecins

Both irinotecan and topotecan contain lactone structures, which can be hydrolysed non-enzymatically into the open-ring form. Under acidic conditions, the equilibrium between the biologically active lactone form and the less active carboxylated form is generally shifted to the lactone form, whereas at physiological or higher values of pH, the lactone form is unstable, because hydrolysis to the open form is favored. In addition, owing to preferential binding of the salt form to serum albumin, the affinity of the carboxylated form for human serum albumin is estimated to be 100 times higher than that of the lactone form. In consequence, when irinotecan is given intravenously, more than 95% of the dose is bound to serum albumin as inactive drug, and is therefore at least transiently unavailable to exert its antineoplastic activity (26–29). Novel camptothecin derivatives, such as exatecan or lurtotecan, are more resistant to rapid hydrolysis because of structural modifications, for example the removal of the 20-OH group (3,10,14,15).

Irinotecan

Irinotecan has been approved for first-line and second-line treatment of advanced colorectal cancer. Conventional dosages range from 350 mg/m^2 intravenously every 3 weeks to 100–125 mg/m^2 intravenously weekly when it is given as a single agent, and 80–180 mg/m^2 intravenously when it is given in combination with 5-fluorouracil and folinic acid weekly (the AIO regimen) or every 14 days (the De Gramont regimen) (4,30).

In contrast to the structurally related topotecan, irinotecan is a prodrug, which has to be converted to its active form, SN-38 (4,30). Cleavage of the side-chain, a bulky piperidino moiety, at the C10 position is rapidly catalysed by carboxylesterases after intravenous administration. SN-38 (7-ethyl-10-hydroxy-camptothecin) is 1000 times more potent than the parent compound. There is an equilibrium between the active lactone and the inactive carboxylated forms in a pH- and protein-dependent manner for both irinotecan and SN-38 (31,32).

The SN-38 is inactivated by conjugation, catalysed by isoforms of uridine diphosphate glucuronosyltransferase, principally UGT 1A7 (33–35). Pharmacogenetic defects in glucuronidation (for example Gilbert's syndrome and Crigler–Najjar syndrome type I) result in impaired glucuronidation. The incidence of Gilbert's syndrome is 0.5–15% in different ethnic groups, and there is significant variability of UGT 1A activity in human livers, with a 17-fold difference between minimum and maximum rates of SN-38 glucuronidation. Patients with Gilbert's syndrome are at increased risk of irinotecan-induced gastrointestinal toxicity and leukopenia if conventional dosages are used (36–40). Paracetamol is a poor predictor of SN-38 glucuronidation capacity based on metabolism by another isozyme (UGT 1A6). However, genotype screening is increasingly becoming feasible. Thus, empirical irinotecan dosage modification or the selection of another anticancer drug is appropriate in patients with poor glucuronidation capacity (36–40).

Both irinotecan and SN-38 are primarily excreted into the bile by the canalicular multispecific organic anion transporter (cMOAT), a member of the ATP cassette of transporters. Therefore, inhibitors of cMOAT, such as ciclosporin, can reduce the clearance of irinotecan and SN-38 (41,42).

The SN-38 glucuronide can be deconjugated in the gut to active SN-38 by bacterial glucuronidases. This enterohepatic circulation of SN-38 results in a further plasma peak, and SN-38 released within the gut lumen has been suggested to be an important cause of delayed intestinal toxicity; in animal experiments constitutive bacterial beta-glucuronidase activity correlated with irinotecan-induced cecal damage. In contrast, the prophylactic use of oral antibiotics (for example aminoglycosides or quinolones) or specific glucuronidase inhibitors resulted in attenuation of intestinal toxicity (43).

Aminopentane-carboxylic acid (APC) is a second major metabolite of irinotecan; it is formed by oxidation of the terminal piperidine ring, catalysed by CYP3A4. APC itself is not hydrolysed to SN-38 and is only a weak inhibitor of topoisomerase I (44–48). However, potent CYP3A4 inducers (for example St. John's wort, carbamazepine, and phenytoin) or inhibitors (for example itraconazole) alter irinotecan pharmacokinetics (49–54). Other identified metabolites include NPC (7-ethyl-10-(4-amino-1-piperidono)-carbonyloxycamptothecin), 5-hydroxyirinotecan, and RPR112526 (a decarboxylated product of the acid form of the irinotecan lactone).

Further drug interactions occur if constitutive SN-38 glucuronidation capacity is modified. For example, phenobarbital may induce UGT 1A activity, whereas valproic acid may inhibit it. Thus, co-administration can alter the clearance of irinotecan.

A half-life of 5–14 hours has been reported after intravenous infusion of irinotecan over 30 and 90 minutes. The half-life of the active metabolite SN-38 (total) is 6–14 hours. However, continuous 5-day intravenous infusion schedules result in prolonged half-lives (about 27 hours and 30 hours for irinotecan and SN-38 respectively). In general, the C_{max} of SN-38 is more than 100 times lower than the corresponding value for irinotecan. Plasma concentrations of SN-38 glucuronide were higher than the corresponding concentrations of SN-38: the AUC of SN-38 glucuronide was at least 10 times higher than that of SN-38 (44–47).

Because of the importance of hepatic metabolism in SN-38 elimination by glucuronidation, the biliary clearance of irinotecan and its metabolites is delayed in patients with impaired hepatic function (55–57), and there is a negative correlation between serum bilirubin concentrations and the total body clearance of irinotecan. In a patient with moderately impaired liver function, it was necessary to reduce the dose to 100 mg/m^2 instead of 350 mg/m^2 intravenously thrice-weekly, in order to achieve half-lives and C_{max} values of irinotecan and SN-38 comparable to those observed in patients with normal liver function (55). However, the corresponding AUCs were still significantly increased, resulting in more severe leukopenia and delayed diarrhea. The authors concluded that to improve tolerance, exposure to the drug in a patient of this kind should not exceed 30 mg/m^2 intravenously.

Detailed studies of irinotecan dose modification in patients with liver dysfunction are warranted. According to the results of pharmacokinetic studies, thrice-weekly intravenous doses of irinotecan have been recommended: 350 mg/m^2 in patients with bilirubin concentrations up to 1.5 times the upper limit of the reference range and 200 mg/m^2 in patients with bilirubin concentrations 1.5–3.0 times the upper limit of the reference range (56).

The systemic availability of oral irinotecan is low and variable (10–20%). Transintestinal transport of irinotecan and SN-38 by P-glycoprotein and cytochrome P$_{450}$-mediated first-pass removal in the intestine accounts for the low absolute availability of irinotecan.

Topotecan

Topotecan has been approved for the treatment of advanced pretreated ovarian and small-cell lung cancer in several countries. After intravenous administration of conventional dosages (for example 1.5 mg/m^2/day for 5 consecutive days) its half-life is 2–4 hours. Prolonged infusion for 3, 5, or 21 days increases drug exposure without affecting the disposition of topotecan (29).

The ratio of the AUCs of the lactone and total topotecan appears to be relatively constant and averages about 0.3, which means that only 30% of the total drug concentration in the plasma represents the closed-ring lactone form. The distribution volume at steady state is 25–75 l/m^2, indicating extensive binding to tissues. Erythrocytes act as a depot for topotecan (lactone), with steady-state concentrations almost 1.7 times those obtained in plasma.

Topotecan is primarily excreted unchanged in the urine. About 49% of the intravenous dose is recovered in the urine as parent drug and 18% in the feces (58). Despite high urinary concentrations, topotecan does not cause urinary toxicity, because of its high water solubility (58,59). Dosage modification is warranted in patients with impaired renal function (60). Reduced doses of 0.75 mg/m^2/day and 0.5 mg/m^2/day have been recommended in untreated and extensively pretreated patients with reduced creatinine clearance (20–40 ml/minute). It has also been suggested that dosage adjustment may even be required if the creatinine clearance is 40–60 ml/minute (61). The recommended starting dose should be 1.2 mg/m^2/day intravenously on five consecutive days, in order to reduce the risk of severe myelosuppression. Because there is no information about topotecan in patients with severe renal insufficiency (creatinine clearance below 20 ml/minute), topotecan should not be given to them (60). There is some evidence that topotecan is hemodialysable (62).

Hepatic metabolism of topotecan, mediated by cytochrome P$_{450}$ isozymes, is of minor quantitative importance (26–29,58). Metabolic pathways include N-dealkylation (producing N-demethyltopotecan) and glucuronidation. There is some evidence that potent inhibitors or inducers of CYP3A4 alter the clearance of topotecan (58).

After conventional intravenous dosages of topotecan (for example 1.5 mg/m^2 as a 30-minute infusion on days 1–5) the mean half-life, plasma clearance, and volume of distribution are respectively 2.7 hours, 1.1 ml/minute, and 170 litres. The plasma protein binding of topotecan is low (7–35%). In contrast to many other anticancer drugs, topotecan can penetrate the central nervous system. If the blood–brain barrier is intact, more than 30% of the plasma concentration can be recovered in the cerebrospinal fluid (26–29,58). Nevertheless, based on case reports and experimental data, intrathecal drug administration has been suggested to be advantageous, in order to achieve higher drug concentrations in the cerebrospinal fluid and to avoid systemic toxicity (63,64).

The systemic availability of oral topotecan is about 30%. Dose-limiting toxicity was reached at a dose of 0.6 mg/m^2 bd and consisted of diarrhea, which started from day 12 to day 20. Other toxic effects, including leukopenia and thrombocytopenia, were mild. The recommended dose for phase II trials was 0.5 mg/m^2 bd for 21 days (65–67).

Podophyllotoxins
Etoposide

At low doses of oral etoposide (for example 50–100 mg), the systemic availability averages 66%, and at higher dosages (100 mg/m^2 and over) 47%. If etoposide phosphate is used, the values are higher (range 66–84%) (68–73).

After intravenous administration of etoposide 150 mg/m^2, the peak plasma concentration averages 20 micrograms/ml and the half-life 7.1 hours. Drug clearance and distribution volume are about 16 ml/minute/m^2 and 17 l/m^2 (6,7,74). With respect to plasma concentrations of etoposide, intravenous etoposide phosphate is equivalent to intravenous etoposide with conventional or intensified dose schedules (75–79). After intravenous administration, the prodrug etoposide phosphate undergoes rapid hydrolysis catalysed by alkaline phosphatase; this conversion is linear even at high intravenous doses of 1200 mg/m^2 infused over 2 hours on days 1 and 2.

About 96% of the dose of etoposide is bound to plasma proteins, the fraction 4% being unbound (80–83). There is a higher risk of myelotoxicity when the unbound fraction is increased by factors such as hyperbilirubinemia or hypoalbuminemia, which is common in patients with hepatic dysfunction or cachexia-inducing tumors (84,85). The variability in unbound drug concentrations has been suggested to be important in the setting of intravenous high-dose etoposide and reinfusion of autologous peripheral blood stem cells. If drug concentrations persist over a longer period of time, the success of engraftment may be severely impaired. Thus, plasma concentration monitoring has been suggested, in order to identify patients at increased risk (86,87).

The renal clearance of etoposide is about 30–40% of the total plasma clearance. Even in patients with nearly normal creatinine concentrations (100–130 µmol/l), there is a slight but significant increase in the AUC, but without more pronounced hematological toxicity. Hepatic etoposide metabolism is mediated by CYP3A4, and results in the production of catechol metabolites. Although these catechols contribute relatively little to the metabolism of etoposide, they may contribute to its late adverse effects, for example secondary malignancies. Further metabolic pathways include glucuronidation and hydroxyacid formation (88). Dosage reductions of 33 and 50% have been recommended for patients with creatinine clearances of 15–25 ml/minute and under 15 ml/minute respectively. In patients with obstructive jaundice and a reduced glomerular filtration rate, a 50% dosage reduction has been recommended empirically (6,7,88,89).

In patients with very severe forms of renal insufficiency, only moderate amounts of etoposide can be eliminated by hemodialysis (90). In patients with brain metastases, high intravenous dosages of etoposide may be needed in order to achieve adequate drug concentrations in the cerebrospinal fluid. In such patients, intrathecal drug administration may be an alternative, in order to reduce systemic toxicity associated with dose-intensive chemotherapy. However, this mode of etoposide administration has not been established (91,92).

There is large interindividual variability in etoposide plasma concentrations with conventional dosages, and some authors have suggested that plasma concentration monitoring would reduce the pharmacokinetic variability and optimize outcomes (93,94).

Teniposide

Teniposide undergoes more extensive metabolic degradation than etoposide, resulting in the catechol derivative 4'-demethyldeoxy-podophyllotoxin. The aglycone and the *trans/cis*-hydroxy acids appear to be formed by pH-dependent hydrolysis reactions (7,95,96).

Plasma concentration monitoring has been proposed to be beneficial in patients receiving teniposide. For example, in one study, maintaining steady-state concentrations above 12 micrograms/ml appeared to be important for clinical responses in patients with recurrent leukemia, lymphoma, or neuroblastoma (95). In 10 patients, whose steady-state concentrations were maintained above 12 micrograms/ml, there was shrinkage of the tumor, whereas only five of 13 patients with lower steady-state concentrations had a response. Teniposide has been used as a continuous infusion over 72 hours in intravenous doses of 300–750 mg/m^2.

The mean systemic availability of teniposide after oral administration is about 42% (range 20–71%). Teniposide capsules 50 mg have been suggested to be useful, but no oral formulation has been approved so far (96).

General adverse effects

The dose-limiting adverse effects of irinotecan depend largely on the dosage schedule. Myelosuppression, particularly leukopenia and neutropenia and rarely thrombocytopenia and anemia, have been observed. Gastrointestinal toxicity (that is, diarrhea) is also common and can be acute or subacute. The most dose-limiting adverse effect of topotecan is myelosuppression, which correlates with individual drug exposure. In contrast, gastrointestinal toxicity is generally mild (97–99).

Common adverse effects of etoposide and teniposide (100) include dose-limiting myelosuppression (causing neutropenia more often than thrombocytopenia), dose-dependent nausea or vomiting, and alopecia. Mucositis can be dose limiting, particularly in patients receiving high doses of etoposide. Hypersensitivity reactions are more common with etoposide and teniposide than with etoposide phosphate, because the formulations of the former contain sensitizing solubilizers. Both drugs have been associated with acute myelogenous leukemia.

Organs and Systems

Cardiovascular

There are reports of myocardial infarction in patients who have received combination chemotherapy containing etoposide. The mechanisms have not been clearly elucidated.

- A 28-year-old man with a non-seminomatous retroperitoneal germ-cell cancer received etoposide (180 mg/day intravenously on days 1–5), bleomycin, and cisplatin (101). He had no cardiac risk factors and no history of cardiac symptoms. On day 3, during infusion of bleomycin, he developed chest pain and dyspnea. The infusion was discontinued and he was given glyceryl trinitrate and diazepam; his symptoms resolved. On day 4 he was given etoposide as scheduled, but four hours later developed severe angina. The electrocardiogram and raised cardiac enzymes were consistent with an acute posterolateral myocardial infarction. He was given heparin, aspirin, and nitrates, and the chemotherapy was discontinued. Within 20 hours his chest pain completely disappeared and his electrocardiogram became normal.

If hypotension occurs during drug administration, it usually subsides when the infusion ends and intravenous fluids or other supportive agents are given. Elderly patients may be particularly susceptible to etoposide-induced hypotension. During a phase I trial of etoposide by continuous infusion, 17 patients were given 75 mg/m^2/day for 5 days and later courses of 100 mg/m^2/day and 150 mg/m^2/day (102). Two patients with pre-existing cardiovascular disease developed myocardial infarctions, one at the 100 mg/m^2/day dose and the other at the 150 mg/m^2/day dose. Another patient developed congestive heart failure at the end of the 5-day infusion and died on day 8; however, this patient also received a saline load of 1500 ml/day for 5 days during etoposide administration and had had previous episodes of congestive cardiac failure. The authors concluded that in patients with underlying cardiovascular disease etoposide must be administered cautiously and that extensive saline loading should be avoided in patients with a history of previous congestive heart failure.

Nervous system

Fatigue is a frequent adverse effect of topotecan and occurs in up to 70% of patients when they receive 1.5 mg/m^2/day (30-minute infusions) for 5 days repeated at day 22; however, only 10% have severe symptoms (4). Topotecan causes headache in some patients.

Rare cases of peripheral neuropathy have been reported after intravenous topotecan, but a causal relation is uncertain.

Neurotoxicity occurs in under 1% of patients who receive teniposide or etoposide, and is more common after high dosages. Adverse nervous system effects, including headache, transient mental confusion, and vertigo, may be related to the blood alcohol concentration, since teniposide and etoposide formulations contain alcohol (103).

Acute neurological dysfunction with exacerbation of pre-existing neurological disorders has been reported after treatment with high-dose etoposide (over 800 mg/m^2/day) given with autologous bone marrow transplantation (104). This happened 9–10 days after the start of treatment, and it abated without sequelae after prompt steroid therapy. Changes in intracranial pressure may explain this acute disturbance.

Peripheral neuropathy, mainly mild and infrequent, has been observed after conventional dosages of etoposide and teniposide. However, during combination therapy with etoposide and vinca alkaloids, more serious forms of peripheral neuropathy have been reported. Of 142 patients with autologous bone marrow transplantation given high-dose etoposide (for example 60 mg/kg combined with melphalan), six developed grade 2–3 polyneuropathy starting 2–8 weeks after transplantation.

About 76% of patients given irinotecan complained of weakness. Grade 3 and 4 weakness has been described in 12–15% with weekly or thrice-weekly administration and during the administration of combination regimens containing fluorouracil.

Hematologic

Myelosuppression, neutropenia, and to a lesser extent thrombocytopenia, are dose-limiting toxic effects of topotecan. Reversible non-cumulative neutropenia usually occurs at between days 8 and 15 after an intravenous dosage of 1.5 mg/m^2 on five consecutive days. The nadir of the neutrophil count occurs on day 11, with recovery on day 21. Neutropenia, with cell counts less than 1.5×10^9/l (grade 2) and 0.5×10^9/l (grade 4), is observed in 70–97% of patients. In addition, 4–33% of patients treated with conventional dosages of topotecan develop neutropenic fever (97–99).

Thrombocytopenia, with platelet counts under 50×10^9/l (grade 3) and 25×10^9/l (grade 4), occurs in 25–77% of patients, with a nadir on day 15 and recovery on day 21. Platelet transfusions are needed in 4–27% of patients. Anemia, defined as a fall in hemoglobin below 8 g/dl (grade 3) or 6.5 g/dl (grade 4), has been reported in 21–41% of patients; erythrocyte transfusions were required in about 25% of treatment courses. More extensive myelosuppression can occur in patients who have been pretreated with cytotoxic drugs. The extent of myelosuppression correlates significantly with both the total topotecan AUC and the topotecan lactone AUC. When prophylactic G-CSF is given, thrombocytopenia is the dose-limiting myelotoxic effect (97–99).

Leukopenia is a dose-limiting adverse effect of irinotecan. Weekly intravenous doses (for example 100–125 mg/m^2) appear to produce a slightly greater incidence of grade 3–4 neutropenia compared with 3-weekly schedules (350 mg/m^2) (16–28 versus 14–22%). The median leukocyte nadir occurs on day 21 (15–27) and recovers 8 days later. Severe anemia (hemoglobin concentrations below 8 g/dl) and severe thrombocytopenia (platelet count below 50×10^9/l) occur in 15 and 2% of patients respectively. There is eosinophilia in up to one-third of patients (2,3).

Myelosuppression is a dose-limiting adverse effect of etoposide and teniposide. Leukopenia is the most common adverse effect associated with oral and intravenous etoposide. Nadirs in neutrophil counts generally occur within 7–14 days. Severe forms following conventional etoposide doses can be expected in about 17% of patients. Thrombocytopenia occurs in 23% of etoposide-treated patients and about 9% are severe (counts below 50×10^9/l). Leukopenia and thrombocytopenia occur respectively in 65 and 80% of patients after administration of teniposide (6,7).

Gastrointestinal

Anorexia, nausea and vomiting, and diarrhea are generally mild after the administration of conventional doses of etoposide and teniposide. Stomatitis is uncommon and mucositis starts to be more severe in patients who receive intravenous doses of etoposide up to 1000 mg/m^2. Gastrointestinal toxicity after topotecan is generally mild to moderate. Under 10% of patients complain of grade 3/4 nausea and vomiting, diarrhea or constipation, abdominal pain, or stomatitis. Mucositis is uncommon and mild after intravenous topotecan.

Besides leukopenia, diarrhea is the major dose-limiting adverse effect of irinotecan (105,106). There are two different forms. The acute form occurs very early and is due to inhibition of acetylcholinesterase. The delayed-onset form occurs simultaneously with the leukocyte nadir and depends on the concentration of the active compound SN-38 in the plasma and bowel.

The acute form of diarrhea is short-lived and can be effectively prevented or rapidly suppressed by concomitant atropine. The cholinergic symptoms are accompanied by abdominal cramps (36%), sweating (57%), salivation (11%), visual disturbances (15%), lacrimation (12%), and piloerection (3%). The recommended dose of atropine is 0.25 mg intravenously for prevention or 0.25–1.0 mg for acute treatment of patients with early cholinergic symptoms. As cholinergic symptoms have not been observed with other camptothecin derivatives, it can be speculated that these adverse effects are restricted to irinotecan, whose piperidino group bears some structural similarity to the potent nicotine receptor stimulant dimethylphenylpiperazinium (106).

Delayed-onset diarrhea of all grades of severity occurs in nearly 90% of patients during the first three treatment cycles with irinotecan. It can resemble a cholera-like syndrome, which occurs several days after completion of the infusion. There is grade 3/4 diarrhea (grade 3 being at least 7–9 stools per day, incontinence, or severe cramps; grade 4 being 10 stools or more per day, grossly bloody stools, or a need for total parenteral nutrition) in 31–37% of patients treated weekly and in 35–39% of patients treated with 3-weekly regimens. The median day of occurrence was day 6 (range days 2–12). Of the four major pathophysiological mechanisms of diarrhea (osmotic, secretory, altered motility, and exudative), irinotecan-induced watery diarrhea appears to be secretory, defined by abnormal ion transport in intestinal epithelial cells (105).

There is increasing evidence that the extent and severity of gastrointestinal toxicity correlates with concentrations of the active compound SN-38 in the plasma and bowel. The role of plasma pharmacokinetics in predicting the severity of irinotecan-induced diarrhea has been highlighted by the introduction of a biliary index, which is the product of the relative area ratio of SN-38 to SN-38 glucuronide and the total AUC. According to preliminary evidence, preventive measures should be considered when the biliary index exceeds 3.484 hours.micrograms/ml (107,108).

Because SN-38 glucuronide undergoes deconjugation by bacteria-derived beta-glucuronidase in the bowel after biliary excretion, a strategy for reducing irinotecan-induced subacute diarrhea has been proposed: inhibition of intestinal microflora by a broad-spectrum antibiotic. In one study, this ameliorated subacute diarrhea in subsequent cycles; in six of seven patients, the prophylactic oral use of neomycin resulted in less severe forms of diarrhea compared with controls (43). About 30% of irinotecan is excreted via the bile unchanged and may be directly converted to SN-38 in the bowel by intestinal carboxyesterases; however, specific non-absorbable inhibitors of intestinal carboxyesterases for oral use are not yet available.

Because the equilibrium between the active lactone form and the ring-opened carboxylate form is pH dependent, oral alkalinization with a mixture consisting of sodium bicarbonate (2.0 g/day), magnesium oxide (2.0–4.0 g/day), water (pH over 7.2, 1.5–2 l/day), and ursodeoxycholic acid (300 mg/day), combined with "controlled" defecation was used in a phase II trial to reduce subacute gastrointestinal toxicity. Anticancer activity was maintained and the incidences of diarrhea and myelosuppression were significantly reduced compared with a non-randomized control group (109–111).

The efficacy of symptomatic antidiarrheal treatment with several drugs, including loperamide, octreotide, racecadodril, and budesonide, has been assessed (105,112,113). Loperamide is recommended when the first signs of subacute, late-onset diarrhea occur; the dose is 4 mg at the start, followed by 2 mg every 2 hours, continued until the diarrhea has stopped for at least 12 hours. Premedication with loperamide is not indicated. Some authors also recommend dosage modification in subsequent cycles. If loperamide alone is insufficient, racecadodril (acetorphane, Tiorfan) 100 mg tds can be added. Racecadodril belongs to a group of drugs that block cAMP-mediated hypersecretion in the gut by inhibiting the intestinal enzyme enkephalinase. The somatostatin analogue octreotide is effective in loperamide-refractory patients with severe diarrhea despite loperamide and/or acetorphane. Subcutaneous doses of 100 micrograms tds up to 500 micrograms every 8 hours for 48–96 hours have produced improvement in diarrhea by one WHO toxicity grade or even more (105).

Oral budesonide has also been proposed to be beneficial in patients with subacute diarrhea. It has 90% first-pass removal in the liver, and so its systemic activity is low. Budesonide controls symptoms of diarrhea in most patients with inflammatory bowel disease. Preliminary data have suggested that the use of budesonide in patients with irinotecan-induced diarrhea could reduce the severity of symptoms. In addition, in a phase III trial budesonide 3 mg tds prevented irinotecan-induced diarrhea to a moderate extent. Budesonide is an option in patients who do not respond to high-dose oral loperamide (113).

The use of oral immunomodulators (for example interleukin-15 and Kampo medicines) has been suggested in order to reduce irinotecan-related diarrhea; however, randomized clinical trials are required, to assess efficacy (42).

Liver

Etoposide has been associated with increased liver enzymes, but a causal relation has not been established (114).

Urinary tract

Camptothecin can cause hemorrhagic cystitis (115), which has not been reported with semisynthetic camptothecin derivatives, supposedly because they are highly soluble in aqueous solutions even at low pH values. However, in a study of the use of camptothecin conjugated to a water-soluble polymer, two of three patients who received 80 mg/m^2/week developed hemorrhagic cystitis (grade 1/3 dysuria and grade 2/3 hematuria) during the second and third cycles; at 120 mg/m^2/week there was grade 1 bladder toxicity in two of three patients (116).

Skin

Skin rashes involving the trunk, scalp, and limbs have been reported in 17–25% of patients receiving topotecan as a short-term infusion, whereas continuous drug infusion appears to be very rarely associated with rashes. These skin reactions typically appear on days 4–8 and resolve on day 15.

- A 45-year-old woman received topotecan and colony-stimulating factor for ovarian cancer and developed erythematous and slightly pruritic plaques on the upper and lower limbs and ear lobes about one week later (117). The lesions subsided spontaneously in about 10 days and recurred after the next dose. A skin biopsy showed neutrophilic eccrine hidradenitis; all skin cultures were negative.

Skin rashes due to podophyllotoxin derivatives may be hypersensitivity reactions and can be related to the drug itself or more commonly to the vehicles used. Dose-related, non-IgE-mediated hypersensitivity has been reported in 16 children receiving teniposide (118). Other published reports of hypersensitivity or anaphylactoid reactions to teniposide include degranulation of basophils (119,120), and eight anaphylactic reactions in children, all associated with the use of intravenous teniposide 150 mg/m^2 (121).

There has been a single report of etoposide-induced hand–foot syndrome (122).

Hair

Reversible alopecia is very common at standard doses of podophyllotoxin derivatives, starting at doses of 500 mg/m^2 of etoposide. It is also common even with low, continuous oral doses of etoposide (for example 50 mg/m^2/day). Partial or complete alopecia occurs in 12–70% of patients taking topotecan or irinotecan (123).

Immunologic

The epipodophyllotoxins etoposide and teniposide can cause hypersensitivity reactions, which appear to be of type I (124). In a review of 93 cases, the characteristic features of the hypersensitivity reactions that occurred after intravenous etoposide included bronchospasm, facial flushing, rashes, dyspnea, fever, chills, tachycardia,

chest tightness, cyanosis, and changes in blood pressure (hypotension and hypertension) (125).

Hypersensitivity to etoposide or tenoposide has been reported in 50 of a series of 108 patients. The risk is related to the cumulative dose, reaching a maximum at 1500–2000 mg/m^2 in the case of tenoposide and 2000–3000 mg/m^2 for etoposide (126). Acute hypersensitivity reactions, characterized by hypotension, bronchospasm, and facial flushing, have been associated with etoposide (127,128). Rechallenge with appropriate prophylactic cover supported the association.

Very severe forms of hypersensitivity reactions, such as Stevens–Johnson syndrome, are very rare (129). Anaphylactic-like reactions have occurred in 0.7–2% of patients after etoposide administration. Some data suggest that the overall frequency of hypersensitivity reactions to teniposide may be as high as 50% if all forms of hypersensitivity are considered. With very few exceptions, patients recover quickly when the drug infusion is stopped immediately (124).

Hypersensitivity reactions to etoposide or teniposide usually occur within minutes after intravenous administration, and are probably related to release of vasoactive substances by basophils and/or mast cells. Several reports have suggested that premedication with an antihistamine and/or a corticosteroid may prevent further hypersensitivity reactions, even in patients with a history of previous reactions. However, this strategy should not be followed when patients have had severe hypersensitivity reactions, such as long-lasting bronchospasm or severe hypotension (130,131). Etoposide was successfully restarted in 78% of patients who had had a hypersensitivity reaction, especially when the drug was infused at a slower rate after premedication with an antihistamine and/or a glucocorticoid (132).

Hypersensitivity reactions to etoposide and teniposide occur in 33–51% of patients (123,124) and are primarily related to adjuvants in the parenteral formulations rather than the drugs themselves. In the case of teniposide, the solubilizing adjuvant polyethoxylated castor oil (Cremophor EL) has been implicated. However, in nine children who had facial edema and flushing after receiving teniposide, the drug alone degranulated basophils in vitro, causing histamine release, while Cremophor did not (119). In addition, etoposide formulations for parenteral use contain several adjuvants, including polysorbate 80, benzyl alcohol, and polyethylene glycol, because it is sparingly soluble in aqueous solutions, and these may contribute to hypersensitivity reactions. Polysorbate 80 may also be implicated in rare cases of hypotension and metabolic acidosis, particularly with high dosages (133).

In contrast, the structurally related etoposide phosphate is highly soluble in aqueous solutions and no solubilizing adjuvants are necessary. Preliminary data suggest that the incidence of hypersensitivity reactions is lower with etoposide phosphate than with etoposide, strengthening the hypothesis that adjuvants have a major role in the development of allergic reactions (123,124). In one case, a patient who had a type I hypersensitivity reaction to etoposide was successfully retreated with etoposide phosphate (134).

On the other hand, cross-reactivity to etoposide has been observed in patients with hypersensitivity reactions to teniposide, suggesting that allergic reactions are not exclusively restricted to the use of the solvents. In addition, hypersensitivity reactions have also been reported after oral etoposide (123,124).

- Hypotension, bronchospasm, and facial flushing occurred in a 38-year-old man with advanced testicular cancer associated with an intravenous infusion of etoposide (127). The reaction began within 3 minutes after the start of the infusion and resolved with intravenous fluids and diphenhydramine. Later, he was given four doses of etoposide after pretreatment with diphenhydramine and dexamethasone, without incident.

Successful rechallenge has been reported after a reaction to etoposide in a 19-year-old man, who was successfully re-treated with etoposide phosphate with only antiemetic doses of glucocorticoids as cover (134). This case tends to support the old assumption that etoposide hypersensitivity is due to the excipients in the formulation.

Long-Term Effects

Mutagenicity

Etoposide and teniposide are mutagenic in various bacterial and mammalian genotoxicity tests (135).

Tumorigenicity

Based on animal experiments, etoposide and teniposide should be classified as potential carcinogens (136).

Exposure to etoposide and teniposide has been reported to be an important risk factor for the development of secondary acute myelogenous leukemia (137–143). Etoposide has been suggested to have considerable leukemogenic activity. Of 119 patients with advanced non-small-cell lung cancers, 24 survived for more than 1 year after treatment with etoposide and cisplatin with or without vindesine (144). Of these 24 patients, four developed secondary acute myelogenous leukemia at 13, 19, 28, and 35 months from the start of treatment, having received a two-fold greater cumulative dose of etoposide (6.8 versus 3.0 g/m^2). Podophyllotoxin-related secondary acute myelogenous leukemia has a rather short latent period (2–3 years), and differs from malignancies caused by other drugs (for example alkylating agents) by its unique molecular marker, a balanced translocation involving the mixed-lineage leukemia (MLL) gene on chromosome 11 ("11q23 abnormalities") (145). Southern blot analysis of enzyme-digested DNA from etoposide-treated cell lines and from peripheral blood cells after treatment with etoposide showed frequent rearrangements of MLL, but not of other genes (146). There are differences between the chromosomal abnormalities and the subsequent acute myeloid leukemia associated with the alkylating agents and those following topoisomerase inhibition by podophyllotoxins (147). The alkylating agents cause abnormalities of chromosomes 5 and 7, singly or together, and the podophyllotoxins damage the 11q23 chromosome locus (145).

- A 15-year-old white girl with stage II Hodgkin's disease, who was treated with a combination of

vincristine, doxorubicin, bleomycin, and etoposide (total dose 2000 mg/m^2) over 4 months followed by radiotherapy, developed secondary acute myelogenous leukemia 16 months after the initial diagnosis (142).
- An 11-year-old boy with virus-associated hemophagocytic syndrome was treated with intravenous and oral etoposide (0.3 g and 2.8 g/m^2 respectively) and developed acute myelogenous leukemia 26 months after the diagnosis (142).

These reports and others confirm that even conventional doses of etoposide can be associated with a risk of secondary acute myelogenous leukemia. The risk appears to be related to both the schedule and the cumulative dose, and it can be aggravated by addition of alkylating agents and/or radiotherapy (148,149).

Two of 21 adults with Hodgkin's disease developed secondary acute myelogenous leukemia after receiving a regimen that included a cumulative dose of etoposide of 945–3640 mg/m^2 given over 3–6 months (141). Both patients also received MOPP after primary treatment failure, and the disease itself is associated with a high risk of secondary malignancies; however, the short latency period before the development of acute myelogenous leukemia (17–32 months) was thought to be typical of podophyllotoxin-associated disease. Altogether the etoposide-related incidence of secondary acute myelogenous leukemia in three retrospective case series was 0.4–8.1%. Secondary leukemia developed 9–68 months after the diagnosis of the first cancer.

Teniposide is about 10 times more potent than etoposide in causing DNA damage in vitro and in vivo. In 21 of 733 children with acute lymphoblastic leukemia in remission, who received maintenance therapy with teniposide once or twice weekly in combination with other anticancer drugs, the risk of secondary acute myelogenous leukemia was about 12 times higher than in patients who had been treated with less intensive schedules (for example a short course of teniposide for induction chemotherapy) (149).

In conclusion, podophyllotoxin-containing regimens carry a small but significant risk of secondary acute myelogenous leukemia. The risk may be increased by higher total cumulative doses (for example etoposide over 2 g/m^2), weekly or twice-weekly schedules, the concomitant administration of drugs that inhibit DNA repair, concomitant radiotherapy, or the use of high doses of cisplatin. It has therefore been recommended that etoposide be used cautiously in low-risk diseases.

Second-Generation Effects

Fertility

The effects on fertility of inhibitors of topoisomerases I and II have not yet been fully elucidated. However, ovarian failure, amenorrhea, anovulatory cycles, and hypomenorrhea have been described in women receiving etoposide (150).

Teratogenicity

Anticancer drugs can be classified as potentially teratogenic and embryocidal, and can cause embryonic resorption, spinal defects, decreased fetal weight, and fetal abnormalities. However, there are no controlled studies of the use of these drugs in pregnant women, and women of childbearing potential should be advised to avoid pregnancy while they are receiving chemotherapy and should be informed about the potential hazards to the fetus (151).

Drug Administration

Drug administration route

The safe intraventricular administration of etoposide has been reported (152).

Drug–Drug Interactions

Ciclosporin

The coadministration of etoposide and high-dose ciclosporin resulted in increased etoposide serum concentrations (153). Lower doses of etoposide were therefore recommended when combined with high-dose ciclosporin.

Cisplatin

Co-administration of cisplatin before topotecan has a sequence-dependent effect on the disposition of topotecan. Cisplatin-related acute changes in glomerular filtration rate can temporarily alter topotecan clearance, causing more severe myelosuppression. Nevertheless, this sequence has been recommended in clinical trials, based on its high antineoplastic efficacy. Patients therefore have to be monitored closely when the two agents are given together (154).

Docetaxel

Topotecan reduced docetaxel clearance by 50% and increased the severity of neutropenia when given over three consecutive days before the combination (155). The underlying reason for this interaction has not been elucidated; however, when combination therapy is used, docetaxel should be scheduled on day 1 and topotecan on days 1–4.

Enzyme inducers

Etoposide and teniposide are substrates of CYP3A4, and their clearance rate is increased by inducers such as carbamazepine, phenobarbital, phenytoin, rifampicin, and St. John's wort (49,51–54,156).

Enzyme inhibitors

Potent inhibitors of CYP3A4, such as ketoconazole or itraconazole, reduce the formation of inactive aminopentane-carboxylic acid from irinotecan, resulting in higher concentrations of the active metabolite SN-38. In seven patients who received irinotecan 350 mg/m^2 alone intravenously for 90 minutes and followed 3 weeks later by irinotecan 100 mg/m^2 in combination with ketoconazole 200 mg orally for 2 days, ketoconazole reduced the formation of aminopentane-carboxylic acid by 87% and increased the formation of SN-38 by 109%; irinotecan

clearance and the formation of SN-38 glucuronide were not affected (50).

Fluorouracil

If irinotecan is combined with 5-fluorouracil and calcium folinate, an infusion regimen of fluorouracil rather than bolus administration is associated with a lower incidence of severe toxicity (leukopenia and life-threatening sepsis) (157).

Neomycin

Diarrhea ameliorated in six of seven patients treated with irinotecan in combination with oral neomycin at 1000 mg tds (43). Neomycin had no effect on the pharmacokinetics of irinotecan and its major metabolites.

Oxaliplatin

Irinotecan (80 mg/m^2 intravenously) given as a 1-hour infusion immediately after oxaliplatin (85 mg/m^2 intravenously) was associated with hypersalivation and abdominal pain (158,159). These symptoms disappeared after an injection of atropine but recurred when irinotecan was given as a single agent or when the two drugs were separated by 24 hours. However, restarting the original schedule once more resulted in extended cholinergic symptoms. It has been postulated that oxaliplatin potentiates the direct inhibitory effect of irinotecan on acetylcholinesterase.

St. John's wort

St. John's wort (300 mg tds, starting 14 days before administration) reduced the AUC of the active metabolite of irinotecan, SN-38, by 42% and the severity of expected myelosuppression (51). Leukocyte and neutrophil counts were reduced by 8.6% and 4.3% after St. John's wort co-administration in contrast to monotherapy (reductions of 56% and 63%). In addition, the AUC of aminopentane-carboxylic acid was reduced by 28%. Whether the concomitant use of dexamethasone had some effect on this interaction has not been elucidated.

Valspodar

Valspodar significantly increased the AUC and half-life of etoposide, and dosage reductions of up to 66% are required to minimize toxicity when these drugs are used together.

References

1. Potmesil M. Camptothecins: from bench research to hospital wards. Cancer Res 1994;54(6):1431–9.
2. Iyer L, Ratain MJ. Clinical pharmacology of camptothecins. Cancer Chemother Pharmacol 1998;42 (Suppl):S31–43.
3. Garcia-Carbonero R, Supko JG. Current perspectives on the clinical experience, pharmacology, and continued development of the camptothecins. Clin Cancer Res 2002;8(3):641–61.
4. Rothenberg ML. Topoisomerase I inhibitors: review and update. Ann Oncol 1997;8(9):837–55.

5. Dennis MJ, Beijnen JH, Grochow LB, van Warmerdam LJ. An overview of the clinical pharmacology of topotecan. Semin Oncol 1997;24(1 Suppl 5):S5–12–5–18.

6. Joel S. The clinical pharmacology of etoposide: an update. Cancer Treat Rev 1996;22(3):179–221.

7. Clark PI, Slevin ML. The clinical pharmacology of etoposide and teniposide. Clin Pharmacokinet 1987;12(4):223–52.

8. Minderman H, Wrzosek C, Cao S, Utsugi T, Kobunai T, Yamada Y, Rustum YM. Mechanism of action of the dual topoisomerase-I and -II inhibitor TAS-103 and activity against (multi)drug resistant cells. Cancer Chemother Pharmacol 2000;45(1):78–84.

9. Rene B, Fosse P, Khelifa T, Jacquemin-Sablon A, Bailly C. Cytotoxicité et interaction de dérivés de l'amsacrine avec l'ADN topo-isomerase II: role du substituant en position 1'du noyau aniline. [Cytotoxicity and interaction of amsacrine derivatives with topoisomerase II: role of the 1'substitute on the aniline nucleus.] Bull Cancer 1997;84(10):941–8.

10. Bailly C. Homocamptothecins: potent topoisomerase I inhibitors and promising anticancer drugs. Crit Rev Oncol Hematol 2003;45(1):91–108.

11. de Jonge MJ, Verweij J, Loos WJ, Dallaire BK, Sparreboom A. Clinical pharmacokinetics of encapsulated oral 9-aminocamptothecin in plasma and saliva. Clin Pharmacol Ther 1999;65(5):491–9.

12. Ellerhorst JA, Bedikian AY, Smith TM, Papadopoulos NE, Plager C, Eton O. Phase II trial of 9-nitrocamptothecin (RFS 2000) for patients with metastatic cutaneous or uveal melanoma. Anticancer Drugs 2002;13(2):169–72.

13. Rowinsky EK, Rizzo J, Ochoa L, Takimoto CH, Forouzesh B, Schwartz G, Hammond LA, Patnaik A, Kwiatek J, Goetz A, Denis L, McGuire J, Tolcher AW. A phase I and pharmacokinetic study of pegylated camptothecin as a 1-hour infusion every 3 weeks in patients with advanced solid malignancies. J Clin Oncol 2003;21(1):148–57.

14. Minami H, Fujii H, Igarashi T, Itoh K, Tamanoi K, Oguma T, Sasaki Y. Phase I and pharmacological study of a new camptothecin derivative, exatecan mesylate (DX-8951f), infused over 30 minutes every three weeks. Clin Cancer Res 2001;7(10):3056–64.

15. Rowinsky EK, Johnson TR, Geyer CE Jr, Hammond LA, Eckhardt SG, Drengler R, Smetzer L, Coyle J, Rizzo J, Schwartz G, Tolcher A, Von Hoff DD, De Jager RL. DX-8951f, a hexacyclic camptothecin analogue, on a daily-times-five schedule: a phase I and pharmacokinetic study in patients with advanced solid malignancies. J Clin Oncol 2000;18(17):3151–63.

16. van Gijn R, ten Bokkel Huinink WW, Rodenhuis S, Vermorken JB, van Tellingen O, Rosing H, van Warmerdam LJ, Beijnen JH. Topoisomerase I/II inhibitor intoplicine administered as a 24 h infusion: phase I and pharmacologic study. Anticancer Drugs 1999;10(1):17–23.

17. Whitacre CM, Zborowska E, Gordon NH, Mackay W, Berger NA. Topotecan increases topoisomerase IIalpha levels and sensitivity to treatment with etoposide in schedule-dependent process. Cancer Res 1997;57(8):1425–8.

18. Bonner JA, Kozelsky TF. The significance of the sequence of administration of topotecan and etoposide. Cancer Chemother Pharmacol 1996;39(1–2):109–12.

19. Dowlati A, Levitan N, Gordon NH, Hoppel CL, Gosky DM, Remick SC, Ingalls ST, Berger SJ, Berger NA. Phase II and pharmacokinetic/pharmacodynamic trial of sequential topoisomerase I and II inhibition with topotecan and etoposide in advanced non-small-cell lung cancer. Cancer Chemother Pharmacol 2001;47(2):141–8.

20. Hammond LA, Eckardt JR, Ganapathi R, Burris HA, Rodriguez GA, Eckhardt SG, Rothenberg ML, Weiss GR, Kuhn JG, Hodges S, Von Hoff DD, Rowinsky EK. A phase I and translational study of sequential administration of the topoisomerase I and II inhibitors topotecan and etoposide. Clin Cancer Res 1998;4(6):1459–67.

21. Caponigro F, Dittrich C, Sorensen JB, Schellens JH, Duffaud F, Paz Ares L, Lacombe D, de Balincourt C, Fumoleau P. Phase II study of XR 5000, an inhibitor of topoisomerases I and II, in advanced colorectal cancer. Eur J Cancer 2002;38(1):70–4.

22. Etievant C, Kruczynski A, Barret JM, Perrin D, van Hille B, Guminski Y, Hill BT. F 11782, a dual inhibitor of topoisomerases I and II with an original mechanism of action in vitro, and markedly superior in vivo antitumour activity, relative to three other dual topoisomerase inhibitors, intoplicin, aclarubicin and TAS-103. Cancer Chemother Pharmacol 2000;46(2):101–13.

23. Malonne H, Atassi G. DNA topoisomerase targeting drugs: mechanisms of action and perspectives. Anticancer Drugs 1997;8(9):811–22.

24. Long BH. Mechanisms of action of teniposide (VM-26) and comparison with etoposide (VP-16). Semin Oncol 1992;19(2 Suppl 6):3–19.

25. Husain I, Mohler JL, Seigler HF, Besterman JM. Elevation of topoisomerase I messenger RNA, protein, and catalytic activity in human tumors: demonstration of tumor-type specificity and implications for cancer chemotherapy. Cancer Res 1994;54(2):539–46.

26. Kollmannsberger C, Mross K, Jakob A, Kanz L, Bokemeyer C. Topotecan—a novel topoisomerase I inhibitor: pharmacology and clinical experience. Oncology 1999;56(1):1–12.

27. Von Pawel J. Topotecan (Hycamtin): potent cytostatic action by selective topoisomerase I inhibition. Onkologie 1997;20:380–6.

28. O'Reilly S. Topotecan: what dose, what schedule, what route? Clin Cancer Res 1999;5(1):3–5.

29. Grochow LB, Rowinsky EK, Johnson R, Ludeman S, Kaufmann SH, McCabe FL, Smith BR, Hurowitz L, DeLisa A, Donehower RC, Noe D. Pharmacokinetics and pharmacodynamics of topotecan in patients with advanced cancer. Drug Metab Dispos 1992;20(5):706–13.

30. Rothenberg ML, Cox JV, DeVore RF, Hainsworth JD, Pazdur R, Rivkin SE, Macdonald JS, Geyer CE Jr, Sandbach J, Wolf DL, Mohrland JS, Elfring GL, Miller LL, Von Hoff DD. A multicenter, phase II trial of weekly irinotecan (CPT-11) in patients with previously treated colorectal carcinoma. Cancer 1999;85(4):786–95.

31. Guemei AA, Cottrell J, Band R, Hehman H, Prudhomme M, Pavlov MV, Grem JL, Ismail AS, Bowen D, Taylor RE, Takimoto CH. Human plasma carboxylesterase and butyrylcholinesterase enzyme activity: correlations with SN-38 pharmacokinetics during a prolonged infusion of irinotecan. Cancer Chemother Pharmacol 2001;47(4):283–90.

32. Hennebelle I, Terret C, Chatelut E, Bugat R, Canal P, Guichard S. Characterization of CPT-11 converting carboxylesterase activity in colon tumor and normal tissues: comparison with p-nitro-phenylacetate converting carboxylesterase activity. Anticancer Drugs 2000;11(6):465–70.

33. Gupta E, Mick R, Ramirez J, Wang X, Lestingi TM, Vokes EE, Ratain MJ. Pharmacokinetic and pharmacodynamic evaluation of the topoisomerase inhibitor irinotecan in cancer patients. J Clin Oncol 1997;15(4):1502–10.

34. Ratain MJ. Insights into the pharmacokinetics and pharmacodynamics of irinotecan. Clin Cancer Res 2000;6(9):3393–4.

35. Lokiec F, Canal P, Gay C, Chatelut E, Armand JP, Roche H, Bugat R, Goncalves E, Mathieu-Boue A. Pharmacokinetics of irinotecan and its metabolites in human blood, bile, and urine. Cancer Chemother Pharmacol 1995;36(1):79–82.

36. Innocenti F, Iyer L, Ratain MJ. Pharmacogenetics of anticancer agents: lessons from amonafide and irinotecan. Drug Metab Dispos 2001;29(4 Pt 2):596–600.

37. Iyer L, King CD, Whitington PF, Green MD, Roy SK, Tephly TR, Coffman BL, Ratain MJ. Genetic predisposition to the metabolism of irinotecan (CPT-11). Role of uridine diphosphate glucuronosyltransferase isoform 1A1 in the glucuronidation of its active metabolite (SN-38) in human liver microsomes. J Clin Invest 1998;101(4):847–54.

38. Kraemer D, Scheurlen M. Morbus Gilbert und Crigler–Najjar-Syndrom Typ I und II beruhen auf mutationen im selben genlocus UGT1A1. [Gilbert disease and type I and II Crigler–Najjar syndrome due to mutations in the same UGT1A1 gene locus.] Med Klin (Munich) 2002;97(9):528–32.

39. Ando Y, Saka H, Asai G, Sugiura S, Shimokata K, Kamataki T. UGT1A1 genotypes and glucuronidation of SN-38, the active metabolite of irinotecan. Ann Oncol 1998;9(8):845–7.

40. Innocenti F, Undevia SD, Iyer L, Das S, Karrison T, Janish L, Ramirez J, Rudin CM, Vokes EE, Ratain MJ. UT1A1*28 polymorphism is a predictor of neutropenia in irinotecan chemotherapy. Proc ASCO 2003;22:A495.

41. Yamamoto W, Verweij J, de Bruijn P, de Jonge MJ, Takano H, Nishiyama M, Kurihara M, Sparreboom A. Active transepithelial transport of irinotecan (CPT-11) and its metabolites by human intestinal Caco-2 cells. Anticancer Drugs 2001;12(5):419–32.

42. Xu Y, Villalona-Calero MA. Irinotecan: mechanisms of tumor resistance and novel strategies for modulating its activity. Ann Oncol 2002;13(12):1841–51.

43. Kehrer DF, Sparreboom A, Verweij J, de Bruijn P, Nierop CA, van de Schraaf J, Ruijgrok EJ, de Jonge MJ. Modulation of irinotecan-induced diarrhea by cotreatment with neomycin in cancer patients. Clin Cancer Res 2001;7(5):1136–41.

44. Slatter JG, Schaaf LJ, Sams JP, Feenstra KL, Johnson MG, Bombardt PA, Cathcart KS, Verburg MT, Pearson LK, Compton LD, Miller LL, Baker DS, Pesheck CV, Lord RS 3rd. Pharmacokinetics, metabolism, and excretion of irinotecan (CPT-11) following I.V. infusion of [(14)C]CPT-11 in cancer patients. Drug Metab Dispos 2000;28(4):423–33.

45. Sparreboom A, de Jonge MJ, de Bruijn P, Brouwer E, Nooter K, Loos WJ, van Alphen RJ, Mathijssen RH, Stoter G, Verweij J. Irinotecan (CPT-11) metabolism and disposition in cancer patients. Clin Cancer Res 1998;4(11):2747–54.

46. Dodds HM, Clarke SJ, Findlay M, Bishop JF, Robert J, Rivory LP. Clinical pharmacokinetics of the irinotecan metabolite 4-piperidinopiperidine and its possible clinical importance. Cancer Chemother Pharmacol 2000;45(1):9–14.

47. Santos A, Zanetta S, Cresteil T, Deroussent A, Pein F, Raymond E, Vernillet L, Risse ML, Boige V, Gouyette A, Vassal G. Metabolism of irinotecan (CPT-11) by CYP3A4 and CYP3A5 in humans. Clin Cancer Res 2000;6(5):2012–20.

48. Sai K, Kaniwa N, Ozawa S, Sawada JI. A new metabolite of irinotecan in which formation is mediated by human hepatic cytochrome P-450 3A4. Drug Metab Dispos 2001;29(11):1505–13.

49. Mansky PJ, Straus SE. St. John's wort: more implications for cancer patients. J Natl Cancer Inst 2002;94(16):1187–8.

50. Kehrer DF, Mathijssen RH, Verweij J, de Bruijn P, Sparreboom A. Modulation of irinotecan metabolism by ketoconazole. J Clin Oncol 2002;20(14):3122–9.

51. Mathijssen RH, Verweij J, de Bruijn P, Loos WJ, Sparreboom A. Effects of St. John's wort on irinotecan metabolism. J Natl Cancer Inst 2002;94(16):1247–9.

52. Murry DJ, Cherrick I, Salama V, Berg S, Bernstein M, Kuttcsch N, Blaney SM. Influence of phenytoin on the disposition of irinotecan: a case report. J Pediatr Hematol Oncol 2002;24(2):130–3.

53. Mathijssen RH, Sparreboom A, Dumez H, van Oosterom AT, de Bruijn EA. Altered irinotecan metabolism in a patient receiving phenytoin. Anticancer Drugs 2002;13(2):139–40.

54. Crews KR, Stewart CF, Jones-Wallace D, Thompson SJ, Houghton PJ, Heideman RL, Fouladi M, Bowers DC, Chintagumpala MM, Gajjar A. Altered irinotecan pharmacokinetics in pediatric high-grade glioma patients receiving enzyme-inducing anticonvulsant therapy. Clin Cancer Res 2002;8(7):2202–9.

55. van Groeningen CJ, Van der Vijgh WJ, Baars JJ, Stieltjes H, Huibregtse K, Pinedo HM. Altered pharmacokinetics and metabolism of CPT-11 in liver dysfunction: a need for guidelines. Clin Cancer Res 2000;6(4):1342–6.

56. Raymond E, Boige V, Faivre S, Sanderink GJ, Rixe O, Vernillet L, Jacques C, Gatineau M, Ducreux M, Armand JP. Dosage adjustment and pharmacokinetic profile of irinotecan in cancer patients with hepatic dysfunction. J Clin Oncol 2002;20(21):4303–12.

57. Ong SY, Clarke SJ, Bishop J, Dodds HM, Rivory LP. Toxicity of irinotecan (CPT-11) and hepato-renal dysfunction. Anticancer Drugs 2001;12(7):619–25.

58. Herben VM, Schoemaker E, Rosing H, van Zomeren DM, ten Bokkel Huinink WW, Dubbelman R, Hearn S, Schellens JH, Beijnen JH. Urinary and fecal excretion of topotecan in patients with malignant solid tumours. Cancer Chemother Pharmacol 2002;50(1):59–64.

59. Loos WJ, Gelderblom HJ, Verweij J, Brouwer E, de Jonge MJ, Sparreboom A. Gender-dependent pharmacokinetics of topotecan in adult patients. Anticancer Drugs 2000;11(9):673–80.

60. O'Reilly S, Rowinsky EK, Slichenmyer W, Donehower RC, Forastiere AA, Ettinger DS, Chen TL, Sartorius S, Grochow LB. Phase I and pharmacologic study of topotecan in patients with impaired renal function. J Clin Oncol 1996;14(12):3062–73.

61. Montazeri A, Culine S, Laguerre B, Pinguet F, Lokiec F, Albin N, Goupil A, Deporte-Fety R, Bugat R, Canal P, Chatelut E. Individual adaptive dosing of topotecan in ovarian cancer. Clin Cancer Res 2002;8(2):394–9.

62. Herrington JD, Figueroa JA, Kirstein MN, Zamboni WC, Stewart CF. Effect of hemodialysis on topotecan disposition in a patient with severe renal dysfunction. Cancer Chemother Pharmacol 2001;47(1):89–93.

63. Blaney SM, Cole DE, Godwin K, Sung C, Poplack DG, Balis FM. Intrathecal administration of topotecan in nonhuman primates. Cancer Chemother Pharmacol 1995;36(2):121–4.

64. Blaney SM, Heideman R, Berg S, Adamson P, Gillespie A, Geyer JR, Packer R, Matthay K, Jaeckle K, Cole D, Kuttcsch N, Poplack DG, Balis FM. Phase I clinical trial of intrathecal topotecan in patients with neoplastic meningitis. J Clin Oncol 2003;21(1):143–7.

65. von Pawel J, Gatzemeier U, Pujol JL, Moreau L, Bildat S, Ranson M, Richardson G, Steppert C, Riviere A, Camlett I, Lane S, Ross G. Phase II comparator study of oral versus intravenous topotecan in patients with chemosensitive small-cell lung cancer. J Clin Oncol 2001;19(6):1743–9.

66. Creemers GJ, Gerrits CJ, Eckardt JR, Schellens JH, Burris HA, Planting AS, Rodriguez GI, Loos WJ, Hudson I, Broom C, Verweij J, Von Hoff DD. Phase I and pharmacologic study of oral topotecan administered twice daily for 21 days to adult patients with solid tumors. J Clin Oncol 1997;15(3):1087–93.

67. Gore M, Oza A, Rustin G, Malfetano J, Calvert H, Clarke-Pearson D, Carmichael J, Ross G, Beckman RA, Fields SZ. A randomised trial of oral versus intravenous topotecan in patients with relapsed epithelial ovarian cancer. Eur J Cancer 2002;38(1):57–63.

68. Jagodic M, Cufer T, Zakotnik B, Cervek J. Selection of candidates for oral etoposide salvage chemotherapy in heavily pretreated breast cancer patients. Anticancer Drugs 2001;12(3):199–204.

69. Harvey VJ, Slevin ML, Joel SP, Johnston A, Wrigley PF. The effect of dose on the bioavailability of oral etoposide. Cancer Chemother Pharmacol 1986;16(2):178–81.

70. Aita P, Robieux I, Sorio R, Tumolo S, Corona G, Cannizzaro R, Colussi AM, Boiocchi M, Toffoli G. Pharmacokinetics of oral etoposide in patients with hepatocellular carcinoma. Cancer Chemother Pharmacol 1999;43(4):287–94.

71. Hande KR, Krozely MG, Greco FA, Hainsworth JD, Johnson DH. Bioavailability of low-dose oral etoposide. J Clin Oncol 1993;11(2):374–7.

72. Millward MJ, Newell DR, Yuen K, Matthews JP, Balmanno K, Charlton CJ, Gumbrell L, Lind MJ, Chapman F, Proctor M, Simmonds D, Cantwell BMJ, Calvert AH. Pharmacokinetics and pharmacodynamics of prolonged oral etoposide in women with metastatic breast cancer. Cancer Chemother Pharmacol 1995;37(1–2):161–7.

73. Chabot GG, Armand JP, Terret C, de Forni M, Abigerges D, Winograd B, Igwemezie L, Schacter L, Kaul S, Ropers J, Bonnay M. Etoposide bioavailability after oral administration of the prodrug etoposide phosphate in cancer patients during a phase I study. J Clin Oncol 1996;14(7):2020–30.

74. Hande KR. Etoposide: four decades of development of a topoisomerase II inhibitor. Eur J Cancer 1998;34(10):1514–21.

75. Schacter LP, Igwemezie LN, Seyedsadr M, Morgenthien E, Randolph J, Albert E, Santabarbara P. Clinical and pharmacokinetic overview of parenteral etoposide phosphate. Cancer Chemother Pharmacol 1994;34(Suppl):S58–63.

76. Kaul S, Igwemezie LN, Stewart DJ, Fields SZ, Kosty M, Levithan N, Bukowski R, Gandara D, Goss G, O'Dwyer P, Schacter LP, Barbhaiya RH. Pharmacokinetics and bioequivalence of etoposide following intravenous administration of etoposide phosphate and etoposide in patients with solid tumors. J Clin Oncol 1995;13(11):2835–41.

77. Budman DR, Igwemezie LN, Kaul S, Behr J, Lichtman S, Schulman P, Vinciguerra V, Allen SL, Kolitz J, Hock K, O'Neill K, Schacter L, Barbhaiya RH. Phase I evaluation of a water-soluble etoposide prodrug, etoposide phosphate, given as a 5-minute infusion on days 1, 3, and 5 in patients with solid tumors. J Clin Oncol 1994;12(9):1902–9.

78. Reif S, Kingreen D, Kloft C, Grimm J, Siegert W, Schunack W, Jaehde U. Bioequivalence investigation of high-dose etoposide and etoposide phosphate in lymphoma patients. Cancer Chemother Pharmacol 2001;48(2):134–40.

79. Kreis W, Budman DR, Vinciguerra V, Hock K, Baer J, Ingram R, Schacter LP, Fields SZ. Pharmacokinetic evaluation of high-dose etoposide phosphate after a 2-hour infusion in patients with solid tumors. Cancer Chemother Pharmacol 1996;38(4):378–84.

80. Joel SP, Shah R, Slevin ML. Etoposide dosage and pharmacodynamics. Cancer Chemother Pharmacol 1994;34(Suppl):S69–75.

81. Joel SP, Shah R, Clark PI, Slevin ML. Predicting etoposide toxicity: relationship to organ function and protein binding. J Clin Oncol 1996;14(1):257–67.

82. Liu B, Earl HM, Poole CJ, Dunn J, Kerr DJ. Etoposide protein binding in cancer patients. Cancer Chemother Pharmacol 1995;36(6):506–12.

83. Nguyen L, Chatelut E, Chevreau C, Tranchand B, Lochon I, Bachaud JM, Pujol A, Houin G, Bugat R, Canal P. Population pharmacokinetics of total and unbound etoposide. Cancer Chemother Pharmacol 1998;41(2):125–32.

84. D'Incalci M, Rossi C, Zucchetti M, Urso R, Cavalli F, Mangioni C, Willems Y, Sessa C. Pharmacokinetics of etoposide in patients with abnormal renal and hepatic function. Cancer Res 1986;46(5):2566–71.

85. Stewart CF, Arbuck SG, Fleming RA, Evans WE. Changes in the clearance of total and unbound etoposide in patients with liver dysfunction. J Clin Oncol 1990;8(11):1874–9.

86. Mross K, Bewermeier P, Kruger W, Stockschlader M, Zander A, Hossfeld DK. Pharmacokinetics of undiluted or diluted high-dose etoposide with or without busulfan administered to patients with hematologic malignancies. J Clin Oncol 1994;12(7):1468–74.

87. Schwinghammer TL, Fleming RA, Rosenfeld CS, Przepiorka D, Shadduck RK, Bloom EJ, Stewart CF. Disposition of total and unbound etoposide following high dose therapy. Cancer Chemother Pharmacol 1993;32(4):273–8.

88. Relling MV, Nemec J, Schuetz EG, Schuetz JD, Gonzalez FJ, Korzekwa KR. O-demethylation of epipodo-phyllotoxins is catalyzed by human cytochrome P450 3A4. Mol Pharmacol 1994;45(2):352–8.

89. Hande KR, Wolff SN, Greco FA, Hainsworth JD, Reed G, Johnson DH. Etoposide kinetics in patients with obstructive jaundice. J Clin Oncol 1990;8(6):1101–7.

90. Holthuis JJ, Van de Vyver FL, van Oort WJ, Verleun H, Bakaert AB, De Broe ME. Pharmacokinetic evaluation of increasing dosages of etoposide in a chronic hemodialysis patient. Cancer Treat Rep 1985;69(11):1279–82.

91. Kiya K, Uozumi T, Ogasawara H, Sugiyama K, Hotta T, Mikami T, Kurisu K. Penetration of etoposide into human malignant brain tumors after intravenous and oral administration. Cancer Chemother Pharmacol 1992;29(5):339–42.

92. van der Gaast A, Sonneveld P, Mans DR, Splinter TA. Intrathecal administration of etoposide in the treatment of malignant meningitis: feasibility and pharmacokinetic data. Cancer Chemother Pharmacol 1992;29(4):335–7.

93. Minami H, Ratain MJ, Ando Y, Shimokata K. Pharmacodynamic modeling of prolonged administration of etoposide. Cancer Chemother Pharmacol 1996;39(1–2):61–6.

94. Hande K, Messenger M, Wagner J, Krozely M, Kaul S. Inter- and intrapatient variability in etoposide kinetics with oral and intravenous drug administration. Clin Cancer Res 1999;5(10):2742–7.

95. Rodman JH, Abromowitch M, Sinkule JA, Hayes FA, Rivera GK, Evans WE. Clinical pharmacodynamics of continuous infusion teniposide: systemic exposure as a determinant of response in a phase I trial. J Clin Oncol 1987;5(7):1007–14.

96. Splinter TA, Holthuis JJ, Kok TC, Post MH. Absolute bioavailability and pharmacokinetics of oral teniposide. Semin Oncol 1992;19(2 Suppl 6):28–34.

97. Breidenbach M, Rein DT, Schondorf T, Schmidt T, Konig E, Valter M, Kurbacher CM. Hematological side-effect profiles of individualized chemotherapy regimen for recurrent ovarian cancer. Anticancer Drugs 2003;14(5):341–6.

98. Rowinsky EK, Grochow LB, Sartorius SE, Bowling MK, Kaufmann SH, Peereboom D, Donehower RC. Phase I

and pharmacologic study of high doses of the topoisomerase I inhibitor topotecan with granulocyte colony-stimulating factor in patients with solid tumors. J Clin Oncol 1996;14(4):1224–35.

99. Saltz L, Sirott M, Young C, Tong W, Niedzwiecki D, Tzy-Jyun Y, Tao Y, Trochanowski B, Wright P, Barbosa K, et al. Phase I clinical and pharmacology study of topotecan given daily for 5 consecutive days to patients with advanced solid tumors, with attempt at dose intensification using recombinant granulocyte colony-stimulating factor. J Natl Cancer Inst 1993;85(18):1499–507.

100. Hande KR. Topoisomerase II inhibitors. In: Giaccone G, Schilsky R, Sondel P, editors. Cancer Chemotherapy and Biological Response Modifiers. Amsterdam: Elsevier, 2003:103–25.

101. Schwarzer S, Eber B, Greinix H, Lind P. Non-Q-wave myocardial infarction associated with bleomycin and etoposide chemotherapy. Eur Heart J 1991;12(6):748–50.

102. Aisner J, Van Echo DA, Whitacre M, Wiernik PH. A phase I trial of continuous infusion VP16–213 (etoposide). Cancer Chemother Pharmacol 1982;7(2–3):157–60.

103. Imrie KR, Couture F, Turner CC, Sutcliffe SB, Keating A. Peripheral neuropathy following high-dose etoposide and autologous bone marrow transplantation. Bone Marrow Transplant 1994;13(1):77–9.

104. Leff RS, Thompson JM, Daly MB, Johnson DB, Harden EA, Mercier RJ, Messerschmidt GL. Acute neurologic dysfunction after high-dose etoposide therapy for malignant glioma. Cancer 1988;62(1):32–5.

105. Saliba F, Hagipantelli R, Misset JL, Bastian G, Vassal G, Bonnay M, Herait P, Cote C, Mahjoubi M, Mignard D, Cvitkovic E. Pathophysiology and therapy of irinotecan-induced delayed-onset diarrhea in patients with advanced colorectal cancer: a prospective assessment. J Clin Oncol 1998;16(8):2745–51.

106. Gandia D, Abigerges D, Armand JP, Chabot G, Da Costa L, De Forni M, Mathieu-Boue A, Herait P. CPT-11-induced cholinergic effects in cancer patients. J Clin Oncol 1993;11(1):196–7.

107. Gupta E, Lestingi TM, Mick R, Ramirez J, Vokes EE, Ratain MJ. Metabolic fate of irinotecan in humans: correlation of glucuronidation with diarrhea. Cancer Res 1994;54(14):3723–5.

108. Castellanos C, Aldaz A, Zufia L, Gurpide A, Navarro V, Quero C, Martin-Algarra S. Biliary index accurately predict the severity of irinotecn-induced delayed diarrea in colorectal cancer patients. Proc ASCO 2003;22:A648.

109. Ikegami T, Ha L, Arimori K, Latham P, Kobayashi K, Ceryak S, Matsuzaki Y, Bouscarel B. Intestinal alkalization as a possible preventive mechanism in irinotecan (CPT-11)-induced diarrhea. Cancer Res 2002;62(1):179–87.

110. Takeda Y, Kobayashi K, Akiyama Y, Soma T, Handa S, Kudoh S, Kudo K. Prevention of irinotecan (CPT-11)-induced diarrhea by oral alkalization combined with control of defecation in cancer patients. Int J Cancer 2001;92(2):269–75.

111. Takasuna K, Hagiwara T, Hirohashi M, Kato M, Nomura M, Nagai E, Yokoi T, Kamataki T. Inhibition of intestinal microflora beta-glucuronidase modifies the distribution of the active metabolite of the antitumor agent, irinotecan hydrochloride (CPT-11) in rats. Cancer Chemother Pharmacol 1998;42(4):280–6.

112. Barbounis V, Koumakis G, Vassilomanolakis M, Demiri M, Efremidis AP. Control of irinotecan-induced diarrhea by octreotide after loperamide failure. Support Care Cancer 2001;9(4):258–60.

113. Karthaus M, Ballo H, Steinmetz T, Geer T, Schimke J, Braumann D, Behrens R, Kindler M, Greinwald R,

Kleeberg U. Budesonide for prevention of CPT-11-induced diarrhea. Results of a double-blind placebo-controlled multicenter randomised phase III study in patients with advanced colorectal cancer. Proc ASCO 2003;22:A2935.

114. Mitchell RB, Wagner JE, Karp JE, Watson AJ, Brusilow SW, Przepiorka D, Storb R, Santos GW, Burke PJ, Saral R. Syndrome of idiopathic hyperammonemia after high-dose chemotherapy: review of nine cases. Am J Med 1988;85(5):662–7.

115. Rivory LP, Robert J. Pharmacologie de la camptothécine et de ses dérivés. [Pharmacology of camptothecin and its derivatives.] Bull Cancer 1995;82(4):265–85.

116. Wachters FM, Groen HJ, Maring JG, Gietema JA, Porro M, Dumez H, de Vries EG, van Oosterom AT. A phase I study with MAG-camptothecin intravenously administered weekly for 3 weeks in a 4-week cycle in adult patients with solid tumours. Br J Cancer 2004;90(12):2261–7.

117. Marini M, Wright D, Ropolo M, Abbruzzese M, Casas G. Neutrophilic eccrine hidradenitis secondary to topotecan. J Dermatolog Treat 2002;13(1):35–7.

118. Carstensen H, Nolte H, Hertz H. Teniposide-induced hypersensitivity reactions in children. Lancet 1989;2(8653):55.

119. Nolte H, Carstensen H, Hertz H. VM-26 (teniposide)-induced hypersensitivity and degranulation of basophils in children. Am J Pediatr Hematol Oncol 1988;10(4):308–12.

120. van de Kerkhof PC, de Vaan GA, Holland R. Pyoderma gangrenosum in acute myeloid leukaemia during immunosuppression. Eur J Pediatr 1988;148(1):34–6.

121. Siddall SJ, Martin J, Nunn AJ. Anaphylactic reactions to teniposide. Lancet 1989;1(8634):394.

122. Schey SA, Cooper J, Summerhayes M. The "handfoot syndrome" occurring with chronic administration of etoposide. Eur J Haematol 1992;48(2):118–19.

123. Alley E, Green R, Schuchter L. Cutaneous toxicities of cancer therapy. Curr Opin Oncol 2002;14(2):212–16.

124. Weiss RB. Hypersensitivity reactions. Semin Oncol 1992;19(5):458–77.

125. Hoetelmans RM, Schornagel JH, ten Bokkel Huinink WW, Beijnen JH, Da Camara C, Dion P. Hypersensitivity reactions to etoposide. Ann Pharmacother 1996;30(4):367–71.

126. Kellie SJ, Crist WM, Pui CH, Crone ME, Fairclough DL, Rodman JH, Rivera GK. Hypersensitivity reactions to epipodophyllotoxins in children with acute lymphoblastic leukemia. Cancer 1991;67(4):1070–5.

127. Cersosimo RJ, Calarese P, Karp DD. Acute hypotensive reaction to etoposide with successful rechallenge: case report and review of the literature. DICP 1989;23(11):876–7.

128. Tester WJ, Cohn JB, Fleekop PD, Rabinowitz MS, Lieberman JS. Successful rechallenge to etoposide after an acute vasomotor response. J Clin Oncol 1990;8(9):1600–1.

129. Jameson CH, Solanki DL. Stevens–Johnson syndrome associated with etoposide therapy. Cancer Treat Rep 1983;67(11):1050–1.

130. Ogle KM, Kennedy BJ. Hypersensitivity reactions to etoposide. A case report and review of the literature. Am J Clin Oncol 1988;11(6):663–5.

131. Bernstein BJ, Troner MB. Successful rechallenge with etoposide phosphate after an acute hypersensitivity reaction to etoposide. Pharmacotherapy 1999;19(8):989–91.

132. Hudson MM, Weinstein HJ, Donaldson SS, Greenwald C, Kun L, Tarbell NJ, Humphrey WA, Rupp C, Marina NM, Wilimas J, Link MP. Acute hypersensitivity reactions to

etoposide in a VEPA regimen for Hodgkin's disease. J Clin Oncol 1993;11(6):1080–4.

133. McLeod HL, Baker DK Jr., Pui CH, Rodman JH. Somnolence, hypotension, and metabolic acidosis following high-dose teniposide treatment in children with leukemia. Cancer Chemother Pharmacol 1991;29(2):150–4.

134. Siderov J, Prasad P, De Boer R, Desai J. Safe administration of etoposide phosphate after hypersensitivity reaction to intravenous etoposide. Br J Cancer 2002;86(1):12–13.

135. Nakanomyo H, Hiraoka M, Shiraya M. [Mutagenicity tests of etoposide and teniposide.] J Toxicol Sci 1986;11(Suppl 1):301–10.

136. Anderson RD, Berger NA. International Commission for Protection Against Environmental Mutagens and Carcinogens. Mutagenicity and carcinogenicity of topoisomerase-interactive agents. Mutat Res 1994;309(1):109–42.

137. Kollmannsberger C, Beyer J, Droz JP, Harstrick A, Hartmann JT, Biron P, Flechon A, Schoffski P, Kuczyk M, Schmoll HJ, Kanz L, Bokemeyer C. Secondary leukemia following high cumulative doses of etoposide in patients treated for advanced germ cell tumors. J Clin Oncol 1998; 16(10):3386–91.

138. Duffner PK, Krischer JP, Horowitz ME, Cohen ME, Burger PC, Friedman HS, Kun LE. Second malignancies in young children with primary brain tumors following treatment with prolonged postoperative chemotherapy and delayed irradiation: a Pediatric Oncology Group study. Ann Neurol 1998;44(3):313–16.

139. Horibe K, Matsushita T, Numata S, Miyajima Y, Katayama I, Kitabayashi T, Yanai M, Sekiguchi N, Egi S. Acute promyelocytic leukemia with t(15;17) abnormality after chemotherapy containing etoposide for Langerhans cell histiocytosis. Cancer 1993;72(12):3723–6.

140. Relling MV, Yanishevski Y, Nemec J, Evans WE, Boyett JM, Behm FG, Pui CH. Etoposide and antimetabolite pharmacology in patients who develop secondary acute myeloid leukemia. Leukemia 1998;12(3):346–52.

141. Zulian GB, Selby P, Milan S, Nandi A, Gore M, Forgeson G, Perren TJ, McElwain TJ. High dose melphalan, BCNU and etoposide with autologous bone marrow transplantation for Hodgkin's disease. Br J Cancer 1989;59(4):631–5.

142. Stine KC, Saylors RL, Sawyer JR, Becton DL. Secondary acute myelogenous leukemia following safe exposure to etoposide. J Clin Oncol 1997;15(4):1583–6.

143. Houck W, Einhorn LH. Secondary leukemias in germ cell tumor patients undergoing autologous stem cell transplantation utilizing high-dose etoposide. Proc ASCO 2003;22:A1566.

144. Ratain MJ, Kaminer LS, Bitran JD, Larson RA, Le Beau MM, Skosey C, Purl S, Hoffman PC, Wade J, Vardiman JW, et al. Acute nonlymphocytic leukemia following etoposide and cisplatin combination chemotherapy for advanced non-small-cell carcinoma of the lung. Blood 1987;70(5):1412–17.

145. Rubin CM, Arthur DC, Woods WG, Lange BJ, Nowell PC, Rowley JD, Nachman J, Bostrom B, Baum ES, Suarez CR, et al. Therapy-related myelodysplastic syndrome and acute myeloid leukemia in children: correlation between chromosomal abnormalities and prior therapy. Blood 1991;78(11):2982–8.

146. Pui CH, Relling MV. Topoisomerase II inhibitor-related acute myeloid leukaemia. Br J Haematol 2000;109(1):13–23.

147. Pedersen-Bjergaard J, Philip P. Two different classes of therapy-related and de-novo acute myeloid leukemia? Cancer Genet Cytogenet 1991;55(1):119–24.

148. Hawkins MM, Wilson LM, Stovall MA, Marsden HB, Potok MH, Kingston JE, Chessells JM. Epipodophyllotoxins, alkylating agents, and radiation and risk of secondary leukaemia after childhood cancer. BMJ 1992;304(6832):951–8.

149. Pui CH, Ribeiro RC, Hancock ML, Rivera GK, Evans WE, Raimondi SC, Head DR, Behm FG, Mahmoud MH, Sandlund JT, Crist W. Acute myeloid leukemia in children treated with epipodophyllotoxins for acute lymphoblastic leukemia. N Engl J Med 1991;325(24):1682–7.

150. Lamont EB, Schilsky RL. Gonadal toxicity and teratogenicity after cytotoxic chemotherapy. In: Lipp HP, editor. Anticancer Drug Toxicity: Prevention, Management and Clinical Pharmacokinetics. New York–Basel: Marcel Dekker Inc, 1999:491–523.

151. Matsui H, Iitsuka Y, Seki K, Sekiya S. Pregnancy outcome after treatment with etoposide (VP-16) for low-risk gestational trophoblastic tumor. Int J Gynecol Cancer 1999;9(2):166–169.

152. Fleischhack G, Reif S, Hasan C, Jaehde U, Hettmer S, Bode U. Feasibility of intraventricular administration of etoposide in patients with metastatic brain tumours. Br J Cancer 2001;84(11):1453–9

153. Lum BL, Kaubisch S, Yahanda AM, Adler KM, Jew L, Ehsan MN, Brophy NA, Halsey J, Gosland MP, Sikic BI. Alteration of etoposide pharmacokinetics and pharmacodynamics by cyclosporine in a phase I trial to modulate multidrug resistance. J Clin Oncol 1992;10(10):1635–42.

154. Rowinsky EK, Kaufmann SH, Baker SD, Grochow LB, Chen TL, Peereboom D, Bowling MK, Sartorius SE, Ettinger DS, Forastiere AA, Donehower RC. Sequences of topotecan and cisplatin: phase I, pharmacologic, and in vitro studies to examine sequence dependence. J Clin Oncol 1996;14(12):3074–84.

155. Zamboni WC, Egorin MJ, Van Echo DA, Day RS, Meisenberg BR, Brooks SE, Doyle LA, Nemieboka NN, Dobson JM, Tait NS, Tkaczuk KH. Pharmacokinetic and pharmacodynamic study of the combination of docetaxel and topotecan in patients with solid tumors. J Clin Oncol 2000;18(18):3288–94.

156. Baker DK, Relling MV, Pui CH, Christensen ML, Evans WE, Rodman JH. Increased teniposide clearance with concomitant anticonvulsant therapy. J Clin Oncol 1992;10(2):311–15.

157. Kohne CH, Van Cutsem E, Wils JA, Bokemeyer C, El-Serafi M, Lutz M, Lorenz M, Anak O, Genicot B, Nordlinger B; the EORTC GI Group. Irinotecan improves the activity of the AIO regimen in metastatic colorectal cancer: results of EORTC GI-group study 40986. Proc Am Soc Clin Oncol 2003;22:A1018.

158. Dodds HM, Bishop JF, Rivory LP. More about: irinotecan-related cholinergic syndrome induced by coadministration of oxaliplatin. J Natl Cancer Inst 1999;91(1):91–2.

159. Wasserman E, Cuvier C, Lokiec F, Goldwasser F, Kalla S, Mery-Mignard D, Ouldkaci M, Besmaine A, Dupont-Andre G, Mahjoubi M, Marty M, Misset JL, Cvitkovic E. Combination of oxaliplatin plus irinotecan in patients with gastrointestinal tumors: results of two independent phase I studies with pharmacokinetics. J Clin Oncol 1999; 17(6):1751–9.

Torasemide

See also Diuretics

General Information

Torasemide is a long-acting loop diuretic promoted for use in hypertension. Like piretanide, it is claimed to be potassium neutral, but the assertion is premature. There is no evidence that torasemide has metabolic advantages over thiazides (SEDA-16, 226) (SEDA-17, 264) (SEDA-18, 237).

Organs and Systems

Skin

Torasemide has been associated with various rashes, including non-specific erythematous lesions, pruritus, and photoallergic lichenoid lesions (SEDA-22, 239).

Immunologic

Two possible cases of vasculitis with renal insufficiency have been reported in patients taking torasemide (1,2). This adverse effect is not surprising, since torasemide is structurally similar to sulfa drugs, which can cause vasculitis.

- A 70-year-old man developed heart failure secondary to ischemic heart disease and severe aortic stenosis (1). Furosemide 20 mg/day was replaced by torasemide 5 mg/day. After the second dose he developed oliguria and an erythematous morbilliform rash with palpable violet petechial lesions on the legs. Chest X-ray showed bilateral alveolar infiltrates. Serum creatinine and potassium were raised (212 µmol/l and 6.7 mmol/l respectively). Skin biopsy showed leukocytoclastic vasculitis. After withdrawal of torasemide, his renal function improved (serum creatinine 97 µmol/l) and the skin lesions resolved (leaving residual pigmented areas) within 8 days.
- An 84-year-old man with ischemic heart disease and hypertension took torasemide 10 mg/day for persistent edema (1). About 24 hours after the first dose of torasemide, he developed painless, non-palpable, petechial lesions on the limbs and trunk, with oliguria. His serum creatinine was 256 µmol/l and his serum potassium 6.2 mmol/l. Skin biopsy showed non-leukocytoclastic vasculitis with a mixed inflammatory infiltrate including eosinophils. He was symptom free 15 days after withdrawal of torasemide.

Neither patient had a previous history of drug hypersensitivity. Both patients had previously tolerated furosemide, another sulfonamide derivative. The temporal correlation with torasemide administration suggested a causal relation, but the mechanism was unclear.

Drug–Drug Interactions

NSAIDs

NSAIDs block the natriuretic effect of torasemide (SEDA-21, 229).

Probenecid

Probenecid blocks the natriuretic effect of torasemide (SEDA-21, 229).

References

1. Palop-Larrea V, Sancho-Calabuig A, Gorriz-Teruel JL, Martinez-Mir I, Pallardo-Mateu LM. Vasculitis with acute kidney failure and torasemide. Lancet 1998;352(9144):1909–10.
2. Sanfelix Genoves J, Benlloch Nieto H, Verdu Tarraga R, Costa Alcaraz AM. Erupcion purpurica compatible con vasculitis y torasemida. [Eruption of purpura compatible with vasculitis and torasemide.] Aten Primaria 1998;21(4):252–3.

Tosufloxacin

See also Fluoroquinolones

General Information

Tosufloxacin is a fluoroquinolone antibacterial with properties similar to those of ciprofloxacin.

Observational studies

In 58 Japanese patients with typhoid fever, 42 with paratyphoid fever, and one with both typhoid fever and paratyphoid fever, almost 80% of whom were treated with tosufloxacin, there were adverse effects (nausea, urticaria, aphthous stomatitis) in 3.6% and raised serum amylase in 8.3% (1). All the adverse reactions resolved with or without a change in drug therapy.

General adverse effects

The most common adverse reactions to tosufloxacin are gastrointestinal disorders, including diarrhea, abdominal discomfort, nausea and vomiting, and skin disorders, including rash and pruritus (2). Central and peripheral nervous system disorders were observed in 0.36% of patients and the most common symptoms were headache and dizziness.

Organs and Systems

Respiratory

- A syndrome of pulmonary infiltration with eosinophilia occurred in an 83-year-old man who was given piperacillin plus tosufloxacin (3).

In vitro blastogenesis of his peripheral blood lymphocytes was strongly enhanced by piperacillin and tosufloxacin, and they generated a large amount of interleukin-5.

Skin

There is a low incidence of phototoxicity with tosufloxacin (2).

Musculoskeletal

Rhabdomyolysis has been reported in 13 patients taking tosufloxacin (2).

Drug–Drug Interactions

Antacids

The C_{max} and AUC of tosufloxacin tosilate 300 mg were significantly reduced by aluminium hydroxide gel fine granules 1 g or magnesium oxide 1 g (2).

References

1. Ohnishi K, Kimura K, Masuda G, Tsunoda T, Obana M, Yoshida H, Goto T, Sakaue Y, Kim YK, Sakamoto M, Sagara H. Oral administration of fluoroquinolones in the treatment of typhoid fever and paratyphoid fever in Japan. Intern Med 2000;39(12):1044–8.
2. Niki Y. Pharmacokinetics and safety assessment of tosufloxacin tosilate. J Infect Chemother 2002;8(1):1–18.
3. Yamamoto T, Tanida T, Ueta E, Kimura T, Doi S, Osaki T. Pulmonary infiltration with eosinophilia (PIE) syndrome induced by antibiotics, PIPC and TFLX during cancer treatment. Oral Oncol 2001;37(5):471–5.

Tosylchloramide sodium

See also Disinfectants and antiseptics

General Information

Tosylchloramide has been used as a wound disinfectant, a general surgical antiseptic, and for the disinfection of water (1).

Organs and Systems

Respiratory

Asthma has been attributed to tosylchloramide (2).

Immunologic

Contact sensitization to tosylchloramide has been reported (3).

- Urticaria, rhinitis, dyspnea, and edema of the face were reported in a female nurse after contact (SEDA-11, 492) (4). Specific IgE antibodies to tosylchloramide were demonstrated.

References

1. Reybrouck G. The bactericidal activity of aqueous disinfectants applied on living tissues. Pharm Weekbl Sci 1985;7(3):100–3.
2. Romeo L, Gobbi M, Pezzini A, Caruso B, Costa G. Asma da tosilcloramide sodica: descrizione di un caso. [Tosylchloramide-induced asthma: description of a case.] Med Lav 1988;79(3):237–40.
3. Metzner HH. Kontaktsensibilisierungen durch Tosylchloramidnatrium (Chloramin) und Hydroxychinolin (Sulfachin). [Contact sensitization caused by tosylchloramide sodium (chloramine) and hydroxyquinoline (Sulfachin).] Dermatol Monatsschr 1987;173(11):674–7.
4. Dooms-Goossens A, Gevers D, Mertens A, Vanderheyden D. Allergic contact urticaria due to chloramine. Contact Dermatitis 1983;9(4):319–20.

Tramadol

General Information

Tramadol is a synthetic opioid analgesic with activity at OP_3 (μ) opioid receptors, but it also inhibits the re-uptake of both 5-HT and noradrenaline and stimulates the pre-synaptic release of 5-HT. It produces a similar analgesic effect to pethidine and is about one-tenth as potent as morphine.

The reported adverse effects of tramadol are nausea, vomiting, sweating, dry mouth, dizziness, sedation, headache, and hypertension (SEDA-17, 84) (SEDA-20, 81). The atypical analgesic effects of tramadol and its associated adverse effects profile have been reviewed (1).

The metabolism of tramadol by CYP2D6 is important for its analgesic effect; tramadol may therefore be a poor analgesic in poor metabolizers by CYP2D6, while extensive metabolizers may have better analgesia and more adverse effects (SEDA-21, 90).

In a review of the use of tramadol in musculoskeletal pain the authors concluded that tramadol can be used at Step 2 of the analgesic ladder, since its efficacy, alone or in conjunction with NSAIDs, in the management of chronic musculoskeletal pain without increasing the frequency of adverse effects has been confirmed (2,3).

Comparative studies

Bupivacaine
In a randomized, controlled study in 60 boys (aged 1–7 years) undergoing unilateral herniorrhaphy, caudal 0.25% bupivacaine 1 mg/kg plus tramadol 1.5 mg/kg resulted in superior analgesia (quality and duration) with no significant increase in opioid-related adverse effects compared with children who received 0.25% bupivacaine 1 mg/kg alone or caudal tramadol 1.5 mg/kg in 0.9% saline alone (4).

Thirty children (1–5 years old) in an open, controlled study were randomly given caudal block with 0.25% bupivacaine 0.8 mg/kg or tramadol 0.8 or 2 mg/kg (5). The duration of analgesia was longer (9.1 hours) in those given tramadol but the incidences of opioid-related adverse effects (gastrointestinal effects and sweating) were significantly higher.

Clomipramine + levomepromazine

Since the monoamine effects of tramadol resemble the effect of antidepressants, it has been compared with clomipramine + levomepromazine in patients with postherpetic neuralgia. The incidence of adverse effects was 77% with tramadol and 83% with clomipramine (SEDA-20, 81).

Codeine

In a 4-week, double-blind, multicenter, randomized study, tramadol plus paracetamol (37.5/325 mg) was as effective as codeine plus paracetamol (co-codamol 30/300 mg) in chronic non-malignant low back pain and osteoarthritis pain, with acceptable tolerability (6).

When tramadol was compared with codeine in 65 patients undergoing elective intracranial surgery, there was a significantly higher incidence of postoperative nausea, vomiting, and sedation with tramadol 75 mg (7). The patients given codeine had significantly lower pain scores over the first 48 hours postoperatively.

Non-steroidal anti-inflammatory drugs

Tramadol and non-steroidal anti-inflammatory drugs have been compared in two studies of patients with joint pain associated with osteoarthritis (8,9). In an open, randomized study 60 patients with osteoarthritis taking NSAIDs were given either modified-release tramadol 100 mg 8-hourly or modified-release dihydrocodeine 60 mg 8-hourly for 4 days; the controls were 30 patients who took an NSAID alone (8). Both opioids provided adequate analgesic adjuncts to NSAIDs, but tramadol caused significantly more minor initial adverse effects.

Diclofenac

In a double-blind, randomized, crossover study in 60 patients with osteoarthritis of the hip or knee, tramadol 50–100 mg up to three times daily was compared with diclofenac (25–50 mg up to three times daily) over 4 weeks (10). Both regimens gave modest pain relief, with no significant differences between the two groups, although within individual patients there were marked differences in analgesic effectiveness. Tramadol was associated with a significantly higher rate of adverse effects (20 versus 3.3%), notably headaches, nausea, constipation, tiredness, and vomiting, but there was no significant difference in adverse events that required withdrawal.

Ketorolac

Intravenous tramadol 1.5 mg/kg has been compared with a single dose of intravenous ketorolac 10 ng in 60 patients scheduled to undergo day-case laparoscopic sterilization in a prospective, randomized, double-blind comparison (11). Tramadol was associated with significantly less postoperative pain. There was no difference in the incidence or severity of nausea and vomiting between the two groups. Dry mouth was significantly more common with tramadol (60 versus 27%).

Opioid analgesics

Fentanyl

In a comparison of tramadol (1 or 2 mg/kg) and fentanyl (2 µg/kg) for postoperative analgesia after pediatric anesthesia, the two drugs had equal analgesic potency and produced similar hemodynamic stability and a similar incidence of adverse effects (12).

Hydrocodone

A randomized, double-blind comparison of the effectiveness of a single dose of tramadol 100 mg with a single dose of hydrocodone 5 mg plus paracetamol 500 mg in acute musculoskeletal pain in 68 subjects after minor trauma has been published (13). Tramadol gave significantly worse analgesia. Adverse effects (nausea and vomiting, drowsiness and dizziness, and anxiety) were uncommon and there was no significant difference between the two drugs.

Morphine

In a comparison of the analgesic effects of intermittent boluses of tramadol or morphine after abdominal surgery in 523 patients, tramadol caused more adverse effects (43 versus 34%), although the difference was not statistically significant. The commonest adverse effects were nausea (32 and 22%), vomiting (4.9 and 3.8%), urinary retention (3.0 and 2.7%), and sweating (3.8 and 0.4%) (SEDA-20, 81).

Tramadol and morphine have been compared in 40 women undergoing hysterectomy (14). At the start of wound closure, patients received either tramadol 3 mg/kg or morphine 0.2 mg/kg intravenously, which did not cause changes in arterial pressure or heart rate. There were no differences in times to spontaneous respiration, awakening, or orientation between the two groups, and ventilation frequency and pain scores were similar throughout 90 minutes. Similar numbers in each group required supplementary analgesia. Performance of the p-deletion test, a measure of psychomotor function, was more rapid in the tramadol group, but the performance of all subjects was impaired at 90 minutes compared with their preoperative scores.

In a randomized, double-blind study in 20 patients with severe postoperative pain given either intravenous tramadol 1 mg/kg or morphine 0.1 mg/kg, both drugs were effective analgesics but higher dosages than those usually administered were necessary (15). Tramadol did not cause any severe adverse effects, but with morphine there was one case each of severe sedation and respiratory depression.

A comparison of tramadol and morphine for subcutaneous patient-controlled analgesia after orthopedic surgery showed that tramadol 40 mg subcutaneously and morphine 2 mg subcutaneously were equally effective in providing analgesia (16). Drug use in the first 24 hours averaged 800 mg for tramadol and 40 mg for morphine. However, mean arterial blood pressure fell significantly in both groups after 24 hours, with a 17% mean maximal fall from baseline concentrations for tramadol and 20% for morphine; heart rate increased by 17 and 15% respectively. Oxygen saturation also fell significantly in both groups, but was not associated with changes in respiratory rate. Nausea and vomiting were more common with tramadol (65%). In this study, patients required significantly more tramadol than had been predicted, and the authors commented that at this dosage, the adverse effects profile was similar to that of morphine.

In a double-blind study 150 patients with post-traumatic musculoskeletal pain were allocated to either tramadol 100 mg, with possible increases to a total of 200 mg, or morphine 5 mg or 10 mg with a total increase to 20 mg (17). Analgesic efficacy and adverse effect profiles were similar in the two groups.

Non-opioid analgesics
In a double-blind, randomized study in 120 patients scheduled to undergo outpatient hand surgery with intravenous regional anesthesia, tramadol 100 mg was compared with either metamizol 1 g or paracetamol 1 g, all 6-hourly (18). Seven patients given tramadol withdrew because of severe nausea and dizziness. Tramadol was the most effective analgesic, but none of the drugs alone provided effective analgesia in all patients and 40% needed rescue analgesia.

Tramadol has been compared with a paracetamol derivative in a double blind, randomized, controlled study in 80 patients undergoing elective thyroidectomy (19). They were randomly assigned to propacetamol (an injectable prodrug of paracetamol) 2 g or intravenous tramadol 1.5 mg/kg. A single dose of tramadol provided better analgesia than propacetamol during the first 6 hours after surgery, but failed to ensure optimal analgesia subsequently. The incidences of nausea, vomiting, and sedation were comparable in the two groups.

Placebo-controlled studies

In two randomized, double-blind studies tramadol provided effective and safe long-term relief of pain in diabetic neuropathy (20) and fibromyalgia (21). The adverse effects (constipation, nausea, and headache) were well tolerated.

The postoperative analgesic efficacy of tramadol 2 mg/kg has been studied in 80 children (aged 1–3 years) undergoing day-case adenoidectomy without premedication in a double-blind, randomized, placebo-controlled study (22). General anesthesia was induced with intravenous alfentanil 10 µg/kg plus lidocaine followed by propofol and mivacurium. The children received intravenous tramadol 2 mg/kg or placebo immediately after induction of anesthesia. Those given tramadol required fewer pethidine rescue medication doses than those given placebo. In fact, 45% of the children who were given tramadol did not require postoperative analgesia at all, compared with 15% of the children who were given placebo. The incidences of adverse effects were similar in the two groups.

The use or addition of tramadol in children undergoing lower abdominal surgery has been examined in three studies (4,5,23). In a double-blind, randomized, controlled study, 125 children undergoing inguinal herniorrhaphy were allocated to receive tramadol 2 mg/kg or morphine sulfate 0.03 mg/kg before surgery; the control group received morphine sulfate 0.03 mg/kg at the end of surgery (23). Caudal tramadol 2 mg/kg provided reliable

postoperative analgesia and there were no inter-group differences in postoperative adverse effects or quality and duration of pain relief.

In 129 patients with severe joint pain associated with osteoarthritis, tramadol was significantly more effective than placebo, but 26 patients taking tramadol and 43 taking placebo withdrew because of ineffectiveness or adverse effects; the main adverse effects of tramadol were nausea and constipation (9).

Tramadol has been used in the treatment of shivering after anesthesia. In one study, 150 patients scheduled for general anesthesia and surgery were randomly allocated to intravenous tramadol 1 or 2 mg/kg or 0.9% saline given at the time of wound closure (24). The authors concluded that both doses of tramadol were effective and safe. Of the patients in the higher-dose group, 2% had shivering, compared with 4% in the lower-dose group and 48% in the control group. In a similar study in 96 patients, the optimal dose of tramadol in preventing shivering after anesthesia was 0.5–1 mg/kg intravenously (25).

Combination studies
Tramadol has been combined with various drugs in order to enhance efficacy or reduce adverse effects.

Aspirin
The analgesic efficacy of tramadol can be further enhanced by adding injectable lysine acetyl salicylate (aspirin) after orthopedic surgery with no significant increase in adverse effects (26).

Dexamethasone
In a randomized, placebo-controlled study, the addition of an intravenous bolus of dexamethasone 150 micrograms/kg with a PCA system programmed to deliver tramadol 20 mg in a 1 ml solution on demand in 50 patients after major abdominal surgery significantly reduced the incidence of nausea, vomiting, and subsequent administration of rescue antiemetic therapy (27).

Droperidol
The use of tramadol for postoperative analgesia by intravenous patient-controlled analgesia (PCA) has gained popularity, mostly because it is less likely to cause sedation and respiratory depression (28). However, it is associated with nausea, vomiting, dry mouth, and sweating. The addition of droperidol to tramadol PCA reduced the incidence of gastrointestinal symptoms without significantly increasing sedation (29). In a double-blind, randomized study, 40 patients undergoing coronary artery bypass grafting and/or valve replacement surgery were given droperidol 0.1 mg/ml plus either tramadol 10 mg/ml or morphine 1 mg/ml. The results in the two groups were comparable in efficacy, adverse effects profiles, and dose requirements, and the authors argued that there may be no advantage in using tramadol rather than morphine in conjunction with droperidol (30).

Ketamine
In 44 patients the addition of ketamine 1 mg/ml to PCA tramadol significantly reduced the consumption of tramadol at 6, 12, and 24 hours postoperatively, with no

differences in the incidence of nausea and sedation (31). Diplopia was reported by two patients.

Magnesium sulfate
In 44 patients the addition of magnesium sulfate 30 mg/ml to PCA tramadol both significantly reduced the consumption of tramadol at 6, 12, and 24 hours postopcratively, with no differences in the incidence of nausea and sedation (31).

Morphine
In a double-blind, randomized, controlled study, the addition of a tramadol infusion to morphine for PCA in 69 patients undergoing elective abdominal surgery resulted in improved analgesic efficacy and reduced morphine requirements, with a relative lack of adverse effects (32).

Observational studies
The role of tramadol in the treatment of rheumatological pain has been reviewed (33). Tramadol causes fewer opioid adverse effects for a given level of analgesia compared with traditional opioids. Common adverse effects, such as nausea and dizziness, usually occur only at the beginning of therapy, abate with time, and are further minimized by up-titrating the dosage over several days (34).

When tramadol 1 mg/kg was given intravenously to 110 adults for postoperative shivering, few adverse effects were reported; two had transient hypotension and two complained of nausea without vomiting. Similarly, mild adverse effects were reported in 20% of patients in a trial of tramadol in cancer pain (SEDA-16, 86), and when it was used to relieve severe pain in sports injuries (SEDA-16, 86).

Organs and Systems

Respiratory

Tramadol is said not to cause respiratory depression (SEDA-17, 84) (SEDA-18, 82), but it has been reported that equipotent doses of tramadol did produce respiratory depression, albeit less severe and for a shorter time than morphine (SEDA-17, 84) (35). This was confirmed in an extensive review of the literature (SEDA-21, 90).

The effect of oral tramadol on the ventilatory response to acute isocapnic hypoxia has been studied in 20 healthy volunteers. Tramadol had a small but significant depressive effect on the hypercapnic ventilatory response but no effect on the hypoxic ventilatory response (36). This is in contrast to morphine, which causes 50–60% suppression of the hypoxic ventilatory response.

Nervous system

Tramadol-associated seizures have been studied retrospectively in 9218 adult tramadol users and 37 232 nonusers (37). Seizures occurred in under 1% of all tramadol users, but the risk of seizure was increased two- to six-fold among users adjusted for selected co-morbidities and polydrug prescription. The risk of seizure was higher in those aged 25–54 years, those who had more than four tramadol prescriptions, and those who had a history of alcohol abuse, stroke, or head injury.

In a nested case-control study of 11 383 patients, there were 21 cases of idiopathic seizures, only three of whom had been exposed to tramadol alone, the other having taken other analgesics (opioids or others) (38). The findings did not suggest an increased risk of seizures among patients taking tramadol alone.

Seizures followed by opioid withdrawal symptoms have been reported in a patient taking tramadol (39).

- A 29-year-old woman took tramadol 50 mg 6-hourly for pain associated with the carpal tunnel syndrome. She slowly increased the dose of tramadol and obtained it from several physicians and different hospitals, so that after 3 years she was taking 30 tramadol 50 mg tablets daily. She had two generalized seizures and stopped taking tramadol; 1 day later she developed severe opioid withdrawal symptoms, including diarrhea, headache, insomnia, and blurred vision. She was detoxified with tapering doses of tramadol and discharged after 6 days.

Psychological, psychiatric

Hallucinations have been attributed to tramadol, both visual (40) and auditory (41).

- A 66-year-old tetraparetic man developed hallucinations while taking tramadol, paroxetine, and dosulepin for chronic pain (40).
- A 74-year-old man with lung cancer took tramadol 200 mg/day for chest pain (41). Soon afterwards (time not specified) he had vivid auditory hallucinations in the form of "two voices singing accompanied by an accordion and a banjo." They resolved 48 hours after withdrawal.

Gastrointestinal

In one study the incidence of nausea was high (30–35%) when tramadol was used for postoperative pain (SEDA-20, 81).

Intravenous tramadol (1.25 mg/kg), codeine (1 mg/kg), morphine (0.125 mg/kg), and saline have been compared for their effect on gastric emptying (using the paracetamol absorption test) in 10 healthy subjects in a randomized, double-blind study (42). Tramadol had a measurable but statistically insignificant inhibitory effect on gastric emptying, whereas morphine and codeine significantly delayed gastric emptying. The implication of this is that the risk of regurgitation is less with tramadol than with the other opioids investigated and that tramadol is less likely to alter the pharmacokinetics of other drugs administered simultaneously.

In mild to moderate postoperative pain, rectal tramadol has been compared with standard treatment with co-codamol (paracetamol plus codeine) suppositories in 40 patients who were given either tramadol 100 mg suppositories 6-hourly or 1000/20 mg of co-codamol 6-hourly (43). Nausea and vomiting were significantly more frequent with tramadol (84%) than with co-codamol (31%).

The effect of tramadol on postoperative nausea and vomiting after ENT surgery has been studied in a prospective, randomized, double-blind comparison with nalbuphine, pethidine, or saline in 281 patients (44). The three opioids caused a similar incidence of postoperative nausea and vomiting (40, 52, and 37% respectively) and more than placebo (32%).

In a randomized, double-blind placebo-controlled study of 76 women undergoing abdominal hysterectomy, tramadol 100 mg was a more effective analgesic than ketorolac 30 mg given every 6 hours intravenously (45). However, of those given tramadol 38% had vomiting compared with only 8% of those who were given ketorolac.

Urinary tract

The Netherlands Pharmacovigilance Foundation (LAREB), has reported five cases of transient difficulty in urinating, which spontaneously resolved on withdrawal of tramadol and was suspected to be induced by tramadol; none needed catheterization (46). In all five cases tramadol had been prescribed for back pain in relatively healthy individuals in a dose range of 50–150 mg.

Skin

- A 47-year-old man taking tramadol 100 mg for low back pain developed a maculopapular rash with secondary erythroderma, which resolved after withdrawal of tramadol (47).

Long-Term Effects

Drug abuse

Tramadol abuse was monitored in the USA during the 3 years (1995–1998) after the drug was marketed there, through the systematic collection and evaluation of reports of suspected abuse in high-risk populations from a network of drug abuse specialists and reports sent through the FDA's Med Watch system (48). The overall conclusion was that experimentation with tramadol during the first 18 months of its introduction peaked at two cases per 100 000 patients exposed. This figure subsequently fell to less than one case per 100 000 patients in the second 18 months of the study period. Of cases of abuse 97% occurred among individuals with a history of substance abuse.

Drug Administration

Drug formulations

The incidence of adverse effects is reduced with the use of an oral, modified-release formulation of tramadol in the treatment of chronic pain (49), starting at the lowest dose, increasing gradually according to the patient's response during chronic oral administration (50,51), and using a loading dose immediately after the start of surgery.

The results of postmarketing surveillance of modified-released tramadol in Germany have been published (52). Modified-release tramadol (mean daily dose 236 mg usually divided into two doses) was used in 3153 patients, of whom most had severe or very severe pain. During the 6-week trial, 316 adverse effects were reported by a total of 206 patients (6.5%). Adverse effects were, in

decreasing order of frequency, nausea (3.4%), dizziness (1.5%), vomiting (1.1%), constipation (0.5%), tiredness (0.5%), sweating (0.4%), dry mouth (0.3%), and pruritus (0.3%). Confusion, hypotension, sleep disturbances, abdominal pain, stomach upset, gastrointestinal hemorrhage, and cerebral hemorrhage were all among the less frequently reported adverse events, and 28% of events were classified as severe. Age did not affect the frequency of events, but women reported a higher frequency of adverse events than men (7.3 versus 5.7%).

The use of modified-release tramadol in chronic malignant pain has been examined in an open, prospective study in 146 patients with moderate to severe cancer pain; 90 patients completed the 6-week trial (53). Dropouts were due to opioid adverse effects (20%), inadequate pain relief (9%), or both (2.5%). There was at least one adverse effect in 86%. Overall, 433 adverse effect events were reported but some reduced in frequency over the 6 weeks. Modified-release tramadol (400 mg/day) provided fast and efficient pain relief in almost 60% of patients both during initial dosing and long-term treatment.

Drug overdose

- A 26-year-old male nurse died of tramadol intoxication (54). The peripheral blood concentration of tramadol was 9.6 micrograms/ml (target concentration 0.1–0.3 micrograms/ml). There was no objective evidence at postmortem of any pre-existing disease or use/overuse of ethanol or other drugs that could have contributed to or caused death.

Drug–Drug Interactions

Ondansetron

Tramadol dosage requirements for patient-controlled analgesia increased when ondansetron was given as a prophylactic antiemetic in 40 patients undergoing lumbar laminectomy in an open, controlled study (55). During the first 4 hours postoperatively tramadol consumption increased by about 30% in those given ondansetron and remained 22–25% higher thereafter. A single dose of ondansetron 4 mg given during induction did not reduce the 24-hour incidence of nausea or vomiting.

In a randomized, controlled study of postoperative PCA using tramadol with or without ondansetron in 59 patients undergoing ear, nose, and throat surgery, ondansetron reduced the overall analgesic effect of tramadol, increased doses of tramadol being needed in the first 12 hours after surgery. This increase in tramadol requirements in those given ondansetron resulted in a significantly higher vomiting scores at 4 and 8 hours postoperatively and an overall increase in the number of episodes of vomiting, despite the use of ondansetron (56).

Oral anticoagulants

Tramadol may increase the anticoagulant effect of phenprocoumon or warfarin (SEDA-22, 103).

Quinidine

Inhibition of the hepatic metabolism of tramadol to morphine by quinidine may reduce its opioid effects (SEDA-21, 90).

Selective serotonin re-uptake inhibitors (SSRIs)

Fluoxetine

Serotonin syndrome and mania occurred in a 72-year-old woman taking fluoxetine 20 mg/day and tramadol 150 mg/day 18 days after she started to take the combination (57). Inhibition of CYP2D6 may have played a part (58).

Sertraline

The serotonin syndrome has been reported after concurrent use of tramadol and sertraline (SEDA-22, 103).

- Serotonin syndrome occurred in an 88-year-old woman who took sertraline 50–100 mg/day and tramadol 200–400 mg/day for 10 days; the symptoms subsided 15 days after withdrawal of tramadol (59).

Venlafaxine

The death of a 36-year-old patient with a history of alcohol dependence who was taking tramadol, venlafaxine, trazodone, and quetiapine has highlighted the increased risk of seizures with concomitant use of tramadol and selective serotonin re-uptake inhibitors (60).

References

1. Budd K, Langford R. Tramadol revisited. Br J Anaesth 1999;82(4):493–5.
2. Reig E. Tramadol in musculoskeletal pain—a survey. Clin Rheumatol 2002;21(Suppl 1):S9–12.
3. Silverfield JC, Kamin M, Wu SC, Rosenthal N; CAPSS-105 Study Group. Tramadol/acetaminophen combination tablets for the treatment of osteoarthritis flare pain: a multi-center, outpatient, randomized, double-blind, placebo-controlled, parallel-group, add-on study. Clin Ther 2002;24(2):282–97.
4. Senel AC, Akyol A, Dohman D, Solak M. Caudal bupivacaine-tramadol combination for postoperative analgesia in pediatric herniorrhaphy. Acta Anaesthesiol Scand 2001;45(6):786–9.
5. Eren GA, Cinar SO, Oba S, Zoylan G. Pediyatrik alt batin cerrahisinde postoperatif analjezi amacli kaudal tramadol kullanimi. Turk Anesteziyol Reanim 2001;29:39–43.
6. Mullican WS, Lacy JR; TRAMAP-ANAG-006 Study Group. Tramadol/acetaminophen combination tablets and codeine/acetaminophen combination capsules for the management of chronic pain: a comparative trial. Clin Ther 2001;23(9):1429–45.
7. Jeffrey HM, Charlton P, Mellor DJ, Moss E, Vucevic M. Analgesia after intracranial surgery: a double-blind, prospective comparison of codeine and tramadol. Br J Anaesth 1999;83(2):245–9.
8. Wilder-Smith CH, Hill L, Spargo K, Kalla A. Treatment of severe pain from osteoarthritis with slow-release tramadol or dihydrocodeine in combination with NSAID's. A randomised study comparing analgesia, antinociception and gastrointestinal effects. Pain 2001;91(1–2):23–31.
9. Fleischmann RM, Caldwell JR, Roth SH, Tesser JRP, Olson W, Kamin M. Tramadol for the treatment of joint pain associated with osteoarthritis: a randomised double-
10. blind, placebo-controlled trial. Curr Ther Res 2001;62:113–28.
11. Pavelka K, Peliskova Z, Stehlikova H, Ratcliffe S, Repas C. Intraindividual differences in pain relief and functional improvement in osteoarthritis with diclofenac or tramadol. Clin Drug Invest 1998;16:421–9.
12. Putland AJ, McCluskey A. The analgesic efficacy of tramadol versus ketorolac in day-case laparoscopic sterilisation. Anaesthesia 1999;54(4):382–5.
13. Joshi GP, Duffy L, Chehade J, Wesevich J, Gajraj N, Johnson ER. Effects of prophylactic nalmefene on the incidence of morphine-related side effects in patients receiving intravenous patient-controlled analgesia. Anesthesiology 1999;90(4):1007–11.
14. Turturro MA, Paris PM, Larkin GL. Tramadol versus hydrocodone–acetaminophen in acute musculoskeletal pain: a randomized, double-blind clinical trial. Ann Emerg Med 1998;32(2):139–43.
15. Coetzee JF, van Loggerenberg H. Tramadol or morphine administered during operation: a study of immediate postoperative effects after abdominal hysterectomy. Br J Anaesth 1998;81(5):737–41.
16. Wiebalck A, Tryba M, Hoell T, Strumpf M, Kulka P, Zenz M. Efficacy and safety of tramadol and morphine in patients with extremely severe postoperative pain. Acute Pain 2000;3:112–18.
17. Hopkins D, Shipton EA, Potgieter D, Van derMerwe CA, Boon J, De Wet C, Murphy J. Comparison of tramadol and morphine via subcutaneous PCA following major orthopaedic surgery. Can J Anaesth 1998;45(5 Pt 1):435–42.
18. Vergnion M, Degesves S, Garcet L, Magotteaux V. Tramadol, an alternative to morphine for treating post-traumatic pain in the prehospital situation. Anesth Analg 2001;92(6):1543–6.
19. Rawal N, Allvin R, Amilon A, Ohlsson T, Hallen J. Postoperative analgesia at home after ambulatory hand surgery: a controlled comparison of tramadol, metamizol, and paracetamol. Anesth Analg 2001;92(2):347–51.
20. Dejonckheere M, Desjeux L, Deneu S, Ewalenko P. Intravenous tramadol compared to propacetamol for postoperative analgesia following thyroidectomy. Acta Anaesthesiol Belg 2001;52(1):29–33.
21. Harati Y, Gooch C, Swenson M, Edelman SV, Greene D, Raskin P, Donofrio P, Cornblath D, Olson WH, Kamin M. Maintenance of the long-term effectiveness of tramadol in treatment of the pain of diabetic neuropathy. J Diabetes Complications 2000;14(2):65–70.
22. Russell IJ, Kamin M, Bennett RM, Schnitzer TJ, Green JA, Katz WA. Efficacy of tramadol in treatment of pain in fibromyalgia. J Clin Rheumatol 2000;6:250–7.
23. Viitanen H, Annila P. Analgesic efficacy of tramadol 2 mg kg^{-1} for paediatric day-case adenoidectomy. Br J Anaesth 2001;86(4):572–5.
24. Ozcengiz D, Gunduz M, Ozbek H, Isik G. Comparison of caudal morphine and tramadol for postoperative pain control in children undergoing inguinal herniorrhaphy. Paediatr Anaesth 2001;11(4):459–64.
25. Mathews S, Al Mulla A, Varghese PK, Radim K, Mumtaz S. Postanaesthetic shivering—a new look at tramadol. Anaesthesia 2002;57(4):394–8.
26. Kaya M, Karakus D, Sariyildiz O, Ozalp G, Kodiogullari N. Genel anestezi sonrasi titreme tedavisinde tramadolum etkinligi. Turk Anesteziyol Reanim Cem Mecmuasi 2002;30:90–3.
27. Pang W, Huang S, Tung CC, Huang MH. Patient-controlled analgesia with tramadol versus tramadol plus lysine acetyl salicylate. Anesth Analg 2000;91(5):1226–9.
28. Tuncer S, Barikaner H, Yosunkaya A, Taulan A. Influence of dexamethasone on nausea and vomiting during patient-

controlled analgesia with tramadol. Clin Drug Invest 2002;22:547–52.

28. Bloch MB, Dyer RA, Heijke SA, James MF. Tramadol infusion for postthoracotomy pain relief: a placebo-controlled comparison with epidural morphine. Anesth Analg 2002;94(3):523–8.

29. Ng KF, Tsui SL, Yang JC, Ho ET. Comparison of tramadol and tramadol/droperidol mixture for patient-controlled analgesia. Can J Anaesth 1997;44(8):810–15.

30. Zimmermann AR, Kibblewhite D, Sleigh J. Comparison of morphine/droperidol and tramadol/droperidol mixture for patient controlled analgesia (PCA) after cardiac surgery: a prospective, randomised, double-blind study. J Acute Pain 2002;4:65–9.

31. Unlugenc H, Gunduz M, Ozalevli M, Akman H. A comparative study on the analgesic effect of tramadol, tramadol plus magnesium, and tramadol plus ketamine for postoperative pain management after major abdominal surgery. Acta Anaesthesiol Scand 2002;46(8):1025–30.

32. Webb AR, Leong S, Myles PS, Burn SJ. The addition of a tramadol infusion to morphine patient-controlled analgesia after abdominal surgery: a double-blinded, placebo-controlled randomized trial. Anesth Analg 2002;95(6):1713–18.

33. Desmeules JA. The tramadol option. Eur J Pain 2000;4(Suppl A):15–21.

34. Schnitzer TJ, Gray WL, Paster RZ, Kamin M. Efficacy of tramadol in treatment of chronic low back pain. J Rheumatol 2000;27(3):772–8.

35. Duthie DJ. Remifentanil and tramadol. Br J Anaesth 1998;81(1):51–7.

36. Warren PM, Taylor JH, Nicholson KE, Wraith PK, Drummond GB. Influence of tramadol on the ventilatory response to hypoxia in humans. Br J Anaesth 2000;85(2):211–16.

37. Gardner JS, Blough D, Drinkard CR, Shatin D, Anderson G, Graham D, Alderfer R. Tramadol and seizures: a surveillance study in a managed care population. Pharmacotherapy 2000;20(12):1423–31.

38. Gasse C, Derby L, Vasilakis-Scaramozza C, Jick H. Incidence of first-time idiopathic seizures in users of tramadol. Pharmacotherapy 2000;20(6):629–34.

39. Yates WR, Nguyen MH, Warnock JK. Tramadol dependence with no history of substance abuse. Am J Psychiatry 2001;158(6):964.

40. Devulder J, De Laat M, Dumoulin K, Renson A, Rolly G. Nightmares and hallucinations after long-term intake of tramadol combined with antidepressants. Acta Clin Belg 1996;51(3):184–6.

41. Keeley PW, Foster G, Whitelaw L. Hear my song: auditory hallucinations with tramadol hydrochloride. BMJ 2000;321(7276):1608.

42. Crighton IM, Martin PH, Hobbs GJ, Cobby TF, Fletcher AJ, Stewart PD. A comparison of the effects of intravenous tramadol, codeine, and morphine on gastric emptying in human volunteers. Anesth Analg 1998;87(2):445–9.

43. Pluim MA, Wegener JT, Rupreht J, Vulto AG. Tramadol suppositories are less suitable for post-operative pain relief than rectal acetaminophen/codeine. Eur J Anaesthesiol 1999;16(7):473–8.

44. van den Berg AA, Halliday E, Lule EK, Baloch MS. The effects of tramadol on postoperative nausea, vomiting and headache after ENT surgery. A placebo-controlled comparison with equipotent doses of nalbuphine and pethidine. Acta Anaesthesiol Scand 1999;43(1):28–33.

45. Olle Fortuny G, Opisso Julia L, Oferil Riera F, Sanchez Pallares M, Calatayud Montesa R, Cabre Roca I. Ketorolaco frente a tramadol: estudio comparativo de la eficaciá analgesica en el dolor postoperatorio de histerectomias abdominal. [Ketorolac versus tramadol: comparative study of analgesic efficacy in the postoperative pain in abdominal hysterectomy.] Rev Esp Anestesiol Reanim 2000;47(4):162–7.

46. Meyboom RH, Brodie-Meijer CC, Diemont WL, van Puijenbroek EP. Bladder dysfunction during the use of tramadol. Pharmacoepidemiol Drug Saf 1999;8(Suppl 1):S63–4.

47. Ghislain PD, Wiart T, Bouhassoun N, Legout L, Alcaraz I, Caron J, Modiano P. Toxidermie au tramadol. [Toxic dermatitis caused by tramadol.] Ann Dermatol Venereol 1999;126(1):38–40.

48. Cicero TJ, Adams EH, Geller A, Inciardi JA, Munoz A, Schnoll SH, Senay EC, Woody GE. A postmarketing surveillance program to monitor Ultram (tramadol hydrochloride) abuse in the United States. Drug Alcohol Depend 1999;57(1):7–22.

49. Raber M, Hofmann S, Junge K, Momberger H, Kuhn D. Analgesic efficacy and tolerability of tramadol 100 mg sustained-release capsules in patients with moderate to severe chronic low back pain. Clin Drug Invest 1999;17:415–23.

50. Ruoff GE. Slowing the initial titration rate of tramadol improves tolerability. Pharmacotherapy 1999;19(1):88–93.

51. Petrone D, Kamin M, Olson W. Slowing the titration rate of tramadol HCl reduces the incidence of discontinuation due to nausea and/or vomiting: a double-blind randomized trial. J Clin Pharm Ther 1999;24(2):115–23.

52. Nossol S, Schwarzbold M, Stadler T. Treatment of pain with sustained-release tramadol 100, 150, 200 mg: results of a post-marketing surveillance study. Int J Clin Pract 1998;52(2):115–21.

53. Petzke F, Radbruch L, Sabatowski R, Karthaus M, Mertens A. Slow-release tramadol for treatment of chronic malignant pain—an open multicenter trial. Support Care Cancer 2001;9(1):48–54.

54. Musshoff F, Madea B. Fatality due to ingestion of tramadol alone. Forensic Sci Int 2001;116(2–3):197–9.

55. De Witte JL, Schoenmaekers B, Sessler DI, Deloof T. The analgesic efficacy of tramadol is impaired by concurrent administration of ondansetron. Anesth Analg 2001;92(5):1319–21.

56. Arcioni R, della Rocca M, Romano S, Romano R, Pietropaoli P, Gasparetto A. Ondansetron inhibits the analgesic effects of tramadol: a possible 5-HT(3) spinal receptor involvement in acute pain in humans. Anesth Analg 2002;94(6):1553–7.

57. Gonzalez-Pinto A, Imaz H, De Heredia JL, Gutierrez M, Mico JA. Mania and tramadol–fluoxetine combination. Am J Psychiatry 2001;158(6):964–5.

58. Ingelman-Sundberg M. Genetic susceptibility to adverse effects of drugs and environmental toxicants. The role of the CYP family of enzymes. Mutat Res 2001;482(1–2):11–19.

59. Sauget D, Franco PS, Amaniou M, Mazere J, Dantoine T. Possible syndrome sérotoninergiques induit par l'association de tramadol à de la sertraline chez une femme agée. [Possible serotonergic syndrome caused by combination of tramadol and sertraline in an elderly woman.] Thérapie. 57(3):309–10.

60. Ripple MG, Pestaner JP, Levine BS, Smialek JE. Lethal combination of tramadol and multiple drugs affecting serotonin. Am J Forensic Med Pathol 2000;21(4):370–4.

Trandolapril

See also Angiotensin converting enzyme inhibitors

General Information

Trandolapril is a non-sulfhydryl ACE inhibitor that has been used in patients with hypertension, congestive heart failure, and myocardial infarction. It is a prodrug that is hydrolyzed to the active diacid trandolaprilat.

Comprehensive reviews and the results of a large trial have shown that trandolapril has a pattern of adverse effects reflecting those usually documented with other ACE inhibitors (1).

Organs and Systems

Respiratory

In 3402 patients with hypertension taking trandolapril, cough, assessed by visual analogue scale, was less common in smokers than in non-smokers (2).

References

1. Kober L, Torp-Pedersen C, Carlsen JE, Bagger H, Eliasen P, Lyngborg K, Videbaek J, Cole DS, Auclert L, Pauly NC. A clinical trial of the angiotensin-converting-enzyme inhibitor trandolapril in patients with left ventricular dysfunction after myocardial infarction. Trandolapril Cardiac Evaluation (TRACE) Study Group. N Engl J Med 1995;333(25):1670–6.
2. Genes N, Vaur L, Etienne S, Clerson P. Evaluation de l'influence du tabac sur la tolérance du trandolapril. [Evaluation of the effect of tobacco on trandolapril tolerance.] Therapie 1999;54(6):693–7.

Tranexamic acid

General Information

During normal fibrinolysis, inactive circulating plasminogen binds to fibrin through an active site that binds lysine. The bound plasminogen is then converted to plasmin by activators (such as tissue plasminogen activator, t-PA) and converted to plasmin, which breaks down the fibrin. Tranexamic acid (Cyklokapron) and aminocaproic acid (ε-aminocaproic acid, EACA, 6-aminohexanoic acid, Amicar) are structural analogues of lysine, which bind irreversibly to the lysine-binding sites on plasminogen, inhibiting binding to fibrin and thus the whole process of fibrinolysis (1,2). These agents inhibit the natural degradation of fibrin and so stabilize clots.

Aminocaproic acid was the first such agent to be used widely, but it has largely been superseded in clinical practice by tranexamic acid, which is about 10 times more potent. Para-aminomethylbenzoic acid (PAMBA) is similar to aminocaproic acid, but is about three times more active in inhibiting plasminogen activators (3). However, it is no longer used despite the fact that it is well tolerated.

Uses

Antifibrinolytic agents are of benefit in the treatment of primary menorrhagia (4–7), recurrent epistaxis (8), oral bleeding in patients with congenital and acquired coagulation disorders (9,10), hemorrhage associated with thrombolytic therapy, and to reduce blood loss associated with surgery (especially cardiac surgery, joint replacement, and orthotopic liver transplantation) (11–14). Antifibrinolytic therapy can be of value in other conditions as well (15–21). It is effective in the bleeding diathesis that can accompany acute promyelocytic leukemia (22,23), but it does not improve outcome after subarachnoid hemorrhage (24).

Tranexamic acid used during cardiopulmonary bypass reduces mediastinal blood losses by about one-third, while transfusion requirements remain unchanged (25). In over 950 patients, not a single thromboembolic complication could be ascribed to it.

General adverse effects

Adverse effects of tranexamic acid are rare and mainly limited to nausea, diarrhea, or abdominal pain (4,5,26–29). These symptoms are usually associated with high doses, and subside if the dose is reduced. The dose of tranexamic acid in patients with renal insufficiency must be reduced to avoid accumulation and associated adverse effects. Hypotension is occasionally observed, typically after rapid intravenous infusion (30). The better safety profile with regard to minor adverse effects of tranexamic acid compared with aminocaproic acid is due to the lower daily dose required for tranexamic acid (3–6 g) compared with aminocaproic acid (18–30 g). Tranexamic acid has very occasionally been associated with skin rashes, including fixed drug eruption (31) and bullous eruptions (32).

Organs and Systems

Sensory systems

Central venous retinopathy was reported in two young women after oral treatment with tranexamic acid for menorrhagia (33).

- A 56-year-old man, who had been undergoing hemodialysis for 1 year after 10 years of peritoneal dialysis, was given intravenous tranexamic acid after an emergency operation for bleeding peptic ulcers; he had gradual loss of sight over about 1 week, and 2 weeks after the operation became blind (34). Retinography was flat and his visual field was narrowed. Fluorescein angiography showed microgranular hyperfluorescence, suggesting malfunction of the pigmented layer of the retina. There were no abnormalities in the brain or optic nerve on MRI scanning. Withdrawal of tranexamic acid restored his sight within a few days. He had received tranexamic acid once before because of a bleeding ulcer, and his sight had been impaired at that time too.

However, in 14 patients who had taken tranexamic acid for an average period of 6 years there was no evidence of ocular damage (35).

Hematologic

Inhibition of plasminogen by tranexamic acid and aminocaproic acid could theoretically facilitate the development of thrombosis, but whether it actually does so has been the subject of contradictory reports. Episodes of venous and arterial thrombosis have been reported in association with treatment using either tranexamic acid or aminocaproic acid. These include thrombosis at unusual sites such as mesenteric thrombosis (36), the aorta (37), retinal artery occlusion (38), and intracranial arterial thrombosis (39–41), as well as deep-vein thrombosis in the legs (42).

- Massive pulmonary thromboembolism was reported in a 62-year-old woman 7 days after treatment with high doses for subarachnoid hemorrhage (43).

However, in a large retrospective study from Sweden, the incidence of thrombosis in women receiving tranexamic acid for menorrhagia was no different to that of the rest of the population (44). During a 9-year period, corresponding to over 238 000 women-years, 11 thromboembolic complications were reported. This corresponds to an annual incidence of 0.005%, which is not higher than the expected incidence in fertile women. Furthermore, a retrospective study of 256 pregnant women treated with tranexamic acid for abruptio placentae or other hemorrhagic problems showed no evidence of a thrombogenic effect of the drug (45), and a study of patients undergoing cardiac surgery who received tranexamic also showed no increased risk of thrombotic complications (46). Thus, the association between use of inhibitors of fibrinolysis and thrombosis appears to be fortuitous and the risk of this potential hazard is very low. However, the data sheet issued by the manufacturers still states that tranexamic acid is contraindicated in patients with a previous history of thromboembolic disease.

Caution should also be exercised in the administration of antifibrinolytic agents in disseminated intravascular coagulation (47,48).

Urinary tract

Acute renal cortical necrosis has been attributed to tranexamic acid in a patient with hemophilia A (49,50).

- A 21-year-old man developed oliguria and uremia after 3 days of treatment with tranexamic acid 3 g/day for epistaxis. He did not recover. Renal angiography showed reduced cortical contrast enhancement, compatible with renal cortical necrosis. No other susceptibility factors for renal cortical necrosis were present.

Renal impairment associated with acute renal cortical necrosis caused by tranexamic acid is rare. The authors found only three previously reported cases in English, of which at least one other was without any known susceptibility factor for acute renal cortical necrosis (49).

Second-Generation Effects

Teratogenicity

There is no evidence of a teratogenic effect with tranexamic acid (51).

Lactation

Tranexamic acid passes into breast milk but reaches a concentration of only about one hundredth of that in maternal blood (51), which should not result in significant inhibition of fibrinolysis in a neonate.

Drug–Drug Interactions

All-*trans* retinoic acid

Tranexamic acid has been used without thrombotic complications for the attempted prophylaxis of hemorrhage in patients with acute promyelocytic leukemia treated with combination chemotherapy, in whom hemorrhage is a significant problem. Since several studies have shown that all-*trans* retinoic acid can produce complete remission, it has become part of standard treatment. Fatal thromboembolism in acute promyelocytic leukemia during all-*trans* retinoic acid therapy combined with antifibrinolytic therapy has been reported (52). Of 31 patients with acute promyelocytic leukemia, treated with different combinations of all-*trans* retinoic acid and chemotherapy, 21 were given tranexamic acid (53). Of the 28 patients who received all-*trans* retinoic acid, 7 died during the study, but of these 7, only 4 were early deaths (within 42 days). All four early deaths were in those who received all-*trans* retinoic acid plus tranexamic acid, and three of the four had sudden and rapid deterioration in their condition; postmortem findings implicated thrombosis in the microvasculature as the predominant cause of death. The authors suggested that in patients taking all-*trans* retinoic acid, tranexamic acid should be used cautiously; supportive therapy with platelets and fresh frozen plasma alone can be used.

References

1. Astedt B. Clinical pharmacology of tranexamic acid. Scand J Gastroenterol Suppl 1987;137:22–5.
2. Hoylaerts M, Lijnen HR, Collen D. Studies on the mechanism of the antifibrinolytic action of tranexamic acid. Biochim Biophys Acta 1981;673(1):75–85.
3. Westlund LE, Lunden R, Wallen P. Effect of EACA, PAMBA, AMCA and AMBOCA on fibrinolysis induced by streptokinase, urokinase and tissue activator. Haemostasis 1982;11(4):235–41.
4. Nilsson L, Rybo G. Treatment of menorrhagia with an antifibrinolytic agent, tranexamic acid (AMCA): a double-blind investigation. Acta Obstet Gynecolog Scand 1967;46:572–80.
5. Vermylen J, Verhaegen-Declercq ML, Verstraete M, Fierens F. A double blind study of the effect of tranexamic acid in essential menorrhagia. Thromb Diath Haemorrh 1968;20(3):583–7.
6. Callender ST, Warner GT, Cope E. Treatment of menorrhagia with tranexamic acid. A double-blind trial. BMJ 1970;4(729):214–16.
7. Prentice A. Fortnightly review. Medical management of menorrhagia. BMJ 1999;319(7221):1343–5.
8. Petruson B. A double-blind study to evaluate the effect in epistaxis with oral administration of the antifibrinolytic drug tranexamic acid (Cyklokapron). Acta Otolaryngol 1974;317(Suppl):57–61.

9. Forbes CD, Barr RD, Reid G, Thomson C, Prentice CR, McNicol GP, Douglas AS. Tranexamic acid in control of haemorrhage after dental extraction in haemophilia and Christmas disease. BMJ 1972;2(809):311–13.

10. Sindet-Pedersen S, Ramstrom G, Bernvil S, Blomback M. Hemostatic effect of tranexamic acid mouthwash in anticoagulant-treated patients undergoing oral surgery. N Engl J Med 1989;320(13):840–3.

11. Jordan D, Delphin E, Rose E. Prophylactic epsilon-amino-caproic acid (EACA) administration minimizes blood replacement therapy during cardiac surgery. Anesth Analg 1995;80(4):827–9.

12. Boylan JF, Klinck JR, Sandler AN, Arellano R, Greig PD, Nierenberg H, Roger SL, Glynn MF. Tranexamic acid reduces blood loss, transfusion requirements, and coagulation factor use in primary orthotopic liver transplantation. Anesthesiology 1996;85(5):1043–8.

13. Benoni G, Fredin H. Fibrinolytic inhibition with tranexamic acid reduces blood loss and blood transfusion after knee arthroplasty: a prospective, randomised, double-blind study of 86 patients. J Bone Joint Surg Br 1996;78(3):434–40.

14. Jansen AJ, Andreica S, Claeys M, D'Haese J, Camu F, Jochmans K. Use of tranexamic acid for an effective blood conservation strategy after total knee arthroplasty. Br J Anaesth 1999;83(4):596–601.

15. Gardner FH, Helmer RE 3rd. Aminocaproic acid. Use in control of hemorrhage in patients with amegakaryocytic thrombocytopenia. JAMA 1980;243(1):35–7.

16. Bartholomew JR, Salgia R, Bell WR. Control of bleeding in patients with immune and nonimmune thrombocytopenia with aminocaproic acid. Arch Intern Med 1989;149(9):1959–61.

17. von Holstein CC, Eriksson SB, Kallen R. Tranexamic acid as an aid to reducing blood transfusion requirements in gastric and duodenal bleeding. BMJ (Clin Res Ed) 1987;294(6563):7–10.

18. Henry DA, O'Connell DL. Effects of fibrinolytic inhibitors on mortality from upper gastrointestinal haemorrhage. BMJ 1989;298(6681):1142–6.

19. Jerndal T, Frisen M. Tranexamic acid (AMCA) and late hyphaema. A double blind study in cataract surgery. Acta Ophthalmol (Copenh) 1976;54(4):417–29.

20. Varnek L, Dalsgaard C, Hansen A, Klie F. The effect of tranexamic acid on secondary haemorrhage after traumatic hyphaema. Acta Ophthalmol (Copenh) 1980;58(5):787–93.

21. Uusitalo RJ, Ranta-Kemppainen L, Tarkkanen A. Management of traumatic hyphema in children. An analysis of 340 cases. Arch Ophthalmol 1988;106(9):1207–9.

22. Schwartz BS, Williams EC, Conlan MG, Mosher DF. Epsilon-aminocaproic acid in the treatment of patients with acute promyelocytic leukemia and acquired alpha-2-plasmin inhibitor deficiency. Ann Intern Med 1986;105(6):873–7.

23. Avvisati G, ten Cate JW, Buller HR, Mandelli F. Tranexamic acid for control of haemorrhage in acute promyelocytic leukaemia. Lancet 1989;2(8655):122–4.

24. Roos Y. Antifibrinolytic treatment in subarachnoid hemorrhage: a randomized placebo-controlled trial. STAR Study Group. Neurology 2000;54(1):77–82.

25. Barrons RW, Jahr JS. A review of post-cardiopulmonary bypass bleeding, aminocaproic acid, tranexamic acid, and aprotinin. Am J Ther 1996;3(12):821–38.

26. Munch EP, Weeke B. Non-hereditary angioedema treated with tranexamic acid. A 6-month placebo controlled trial with follow-up 4 years later. Allergy 1985;40(2):92–7.

27. Hedlund PO. Antifibrinolytic therapy with Cyklokapron in connection with prostatectomy. A double blind study. Scand J Urol Nephrol 1969;3(3):177–82.

28. Sheffer AL, Austen KF, Rosen FS. Tranexamic acid therapy in hereditary angioneurotic edema. N Engl J Med 1972;287(9):452–4.

29. Westrom L, Bengtsson LP. Effect of tranexamic acid (AMCA) in menorrhagia with intrauterine contraceptive devices. J Reprod Med 1970;5(4):154–61.

30. Dunn CJ, Goa KL. Tranexamic acid: a review of its use in surgery and other indications. Drugs 1999;57(6):1005–32.

31. Kavanagh GM, Sansom JE, Harrison P, Warwick JA, Peachey RD. Tranexamic acid (Cyklokapron)-induced fixed-drug eruption. Br J Dermatol 1993;128(2):229–30.

32. Carrion-Carrion C, del Pozo-Losada J, Gutierrez-Ramos R, de Lucas-Laguna R, Garcia-Diaz B, Casado-Jimenez M, Esperanza-Jimenez Caballero ME. Bullous eruption induced by tranexamic acid. Ann Pharmacother 1994;28(11):1305–6.

33. Snir M, Axer-Siegel R, Buckman G, Yassur Y. Central venous stasis retinopathy following the use of tranexamic acid. Retina 1990;10(3):181–4.

34. Kitamura H, Matsui I, Itoh N, Fujii T, Aizawa M, Yamamoto R, Okuno A, Okazaki Y, Fujita Y, Kuwayama Y, Imai E, Fujii M. Tranexamic acid-induced visual impairment in a hemodialysis patient. Clin Exp Nephrol 2003;7(4):311–14.

35. Theil PL. Ophthalmological examination of patients in long-term treatment with tranexamic acid. Acta Ophthalmol (Copenh) 1981;59(2):237–41.

36. Razis PA, Coulson IH, Gould TR, Findley IL. Acquired C1 esterase inhibitor deficiency. Anaesthesia 1986;41(8):838–40.

37. Hocker JR, Saving KL. Fatal aortic thrombosis in a neonate during infusion of epsilon-aminocaproic acid. J Pediatr Surg 1995;30(10):1490–2.

38. Parsons MR, Merritt DR, Ramsay RC. Retinal artery occlusion associated with tranexamic acid therapy. Am J Ophthalmol 1988;105(6):688–9.

39. Davies D, Howell DA. Tranexamic acid and arterial thrombosis. Lancet 1977;1(8001):49.

40. Agnelli G, Gresele P, De Cunto M, Gallai V, Nenci GG. Tranexamic acid, intrauterine contraceptive devices and fatal cerebral arterial thrombosis. Case report. Br J Obstet Gynaecol 1982;89(8):681–2.

41. Humbert P, Gutknecht J, Mallet H, Dupond JL, Leconte des Floris R. Acide tranéxamique et thrombose du sinus londitudinal supérieur. [Tranexamic acid and thrombosis of the superior longitudinal sinus.] Therapie 1987;42(1):65–6.

42. Endo Y, Nishimura S, Miura A. Deep-vein thrombosis induced by tranexamic acid in idiopathic thrombocytopenic purpura. JAMA 1988;259(24):3561–2.

43. Woo KS, Tse LK, Woo JL, Vallance-Owen J. Massive pulmonary thromboembolism after antifibrinolytic therapy. Ann Emerg Med 1989;18(1):116–17.

44. Rybo, G. Tranexamic acid therapy is effective treatment in heavy menstrual bleeding. Clinical update on safety. Therapeutic Adv 1991;4:1–8.

45. Lindoff C, Rybo G, Astedt B. Treatment with tranexamic acid during pregnancy, and the risk of thrombo-embolic complications. Thromb Haemost 1993;70(2):238–40.

46. Rousou JA, Engelman RM, Flack JE 3rd, Deaton DW, Owen SG. Tranexamic acid significantly reduces blood loss associated with coronary revascularization. Ann Thorac Surg 1995;59(3):671–5.

47. Giles AR. Disseminated intravascular coagulation. Edinburgh: Churchill Livingston, 1994.

48. Asakura H, Sano Y, Yamazaki M, Morishita E, Miyamoto K, Nakao S. Role of fibrinolysis in tissue-factor-induced disseminated intravascular coagulation in rats—an effect of tranexamic acid. Haematologica 2004;89(6):757–8.

49. Koo JR, Lee YK, Kim YS, Cho WY, Kim HK, Won NH. Acute renal cortical necrosis caused by an antifibrinolytic drug (tranexamic acid). Nephrol Dial Transplant 1999;14(3):750–2.

50. Odabas AR, Cetinkaya R, Selcuk Y, Kaya H, Coskun U. Tranexamic-acid-induced acute renal cortical necrosis in a patient with haemophilia A. Nephrol Dial Transplant 2001;16(1):189–90.

51. Briggs GG, Freeman RK, Jaffe SJ. Drugs in Pregnancy and Lactation. 5th ed. Baltimore: Williams and Wilkins, 1998.

52. Hashimoto S, Koike T, Tatewaki W, Seki Y, Sato N, Azegami T, Tsukada N, Takahashi H, Kimura H, Ueno M, Arakawa M, Shibata A. Fatal thromboembolism in acute promyelocytic leukemia during all-trans retinoic acid therapy combined with antifibrinolytic therapy for prophylaxis of hemorrhage. Leukemia 1994;8(7):1113–15.

53. Brown JE, Olujohungbe A, Chang J, Ryder WD, Morganstern GR, Chopra R, Scarffe JH. All-trans retinoic acid (ATRA) and tranexamic acid: a potentially fatal combination in acute promyelocytic leukaemia. Br J Haematol 2000;110(4):1010–12.

Tranilast

General Information

Tranilast is an orally active antiallergic agent. It may have a similar mechanism of action to that of cromoglicate.

Its adverse reactions include liver function abnormalities, anorexia, nausea, vomiting, abdominal pain, reduced hemoglobin, headache, drowsiness, insomnia, dizziness, and general malaise (1).

Organs and Systems

Urinary tract

Some patients taking tranilast develop severe bladder symptoms, unrelieved by antibiotic treatment (2). Fourteen patients have been reported in detail. In patients whose bladder wall was biopsied there was eosinophilic inflammation. Drug-induced lymphocyte stimulation showed that tranilast and its major metabolite are causative agents. The symptoms disappear within a few days of stopping the drug (SEDA-12, 145) (SEDA-14, 139) (SEDA-17, 205) (3).

- A 59-year-old man who had been taking tranilast 600 mg/day for 15 weeks developed bladder irritability (4). Cystoscopy showed extensive mucosal edema, strongly suggestive of drug-induced cystitis. He stopped taking tranilast and the symptoms disappeared within 3 weeks.

Immunologic

Immune thrombocytopenia caused by tranilast has been reported in a 17-year-old man. The drug was withdrawn and oral prednisolone was started. He recovered within 1 week. Antiplatelet antibodies were not detected, but there was a platelet-associated IgG, which increased when a sample of his serum was incubated with tranilast in vitro (5).

References

1. Anonymous. Tranilast. Drugs Today 1983;19:485.
2. Nishida T, Kusakai Y, Ogoshi R. [Four cases of cystitis induced by the anti-allergic drug tranilast.] Hinyokika Kiyo 1985;31(10):1813–17.
3. Sakai N, Yamada T, Murayama T. [Eosinophilic cystitis induced by tranilast: a case report.] Hinyokika Kiyo 1998;44(1):45–7.
4. Saito M, Yoshimura S, Fujii A, Iwai A. Bladder irritability caused by tranilast. Iryo Jpn J Natl Med Serv 2000;54:361–4.
5. Nagae S, Hori Y. Immune thrombocytopenia due to tranilast (Rizaben): detection of drug-dependent platelet-associated IgG. J Dermatol 1998;25(11):706–9.

Tranylcypromine

See also Monoamine oxidase inhibitors

General Information

Tranylcypromine is a non-hydrazine monoamine oxidase (MAO) inhibitor with actions and uses similar to those of phenelzine, but with less prolonged inhibition. Its half-life is 90–190 minutes. It is structurally related to amfetamine, to which it is metabolized in overdose (1).

Long-Term Effects

Drug abuse

Four cases of addiction to tranylcypromine have been described, in addition to the three reported since 1965 (2). The dosage was 150–300 mg/day. The mild euphoriant properties of tranylcypromine reflect its structural resemblance to amfetamine, and probably account for tolerance and addiction in predisposed individuals. Tranylcypromine abuse in 18 patients has been reviewed (3), and two further reports have appeared (SEDA-17, 17) (4). In one case (5), the patient took 440 mg/day without any adverse effects. The patient reported that she was longing for the "energizing" effect of the drug and for the feeling of "freedom and power." Withdrawal resulted in repeated generalized seizures and status epilepticus.

Susceptibility Factors

Hepatic disease

A carefully controlled study showed that patients with impaired liver function are especially sensitive to tranylcypromine, sometimes developing obtunded consciousness and slow electroencephalograms similar to those found in hepatic encephalopathy (6).

Drug Administration

Drug overdose

The fatal effects of antidepressants in England, Scotland, and Wales during 1975–1984 and 1985–1989 have been compared in retrospective epidemiological studies (7,8). There were 24 deaths due to tranylcypromine, the fatality index for which was significantly higher than the mean for all antidepressants, while that for the other MAO inhibitors was lower.

References

1. Youdim MB, Aronson JK, Blau K, Green AR, Grahame-Smith DG. Tranylcypromine ("Parnate") overdose: measurement of tranylcypromine concentrations and MAO inhibitory activity and identification of amphetamines in plasma. Psychol Med 1979;9(2):377–82.
2. Griffin N, Draper RJ, Webb MG. Addiction to tranylcypromine. BMJ (Clin Res Ed) 1981;283(6287):346.
3. Briggs NC, Jefferson JW, Koenecke FH. Tranylcypromine addiction: a case report and review. J Clin Psychiatry 1990;51(10):426–9.
4. Shepherd JT, Whiting B. Beta-adrenergic blockade in the treatment of M.A.O.I. self-poisoning. Lancet 1974;2(7887):1021.
5. Vartzopoulos D, Krull F. Dependence on monoamine oxidase inhibitors in high dose. Br J Psychiatry 1991;158:856–7.
6. Morgan MH, Read AE. Antidepressants and liver disease. Gut 1972;13(9):697–701.
7. Cassidy S, Henry J. Fatal toxicity of antidepressant drugs in overdose. BMJ (Clin Res Ed) 1987;295(6605):1021–4.
8. Henry JA, Antao CA. Suicide and fatal antidepressant poisoning. Eur J Med 1992;1(6):343–8.

Trastuzumab

See also Monoclonal antibodies

General Information

Trastuzumab is a recombinant humanized monoclonal antibody that binds to the proto-oncogene, HER-2/neu gene product, which is expressed in 25–30% of primary breast cancers. It has been used to treat selected patients with metastatic breast cancer whose tumors overexpress the HER2 protein, which is amplified in 25–30% of breast cancers and is associated with an aggressive form of disease (1). Adverse effects mostly consisted of infusion-related constitutional symptoms, digestive disorders (diarrhea, vomiting), pain, cough, headache, dyspnea, mild infections, and insomnia. Compared with chemotherapy alone, the addition of trastuzumab more often produced moderately severe adverse hematological effects (leukopenia and anemia) and diarrhea. Severe congestive cardiac failure is a major adverse effect of trastuzumab. According to the product labelling, severe cardiac failure was observed in 5–19% of patients (trastuzumab alone versus trastuzumab plus anthracycline and cyclophosphamide). Other serious adverse events, including death, have occurred in 0.25% of patients treated with

trastuzumab. They fall into three categories: infusion reactions; hypersensitivity reactions, including fatal anaphylaxis; and pulmonary events, including adult respiratory distress syndrome.

Organs and Systems

Cardiovascular

Cardiotoxicity is a major concern with trastuzumab, particularly as it is often used in patients who are receiving or who have previously received anthracycline antibiotics (2). It occurs in 5% of patients given trastuzumab alone, in 13% of patients given trastuzumab with paclitaxel, and in 27% of patients given trastuzumab in combination with anthracyclines and cyclophosphamide (3).

The efficacy and safety of trastuzumab have been evaluated in 235 women with metastatic breast cancer receiving standard chemotherapy (4). The most important adverse event was cardiac failure, which occurred in 27% of those who were given anthracycline, cyclophosphamide, and trastuzumab, 8% of those who were given anthracycline and cyclophosphamide alone, 13% of those who were given paclitaxel and trastuzumab, and 1% of those who were given paclitaxel alone. The incidence of cardiac failure of New York Heart Association class III or class IV was highest among patients who had received an anthracycline, cyclophosphamide, and trastuzumab. The mechanism is unknown. In a retrospective analysis of all patients with cardiac failure by an independent review and evaluation committee, the only significant risk factor was older age. Although the cardiotoxicity was severe, and in some cases life-threatening, the symptoms improved with standard medical management.

Seven phase II and III clinical trials of trastuzumab in patients with metastatic breast cancer have been reviewed (5). The physiopathology of trastuzumab-associated cardiac disease is poorly understood, and baseline MUGA scanning is recommended to identify cardiac disease. The rates of cardiac disease were highest when trastuzumab was given in combination with anthracyclines or when there had been previous exposure to anthracyclines. Given the 25% improvement in overall survival in these patients with metastatic disease, the use of trastuzumab is justified.

- A 60-year-old woman with coronary heart disease and hypertension developed breast cancer and a core biopsy showed ER+/PR+/HER2–3+ (3). She enrolled in an institutional study with neoadjuvant trastuzumab with docetaxel. A pretreatment blood pool radionuclide angiography (MUGA) scan revealed a left ventricular ejection fraction of 56%. She had a good clinical response to treatment at 3 months. Before surgery a repeat MUGA showed a dilated left ventricle and a reduced ejection fraction (35%). She underwent surgery and 2 months later her ejection fraction was 44%.
- An overweight 59-year-old woman with hypertension and asthma developed breast cancer (ER+/PR+/HER2–2+) (3). Her MUGA scan showed a left ventricular ejection fraction of 57%. She was given trastuzumab with docetaxel and had a good response after 4 months. Before surgery she became dyspneic, and a

MUGA scan showed an ejection fraction of 24%; even 7 months after surgery her MUGA scan showed no improvement.

The efficacy and tolerability of trastuzumab in clinical trials has been reviewed (6). Of the first 48 patients treated in Sweden with or without chemotherapy, two had serious cardiac events and both had previously been treated with an anthracycline. As not all patients who received trastuzumab had echocardiography, the number of cardiac events was probably underestimated. It has been postulated that HER2 pathways may be involved in myocyte repair, and that concomitant administration of trastuzumab may interfere with the repair of anthracycline-damaged myocytes (7). Evidence from 20 patients has shown that cardiotoxicity is related to trastuzumab uptake in the myocardium, suggesting that the extent of HER2 receptor expression, or a related cross-reactive antigen in the myocardium, may be the underlying mechanism.

Respiratory

The toxicity of five escalating doses of trastuzumab (1–8 mg/kg) when combined with a fixed dose of interleukin-2 has been determined in 45 patients with non-hematological malignancies that overexpressed HER2 (8). There was no evidence of increasing toxicity related to the dose of trastuzumab. Five patients had pulmonary toxicity of grade 3 or higher; these were primarily attributed to interleukin-2, as the patients improved on reduction of the dose of interleukin-2.

Drug–Drug Interactions

Paclitaxel

In primates, trastuzumab clearance was reduced when it was administered with paclitaxel (9).

References

1. Goldenberg MM. Trastuzumab, a recombinant DNA-derived humanized monoclonal antibody, a novel agent for the treatment of metastatic breast cancer. Clin Ther 1999;21(2):309–18.
2. Seidman AD, Fornier MN, Esteva FJ, Tan L, Kaptain S, Bach A, Panageas KS, Arroyo C, Valero V, Currie V, Gilewski T, Theodoulou M, Moynahan ME, Moasser M, Sklarin N, Dickler M, D'Andrea G, Cristofanilli M, Rivera E, Hortobagyi GN, Norton L, Hudis CA. Weekly trastuzumab and paclitaxel therapy for metastatic breast cancer with analysis of efficacy by HER2 immunophenotype and gene amplification. J Clin Oncol 2001;19(10):2587–95.
3. Tham YL, Verani MS, Chang J. Reversible and irreversible cardiac dysfunction associated with trastuzumab in breast cancer. Breast Cancer Res Treat 2002;74(2):131–4.
4. Slamon DJ, Leyland-Jones B, Shak S, Fuchs H, Paton V, Bajamonde A, Fleming T, Eiermann W, Wolter J, Pegram M, Baselga J, Norton L. Use of chemotherapy plus a monoclonal antibody against HER2 for metastatic breast cancer that overexpresses HER2. N Engl J Med 2001;344(11):783–92.
5. Seidman A, Hudis C, Pierri MK, Shak S, Paton V, Ashby M, Murphy M, Stewart SJ, Keefe D. Cardiac dysfunction in the trastuzumab clinical trials experience. J Clin Oncol 2002;20(5):1215–21.
6. Andersson J, Linderholm B, Greim G, Lindh B, Lindman H, Tennvall J, Tennvall-Nittby L, Pettersson-Skold D, Sverrisdottir A, Soderberg M, Klaar S, Bergh J. A population-based study on the first forty-eight breast cancer patients receiving trastuzumab (Herceptin) on a named patient basis in Sweden. Acta Oncol 2002;41(3):276–81.
7. Leonard DS, Hill AD, Kelly L, Dijkstra B, McDermott E, O'Higgins NJ. Anti-human epidermal growth factor receptor 2 monoclonal antibody therapy for breast cancer. Br J Surg 2002;89(3):262–71.
8. Fleming GF, Meropol NJ, Rosner GL, Hollis DR, Carson WE 3rd, Caligiuri M, Mortimer J, Tkaczuk K, Parihar R, Schilsky RL, Ratain MJ. A phase I trial of escalating doses of trastuzumab combined with daily subcutaneous interleukin 2: report of cancer and leukemia group B 9661. Clin Cancer Res 2002;8(12):3718–27.
9. McKeage K, Perry CM. Trastuzumab: a review of its use in the treatment of metastatic breast cancer overexpressing HER2. Drugs 2002;62(1):209–43.

Travoprost

See also Prostaglandins

General Information

Travoprost is a derivative of fluprostenol and $PGF_{2\alpha}$ and has intraocular pressure-lowering activity.

Organs and Systems

Sensory systems

Travoprost causes changes in iris pigmentation (3.1–5.0%) and changes in eyelash characteristics, including length, thickness, density, and color (44–57%), similar to those described with latanoprost, after 12 months (1).

Reference

1. Netland PA, Landry T, Sullivan EK, Andrew R, Silver L, Weiner A, Mallick S, Dickerson J, Bergamini MV, Robertson SM, Davis AA; Travoprost Study Group. Travoprost compared with latanoprost and timolol in patients with open-angle glaucoma or ocular hypertension. Am J Ophthalmol 2001;132(4):472–84.

Trazodone

See also Antidepressants, second-generation

General Information

Trazodone (SEDA-7, 19–21) is a triazolopyridine derivative that selectively but weakly inhibits 5-hydroxytryptamine (5-HT) re-uptake and is an alpha-adrenoceptor antagonist at both presynaptic and postsynaptic receptors

(1). During long-term administration it down-regulates serotonin receptors (2).

Experience with therapeutic and toxic dose ranges of trazodone has thrown much doubt on earlier claims for its greater safety, and some unanticipated problems have surfaced.

Trazodone is rapidly absorbed, with peak plasma concentrations at 0.5–2 hours. It is extensively metabolized and eliminated mainly via the kidneys, with a half-life of 13 hours for total drug and metabolites.

A review of controlled clinical studies in depressed patients in Europe and the USA showed that trazodone is superior to placebo (3) and can be as effective as imipramine or amitriptyline (3,4). The doses needed to secure an equivalent effect (150–800 mg/day) were generally double those of the tricyclic antidepressants.

In 28 depressed patients treated with up to 600 mg/day for 4 weeks, plasma concentrations varied eightfold (5). There was a significant correlation between dosage and plasma concentration, but no association with outcome and no significant difference between the mean plasma concentrations in responders (1.51 µg/ml) and non-responders (1.64 µg/ml).

The short half-life of trazodone naturally raises the question of the optimal dosage frequency. The General Practitioner Research Group in Britain (6) has conducted a series of comparisons of trazodone given once, twice, and thrice a day to anxious and depressed patients taking up to 200 mg/day. Efficacy was the same with all three regimens, although there were more complaints of dizziness and fewer of drowsiness with the thrice-daily regimen.

Organs and Systems

Cardiovascular

Based on animal research and restricted experience in overdosage (SEDA-7, 19–21), early attempts to differentiate trazodone from tricyclic antidepressants suggested that it might be relatively free of cardiotoxic effects. However, a preliminary report of a study of the effects of trazodone on the cardiovascular system in 20 subjects mentioned two patients who had ventricular dysrhythmias (7). Others have reported ventricular tachycardia (8–10), atrial fibrillation (11), and complete heart block (12).

Additive hypotensive effects of trazodone and phenothiazines have been reported (13).

Trazodone can cause peripheral edema, as outlined in a report of 10 cases (14).

Nervous system

Trazodone is markedly sedative, very similar in profile to amitriptyline. It produces marked sedation and lethargy within an hour, lasting up to 6 hours, and is about half as potent as imipramine (4).

Although it is claimed to be relatively free of effects usually attributed to anticholinergic activity, trazodone does cause complaints of dry mouth and blurred vision, which may be mediated through its actions on alpha-adrenoceptors. Urinary retention has been reported in a

69-year-old woman taking a combination of trazodone and an anticholinergic drug (isopropamide iodide) (15). Cholinergic overactivity has also been described in two patients after withdrawal (16).

The manufacturers of trazodone received 30 unpublished reports of seizures in patients, most of whom had evidence of seizure predisposition or concurrent contributory conditions. Two reports are detailed here (17,18).

- A 50-year-old woman with an electroencephalographic abnormality but no history of epilepsy, who had taken amitriptyline and perphenazine uneventfully for years, suffered two seizures 18 days after switching to trazodone 50 mg/day.
- A 47-year-old man developed 30-second episodes of facial contortions, aphasia, garbled speech, neologism, nocturnal episodes of deep breathing, swallowing, and incomprehensible speech after taking trazodone 150 mg/day for 3 weeks. On withdrawal of trazodone, his symptoms abated, but an electroencephalogram showed a left anterior lobe spike. He was treated with carbamazepine and within 6 months was not depressed and had no further convulsive symptoms.

Sensory systems

Three cases of palinopsia (the persistence or reappearance of an image of a recently viewed object) have been reported (SEDA-17, 22); the authors speculated that this may have been due to pharmacological effects resembling those of LSD and mescaline.

Psychological, psychiatric

Conversion to mania has been reported in patients with unipolar depression (19,20) and bipolar illness (20).

Delirium, which also occurs with tricyclic antidepressants, has been reported with trazodone (21).

Liver

Hepatotoxicity, a known hazard of tricyclic compounds, has been reported with trazodone (22,23).

Skin

Trazodone has caused generalized erythematous maculo-papular eruptions (24), erythema multiforme (although the patient was also taking lithium) (25), and generalized pustular psoriasis in a patient who had had stable plaque psoriasis for 19 years (26).

Sexual function

Inhibition of ejaculation was reported in a middle-aged man 1 week after he started taking trazodone 100 mg at night (27). The symptoms abated 3 days after withdrawal and did not return when treatment was changed to doxepin 50 mg/day. Because trazodone has relatively more alpha-adrenoceptor blocking action and less anticholinergic activity than doxepin, the author speculated that this was the mechanism.

Trazodone can cause severe and persistent priapism. In a communication from the manufacturers in 1987, it was noted that there had been 136 reports of "increased penile tumescence" in patients taking trazodone. These included all reports of abnormal erectile activity. The company reported that the incidence of all abnormal erectile activity was about one in 6000 men, that in 36 of the 136 patients surgical interventions had been performed, and that at least nine of these patients were impotent. They suggested that early intervention is the treatment of choice, and that trazodone should be withdrawn immediately at the first signs of prolonged erections. They recommended that if conservative measures fail, intracavernosal irrigation with a weak solution of adrenaline should be considered (28). This rare adverse effect has been reported previously with a number of psychoactive and antihypertensive drugs (phenothiazines, guanethidine, prazosin, hydralazine) and has been ascribed to their alpha-adrenoceptor antagonist activity. The same mechanism probably explains the effect of trazodone.

Increased libido (29) and anorgasmia (30) have been reported with trazodone.

Drug Administration

Drug overdose

In a 1980 review there were 68 cases of trazodone overdosage in amounts ranging up to 5 g (12 times the maximum therapeutic dose) (31). The predominant symptoms were drowsiness, dizziness, and rarely coma. There were no deaths in patients who took trazodone alone, and only two in those who took it in combination with other potentially lethal drugs. A brief review of data obtained from 46 cases of trazodone overdose reported to the National Poisons Information Service in London showed that 25 of the patients took overdoses of trazodone alone, while 21 took trazodone in combination with other drugs (32). This retrospective questionnaire study had inherent methodological flaws, but it did lend credence to the belief that trazodone is safe in overdose.

Trazodone is less cardiotoxic than tricyclic antidepressants, although it has rarely been reported to cause ventricular tachycardia. QT interval prolongation has been reported in overdose (33).

- A patient who took an overdose of trazodone (3 g) had sinus bradycardia (57 beats/minute) and a prolonged QT_c interval (60 msec). The abnormal QT_c interval gradually normalized over the next 3 days with supportive hospital treatment.

Drug–Drug Interactions

Amiodarone

A patient taking both trazodone and amiodarone developed prolongation of the QT interval and a polymorphous ventricular tachycardia, perhaps by mutual potentiation (34).

Carbamazepine

In a 53-year-old man, trazodone produced a clinically significant increase in carbamazepine concentrations (35). This suggests that trazodone inhibits CYP3A4. It should be used with caution in combination with carbamazepine.

MAOIs and SSRIs

Although trazodone is related to nefazodone it probably potentiates 5-HT neurotransmission less. Trazodone is often added to monoamine oxidase inhibitors and serotonin re-uptake inhibitors at low doses (50–150 mg/day) as a hypnotic. In one case the combination of trazodone with nefazodone provoked the serotonin syndrome (36).

- When a 60-year-old woman taking nefazodone 500 mg/day also took trazodone 50 mg/day she developed confusion, restlessness, sweating, and nausea after 3 days. Her symptoms settled quickly on withdrawal of both antidepressants.

References

1. Riblet LA, Taylor DP. Pharmacology and neurochemistry of trazodone. J Clin Psychopharmacol 1981;1(Suppl):175.
2. Subhash MN, Srinivas BN, Vinod KY. Alterations in 5-HT (1A) receptors and adenylyl cyclase response by trazodone in regions of rat brain. Life Sci 2002;71(13):1559–67.
3. Davis JM, Vogel C. Efficacy of trazodone: data from European and United States studies. J Clin Psychopharmacol 1981;1(Suppl.):275.
4. Brogden RN, Heel RC, Speight TM, Avery GS. Trazodone: a review of its pharmacological properties and therapeutic use in depression and anxiety. Drugs 1981;21(6):401–29.
5. Mann JJ, Georgotas A, Newton R, Gershon S. A controlled study of trazodone, imipramine, and placebo in outpatients with endogenous depression. J Clin Psychopharmacol 1981;1(2):75–80.
6. Wheatley D. Trazodone in depression. Int Pharmacopsychiatry 1980;15(4):240–6.
7. Janowsky D, Curtis G, Zisook S, Kuhn K, Resovsky K, Le Winter M. Trazodone-aggravated ventricular arrhythmias. J Clin Psychopharmacol 1983;3(6):372–6.
8. Vlay SC, Friedling S. Trazodone exacerbation of VT. Am Heart J 1983;106(3):604.
9. Vitullo RN, Wharton JM, Allen NB, Pritchett EL. Trazodone-related exercise-induced nonsustained ventricular tachycardia. Chest 1990;98(1):247–8.
10. Aronson MD, Hafez H. A case of trazodone-induced ventricular tachycardia. J Clin Psychiatry 1986;47(7):388–9.
11. White WB, Wong SH. Rapid atrial fibrillation associated with trazodone hydrochloride. Arch Gen Psychiatry 1985;42(4):424.
12. Rausch JL, Pavlinac DM, Newman PE. Complete heart block following a single dose of trazodone. Am J Psychiatry 1984;141(11):1472–3.
13. Asayesh K. Combination of trazodone and phenothiazines: a possible additive hypotensive effect. Can J Psychiatry 1986;31(9):857–8.
14. Barrnett J, Frances A, Kocsis J, Brown R, Mann JJ. Peripheral edema associated with trazodone: a report of ten cases. J Clin Psychopharmacol 1985;5(3):161–4.
15. Chan CH, Ruskiewicz RJ. Anticholinergic side effects of trazodone combined with another pharmacologic agent. Am J Psychiatry 1990;147(4):533.
16. Montalbetti DJ, Zis AP. Cholinergic rebound following trazodone withdrawal? J Clin Psychopharmacol 1988;8(1):73.
17. Lefkowitz D, Kilgo G, Lee S. Seizures and trazodone therapy. Arch Gen Psychiatry 1985;42(5):523.

18. Tasini M. Complex partial seizures in a patient receiving trazodone. J Clin Psychiatry 1986;47(6):318–19.

19. Warren M, Bick PA. Two case reports of trazodone-induced mania. Am J Psychiatry 1984;141(9):1103–4.

20. Knobler HY, Itzchaky S, Emanuel D, Mester R, Maizel S. Trazodone-induced mania. Br J Psychiatry 1986;149:787–9.

21. Damlouji NF, Ferguson JM. Trazodone-induced delirium in bulimic patients. Am J Psychiatry 1984;141(3):434–5.

22. Sheikh KH, Nies AS. Trazodone and intrahepatic cholestasis. Ann Intern Med 1983;99(4):572.

23. Chu AG, Gunsolly BL, Summers RW, Alexander B, McChesney C, Tanna VL. Trazodone and liver toxicity. Ann Intern Med 1983;99(1):128–9.

24. Rongioletti F, Rebora A. Drug eruption from trazodone. J Am Acad Dermatol 1986;14(2 Part 1):274–5.

25. Ford HE, Jenike MA. Erythema multiforme associated with trazodone therapy: case report. J Clin Psychiatry 1985;46(7):294–5.

26. Barth JH, Baker H. Generalized pustular psoriasis precipitated by trazodone in the treatment of depression. Br J Dermatol 1986;115(5):629–30.

27. Jones SD. Ejaculatory inhibition with trazodone. J Clin Psychopharmacol 1984;4(5):279–81.

28. Goldstein I, Payton TR. Pharmacologic detumescence – the alternative to surgical shunting. J Urol 1986;135:308A.

29. Gartrell N. Increased libido in women receiving trazodone. Am J Psychiatry 1986;143(6):781–2.

30. Garvey MJ, Tollefson GD. Occurrence of myoclonus in patients treated with cyclic antidepressants. Arch Gen Psychiatry 1987;44(3):269–72.

31. Faillace LA. Antidepressant therapy: risks and alternatives. Emerg Med Spec 1983;(Suppl):20.

32. Ali CJ, Henry JA. Trazodone overdosage: experience over 5 years. Neuropsychobiology 1986;15(Suppl 1):44–5.

33. Levenson JL. Prolonged QT interval after trazodone overdose. Am J Psychiatry 1999;156(6):969–70.

34. Mazur A, Strasberg B, Kusniec J, Sclarovsky S. QT prolongation and polymorphous ventricular tachycardia associated with trasodone-amiodarone combination. Int J Cardiol 1995;52(1):27–9.

35. Romero AS, Delgado RG, Pena MF. Interaction between trazodone and carbamazepine. Ann Pharmacother 1999;33(12):1370.

36. Margolese HC, Chouinard G. Serotonin syndrome from addition of low-dose trazodone to nefazodone. Am J Psychiatry 2000;157(6):1022.

Trecovirsen

General Information

Trecovirsen is a 25-met antisense phosphorothioate oligonucleotide, which is targeted at the gag site of the HIV gene. In an early clinical experiment it was given to HIV-positive volunteers by intravenous infusion in single escalating doses of 0.1–2.5 mg/kg in groups of 6–12 subjects (1). The only significant adverse event was an isolated transitory increase in activated partial thromboplastin time at doses of 2.0 mg/kg or more; it was related to plasma trecovirsen concentrations and was attributed to the polyanionic character of the molecule. Headache occurred in 12% of subjects, and there were some cases of abdominal pain, back pain, diarrhea, and weakness.

Reference

1. Sereni D, Tubiana R, Lascoux C, Katlama C, Taulera O, Bourque A, Cohen A, Dvorchik B, Martin RR, Tournerie C, Gouyette A, Schechter PJ. Pharmacokinetics and tolerability of intravenous trecovirsen (GEM 91), an antisense phosphorothioate oligonucleotide, in HIV-positive subjects. J Clin Pharmacol 1999;39(1):47 54.

Triamterene

See also Diuretics

General Information

Triamterene is a potassium-sparing diuretic that acts in the distal convoluted tubule independently of the action of aldosterone, inhibiting sodium channels (1).

Patients with congenital nephrogenic diabetes insipidus are often treated with a combination of a thiazide and a potassium-sparing diuretic, without consensus on the preferred potassium-sparing diuretic. A Japanese adult was systematically studied to determine the renal effects of hydrochlorothiazide plus amiloride and hydrochlorothiazide plus triamterene (2). The combination with amiloride was superior to that with triamterene in preventing excessive urinary potassium loss, hypokalemia, and metabolic alkalosis. These results suggest that amiloride is the preferred add-on therapy to hydrochlorothiazide in nephrogenic diabetes insipidus.

Organs and Systems

Hematologic

Triamterene blocks dihydrofolate reductase and can cause folate deficiency with megaloblastic anemia and pancytopenia, particularly in patients with hepatic cirrhosis, who have reduced clearance of the drug (SED-11, 431). When this has been reported, all patients were taking doses of 150–600 mg/day for ascites and all had hepatic cirrhosis, often due to alcohol abuse (SEDA-17, 269). It is advisable to use spironolactone rather than triamterene in patients with cirrhosis.

Gastrointestinal

Of the milder adverse effects of triamterene, nausea, vomiting, and diarrhea are fairly common (3).

Urinary tract

Like other diuretics, triamterene occasionally causes interstitial nephritis (4), but it has also been responsible for other renal problems, notably reversible non-oliguric renal insufficiency when it is given along with indomethacin (or presumably any other inhibitor of prostaglandin synthesis) (5).

Triamterene can cause transient asymptomatic crystalluria in acidic urine (6). In most cases, the crystals are associated with brown casts, also due to triamterene.

Triamterene crystals should be regarded as a potential cause of severe tubular injury.

Triamterene can cause nephrolithiasis. Microcrystals of the parahydroxy metabolite form a particularly suitable nucleus for crystalline calcium oxalate deposition (7). However, a cause-and-effect relation has been questioned on epidemiological grounds and in the light of a controlled study that found no link (8), and triamterene could be an innocent bystander in stone formation (SEDA-11, 200). Nevertheless, triamterene is sometimes detected in urinary calculi. In a French analysis of 22 510 urinary calculi performed by infrared spectroscopy, drug-induced urolithiasis was divided into two categories: first, stones with drugs physically embedded ($n = 238$; 1.0%), notably indinavir monohydrate ($n = 126$; 53%), followed by triamterene ($n = 43$; 18%), sulfonamides ($n = 29$; 12%), and amorphous silica ($n = 24$; 10%); secondly, metabolic nephrolithiasis induced by drugs ($n = 140$; 0.6%), involving mainly calcium/vitamin D supplementation ($n = 56$; 40%) and carbonic anhydrase inhibitors ($n = 33$; 24%) (9). Drug-induced stones are responsible for about 1.6% of all calculi in France. Physical analysis and a thorough drug history are important elements in the diagnosis.

Skin

Rashes, including photodermatitis (10), sometimes occur with triamterene.

Pseudoporphyria has been attributed to co-triamterzide (hydrochlorothiazide plus triamterene, Dyazide) in a patient with vitiligo (11). It is uncertain which constituent was responsible.

Body temperature

Drug fever has been attributed to triamterene (12).

Second-Generation Effects

Pregnancy

Because of the potential risk of folate deficiency it is sensible to avoid triamterene in pregnancy (13).

Teratogenicity

Neural tube defects, characterized by a failure of the neural tube to close properly after conception, affect about one in 1000 live births in the USA. Periconceptional folic acid supplementation reduces the risk. To determine whether periconceptional exposure to folic acid antagonists might therefore increase the risk of neural tube defects, data from a case-control study of birth defects (1979–98) in the USA and Canada have been examined (14). Data on 1242 infants with neural tube defects (spina bifida, anencephaly, and encephalocele) were compared with data from a control group of 6660 infants with malformations not related to vitamin supplementation. Triamterene is a folic acid antagonist and in this series was associated with the development of neural tube defects, but there were too few cases to estimate an odds ratio.

Susceptibility Factors

Age

Triamterene is often given in combination with the thiazide diuretic bemetizide. The pharmacokinetics and the pharmacodynamics of a fixed combination of bemetizide 25 mg and triamterene 50 mg have been evaluated in 15 elderly patients (aged 70–84 years) and 10 young volunteers (aged 18–30 years) after single doses (on day 1) and multiple doses (at steady state on day 8) (15). Mean plasma concentrations of bemetizide, triamterene, and the active metabolite of triamterene, hydroxytriamterene, were significantly higher in the elderly subjects after single and multiple doses and urine flow and sodium excretion rates fell in tandem with the accumulation of these drugs. The glomerular filtration rate, known to be reduced in elderly people, was further reduced at higher concentrations of bemetizide and triamterene, which may explain why there were limited diuretic and saliuretic effects after multiple doses. This study clearly points to a modulating effect of the degree of renal function on the diuretic actions of these compounds in the elderly.

Drug–Drug Interactions

Methotrexate

An interaction between triamterene and methotrexate (also an inhibitor of dihydrofolate reductase), leading to pancytopenia, has been reported (16). Dehydration due to diuretic treatment may have contributed to renal impairment and reduced clearance of methotrexate, further increasing the risk of bone marrow suppression.

References

1. Sica DA, Gehr TW. Triamterene and the kidney. Nephron 1989;51(4):454–61.
2. Konoshita T, Kuroda M, Kawane T, Koni I, Miyamori I, Tofuku Y, Mabuchi H, Takeda R. Treatment of congenital nephrogenic diabetes insipidus with hydrochlorothiazide and amiloride in an adult patient. Horm Res 2004;61(2):63–7.
3. Bender AD, Carter CL, Hansen KB. Use of a diuretic combination of triamterene and hydrochlorothiazide in elderly patients. J Am Geriatr Soc 1967;15(2):166–73.
4. Bailey RR, Lynn KL, Drennan CJ, Turner GA. Triamterene-induced acute interstitial nephritis. Lancet 1982;1(8265):226.
5. Favre L, Glasson P, Vallotton MB. Reversible acute renal failure from combined triamterene and indomethacin: a study in healthy subjects. Ann Intern Med 1982;96(3):317–20.
6. Fogazzi GB. Crystalluria: a neglected aspect of urinary sediment analysis. Nephrol Dial Transplant 1996;11(2):379–87.
7. White DJ, Nancollas GH. Triamterene and renal stone formation. J Urol 1982;127(3):593–7.
8. Jick H, Dinan BJ, Hunter JR. Triamterene and renal stones. J Urol 1982;127(2):224–5.
9. Cohen-Solal F, Abdelmoula J, Hoarau MP, Jungers P, Lacour B, Daudon M. Les lithiases urinaires d'origine médicamenteuse. [Urinary lithiasis of medical origin.] Therapie 2001;56(6):743–50.

10. Fernandez de Corres L, Bernaola G, Fernandez E, Leanizbarrutia I, Munoz D. Photodermatitis from triamterene. Contact Dermatitis 1987;17(2):114–15.
11. Motley RJ. Pseudoporphyria due to Dyazide in a patient with vitiligo. BMJ 1990;300(6737):1468.
12. Safdi MA. Fever secondary to triamterene therapy. N Engl J Med 1980;303(12):701.
13. Corcino J, Waxman S, Herbert V. Mechanism of triamterene-induced megaloblastosis. Ann Intern Med 1970;73(3):419–24.
14. Hernandez-Diaz S, Werler MM, Walker AM, Mitchell AA. Neural tube defects in relation to use of folic acid antagonists during pregnancy. Am J Epidemiol 2001;153(10):961–8.
15. Muhlberg W, Mutschler E, Hofner A, Spahn-Langguth H, Arnold O. The influence of age on the pharmacokinetics and pharmacodynamics of bemetizide and triamterene: a single and multiple dose study. Arch Gerontol Geriatr 2001;32(3):265–73.
16. Richmond R, McRorie ER, Ogden DA, Lambert CM. Methotrexate and triamterene—a potentially fatal combination? Ann Rheum Dis 1997;56(3):209–10.

Triazolam

See also Benzodiazepines

General Information

The history of the introduction of triazolam has been reviewed (SEDA-4, v). Triazolam continues to be controversial (1) and much of the controversy has been reviewed (2–5).

Much of the literature on the adverse effects of triazolam is based on doses of 0.25 mg and above; the reduction in recommended dose to 0.125 mg may improve therapeutic safety, at the cost of compromising hypnotic efficacy in most patients. A low therapeutic index is also suggested by the possibility of amnesia, even after a single dose (6), and triazolam appears to be associated with a greater incidence of behavioral disturbances than other hypnotic benzodiazepine agonists, such as temazepam and zopiclone.

A case of recurrent iatrogenic Kleine–Levin syndrome with irritability, hyperphagia, and amnesia (7) has provided a further example of the bizarre behavior not infrequently seen with triazolam in a high dose (0.5 mg); see also the monograph on flunitrazepam. At this dose, triazolam produces too many adverse effects on sleep, memory, and judgement to be useful to the military or to commercial airline pilots; elderly patients are particularly sensitive, even to lower doses, owing in part to reduced drug clearance (SED-12, 99). Amnesia and confusion, which can occur even after single doses of triazolam, are accentuated by continued use, and frank psychopathology occurred in psychiatric patients during 2 weeks' use and during withdrawal (8).

The demonstrated ability of triazolam to impair acetylcholine release (SEDA-19, 36) suggests a mechanism for its amnestic effects, and should further caution prescribers about its use in elderly people, particularly those with pre-existing cognitive impairment. The extent to which this anticholinergic effect is shared by other benzodiazepines is yet to be established. The ability of triazolobenzodiazepines, such as triazolam and alprazolam, to inhibit the noradrenergic neurons of the locus ceruleus is unlikely to explain the prominent adverse effects of these drugs (SEDA-21, 37). For one thing, all GABA enhancers share this property; for another, a far more specific and selective inhibitor in the locus ceruleus (clonidine) has an adverse effects profile that is dramatically different from that of the benzodiazepines, whose adverse effects probably relate to their actions at a far wider range of GABA-ergic synapses.

Organs and Systems

Psychological, psychiatric

The effect of triazolam on muscarinic acetylcholine receptor binding has been investigated in living brain slices by the use of a positron-based imaging technique (9). Stimulation of GABA/benzodiazepine binding sites lowered the affinity of the muscarinic acetylcholine cholinergic receptor for its ligand, which may underlie benzodiazepine-induced amnesia, a serious clinical adverse effect of benzodiazepines.

Ten healthy men participated in a randomized, double-blind, crossover study involving placebo and triazolam 0.125 mg (10). Resting electroencephalography and event-related potentials under an oddball paradigm were recorded before drug administration, and at 1, 2, 4, 6, and 8 hours after. P300 waveforms were analysed by peak amplitudes. Triazolam can cause cognitive dysfunction without general sedation or apparent sleepiness, and this effect appeared up to 6 hours after administration of a low dose of triazolam.

The subjective and behavioral effects of triazolam were investigated in 20 healthy women, who took oral triazolam 0.25 mg or placebo at the follicular, periovulatory, and luteal phases of their menstrual cycle in a within-subject design (11). After triazolam most of them reported the expected increases in fatigue and decreases in arousal and psychomotor performance. Neither plasma concentrations of triazolam nor mood and performance differed across the three phases. This study shows that the effects of triazolam are highly stable across the menstrual cycle.

Liver

Liver damage has been attributed to triazolam (12).

- A 64-year-old woman developed anorexia, fatigue, and jaundice. She had occasionally taken triazolam 0.25 mg for insomnia, and her liver function tests had been normal 5 months before. There was no history of liver disease or alcohol misuse or other serious medical history. She was jaundiced, with spider angiomata, and gradually deteriorated over the next 16 days, finally losing consciousness. Liver histology was consistent with submassive necrosis, extensive coagulation necrosis, and marked inflammation secondary to triazolam. She had a liver transplant 31 days after the initial presentation and 2 years later was in good health.

Drug Administration

Drug overdose

Death has been attributed to an overdose of triazolam (13).

- A 77-year-old woman was found dead in her bathtub. She had a history of depression, liver disease, spinal stenosis, and diabetes mellitus. An empty bottle of triazolam was found in the bin. At autopsy there was no injury or evidence of drowning. There was triazolam 0.12 mg/l in the heart blood.

Drug–Drug Interactions

Fluconazole

Fluconazole increases blood concentrations of triazolam (14).

Grapefruit juice

In a randomized, four-phase, crossover study, the effect of grapefruit juice on the metabolism of triazolam interaction was investigated. Even one glass of grapefruit juice increased plasma triazolam concentrations, and chronic consumption produced a significantly greater increase. The half-life of triazolam is prolonged by repeated consumption of grapefruit juice, probably due to inhibition of hepatic CYP3A4 activity (15).

Isoniazid

Isoniazid is a potent hepatic enzyme inhibitor and interferes with the metabolism of many drugs (SEDA-8, 287) (SEDA-11, 271). In healthy volunteers the half-life of triazolam was prolonged from 2.5 to 3.3 hours when it was given with isoniazid, whereas isoniazid did not affect the kinetics of oxazepam (SEDA-9, 267).

Ketoconazole

Ketoconazole can increase the concentrations of triazolam through inhibition of CYP3A4 (16).

If erythromycin, also a CYP3A4 inhibitor, is given in combination with ketoconazole, there is an even more dramatic effect on triazolam concentrations.

In a double-blind, crossover kinetic and dynamic study of the interaction of ketoconazole with alprazolam and triazolam, two CYP3A4 substrate drugs with different kinetic profiles, impaired clearance by ketoconazole had more profound clinical consequences for triazolam than for alprazolam (17).

Macrolide antibiotics

Interactions of macrolides with triazolam are clinically relevant. Increases in serum concentration, AUC, and half-life, and a reduction in clearance have been documented (18–20). These changes can result in clinical effects, such as prolonged psychomotor impairment, amnesia, or loss of consciousness.

In a randomized, double-blind, pharmacokinetic–pharmacodynamic study, 12 volunteers took placebo or triazolam 0.125 mg orally, together with placebo, azithromycin, erythromycin, or clarithromycin. The apparent oral clearance of triazolam was significantly reduced by erythromycin and clarithromycin. The peak plasma concentration was correspondingly increased, and the half-life was prolonged. The effects of triazolam on dynamic measures were nearly identical when triazolam was given with placebo or azithromycin, but benzodiazepine agonist effects were enhanced by erythromycin and clarithromycin (21).

Erythromycin

Erythromycin can increase concentrations of triazolam by inhibition of CYP3A4, and dosage reductions of 50% have been proposed if concomitant therapy is unavoidable (22).

Miocamycin

CYP3A4 is mainly responsible for catalyzing the hydroxylation of miocamycin metabolites, which can alter the metabolism of concomitantly administered drugs by the formation of a metabolic intermediate complex with CYP450 or by competitive inhibition of CYP450 (23). This can cause excessive sedation with benzodiazepines such as triazolam.

Nefazodone

Nefazodone is a weak inhibitor of CYP2D6, but a potent inhibitor of CYP3A4, and increases plasma concentrations of drugs that are substrates of CYP3A4, such as triazolam (24,25).

Ritonavir

The inhibitory effect of ritonavir on the biotransformation of triazolam and zolpidem has been investigated (26). Short-term low-dose ritonavir produced a large and significant impairment of triazolam clearance and enhancement of its clinical effects. In contrast, ritonavir produced small and clinically unimportant reductions in zolpidem clearance. The findings are consistent with the complete dependence of triazolam clearance on CYP3A activity, compared with the partial dependence of zolpidem clearance on CYP3A.

References

1. O'Donovan MC, McGuffin P. Short acting benzodiazepines. BMJ 1993;306(6883):945–6.
2. Ashton H. Guidelines for the rational use of benzodiazepines. When and what to use. Drugs 1994;48(1):25–40.
3. Schneider PJ, Perry PJ. Triazolam—an "abused drug" by the lay press? DICP 1990;24(4):389–92.
4. Abraham J. Transnational industrial power, the medical profession and the regulatory state: adverse drug reactions and the crisis over the safety of Halcion in the Netherlands and the UK. Soc Sci Med 2002;55(9):1671–90.
5. Te Lintelo J, Pieters T. Halcion: de lotgevallen van de "Dutch Hysteria". Historie biedt lessen voor farmaceutische patiëntenzorg. Pharm Wkblad 2003;138(46):1600–5.
6. Bixler EO, Kales A, Manfredi RL, Vgontzas AN, Tyson KL, Kales JD. Next-day memory impairment with triazolam use. Lancet 1991;337(8745):827–31.
7. Menkes DB. Triazolam-induced nocturnal bingeing with amnesia. Aust NZ J Psychiatry 1992;26(2):320–1.
8. Soldatos CR, Sakkas PN, Bergiannaki JD, Stefanis CN. Behavioral side effects of triazolam in psychiatric inpatients: report of five cases.. Drug Intell Clin Pharm 1986;20(4):294–7.
9. Mendelson WB, Jain B. An assessment of short-acting hypnotics. Drug Saf 1995;13(4):257–70.

10. Hayakawa T, Uchiyama M, Urata J, Enomoto T, Okubo J, Okawa M. Effects of a small dose of triazolam on P300. Psychiatry Clin Neurosci 1999;53(2):185–7.

11. Rukstalis M, de Wit H. Effects of triazolam at three phases of the menstrual cycle. J Clin Psychopharmacol 1999;19(5):450–8.

12. Kanda T, Yokosuka O, Fujiwara K, Saisho H, Shiga H, Oda S, Okuda K, Sugawara Y, Makuuchi M, Hirasawa H. Fulminant hepatic failure associated with triazolam. Dig Dis Sci 2002;47(5):1111–14.

13. Levine B, Grieshaber A, Pestaner J, Moore KA, Smialek JE. Distribution of triazolam and alpha-hydroxytriazolam in a fatal intoxication case. J Anal Toxicol 2002;26(1):52–4.

14. Varhe A, Olkkola KT, Neuvonen PJ. Effect of fluconazole dose on the extent of fluconazole–triazolam interaction. Br J Clin Pharmacol 1996;42(4):465–70.

15. Lilja JJ, Kivisto KT, Backman JT, Neuvonen PJ. Effect of grapefruit juice dose on grapefruit juice–triazolam interaction: repeated consumption prolongs triazolam half-life. Eur J Clin Pharmacol 2000;56(5):411–15.

16. Bickers DR. Antifungal therapy: potential interactions with other classes of drugs. J Am Acad Dermatol 1994;31(3 Pt 2):S87–90.

17. Greenblatt DJ, Wright CE, von Moltke LL, Harmatz JS, Ehrenberg BL, Harrel LM, Corbett K, Counihan M, Tobias S, Shader RI. Ketoconazole inhibition of triazolam and alprazolam clearance: differential kinetic and dynamic consequences. Clin Pharmacol Ther 1998;64(3):237–47.

18. Warot D, Bergougnan L, Lamiable D, Berlin I, Bensimon G, Danjou P, Puech AJ. Troleandomycin–triazolam interaction in healthy volunteers: pharmacokinetic and psychometric evaluation. Eur J Clin Pharmacol 1987;32(4):389–93.

19. Phillips JP, Antal EJ, Smith RB. A pharmacokinetic drug interaction between erythromycin and triazolam. J Clin Psychopharmacol 1986;6(5):297–9.

20. Gascon MP, Dayer P, Waldvogel F. Les interactions médicamenteuses du midazolam. [Drug interactions of midazolam.] Schweiz Med Wochenschr 1989;119(50):1834–6.

21. Laux G. Aktueller stand der Behand lung mit Benzodiazepinen. [Current status of treatment with benzodiazepines.] Nervenarzt 1995;66(5):311–22.

22. Amsden GW. Macrolides versus azalides: a drug interaction update. Ann Pharmacother 1995;29(9):906–17.

23. Rubinstein E. Comparative safety of the different macrolides. Int J Antimicrob Agents 2001;18(Suppl 1):S71–6.

24. Ereshefsky L, Riesenman C, Lam YW. Serotonin selective reuptake inhibitor drug interactions and the cytochrome P450 system. J Clin Psychiatry 1996;57(Suppl 8):17–25.

25. Nemeroff CB, DeVane CL, Pollock BG. Newer antidepressants and the cytochrome P450 system. Am J Psychiatry 1996;153(3):311–20.

26. Greenblatt DJ, von Moltke LL, Harmatz JS, Durol AL, Daily JP, Graf JA, Mertzanis P, Hoffman JL, Shader RI. Differential impairment of triazolam and zolpidem clearance by ritonavir. J Acquir Immune Defic Syndr 2000;24(2):129–36.

Tribenoside

General Information

Tribenoside, ethyl-3,5,6-tri-O-benzyl-D-glucofuranoside, is used as an anti-hemorrhoidal in oral and suppository formulations.

Organs and Systems

Skin

- A 57-year-old woman developed erythema exsudativum multiforme after using tribenoside 200 mg tds orally for 10 days (1). Patch tests with tribenoside (1% and 10% in petrolatum) showed erythema on days 2 and 3. Five controls were negative.

Reference

1. Endo H, Kawada A, Yudate T, Aragane Y, Yamada H, Tezuka T. Drug eruption due to tribenoside. Contact Dermatitis 1999;41(4):223.

Tribuzone

See also Non-steroidal anti-inflammatory drugs

General Information

The usual adverse effects of NSAIDs have been observed with tribuzone, namely gastric effects, fluid retention, and headache (SED-9, 145) (1).

Reference

1. Pavelka K, Vojtisek O, Bremova A, Kaukova D, Handlova D. A new pyrazolidine derivative—Benetazone Spofa—in short- and medium-term treatment of rheumatoid arthritis. (Double-blind comparative study with phenylbutazone). Int J Clin Pharmacol Biopharm 1976;14(1):20–8.

Trichloroethylene

See also General anesthetics

General Information

Trichloroethylene is a volatile halogenated anesthetic with weak anesthetic properties compared with other halogenated anesthetics and poor muscle relaxant activity. It has been used in dry cleaning, for metal degreasing, and as a solvent for oils and resins.

Long-Term Effects

Tumorigenicity

The incidence of cancer among 803 Danish workers exposed to trichloroethylene has been evaluated (1). There was no overall increase. However, the standardized incidence ratio was significantly higher in men with non-Hodgkin's lymphoma or esophageal cancer and in women with cervical cancer.

Reference

1. Hansen J, Raaschou-Nielsen O, Christensen JM, Johansen I, McLaughlin JK, Lipworth L, Blot WJ, Olsen JH. Cancer incidence among Danish workers exposed to trichloroethylene. J Occup Environ Med 2001;43(2):133–9.

Triclabendazole

See also Benzimidazoles

General Information

Triclabendazole is a benzimidazole derivative primarily used in veterinary medicine but has also been used experimentally in man. Chills, fever, leukopenia, and upper abdominal colic have been described (SEDA-14, 263).

Several reports have suggested that triclabendazole may be of use in the treatment of *Fasciola hepatica* infection. In 20 patients with fascioliasis treated with two single doses of triclabendazole 10 mg/kg, the plasma concentrations of triclabendazole, its active metabolite triclabendazole-SO, and its sulfone metabolite were doubled by food (1). There were no serious adverse effects, except for some right-sided upper abdominal pain in several patients, which was relieved by oral spasmolytics. Triclabendazole should be administered with food.

Reference

1. Lecaillon JB, Godbillon J, Campestrini J, Naquira C, Miranda L, Pacheco R, Mull R, Poltera AA. Effect of food on the bioavailability of triclabendazole in patients with fascioliasis. Br J Clin Pharmacol 1998;45(6):601–4.

Triclocarban

See also Disinfectants and antiseptics

General Information

Triclocarban is mainly used as an antibacterial agent in soaps and antiperspirants (1).

Organs and Systems

Hematologic

Methemoglobinemia was attributed to triclocarban in seven neonates (2). There was no history of familial methemoglobinemia, but in one case the mother had been taking phenacetin before labor and this was most probably the cause. In five of the six other cases the methemoglobinemia was thought to be due to the use of disinfecting solutions or ointments containing triclocarban that had been used as a vaginal disinfectant in four cases and as a powder for the umbilicus in one case. The authors advised against the use of triclocarban in maternity units and by those dealing with neonates.

Skin

Several patients developed relatively minor dermatological problems after treatment with triclocarban (3). Three developed very extensive erosive cutaneomucosal lesions after using triclocarban for periods ranging from 20 days to 3 months.

Immunologic

There have been several cases of allergic contact dermatitis after the use of antiperspirants containing triclocarban and propylene glycol (4).

References

1. Bodey GP, Arnett J, De Salva S. Comparative trial of bacteriostatic soap preparations: Hexachlorophene versus triclosan and triclocarbon. Curr Ther Res 1978;24:542.
2. Ponte G, Richard J, Bonte C, et al. Méthémoglobinèmes chez le nouveau-né: discussion du rôle étiologique du trichlorcarbanilide. Ann Pédiatr 1974;21:359.
3. Barriere H. La dermite cutanéomuqueuse caustique du trichloro carbanilide. [Caustic cutaneo-mucosal dermatitis caused by trichlorcarbanilide.] Therapeutique 1973;49(10):685–7.
4. Osmundsen PE. Concomitant contact allergy to propantheline bromide and TCC. Contact Dermatitis 1975;1(4):251–2.

Tricyclic antidepressants

See also Individual agents

General Information

There are no accurate data on the worldwide use of the many tricyclic compounds listed in Table 1, and the availability of particular drugs varies from country to country. The dosage range for all these compounds is 50–300 mg/day, with the exception of nortriptyline, which has an upper limit of 200 mg, and protriptyline, which is more potent (range 10–60 mg/day). Well-controlled comparisons are few, but it is clear that these drugs resemble each other more than they differ. Their adverse effects will be discussed for the class as a whole, with distinguishing features of specific compounds mentioned when appropriate.

Tricyclic antidepressants interfere with the activity of at least five putative neurotransmitters by several different potential mechanisms at both central and peripheral sites. This gives rise to uncertainty in understanding the mechanisms that underlie a bewildering variety of untoward effects, which are in turn further modified by temporal factors, probably related to changes in receptor sensitivity. Differences between drugs are often inferred on the basis of selective effects on isolated organs in specific species, but their relevance to actions in man is largely unsubstantiated, owing to a lack of early clinical

Table 1 Tricyclic antidepressants that have been widely studied or are currently available for treating depression (all rINNs)

Compound	Structure	Comments
Imipramine	Dibenzapine; tertiary amine	Prototype compound
Desipramine	Secondary amine	First metabolite of imipramine
Amitriptyline	Dibenzocycloheptene; tertiary amine	Meta-analyses suggest the most effective
Nortriptyline	Secondary amine	First metabolite of amitriptyline
Protriptyline	Secondary amine	Most potent; least sedative
Doxepin	Dibenzoxepine ring	Sedative
Clomipramine	Halogenated ring	Available for intravenous use
Dimetacrine	Acridine ring	
Lofepramine	Propylamine side-chain	Relatively safe in overdose
Noxiptiline	Oxyimino side-chain	
Butriptyline	Isobutyl side-chain	More potent dopamine effects
Imipramine oxide	Oxygenated ring	Metabolite of imipramine
Amitriptyline oxide	Oxygenated ring	Metabolite of amitriptyline
Dibenzepin	Dibenzodiazepine ring	
Melitracen	Anthracene ring	
Amoxapine	Dibenzoxazepine ring; piperazine side-chain	Less potent than other tricyclics; dopamine D_2 receptor antagonist
Iprindole	6,5,8 ring structure	Weak action on amino pump mechanism
Dosulepin	Dibenzothiepine ring	
Trimipramine	Propyl side-chain	Little effect on monoamine re-uptake
Amineptine	Seven-carbon side-chain	Less sedative than other tricyclics

pharmacology studies. There is a high base rate for spontaneously occurring complaints or placebo-induced adverse effects in psychiatric populations, which complicates interpretation, even in controlled studies. There is also a wide range of interindividual sensitivity and susceptibility between patients, and very little consistent correlation between plasma concentrations and particular adverse effects.

All tricyclic compounds (with the possible exception of protriptyline) have sedative effects, and this may be desirable or undesirable, depending on a particular patient's state of apathy or agitation. They have a spectrum of anticholinergic activity, presenting as troublesome adverse effects, such as dry mouth, sweating, confusion, constipation, blurred vision, and urinary hesitancy, depending on individual patient susceptibility. Weight gain is a common and troublesome adverse effect; it is mediated in part by histamine H_1 receptor antagonism.

The adverse effects of most serious concern relate to the cardiovascular system and seizure threshold. Actions on the adrenergic and cholinergic systems probably contribute to both hypotensive and direct cardiac effects, including alterations in heart rate, quinidine-like delays in conduction, and reduced myocardial contractility. The seizure threshold is lowered, increasing the frequency of epileptic seizures. All of these adverse effects can occur at therapeutic dosages in susceptible populations, such as elderly people, children, and people with cardiac problems or epilepsy, but are also a major cause of morbidity and mortality in accidental or intentional overdosage. Doses in excess of 500 mg can be seriously toxic, and death is fairly common when doses of 2 g or more are taken.

Tricyclic antidepressants rarely cause cholestatic jaundice and agranulocytosis due to hypersensitivity reactions. The rare liver necrosis may reflect severe hypersensitivity. Two fatal cases of hypersensitivity myocarditis and hepatitis have been described (1). A variety of dermatological manifestations have been reported (rash, urticaria,

vasculitis), but their relation to drug ingestion is often uncertain. A single case of pulmonary hypersensitivity with pleural effusions and eosinophilia has been reported with desipramine (2).

Tumor-inducing effects have not been reported.

Plasma concentrations and adverse effects

Plasma concentrations of antidepressants are influenced by pharmacogenetic factors, age, and drug interactions. Several studies have attempted to define the relation between plasma concentrations of tricyclic antidepressants and their therapeutic or adverse effects. However, the results are conflicting (SEDA-3, 12) (SEDA-5, 15) (3). Sometimes there is a clear relation between cardiac toxicity and high plasma concentrations (4–6), but in some individuals cardiotoxic effects occur at presumed therapeutic concentrations. Sporadic reports of severe adverse effects, mostly of the anticholinergic type, have often been associated with high plasma concentrations of amitriptyline or nortriptyline (7,8), although these vary with each drug and from patient to patient. The risk of central nervous system toxicity in patients treated with tricyclic antidepressants may be correlated with plasma concentrations, age, and sex (SEDA-16, 8) (SEDA-17, 17). It can be concluded that routine plasma concentration monitoring is generally of little practical value in managing patients with adverse effects, but in view of the great interindividual variability in the pharmacokinetics of the tricyclic antidepressants, monitoring may be useful in those patients who report adverse effects at low doses.

Once-daily dosage

Most comparisons of once-daily with divided regimens for a variety of tricyclic compounds have shown equal efficacy and reduced adverse effects with once-daily regimens (SEDA-3, 10). However, the significance of such regimens for compliance may have been exaggerated.

Multiple drugs have a much clearer impact on compliance than do multiple dosages of a single drug. Compliance is not usually impaired until more than three tablets a day are prescribed (9). A patient who forgets to take a single dose of a once-daily regimen loses more therapeutic effect than a patient who is equally forgetful about a divided regimen. Divided regimens may also be useful for patients who benefit from short-term sedation during the daytime.

Some adverse effects are more marked with single large doses, particularly in vulnerable patients. One study showed an increased frequency of frightening dreams when tricyclic antidepressants were given in a single bedtime dose (10). Elderly patients who take large single doses at bedtime may be at risk of dizziness, ataxia, and confusion caused by postural hypotension when they attempt to get out of bed in the dark (8).

Compatibility with electroconvulsive therapy

An important practical question concerns the compatibility of tricyclic antidepressants and electroconvulsive therapy (ECT). This has been studied in 15 patients taking 150–250 mg/day of imipramine or amitriptyline who received 4–16 ECT treatments (11). Continuous monitoring of cardiac function by oscilloscopy showed dysrhythmias in 40% of the ECT sessions. There were single extra atrial beats in 46 of 151 sessions and 1–3 premature ventricular beats in 12 sessions. Transient ventricular tachycardia occurred in one 32-year-old woman taking amitriptyline 250 mg/day who received 12 ECT treatments. The authors concluded that the cardiac effects are similar to those observed in previous studies of electrocardiographic changes during ECT in patients not taking antidepressants, and expressed the opinion that combined therapy does not involve any increased risk of serious cardiac dysrhythmias. A controlled comparison of ECT given to 19 patients taking tricyclic antidepressants and 27 control patients showed no differences in heart rate, blood pressure, or ectopic heart beats (12).

Tricyclic antidepressants in the treatment of enuresis

Although pediatric psychopharmacology is much neglected, nocturnal enuresis is an area of extensive research. An earlier review catalogued almost 100 publications on the topic (13). The tricyclic antidepressants have been shown to be effective in well-controlled trials, and over 40 publications had appeared before 1970. At that time adverse effects in children appeared to be minimal and comparable to those in adults. Since then considerable concern has developed over cardiotoxic effects and the risks of accidental overdose in children. The earlier reports have been summarized (SEDA-1, 10); managing overdose in children has been reviewed (SEDA-2, 10); death in a 16-month-old infant has been reported (SEDA-3, 9).

Sudden death, possibly related to cardiac effects in children and adolescents, has been discussed (SEDA-15, 13) (SEDA-16, 9) (SEDA-18, 18); it was concluded that children taking tricyclic antidepressants require careful monitoring of the electrocardiogram, even when relatively low doses are used (SEDA-18, 18).

Symptoms of intoxication in children taking tricyclic antidepressants may fail to be recognized in time, as shown by a number of cases published in the former German Democratic Republic (14), which led to serious consideration of the abandonment of such treatment there.

The British Committee on Review of Medicines recommended that these drugs should not be used in children under 6 years of age and should be given for periods not exceeding 3 months, and then only after a full examination (including electrocardiography) and consideration of other treatment options.

Long-term adverse effects

Treatment guidelines for depression and anxiety increasingly emphasize the value of longer-term maintenance treatment with antidepressants in order to prevent recurrence of illness. It is therefore important to assess the adverse effects burden of longer-term medication. The change in adverse effects profile over 1 year of treatment has been studied in a double-blind, placebo-controlled study of maintenance treatment with imipramine (average daily dose 160 mg) in 53 patients with panic disorder (15). Adverse effects of imipramine, such as sweating, dry mouth, and increased heart rate, persisted over the year of treatment, while rates of sexual dysfunction fell. Weight gain became increasingly problematic, and by the end of the trial imipramine-treated patients had a mean increase in weight of 4.5 kg, significantly more than the placebo-treated subjects, who gained only 1.3 kg. Data of this kind are helpful when advising patients on which adverse effects may remit and which are likely to persist during longer-term treatment. These data suggest that relative to SSRIs, such as fluoxetine and sertraline, maintenance treatment with imipramine is less likely to cause sexual dysfunction but has a greater risk of weight gain.

Organs and Systems

Cardiovascular

The cardiac toxicity of tricyclic antidepressants in overdose has been a source of continued concern. Undesirable cardiovascular effects, besides representing a major therapeutic limitation for this category of drugs, delineate an area in which tricyclic compounds with novel structures, as well as second-generation antidepressants, may have significant advantages. The cardiovascular effects of tricyclic antidepressants and the new generation of antidepressants have been reviewed (SEDA-18, 16) (16).

Since the inception of SEDA in 1977, each volume has included a review of the evolving literature, focusing on specific aspects, including direct myocardial actions (SEDA-12, 13), hypotension (SEDA-12, 13), and the incidence, severity, and management of overdosage in adults and children (SEDA-10, 19) (SEDA-11, 16) (4,17–21).

Direct myocardial actions

Tricyclic antidepressants are highly concentrated in the myocardium; this may account for the vulnerability of the heart as a target organ as well as for inconsistently and inconclusively reported relations between plasma drug concentrations and specific manifestations of cardiac toxicity. These drugs interfere with the normal rate, rhythm, and contractility of the heart through actions on both nerve and muscle that are mediated by at least four different mechanisms (singly, in combination, or due to imbalance), including an anticholinergic action, interference with re-uptake of catecholamines, direct myocardial depression, and alterations in membrane permeability due to lipophilic and surfactant properties.

Acute experiments in dogs have shown a negative inotropic effect sufficient to cause congestive cardiac failure, but a carefully conducted long-term study in man did not show impaired left ventricular function in depressed patients with concurrent congestive failure (SEDA-9, 18). In another study (22) nortriptyline (mean dose 76 mg/day, mean plasma concentration 107 ng/ml) was given to 21 depressed patients with either congestive heart failure or enlarged hearts. In this study, nortriptyline was effective and well tolerated, producing only one episode of intolerable hypotension.

The most readily observable change in cardiac function is sinus tachycardia, which occurs to a greater or lesser extent in more patients and which correlates weakly or inconsistently with plasma concentrations (4,17,18). The mechanism may be related to both central and peripheral effects on cholinergic and adrenergic systems, but is not simply a reflex response to hypotension (4). The presence of tachycardia can serve as an indirect measure of compliance (4), but it is seldom a cause for concern, except in individuals who anxiously monitor their own physiological functions.

The complex changes that occur in cardiac rhythm have been intensively studied using 24-hour high-speed and high-fidelity cardiographic tracings, His bundle electrocardiography (23,24), and cardiac catheterization (25,26). Changes in conduction and repolarization cause prolongation of the PR, QRS, and QT intervals and flattening or inversion of T-waves on routine electrocardiograms; conduction delay occurs distal to the atrioventricular node and is apparent as a prolonged HV interval (the time from activation of the bundle of His to contraction of the ventricular muscle). This effect resembles that due to type I cardiac antidysrhythmic drugs, such as quinidine and procainamide. These conduction changes can cause atrioventricular or bundle branch block and can predispose to re-entrant excitation currents with ventricular extra beats, tachycardia, or fibrillation.

The implications and complications of these changes in cardiac function and rhythm are less clear; knowledge of their existence provoked concern about the incidence of sudden death in patients with cardiovascular disease, but the evidence from epidemiological sources is equivocal (19). General guidelines for the use of these drugs in the elderly have been discussed above, and a review of studies on the cardiovascular effects of therapeutic doses of tricyclic antidepressants has supported their use in elderly patients and those with pre-existing cardiovascular disease, provided precautions are taken. Atrial fibrillation has been reported in predisposed elderly subjects (SEDA-18, 19). In children taking desipramine there have been reports of sudden death (27,28) and

tachycardia, and cardiographic evidence of an intraventricular conduction defect (SEDA-18, 18) (29).

The antidysrhythmic effect of imipramine was first reported in 1977 during treatment of two depressed patients whose ventricular extra beats improved during treatment (30). Tricyclic compounds can trigger serious dysrhythmias at high doses and perhaps also when the myocardium is sensitized.

Care should be taken in patients with a recent myocardial infarction who show evidence of impaired conduction (first-degree heart block, bundle-branch block, or prolongation of the QT_c interval), since tricyclic antidepressants can theoretically add to the already increased risk of ventricular fibrillation in such patients (31). Reviews in earlier editions of Meyler's *Side Effects of Drugs* discussed these effects and gave practical guidelines on the use of tricyclic antidepressants in patients with heart disease (32).

There is sometimes a clear-cut correlation between cardiac toxicity and high plasma concentrations (SEDA-18, 18) (4–6), but this may not always be so in individuals who are highly sensitive to the drug or in whom prolonged treatment may have led to drug accumulation in the myocardium, despite plasma concentrations in the usual target range. Routine plasma concentration monitoring does not seem indicated, since plasma concentrations account for only a small part of the variance in cardiac effects (17). If an individual shows significant changes clinically or cardiographically, a spot measurement may show a high plasma concentration, requiring dosage reduction.

To date there have been no prospective studies that clearly show increased mortality in cardiac patients who use tricyclic antidepressants. It has been suggested that overall mortality due to cardiac disease may be higher in depressed patients who remain untreated than in those who receive either an antidepressant or electroconvulsive therapy (33). Even in patients who have chronic heart disease, the risks of effective treatment with a tricyclic appear to be minimal (34).

Hypotension

As many as 20% of patients taking adequate doses of a tricyclic antidepressant experience marked postural hypotension. This effect is not consistently correlated with plasma concentrations and tolerance does not develop during treatment (35–37). The mechanism for this effect is uncertain; it has been attributed to a peripheral antiadrenergic action, to a myocardial depressant effect, and to an action mediated by alpha-adrenoceptors in the central nervous system (38). Studies of left ventricular function in man are conflicting. One study of systolic time intervals showed a decrement in left ventricular function with therapeutic doses (39), while two in which cardiac function was observed directly during cardiac catheterization after overdosage showed no evidence of impaired myocardial efficiency, whereas the hypotension persisted after left ventricular filling pressures and cardiac output had returned to normal (40,41).

Postural hypotension can lead to falls. Its occurrence may be predictable, since patients who have raised systolic pressures and who have a pronounced postural drop before treatment are most likely to experience drug-induced hypotension (37). Such patients should be cautioned to rise slowly from sitting positions and, since elderly people are especially at risk of falling at night, single large bedtime doses of sedative tricyclic drugs should be avoided. These preventive measures are the most helpful, since the hypotensive effect is not directly related to plasma drug concentrations and may not improve with dosage reduction. The wisdom of using sympathomimetic drugs to counter this undesirable effect is questionable (42).

Use in patients with cardiac disease

The diagnosis of depression and the use of antidepressant medication are both associated with an increased risk of myocardial infarction. The relative contribution of these two factors is uncertain. In a case-control study of 2247 subjects, taking antidepressants was associated with a 2.2-fold (CI = 1.3, 3.7) increase in the risk of myocardial infarction (43). This increased risk seemed to be accounted for entirely by the use of tricyclic antidepressants, because selective serotonin re-uptake inhibitors were not associated with an increased risk, although the confidence intervals were wide (relative risk 0.8; CI = 0.2, 3.5). These findings support the usual clinical advice that tricyclic antidepressants are best avoided in those with known cardiovascular disease or significant risk factors.

Cardiovascular complications of overdosage

The relation between the dosage of a tricyclic antidepressant and the development of life-threatening cardiovascular complications is unclear and individually variable (44,45), although plasma concentrations above 1000 ng/ml give cause for serious concern. Plasma concentrations vary widely, and absorption can be delayed or deceptive, owing to gastric stasis and enterohepatic recycling (46). Dysrhythmias can occur for the first time up to 36 hours after drug ingestion or admission to hospital (46). The frequency of serious cardiac conditions in one series of 68 cases (47) was 46% in patients who took over 2000 mg of imipramine or its equivalent, almost twice that of those who took less (25%). An intensive study of cardiovascular complications among 35 overdose patients showed that 51% had significant hypotension and 80% had abnormal electrocardiograms (40). The latter consisted of sinus tachycardia (71%) and various abnormalities that reflect impaired conduction, including prolongation of the QT_c interval (86%), QRS complex (29%), and PR interval (11%). The ST segments and T-waves were abnormal in 28% of patients. Despite these manifestations of disturbed conduction and repolarization, there were relatively few dysrhythmias; 13 patients (37%) had ventricular extra beats, which lasted up to 72 hours after admission and subsided within 36 hours in 10 cases. No patients developed sustained repeated ventricular tachydysrhythmias, and the authors speculated that bizarre wide QRS complexes seen in aberrantly conducted supraventricular tachycardia (present in some cases) may sometimes be misinterpreted as ventricular tachycardia.

The basic principles of intensive supportive care should be applied early, and artificial ventilation is often necessary, since respiratory depression is more frequent than is commonly supposed (48,49). Patients should be monitored for 24 hours if the initial (or subsequent) electrocardiogram shows a dysrhythmia. Among 75 patients with overdose, none who had a normal electrocardiogram and level of consciousness for 24 hours went on to develop any significant dysrhythmia (50). However, a case was subsequently reported of a patient who died an acute cardiac death 57 hours after admission and 33 hours after normalization of the electrocardiogram (51). The authors suggested that prolonged monitoring may be justified in individuals who have taken antidepressants for prolonged periods, compared with those who overdose early in treatment.

More specific treatment to combat cardiotoxic effects is usually necessary in only a minority of instances; in the series reported above (40), five patients (14%) had marked hypotension. Initial low left ventricular filling pressures were corrected within 3 hours by infusion of isotonic saline. Systemic hypotension persisted and was corrected by infusion of sympathomimetic amines. Routine insertion of a pulmonary artery catheter, with continuous monitoring of blood gases, pulmonary arterial pressure, left atrial wedge pressure, and cardiac output have been recommended (40). Volume expansion is suggested for low left atrial pressure, with dopamine infusion to improve myocardial contractility if cardiac output remains low.

The management of ventricular extra beats is based on recognition of the quinidine-like basis of the conduction defect. In the series reported above (40) all 13 patients with ventricular arrhythmias responded to intravenous infusion of lidocaine (mean dose 2.0 mg/minute). This alone might account for the absence of deaths in this series.

Another indirect method of benefiting the patient with cardiotoxic effects has been the alkalinization of plasma to a pH of 7.50–7.55 using sodium bicarbonate infusion (52). This enhances plasma protein binding, making the drug less available to the tissues. It is claimed that this technique reverses both hypotension and cardiac dysrhythmias without the risk of the undesirable effects of antidysrhythmic drugs (46). Recommendations for the management of poisoning with tricyclic antidepressants given in a recent review have been summarized (SEDA-16, 8).

Differences among tricyclic compounds

There is evidence that doxepin is significantly less cardiotoxic than other tricyclic compounds (53). However, a complete review of all the animal and clinical data has suggested that doxepin overdose can still cause lethal dysrhythmias in man, probably by producing more marked respiratory depression.

Three different studies have shown that there is less risk of hypotension in patients treated with nortriptyline (54–56) than with other tricyclic compounds. However, a similar claim has been made for doxepin (57).

Increased pulse rate and blood pressure have been associated with desipramine in the treatment of bulimia nervosa (SEDA-17, 18).

Respiratory

There has been one case report of reduced ventilatory response to hypercapnia after nortriptyline in a woman with chronic obstructive pulmonary disease (SEDA-18, 19).

Nervous system

Miscellaneous symptoms that have been attributed to the tricyclic antidepressants include fatigue, weakness, dizziness, headache, and tremor; patients are likely to fall because of these disturbances.

Seizures are serious adverse events associated with the use of antidepressants, and the relative frequencies for different antidepressants have for a long time been a matter of controversy. The literature has been critically evaluated, taking into account predisposing factors, drug doses, plasma drug concentrations, and the duration of treatment (58). A significant proportion of seizures occurred in predisposed individuals, and the risk of seizure for most antidepressants increased with dose or blood concentration. After overdose the risk was higher for amoxapine and the tetracyclic drug maprotiline than for other antidepressants, but for several drugs there are not enough data to estimate the risk. Imipramine was the most frequently studied tricyclic, with a seizure risk of 0.3–0.6% at effective doses. For several of the second-generation antidepressants, a lower seizure risk has been reported in large clinical trials. Caution with all antidepressants should certainly be exercised in people who are predisposed to seizure activity because of brain damage or alcohol or drug abuse.

Concurrent use of lithium may be a risk factor for neurological adverse effects.

- A 34-year-old woman took amitriptyline 300 mg each night for several years. Six days after starting lithium 300 mg tds she had several generalized tonic-clonic seizures. A second episode occurred on re-exposure to lithium (59).

Patients with phobias or panic disorders are extremely sensitive to the adverse effects of tricyclic drugs early in treatment. They often have a syndrome of fine tremor, insomnia, and anxiety, which can be characterized as "jitteriness" and which is sometimes attributed to adrenergic hypersensitivity (SEDA-13, 9). Serum iron concentrations were significantly lower in jittery patients than in those who were not affected (SEDA-17, 19) (60). The authors suggested that this may be related to the role of iron as a co-factor for tyrosine hydroxylase.

Because tricyclic antidepressants suppress REM sleep, they have been used in the management of narcolepsy and cataplexy when amphetamines fail or abuse potential is high. Clomipramine is the most effective, possibly because it has more pronounced actions on serotonergic mechanisms (61).

Three reports have referred to a type of difficulty in articulation described as "speech blockage" or "dysarthria" (62–64). The disturbance was described as a delay in thinking and speech, in which the patient has difficulty in conceptualizing or transferring the next logical thought into words. The effect resembles stammering.

There have been sporadic reports of bilateral foot-drop with peroneal nerve involvement (65). A major neuropathy, with high stepping gait and inability to dorsiflex the foot, occurred in an 84-year-old woman; this presumed adverse effect remitted 8 weeks after withdrawal (66).

Unusual neurological reactions have been observed in some patients, generally when combinations of drugs (often including maprotiline) have been used (67). The symptoms were ataxia, akathisia, hypokinetic disorders of speech and motion, a dream-like state, and transiently impaired memory.

Confusion was observed in 13% of 150 patients taking tricyclic drugs, and in as many as 35% of patients over 40 years of age. All responded rapidly to drug withdrawal (SEDA-9, 26).

Aggressiveness during treatment in patients taking imipramine and amitriptyline in relatively low doses has been described (68). Violent behavior has also been attributed to amitriptyline (SEDA-17, 18).

Anticholinergic actions

Several organs are the target for the anticholinergic (antimuscarinic) activity of the tricyclic antidepressants. They constitute the most common and troublesome adverse effects of the tricyclic antidepressants, but the peripheral anticholinergic actions can also be put to therapeutic use in conditions such as irritable bowel syndrome, premature ejaculation, and nocturnal enuresis.

Experiments on receptor binding in rat brain and guinea-pig ileum have shown a spectrum of activity at muscarinic acetylcholine receptors for different tricyclic antidepressants (69). A comparison of five compounds showed that amitriptyline and doxepin were the most and desipramine the least potent, imipramine and nortriptyline being intermediate. Single-dose experiments in volunteers (given up to 100 mg of each drug) have confirmed the same rank order for both the peripheral anticholinergic actions (on salivary flow) and the central effects (sedation and other measures on a mood scale) (70). The significance of these differences between relatively low single doses of these drugs in healthy volunteers should not be uncritically extrapolated to clinical practice. However, they do provide a rationale for selecting among the different drugs for patients in whom either a high degree of sedation is desirable or anticholinergic effects are likely to be troublesome. No tricyclic is entirely free of anticholinergic action, and individual differences in susceptibility or metabolism can still cause serious problems in some patients. It is also difficult to predict which particular organ will become the major target for anticholinergic activity; some patients complain bitterly of a dry mouth, others report blurred vision, and some develop bowel or bladder symptoms. Careful history taking and physical examination will often reveal a possible cause for concern, based on the patient's previous response to similar drugs, existing disease (such as narrow-angle glaucoma, enlarged prostate, constipation), or advancing age.

Older people are supposedly susceptible to delirium caused by centrally acting anticholinergic drugs. This can take the form of anxiety, agitation, or frank hypomania. Such difficulties are more likely if the patient is also taking antipsychotic drugs (many of which also have anticholinergic effects) or anticholinergic antiparkinsonian drugs. Although such effects have long been recognized as a risk associated with the anticholinergic properties of these drugs, it has been suggested that their incidence may be lower than is often assumed (71). In an epidemiological study from a West German multicenter drug surveillance system in almost 14 000 patients for 5 years, exposure-related incidence rates were 1.2% for tricyclic antidepressants compared with 0.8% for both tranylcypromine and neuroleptic drugs (72). The risk increased steadily with age in both sexes and all diagnostic subgroups, and was six-fold higher (3.4%) in those over 60 years. Also at greater risk were women and patients with affective psychosis.

Adverse anticholinergic effects can occur immediately after the first dose of a tricyclic antidepressant. They are a major cause of poor compliance in patients who expect immediate relief, but who are not properly prepared for the delay that can occur in the beneficial effects of these drugs on mood and energy.

Sensory systems
Loss of accommodation and blurred vision are common inconveniences that can usually be tolerated in the knowledge that they lessen with the duration of treatment. Exacerbation of narrow-angle glaucoma in the elderly can occur, but is not an absolute contraindication to treatment with a tricyclic antidepressant, since the anticholinergic effects can be balanced by judicious use of pilocarpine (73,74).

Damage can occur to the corneal epithelium, due to reduced lacrimation and relative accumulation of mucoid secretions in patients who wear contact lenses (75).

Mouth and teeth
Rampant dental caries due to xerostomia occurred in a patient who took doxepin up to 300 mg/day for over 2 years (76). The author warned of the need to counsel patients to carry out rigorous and regular dental hygiene, as well as simple measures to promote increased salivation, such as sugarless lemon drops or chewing gum. In another study there was an increase in the number of decayed teeth in 35 children treated with amitriptyline or nortriptyline for enuresis, compared with a smaller group of untreated children with enuresis and a larger matched population control group (77).

Gastrointestinal
Simple dietary advice about bulk foods can mitigate minor bowel disturbances. More serious complications that can arise include paralytic ileus, which can be life-threatening, especially in the elderly (78). A less well-known adverse effect is the potential for aggravating or even possibly inducing a hiatus hernia, presumably due to an anticholinergic effect on the cardiac sphincter (79).

Urinary tract
The tricyclic antidepressants increase bladder sphincter tone and the volume of fluid necessary to trigger detrusor contraction (80). Such effects may account for their efficacy in nocturnal enuresis, in which the benefit occurs early and at a low dosage, consistent with anticholinergic activity. However, this pharmacological action can cause hesitancy and urinary retention, especially in predisposed men who have prostatic hyperplasia.

Renal damage from tricyclic antidepressants has been suggested on only one occasion.

- A 65-year-old man taking imipramine 300 mg/day developed toxic psychosis, anorexia, and nausea after 24 days. He was mildly azotemic, but these changes quickly reverted after withdrawal. No biopsy or renal function tests were reported.

The findings are entirely compatible with prerenal azotemia associated with diminished fluid intake during a drug-induced psychosis (81).

Neuroleptic malignant syndrome
The neuroleptic malignant syndrome, which is classically associated with antipsychotic drugs and is usually attributed to excessive dopamine D2 receptor blockade, can rarely occur with other medications, including tricyclic antidepressants.

- A 62-year-old man was found unresponsive in his apartment. He had a past history of bipolar disorder, for which he was taking nortriptyline and sodium valproate (dosages not stated). On admission to hospital his rectal temperature was 107.1 °F and he had increased muscle tone. He was intubated and cooled with ice packs. His creatine kinase activity was raised (1046 IU/l) but valproate and nortriptyline concentrations were within the target ranges. Extensive investigations, including biochemical screens and brain scans, showed no clear cause for his condition. Shortly afterwards he developed disseminated intravenous coagulation and died.

The authors concluded that the features of the illness were consistent with nortriptyline-induced neuroleptic malignant syndrome (82). However, a contributory role for sodium valproate was also possible.

The neuroleptic malignant syndrome has also been reported in association with the antidepressants trimipramine (SEDA-21, 11) (83), desipramine (SEDA-17, 18), and amoxapine (SEDA-16, 9) (SEDA-17, 18) (84). Amoxapine in particular has significant dopamine D2 receptor antagonistic properties. In most cases the patients were taking several other drugs, but there have been reports of the syndrome in association with amoxapine or desipramine alone.

Serotonin syndrome
The serotonin syndrome is usually associated with the use of combinations of drugs that potentiate brain serotonin function. This syndrome has been associated with several tricyclic antidepressants when used in combination with monoamine oxidase (MAO) inhibitors (85). Rarely it can be associated with the use of a single agent, such as clomipramine, a tricyclic antidepressant with potent serotonin re-uptake inhibitor properties (86).

- A 60-year-old woman, with a history of hypertension, type 2 diabetes mellitus, and depression, took clomipramine 200 mg/day for 8 months and then 250 mg/day for 3 months. Her other medications were glibenclamide 7.5 mg/day, lisinopril 5 mg/day, and clonazepam 0.5 mg/day. Without any change in medications or other precipitants, she began to feel confused and weak. She became pyrexial (41.6°C), confused, and tremulous, with myoclonic jerking. The combined plasma concentrations of clomipramine and desmethylclomipramine were 2230 nmol/l, somewhat over the usual target range (below 1900 nmol/l). Within hours her condition deteriorated, with seizures, ventricular tachycardia, and disseminated intravascular coagulation. Rhabdomyolysis led to acute renal insufficiency, which required dialysis. She remained severely ill over the next 4 weeks and eventually died of opportunistic Gram-negative infections.

This case illustrates that the serotonin syndrome can occasionally occur apparently spontaneously in patients taking a single serotonergic drug. The authors were unable to find any reason why the syndrome developed so catastrophically when it did, except for the modestly increased concentrations of clomipramine and its metabolite.

Extrapyramidal symptoms

Tricyclic antidepressants are often listed among the many drugs that can produce buccofaciolingual or choreoathetoid movements (87). A putative mechanism is a central anticholinergic action, which upsets the balance between the dopaminergic and cholinergic systems. The spontaneous occurrence of this syndrome makes it difficult to establish a cause-and-effect relation, although both patients described in the above report had symptoms again when rechallenged.

There is a more clear-cut cause-and-effect relation in the parkinsonian symptoms that occasionally occur with high-dosage tricyclic therapy in susceptible individuals (particularly elderly women). Because of its piperazine side-chain and structural resemblance to the phenothiazines, amoxapine has antidopaminergic properties that appear to produce typical dystonic reactions (88), but other tricyclic antidepressants may also be implicated in producing the full range of so-called extrapyramidal syndromes, including akathisia, dystonic reactions, parkinsonism, and tardive dyskinesia. Case reports have been described before (SEDA-16, 9) (SEDA-17, 18) (SEDA-18, 18). In the reports of tardive dyskinesia the problem is often that these patients have taken many different drugs.

Sensory systems

Eyes

Loss of accommodation and blurred vision are common inconveniences that can usually be tolerated, in the knowledge that they lessen with the duration of treatment. Exacerbation of narrow-angle glaucoma in the elderly can occur, but is not an absolute contraindication to treatment with a tricyclic antidepressant, since the anticholinergic effects can be balanced by judicious use of pilocarpine (73,74).

Treatment with bright light is used for mood disorders, and it has been suggested that antidepressants, which may act as photosensitizers, could enhance the effect of bright light on the eye, giving rise to adverse effects (SEDA-18, 17).

Ears

Tinnitus can occur after prolonged treatment with tricyclic antidepressants. In an early trial of imipramine (89)

there were two cases of transient deafness, but in the subsequent 20 years no auditory effects have been recorded. In 1980, a report appeared (90) concerning four patients, all taking imipramine in dosages below 150 mg/day. Each complained of buzzing or ringing in the ears. In each case the symptoms improved or disappeared on dosage reduction, with maintenance of therapeutic benefit, and in one case the patient was switched to an equivalent dosage of desipramine without recurrence. A further report concerned a patient taking protriptyline 45 mg/day who developed ringing in both ears after 12 days (91). Symptom severity fell with dosage reduction and disappeared entirely after desipramine 100 mg/day was substituted. The authors postulated that non-vibratory tinnitus had originated from either neurological factors or changes in blood flow. In a chart review of 475 patients treated with tricyclic antidepressants there were five patients with tinnitus. Each developed the symptom in the second or third week of treatment at dosages of imipramine of 150–250 mg/day, with plasma concentrations of 200–400 ng/ml (92). In every case tinnitus subsided spontaneously within a further 2–4 weeks after onset, even though dosage and plasma concentrations remained constant.

Another unusual disturbance of hearing has been reported in a child taking tricyclic antidepressants (93). Auditory acuity was normal, but discriminative ability for both clear and distorted speech was depressed. The disorder cleared within some days of withdrawal.

Psychological, psychiatric

Cognitive impairment has been associated with nortriptyline in elderly subjects (SEDA-17, 19).

Musical hallucinations have been reported in association with clomipramine (SEDA-17, 18).

Mania

It is widely believed that there is a significant risk that tricyclic antidepressants can precipitate mania or rapid cycling in up to 10% of patients, and that various factors increase this possibility, including being female or younger, having an earlier onset of illness, and having a positive first-degree family history (SED-11, 40). Biochemical risk factors have been alleged to include patients with a low urinary excretion of the noradrenaline metabolite methoxyhydroxyphenol glycol (MHPG); the risk is possibly greater in patients taking tricyclic antidepressants rather than MAO inhibitors, and particularly in the case of clomipramine. The data on which these conclusions were based have now been rigorously analysed (94) in a review of the controversy surrounding the alternative suggestion that the so-called switch effect is a random manifestation of bipolar illness. There is a paucity of both prospective and long-term placebo-controlled studies, and existing research has suffered from unrepresentative samples and poor definition of manic outcomes. The reviewers concluded that "...some bipolar patients and few, if any, unipolar patients become manic when they are treated with antidepressants. A small number of patients develop rapid cycling."

This more cautious conclusion is supported by the results of a prospective study of 230 carefully selected patients with recurrent depression (at least two episodes, with an average of six) who took imipramine (200 mg/day) for an average of over 46 weeks (95). Mania and hypomania were defined and measured by the Raskin rating scale. Only six patients (2.6%) developed hypomania, and four of these did so after withdrawal. Younger patients, women, and those with a previous history of hypomania (bipolar II) were no more likely to switch than unipolar patients.

These results suggest that the risk of mania or hypomania in the long-term treatment of recurrent unipolar depressed patients is relatively small. The 12 placebo-controlled studies of acute treatment in less carefully defined samples support higher incidence rates (around 6–7% for hypomania and 1–2% for mania), but these figures may be inflated owing to the inclusion of bipolar patients with a high risk of a spontaneous switch (94).

Metabolism

Weight gain has long been recognized as a concomitant of antidepressant and antipsychotic drug therapy. This may in part reflect improvement in mental state, but there also appears to be a physiological component, with an increased craving for sweets (96). No abnormalities have been found in fasting glucose and insulin concentrations or in intravenous insulin tolerance tests (96,97). Another possible suggestion for weight gain is that taste perception in depression improves after therapy with tricyclic antidepressants (98). A study of 50 depressed patients attempted to address some of these issues (99). Increased energy efficiency during antidepressant treatment has also been suggested as a reason for weight gain (SEDA-17, 8). A warning to patients with diabetes that hypoglycemia can be masked seems appropriate (100).

Endocrine

The "Division of Drug Experience" of the US Department of Health and Welfare issued a note on five cases of the syndrome of inappropriate antidiuretic hormone secretion and drugs to which it has been attributed (101). All involved drugs with a tricyclic structure; one patient was taking imipramine, three carbamazepine, and the others the closely related muscle relaxant cyclobenzaprine. The dosage of imipramine was 50 mg/day for 3 weeks and the patient was a 72-year-old woman. Other cases have been reported, involving amitriptyline (101), imipramine, and protriptyline (SEDA-17, 17).

Tricyclic antidepressants, presumably through blocking the re-uptake of noradrenaline, can cause a crisis in a patient with a pheochromocytoma (SEDA-21, 11) (102).

Prolactin concentrations are very rarely altered during treatment with tricyclic antidepressants, but this is more likely to occur and to produce galactorrhea or amenorrhea with clomipramine and amoxapine and when there are other contributory factors that may stimulate prolactin secretion, such as stress or electroconvulsive therapy (103).

Hematologic

Occasional cases of blood dyscrasias with tricyclic antidepressants continue to be reported (SEDA-12, 46) (SEDA-18, 18) (SEDA-21, 10). Antidepressant-induced blood dyscrasias have recently been reviewed (104).

Agranulocytosis has been associated with tricyclic antidepressants (105). Of 20 cases, eight were fatal and 12 recovered after 3–20 days.

Two cases of non-thrombocytopenic purpura occurred in patients taking tricyclic antidepressants. Both improved on withdrawal (106). True thrombocytopenia, with platelets counts as low as 120×10^{12}/l, occurred in a 79-year-old woman taking doxepin. During later treatment with amitriptyline, thrombocytopenia recurred, but not when she took imipramine (107). Cross-sensitivity must be highly specific to chemical structure, doxepin and amitriptyline being more like each other than imipramine.

Liver

Cholestasis was among the first adverse effects reported with phenothiazines, tricyclic antidepressants, and MAO inhibitors. Its incidence appears to have fallen, for reasons that are not understood, but under-reporting may be a factor. Increases in liver enzymes, especially transaminases and alkaline phosphatase, are quite common during treatment with both phenothiazines and tricyclic antidepressants. Such effects are usually benign, but one careful study of a patient taking amitriptyline showed biopsy findings of mononuclear and eosinophilic infiltration; cholestasis and jaundice were absent (108). In a controlled comparison of lofepramine and fluoxetine, there were significant increases in alkaline phosphatase, alanine aminotransferase, and gammaglutamyl transferase in patients taking lofepramine but not fluoxetine (109).

More serious and sometimes fatal liver necrosis has been reported with a number of different tricyclic structures and probably represents an extreme form of hypersensitivity (110,111). Liver necrosis in a 33-year-old woman who took imipramine 300 mg/day for over 1 month led the authors to suggest that once-daily dosage may pose a special hazard, because peak concentrations can exceed the toxic concentration, even though steady-state plasma concentrations are in the usual target range (112). A particular hazard appears to be posed by amineptine (qv).

There is no indication for routine liver function tests in patients taking tricyclic antidepressants; raised transaminases and alkaline phosphatase within the limits of the reference ranges are not a cause for serious concern, unless they are accompanied by clinical signs or symptoms indicative of liver dysfunction.

Skin

Skin rashes are so common that it is difficult to determine a cause-and-effect relation. A choice must be made between waiting to see if the rash clears despite continued treatment or switching to a different compound and, if necessary, rechallenging at a later date. Serious reported skin reactions include cutaneous vasculitis, urticaria, and photosensitivity. A grey discoloration of the skin in light-exposed areas has been associated with long-term therapy with imipramine and desipramine (SEDA-17, 19) (SEDA-18, 18). Pigmentary changes in the iris were also reported in one of the cases. Amineptine has been reported (113) to cause a particularly active acne, occurring beyond the usual distribution on the body and beyond the usual age, especially in women. The remedy recommended is withdrawal of amineptine. A single case of a rosacea-like eruption on the face of a 76-year-old woman was also caused by this drug, and the association was confirmed by re-challenge (114).

Hyperpigmentation is a recognized adverse effect of the antipsychotic drug chlorpromazine. Four cases of hyperpigmentation have been described in patients taking the structurally related tricyclic antidepressant imipramine (115). All were women and had taken imipramine for at least 2 years. The hyperpigmentation occurred in a photodistribution on the face, arms, and the backs of the hands. In two patients who discontinued imipramine the hyperpigmentation resolved within 1 year. The authors speculated that the pigmentation might have been due to deposition of melanin in an unusual form, possibly in a complex with a metabolite of imipramine.

Sexual function

A review of sexual dysfunction due to antidepressant drugs in men, citing both published findings and reports provided by the manufacturers, drew a distinction between erectile dysfunction, ejaculatory problems, and changes in libido (116). A complicating factor is the lack of information concerning the base rate of these problems in depression itself. Erectile impotence has been reported with all of the commonly used tricyclic compounds in low normal dosages. Delayed and occasionally painful ejaculation occurs, and four cases of painful ejaculation in association with imipramine and clomipramine have been reported (SEDA-17, 18). Priapism can occur (116). Both increased and decreased libido have been reported, but it is virtually impossible to distinguish drug relatedness from the natural history of the condition. A small number of uncontrolled studies have shown therapeutic benefits in patients with premature ejaculation or disturbed sexual function accompanied by depression (117).

Delayed orgasm or loss of ability to obtain orgasm has been reported in women taking desipramine (118).

The sexual dysfunction is probably due to 5-HT re-uptake blockade, because similar effects are seen in patients taking SSRIs.

Long-Term Effects

Drug withdrawal

There is compelling evidence for a withdrawal syndrome due to abrupt discontinuation of tricyclic antidepressants (SEDA-5, 16), and the literature has been reviewed (119). Reports have involved both imipramine and doxepin (120). Symptoms occur as early as the morning after a missed dose (121), but more often after 48 hours and up to 2 weeks after withdrawal. They include anxiety, restlessness, sweating, diarrhea, hot or cold flushes, and piloerection. Amitriptyline withdrawal was followed by similar physical symptoms 36 hours after the last dose, followed by severe depressive illness (SEDA-17, 18).

Delirium after withdrawal of doxepin has been reported (122), as well as instances of mania (123). Pronounced neurological symptoms have been described after sudden withdrawal of amitriptyline (SEDA-18, 18).

The existence of a withdrawal syndrome was subjected to a controlled test (120) in seven patients who had been taking long-term amitriptyline up to 250 mg/day, imipramine 200 mg/day, or desipramine 250 mg/day. After 4 weeks placebo was substituted double-blind for 10–21 days. Both plasma and urine MHPG concentrations increased by an average of 74% above baseline, starting within 36 hours and reaching a peak 3 weeks after withdrawal. Despite these pronounced neurochemical changes there were no alterations in pulse rate or heart beat, and only two patients had definitely worse anxiety.

There is clearly a need for larger controlled studies to determine the incidence and severity of withdrawal effects after withdrawal of tricyclic antidepressants. Based on uncontrolled observations, it has been suggested that the incidence varies from under a quarter to over half of all patients.

A report of three cases (124) has suggested that central cholinergic overactivity is implicated, and that atropine sulfate 3 mg/day or synthetic anticholinergic agents (such as benzatropine mesylate 4 mg/day) ameliorate withdrawal symptoms within a few hours. The authors suggested that this technique may be especially useful in patients in whom tricyclic antidepressants must be abruptly withdrawn because of allergic or idiosyncratic reactions.

Second-Generation Effects

Teratogenicity

In chick embryos there was a high prevalence of abnormalities, including microphthalmia, micromelia, and reduced body size, after the administration of imipramine, but the dosages of imipramine were close to lethal (125).

The issue of dysmorphogenesis due to these drugs was first seriously discussed after a report on three possible cases from Australia in 1972 (126). Although the data underlying this report were later discredited, it led to a careful study of the case records of women who had taken tricyclic antidepressants in pregnancy, and more than 300 cases were rapidly identified in which such treatment had been followed by the birth of a normal infant. Other negative reports exonerating the drugs have appeared since (127–130), although sporadic case reports continue to appear (131).

In spite of these reports, which negate a possible association between tricyclic antidepressants and teratogenicity, it may be advisable to avoid these drugs during pregnancy, especially in the early stages, unless there is a compelling need. In many of the reports the drugs were given in low doses or for indications not justifying their use.

Fetotoxicity

Instances of distress in the newborn have been reported after treatment of their mothers with tricyclic antidepressants in the period before delivery (132). In one case, a neonate had signs of congestive heart failure without cardiac abnormality; another had tachycardia and myoclonus; a third had respiratory distress and neuromuscular spasms. These effects were thought to have resulted from both the adrenergic and anticholinergic effects of the tricyclic antidepressants, which readily pass the placenta and should be avoided during the perinatal period.

Infants born to mothers taking tricyclic antidepressants can become jittery in the first few days of life (133).

- A healthy boy (weight 3370 g) was born to a mother who had taken clomipramine 100 mg/day throughout pregnancy. On the second day after delivery, the child was jittery and on the fifth day he developed myoclonic jerking of his arms and legs. There was no epileptic activity on a 10-channel electroencephalogram, and clonazepam and phenobarbital did not suppress the movements. However, the movements were suppressed by a single dose of intravenous clomipramine 0.5 mg. The myoclonus recurred only occasionally over the next 4 days. Examination at one month later was normal, apart from mild jitteriness in response to touch.

Maternal clomipramine use is associated with seizures in neonates but this case appears to have been caused by a withdrawal state that was relieved by clomipramine administration.

Another report has suggested that effects in the neonate may be due to withdrawal from maternal antidepressants after birth (134). Two cases of neonatal convulsions have been reported in infants whose mothers had been treated with clomipramine. In both cases the seizures occurred on the first day of life coincident with a fall in plasma clomipramine concentrations. In one case the convulsions were controlled by administration of clomipramine followed by tapered withdrawal.

Hypotonia has been described in four children, one of whom also developed jitteriness (SEDA-17, 18).

Lactation

There are few reports on the excretion of antidepressant drugs in breast milk, even though postpartum depression is relatively common. In a 32-year-old woman who took imipramine 200 mg/day from 1 month postpartum imipramine and desipramine were detectable in breast milk (135). There have also been reports that amitriptyline (136), desipramine (137), and nortriptyline (138,139) were detectable in the milk of nursing mothers and in the plasma of the mothers and infants. Neither parent compound nor metabolite were detected in infants' serum, except for two infants who had low concentrations of 10-hydroxynortriptyline. There were no adverse effects in any of the infants. The use of antidepressants during lactation has been reviewed, including 15 studies in which serum concentrations of antidepressants were obtained from nursing infants (140).

There has been a report of an 8-week-old breast-fed infant whose mother was taking doxepin (141). Four days after an increase in the daily dosage from 10 to 75 mg the infant developed respiratory depression; desmethyldoxepin was detected in the baby's plasma.

Susceptibility Factors

Age

Elderly people

Elderly people have high rates of depression but tend to be excluded from randomized trials of antidepressant treatment. In general, older people metabolize tricyclic antidepressants more slowly and have higher steady-state plasma concentrations. There is an increased risk of adverse effects of tricyclic antidepressants in elderly patients (SEDA-18, 17). Elderly people often take other drugs that can cause depression or interact with its treatment (142). These potential sources of variation are superimposed on the wide range of plasma concentrations reported among individuals, and on the differences between drugs in dose–response profiles. The dictates of safe practice are that treatment in elderly people be begun with low dosages (50 mg/day of imipramine or equivalent) in divided amounts, with dosage increases in small increments (50 mg/day of imipramine each week) and a reduced total dose range (75–150 mg/day, except in exceptional circumstances) (143). Close attention should be paid to the potential anticholinergic, neurological, or cardiovascular complications to which elderly people are especially vulnerable (31).

The adverse effects profile of fixed-dose clomipramine (150 mg/day) has been assessed in 112 hospitalized depressed patients (aged 22–70 years), of whom 38 were over 55 years of age (144). The only adverse effect that distinguished patients over 55 years was orthostatic hypotension: older subjects had a significantly greater fall in systolic blood pressure on standing. Orthostatic hypotension can lead to falls and injuries, particularly in patients being treated at home, and this suggests that blood pressure should be monitored in older patients who are taking psychiatric doses of tricyclic antidepressants. It is also worth noting that the upper age limit of patients in this study was only 70 years, so it is unclear how more elderly patients would fare with this rather substantial dose of clomipramine.

Drug Administration

Drug overdose

Both accidental and intentional overdose are relatively frequent and pose difficult management problems. Particular concern has been expressed for children, either because they gain access to parents' tablets or have been treated for enuresis. During one year a Melbourne hospital admitted 35 children poisoned with tricyclic antidepressants (145). In 1979 it was reported that tricyclic antidepressants had replaced salicylates as the most common cause of accidental death in English children under the age of five. Concern was expressed about this (146), and Swiss federal statistics raised similar worries (147).

The majority of all deaths from antidepressant poisoning in Scotland, England, and Wales, during 1975–1984 and 1985–1989 were due to two tricyclic drugs, amitriptyline and dosulepin, and they, as well as the entire group of older tricyclic antidepressants, had a fatality index (deaths per million prescriptions) significantly higher than the mean (148).

A nation-wide analysis of suicide mortality in Finland showed that between 1990 and 1995 the overall suicide mortality fell significantly from 30 per 100 000–27 (149). However, the use of antidepressants in completed suicide showed an upward trend, while the use of more violent methods (gassing, hanging) fell. During this time prescription of moclobemide and two SSRIs (citalopram and fluoxetine) increased, while that of tricyclics (mainly doxepin and amitriptyline) remained steady. The mean annual fatal toxicity index was highest for tricyclics, such as doxepin, trimipramine, and amitripyline, and lowest for SSRIs.

Educational policies and commercial marketing of antidepressant drugs have led to an increase in the detection and treatment of depression. Conceivably this may be associated with the fall in suicide rates noted in Finland. However, overdosage of tricyclic antidepressants continues to contribute to deaths from suicide. Whether completely replacing tricyclics with less toxic compounds would lower overall suicide rate remains controversial.

The results of a British survey of all deaths due to acute poisoning due to antidepressants are shown in Table 2 (150).

A major problem in evaluating the incidence and severity of complications due to overdosage in adults has been the reporting of individual cases or selected samples, often with the inclusion of patients who have taken

several drugs or who have concurrent physical disease. More reliable epidemiological surveys from different countries (45,151,152) have suggested that the mean ingested overdose of a tricyclic antidepressant in adults is around 1000 mg, and that only about 3% of patients take enough to cause fatal complications. There is considerable individual variability in response to overdosage, and there are conflicting reports concerning the degree of correlation between plasma concentrations and complications. One large study showed that plasma concentrations in excess of 1000 ng/ml were associated with coma, convulsions, cardiac dysrhythmias, and a need for supportive measures (21). In other studies there was no clear-cut correlation between plasma concentration and the incidence of toxic complications (153). Cardiac complications have been reviewed above and are serious, but should not deflect attention from other serious effects. A review of all deaths due to these drugs in Britain during 1976 showed that dysrhythmias were less common than supposed (11 of 113 patients who died in hospitals), but that respiratory depression was more frequent (54 of 113

Table 2 Deaths per million prescriptions for antidepressants in the UK

Drug	No. of prescriptions	Total deaths	Deaths per million prescriptions (95% CI)
Tricyclic antidepressants and related drugs	74 598 000	2598	35 (34, 36)
Desipramine	45 000	9	201 (92, 382)
Amoxapine	107 000	10	94 (45, 172)
Dosulepin	26 210 000	1398	53 (51, 56)
Amitriptyline	23 844 000	906	38 (36, 41)
Imipramine	3 354 000	110	33 (27, 40)
Doxepin	1 587 000	40	25 (18, 34)
Trimipramine	2 370 000	39	17 (12, 23)
Clomipramine	4 315 000	54	13 (9.4, 16)
Nortriptyline	1 269 000	7	5.5 (2.2, 11)
Maprotiline	201 000	1	5.0 (0.1, 28)
Trazodone	2 753 000	11	4.0 (2.0, 7.1)
Mianserin	922 000	3	3.3 (0.7, 9.5)
Mirtazapine	324 000	1	3.1 (0.1, 17)
Lofepramine	7 189 000	9	1.3 (0.6, 2.4)
Butriptyline	1000	0	0 (0, 3372)
Iprindole	3000	0	0 (0, 1218)
Viloxazine	10 000	0	0 (0, 357)
Protriptyline	94 000	0	0 (0, 39)
Serotonin re-uptake inhibitors	47 329 000	77	1.6 (1.3, 2.0)
Venlafaxine	2 570 000	34	13 (9.2, 19)
Fluvoxamine	660 000	2	3.0 (0.3, 11)
Citalopram	2 603 000	5	1.9 (0.6, 4.5)
Sertraline	5 964 000	7	1.2 (0.5, 2.4)
Fluoxetine	19 926 000	18	0.9 (0.5, 1.4)
Paroxetine	15 031 000	11	0.7 (0.4, 1.3)
Nefazodone	576 000	0	0 (0, 6.4)
Monoamine oxidase inhibitors	1 203 000	24	20 (13, 30)
Tranylcypromine	367 000	16	44 (25, 71)
Phenelzine	404 000	6	15 (5.5, 32)
Moclobemide	365 000	2	5.5 (0.6, 20)
Iproniazid	200	0	0 (0, 18 444)
Isocarboxazid	68 000	0	0 (0, 55)
Other antidepressants	2 523 000	1	0.4 (0, 2.2)
Flupentixol	28 000	0	0 (0, 2.4)
Tryptophan	28 000	0	0 (0, 133)
Reboxetine	175 000	0	0 (0, 21)
Lithium	5 106 000	37	7.2 (5.1, 10)

Numbers may not add up to the total because of rounding.

patients) (48). Some such deaths might have been avoided by more frequent artificial ventilation and better attention to the principles of supportive care.

Management of overdose

The literature on poisoning with tricyclic antidepressants has been reviewed and recommendations for the management of overdose proposed (SEDA-16, 8) (154). In overdose, physostigmine can reverse life-threatening dysrhythmias, but its effect is short-lasting and it has adverse effects of its own; it should be avoided (154).

Drug–Drug Interactions

General

The large number of drugs with which tricyclic antidepressants interact are summarized in Table 3; those of major concern are discussed in more detail below.

Table 3 Interactions of tricyclic antidepressants with other substances

Interacting substance(s)	Type of interaction(s)	Comments
Alcohol	Additive sedative effects	May be more pronounced with more sedative tricyclic compounds
Anticholinergic drugs	Additive effects on pupils, nervous system, bowel, and bladder	Particularly likely to occur when a tricyclic drug, a phenothiazine, and a antiparkinsonian drug are prescribed concurrently
Anticoagulants	Increased serum concentrations of oral anticoagulant	Tricyclic drugs can interfere with the metabolism of oral anticoagulants
Antiepileptic drugs	Antagonism	Convulsive threshold lowered
	Decreased plasma concentrations of some tricyclic drugs	Hepatic microsomal enzyme induction
Antihypertensive agents	Reversal of hypotensive effects of clonidine, reserpine, α-methyldopa, and guanethidine	Hypertension should be controlled with diuretics, β-blockers, or vasodilators before treatment of depression
Barbiturates	Reduced plasma concentrations of tricyclic drugs	Hepatic microsomal enzyme induction
Calcium channel blockers	Increased plasma concentrations of imipramine and possibly other drugs	
Cigarette smoking	Decreased plasma concentrations of tricyclic drugs	Probably increased metabolism
Cimetidine	Increased systemic availability of tricyclic drugs	Probably due to impaired hepatic extraction
Disulfiram	Increased plasma concentrations of tricyclic drugs	Probably inhibition of metabolism
Diuretics	Increased risk of postural hypotension	Pharmacodynamic interaction
Halofantrine	Increased risk of ventricular dysrhythmias	Prolonged QT interval
Levodopa	Impaired gastrointestinal absorption	May apply to other drugs metabolized in the gut
Monoamine oxidase inhibitors	Increased incidence of weight gain	See text; see also monograph on Monoamine oxidase inhibitors
	Increased anticholinergic effects	
	Hyperthermia, hyper-reflexia, convulsions, death (very rare)	
Membrane-stabilizing drugs (quinidine type)	Synergism	
Methylphenidate	Increased plasma concentrations of tricyclic drugs	Probably inhibition of metabolism
Morphine	Potentiation of analgesic effect of morphine	May be partly due to increased systemic availability of morphine
Nitrates	Reduced effect of sublingual nitrates	Owing to dry mouth
Phenothiazines	Increased plasma concentrations of tricyclic drugs	Due to inhibition of metabolism
	Possible potentiation and/or increased speed of onset of antidepressant effect	
	Enhanced cardiotoxic effects with thioridazine	Presynaptic α₂-adrenoceptor blockade (animal studies)
		Ventricular dysrhythmias can occur
Rifampicin	Decreased plasma concentrations of some tricyclic drugs	Hepatic microsomal enzyme induction
Ritonavir	Possibly increased plasma concentrations of tricyclic drugs	Inhibition of metabolism
SSRIs	Increased plasma concentrations of tricyclic drugs	Inhibition of metabolism
Corticosteroids	Altered systemic availability of tricyclic drugs	Inhibition of metabolism
	Akathisia	Receptor interaction
	Exacerbation of psychosis	
Sympathomimetic agents	Potentiation of hypertensive effects with phenylephrine, noradrenaline, methylphenidate	
	Potentiation of effects of pheochromocytoma	
Thyroid hormones	Can manifest as spurious hyperthyroidism, cardiac dysrhythmias, or, in some cases, enhanced therapeutic actions of tricyclics	Increased receptor sensitivity to catecholamines

Alcohol

Alcohol in combination with tricyclic antidepressants impairs performance, and it is customary to caution patients about the risk of impairment in their ability to drive or handle machinery. Not only can additive impairment occur (mediated at the receptor level), but alcohol can also alter the metabolism of the antidepressant (SEDA-8, 24).

Amines

Tricyclic antidepressants act on both presynaptic and postsynaptic neurons, as well as on alpha- and beta-adrenoceptors. Because their principal action is to block the re-uptake of noradrenaline at the presynaptic neuron, they potentiate the hypertensive effects of both directly acting and indirectly acting amines (155,156). The hypertensive effects of phenylephrine are increased by a factor of 2–3, and of noradrenaline by a factor of 4–8. Even the administration of local anesthetics containing noradrenaline as a vasoconstrictor has proven fatal. The types of compound that can produce this interaction and the symptoms that result have been previously reviewed in detail (SEDA-1, 11).

Anesthetics

In 190 patients taking tricyclic antidepressants that could not be discontinued before surgery, who underwent general and 61 local or regional anesthesia, there were no changes in the cardiovascular effect of halothane, induction time with pentobarbital, propanidid, or ketamine, or the duration of depolarization or recovery time (157). The general conclusion was that it is safer to continue treatment with tricyclic antidepressants than to risk potential disruption from withdrawal before surgery.

Anticoagulants

Tricyclic antidepressants can interfere with the metabolism of oral anticoagulants, increase their serum concentrations, and prolong their half-lives by as much as 300% (SEDA-21, 10) (158). Prothrombin activity should be carefully monitored in patients taking oral anticoagulants.

Antidysrhythmic drugs

Because of their similar lipophilic and surfactant properties, tricyclic antidepressants interact with antidysrhythmic drugs of the quinidine type, interfering with the voltage-dependent stimulus and producing dose-related synergy (159). Cardiac glycosides and beta-blockers are free of this interaction, although animal studies have suggested increased lethality of digoxin in rats pretreated with tricyclic antidepressants (160), while propranolol may potentiate direct depression of myocardial contractility due to tricyclic antidepressants. For all of these reasons, the preferred treatment for tricyclic-induced dysrhythmias is lidocaine, but even this is reported to be only variably effective and possibly to potentiate the hypotensive effects of tricyclic drugs (46).

Antipsychotic drugs

Tricyclic antidepressants lower the seizure threshold and should therefore be used with caution with other agents that can also lower seizure threshold, such as antipsychotic drugs (161).

- A 34-year-old man with schizophrenia responded well to olanzapine 20 mg/day. However, he then had obsessional hand washing and was given clomipramine, which was increased to a dosage of 250 mg/day. He then reported myoclonic jerks with some dizziness, and 10 days later had a generalized tonic-clonic seizure. The combined clomipramine + desmethylclomipramine concentration was 2212 nmol/l, higher than the upper end of the usual target range (1300 nmol/l). An electroencephalogram showed paroxysmal slowing and spike-and-wave activity. Both olanzapine and clomipramine were withdrawn. Later the clomipramine was restarted as monotherapy and a dose of 300 mg/day was reached, which led to an even higher clomipramine + desmethylclomipramine concentration (3234 nmol/l), but there was no clinical or electroencephalographic evidence of seizure activity. However, when olanzapine was added in a dosage of 15 mg/day, myoclonic jerking and abnormal electroencephalographic activity recurred within 7 days.

The seizures occurred in the presence of high concentrations of clomipramine in this case, suggesting a pharmacodynamic drug interaction, since neither agent given alone provoked seizure activity, whereas the combination did. It is, however, possible that clomipramine might have caused a rise in olanzapine blood concentrations, which were not measured.

Benzodiazepines

Four patients developed adverse effects attributable to combinations of benzodiazepines with tricyclic antidepressants, including exacerbations of delusional thought disorders (162).

Corticosteroids

Patients taking prednisone have experienced psychosis, perhaps due to an interaction at dopamine receptor sites (163,164).

Fluconazole

Fluconazole can increase plasma concentrations of amitriptyline, presumably by inhibiting cytochrome P450 isozymes (CYP3A4 and CYP2C19), preventing its demethylation. Two patients taking amitriptyline and fluconazole developed syncope and in one concomitant electrocardiographic monitoring showed a prolonged QT interval and torsade de pointes (165,166). In neither case were serum amitriptyline concentrations measured, but the symptoms were consistent with tricyclic antidepressant toxicity. These case reports suggest that this combination should be used with caution and probably with monitoring of amitriptyline concentrations.

Levodopa

The anticholinergic effects of imipramine and other tricyclic antidepressants can delay gastrointestinal motility enough to interfere with the absorption of various other drugs. Such was the case in an experimental study of the absorption of levodopa in four healthy subjects (167). It is likely that this effect may interfere with absorption of other drugs, especially those, such as chlorpromazine, that are extensively metabolized in the gut.

Methylphenidate

The interaction with methylphenidate may be of particular significance, because of claims that tricyclic antidepressants and methylphenidate have a synergistic effect on mood, owing to interference by methylphenidate with the metabolism of imipramine, resulting in increased blood imipramine concentrations (168). The occurrence of this hypertensive interaction calls for caution in the use of such combinations, for which there is no established evidence.

Monoamine oxidase inhibitors

The interactions of tricyclic antidepressants with MAO inhibitors are so dangerous that they constitute a formidable barrier to their combined clinical use. The temptation to treat refractory patients with this combination is great, but considerable care should be taken (169,170), and it should be remembered that there is no firm proof of the superiority of such combinations. Several reviewers (171–173) have concluded that the dangers of these interactions have been overstated and the potential therapeutic advantages underestimated. On the other hand, reports of serious and fatal complications continue to appear (174,175). Specialists have advised that the combination of an MAO inhibitor with trimipramine or amitriptyline is usually safe, but that imipramine and clomipramine must be avoided.

Phenothiazines

Two Scandinavian patients taking combinations of neuroleptic drugs and tricyclic antidepressants developed epileptic seizures (176). The risk of seizures is greater in patients with brain damage or epilepsy and with high dosages, sudden increases in dosage, or shortly after the introduction of a second compound.

The possible mechanism for these interactions with phenothiazines is raised plasma concentrations of the tricyclic compounds due to competition for the hepatic cytochrome P450 that metabolizes both types of compound (SEDA-9, 30) (177). Antidepressant plasma concentrations may increase by up to 70% (178).

Postganglionic blockers

Tricyclic antidepressants reverse the hypotensive effects of postganglionic blocking agents, guanethidine, reserpine, clonidine, and alpha-methyldopa, and the addition of a tricyclic can result in loss of blood pressure control (159,179). Sudden withdrawal of a tricyclic compound from a patient stabilized with these compounds can also result in serious hypotension. An additional reason for avoiding drugs such as reserpine, methyldopa, and propranolol in depressed cardiovascular patients is that these drugs can also cause or aggravate depression.

Psychotropic drugs

The evidence for interactions with other commonly prescribed psychotropic drugs has been reviewed extensively (SEDA-8, 25).

Salicylates

Tricyclic antidepressants are highly bound to plasma proteins. Theoretically, other drugs that are highly protein bound could displace tricyclic antidepressants from protein binding sites; this would be expected to lead to increased plasma concentrations of unbound antidepressant and a greater likelihood of adverse effects. In practice, however, important interactions of this kind are unusual, probably because these drugs have high apparent volumes of distribution, and the amount of drug that can be displaced from plasma proteins is very small compared with tissue concentrations. Salicylates are highly protein bound, and the effect of adding acetylsalicylic acid 1 g/day for 2 days on the plasma availability of imipramine (150 mg/day) has been studied in 20 depressed patients (180). Acetylsalicylic acid reduced the protein binding of imipramine and while the total plasma concentration of imipramine was not altered, the unbound concentration rose almost four-fold. The number of characteristic adverse effects of imipramine also increased significantly. However, this study was not blind and the results must be in doubt, since it is unlikely that brain concentrations of the drug changed significantly.

Sex hormones

Oral contraceptives have a complex effect on the metabolism of tricyclic drugs, resulting in reduced systemic availability (181). Conjugated estrogens also cause akathisia in some patients taking tricyclic drugs, perhaps due to an interaction at dopamine receptor sites (182).

Sodium valproate

Sodium valproate can increase serum tricyclic drug concentrations (SEDA-21, 22).

- In a 46-year-old woman, in whom valproate 1 g/day was added to clomipramine 150 mg/day, there was a substantial increase in serum clomipramine concentrations (from 185 ng/ml to 447 ng/ml); she had feelings of numbness and sleep disturbance, which disappeared when the dose of clomipramine was reduced (183).

The increase in tricyclic concentrations following valproate is probably partly due to inhibition of CYP2C isozymes, preventing demethylation of tertiary tricyclic antidepressants to the corresponding secondary amines (desmethylimipramine in the case of clomipramine). However, valproate can also increase the plasma concentrations of secondary amine tricyclics, such as nortriptyline (183). The current data suggest that the combined use of tricyclic antidepressants and valproate should be undertaken with caution.

SSRIs

Fluoxetine can increase blood concentrations of desipramine and nortriptyline (184–187).

St John's wort

St John's wort can cause drug interactions by inducing hepatic microsomal drug-metabolizing enzymes or the drug transporter P-glycoprotein, which causes a net efflux of substrates, such as amitriptyline, from intestinal epithelial cells into the gut lumen (SEDA-24, 12). In 12 patients (9 women, 3 men) the addition of St John's wort 900 mg/day to amitriptyline 150 mg/day led to a 20% reduction in plasma amitriptyline concentrations, while nortriptyline concentrations were almost halved (188).

Thioridazine

The interaction of thioridazine with a tricyclic antidepressant is particularly dangerous, since both cause cardiac toxicity. One report concerned two young patients who developed ventricular dysrhythmias, from which they recovered (189).

Thyroid hormone

Spurious hyperthyroidism occurred in a child taking thyroid hormone and imipramine for enuresis (190). The ability of thyroid hormone to increase receptor sensitivity to catecholamines has long been known, and has been used to enhance the clinical response in some refractory patients, especially women.

Yohimbine

Yohimbine can cause hypertension in patients taking tricyclic antidepressants. A drug history should include the use of herbal remedies before conventional treatments are prescribed.

References

1. Morrow PL, Hardin NJ, Bonadies J. Hypersensitivity myocarditis and hepatitis associated with imipramine and its metabolite, desipramine. J Forensic Sci 1989;34(4):1016–20.
2. Carlson DH, Healy J. Pulmonary hypersensitivity to imipramine. South Med J 1982;75(4):514.
3. Anonymous. Tricyclic antidepressants—blood level measurements and clinical outcome: an APA Task Force report. Task Force on the Use of Laboratory Tests in Psychiatry. Am J Psychiatry 1985;142(2):155–62.
4. Ziegler VE, Co BT, Biggs JT. Plasma nortriptyline levels and ECG findings. Am J Psychiatry 1977;134(4):441–3.
5. Kantor SJ, Glassman AH, Bigger JT Jr, Perel JM, Giardina EV. The cardiac effects of therapeutic plasma concentrations of imipramine. Am J Psychiatry 1978;135(5):534–8.
6. Kantor SJ, Bigger JT Jr, Glassman AH, Macken DL, Perel JM. Imipramine-induced heart block. A longitudinal case study. JAMA 1975;231(13):1364–6.
7. Preskorn SH, Biggs JT. Use of tricyclic antidepressant blood levels. N Engl J Med 1978;298(3):166.
8. Carr AC, Hobson RP. High serum concentrations of antidepressants in elderly patients. BMJ 1977; 2(6095):1151.
9. Blackwell B. The drug regimen and treatment compliance. In: Haynes RB, Taylor DW, Sacket DL, editors. Compliance in Health Care. Baltimore: Johns Hopkins University Press, 1979:144.
10. Flemenbaum A. Pavor nocturnus: a complication of single daily tricyclic or neuroleptic dosage. Am J Psychiatry 1976;133(5):570–2.
11. Hoppe E, Kramp P, Sandoe E, Bolwig TG. Elektrokonvulsiv behandling og tricykliske antidepressiva: risiko for udvikling af hjertearitmi. [Electroconvulsive therapy and tricyclic antidepressants: risk of development of cardiac arrythmia.] Ugeskr Laeger 1977;139(44):2636–8
12. Azar I, Lear E. Cardiovascular effects of electroconvulsive therapy in patients taking tricyclic antidepressants. Anesth Analg 1984;63(12):1140.
13. Blackwell B, Currah J. The psychopharmacology of nocturnal enuresis. In: Kolvin IL, MacKeith RC, Meadow SR, editors. Bladder Control and Enuresis. London: William Heinemann Medical Books, 1973:231.
14. Ratzman GW, Seer OR. Zur Symptomatologie toxischer Nebenwirkungen bei der Therapie der Enuresis im Kindesalter mit Imipramin (Pryleugan). [On the symptomatology of toxic adverse effects of imipramine (Pryleugan) in the treatment of enuresis in children.] Dtsch Gesundheitswes 1978;33:XII
15. Mavissakalian M, Perel J, Guo S. Specific side effects of long-term imipramine management of panic disorder. J Clin Psychopharmacol 2002;22(2):155–61.
16. Glassman AH, Preud'homme XA. Review of the cardiovascular effects of heterocyclic antidepressants. J Clin Psychiatry 1993;54(Suppl):16–22.
17. Veith RC, Friedel RO, Bloom V, Bielski R. Electrocardiogram changes and plasma desipramine levels during treatment of depression. Clin Pharmacol Ther 1980;27(6):796–802.
18. Spiker DG, Weiss AN, Chang SS, Ruwitch JF Jr, Biggs JT. Tricyclic antidepressant overdose: clinical presentation and plasma levels. Clin Pharmacol Ther 1975;18(5 Part 1):539–46.
19. Burrows GD, Vohra J, Hunt D, Sloman JG, Scoggins BA, Davies B. Cardiac effects of different tricyclic antidepressant drugs. Br J Psychiatry 1976;129:335–41.
20. Hallstrom C, Gifford L. Antidepressant blood levels in acute overdose. Postgrad Med J 1976;52(613):687–8.
21. Petit JM, Spiker DG, Ruwitch JF, Ziegler VE, Weiss AN, Biggs JT. Tricyclic antidepressant plasma levels and adverse effects after overdose. Clin Pharmacol Ther 1977;21(1):47–51.
22. Roose SP, Glassman AH, Giardina EG, Johnson LL, Walsh BT, Woodring S, Bigger JT Jr. Nortriptyline in depressed patients with left ventricular impairment. JAMA 1986;256(23):3253–7.
23. Bigger JT, Kantor SJ, Glassman AH, et al. Cardiovascular effects of tricyclic antidepressant drugs. In: Lipton MA, Dimascio A, Killam KF, editors. Psychopharmacology: a Generation of Progress. New York: Raven Press, 1978:1033.
24. Burrows GD, Vohra J, Dumovic P, et al. Tricyclic antidepressant drugs and cardiac conduction. Prog Neuropsychopharmacol 1977;1:329.
25. Brorson L, Wennerblom B. Electrophysiological methods in assessing cardiac effects of the tricyclic antidepressant imipramine. Acta Med Scand 1978;203(5):429–32.
26. Scherlag BJ, Lau SH, Helfant RH, Berkowitz WD, Stein E, Damato AN. Catheter technique for recording His bundle activity in man. Circulation 1969;39(1):13–18.
27. Anonymous. Sudden death in children treated with a tricyclic antidepressant. Med Lett Drugs Ther 1990;32(819):53.

28. Riddle MA, Nelson JC, Kleinman CS, Rasmusson A, Leckman JF, King RA, Cohen DJ. Sudden death in children receiving Norpramin: a review of three reported cases and commentary. J Am Acad Child Adolesc Psychiatry 1991;30(1):104–8.

29. Biederman J, Baldessarini RJ, Wright V, Knee D, Harmatz JS, Goldblatt A. A double-blind placebo controlled study of desipramine in the treatment ADD. II. Serum drug levels and cardiovascular findings. J Am Acad Child Adolesc Psychiatry 1989;28(6):903–11.

30. Bigger JT, Giardina EG, Perel JM, Kantor SJ, Glassman AH. Cardiac antiarrhythmic effect of imipramine hydrochloride. N Engl J Med 1977;296(4):206–8.

31. Wasylenki D. Depression in the elderly. Can Med Assoc J 1980;122(5):525–32.

32. Todd RD, Faber R. Ventricular arrhythmias induced by doxepin and amitriptyline: case report. J Clin Psychiatry 1983;44(11):423–5.

33. Avery D, Winokur G. Mortality in depressed patients treated with electroconvulsive therapy and antidepressants. Arch Gen Psychiatry 1976;33(9):1029–37.

34. Veith RC, Raskind MA, Caldwell JH, Barnes RF, Gumbrecht G, Ritchie JL. Cardiovascular effects of tricyclic antidepressants in depressed patients with chronic heart disease. N Engl J Med 1982;306(16):954–9.

35. Ziegler VE, Taylor JR, Wetzel RD, Biggs JT. Nortriptyline plasma levels and subjective side effects. Br J Psychiatry 1978;132:55.

36. Reisby N, Gram LF, Bech P, Nagy A, Petersen GO, Ortmann J, Ibsen I, Dencker SJ, Jacobsen O, Krautwald O, Sondergaard I, Christiansen J. Imipramine: clinical effects and pharmacokinetic variability. Psychopharmacology (Berl) 1977;54(3):263–72.

37. Glassman AH, Bigger JT Jr, Giardina EV, Kantor SJ, Perel JM, Davies M. Clinical characteristics of imipramine-induced orthostatic hypotension. Lancet 1979;1(8114):468–72.

38. van Zwieten PA. The central action of antihypertensive drugs, mediated via central alpha-receptors. J Pharm Pharmacol 1973;25(2):89–95.

39. Taylor DJ, Braithwaite RA. Cardiac effects of tricyclic antidepressant medication. A preliminary study of nortriptyline. Br Heart J 1978;40(9):1005–9.

40. Langou RA, Van Dyke C, Tahan SR, Cohen LS. Cardiovascular manifestations of tricyclic antidepressant overdose. Am Heart J 1980;100(4):458–64.

41. Thorstrand C. Cardiovascular effects of poisoning with tricyclic antidepressants. Acta Med Scand 1974;195(6):505–14.

42. Sternon J, Owieczka J. La prophylaxie de l'hypotension orthostatique induite par les antidepresseurs tricycliques. [The prophylaxis of orthostatic hypotension caused by tricyclic antidepressants.] Ars Med (Brux) 1979;34:641

43. Cohen HW, Gibson G, Alderman MH. Excess risk of myocardial infarction in patients treated with antidepressant medications: association with use of tricyclic agents. Am J Med 2000;108(1):2–8.

44. Siddiqui JH, Vakassi MM, Ghani MF. Cardiac effects of amitriptyline overdose. Curr Ther Res Clin Exp 1977;22:321.

45. O'Brien JP. A study of low-dose amitriptyline overdoses. Am J Psychiatry 1977;134(1):66–8.

46. Hoffman JR, McElroy CR. Bicarbonate therapy for dysrhythmia hypotension in tricyclic antidepressant overdose. West J Med 1981;134(1):60–4.

47. Serafimovski N, Thorball N, Asmussen I, Lunding M. Tricyclic antidepressive poisoning with special reference to cardiac complications. Acta Anaesthesiol Scand Suppl 1975;57:55–63.

48. Crome P, Newman B. Fatal tricyclic antidepressant poisoning. J R Soc Med 1979;72(9):649–53.

49. Nogue Xarau S, Nadal Trias P, Bertran Georges A, Mas Ordeig A, Munne Mas P, Milla Santos J. Intoxicacion agoda grave por antidepresivos triciclcos. Estudio retrospective de is casos. [Severe acute poisoning following the ingestion of tricyclic antidepressants.] Med Clin (Barc) 1980;74(7):257–62.

50. Goldberg RJ, Capone RJ, Hunt JD. Cardiac complications following tricyclic antidepressant overdose. Issues for monitoring policy. JAMA 1985;254(13):1772–5.

51. McAlpine SB, Calabro JJ, Robinson MD, Burkle FM Jr. Late death in tricyclic antidepressant overdose revisited. Ann Emerg Med 1986;15(11):1349–52.

52. Brown TC, Barker GA, Dunlop ME, Loughnan PM. The use of sodium bicarbonate in the treatment of tricyclic antidepressant-induced arrhythmias. Anaesth Intensive Care 1973;1(3):203–10.

53. Pinder RM, Brogden RN, Speight TM, Avery GS. Doxepin up-to-date: a review of its pharmacological properties and therapeutic efficacy with particular reference to depression. Drugs 1977;13(3):161–218.

54. Reed K, Smith RC, Schoolar JC, Hu R, Leelavathi DE, Mann E, Lippman L. Cardiovascular effects of nortriptyline in geriatric patients. Am J Psychiatry 1980;137(8):986 9.

55. Roose SP, Glassman AH, Siris SG, Walsh BT, Bruno RL, Wright LB. Comparison of imipramine- and nortriptyline-induced orthostatic hypotension: a meaningful difference. J Clin Psychopharmacol 1981;1(5):316–19.

56. Thayssen P, Bjerre M, Kragh-Sorensen P, Moller M, Petersen OL, Kristensen CB, Gram LF. Cardiovascular effect of imipramine and nortriptyline in elderly patients. Psychopharmacology (Berl) 1981;74(4):360–4.

57. Neshkes RE, Gerner R, Jarvik LF, Mintz J, Joseph J, Linde S, Aldrich J, Conolly ME, Rosen R, Hill M. Orthostatic effect of imipramine and doxepin in depressed geriatric outpatients. J Clin Psychopharmacol 1985;5(2):102–6.

58. Rosenstein DL, Nelson JC, Jacobs SC. Seizures associated with antidepressants: a review. J Clin Psychiatry 1993;54(8):289–99.

59. Solomon JG. Seizures during lithium-amitriptyline therapy. Postgrad Med 1979;66(3):145–6.

60. Yeragani VK, Pohl R, Balon R, Kulkarni A, Keshavan M. Low serum iron levels and tricyclic antidepressant-induced jitteriness. J Clin Psychopharmacol 1989;9(6):447–8.

61. Bental E, Lavie P, Sharf B. Severe hypermotility during sleep in treatment of cataplexy with clomipramine. Isr J Med Sci 1979;15(7):607–9.

62. Schatzberg AF, Cole JO, Blumer DP. Speech blockage: a tricyclic side effect. Am J Psychiatry 1978;135(5):600–1.

63. Quader SE. Dysarthria: an unusual side effect of tricyclic antidepressants. BMJ 1977;2(6079):97.

64. Saunders M. Dysarthria: an unusual side effect of tricyclic antidepressants. BMJ 1977;2:317.

65. Casarino JP. Neuropathy associated with amitriptyline. Bilateral footdrop. NY State J Med 1977;77(13):2124–6.

66. Yeragani VK, Meiri P, Balon R, Pohl R, Golec S. Effect of imipramine treatment on changes in heart rate and blood pressure during postural and isometric handgrip tests. Eur J Clin Pharmacol 1990;38(2):139–44.

67. Davies RK, Tucker GJ, Harrow M, Detre TP. Confusional episodes and antidepressant medication. Am J Psychiatry 1971;128(1):95–9.

68. Rampling D. Aggression: a paradoxical response to tricyclic antidepressants. Am J Psychiatry 1978;135(1):117–18.

69. Snyder SH, Yamamura HI. Antidepressants and the muscarinic acetylcholine receptor. Arch Gen Psychiatry 1977;34(2):236–9.

70. Blackwell B, Peterson GR, Kuzma RJ, Hostetler RM, Adolphe AB. The effect of five tricyclic antidepressants on salivary flow and mood in healthy volunteers. Commun Psychopharmacol 1980;4(4):255–61.

71. Meyers BS, Mei-Tal V. Psychiatric reactions during tricyclic treatment of the elderly reconsidered. J Clin Psychopharmacol 1983;3(1):2–6.

72. Schmidt LG, Grohmann R, Strauss A, Spiess-Kiefer C, Lindmeier D, Muller-Oerlinghausen B. Epidemiology of toxic delirium due to psychotropic drugs in psychiatric hospitals. Compr Psychiatry 1987;28(3):242–9.

73. Nouri A, Cuendet JF. Atteintes oculaires au cours des traitements aux thymoleptiques. [Ocular disturbances during treatment with thymoleptics.] Schweiz Med Wochenschr 1971;101(32):1178–80.

74. Reid WH, Blouin P, Schermer M. A review of psychotropic medications and the glaucomas. Int Pharmacopsychiatry 1976;11(3):163–74.

75. Litovitz GL. Amitriptyline and contact lenses. J Clin Psychiatry 1984;45(4):188.

76. Slome BA. Rampant caries: a side effect of tricyclic antidepressant therapy. Gen Dent 1984;32(6):494–6.

77. von Knorring AL, Wahlin YB. Tricyclic antidepressants and dental caries in children. Neuropsychobiology 1986;15(3–4):143–5.

78. Clarke IM. Adynamic ileus and amitriptyline. BMJ 1971;2(760):531.

79. Tyber MA. The relationship between hiatus hernia and tricyclic antidepressants: a report of five cases. Am J Psychiatry 1975;132(6):652–3.

80. Appel P, Eckel K, Harrer G. Veränderungen des Blasen- und Blasensphinktertonus durch Thymoleptika. [Changes in tonus of the bladder and its sphincter under thymoleptic treatment. Cystomanometric measurements in man.] Int Pharmacopsychiatry 1971;6(1):15–22.

81. Sathananthan G, Gershon S. Renal damage due to imipramine. Lancet 1973;1(7807):833–4.

82. June R, Yunus M, Gossman W. Neuroleptic malignant syndrome associated with nortriptyline. Am J Emerg Med 1999;17(7):736–7.

83. Langlow JR, Alarcon RD. Trimipramine–induced neuroleptic malignant syndrome after transient psychogenic polydipsia in one patient. J Clin Psychiatry 1989;50(4):144–5.

84. Washington C, Haines KA, Tam CW. Amoxapine-induced neuroleptic malignant syndrome. DICP 1989;23(9):713.

85. Sporer KA. The serotonin syndrome. Implicated drugs, pathophysiology and management. Drug Saf 1995;13(2):94–104.

86. Rosebush PI, Margetts P, Mazurek MF. Serotonin syndrome as a result of clomipramine monotherapy. J Clin Psychopharmacol 1999;19(3):285–7.

87. Fann WE, Sullivan JL, Richman BW. Dyskinesias associated with tricyclic antidepressants. Br J Psychiatry 1976;128:490–3.

88. Steele TE. Adverse reactions suggesting amoxapine-induced dopamine blockade. Am J Psychiatry 1982;139(11):1500–1.

89. Barker PA, Ashcroft GW, Binns JK. Imipramine in chronic depression. J Ment Sci 1960;106:1447–51.

90. Racy J, Ward-Racy EA. Tinnitus in imipramine therapy. Am J Psychiatry 1980;137(7):854–5.

91. Evans DL, Golden RN. Protriptyline and tinnitus. J Clin Psychopharmacol 1981;1(6):404–6.

92. Tandon R, Grunhaus L, Greden JF. Imipramine and tinnitus. J Clin Psychiatry 1987;48(3):109–11.

93. Smith EE, Reece CA, Kauffman R. Ototoxic reaction associated with use of nortriptyline hydrochloride: case report. J Pediatr 1972;80(6):1046–8.

94. Wehr TA, Goodwin FK. Can antidepressants cause mania and worsen the course of affective illness? Am J Psychiatry 1987;144(11):1403–11.

95. Kupfer DJ, Carpenter LL, Frank E. Possible role of antidepressants in precipitating mania and hypomania in recurrent depression. Am J Psychiatry 1988;145(7):804–8.

96. Paykel ES, Mueller PS, De la Vergne PM. Amitriptyline, weight gain and carbohydrate craving: a side effect. Br J Psychiatry 1973;123(576):501–7.

97. Nakra BR, Rutland P, Verma S, Gaind R. Amitriptyline and weight gain: a biochemical and endocrinological study. Curr Med Res Opin 1977;4(8):602–6.

98. Steiner JE, Rosenthal-Zifroni A, Edelstein EL. Taste perception in depressive illness. Isr Ann Psychiatr Relat Discip 1969;7(2):223–32.

99. Fernstrom MH, Krowinski RL, Kupfer DJ. Appetite and food preference in depression: effects of imipramine treatment. Biol Psychiatry 1987;22(5):529–39.

100. Sherman KE, Bornemann M. Amitriptyline and asymptomatic hypoglycemia. Ann Intern Med 1988;109(8):683–4.

101. Luzecky MH, Burman KD, Schultz ER. The syndrome of inappropriate secretion of antidiuretic hormone associated with amitriptyline administration. South Med J 1974;67(4):495–7.

102. Kuhs H. Demaskierung eines Phäochromozytoms durch Amitriptylin. [Unmasking pheochromocytoma by amitriptyline.] Nervenarzt 1998;69(1):76–7.

103. Anand VS. Clomipramine–induced galactorrhoea and amenorrhoea. Br J Psychiatry 1985;147:87–8.

104. Levin GM, DeVane CL. A review of cyclic antidepressant-induced blood dyscrasias. Ann Pharmacother 1992;26(3):378–83.

105. Albertini RS, Penders TM. Agranulocytosis associated with tricyclics. J Clin Psychiatry 1978;39(5):483–5.

106. Kozakova M. Liekova purpura po antidepresivach. [Drug-induced purpura due to antidepressive drugs.] Cesk Dermatol 1971;46(4):158–60.

107. Nixon DD. Thrombocytopenia following doxepin treatment. JAMA 1972;220(3):418.

108. Yon J, Anuras S. Hepatitis caused by amitriptyline therapy. JAMA 1975;232(8):833–4.

109. Robertson MM, Abou Saleh MR, Harrison DA, et al. A double blind controlled comparison of fluoxetine and lofepramine in major depressive illness. J Psychopharmacol 1994;8:98–103.

110. Schiff L, editor. Diseases of the Liver. Philadelphia: Lippinc-ott, 1982:604.

111. van Vliet AC, Frenkel M, Wilson JH. Acute leverinsufficientie na opipramolgebruik. [Acute liver necrosis after treatment with opipramol.] Ned Tijdschr Geneeskd 1977;121(34):1325–7.

112. Moskovitz R, DeVane CL, Harris R, Stewart RB. Toxic hepatitis and single daily dosage imipramine therapy. J Clin Psychiatry 1982;43(4):165–6.

113. Thioly-Bensoussan D, Charpentier A, Triller R, Thioly F, Blanchet P, Tricoire N, Noury JY, Grupper C. Acne iatrogène à l'amineptine (Survector): à propos de 8 cas. [Iatrogenic acne caused by amineptin (Survector): apropos 8 cases.] Ann Dermatol Venereol 1988;115(11):1177–80.

114. Jeanmougin M, Civatte J, Cavelier-Balloy B. Toxidermie rosacéiforme à l'amineptine (Survector). [Rosaceous drug eruption caused by amineptin (Survector).] Ann Dermatol Venereol 1988;115(11):1185–6.

115. Ming ME, Bhawan J, Stefanato CM, McCalmont TH, Cohen LM. Imipramine-induced hyperpigmentation: four cases and a review of the literature. J Am Acad Dermatol 1999;40(2 Part 1):159–66.

116. Mitchell JE, Popkin MK. Antidepressant drug therapy and sexual dysfunction in men: a review. J Clin Psychopharmacol 1983;3(2):76–9.

117. Renshaw DC. Doxepin treatment of sexual dysfunction associated with depression. In: Sinequan: a monograph of clinical studies. Amsterdam: Excerpta Medica; 1975.

118. Yeragani VK. Anorgasmia associated with desipramine. Can J Psychiatry 1988;33(1):76.

119. Dilsaver SC. Antidepressant withdrawal syndromes: phenomenology and pathophysiology. Acta Psychiatr Scand 1989;79(2):113–17.

120. Charney DS, Heninger GR, Sternberg DE, Landis H. Abrupt discontinuation of tricyclic antidepressant drugs: evidence for noradrenergic hyperactivity. Br J Psychiatry 1982;141:377–86.

121. Stern SL, Mendels J. Withdrawal symptoms during the course of imipramine therapy. J Clin Psychiatry 1980;41(2):66–7.

122. Santos AB Jr, Mccurdy L. Delirium after abrupt withdrawal from doxepin: case report. Am J Psychiatry 1980;137(2):239–40.

123. Mirin SM, Schatzberg AF, Creasey DE. Hypomania and mania after withdrawal of tricyclic antidepressants. Am J Psychiatry 1981;138(1):87–9.

124. Dilsaver SC, Feinberg M, Greden JF. Antidepressant withdrawal symptoms treated with anticholinergic agents. Am J Psychiatry 1983;140(2):249–51.

125. Gilani SH. Imipramine and congenital abnormalities. Pathol Microbiol (Basel) 1974;40(1):37–42.

126. McBride WG. Limb deformities associated with iminodibenzyl hydrochloride. Med J Aust 1972;1(10):492.

127. Crombie DL, Pinsent RJ, Fleming D. Imipramine in pregnancy. BMJ 1972;1(5802):745.

128. Kuenssberg EV, Knox JD. Imipramine in pregnancy. BMJ 1972;2(808):292.

129. Idanpaan-Heikkila J, Saxen L. Possible teratogenicity of imipramine–chloropyramine. Lancet 1973;2(7824):282–4.

130. Fu TK, Jarvik LF, Yen FS, Matsuyama SS, Glassman AH, Perel JM, Maltiz S. Effects of imipramine on chromosomes in psychiatric patients. Neuropsychobiology 1978;4(2):113–20.

131. Anonymous. Report on clomipramine H. Kuwait University Drug Adverse React Series 1983;2:14.

132. Eggermont E, Raveschot J, Deneve V, Casteels-van Daele M. The adverse influence of imipramine on the adaptation of the newborn infant to extrauterine life. Acta Paediatr Belg 1972;26(4):197–204.

133. Bloem BR, Lammers GJ, Roofthooft DW, De Beaufort AJ, Brouwer OF. Clomipramine withdrawal in newborns. Arch Dis Child Fetal Neonatal Ed 1999;81(1):F77.

134. Cowe L, Lloyd DJ, Dawling S. Neonatal convulsions caused by withdrawal from maternal clomipramine. BMJ (Clin Res Ed) 1982;284(6332):1837–8.

135. Sovner R, Orsulak PJ. Excretion of imipramine and desipramine in human breast milk. Am J Psychiatry 1979;136(4A):451–2.

136. Pittard WB 3rd, O'Neal W Jr. Amitriptyline excretion in human milk. J Clin Psychopharmacol 1986;6(6):383–4.

137. Stancer HC, Reed KC. Desipramine and 2-hydroxydesipramine in human breast milk and the nursing infants serum. Am J Psychiatry 1986;143(12):1597–600.

138. Wisner KL, Perel JM, Findling RL, Hinnes RL. Nortriptyline and its hydroxymetabolites in breastfeeding mothers and newborns. Psychopharmacol Bull 1997;33(2):249–51.

139. Wisner KL, Perel JM. Serum nortriptyline levels in nursing mothers and their infants. Am J Psychiatry 1991;148(9):1234–6.

140. Wisner KL, Perel JM, Findling RL. Antidepressant treatment during breast-feeding. Am J Psychiatry 1996;153(9):1132–7.

141. Matheson I, Pande H, Alertsen AR. Respiratory depression caused by N-desmethyldoxepin in breast milk. Lancet 1985;2(8464):1124.

142. Salzman C, Shader RI. Drugs that may contribute to depression in the elderly. In: Raskin A, Jarvik LF, editors. Psychiatric Symptoms and Cognitive Loss in the Elderly. New York: Wiley and Sons, 1979:57.

143. Gulevich G. Psychopharmacological treatment of the aged. In: Barelos ID, et al., editor. Psychopharmacology. Oxford: Oxford University Press, 1977:448.

144. Stage KB, Kragh-Sorensen PB; Danish University Antidepressant Group. Age-related adverse drug reactions to clomipramine. Acta Psychiatr Scand 2002;105(1):55–9.

145. Brown TC, Dwyer ME, Stocks JG. Antidepressant overdosage in children—a new menace. Med J Aust 1971;2(17):848–51.

146. Anonymous. Tricyclic antidepressant poisoning in children. Lancet 1979;2(8141):511.

147. Haner H, Brandenberger H, Pasi A, Moccetti T, Hartmann H. Ausserg ewohnliche Todesfalle durch trizyclische Antidepressivo. [Tricyclic antidepressants (TAD) as a cause of unexpected death.] Z Rechtsmed 1980;84(4):255–62.

148. Henry JA, Antao CA. Suicide and fatal antidepressant poisoning. Eur J Med 1992;1(6):343–8.

149. Ohberg A, Vuori E, Klaukka T, Lonnqvist J. Antidepressants and suicide mortality. J Affect Disord 1998;50(2–3):225–33.

150. Buckley NA, McManus PR. Fatal toxicity of serotoninergic and other antidepressant drugs: analysis of United Kingdom mortality data. BMJ 2002;325(7376):1332–3.

151. Biggs JT. Clinical pharmacology and toxicology of antidepressants. Hosp Pract 1978;13(2):79–84.

152. van de Ree JK, Zimmerman AN, van Heijst AN. Intoxication by tricyclic antidepressant drugs: experimental study and therapeutic considerations. Neth J Med 1977;20(4–5):149–55.

153. Hulten BA, Adams R, Askenasi R, Dallos V, Dawling S, Volans G, Heath A. Predicting severity of tricyclic antidepressant overdose. J Toxicol Clin Toxicol 1992;30(2):161–70.

154. Dziukas LJ, Vohra J. Tricyclic antidepressant poisoning. Med J Aust 1991;154(5):344–50.

155. Rumack BH, Anderson RJ, Wolfe R, Fletcher EC, Vestal BK. Ornade and anticholinergic toxicity. Hypertension, hallucinations, arrhythmias. Clin Toxicol 1974;7(6):573–81.

156. Kadar D. Letter: Amitriptyline and isoproterenol: fatal drug combination. Can Med Assoc J 1975;112(5):556–7.

157. Meignan L. Anesthésie et anti-dépresseurs tricycliques. [Anesthesia and tricyclic antidepressants.] Cah Anesthesiol 1977;25:735.

158. Vesell ES, Passananti GT, Greene FE. Impairment of drug metabolism in man by allopurinol and nortriptyline. N Engl J Med 1970;283(27):1484–8.

159. Cocco G, Ague C. Interactions between cardioactive drugs and antidepressants. Eur J Clin Pharmacol 1977;11(5):389–93.

160. Attree T, Sawyer P, Turnbull MJ. Interaction between digoxin and tricyclic antidepressants in the rat. Eur J Pharmacol 1972;19(2):294–6.

161. Deshauer D, Albuquerque J, Alda M, Grof P. Seizures caused by possible interaction between olanzapine and clomipramine. J Clin Psychopharmacol 2000;20(2):283–4.

162. Beresford TP, Feinsilver DL, Hall RC. Adverse reactions to benzodiazepine–tricyclic antidepressant compound. J Clin Psychopharmacol 1981;1(6):392–4.

163. Hall RC, Popkin MK, Kirkpatrick B. Tricyclic exacerbation of steroid psychosis. J Nerv Ment Dis 1978;166(10):738–42.

164. Malinow KL, Dorsch C. Tricyclic precipitation of steroid psychosis. Psychiatr Med 1984;2(4):351–4.

165. Dorsey ST, Biblo LA. Prolonged QT interval and torsades de pointes caused by the combination of fluconazole and amitriptyline. Am J Emerg Med 2000;18(2):227–9.

166. Robinson RF, Nahata MC, Olshefski RS. Syncope associated with concurrent amitriptyline and fluconazole therapy. Ann Pharmacother 2000;34(12):1406–9.

167. Messiha FS, Morgan JP. Imipramine-mediated effects on levodopa metabolism in man. Biochem Pharmacol 1974;23(10):1503–7.

168. Flemenbaum A. Hypertensive episodes after adding methylphenidate (Ritalin) to tricyclic antidepressants. (Report of three cases and review of clinical advantages.) Psychosomatics 1972;13(4):265–8.

169. Frejaville JP. De mauvais mélanges d'antidépresseurs. [Bad combinations of antidepressant drugs.] Concours Med 1972;94:8543.

170. Ponto LB, Perry PJ, Liskow BI, Seaba HH. Drug therapy reviews: tricyclic antidepressant and monoamine oxidase inhibitor combination therapy. Am J Hosp Pharm 1977;34(9):954–61.

171. Goldberg RS, Thornton WE. Combined tricyclic–MAOI therapy for refractory depression: a review, with guidelines for appropriate usage. J Clin Pharmacol 1978;18(2–3):143–7.

172. Anath J, Luchins DJ. Combined MAOI–tricyclic therapy (a critical review). Indian J Psychiatry 1976;18:26.

173. White K, Simpson G. Combined MAOI–tricyclic antidepressant treatment: a reevaluation. J Clin Psychopharmacol 1981;1(5):264–82.

174. Anonymous. Antidepressant interaction led to death. Pharm J 1982;13:191.

175. Graham PM, Potter JM, Paterson J. Combination monoamine oxidase inhibitor/tricyclic antidepressants interaction. Lancet 1982;2(8295):440.

176. Waehrens J. Krampeanfald ved samtidig behandling med neuroleptika og antidepressiva. [Convulsions during simultaneous treatment with neuroleptics and antidepressive agents.] Ugeskr Laeger 1982;144(2):106–8.

177. Siris SG, Cooper TB, Rifkin AE, Brenner R, Lieberman JA. Plasma imipramine concentrations in patients receiving concomitant fluphenazine decanoate. Am J Psychiatry 1982;139(1):104–6.

178. Linnoila M, George L, Guthrie S. Interaction between antidepressants and perphenazine in psychiatric inpatients. Am J Psychiatry 1982;139(10):1329–31.

179. Reda G, Lacerna F, Reda M, Lauro R. Interazioni tra farmaci antidepressi ed antipertensivi. Riv Psichiatr 1977;XII:309.

180. Juarez-Olguin H, Jung-Cook H, Flores-Perez J, Asseff IL. Clinical evidence of an interaction between imipramine and acetylsalicylic acid on protein binding in depressed patients. Clin Neuropharmacol 2002;25(1):32–6.

181. Abernethy DR, Greenblatt DJ, Shader RI. Imipramine disposition in users of oral contraceptive steroids. Clin Pharmacol Ther 1984;35(6):792–7.

182. Krishnan KR, France RD, Ellinwood EH Jr. Tricyclic-induced akathisia in patients taking conjugated estrogens. Am J Psychiatry 1984;141(5):696–7.

183. Fehr C, Grunder G, Hiemke C, Dahmen N. Increase in serum clomipramine concentrations caused by valproate. J Clin Psychopharmacol 2000;20(4):493–4.

184. Goodnick PJ. Influence of fluoxetine on plasma levels of desipramine. Am J Psychiatry 1989;146(4):552.

185. Bell IR, Cole JO. Fluoxetine induces elevation of desipramine level and exacerbation of geriatric nonpsychotic depression. J Clin Psychopharmacol 1988;8(6):447–8.

186. Vaughan DA. Interaction of fluoxetine with tricyclic antidepressants. Am J Psychiatry 1988;145(11):1478.

187. von Ammon Cavanaugh S. Drug–drug interactions of fluoxetine with tricyclics. Psychosomatics 1990;31(3):273–6.

188. Johne A, Schmider J, Brockmoller J, Stadelmann AM, Stormer E, Bauer S, Scholler G, Langheinrich M, Roots I. Decreased plasma levels of amitriptyline and its metabolites on comedication with an extract from St. John's wort (*Hypericum perforatum*). J Clin Psychopharmacol 2002;22(1):46–54.

189. Heiman EM. Cardiac toxicity with thioridazine–tricyclic antidepressant combination. J Nerv Ment Dis 1977;165(2):139–43.

190. Colantonio L, Orson J. Hyperthyroidism with normal T4-induction by imipramine. Clin Pharmacol Ther 1975;15:203.

Trientine

General Information

Trientine is a copper chelator that is used as an alternative to penicillamine in Wilson's disease, although experience with it is limited (1–4).

Organs and Systems

Nervous system

Trientine can, like penicillamine, initially worsen the neurological manifestations of Wilson's disease, presumably by mobilizing and redistributing copper (5,6). It should be started in small doses followed by gradual increases.

Metal metabolism

Excessive excretion of metals (zinc, iron) can occur in patients taking trientine, and can cause deficiency symptoms (7).

Hematologic

There have been several cases of sideroblastic anemia, characterized by an excess of ringed sideroblasts in the bone marrow, as a suspected adverse effect of trientine (8,9).

Gastrointestinal

In two patients the use of trientine was associated with serious colitis (with concomitant duodenitis in one), raising the suspicion of a possible causal relation (6).

Immunologic

- A 44-year-old woman developed antinuclear and anti-double-stranded-DNA antibodies (without clinical signs) while taking penicillamine; the antibodies disappeared after withdrawal, but recurred when she was subsequently given trientine (10).

References

1. Dubois RS, Rodgerson DO, Hambidge KM. Treatment of Wilson's disease with triethylene tetramine hydrochloride (Trientine). J Pediatr Gastroenterol Nutr 1990;10(1):77–81.
2. Siegemund R, Lossner J, Gunther K, Kuhn HJ, Bachmann H. Mode of action of triethylenetetramine dihydrochloride on copper metabolism in Wilson's disease. Acta Neurol Scand 1991;83(6):364–6.
3. Kiechl SG, Willeit J, Aichner F, Felber S. Treatment of Wilson's disease: penicillamine or triene. Acta Neurol Scand 1991;84:154–5.
4. Siegemund R. Reply. Acta Neurol Scand 1991;84:155–7.
5. Saito H, Watanabe K, Sahara M, Mochizuki R, Edo K, Ohyama Y. Triethylene-tetramine (trien) therapy for Wilson's disease. Tohoku J Exp Med 1991;164(1):29–35.
6. Dàhlman T, Hartvig P, Lofholm M, Nordlinder H, Loof L, Westermark K. Long-term treatment of Wilson's disease with triethylene tetramine dihydrochloride (Trientine). QJM 1995;88(9):609–16.
7. Walshe JM. Treatment of Wilson's disease with Trientine (triethylene tetramine) dihydrochloride. Lancet 1982;1(8273):643–7.
8. Condamine L, Hermine O, Alvin P, Levine M, Rey C, Courtecuisse V. Acquired sideroblastic anaemia during treatment of Wilson's disease with triethylene tetramine dihydrochloride. Br J Haematol 1993;83(1):166–8.
9. Walshe JM, Yealland M. Chelation treatment of neurological Wilson's disease. Q J Med 1993;86(3):197–204.
10. Demelia L, Vallebona E, Perpignano G, Pitzus F. Positivizzazione di sierologia lupica in corso di morbo di Wilson in trattamento con penicillamina. Reumatismo 1991;43:119–24.

Trifluoromethane

General Information

Research in animals, including primates, has shown that the inhaled fluorine gas, trifluoromethane (FC-23) can be used as an indicator of cerebral blood flow measured by magnetic resonance imaging (MRI) (1,2). The development of a fluorinated indicator to measure cerebral blood flow with MRI would allow the interleaving of images of cerebral anatomy and metabolism with images of regional cerebral blood flow, all obtainable in one setting by magnetic resonance methods. However, trifluoromethane is not inert and humans do not tolerate concentrations suitable for current MRI technology. Five healthy volunteers inhaled trifluoromethane at concentrations of 10–60% in a double fluid study (3). Concentrations over 30% produced impairment of neuropsychological function.

Organs and Systems

Psychological, psychiatric

In a phase 1, dose-ranging study, trifluoromethane 10–60% impaired neuropsychological function in five healthy men. Symptoms that occurred more often at higher doses included tiredness, difficulty in concentrating, tingling, dry mouth, and loss of appetite (3).

References

1. Branch CA, Helpern JA, Ewing JR, Welch KM. ^{19}F NMR imaging of cerebral blood flow. Magn Reson Med 1991;20(1):151–7.
2. Branch CA, Ewing JR, Helpern JA, Ordidge RJ, Butt S, Welch KM. Atraumatic quantitation of cerebral perfusion in cats by ^{19}F magnetic resonance imaging. Magn Reson Med 1992;28(1):39–53.
3. Rahill AA, Brown GG, Fagan SC, Ewing JR, Branch CA, Balakrishnan G. Neuropsychological dose effects of a freon, trifluoromethane (FC-23), compared to N_2O. Neurotoxicol Teratol 1998;20(6):617–26.

Trifluridine

General Information

Trifluridine, which is active against *Herpes simplex* and *Varicella zoster*, has only been used in topical antiherpetic solutions. It is twice as potent as idoxuridine in 1% solution and 10 times more soluble. Trifluridine has been reported to heal dendritic keratitis faster than idoxuridine, to be as effective as vidarabine when used five times a day, to have no cross-toxicity with idoxuridine or vidarabine, to heal stromal corneal defects more effectively than idoxuridine, and to produce topical allergy, punctal narrowing, and punctal keratitis only rarely. Furthermore, it gives excellent results in herpetic ulcers previously treated with topical glucocorticoids and in idoxuridine-unresponsive ulcers.

Organs and Systems

Immunologic

Trifluridine can cause allergic reactions (1).

Reference

1. Cirkel PK, van Ketel WG. Allergic contact dermatitis to trifluorothymidine eyedrops. Contact Dermatitis 1981;7(1):49–50.

Trihexyphenidyl

See also Anticholinergic drugs

General Information

Trihexyphenidyl (benzhexol) is an anticholinergic drug. It is given in oral doses rising from 2 to 20 mg/day, and even higher doses are used in dystonic patients. A wide range of anticholinergic adverse reactions can occur, but trihexyphenidyl is apparently particularly likely to cause excitement.

Organs and Systems

Cardiovascular

Paradoxical bradycardia has been reported; the reaction was specific to trihexyphenidyl and was not observed when the patient took other anticholinergic drugs (SEDA-12, 125).

Nervous system

Orofacial dyskinesia has been described with trihexyphenidyl in a patient who did not experience this reaction with levodopa (SEDA-18, 160).

Sensory systems

Trihexyphenidyl can precipitate glaucoma in predisposed patients, and blindness has resulted (1).

Psychological, psychiatric

Although it has been thought that high doses of trihexyphenidyl might impair learning in children, a careful study of this question suggested that there is in practice little interference (2).

As little as 8 mg/day combined with levodopa has caused an acute toxic confusional state in some patients.

- A 75-year-old man with a 10-year history of parkinsonism developed fever and acute delirium after taking levodopa plus trihexyphenidyl (3). He had visual hallucinations, was disoriented in time and place, and could respond only to simple questions. He was unable to stand or walk and had paratonic rigidity in all limbs and marked bradykinesia. There were occasional myoclonic jerks in the arms and legs. Deep reflexes were reduced bilaterally, and the plantar reflexes were absent.

Impairment of memory was attributed to trihexyphenidyl in healthy volunteers (SEDA-13, 115).

Long-Term Effects

Drug withdrawal

Acute withdrawal of trihexyphenidyl after a patient has become adapted to it can trigger an encephalopathy, requiring readministration (SEDA-22, 157).

Drug Administration

Drug overdose

Trihexyphenidyl has been misused by drug addicts to produce elation or relieve depression. One patient who took 300 mg with suicidal intent survived the resulting toxic psychosis (4).

References

1. Friedman Z, Neumann E. Benzhexol-induced blindness in Parkinson's disease. BMJ 1972;1(800):605.
2. Marsden CD, Marion MH, Quinn N. The treatment of severe dystonia in children and adults. J Neurol Neurosurg Psychiatry 1984;47(11):1166–73.
3. Tanabe K, Yokochi F, Hirai S, Mori H, Suda K, Kondo T, Mizuno Y. [A 75-year-old man with parkinsonism and delirium.] No To Shinkei 1994;46(1):85–92.
4. Ananth JV, Lehmann HE, Ban TA. Toxic psychosis induced by benzhexol hydrochloride. Can Med Assoc J 1970; 103(7):771.

Trimethoprim and co-trimoxazole

General Information

Trimethoprim is a 2,4-diamino-5-(3′,4′,5′-trimethoxybenzyl) pyrimidine that inhibits dihydrofolate reductase, the enzyme in folate synthesis after the step that is blocked by sulfonamides (1). Trimethoprim therefore inhibits the conversion of dihydrofolate to tetrahydrofolate. It has been combined with sulfonamides, including sulfamethoxazole, sulfametrol, sulfadiazine, sulfamoxole, and sulfadimidine (2,3).

A widely available fixed combination is co-trimoxazole (Bactrim, Eusaprim, Septrin), which contains trimethoprim and sulfamethoxazole in a ratio of 1:5. Both trimethoprim and sulfamethoxazole have favorable and comparable pharmacokinetics and the combination is bactericidal (4). Synergy between trimethoprim and sulfonamides has conventionally been ascribed to sequential inhibition of dihydropteroate synthetase by sulfonamides (in competition with *para*-aminobenzoic acid) and of dihydrofolate reductase by trimethoprim (in competition with dihydrofolate). However, sulfonamides in high concentrations also inhibit dihydrofolate reductase. Thus, an initial partial sequential blockade by trimethoprim (inhibition of dihydrofolate reductase) and sulfonamides (inhibition of dihydropteroate synthetase) leads to defective protein synthesis and cytoplasmic damage, which in turn results in marked increases in the uptake of both agents and "double strength" inhibition of dihydrofolate reductase (5).

Trimethoprim is fairly active against a variety of Gram-positive cocci and Gram-negative rods. Established indications for co-trimoxazole are infections of the sinuses, ears, lungs, and urinary tract, and infections due to *Salmonella*, *Nocardia*, *Brucella*, *Stenotrophomonas maltophilia*, *Pneumocystis jiroveci*, and *Toxoplasma* (1,6). Co-trimoxazole is also used in the treatment of Wegener's granulomatosis, for prevention of spontaneous bacterial peritonitis, and in patients with advanced HIV infection for the prophylaxis of opportunistic infections (1,6).

There have been few comparisons of the efficacy of trimethoprim and co-trimoxazole. In uncomplicated urinary tract, bronchopulmonary, and ear infections, no advantage of co-trimoxazole over trimethoprim has been documented (7,8). However, in complicated urinary tract infections most studies have shown better results with co-trimoxazole than with trimethoprim alone (9). Despite the widespread use of co-trimoxazole for about 35 years, bacterial resistance has not emerged as a major problem (10,11).

The adverse effects of co-trimoxazole are mostly ascribed to the sulfamethoxazole component. However, adverse effects can also be caused by trimethoprim or by the combination. It is important to realize that the culprit agent can only be definitely determined by re-exposure of the single drugs in the individual patient. Thus, in clinical practice it may be impossible to determine the causative compound.

Tetroxoprim is another 2,4-diaminopyrimidine derivative with comparable actions to those of trimethoprim. It is exclusively used in combinations with sulfonamides.

General adverse effects

Severe adverse drug reactions with trimethoprim and co-trimoxazole are rare (12–14). This also applies to children (15). The adverse effects of co-trimoxazole correspond to those expected from a sulfonamide (16). In HIV-infected patients, adverse effects of co-trimoxazole are more frequent and more severe (17–19). Hematological disturbances due to co-trimoxazole include mild anemia, leukopenia, and thrombocytopenia, which may be due to folic acid antagonism. Serious metabolic disturbances that are associated with trimethoprim include hyperkalemia and metabolic acidosis. Trimethoprim can cause hypersensitivity reactions. However, with co-trimoxazole, the sulfonamide is generally believed to be more allergenic (12). Generalized skin reactions predominate. Other effects, such as anaphylactic shock, are extremely rare (20–22). Carcinogenicity due to trimethoprim or co-trimoxazole has not been reported.

Organs and Systems

Respiratory

Cases of allergic pneumonitis and pulmonary infiltrates with eosinophilia have been described with co-trimoxazole (23). Such reactions have not been reported with trimethoprim alone. Pulmonary infiltrates due to co-trimoxazole hypersensitivity in patients with AIDS are particularly worrisome, since they mimic progression of underlying opportunistic pulmonary infections.

- Pneumonitis developed after the administration of co-trimoxazole in a patient with intractable ulcerative colitis complicated by *P. jiroveci* pneumonia. This patient had also previously had sulfasalazine-induced pneumonitis (24).
- A 33-year-old man taking co-trimoxazole developed bilateral pulmonary infiltrates and a fever of 39°C after 2 weeks (25). Co-trimoxazole was withdrawn. The fever resolved 6 days later. A lung biopsy showed non-specific interstitial pneumonia. A lymphocyte stimulation test for co-trimoxazole was positive.

Nervous system

Co-trimoxazole can cause tremor (26), which has been described in patients with AIDS taking co-trimoxazole (27,28).

- A 66-year-old man with pulmonary fibrosis and cor pulmonale was given intravenous co-trimoxazole for 3 weeks followed by oral treatment for an infection with Nocardia farcinica. On day 3 of oral treatment, he developed a tremor in both arms and legs, exacerbated by trying to stay calm. The symptoms resolved 3 days after drug withdrawal.

Aseptic meningitis and meningoencephalitis occur with trimethoprim and co-trimoxazole (29–39). The pathogenetic mechanism is still uncertain.

- A 15-year-old boy developed aseptic meningitis while taking trimethoprim 200 mg in the morning and 100 mg in the evening (40).

Immune complex deposition, immediate hypersensitivity, direct drug toxicity, and induction of anti-tissue antibodies have all been suggested. Interleukin-6 may be an important mediator of trimethoprim-induced aseptic meningitis in some patients. A case with three episodes after re-exposure to co-trimoxazole has been reported (41). Polymorphonuclear or mononuclear cells may preponderate (42). Interleukin-6 may be an important mediator of trimethoprim-induced aseptic meningitis in some patients (43,44).

Ataxia has been described in two patients with AIDS after intravenous use of co-trimoxazole (45).

Extrapyramidal symptoms developed with co-trimoxazole in a girl with dihydropteridine reductase deficiency and rapidly disappeared after withdrawal. This variant of phenylketonuria should be considered in all infants found to have raised phenylalanine concentrations during the neonatal period (46).

Sensory systems

Uveitis in combination with meningitis (47) and uveitis in combination with arthritis and Stevens–Johnson syndrome (48) have been reported with trimethoprim. Uveitis with retinal hemorrhages has also been described (49).

In unmedicated young and elderly volunteers and unmedicated HIV-infected patients, trimethoprim applied to the tongue was primarily described as bitter and medicinal (50).

Psychological, psychiatric

- Delirium occurred after treatment with co-trimoxazole in a patient with AIDS; the episode completely resolved within 72 hours of drug withdrawal (51).

Endocrine

In a child, co-trimoxazole was the probable cause of growth failure (52).

Co-trimoxazole has been suggested to have some antithyroid activity. However, whether this effect is due to trimethoprim alone is still unclear (53,54). Co-trimoxazole 27–31 mg/kg bd orally substantially altered serum total T4 and TSH concentrations and neutrophil counts in dogs within as short a time as a few weeks (55).

Metabolism

Co-trimoxazole can cause reversible hypoglycemia, which may be prolonged, particularly in patients with risk factors for hypoglycemia. Common risk factors include compromised renal function, prolonged fasting, malnutrition, and the use of excessive doses. It has been postulated that the sulfonamide mimics the action of sulfonylureas, stimulating pancreatic islet cells to secrete insulin. In elderly people, co-trimoxazole-induced hypoglycemia can cause altered mental state (56,57).

Metabolic acidosis has been observed in patients with AIDS after intravenous co-trimoxazole (58). The acidosis developed 3–5 days after the start of treatment and had a favorable course. It is likely that the sulfonamide was responsible, because of renal loss of bicarbonate.

Nutrition

A median increase in serum homocysteine of 50% (range 27–333%) was found in seven healthy male volunteers after a 2-week course of trimethoprim 300 mg bd (59). Concomitantly, serum folate concentrations fell significantly. By day 50, baseline values of homocysteine and folate were regained. Since tetrahydrofolate serves as a methyl group carrier in the remethylation of homocysteine to methionine, the inhibitory effect of trimethoprim on dihydrofolate reductase may be most important, but other mechanisms could not be excluded.

Electrolyte balance

Hyperkalemia is a relatively common complication of trimethoprim therapy and occurs at both high and standard dosages. It is thought to be caused by a potassium-sparing effect, to which elderly people appear to be particularly vulnerable (60–63). However, pre-existing renal impairment and concomitant potassium sparing diuretics may also contribute (60). In almost all cases the electrolyte changes resolve on withdrawal. Trimethoprim reduces renal potassium excretion by competitively inhibiting epithelial sodium channels in the distal nephron like triamterene. Higher dosages and pre-existing renal dysfunction are associated with an increased risk of hyperkalemia, as are probably other disturbances in potassium homeostasis, such as hypoaldosteronism and treatment with drugs that impair renal potassium excretion. Conversely, alkalinization of the urine and induction of high urinary flow rates block the antikaliuretic effect of trimethoprim in the distal nephron (64).

Co-trimoxazole can reduce potassium excretion and cause life-threatening hyperkalemia (65,66), even in therapeutic doses. In one study with standard dosages of co-trimoxazole, up to 62% of patients developed a peak serum potassium concentration of over 5.0 mmol/l and 21% a peak concentration of over 5.5.mmol/l (12,60,66). About 20–53% of patients with AIDS taking high-dosage co-trimoxazole for *P. jiroveci* pneumonia also develop hyperkalemia, and around 10% reach dangerously high concentrations (over 6.0 mmol/l). Withdrawal of trimethoprim is often required. Alkalinization of the urine and the induction of high urinary flow rates with intravenous fluids and loop diuretics block the antikaliuretic effect of trimethoprim on distal nephron cells (67,68).

Life-threatening hyperkalemia secondary to the use of standard doses of co-trimoxazole has been reported in two renal transplant recipients who developed end-stage renal disease secondary to familial Mediterranean fever, who may be at increased risk of hyperkalemia because of concurrent renal insufficiency, concomitant use of

ciclosporin, and associated tubulointerstitial disease (69). In one patient, underlying adrenal insufficiency might have contributed to the hyperkalemia.

- Hyperkalemia due to high doses of co-trimoxazole (14 mg/kg/day trimethoprim and 70 mg/kg/day sulfamethoxazole) occurred in an HIV-positive patient with *P. jiroveci* pneumonia (70).
- Life-threatening hyperkalemia secondary to the use of standard oral doses of co-trimoxazole (trimethoprim 320 mg/day and sulfamethoxazole 1600 mg/day) occurred in a 77-year-old man with moderate chronic renal insufficiency from diabetic nephropathy (71). In addition to hyperkalemia, he developed severe metabolic acidosis; both resolved on appropriate medical intervention and withdrawal of co-trimoxazole.
- A 41-year-old black man with AIDS and sickle cell anemia was treated on two separate occasions with co-trimoxazole and prednisone 40 mg/day for *P. jiroveci* pneumonia (72). On both occasions he developed a hyperkalemic metabolic acidosis together with renal tubular acidosis after several days of therapy.

Concurrent acidosis in patients with trimethoprim-induced hyperkalemia is uncommon, which could be explained if the action of trimethoprim, like that of amiloride, is limited to the cortical collecting tubule but does not affect the medullary collecting tubule, which has a large capacity to secrete hydrogen ions and may therefore prevent the development of acidosis. Predisposing factors for the rare adverse effect of renal tubular acidosis in this case may have been aldosterone deficiency or resistance, medullary dysfunction of sickle cell anemia, and renal insufficiency. All these factors could contribute to impaired renal handling of secretion of hydrogen ions (72).

According to studies on animals, tetroxoprim, which is structurally similar to trimethoprim, has stronger antikaliuretic effects than trimethoprim. Tetroxoprim-induced hyperkalemia has not been described yet. However, tetroxoprim is only rarely used and dosages are low (73).

Trimethoprim uncommonly causes hyponatremia.

- A 78-year-old woman developed severe symptomatic hyponatremia after treatment with anhydrous theophylline and 6 months later developed hyponatremia after treatment with co-trimoxazole for a presumptive urinary tract infection (74).

Hematologic

Most hematological adverse effects associated with trimethoprim have been reported with co-trimoxazole. These include macrocytic and megaloblastic anemia, aplastic anemia, neutropenia, hypersegmentation of leukocytes, thrombocytopenia, and pancytopenia (12,61–63,75–79). Sulfonamides alone have not been associated with folate deficiency, but in combination with trimethoprim they can deplete folate stores in patients with pre-existing deficiency of folate or vitamin B_{12} (80). Treatment with co-trimoxazole can impair the function of mobilized autologous peripheral blood stem cells (81).

Mild hemopoietic suppression due to co-trimoxazole in an immunocompromised host is common, even with low-dose regimens. This effect is notable in combination with other marrow-suppressive agents (for example azathioprine, ganciclovir, cyclophosphamide, and allopurinol), malnutrition, or infection (CMV and hepatitis C virus) (82).

Pancytopenia in the setting of severe drug hypersensitivity syndrome due to co-trimoxazole has been reported (83).

- A 53-year-old woman with congenital dyskeratosis took six co-trimoxazole double-strength tablets a day (trimethoprim 960 mg/day and sulfamethoxazole 4800 mg/day) for *P. jiroveci*, plus folic acid, and after 9 days developed a fever (39°C) accompanied by a morbilliform rash and painful cervical lymphadenopathy. She had a white blood cell count of $1.7 \times 10^9/l$, with $0.5 \times 10^9/l$ neutrophils; hemoglobin 7.3 g/dl; platelets $17 \times 10^9/l$; and hemolysis. A myelogram showed extensive hemophagocytosis. Polyvalent intravenous immunoglobulin (1 g/kg/day) was given for 2 days. She became apyrexial within 48 hours, accompanied by marked clinical improvement, and recovered within 1 month.

Erythrocytes

Megaloblastic anemia and aplastic anemia occur in very few patients (78,84,85). They develop particularly in patients who have pre-existing low folic acid concentrations and who are not taking folic acid supplements (79,85–87). Patients with megaloblastic anemia should not be treated with co-trimoxazole. Other predisposing factors include other drugs with antimetabolite properties or anticonvulsants (88). In patients with pre-existing folic acid deficiency or with HIV infection, the administration of folinic acid has been advised, in order to reduce the hematological adverse effects. However, preliminary data suggest that adjunctive folinic acid may be associated with an increased risk of therapeutic failure and death (89).

Leukocytes

Agranulocytosis is very rare. If leukocytes are routinely monitored during treatment (more often than clinically indicated), mild leukopenia is encountered in 0.4–10% of patients taking either co-trimoxazole (13,84,90–92) or trimethoprim alone (93).

Platelets

Mild thrombocytopenia is quite common with co-trimoxazole, affecting 0.1% to several% of patients treated (8,9,85,90,92–94). In a retrospective review in Denmark, co-trimoxazole was one of the commonest reported causes of drug-induced thrombocytopenia (11% of reports), with the exception of cytotoxic drugs (95). In a similar review in Sweden from 1985 to 1994 of all drug-induced blood dyscrasias, thrombocytopenia occurred most frequently, the major causes being furosemide (17%) and co-trimoxazole (9%) (96). Older patients were most at risk. However, clinically significant thrombocytopenia is only rarely seen. Although folic acid deficiency may contribute to thrombocytopenia, immunological reactions to either the sulfonamide (75,97) or trimethoprim (98) have been proposed (99,100).

Severe, life-threatening thrombocytopenia associated with co-trimoxazole has been reported (101).

- A 54-year-old white woman took a 10-day course of co-trimoxazole (trimethoprim 160 mg, sulfamethoxazole 800 mg) for chronic sinusitis. One day after finishing the course she developed scattered petechiae on both hands and blood blisters in her mouth. She had a low platelet count of $20 \times 10^9/l$. Other laboratory tests were normal, except for a raised blood glucose concentration. She was treated successfully with a transfusion of two units of platelets and oral prednisone. Four days after withdrawal of co-trimoxazole her platelet count increased to $110 \times 10^9/l$.

Reports of drug-induced thrombocytopenia have been systematically reviewed (102). Among the 98 different drugs described in 561 articles the following antibiotics were found with level I (definite) evidence: co-trimoxazole, rifampicin, vancomycin, sulfisoxazole, cefalothin, piperacillin, methicillin, novobiocin. Drugs with level II (probable) evidence were oxytetracycline and ampicillin.

In another retrospective analysis of drug-induced thrombocytopenia reported to the Danish Committee on Adverse Drug Reactions, 192 cases caused by the most frequently reported drugs were included and analysed (103). There were pronounced drug-specific differences in the clinical appearance. Early thrombocytopenia was characteristic of cases caused by sulfonamides and co-trimoxazole. These drugs also often caused hemorrhage. Accompanying leukopenia was observed in some cases associated with co-trimoxazole. There were no patient-specific factors responsible for the heterogeneity of the clinical appearance, and factors related to the physician seemed to be of little significance.

Gastrointestinal

Nausea and possibly vomiting occur in a few to 20% of adult patients taking normal dosages of co-trimoxazole (13,94). With trimethoprim alone in a dose of up to 400 mg/day, gastrointestinal tolerance was better and skin reactions were less frequent than with the combination (3). A review of the data from five different centers has shown that gastrointestinal complaints are less frequent with trimethoprim than with the combination (9).

Drug-induced esophagitis is rare, accounting for about 1% of all cases of esophagitis. An incidence of 3.9 in 100 000 has been reported. After the first description, there have been more than 250 observations, with more than 50 different drugs. Among those, the principal antibiotics included tetracyclines (doxycycline, metacycline, minocycline, oxytetracycline, and tetracycline), penicillins (amoxicillin, cloxacillin, penicillin V, and pivmecillinam), clindamycin, co-trimoxazole, erythromycin, lincomycin, spiramycin, and tinidazole. Doxycycline alone was involved in one-third of all cases. Risk factors included prolonged esophageal passage, due to motility disorders, stenosis, cardiomegaly, the formulation, supine position during drug ingestion, and failure to use liquid to wash down the tablet. Direct toxic effects of the drug (pH, accumulation in epithelial cells, non-uniform dispersion) also seem to contribute to the development of drug-induced esophagitis (104).

Antibiotic-associated colitis is only very rarely seen with co-trimoxazole (105,106).

Liver

Intrahepatic cholestasis associated with phospholipidosis has been reported with trimethoprim (107). In one case trimethoprim caused cholestatic hepatitis after re-exposure (108).

The same types of liver disease occur with co-trimoxazole as with sulfonamides alone (109–111). Mild rises in serum transaminases and cholestatic hepatotoxicity are well reported, usually starting after a latent period of several weeks, and associated with a rash. There have been very few case reports of fulminant hepatic failure associated with co-trimoxazole.

- A 32-year-old woman developed a pruritic maculopapular rash and fever (112). She had taken a 12-day course of co-trimoxazole that had finished 5 days before and was taking no other drugs. She had normal hematological indices but a raised alkaline phosphatase and aspartate transaminase. Serological testing for Epstein-Barr virus, hepatitis A, B, and C, cytomegalovirus, echo virus, rubella, and measles showed no evidence of recent infection. Her rash improved but her general condition worsened and steroids were started. An abdominal CT scan showed a large liver with a moderate amount of ascites. The aspartate transaminase rose to 1330 IU/l and the prothrombin time increased. She developed progressive liver failure and died while awaiting liver transplant. At autopsy the liver showed signs of massive hepatic necrosis with no other abnormalities.
- Hepato-renal insufficiency combined with pancytopenia followed the administration of co-trimoxazole for 10 days for suspected pyelonephritis in a 48-year-old man (113). Hemodialysis was temporarily required, and renal and liver function and blood counts returned to normal afterwards.

Pancreas

Acute pancreatitis, with relapse on re-exposure, has been observed in a patient taking co-trimoxazole (114).

Urinary tract

Trimethoprim interferes with the tubular secretion of creatinine, causing an increased serum creatinine concentration and a reduced creatinine clearance, without affecting true glomerular filtration rate (115–118). Thus, a small increase in serum creatinine concentration at the beginning of treatment is not necessarily indicative of impaired renal function (119,120). Nevertheless, co-trimoxazole may have a direct nephrotoxic effect, mainly in patients with pre-existing renal impairment taking large dosages (115,116,121). This can be prevented by reducing the dose (117,118). If creatinine clearance is reduced to 15–25 ml/minute, the standard dose of co-trimoxazole should be reduced by half after an initial 3 days of treatment with the usual dose.

Treatment with co-trimoxazole (or other antibiotics) can increase the risk of the hemolytic-uremic syndrome in children with gastrointestinal infections caused by *Escherichia coli* O157:H7 compared with children with no antibiotic treatment (122).

Extremely rare instances of crystalluria followed by renal insufficiency due to obstruction have been described in patients taking trimethoprim (123).

Skin

The skin reactions observed with co-trimoxazole can be due to trimethoprim or to the sulfonamide. Data collected from five different centers have shown that skin rashes are less frequent with trimethoprim than with co-trimoxazole (9).

- Generalized erythematous skin eruptions have now been reported in a 20-year-old Japanese woman and a 70-year-old Japanese man taking co-trimoxazole (124). Patch tests showed that trimethoprim alone was responsible for the erythematous popular-type skin eruption in the young woman. The old man's skin responded to both trimethoprim and sulfamethoxazole.

The skin rashes due to trimethoprim and co-trimoxazole are mostly maculopapular and are related to the duration of treatment (125). They occur with a frequency of 1.3–5.9% (94,126–128).

In a randomized, open trial of long-term intermittent co-trimoxazole on recurrences of toxoplasmic retinochoroiditis, four of 54 patients who took a single tablet of co-trimoxazole (trimethoprim 160 mg, sulfamethoxazole 800 mg) withdrew when they developed mild cutaneous erythema that resolved when drug treatment was stopped (129).

Fixed drug eruptions

Fixed drug eruptions have been analysed in 450 patients (130). The ratio of men to women was 10:11. The mean age of the men was 30 years, and that of the women 31 years. In 13% the fixed drug eruption had occurred for the first time, 2.7% had had more than 40 episodes. There was atopy in 11%, and 23% had a positive family history of drug reactions. Co-trimoxazole was the most common cause of fixed drug eruptions. Other antibiotics included tetracycline, metronidazole, amoxicillin, ampicillin, erythromycin, and clindamycin.

Co-trimoxazole was the offender in 75% of 64 cases of fixed drug eruption. The eruption was mainly located on male genitalia, but unusual findings included familial occurrence, symmetrical and asymmetrical non-pigmented lesions, linear lesions, a solitary plaque on the cheek, and wandering lesions (131).

There may be an association between fixed drug eruption and HLA class I antigens. In 42 of 67 patients with fixed drug eruptions caused by co-trimoxazole there were significantly higher frequencies of the A30 antigen and A30 B13 Cw6 haplotype than in 2378 control subjects (132). HLA-B55 (split of B22) was present exclusively in co-trimoxazole fixed drug eruption, and in a higher frequency than in control subjects.

Topical provocation of fixed drug eruption and positive reactions with co-trimoxazole are extremely rare and have never been seen on unaffected skin.

- In a 42-year-old Caucasian woman with histopathologically confirmed fixed drug eruption induced by co-trimoxazole, positive topical provocation by trimethoprim was obtained on both involved and uninvolved skin (133).

Cross-sensitivity to co-trimoxazole and nimesulide has been reported (134).

- A 10-year-old-boy developed an extensive fixed drug eruption when he took co-trimoxazole (trimethoprim 200 mg, sulfamethoxazole 40 mg bd) 8 weeks after having had a fixed drug eruption due to nimesulide. An oral provocation test with co-trimoxazole 1 month later showed reactivation within 12 hours in the form of severe itching and erythema at the sites of the lesions with one-quarter of the dose.

Erythema multiforme

Erythema multiforme and its related syndromes (Stevens–Johnson syndrome and toxic epidermal necrolysis) are well recognized with co-trimoxazole and can be caused by trimethoprim as a single drug (135). A European review identified sulfonamides (and particularly co-trimoxazole) as a major causative factor in Stevens–Johnson syndrome and toxic epidermal necrolysis, the crude relative risk being far in excess of any other implicated drug (136). In a histopathological study of 111 cases from Germany, co-trimoxazole accounted for 22 cases (20%) (137). There were no histological features that could have discriminated between the different causes of this severe reaction.

- A 34-year-old Asian woman developed toxic epidermal necrolysis associated with co-trimoxazole (160/800 mg bd) (138). She recovered completely without serious sequelae.
- Toxic epidermal necrolysis, associated with co-trimoxazole for sinusitis in a 16-year-old woman, was successfully treated with intravenous immunoglobulins (0.4 g/kg for 5 days) (139).
- Toxic epidermal necrolysis, associated with treatment with co-trimoxazole (480/2400 mg/day) for sepsis in a 66-year-old Caucasian man, was successfully treated with intravenous immunoglobulin (0.75 g/kg for 5 days) (140).
- An 86-year-old man developed severe and extensive toxic epidermal necrolysis within 24 hours of taking co-trimoxazole for a urinary infection (141). He had had an allergic reaction to co-trimoxazole a few years before. He recovered completely without serious sequelae.
- A 50-year-old man took oral co-trimoxazole (trimethoprim 160 mg, sulfamethoxazole 800 mg) and developed toxic epidermal necrolysis 13 days later (142).

In 20 Indian patients (of whom 70% were women) with Steven–Johnson syndrome and ocular involvement, co-trimoxazole was the commonest identifiable risk factor (143). Conjunctival involvement and its sequelae were the major ocular manifestations.

Susceptibility factors

Skin reactions occur with high frequency during co-trimoxazole therapy in patients with AIDS (18,19). Other symptoms in such patients have been described in association with skin eruptions, including fever, neutropenia, thrombocytopenia, and rises in transaminase activities (18,79). The high dosages used to treat *P. jiroveci* in these patients may partly be responsible for the high

frequency of adverse effects, since low-dose co-trimoxazole for the prevention of *P. jiroveci* pneumonia reduced the adverse effects from 28 to 9% (144).

Nails

- Co-trimoxazole was suggested to have caused loss of fingernails and toenails in a 3-year-old boy (145). He was initially treated with gentamicin 2 mg/kg intravenously every 8 hours for *E. coli* urinary tract infection, and co-trimoxazole was given once daily in a prophylactic dose. After 2 weeks his fingernails and toenails began to slough. Co-trimoxazole was withdrawn, and within 2 weeks his nails had returned to normal.

Immunologic

The sulfonamide component of co-trimoxazole is generally believed to be more allergenic than trimethoprim. However, trimethoprim alone can cause hypersensitivity reactions more commonly than has previously been thought. Most of these reactions present as generalized skin reactions. The hydroxylamine and other metabolites of sulfamethoxazole can bind covalently to proteins because of their chemical reactivity, resulting in the induction of specific adverse immune responses. Therefore, changes in the activity of detoxification pathways are associated with a greater risk of allergic reactions to sulfonamides. Allergies to sulfonamides, particularly sulfamethoxazole, are more frequent in patients with AIDS, but the reason for this increased risk is not fully understood. No tools are available to predict which patients have a greater risk for developing allergies to sulfonamides. In a small study in HIV-positive patients with hypersensitivity syndrome reaction, the lymphocyte toxicity assay has a strong potential for use as a diagnostic tool to assess co-trimoxazole hypersensitivity (146). Diagnosis is essential to avoid possible progression to severe reactions and readministration of the offending drug.

In patients who absolutely require further treatment, successful desensitization can be achieved (147). Two patients with chronic granulomatous disease who had previously been intolerant of co-trimoxazole completed a 5-day desensitization protocol with a good clinical outcome (148).

Anaphylactic shock is rare, but has been reported with co-trimoxazole (20). However, it is possible that this reaction was due to the sulfonamide compound (21). The case histories of 13 patients (12 women, one man, aged 22–68 years) with anaphylactic reactions to trimethoprim alone that were reported to a national drug safety unit have been analysed (20). Nine were classified as probable anaphylaxis. The casual relation between exposure to trimethoprim and anaphylaxis was classified as definite in three reports, possible in four, and probable in six. In one patient, IgE antibodies against trimethoprim were demonstrated.

- Culture-negative arthritis, bilateral uveitis, mucocutaneous Stevens–Johnson syndrome, and eosinophilia developed in a 31-year-old woman after 3 days of therapy with oral trimethoprim 160 mg bd for a lower urinary tract infection (48). At the start of antibiotic therapy, glucocorticoids and local anesthetics were injected into the lateral aspect of the right knee. Recovery was rapid after trimethoprim was withdrawn. Two months later she developed headache, nausea, malaise, and bilateral uveitis after taking trimethoprim again.

With sera from patients with known hypersensitivity to trimethoprim, IgE-specific recognition of three different but related metabolites has been demonstrated, including the entire molecule itself, the 3,4-dimethoxybenzyl group, and the 2,4-diamino-5-(3′,4′-dimethoxybenzyl) pyrimidine group (149). The incidence of adverse reactions in patients with AIDS is higher than in others (12). Most of these effects are not true allergic reactions, but are related to high doses of co-trimoxazole, and include rashes, nausea, and vomiting. They can be reduced in both frequency and severity by corticosteroids, which are often given in moderate to severe *P. jiroveci* pneumonia. The risk of hypersusceptibility reactions (Stevens–Johnson syndrome, neutropenia, hepatotoxicity, aseptic meningitis, thrombocytopenia) is also higher than in other patients. Since many rashes with co-trimoxazole are not necessarily due to allergic mechanisms, a previous rash should not prevent later re-administration. It may be prudent, however, to use a rapid test dose when co-trimoxazole is the treatment of choice (150).

The incidence of adverse reactions to co-trimoxazole in HIV-infected patients is high. Several reports have shown that an incremental increase in drug dosage may allow a significant proportion of patients to tolerate prophylactic dosages of co-trimoxazole. Eight of 14 selected HIV-infected patients (13 men, 1 woman; patients who experienced severe reactions such as anaphylaxis or Stevens–Johnson syndrome were excluded) were successfully desensitized and after a regimen of gradual incremented exposure over 11 days as an outpatient procedure could continue to take co-trimoxazole (151). *N*-acetylcysteine (3 g of a 20% liquid solution bd) did not prevent hypersensitivity reactions to co-trimoxazole in HIV-infected patients (152). Although cross-reactivity can occur, dapsone can be used for patients with mild hypersensitivity reactions to co-trimoxazole for prophylaxis of *P. jiroveci* pneumonia (153).

A syndrome that resembles bacterial sepsis is well recognized in patients with AIDS (154). This reaction can occur within hours of a large dose of co-trimoxazole, but most often occurs on rechallenge.

- A sepsis-like hypersensitivity reaction occurred in 38-year-old HIV-positive Hispanic man after a 14-day course of co-trimoxazole (155).

The mechanism of this unusual reaction is unclear.

Desensitization

Desensitization can be efficient in a large proportion of patients (88%) using a 5-day protocol, in which co-trimoxazole is administered orally in a granular formulation in increasing doses, beginning with trimethoprim 0.4 mg and sulfamethoxazole 2 mg and doubling the dose every 12 hours until the therapeutic dose is achieved (156). Another dosage regimen (12 doses of increasing amounts of co-trimoxazole at half-hour intervals) resulted

in an overall success rate of 91% at 1 month in 44 patients (157). Such tolerance induction protocols can be adopted, even during pregnancy without risk to the mother or to the fetus (158).

Another uncontrolled trial of a 6-day desensitization procedure in 33 cases has been reported (159). The protocol started with a dose of 0.2 mg rising to 800 mg over 6 days and 32 of the subjects successfully completed the course. In addition, 12 of 14 cases were successfully re-challenged with co-trimoxazole. However, this study lacked a clear description of follow-up or the reasons for the selection of subjects for desensitization or re-challenge, and cannot be used as a basis for recommending this desensitization technique.

Oral desensitization to co-trimoxazole was successfully achieved in patients with AIDS suffering from fever, rash, and wheezing due to the drug (160–163). In a randomized study of desensitization with rechallenge in HIV-positive patients with previous adverse effects of co-trimoxazole 73 patients were given a 14-day course of trimethoprim 200 mg/day (164). Fourteen had adverse reactions to trimethoprim. The remaining 59 subjects were randomized to a 2-day desensitization technique (34 subjects) or rechallenge (25 subjects). There were seven hypersensitivity reactions in both groups. Clearly there is no advantage of this 2-day desensitization technique over rechallenge with co-trimoxazole in HIV-positive individuals.

In a randomized, double-blind study in HIV patients, gradual introduction of co-trimoxazole was associated with significantly fewer adverse drug reactions compared with standard initiation of therapy (165).

Overall it appears that desensitization to co-trimoxazole is safe in the absence of previous serious adverse events, although it is not yet certain whether desensitization is better than re-challenge or indeed what the ideal desensitization method should be.

Infection risk

There have been rare reports of an association between sulfonamide antibiotics and increased severity of rickettsial infections. Sulfonamides do not increase the pathogenicity of *Ehrlichia* species, but a case of human monocytic ehrlichiosis complicated by ARDS has previously been reported in a patient who had taken oral co-trimoxazole. It has been speculated that oral co-trimoxazole, given for acne, may have contributed to the unusual severity of *Ehrlichia chaffeensis* infection that progressed to respiratory failure in a previously healthy 16-year-old boy (166).

Long-Term Effects

Drug tolerance

Bacteria have developed several mechanisms that make them resistant to trimethoprim. Resistance can occur rapidly, and has been reported in Europe, the USA, Asia, and South America, which may account for the fact that trimethoprim is usually used in combination (1,167,168). However, the clinical significance of resistance to trimethoprim has been debated (1,7,16,169).

From a total of 31 319 *Shigella* strains isolated in Israel between 1990 and 1996, the rates of resistance of *Shigella sonnei*, *Shigella flexneri*, and *Shigella boydii* to co-trimoxazole were 94%, 51%, and 62% respectively; the proportion of strains that exhibited multiple drug resistance was higher for *S. sonnei* than for the other serotypes studied (170).

Among 12 045 isolates of *Streptococcus pneumoniae* collected between 1995 and 1998, resistance to co-trimoxazole increased slightly, from 25% to 29% (171).

Mutagenicity

Genotoxic effects of trimethoprim on cultured human lymphocytes have been described (172). Chromosome studies performed in cultures of peripheral blood lymphocytes did not show significant differences before and after treatment. Cytogenetic studies on bone marrow cells from 12 patients with urinary tract infections treated with co-trimoxazole did not show structural chromosomal aberrations; however, there was an increased number of micronuclei in these patients compared with controls (173).

Second-Generation Effects

Fertility

Whether reported cases of impaired male fertility were due to co-trimoxazole is not clear, since most of the men were being treated for underlying urogenital infections, which may have contributed to reduced fertility (174,175).

Teratogenicity

An early review of newer case reports and placebo-controlled trials involving several hundred patients did not show an increase in fetal abnormalities (176). However, the relative risks of cardiovascular defects and oral clefts in infants whose mothers were exposed to dihydrofolate reductase inhibitors, such as trimethoprim, during the second or third month after the last menstrual period, compared with infants whose mothers had no such exposure, are 3.4 (95% CI = 1.8, 6.4) and 2.6 (1.1, 6.1) respectively (177). Multivitamin supplements containing folic acid reduced the adverse effects of dihydrofolate reductase inhibitors. There have been two reports of severe spinal malformations in the fetuses of HIV-positive women treated with combination antiretroviral therapy and co-trimoxazole (178).

Susceptibility Factors

Renal disease

In renal insufficiency, co-trimoxazole should be used with caution, particularly when there is hyperkalemia (66,115).

Other features of the patient

Co-trimoxazole should not be given to patients with malnutrition, pregnancy, severe liver damage, megaloblastic anemia, agranulocytosis, or bone marrow failure (12,14,87).

HIV infection

The use of co-trimoxazole in HIV-positive patients has been associated with a high rate of hypersensitivity reactions (40–80%), attributed to the bioactivation of the sulfonamide component, sulfamethoxazole, to its toxic hydroxylamine and nitroso metabolites. In a study of HIV-positive patients with ($n = 56$) and without ($n = 89$) hypersensitivity to co-trimoxazole, functionally significant polymorphisms in the genes coding for enzymes involved in co-trimoxazole metabolism were unlikely to have been major predisposing factors in determining individual susceptibility to co-trimoxazole hypersensitivity (179).

In a randomized, double-blind study in 372 HIV-positive patients with CD4+ counts below 250×10^6/l, gradual initiation of co-trimoxazole treatment was associated with significantly fewer adverse drug reactions compared with standard initiation (180).

The relation between the onset of adverse reactions to co-trimoxazole in HIV-infected patients and the subsequent development of toxoplasmosis, other AIDS-defining events, and survival has been studied in 592 French patients (181). A low CD4 cell count when co-trimoxazole was introduced was the only factor associated with the onset of adverse reactions. The occurrence of toxoplasmosis and first AIDS-defining events was significantly and independently linked to a low CD4 cell count when co-trimoxazole was introduced and to previous co-trimoxazole withdrawal for adverse events, but not to previous co-trimoxazole withdrawal for reasons other than adverse events, compared with patients who did not stop taking co-trimoxazole. The survival rate was significantly shorter among patients who stopped taking co-trimoxazole for adverse events and for other reasons, compared with patients who continued to take it.

Drug–Drug Interactions

Anticonvulsants

Most interactions of trimethoprim and co-trimoxazole with other drugs are due to folic acid antagonism. This may be more pronounced with co-trimoxazole than with either drug alone. Such interactions have previously been suspected with anticonvulsants, such as barbiturates, phenytoin, and primidone, which themselves produce folic acid deficiency and megaloblastic anemia (88). In order to circumvent the risk of folate deficiency, folic acid or folinic acid can be given. There is some concern that folate replacement may antagonize the desired antimicrobial effect, particularly in some protozoal parasites, but this concern has been debated (89).

Azathioprine

In renal transplant patients, combining azathioprine with co-trimoxazole was followed by neutropenia and thrombocytopenia (92).

Coumarin anticoagulants

Co-trimoxazole can significantly augment the hypoprothrombinemic effect of warfarin (182,183), acenocoumarol (184,185), and phenprocoumon (185).

Cytotoxic drugs

Most interactions of trimethoprim and co-trimoxazole with other drugs are due to folic acid antagonism. This may be more pronounced with co-trimoxazole than with either drug alone. Such interactions have been suspected with cytotoxic drugs (186,187). In order to circumvent the risk of folate deficiency, folic acid or folinic acid can be given. There is some concern that folate replacement may antagonize the desired antimicrobial effect, particularly in some protozoal parasites, but this concern has been debated (89).

In children with acute lymphoblastic leukemia co-trimoxazole inhibited 6-mercaptopurine metabolism (186).

In another study, co-trimoxazole produced a 66% increase in systemic exposure to methotrexate (187).

Prolonged treatment with co-trimoxazole can reduce cyclophosphamide requirements in patients with Wegener's granulomatosis (188).

Glucocorticoids

Prolonged treatment with co-trimoxazole can reduce glucocorticoid requirements in patients with Wegener's granulomatosis (188).

HIV protease inhibitors

In an animal model, indinavir nephrotoxicity was potentiated by co-trimoxazole, but nelfinavir alone or in combination with co-trimoxazole was not nephrotoxic (189).

Immunosuppressants

Most interactions of trimethoprim and co-trimoxazole with other drugs are due to folic acid antagonism. This may be more pronounced with co-trimoxazole than with either drug alone. Such interactions have previously been suspected with immunosuppressant drugs (186,187). In order to circumvent the risk of folate deficiency, folic acid or folinic acid can be given. There is some concern that folate replacement may antagonize the desired antimicrobial effect, particularly in some protozoal parasites, but this concern has been debated (89).

Pronounced nephrotoxicity resulted from the interaction of co-trimoxazole with ciclosporin in patients with a renal transplant (190,191).

Lithium

Trimethoprim has the same effect on the kidney as amiloride, whose combined use with lithium can cause a raised serum lithium concentration.

- The addition of trimethoprim caused severe lithium toxicity in a 40-year-old woman with a schizoaffective disorder; following rehydration, she made a good recovery (192).

Methotrexate

Methotrexate, a folic acid antagonist, is used in the treatment of several disorders. Its major action is inhibition of dihydrofolate reductase, a critical enzyme in intracellular folate metabolism. Co-trimoxazole competes with methotrexate in inhibiting dihydrofolate reductase and further impairs DNA synthesis.

- A fatal case of toxic epidermal necrolysis that involved 90% of the total body surface has been described in a 15-year-old boy with T cell acute lymphoblastic leukemia treated concomitantly with co-trimoxazole and methotrexate (193).

The authors suggested that methotrexate toxicity was precipitated by co-trimoxazole.

- Fatal bone marrow suppression has been reported in an 82-year-old woman who took methotrexate 7.5 mg/week for one year for rheumatoid arthritis without hematological problems. She was given trimethoprim 100 mg/day at first and later 200 mg/day. One week later, she developed severe pancytopenia. The bone marrow failed to recover despite treatment with folinic acid and G-CSF, and she died of bronchopneumonia.

In a literature review, the authors found two other cases of bone marrow suppression after treatment with methotrexate and trimethoprim with full recovery of both. This interaction is also listed in the British National Formulary 1997 (194,195).

Oral contraceptives

Some antibiotics interfere with the effects of oral contraceptives, putatively by inhibiting bacterial deconjugation in the bowel and thus reducing their reabsorption after biliary excretion. However, in women taking oral contraceptives, short courses of co-trimoxazole are unlikely to cause any adverse effects on contraceptive control (196).

Phenytoin

Massive hepatic necrosis after exposure to phenytoin and co-trimoxazole is rare.

- Acute liver failure has been reported in a 60-year-old woman after concomitant ingestion of phenytoin and co-trimoxazole over 9 days (197). Autopsy showed acute fulminant hepatic failure.

Drug interactions can potentiate the hepatotoxicity of single agents; withdrawal of co-trimoxazole may be needed in the presence of early liver injury.

Procainamide

Trimethoprim inhibits the active tubular secretion of procainamide (198).

Rifamycins

In 10 HIV-positive patients who had been taking one double-strength tablet of co-trimoxazole daily for more than 1 month, the concentrations of trimethoprim and sulfamethoxazole in serum were significantly reduced after the administration of rifampicin (199).

Trimeprazine

The antihistaminic phenothiazine trimeprazine has significant antibacterial activity in vitro and in vivo, and a combination with trimethoprim is highly synergistic, as shown in vivo in Swiss white mice using *Salmonella typhimurium* as the challenge bacterium (200).

Zidovudine

In one pharmacokinetic study in eight HIV-infected subjects, the renal clearance of zidovudine was significantly reduced by trimethoprim (201). The authors concluded that zidovudine dosages may need to be reduced if trimethoprim is given to patients with impairment of liver function or glucuronidation. Zidovudine, on the other hand, did not alter the pharmacokinetics of trimethoprim.

Interference with Diagnostic Tests

Serum folate concentration

Serum folate concentrations should not be measured by the radioisotope method in patients taking trimethoprim (202).

References

1. Zinner SH, Mayer KH. Basic principles in the diagnosis and management of infectious diseases: sulfonamides and trimethoprim. In: Mandell GL, Douglas RG, Bennett JE, editors. Principles and Practice of Infectious Diseases. 4th ed. Edinburgh: Churchill Livingstone, 1996:354.
2. Finland M. Editorial: Combinations of antimicrobial drugs: trimethoprim–sulfamethoxazole. N Engl J Med 1974;291(12):624–7.
3. Garg SK, Ghosh SS, Mathur VS. Comparative pharmacokinetic study of four sulfonamides in combination with trimethoprim in human volunteers. Int J Clin Pharmacol Ther Toxicol 1986;24(1):23–5.
4. Bushby SR, Hitchings GH. Trimethoprim, a sulphonamide potentiator. Br J Pharmacol Chemother 1968;33(1):72–90.
5. Richards RM, Taylor RB, Zhu ZY. Mechanism for synergism between sulphonamides and trimethoprim clarified. J Pharm Pharmacol 1996;48(9):981–4.
6. Gruneberg RN. The microbiological rationale for the combination of sulphonamides with trimethoprim. J Antimicrob Chemother 1979;5(B):27–36.
7. Brumfitt W, Hamilton-Miller JM. Co-trimoxazole or trimethoprim alone? A viewpoint on their relative place in therapy. Drugs 1982;24(6):453–8.
8. Brumfitt W, Hamilton-Miller JM. Combinations of sulphonamides with diaminopyrimidines: how, when and why? J Chemother 1995;7(2):136–9.
9. Brogden RN, Carmine AA, Heel RC, Speight TM, Avery GS. Trimethoprim: a review of its antibacterial activity, pharmacokinetics and therapeutic use in urinary tract infections. Drugs 1982;23(6):405–30.
10. Dornbusch K, Toivanen P. Effect of trimethoprim or trimethoprim/sulphamethoxazole usage on the emergence of trimethoprim resistance in urinary tract pathogens. Scand J Infect Dis 1981;13(3):203–10.
11. Wust J, Kayser FH. Die Empfindlichkeit von Bakterieu gegen chemo therapeutika (zürich, 1993). [Sensitivity of bacteria to chemotherapeutic agents (Zurich, 1993).] Schweiz Rundsch Med Prax 1995;84(4):98–105.
12. Cribb AE, Lee BL, Trepanier LA, Spielberg SP. Adverse reactions to sulphonamide and sulphonamide–trimethoprim antimicrobials: clinical syndromes and pathogenesis. Adverse Drug React Toxicol Rev 1996;15(1):9–50.
13. Jick H. Adverse reactions to trimethoprim–sulfamethoxazole in hospitalized patients. Rev Infect Dis 1982; 4(2):426–8.
14. Lawson DH, Jick H. Adverse reactions to co-trimoxazole in hospitalized medical patients. Am J Med Sci 1978;275(1):53–7.
15. Gutman LT. The use of trimethoprim–sulfamethoxazole in children: a review of adverse reactions and indications. Pediatr Infect Dis 1984;3(4):349–57.
16. Martin AJ, Lacey RW. A blind comparison of the efficacy and incidence of unwanted effects of trimethoprim and co-trimoxazole in the treatment of acute infection of the urinary tract in general practice. Br J Clin Pract 1983;37(3):105–11.
17. Coopman SA, Johnson RA, Platt R, Stern RS. Cutaneous disease and drug reactions in HIV infection. N Engl J Med 1993;328(23):1670–4.
18. Gordin FM, Simon GL, Wofsy CB, Mills J. Adverse reactions to trimethoprim–sulfamethoxazole in patients with the acquired immunodeficiency syndrome. Ann Intern Med 1984;100(4):495–9.
19. Mitsuyasu R, Groopman J, Volberding P. Cutaneous reaction to trimethoprim–sulfamethoxazole in patients with AIDS and Kaposi's sarcoma. N Engl J Med 1983;308(25):1535–6.
20. Bijl AM, Van der Klauw MM, Van Vliet AC, Stricker BH. Anaphylactic reactions associated with trimethoprim. Clin Exp Allergy 1998;28(4):510–12.
21. Johnson MP, Goodwin SD, Shands JW Jr. Trimethoprim–sulfamethoxazole anaphylactoid reactions in patients with AIDS: case reports and literature review. Pharmacotherapy 1990;10(6):413–16.
22. Cabanas R, Caballero MT, Vega A, Martin-Esteban M, Pascual C. Anaphylaxis to trimethoprim. J Allergy Clin Immunol 1996;97(1 Pt 1):137–8.
23. Silvestri RC, Jensen WA, Zibrak JD, Alexander RC, Rose RM. Pulmonary infiltrates and hypoxemia in patients with the acquired immunodeficiency syndrome re-exposed to trimethoprim–sulfamethoxazole. Am Rev Respir Dis 1987;136(4):1003–4.
24. Oshitani N, Matsumoto T, Moriyama Y, Kudoh S, Hirata K, Kuroki T. Drug-induced pneumonitis caused by sulfamethoxazole, trimethoprim during treatment of *Pneumocystis carinii* pneumonia in a patient with refractory ulcerative colitis. J Gastroenterol 1998;33(4):578–81.
25. Hashizume T, Numata H, Matsushita K. [Drug-induced pneumonitis caused by sulfamethoxazole–trimethoprim.] Nihon Kokyuki gakkai Zasshi 2001;39(9):664–7.
26. de Arce Borda AM, Goenaga Sanchez MA. Tremblor producids pox trimetoprim–sulfamethoxazole. [Tremor produced by trimethoprim–sulfamethoxazole.] Neurologia 2000;15(6):264–5.
27. Borucki MJ, Matzke DS, Pollard RB. Tremor induced by trimethoprim-sulfamethoxazole in patients with the acquired immunodeficiency syndrome (AIDS). Ann Intern Med 1988;109(1):77–8.
28. Slavik RS, Rybak MJ, Lerner SA. Trimethoprim/sulfamethoxazole-induced tremor in a patient with AIDS. Ann Pharmacother 1998;32(2):189–92.
29. Whalström B, Nyström-Rosander C, Åberg H, Friman G. Upprepad meningit och perimyokardit efter intag ar trimetoprim. [Recurrent meningitis and perimyocarditis after trimethoprim.] Lakartidningen 1982;79(51):4854–5.
30. Haas EJ. Trimethoprim–sulfamethoxazole: another cause of recurrent meningitis. JAMA 1984;252(3):346.
31. Kremer I, Ritz R, Brunner F. Aseptic meningitis as an adverse effect of co-trimoxazole. N Engl J Med 1983;308(24):1481.
32. Joffe AM, Farley JD, Linden D, Goldsand G. Trimethoprim–sulfamethoxazole-associated aseptic meningitis: case reports and review of the literature. Am J Med 1989;87(3):332–8.

33. Carlson J, Wiholm BE. Trimethoprim associated aseptic meningitis. Scand J Infect Dis 1987;19(6):687–91.

34. Derbes SJ. Trimethoprim-induced aseptic meningitis. JAMA 1984;252(20):2865–6.

35. Hedlund J, Aurelius E, Andersson J. Recurrent encephalitis due to trimethoprim intake. Scand J Infect Dis 1990;22(1):109–12.

36. Capra C, Monza GM, Meazza G, Ramella G. Trimethoprim–sulfamethoxazole-induced aseptic meningitis: case report and literature review. Intensive Care Med 2000;26(2):212–14.

37. Meng MV, St Lezin M. Trimethoprim–sulfamethoxazole induced recurrent aseptic meningitis. J Urol 2000;164(5):1664–5.

38. Antonen J, Hulkkonen J, Pasternack A, Hurme M. Interleukin 6 may be an important mediator of trimethoprim-induced systemic adverse reaction resembling aseptic meningitis. Arch Intern Med 2000;160(13):2066–7.

39. Andrade A, Hilmas E, Walter C. A rare occurrence of trimethoprim/sulfamethoxazole (TMP/SMX)-induced aseptic meningitis in an older woman. J Am Geriatr Soc 2000;48(11):1537–8.

40. Redman RC 4th, Miller JB, Hood M, DeMaio J. Trimethoprim-induced aseptic meningitis in an adolescent male. Pediatrics 2002;110(2 Pt 1):e26.

41. Auxier GG. Aseptic meningitis associated with administration of trimethoprim and sulfamethoxazole. Am J Dis Child 1990;144(2):144–5.

42. Biosca M, de la Figuera M, Garcia-Bragado F, Sampol G. Aseptic meningitis due to trimethoprim–sulfamethoxazole. J Neurol Neurosurg Psychiatry 1986;49(3):332–3.

43. Muller MP, Richardson DC, Walmsley SL. Trimethoprim-sulfamethoxazole induced aseptic meningitis in a renal transplant patient. Clin Nephrol 2001;55(1):80–4.

44. Antonen JA, Saha HH, Hurme M, Pasternack AI. IL-6 may be the key mediator in trimethoprim-induced systemic adverse reaction and aseptic meningitis: a reply to Muller et al. Clin Nephrol 2001;55(6):489–90.

45. Liu LX, Seward SJ, Crumpacker CS. Intravenous trimethoprim–sulfamethoxazole and ataxia. Ann Intern Med 1986;104(3):448.

46. Woody RC, Brewster MA. Adverse effects of trimethoprim–sulfamethoxazole in a child with dihydropteridine reductase deficiency. Dev Med Child Neurol 1990;32(7):639–42.

47. Gilroy N, Gottlieb T, Spring P, Peiris O. Trimethoprim-induced aseptic meningitis and uveitis. Lancet 1997;350(9071):112.

48. Arola O, Peltonen R, Rossi T. Arthritis, uveitis, and Stevens–Johnson syndrome induced by trimethoprim. Lancet 1998;351(9109):1102.

49. Kristinsson JK, Hannesson OB, Sveinsson O, Thorleifsson H. Bilateral anterior uveitis and retinal haemorrhages after administration of trimethoprim. Acta Ophthalmol Scand 1997;75(3):314–15.

50. Schiffman SS, Zervakis J, Westall HL, Graham BG, Metz A, Bennett JL, Heald AE. Effect of antimicrobial and anti-inflammatory medications on the sense of taste. Physiol Behav 2000;69(4–5):413–24.

51. Salkind AR. Acute delirium induced by intravenous trimethoprim–sulfamethoxazole therapy in a patient with the acquired immunodeficiency syndrome. Hum Exp Toxicol 2000;19(2):149–51.

52. Murphy JL, Griswold WR, Reznik VM, Mendoza SA. Trimethoprim/sulfamethoxazole-induced renal tubular acidosis. Child Nephrol Urol 1990;10(1):49–50.

53. Cohen HN, Pearson DW, Thomson JA, Ratcliffe WA, Beastall GH. Trimethoprim and thyroid function. Lancet 1981;1(8221):676–7.

54. Smellie JM, Bantock HM, Thompson BD. Co-trimoxazole and the thyroid. Lancet 1982;2(8289):96.

55. Williamson NL, Frank LA, Hnilica KA. Effects of short-term trimethoprim–sulfamethoxazole administration on thyroid function in dogs. J Am Vet Med Assoc 2002;221(6):802–6.

56. Fox GN. Trimethoprim–sulfamethoxazole-induced hypoglycemia. J Am Board Fam Pract 2000;13(5):386.

57. Mathews WA, Manint JE, Kleiss J. Trimethoprim–sulfamethoxazole-induced hypoglycemia as a cause of altered mental status in an elderly patient. J Am Board Fam Pract 2000;13(3):211–12.

58. Porras MC, Lecumberri JN, Castrillon JL. Trimethoprim–sulfamethoxazole and metabolic acidosis in HIV-infected patients. Ann Pharmacother 1998;32(2):185–9.

59. Smulders YM, de Man AM, Stehouwer CD, Slaats EH. Trimethoprim and fasting plasma homocysteine. Lancet 1998;352(9143):1827–8.

60. Bugge JF. Severe hyperkalaemia induced by trimethoprim in combination with an angiotensin-converting enzyme inhibitor in a patient with transplanted lungs. J Intern Med 1996;240(4):249–51.

61. Velazquez H, Perazella MA, Wright FS, Ellison DH. Renal mechanism of trimethoprim-induced hyperkalemia. Ann Intern Med 1993;119(4):296–301.

62. Reiser IW, Chou SY, Brown MI, Porush JG. Reversal of trimethoprim-induced antikaliuresis. Kidney Int 1996;50(6):2063–9.

63. Eiam-Ong S, Kurtzman NA, Sabatini S. Studies on the mechanism of trimethoprim-induced hyperkalemia. Kidney Int 1996;49(5):1372–8.

64. Schreiber M, Schlanger LE, Chen CB, Lessan-Pezeshki M, Halperin ML, Patnaik A, Ling BN, Kleyman TR. Antikaliuretic action of trimethoprim is minimized by raising urine pH. Kidney Int 1996;49(1):82–7.

65. Greenberg S, Reiser IW, Chou SY, Porush JG. Trimethoprim–sulfamethoxazole induces reversible hyperkalemia. Ann Intern Med 1993;119(4):291–5.

66. Alappan R, Perazella MA, Buller GK. Hyperkalemia in hospitalized patients treated with trimethoprim–sulfamethoxazole. Ann Intern Med 1996;124(3):316–20.

67. Perazella MA. Trimethoprim-induced hyperkalaemia: clinical data, mechanism, prevention and management. Drug Saf 2000;22(3):227–36.

68. Gabriels G, Stockem E, Greven J. Potassium-sparing renal effects of trimethoprim and structural analogues. Nephron 2000;86(1):70–8.

69. Koc M, Bihorac A, Ozener CI, Kantarci G, Akoglu E. Severe hyperkalemia in two renal transplant recipients treated with standard dose of trimethoprim–sulfamethoxazole. Am J Kidney Dis 2000;36(3):E18.

70. Brazille P, Benveniste O, Herson S, Cherin P. Une cause meconnue d'hyperkaliemie: le trimethoprime-sulfamethoxazole. [A cause of unexplained hyperkalemia: trimethoprim–sulfamethoxazole.] Rev Med Interne 2001;22(1):82–3.

71. Margassery S, Bastani B. Life threatening hyperkalemia and acidosis secondary to trimethoprim–sulfamethoxazole treatment. J Nephrol 2001;14(5):410–14.

72. Sheehan MT, Wen SF. Hyperkalemic renal tubular acidosis induced by trimethoprim–sulfamethoxazole in an AIDS patient. Clin Nephrol 1998;50(3):188–93.

73. Gabriels G, Stockem E, Greven J. Hyperkaliämie nach Trimethoprim oder Pentamidin. Eine bisher wenig beachtete Nebenwirkung antimikrobieller Therapiemassnahmen bei AIDS-Patienten. [Hyperkalemia after trimethoprim or pentamidine. Until now, a little noticed side effect of antimicrobial therapeutic measures in AIDS patients.] Dtsch Med Wochenschr 1998;123(45):1351–5.

74. Dreiher J, Porath A. Severe hyponatremia induced by theophylline and trimethoprim. Arch Intern Med 2001;161(2):291–2.

75. Kiefel V, Santoso S, Schmidt S, Salama A, Mueller-Eckhardt C. Metabolite-specific (IgG) and drug-specific antibodies (IgG, IgM) in two cases of trimethoprim–sulfamethoxazole-induced immune thrombocytopenia. Transfusion 1987;27(3):262–5.

76. Stricker RB, Goldberg B. AIDS and pure red cell aplasia. Am J Hematol 1997;54(3):264.

77. Keisu M, Wiholm BE, Palmblad J. Trimethoprim–sulfamethoxazole-associated blood dyscrasias. Ten years' experience of the Swedish spontaneous reporting system. J Intern Med 1990;228(4):353–60.

78. Blackwell EA, Hawson GA, Leer J, Bain B. Acute pancytopenia due to megaloblastic arrest in association with co-trimoxazole. Med J Aust 1978;2(1):38–41.

79. Tulloch AL. Pancytopenia in an infant associated with sulfamethoxazole–trimethoprim therapy. J Pediatr 1976;88(3):499–500.

80. Epstein JH. Photoallergy. A review. Arch Dermatol 1972;106(5):741–8.

81. Fuchs M, Scheid C, Schulz A, Diehl V, Sohngen D. Trimethoprim/sulfamethoxazole prophylaxis impairs function of mobilised autologous peripheral blood stem cells. Bone Marrow Transplant 2000;26(7):815–16.

82. Fishman JA. Prevention of infection caused by Pneumocystis carinii in transplant recipients. Clin Infect Dis 2001;33(8):1397–405.

83. Lambotte O, Costedoat-Chalumeau N, Amoura Z, Piette JC, Cacoub P. Drug-induced hemophagocytosis. Am J Med 2002;112(7):592–3.

84. Muller U. Hämatologische Nebenwirkungen von Medikamenten. [Hematologic side effects of drugs.] Ther Umsch 1987;44(12):942–8.

85. Asmar BI, Maqbool S, Dajani AS. Hematologic abnormalities after oral trimethoprim–sulfamethoxazole therapy in children. Am J Dis Child 1981;135(12):1100–3.

86. Deen JL, von Seidlein L, Pinder M, Walraven GE, Greenwood BM. The safety of the combination artesunate and pyrimethamine–sulfadoxine given during pregnancy. Trans R Soc Trop Med Hyg 2001;95(4):424–8.

87. Poskitt EM, Parkin JM. Effect of trimethoprim–sulphamethoxazole combination on folate metabolism in malnourished children. Arch Dis Child 1972;47(254):626–30.

88. Reynolds EH. Anticonvulsants, folic acid, and epilepsy. Lancet 1973;1(7816):1376–8.

89. Safrin S, Lee BL, Sande MA. Adjunctive folinic acid with trimethoprim-sulfamethoxazole for Pneumocystis carinii pneumonia in AIDS patients is associated with an increased risk of therapeutic failure and death. J Infect Dis 1994;170(4):912–17.

90. Baumgartner A, Hoigné R, Müller U, et al. Medikamentöse Schäden des Blutbildes: Erfahrungen aus dem Komprehensiven Spital-Drug-Monitoring Bern, 1974–1979. Schweiz Med Wochenschr 1982;112:1530.

91. Wang KK, Bowyer BA, Fleming CR, Schroeder KW. Pulmonary infiltrates and eosinophilia associated with sulfasalazine. Mayo Clin Proc 1984;59(5):343–6.

92. Bradley PP, Warden GD, Maxwell JG, Rothstein G. Neutropenia and thrombocytopenia in renal allograft recipients treated with trimethoprim–sulfamethoxazole. Ann Intern Med 1980;93(4):560–2.

93. Hoigne R, Klein U, Muller U. Results of four-week course of therapy of urinary tract infections: a comparative study using trimethoprim with sulfamethoxazole (Bactrim; Roche) and trimethoprim alone. In: Hejzlar M, Semonsky M, Masak S, editors. Advances in Antimicrobial and Antineoplastic Chemotherapy. Munchen-Berlin-Wien: Urban and Schwarzenberg, 1972:1283.

94. Havas L, Fernex M, Lenox-Smith I. The clinical efficacy and tolerance of co-trimoxazole (Bactrim; Septrim). Clin Trials J 1973;3:81.

95. Pedersen-Bjergaard U, Andersen M, Hansen PB. Thrombocytopenia induced by noncytotoxic drugs in Denmark 1968–91. J Intern Med 1996;239(6):509–15.

96. Wiholm BE, Emanuelsson S. Drug-related blood dyscrasias in a Swedish reporting system, 1985–1994. Eur J Haematol Suppl 1996;60:42–6.

97. Barr AL, Whineray M. Immune thrombocytopenia induced by cotrimoxazole. Aust NZ J Med 1980;10(1):54–5.

98. Claas FH, van der Meer JW, Langerak J. Immunological effect of co-trimoxazole on platelets. BMJ 1979;2(6195):898–9.

99. Moeschlin S. Immunological granulocytopenia and agranulocytosis; clinical aspects. Sang 1955;26(1):32–51.

100. Rios Sanchez I, Duarte L, Sanchez Medal L. Agranulocitosis: analisis de 29 episodios en 19 pacientes. [Agranulocytosis. Analysis of 29 episodes in 19 patients.] Rev Invest Clin 1971;23(1):29–42.

101. Yamreudeewong W, Fosnocht BJ, Weixelman JM. Severe thrombocytopenia possibly associated with TMP/SMX therapy. Ann Pharmacother 2002;36(1):78–82.

102. George JN, Raskob GE, Shah SR, Rizvi MA, Hamilton SA, Osborne S, Vondracek T. Drug-induced thrombocytopenia: a systematic review of published case reports. Ann Intern Med 1998;129(11):886–90.

103. Pedersen-Bjergaard U, Andersen M, Hansen PB. Drug-specific characteristics of thrombocytopenia caused by non-cytotoxic drugs. Eur J Clin Pharmacol 1998;54(9–10):701–6.

104. Zerbib F. Les oesophagites médicamenteuses. Hepato-Gastro 1998;5:115–20.

105. Cameron A, Thomas M. Pseudomembranous colitis and co-trimoxazole. BMJ 1977;1(6072):1321.

106. Zehnder D, Kunzi UP, Maibach R, Zoppi M, Halter F, Neftel KA, Muller U, Galeazzi RL, Hess T, Hoigne R. Die Häufigkeit der Antibiotika-assoziierten Kolitis bei hospitalisierten Patienten der Jahre 1974–1991 im 'Comprehensive Hospital Drug Monitoring' Bern/St Gallen. [Frequency of antibiotics-associated colitis in hospitalized patients in 1974–1991 in "Comprehensive Hospital Drug Monitoring," Bern/St. Gallen.] Schweiz Med Wochenschr 1995;125(14):676–83.

107. Munoz SJ, Martinez-Hernandez A, Maddrey WC. Intrahepatic cholestasis and phospholipidosis associated with the use of trimethoprim–sulfamethoxazole. Hepatology 1990;12(2):342–7.

108. Tanner AR. Hepatic cholestasis induced by trimethoprim. BMJ (Clin Res Ed) 1986;293(6554):1072–3.

109. Horak J, Mertl L, Hrabal P. Severe liver injuries due to sulfamethoxazole–trimethoprim and sulfamethoxydiazine. Hepatogastroenterology 1984;31(5):199–200.

110. Ransohoff DF, Jacobs G. Terminal hepatic failure following a small dose of sulfamethoxazole–trimethoprim. Gastroenterology 1981;80(4):816–19.

111. Thies PW, Dull WL. Trimethoprim–sulfamethoxazole-induced cholestatic hepatitis. Inadvertent rechallenge. Arch Intern Med 1984;144(8):1691–2.

112. Tse W, Singer C, Dominick D. Acute fulminant hepatic failure caused by trimethoprim–sulfamethoxazole. Infect Dis Clin Pract 2000;9:302–3.

113. Windecker R, Steffen J, Cascorbi I, Thurmann PA. Co-trimoxazole-induced liver and renal failure. Case report. Eur J Clin Pharmacol 2000;56(2):191–3.

114. Antonow DR. Acute pancreatitis associated with trimethoprim–sulfamethoxazole. Ann Intern Med 1986;104(3):363–5.

115. Bailey RR, Little PJ. Deterioration in renal function in association with co-trimoxazole therapy. Med J Aust 1976;1(24):914, 916.

116. Kalowski S, Nanra RS, Mathew TH, Kincaid-Smith P. Deterioration in renal function in association with co-trimoxazole therapy. Lancet 1973;1(7800):394–7.

117. Horn B, Cottier P. Kreatininkonzentration im Serum vor und unter Behandlung mit Trimethoprim–Sulfamethoxazol. [Serum creatinine concentration prior to and following trimethoprim–sulfamethoxazole (Bactrim) treatment.] Schweiz Med Wochenschr 1974;104(49):1809–12.

118. Naderer O, Nafziger AN, Bertino JS Jr.. Effects of moderate-dose versus high-dose trimethoprim on serum creatinine and creatinine clearance and adverse reactions. Antimicrob Agents Chemother 1997;41(11):2466–70.

119. Trollfors B, Wahl M, Alestig K. Co-trimoxazole, creatinine and renal function. J Infect 1980;2(3):221–6.

120. Kainer G, Rosenberg AR. Effect of co-trimoxazole on the glomerular filtration rate of healthy adults. Chemotherapy 1981;27(4):229–32.

121. Craig WA, Kunin CM. Trimethoprim–sulfamethoxazole: pharmacodynamic effects of urinary pH and impaired renal function. Studies in humans. Ann Intern Med 1973;78(4):491–7.

122. Wong CS, Jelacic S, Habeeb RL, Watkins SL, Tarr PI. The risk of the hemolytic–uremic syndrome after antibiotic treatment of *Escherichia coli* O157:H7 infections. N Engl J Med 2000;342(26):1930–6.

123. Siegel WH. Unusual complication of therapy with sulfamethoxazole-trimethoprim. J Urol 1977;117(3):397.

124. Hattori N, Hino H. Generalized erythematous skin eruptions due to trimethoprim itself and co-trimoxazole. J Dermatol 1998;25(4):269–71.

125. Hoigne R, Sonntag MR, Zoppi M, Hess T, Maibach R, Fritschy D. Occurrence of exanthema in relation to aminopenicillin preparations and allopurinol. N Engl J Med 1987;316(19):1217.

126. Bigby M, Jick S, Jick H, Arndt K. Drug-induced cutaneous reactions. A report from the Boston Collaborative Drug Surveillance Program on 15,438 consecutive inpatients, 1975 to 1982. JAMA 1986;256(24):3358–63.

127. Sonntag MR, Zoppi M, Fritschy D, Maibach R, Stocker F, Sollberger J, Buchli W, Hess T, Hoigne R. Exantheme unter häufig angewandten Antibiotika und anti-bakteriellen Chemotherapeutika (Penicilline, speziell Aminopenicilline, Cephalosporine und Cotrimoxazol) sowie Allopurinol. [Exanthema during frequent use of antibiotics and antibacterial drugs (penicillin, especially aminopenicillin, cephalosporin and cotrimoxazole) as well as allopurinol. Results of The Berne Comprehensive Hospital Drug Monitoring Program.] Schweiz Med Wochenschr 1986;116(5):142–5.

128. Arndt KA, Jick H. Rates of cutaneous reactions to drugs. A report from the Boston Collaborative Drug Surveillance Program. JAMA 1976;235(9):918–23.

129. Silveira C, Belfort R Jr, Muccioli C, Holland GN, Victora CG, Horta BL, Yu F, Nussenblatt RB. The effect of long-term intermittent trimethoprim/sulfamethoxazole treatment on recurrences of toxoplasmic retinochoroiditis. Am J Ophthalmol 2002;134(1):41–6.

130. Mahboob A, Haroon TS. Drugs causing fixed eruptions: a study of 450 cases. Int J Dermatol 1998;37(11):833–8.

131. Ozkaya-Bayazit E, Bayazit H, Ozarmagan G. Drug related clinical pattern in fixed drug eruption. Eur J Dermatol 2000;10(4):288–91.

132. Ozkaya-Bayazit E, Akar U. Fixed drug eruption induced by trimethoprim–sulfamethoxazole: evidence for a link to HLA-A30 B13 Cw6 haplotype. J Am Acad Dermatol 2001;45(5):712–17.

133. Ozkaya-Bayazit E, Gungor H. Trimethoprim-induced fixed drug eruption: positive topical provocation on previously involved and uninvolved skin. Contact Dermatitis 1998;39(2):87–8.

134. Sarkar R, Kaur C, Kanwar AJ. Extensive fixed drug eruption to nimesulide with cross-sensitivity to sulfonamides in a child. Pediatr Dermatol 2002;19(6):553–4.

135. Nwokolo C, Byrne L, Misch KJ. Toxic epidermal necrolysis occurring during treatment with trimethoprim alone. BMJ (Clin Res Ed) 1988;296(6627):970.

136. Revuz JE, Roujeau JC. Advances in toxic epidermal necrolysis. Semin Cutan Med Surg 1996;15(4):258–66.

137. Rzany B, Hering O, Mockenhaupt M, Schroder W, Goerttler E, Ring J, Schopf E. Histopathological and epidemiological characteristics of patients with erythema exudativum multiforme major, Stevens–Johnson syndrome and toxic epidermal necrolysis. Br J Dermatol 1996;135(1):6–11.

138. See S, Mumford JM. Trimethoprim/sulfamethoxazole-induced toxic epidermal necrolysis. Ann Pharmacother 2001;35(6):694–7.

139. Magina S, Lisboa C, Goncalves E, Conceicao F, Leal V, Mesquita-Guimaraes J. A case of toxic epidermal necrolysis treated with intravenous immunoglobin. Br J Dermatol 2000;142(1):191–2.

140. Paquet P, Jacob E, Damas P, Pierard GE. Treatment of drug-induced toxic epidermal necrolysis (Lyell's syndrome) with intravenous human immunoglobulins. Burns 2001;27(6):652–5.

141. Lipozencic J, Milavec-Puretic V, Kotrulja L, Tomicic H, Stulhofer Buzina D. Toxic epidermal necrolysis due to cotrimoxazole. J Eur Acad Dermatol Venereol 2002;16(2):182–3.

142. Nassif A, Bensussan A, Dorothee G, Mami-Chouaib F, Bachot N, Bagot M, Boumsell L, Roujeau JC. Drug specific cytotoxic T cells in the skin lesions of a patient with toxic epidermal necrolysis. J Invest Dermatol 2002;118(4):728–33.

143. Pushker N, Tandon R, Vajpayee RB. Stevens-Johnson syndrome in India — risk factors, ocular manifestations and management. Ophthalmologica 2000;214(4):285–8.

144. Wormser GP, Horowitz HW, Duncanson FP, Forseter G, Javaly K, Alampur SK, Gilroy SA, Lenox T, Rappaport A, Nadelman RB. Low-dose intermittent trimethoprim–sulfamethoxazole for prevention of *Pneumocystis carinii* pneumonia in patients with human immunodeficiency virus infection. Arch Intern Med 1991;151(4):688–92.

145. Canning DA. A suspected case of trimethoprim–sulfamethoxazole-induced loss of fingernails and toenails. J Urol 2000;163(4):1386–7.

146. Neuman MG, Malkiewicz IM, Phillips EJ, Rachlis AR, Ong D, Yeung E, Shear NH. Monitoring adverse drug reactions to sulfonamide antibiotics in human immunodeficiency virus-infected individuals. Ther Drug Monit 2002;24(6):728–36.

147. Choquet-Kastylevsky G, Vial T, Descotes J. Allergic adverse reactions to sulfonamides. Curr Allergy Asthma Rep 2002;2(1):16–25.

148. Hasui M, Kotera F, Tsuji S, Yamamoto A, Taniuchi S, Fujikawa Y, Nakajima M, Yoshioka A, Kobayashi Y. Successful resumption of trimethoprim–sulfamethoxazole after oral desensitisation in patients with chronic granulomatous disease. Eur J Pediatr 2002;161(6):356–7.

149. Pham NH, Baldo BA, Manfredi M, Zerboni R. Fine structural specificity differences of trimethoprim allergenic determinants. Clin Exp Allergy 1996;26(10):1155–60.

150. Greenberger PA, Patterson R. Management of drug allergy in patients with acquired immunodeficiency syndrome. J Allergy Clin Immunol 1987;79(3):484–8.

151. Theodore CM, Holmes D, Rodgers M, McLean KA. Co-trimoxazole desensitization in HIV-seropositive patients. Int J STD AIDS 1998;9(3):158–61.

152. Walmsley SL, Khorasheh S, Singer J, Djurdjev O, Schlech W, Thompson W, Duperval R, Toma E, Tsoukas C, Senay H, Wells P, Uetrecht J, Shear N, Rachlis A, Fong B, McGreer A, Smaill F, Cohen J, Ford P, Gilmour J, Mackie I, Williams K, Montaner J, Zarowny D. A randomized trial of N-acetylcysteine for prevention of trimethoprim-sulfamethoxazole hypersensitivity reactions in Pneumocystis carinii pneumonia prophylaxis (CTN 057). Canadian HIV Trials Network 057 Study Group. J Acquir Immune Defic Syndr Hum Retrovirol 1998;19(5):498–505.

153. Holtzer CD, Flaherty JF Jr, Coleman RL. Cross-reactivity in HIV-infected patients switched from trimethoprim–sulfamethoxazole to dapsone. Pharmacotherapy 1998;18(4):831–5.

154. O'Kane EB, Schneeweiss R. Trimethoprim–sulfamethoxazole-induced sepsis-like syndrome in a patient with AIDS. J Am Board Fam Pract 1996;9(6):448–50.

155. Moran KA, Ales NC, Hemmer PA. Newly diagnosed human immunodeficiency virus after sepsis-like reaction of trimethoprim–sulfamethoxazole. South Med J 2001;94(3):350–2.

156. Yoshizawa S, Yasuoka A, Kikuchi Y, Honda M, Gatanaga H, Tachikawa N, Hirabayashi Y, Oka S. A 5-day course of oral desensitization to trimethoprim/sulfamethoxazole (T/S) in patients with human immunodeficiency virus type-1 infection who were previously intolerant to T/S. Ann Allergy Asthma Immunol 2000;85(3):241–4.

157. Demoly P, Messaad D, Reynes J, Faucherre V, Bousquet J. Trimethoprim–sulfamethoxazole-graded challenge in HIV-infected patients: long-term follow-up regarding efficacy and safety. J Allergy Clin Immunol 2000;105(3):588–9.

158. Nucera E, Schiavino D, Buonomo A, Del Ninno M, Sun JY, Patriarca G. Tolerance induction to cotrimoxazole. Allergy 2000;55(7):681–2.

159. Lopez-Serrano MC, Moreno-Ancillo A. Drug hypersensitivity reactions in HIV-infected patients. Induction of cotrimoxazole tolerance. Allergol Immunol Clin 2000;15:347–51.

160. Sher MR, Suchar C, Lockey RF. Anaphylactic shock induced by oral desensitization to trimethoprim/sulfmethoxazole. J Allergy Immunol 1986;77:133.

161. Torgovnick J, Arsura E. Desensitization to sulfonamides in patients with HIV infection. Am J Med 1990;88(5):548–9.

162. Finegold I. Oral desensitization to trimethoprim–sulfamethoxazole in a patient with acquired immunodeficiency syndrome. J Allergy Clin Immunol 1986;78(5 Pt 1):905–8.

163. Papakonstantinou G, Fuessl H, Hehlmann R. Trimethoprim–sulfamethoxazole desensitization in AIDS. Klin Wochenschr 1988;66(8):351–3.

164. Bonfanti P, Pusterla L, Parazzini F, Libanore M, Cagni AE, Franzetti M, Faggion I, Landonio S, Quirino T. The effectiveness of desensitization versus rechallenge treatment in HIV-positive patients with previous hypersensitivity to TMP–SMX: a randomized multicentric study. C.I.S.A.I. Group. Biomed Pharmacother 2000;54(1):45–9.

165. Leoung GS, Stanford JF, Giordano MF, Stein A, Torres RA, Giffen CA, Wesley M, Sarracco T, Cooper EC, Dratter V, Smith JJ, Frost KR; American Foundation for AIDS Research (amfAR) Community-Based Clinical Trials Network. Trimethoprim–sulfamethoxazole (TMP-SMZ) dose escalation versus direct rechallenge for Pneumocystis carinii pneumonia prophylaxis in human immunodeficiency virus-infected patients with previous adverse reaction to TMP–SMZ. J Infect Dis 2001;184(8):992–7.

166. Peters TR, Edwards KM, Standaert SM. Severe ehrlichiosis in an adolescent taking trimethoprim–sulfamethoxazole. Pediatr Infect Dis J 2000;19(2):170–2.

167. Konttinen A, Perasalo JO, Eisalo A. Sulfonamide hepatitis. Acta Med Scand 1972;191(5):389–91.

168. Huovinen P, Toivanen P. Trimethoprim resistance in Finland after five years' use of plain trimethoprim. BMJ 1980;280(6207):72–4.

169. Turnidge JD. A reappraisal of co-trimoxazole. Med J Aust 1988;148(6):296–305.

170. Mates A, Eyny D, Philo S. Antimicrobial resistance trends in Shigella serogroups isolated in Israel, 1990–1995. Eur J Clin Microbiol Infect Dis 2000;19(2):108–11.

171. Whitney CG, Farley MM, Hadler J, Harrison LH, Lexau C, Reingold A, Lefkowitz L, Cieslak PR, Cetron M, Zell ER, Jorgensen JH, Schuchat A; Active Bacterial Core Surveillance Program of the Emerging Infections Program Network. Increasing prevalence of multidrug-resistant Streptococcus pneumoniae in the United States. N Engl J Med 2000;343(26):1917–24.

172. Abou-Eisha A, Creus A, Marcos R. Genotoxic evaluation of the antimicrobial drug, trimethoprim, in cultured human lymphocytes. Mutat Res 1999;440(2):157–62.

173. Sorensen PJ, Jensen MK. Cytogenetic studies in patients treated with trimethoprim–sulfamethoxazole. Mutat Res 1981;89(1):91–4.

174. Guillebaud J. Sulpha–trimethoprim combinations and male infertility. Lancet 1978;2(8088):523.

175. Murdia A, Mathur V, Kothari LK, Singh KP. Sulpha–trimethoprim combinations and male fertility. Lancet 1978;2(8085):375–6.

176. Brigg GG, Freedman RK, Jaffe SJ. A Reference Guide to Fetal and Neonatal Risk: Drugs in Pregnancy and Lactation. 3rd ed. Baltimore-Hong Kong-London-Sydney: Williams and Wilkins, 1990:621.

177. Hernandez-Diaz S, Werler MM, Walker AM, Mitchell AA. Folic acid antagonists during pregnancy and the risk of birth defects. N Engl J Med 2000;343(22):1608–14.

178. Richardson MP, Osrin D, Donaghy S, Brown NA, Hay P, Sharland M. Spinal malformations in the fetuses of HIV infected women receiving combination antiretroviral therapy and co-trimoxazole. Eur J Obstet Gynecol Reprod Biol 2000;93(2):215–17.

179. Pirmohamed M, Alfirevic A, Vilar J, Stalford A, Wilkins EG, Sim E, Park BK. Association analysis of drug metabolizing enzyme gene polymorphisms in HIV-positive patients with co-trimoxazole hypersensitivity. Pharmacogenetics 2000;10(8):705–13.

180. Para MF, Finkelstein D, Becker S, Dohn M, Walawander A, Black JR. Reduced toxicity with gradual initiation of trimethoprim–sulfamethoxazole as primary prophylaxis for Pneumocystis carinii pneumonia: AIDS Clinical Trials Group 268. J Acquir Immune Defic Syndr 2000;24(4):337–43.

181. Rabaud C, Charreau I, Izard S, Raffi F, Meiffredy V, Leport C, Guillemin F, Yeni P, Aboulker JP, Delta trial group. Adverse reactions to cotrimoxazole in HIV-infected patients: predictive factors and subsequent HIV disease progression. Scand J Infect Dis 2001;33(10):759–64.

182. O'Reilly RA, Motley CH. Racemic warfarin and trimethoprim–sulfamethoxazole interaction in humans. Ann Intern Med 1979;91(1):34–6.

183. Chafin CC, Ritter BA, James A, Self TH. Hospital admission due to warfarin potentiation by TMP-SMX. Nurse Pract 2000;25(12):73–5.

184. Penning-van Beest FJ, van Meegen E, Rosendaal FR, Stricker BH. Drug interactions as a cause of

overanticoagulation on phenprocoumon or acenocoumarol predominantly concern antibacterial drugs. Clin Pharmacol Ther 2001;69(6):451–7.

185. Visser LE, Penning-van Bees FJ, Kasbergen AA, De Smet PA, Vulto AG, Hofman A, Stricker BH. Overanticoagulation associated with combined use of anti-bacterial drugs and acenocoumarol or phenprocoumon anticoagulants. Thromb Haemost 2002;88(5):705–10.

186. Rees CA, Lennard L, Lilleyman JS, Maddocks JL. Disturbance of 6-mercaptopurine metabolism by cotrimoxazole in childhood lymphoblastic leukaemia. Cancer Chemother Pharmacol 1984;12(2):87–9.

187. Ferrazzini G, Klein J, Sulh H, Chung D, Griesbrecht E, Koren G. Interaction between trimethoprim–sulfamethoxazole and methotrexate in children with leukemia. J Pediatr 1990;117(5):823–6.

188. Rusterholz D, Schlegel C. Infektiose Aspekte des Morbus Wegener. [Infectious aspects of Wegener's granulomatosis.] Schweiz Med Wochenschr 2000;(Suppl 125):41S–3S.

189. de Araujo M, Seguro AC. Trimethoprim–sulfamethoxazole (TMP/SMX) potentiates indinavir nephrotoxicity. Antivir Ther 2002;7(3):181–4.

190. Ringden O, Myrenfors P, Klintmalm G, Tyden G, Ost L. Nephrotoxicity by co-trimoxazole and cyclosporin in transplanted patients. Lancet 1984;1(8384):1016–17.

191. Thompson JF, Chalmers DH, Hunnisett AG, Wood RF, Morris PJ. Nephrotoxicity of trimethoprim and cotrimoxazole in renal allograft recipients treated with cyclosporine. Transplantation 1983;36(2):204–6.

192. de Vries PL. Lithiumintoxicatie bij gelijktijdig gebruik van trimethoprim. [Lithium intoxication due to simultaneous use of trimethoprim.] Ned Tijdschr Geneeskd 2001;145(11):539–40.

193. Yang CH, Yang LJ, Jaing TH, Chan HL. Toxic epidermal necrolysis following combination of methotrexate and trimethoprim-sulfamethoxazole. Int J Dermatol 2000;39(8):621–3.

194. Steuer A, Gumpel JM. Methotrexate and trimethoprim: a fatal interaction. Br J Rheumatol 1998;37(1):105–6.

195. Richards AJ. Re: Interaction between methotrexate and trimethoprim. Br J Rheumatol 1998;37(7):806.

196. Grimmer SF, Allen WL, Back DJ, Breckenridge AM, Orme M, Tjia J. The effect of cotrimoxazole on oral contraceptive steroids in women. Contraception 1983;28(1):53–9.

197. Ilario MJ, Ruiz JE, Axiotis CA. Acute fulminant hepatic failure in a woman treated with phenytoin and trimethoprim–sulfamethoxazole. Arch Pathol Lab Med 2000;124(12):1800–3.

198. Trujillo TC, Nolan PE. Antiarrhythmic agents: drug interactions of clinical significance. Drug Saf 2000;23(6):509–32.

199. Ribera E, Pou L, Fernandez-Sola A, Campos F, Lopez RM, Ocana I, Ruiz I, Pahissa A. Rifampin reduces concentrations of trimethoprim and sulfamethoxazole in serum in human immunodeficiency virus-infected patients. Antimicrob Agents Chemother 2001;45(11):3238–41.

200. Guha Thakurta A, Mandal SK, Ganguly K, Dastidar SG, Chakrabarty AN. A new powerful antibacterial synergistic combination of trimethoprim and trimeprazine. Acta Microbiol Immunol Hung 2000;47(1):21–8.

201. Lee BL, Safrin S, Makrides V, Gambertoglio JG. Zidovudine, trimethoprim, and dapsone pharmacokinetic interactions in patients with human immunodeficiency virus infection. Antimicrob Agents Chemother 1996;40(5):1231–6.

202. Streeter AM, Shum HY, O'Neill BJ. The effect of drugs on the microbiological assay of serum folic acid and vitamin B12 levels. Med J Aust 1970;1(18):900–1.

Trimetrexate

General Information

Trimetrexate is a lipid-soluble analogue of methotrexate that has been used in the management of *Pneumocystis jiroveci* in patients with AIDS when other therapy has proved ineffective. It has also been used as an antineoplastic drug in the management of various solid tumors. It is given with leucovorin (folinic acid) to minimize hematological toxicity. Trimetrexate can cause neutropenia and/or thrombocytopenia (SEDA-12, 704) (1,2). Fever and raised liver transaminases, while uncommon, have been noticed. The efficacy of trimetrexate is not as high as that of co-trimoxazole and the recurrence rate is markedly higher (3).

References

1. Hughes WT. *Pneumocystis carinii* pneumonitis. N Engl J Med 1987;317(16):1021–3.
2. Allegra CJ, Chabner BA, Tuazon CU, Ogata-Arakaki D, Baird B, Drake JC, Simmons JT, Lack EE, Shelhamer JH, Balis F, et al. Trimetrexate for the treatment of *Pneumocystis carinii* pneumonia in patients with the acquired immunodeficiency syndrome. N Engl J Med 1987;317(16):978–85.
3. Masur H. Prevention and treatment of *pneumocystis* pneumonia. N Engl J Med 1992;327(26):1853–60.

Trimipramine

See also Tricyclic antidepressants

General Information

Trimipramine is a sedating tricyclic antidepressant that has been used as a hypnotic (1); it shares this activity with other drugs of its class, notably amitriptyline, dosulepin, doxepin, and trazodone, and with the tetracyclics mianserin and mirtazapine. Trimipramine may be preferred for this purpose, since it has less effect on sleep architecture, including REM sleep (2), and has only a modest propensity to produce rebound insomnia in a subset of patients (3). Sedative antidepressants may be particularly appropriate for individuals at risk of benzodiazepine abuse and patients with chronic pain (4). The usual pattern of tricyclic adverse effects, especially antimuscarinic and hypotensive effects and weight gain, can be expected. Some authors, enthusiastic about GABA enhancers, contend that antidepressants are not useful hypnotic alternatives (5).

Antidepressant drugs of various classes (tricyclics, monoamine oxidase inhibitors, SSRIs) have broad efficacy in generalized anxiety and in panic disorder, for which they are the treatments of choice (6,7). While not likely to cause benzodiazepine-like dependence or abuse, they do have a significant therapeutic latency, and the older drugs are very toxic in overdose.

References

1. Settle EC Jr, Ayd FJ Jr. Trimipramine: twenty years' worldwide clinical experience. J Clin Psychiatry 1980;41(8):266–74.
2. Dunleavy DL, Brezinova V, Oswald I, Maclean AW, Tinker M. Changes during weeks in effects of tricyclic drugs on the human sleeping brain. Br J Psychiatry 1972;120(559):663–72.
3. Hohagen F, Montero RF, Weiss E, Lis S, Schonbrunn E, Dressing H, Riemann D, Berger M. Treatment of primary insomnia with trimipramine: an alternative to benzodiazepine hypnotics? Eur Arch Psychiatry Clin Neurosci 1994;244(2):65–72.
4. Stiefel F, Stagno D. Management of insomnia in patients with chronic pain conditions. CNS Drugs 2004;18(5):285–96.
5. Laux G. [Current status of treatment with benzodiazepines.] Nervenarzt 1995;66(5):311–22.
6. Lader M. Psychiatric disorders. In: Speight T, Holford N, editors. Avery's Drug Treatment. 4th ed. Auckland: ADIS International Press, 1997:1437.
7. Menkes DB. Antidepressant drugs. New Ethicals 1994;31:101.

Triperaqulne

General Information

Triperaquine is a 4-aminoquinoline derivative, the adverse reaction pattern of which is unknown. The WHO Scientific Group's report concerning this drug dates from 1984 and there seems to be little or no later information about it in humans.

Triptans

General Information

The triptans are agonists at 5-hydroxytryptamine (5-HT$_{1b/1d}$) receptors, used in the treatment of migraine. They include almotriptan, avitriptan, eletriptan, frovatriptan, naratriptan, rizatriptan, sumatriptan, and zolmitriptan (all rINNs). The way in which the triptans produce their therapeutic effect is not clear. Sumatriptan penetrates the blood–brain barrier poorly and presumably acts peripherally on extracranial blood vessels.

Sumatriptan

Sumatriptan was the first drug of its type to be introduced and has been reviewed (SEDA-18, 171). Most of the information about drugs in this group relates to sumatriptan.

Sumatriptan is effective in the treatment of all features of the headache phase of an acute attack of migraine (SEDA-18, 171) (1). It is available as tablets and suppositories, as prefilled syringes for self-administered subcutaneous injection, and as intranasal spray. Its systemic availability is high (96%) after subcutaneous injection, but rather low (14%) after oral administration because of first-pass metabolism. Its half-life is short (2 hours) and 80% is removed by metabolism. The principal metabolite is an inactive indoleacetic acid analogue. Propranolol, flunarizine, and pizotifen, drugs that are all commonly used in migraine prophylaxis, do not affect the pharmacokinetics of sumatriptan (2,3).

A high proportion of patients respond to a single standard dose of therapy, with minor or mild adverse effects. Because of the short half-life, recurrence of headache within 24 hours is common (50%) but can be effectively treated by a second dose. Any adverse effect is also likely to be brief. The most common adverse effects are a feeling of pressure/stiffness in the neck and throat or of pressure/tightness or pain in the chest. Tingling sensations in the head and arms, dizziness, and tiredness are also commonly reported. Dyspnea can occur in patients with obstructive lung disease. Local reactions at the injection site are usually mild. The reported frequencies of these adverse effects vary widely between clinical trials and postmarketing surveys; this may be attributable to selection of patients in trials and differences in the questionnaires used to evaluate unwanted effects (4,5). Allergic reactions are rare.

Rizatriptan

The available data on rizatriptan have been reviewed. Only safety aspects are mentioned here. With oral administration, adverse effects were mild and transient in placebo controlled trials. Digestive intolerance, dizziness, somnolence, weakness and fatigue, and pain or pressure sensations were the most commonly mentioned (6).

Zolmitriptan

The available data on zolmitriptan have been reviewed. Only safety aspects are mentioned here. Orally administered zolmitriptan appears to have been generally well tolerated in placebo-controlled studies (7). The most commonly reported adverse events are weakness, heaviness or tightness (other than in the chest), dry mouth, nausea, dizziness, somnolence, paresthesia, a sensation of warmth, and chest pain. They were mild to moderate and resolved without the need for intervention or drug withdrawal. Electrocardiographic changes were as frequent with placebo as with zolmitriptan and were not associated with chest tightness or pressure; changes suggesting an ischemic event were not recorded. Nevertheless, zolmitriptan is not recommended in patients with ischemic heart disease.

A spinal cord infarct temporarily related to zolmitriptan use has been reported after the use of zolmitriptan in a 50-year-old woman with a history of migraine (8).

Comparisons between triptans

Four randomized, double-blind clinical trials in which rizatriptan was compared with sumatriptan have been reviewed (9). The two drugs have similar safety profiles, but the frequency of adverse effects depends largely on the dose, which varied from trial to trial. Adverse events reported in over 5% of patients were somnolence, dizziness, weakness/fatigue, nausea and vomiting, abdominal pain, and chest pain.

Seven triptans have been compared and rated as generally very well tolerated (10). Naratriptan, almotriptan, and frovatriptan were considered to have the best safety profiles, although the differences are minor. Coronary vasoconstriction is a potential risk of the entire class, but the risk is minimal in the absence of coronary artery disease or uncontrolled hypertension; significant vascular disease is therefore a hazard of using any of the triptans. Patient preference, however, appears to be more closely related to efficacy than to tolerance.

Organs and Systems

Cardiovascular

Particularly when injected, sumatriptan can cause a transient increase in both systolic and diastolic blood pressures; oral doses, which are usually higher, have this effect to a lesser extent. It is unwise to use sumatriptan in patients with uncontrolled severe hypertension.

Some of the minor discomfort often experienced (tingling, flushing, sensations of heat or cold) may also reflect cardiovascular effects.

Coronary vasoconstriction is a potential risk of all triptans, but the risk is minimal in the absence of coronary artery disease or uncontrolled hypertension. Chest tightness and pain are reported in up to 15% of patients taking sumatriptan and are presumed to be due to vasoconstriction of the coronary arteries. Myocardial infarction has been reported and as a consequence sumatriptan should not be used in patients with cardiovascular disease (11). Intravenous sumatriptan causes some coronary vasoconstriction during diagnostic angiography. Myocardial infarction occurred in a patient who had received sumatriptan 6 mg subcutaneously, but the causal association was not clear.

Cardiac dysrhythmias can occur occasionally.

- A 41-year-old otherwise perfectly healthy woman developed the typical symptoms of a migraine attack after an aerobics class followed by a sauna and took sumatriptan 100 mg (12). She collapsed half an hour later and a resuscitation team diagnosed ventricular fibrillation, which was converted to ventricular tachycardia and later to sinus rhythm. Neither the electrocardiogram nor enzyme changes suggested myocardial infarction. She remained comatose and died 6 weeks later. At autopsy there was no evidence of atherosclerotic coronary disease or any other underlying cardiac disorder.
- A 34-year-old man with migraine had palpitation after taking sumatriptan by nasal spray for a severe headache (13). A similar episode had occurred after he had previously taken sumatriptan. He had atrial fibrillation with a rapid ventricular rate. Sinus rhythm returned spontaneously within a few hours. No structural cardiac abnormality was detected.

Myocardial ischemia secondary to coronary spasm was the putative trigger of atrial fibrillation in the latter case.

Vasoconstriction leading to organ ischemia has been repeatedly reported with triptans. The risk is very low in the absence of pre-existing arterial disease.

Nevertheless, cases of myocardial infarction, mesenteric ischemia, and ischemic colitis have been described, as has splenic infarction (14).

- A 48-year-old woman with a low risk of atherosclerotic disease who was not taking oral contraception was admitted with sudden heavy pain in the left hypochondrium. Routine tests were normal, but there was a triangular hypodensity in the spleen on computerized tomography consistent with a splenic infarct. There was a history of postoperative venous thrombosis 15 years before, but tests for thrombophilia were all normal. No source of embolism was identified in the heart or proximal arteries. She had repeatedly taken zolmitriptan over the previous few months for migraine, and the symptoms started 3 hours after the most recent dose.

The temporal relation and the absence of an alternative cause to explain the infarct led the authors to conclude that zolmitriptan had been causative.

Nervous system

One of the main drawbacks of acute migraine therapies, including 5-HT$_{1a}$ receptor agonists, is that headache recurs within 24 hours in about one-third of patients who initially experienced relief after first dosing. Similar recurrence rates and mean time to recurrence are observed for the new triptans as for sumatriptan (15). An increase in migraine frequency is usually the first sign of a developing drug-induced headache. It occurs with sumatriptan and is also reported with the new triptans (16). Headache has also been reported with chronic sumatriptan use and abuse (SEDA-20, 193).

The role of sumatriptan and ergotamine in drug-induced headache has been surveyed in over 2000 patients at a regional headache clinic (17). About 600 had taken ergot derivatives previously and a similar number had used sumatriptan, while nearly 250 had experience of both. Drug overuse was defined as the use of at least one dose of either drug on 18 or more days every month for at least 3 months. By these criteria the rates of ergotamine and sumatriptan overuse were estimated at 14 and 3.5% respectively. Drug-induced headache was much more common among ergotamine overusers than sumatriptan overusers (68 versus 32%).

Fatal cerebellar infarction has been described in a 39-year-old man who took sumatriptan 100 mg for an acute attack of migraine. The cerebellar infarct was diagnosed at autopsy, and intracranial vasospasm was thought to be the likely mechanism (18). It should be noted that stroke has also been documented in patients with migraine, independently of drug treatment.

Akathisia occurred in five fairly young patients after subcutaneous or oral sumatriptan (19). The symptoms were short-lived. Increased serotonergic activity, leading to inhibition of nigrostriatal dopaminergic neurons and extrapyramidal symptoms, was the postulated mechanism. A similar mechanism has been thought to provoke the same symptoms with serotonin re-uptake inhibitors.

Sensory systems

Nasal spray sumatriptan can cause taste disturbance, described as a bad, bitter, unpleasant, or unusual taste (20).

Gastrointestinal

Ischemic colitis has been associated with the use of sumatriptan. Retrospective review and analysis of postmarketing reports showed seven confirmed cases (colonoscopy and/or biopsy) and another has been reported (21). Seven of the patients were women. Sumatriptan was mainly given subcutaneously, the dosages were not excessive, and the median time between the last administration to the onset of symptoms was less than 24 hours in only four patients. All the patients recovered on withdrawal of sumatriptan. Although many of these patients were using other drugs, particularly beta-blocking and NSAIDs, confusing the analysis, the authors suggested that vasoconstrictor effects in the mesenteric circulation associated with the use of sumatriptan played a causative role in inducing the ischemia.

- Two women were investigated for cramping abdominal pain and bloody diarrhea (22). In only one did the episodes completely disappear after withdrawal of sumatriptan. The other underwent an exploratory laparotomy and right hemicolectomy for transmural bowel necrosis.

Nausea, vomiting, and taste disturbances are more common with sumatriptan than placebo (SEDA-19, 207).

Second-Generation Effects

Teratogenicity

There are data from the Swedish Medical Birth Registry relating to 912 infants, whose mothers, at their first antenatal visit, had reported using migraine therapies, in most cases (658) sumatriptan (23). There was no increase in the rate of congenital malformations; slightly more infants than expected were preterm and had a birth weight lower than 2500 g, but none of the differences was statistically significant. These data suggest that sumatriptan is not teratogenic.

Susceptibility Factors

Age

Because of limited experience, sumatriptan is best avoided in children and elderly people.

Other features of the patient

Significant vascular disease is a contraindication to the use of any of the triptans (SEDA-20, 192).

It has been suggested that triptans should not be used in patients with basilar or familial hemiplegic migraine, although some successes have been reported without adverse effects (24).

Drug Administration

Drug formulations

Sumatriptan is available as film-coated tablets, as prefilled syringes for self-administered subcutaneous injection, as intranasal spray, and in a formulation for rectal

use. Sumatriptan suppositories appear to be well tolerated: reported adverse events were similar to those during oral or subcutaneous treatment of patients with migraine. Local events involving the anus or rectum were rarely observed (25,26).

Drug–Drug Interactions

Beta-blockers

In four double-blind, placebo-controlled, randomized, crossover studies in 51 healthy subjects a single dose of rizatriptan 10 mg was administered after administration of propranolol 60 and 120 mg bd, nadolol 80 mg bd, metoprolol 100 mg bd, or placebo for 7 days (27). Propranolol 60 or 120 mg bd increased the AUC of rizatriptan by about 67% and the C_{max} by about 75%. Nadolol and metoprolol had no effects.

Similarly, in healthy volunteers co-administration of propranolol resulted in a 56% increase in the AUC of zolmitriptan and a 11% decrease in the AUC of its active metabolite (28).

Clarithromycin

In an open, randomized, 2-way crossover study in 24 healthy volunteers clarithromycin 500 mg orally every 12 hours for 4 days had no effects on the pharmacokinetics of a single oral dose of sumatriptan 50 mg (29).

Ergot alkaloids

The use of sumatriptan is discouraged and even considered contraindicated together with or within 24 hours after ergotamine or ergotamine-type medications, such as methysergide. The contraindication is based on the possibility of severe prolonged vasospasm with the combined use of agents with agonist properties at the same receptors.

- A 20-year-old woman developed generalized tonic–clonic seizures after she took sumatriptan 6 mg followed by three tablets of ergonovine for postpartum headache (30). Cerebral angiography 1 day later showed multiple narrowed segments in the vertebrobasillar and middle cerebral arteries.
- A myocardial infarction occurred in a 43-year-old woman with no known coronary artery disease who was taking methysergide and injected herself with sumatriptan 6 mg because of persisting headache (31).

5-HT re-uptake inhibitors

On theoretical grounds, sumatriptan should not be used with 5-HT re-uptake inhibitors, since this combination could theoretically cause serotonin toxicity. Although case series have suggested that sumatriptan can be safely combined with SSRIs, there are occasional reports of toxicity (SEDA-22, 14).

Treatment of 12 healthy volunteers with paroxetine (20 mg/day for 14 days) did not alter the pharmacokinetics or pharmacodynamic effects of an acute dose of rizatriptan (10 mg orally) (32). These data are reassuring, but it is possible that sporadic cases of 5-HT neurotoxicity could still occur when a triptan is combined with an SSRI.

Lithium

On theoretical grounds, sumatriptan should not be used with lithium. However, a review of the subject found little substantiation for a severe interaction between sumatriptan and lithium (33).

Monoamine oxidase inhibitors

Some of the triptans are metabolized by monoamine oxidase and they should not be used with monoamine oxidase inhibitors. This includes almotriptan (34), rizatriptan (35), sumatriptan (36), and zolmitriptan (28). The effect of moclobemide on the pharmacokinetics of almotriptan was less than with other triptans (34).

References

1. Morley J. Beta agonists and asthma mortality: déja vu. Clin Exp Allergy 1992;22(7):724–5.
2. Rose FC. Sumatriptan: an overview. Headache Q 1993;4(Suppl 2):37.
3. Scott AK. Sumatriptan clinical pharmacokinetics. Clin Pharmacokinet 1994;27(5):337–44.
4. Dahlof C, Ekbom K, Persson L. Clinical experiences from Sweden on the use of subcutaneously administered sumatriptan in migraine and cluster headache. Arch Neurol 1994;51(12):1256–61.
5. Ottervanger JP, van Witsen TB, Valkenburg HA, Grobbee DE, Stricker BH. Adverse reactions attributed to sumatriptan. A postmarketing study in general practice. Eur J Clin Pharmacol 1994;47(4):305–9.
6. Fink HA, MacDonald R, Rutks IR, Nelson DB, Wilt TJ. Sildenafil for male erectile dysfunction: a systematic review and meta-analysis. Arch Intern Med 2002;162(12):1349–60.
7. Evers S, Gralow I, Bauer B, Suhr B, Buchheister A, Husstedt IW, Ringelstein EB. Sumatriptan and ergotamine overuse and drug-induced headache: a clinicoepidemiologic study. Clin Neuropharmacol 1999;22(4):201–6.
8. Vijayan N, Peacock JH. Spinal cord infarction during use of zolmitriptan: a case report. Headache 2000;40(1):57–60.
9. Tfelt-Hansen P, Ryan RE Jr. Oral therapy for migraine: comparisons between rizatriptan and sumatriptan. A review of four randomized, double-blind clinical trials. Neurology 2000;55(9 Suppl 2):S19–24.
10. Stauffer JC, Ruiz V, Morard JD. Subaortic obstruction after sildenafil in a patient with hypertropic cardiomyopathy. N Engl J Med 1999;341(9):700–1.
11. Committee on Safety of Medicines. Sumatriptan (Imigran) and chest pain. Curr Probl 1992;34:2.
12. Hicklin LA, Ryan C, Wong DK, Hinton AC. Nose-bleeds after sildenafil (Viagra). J R Soc Med 2002;95(8):402–3.
13. Morgan DR, Trimble M, McVeigh GE. Atrial fibrillation associated with sumatriptan. BMJ 2000;321(7256):275.
14. Bellaiche G, Radu B, Boucard M, Ley G, Slama JL. Infarctus splénique associé à la prise de zolmitriptan. [Splenic infarction associated with zolmitriptan use.] Gastroenterol Clin Biol 2002;26(3):298.
15. Monastero R, Pipia C, Camarda LK, Camarda R. Intracerebral haemorrhage associated with sildenafil citrate. J Neurol 2001;248(2):141–2.
16. Langtry HD, Markham A. Sildenafil: a review of its use in erectile dysfunction. Drugs 1999;57(6):967–89.
17. Smith MA, Ross MB. Oral 5-HT$_1$ receptor agonists for migraine: comparative considerations. Formulary 1999;34:324–8.
18. Jayamaha JE, Street MK. Fatal cerebellar infarction in a migraine sufferer whilst receiving sumatriptan. Intensive Care Med 1995;21(1):82–3.
19. Lopez-Alemany M, Ferrer-Tuset C, Bernacer-Alpera B. Akathisia and acute dystonia induced by sumatriptan. J Neurol 1997;244(2):131–2.
20. Limmroth V, Kazarawa Z, Fritsche G, Diener HC. Headache after frequent use of serotonin agonists zolmitriptan and naratriptan. Lancet 1999;353(9150):378.
21. Knudsen JF, Friedman B, Chen M, Goldwasser JE. Ischemic colitis and sumatriptan use. Arch Intern Med 1998;158(17):1946–8.
22. Liu JJ, Brandhagen DJ, Ardolf JC. Sumatriptan-associated mesenteric ischemia. Ann Intern Med 2000;132(7):597.
23. Kallen B, Lygner PE. Delivery outcome in women who used drugs for migraine during pregnancy with special reference to sumatriptan. Headache 2001;41(4):351–6.
24. Klapper J, Mathew N, Nett R. Triptans in the treatment of basilar migraine and migraine with prolonged aura. Headache 2001;41(10):981–4.
25. Perry CM, Markham A. Sumatriptan. An updated review of its use in migraine. Drugs 1998;55(6):889–922.
26. Tepper SJ, Cochran A, Hobbs S, Woessner M, Saiers J. Sumatriptan suppositories for the acute treatment of migraine. S2B351 Study Group. Int J Clin Pract 1998;52(1):31–5.
27. Goldberg MR, Sciberras D, De Smet M, Lowry R, Tomasko L, Lee Y, Olah TV, Zhao J, Vyas KP, Halpin R, Kari PH, James I. Influence of beta-adrenoceptor antagonists on the pharmacokinetics of rizatriptan, a 5-HT$_{1B/1D}$ agonist: differential effects of propranolol, nadolol and metoprolol. Br J Clin Pharmacol 2001;52(1):69–76.
28. Rolan P. Potential drug interactions with the novel antimigraine compound zolmitriptan (Zomig, 311C90). Cephalalgia 1997;17(Suppl 18):21–7.
29. Moore KH, Leese PT, McNeal S, Gray P, O'Quinn S, Bye C, Sale M. The pharmacokinetics of sumatriptan when administered with clarithromycin in healthy volunteers. Clin Ther 2002;24(4):583–94.
30. Dooley M, Faulds D. Rizatriptan: a review of its efficacy in the management of migraine. Drugs 1999;58(4):699–723.
31. Laine K, Raasakka T, Mantynen J, Saukko P. Fatal cardiac arrhythmia after oral sumatriptan. Headache 1999;39(7):511–12.
32. Goldberg MR, Lowry RC, Musson DG, Birk KL, Fisher A, De Puy ME, Shadle CR. Lack of pharmacokinetic and pharmacodynamic interaction between rizatriptan and paroxetine. J Clin Pharmacol 1999;39(2):192–9.
33. Gardner DM, Lynd LD. Sumatriptan contraindications and the serotonin syndrome. Ann Pharmacother 1998;32(1):33–8.
34. Fleishaker JC, Ryan KK, Jansat JM, Carel BJ, Bell DJ, Burke MT, Azie NE. Effect of MAO-A inhibition on the pharmacokinetics of almotriptan, an antimigraine agent in humans. Br J Clin Pharmacol 2001;51(5):437–41.
35. Van Haarst AD, Van Gerven JM, Cohen AF, De Smet M, Sterrett A, Birk KL, Fisher AL, De Puy ME, Goldberg MR, Musson DG. The effects of moclobemide on the pharmacokinetics of the 5-HT$_{1B/1D}$ agonist rizatriptan in healthy volunteers. Br J Clin Pharmacol 1999;48(2):190–6.
36. Blier P, Bergeron R. The safety of concomitant use of sumatriptan and antidepressant treatments. J Clin Psychopharmacol 1995;15(2):106–9.

Tritiozine

General Information

Tritiozine is a non-anticholinergic, antisecretory agent. It has been associated with drowsiness and occasional slight increases in transaminases (1).

Organs and Systems

Nervous system

Predominantly sensory neuropathies with Wallerian degeneration of the myelinated fibers occurred in three patients taking tritiozine (2).

Liver

Acute hepatitis has been attributed to tritiozine (3,4).

References

1. Pellegrini R. Clinical effects of trithiozine, a newer gastric anti-secretory agent. J Int Med Res 1979;7(5):452–8.
2. Littman A. Potent acid reduction and risk of enteric infection. Lancet 1990;335(8683):222.
3. Navarro Izquierdo A, Perez Gomez A, Hernandez Guio C. Hepatitis aguda por tritiozine. [Acute hepatitis caused by trithiozine.] Rev Clin Esp 1982;164(2):129–30.
4. Vazquez Cruz DJ, Nieto Calvet M, Rodriguez Galipienzo JM, Alvarez Fernandez F, Serrano Figueras S. Hepatitis aguda tras la administracion de tritiozina. A proposito de un caso. [Acute hepatitis following the administration of trithiozine. Apropos of a case.] Rev Esp Enferm Apar Dig 1983;63(2):188–92.

Troleandomycin

See also Macrolide antibiotics

General Information

Troleandomycin is a macrolide antibiotic with actions and uses similar to those of erythromycin.

Organs and Systems

Endocrine

Serum TSH concentrations are moderately but significantly reduced by troleandomycin compared with josamycin or placebo given over 10 days. At the same time serum estradiol concentration was significantly increased (1).

Liver

Most reports associating cholestatic jaundice with the concomitant use of oral contraceptives and macrolides have implicated troleandomycin (2–5). The exact mechanism of this interaction has not been established.

Troleandomycin possibly inhibits the metabolism of estrogens and progestogens (6). In most patients jaundice persisted for more than a month after the antibiotic was withdrawn.

Drug–Drug Interactions

Alprazolam

Troleandomycin may inhibit the metabolism of alprazolam by inhibiting CYP3A4 (7).

Carbamazepine

Troleandomycin can cause carbamazepine toxicity by inhibiting CYP3A4 (8).

Ecabapide

Troleandomycin may inhibit the metabolism of ecabapide, a gastric prokinetic drug, by inhibiting CYP3A4 (9).

Ergot alkaloids

Clinically severe interactions between troleandomycin and ergotamine (10–13), resulting in ischemia of the extremities, probably result from inhibition of the metabolism of the ergopeptides (14,15), with raised serum concentrations of dihydroergotamine (16,17).

Quinine

Troleandomycin is an in vitro competitive inhibitor of quinine 3-hydroxylation, which is mediated by CYP3A4, and may therefore interact when co-administered with quinine (18).

References

1. Uzzan B, Nicolas P, Perret G, Vassy R, Tod M, Petitjean O. Effects of troleandomycin and josamycin on thyroid hormone and steroid serum levels, liver function tests and microsomal monooxygenases in healthy volunteers: a double blind placebo-controlled study. Fundam Clin Pharmacol 1991;5(6):513–26.
2. Claudel S, Euvrard P, Bory R, Chavaillon A, Paliard P. Cholestase intrahépatique apres aasociation triacetyloleandomycine–estroprogestatif. [Intra-hepatic cholestasis after taking a triacetyloleandomycin-estroprogestational combination.] Nouv Presse Méd 1979;8(14):1182.
3. Fevery J, Van Steenbergen W, Desmet V, Deruyttere M, De Groote J. Severe intrahepatic cholestasis due to the combined intake of oral contraceptives and triacetyloleandomycin. Acta Clin Belg 1983;38(4):242–5.
4. Haber I, Hubens H. Cholestatic jaundice after triacetyloleandomycin and oral contraceptives. The diagnostic value of gamma-glutamyl transpeptidase. Acta Gastroenterol Belg 1980;43(11–12):475–82.
5. Miguet JP, Vuitton D, Pessayre D, Allemand H, Metreau JM, Poupon R, Capron JP, Blanc F. Jaundice from troleandomycin and oral contraceptives. Ann Intern Med 1980;92(3):434.
6. Watkins PB, Murray SA, Winkelman LG, Heuman DM, Wrighton SA, Guzelian PS. Erythromycin breath test as an assay of glucocorticoid-inducible liver cytochromes

P-450. Studies in rats and patients. J Clin Invest 1989;83(2):688–97.

7. Gorski JC, Jones DR, Hamman MA, Wrighton SA, Hall SD. Biotransformation of alprazolam by members of the human cytochrome P4503A subfamily. Xenobiotica 1999;29(9):931–44.

8. Pauwels O. Factors contributing to carbamazepine–macrolide interactions. Pharmacol Res 2002;45(4):291–8.

9. Fujimaki Y, Arai N, Inaba T. Identification of cytochromes P450 involved in human liver microsomal metabolism of ecabapide, a prokinetic agent. Xenobiotica 1999;29(12):1273–82.

10. Bacourt F, Couffinhal JC. Ischémie des membres par association dihydroergotamine-triacetyloléandomycin. [Ischemia of the extremities caused by a combination of dihydroergotamine and triacetyloleandomycin. New case report.] Nouv Presse Méd 1978;7(18):1561.

11. Franco A, Bourlard P, Massot C, Lecoeur J, Guidicelli H, Bessard G. Ergotamine par association dihydroergotamine–triacetyloléandomycin. [Acute ergotism caused by dihydroergotamine–triacetyloleandomycin association.] Nouv Presse Méd 1978;7(3):205.

12. Hayton AC. Precipitation of acute ergotism by triacetyloleandomycin. NZ Med J 1969;69(440):42.

13. Matthews NT, Havill JH. Ergotism with therapeutic doses of ergotamine tartrate. NZ Med J 1979;89(638):476–7.

14. Pea F, Furlanut M. Pharmacokinetic aspects of treating infections in the intensive care unit: focus on drug interactions. Clin Pharmacokinet 2001;40(11):833–68.

15. Eadie MJ. Clinically significant drug interactions with agents specific for migraine attacks. CNS Drugs 2001;15(2):105–18.

16. Azria M, Kiechel J, Lavenne D. Contribution à l'étude de l'interaction de la triacetyloléandomycine avec l'ergotamine ou la dihydroergotamine. J Pharmacol 1979;10:431.

17. Martinet M, Kiechel JR. Interaction of dihydroergotamine and triacetyloleandomycin in the minipig. Eur J Drug Metab Pharmacokinet 1983;8(3):261–7.

18. Zhao XJ, Ishizaki T. A further interaction study of quinine with clinically important drugs by human liver microsomes: determinations of inhibition constant (Ki) and type of inhibition. Eur J Drug Metab Pharmacokinet 1999;24(3):272–8.

Tropicamide

General Information

Tropicamide is an anticholinergic drug that tends to have a greater mydriatic than cycloplegic effect. It is a short-acting atropine-like derivative and has been regarded as an effective and safe mydriatic, used for pupillary dilatation by professionals, who are not always medical doctors.

Organs and Systems

Cardiovascular

A transient ischemic attack occurred in a 64-year-old patient with cardiovascular risk factors who used topical tropicamide (1).

Nervous system

Near fatal anticholinergic intoxication has been reported after routine fundoscopy with tropicamide (2).

- A 62-year-old man underwent fundoscopy after pupillary dilatation with tropicamide eye-drops. Half an hour after fundoscopic examination he had two generalized seizures with respiratory arrest and required intubation and mechanical ventilation. He was treated with physostigmine and made a full recovery.

Immunologic

A solution containing tropicamide 1% and benzalkonium chloride 0.01% (Mydriaticum) was introduced in 1979 to obtain mydriasis and cycloplegia for diagnostic purposes. Contact dermatitis from ophthalmic formulations is common, preservatives being the most frequent causes (3). Allergic contact dermatitis has been reported, implicating tropicamide as a sensitizer (4).

References

1. Vicedo CMF, Garcia MB, Bellver MJG, Bustamante AP. Conjunctival tropicamide and transitory ischemic accident (TIA). Farm Clin 1998;15:115–18.

2. Brunner GA, Fleck S, Pieber TR, Lueger A, Kaufmann P, Smolle KH, Brussee H, Krejs GJ. Near fatal anticholinergic intoxication after routine fundoscopy. Intensive Care Med 1998;24(7):730–1.

3. Herbst RA, Maibach HI. Allergic contact dermatitis from ophthalmics: update 1997. Contact Dermatitis 1997;37(5):252–3.

4. Boukhman MP, Maibach HI. Allergic contact dermatitis from tropicamide ophthalmic solution. Contact Dermatitis 1999;41(1):47–8.

Troxerutin

General Information

Troxerutin, a flavonoid derivative, is claimed to reduce capillary fragility. It is generally well tolerated (SEDA-19, 207), but ineffective (1).

Organs and Systems

Skin

Troxerutin is a yellow substance (SEDA-13, 170), and a few cases of yellow discoloration of the skin, but not of the sclerae, have been observed. The discoloration, which can be mistaken for jaundice, vanishes when the drug is withdrawn.

Reference

1. Anonymous. Paroven: not much effect in trials. Drug Ther Bull 1992;30(2):7–8.

Tryptophan

General Information

The possibility that mental illness may be alleviated by biogenic amine precursors is an appealing one (SEDA-4, 18). Tryptophan is a naturally-occurring essential amino acid, which has been advocated as an innocuous health food for the treatment of depression, insomnia, stress, behavioral disorders, and premenstrual syndrome. The availability of amino acids in health food stores and a contemporary interest in natural remedies led to reported widespread use of tryptophan to treat depression. It was estimated in 1976 that up to that time several hundred patients with affective disorders had been studied, with results reported in at least 21 papers (1). However, the results of clinical trials with L-tryptophan in the treatment of depressive disorders are inconsistent (2).

It has been suggested that there may be some benefit of using tryptophan in selected patients, particularly those with psychomotor retardation (3). Unfortunately, most of these reports have appeared as letters to the editors of journals (4–6) or as preliminary communications (7). In addition to the possible absence of any consistent effect, there are many plausible reasons to explain the variability in response. Tryptophan has been given in both the racemic and monomeric (levorotatory) forms, both alone and together with a number of substances intended to increase the synthesis or availability of serotonin, including mono-amine oxidase (MAO) inhibitors (8), potassium or carbohydrate supplements (9), and co-enzymes such as pyridoxine or ascorbic acid (10). It has also been suggested that tryptophan plasma concentrations have a therapeutic window (4), and that repeated administration induces hepatic tryptophan pyrrolase, resulting in lowered plasma concentrations and loss of therapeutic effect after 2 weeks of treatment (8). Attempts have been made to ameliorate this problem by coadministration of nicotinamide (4).

In addition to the difficulty of interpreting possible benefits due to tryptophan, there is a paucity of information on its adverse effects. This may be partly accounted for by the assumed safety of a natural substance, but it is also contributed to by the preliminary nature of many communications. In at least two studies (5,7) in which tryptophan was compared with a tricyclic antidepressant, inquiry about adverse effects was deliberately avoided, in order to protect the double-blind integrity of the study. Two studies have reported the lack of any consistent or definite changes in hematological values, serum electrolytes, plasma proteins, or liver function tests after 4 weeks of treatment with L-tryptophan up to 8 g/day (7,10). Nausea early in treatment (11), light-headedness, which does not appear to be related to postural hypotension (12), and deterioration in mental status (13,14) have been reported. Hypomania on combining tryptophan with a MAO inhibitor has been reported (14) and toxic effects, including muscle tremor, hypomanic mood, hyper-reflexia, and bilateral Babinski signs, were seen in a patient taking phenelzine and tryptophan.

Eosinophilia–myalgia syndrome

No severe or irreversible adverse effects of tryptophan were reported until 1989, when an eosinophilia–myalgia syndrome was described, and L-tryptophan-containing products were withdrawn from the market (SEDA-15, 518). This syndrome was characterized by an eosinophil count of at least 1×10^9/l and intense generalized myalgia. Other relatively frequent signs and symptoms were fatigue, arthralgia, skin rash, cough and dyspnea, edema of the limbs, fever, scleroderma-like skin abnormalities, increased hair loss, xerostomia, neuropathy, and pneumonia or pneumonitis with or without pulmonary vasculitis. About one-third of the cases required hospitalization, and a substantial number of patients died. The syndrome is suspected to have been due to an unidentified impurity in products from one manufacturer (SEDA-18, 22).

The syndrome appears to be only part of a spectrum of adverse effects associated with tryptophan (15). There has been much discussion, but finally it appears that the links are causal, as consistent findings were found in multiple independently conducted studies and the incidence of eosinophilia–myalgia syndrome in the USA fell abruptly once tryptophan-containing products were recalled (16).

Although L-tryptophan was withdrawn in many countries, in 1994 it became available again in the UK for combination treatment of patients with long-standing refractory depression, on the strict condition that it should only be prescribed by hospital specialists for patients with long-standing resistant depression (SEDA-18, 22). It is also still in use in Canada but not in the USA.

Organs and Systems

Respiratory

A case of interstitial pneumonitis and pulmonary vasculitis was ascribed to L-tryptophan, and unintended rechallenge supported a causal relation (17).

References

1. Farkas T, Dunner DL, Fieve RR. L-tryptophan in depression. Biol Psychiatry 1976;11(3):95–302.
2. Mendels J, Stinnett JL, Burns D, Frazer A. Amine precursors and depression. Arch Gen Psychiatry 1975;32(1):22–30.
3. Cooper AJ. Tryptophan antidepressant "physiological sedative": fact or fancy? Psychopharmacology (Berl) 1979;61(1):97–102.
4. Chouinard G, Young SN, Annable L, Sourkes TL. Tryptophan dosage critical for its antidepressant effect. BMJ 1978;1(6124):1422.
5. Rao B, Broadhurst AD. Letter: Tryptophan and depression. BMJ 1976;1(6007):460.
6. Jensen K, Fruensgaard K, Ahlfors UG, Pihkanen TA, Tuomikoski S, Ose E, Dencker SJ, Lindberg D, Nagy A. Letter: Tryptophan/imipramine in depression. Lancet 1975;2(7941):920.
7. Herrington RN, Bruce A, Johnstone EC, Lader MH. Comparative trial of L-tryptophan and amitriptyline in depressive illness. Psychol Med 1976;6(4):673–8.
8. Coppen A, Shaw DM, Farrell JP. Potentiation of the antidepressive effect of a monoamine-oxidase inhibitor by tryptophan. Lancet 1963;1:79–81.

9. Coppen A, Shaw DM, Herzberg B, Maggs R. Tryptophan in the treatment of depression. Lancet 1967;2(7527):1178–80.
10. Herrington RN, Bruce A, Johnstone EC. Comparative trial of L-tryptophan and E.C.T. in severe depressive illness. Lancet 1974;2(7883):731–4.
11. Broadhurst AD. L-tryptophan verses E.C.T. Lancet 1970;1(7661):1392–3.
12. Carroll BJ, Mowbray RM, Davies B. Sequential comparison of L-tryptophan with E.C.T. in severe depression. Lancet 1970;1(7654):967–9.
13. Murphy DL, Baker M, Goodwin FK, Miller H, Kotin J, Bunney WE Jr. L-tryptophan in affective disorders: indoleamine changes and differential clinical effects. Psychopharmacologia 1974;34(1):11–20.
14. Gayford JJ, Parker AL, Phillips EM, Rowsell AR. Whole blood 5-hydroxytryptamine during treatment of endogenous depressive illness. Br J Psychiatry 1973;122(570):597–8.
15. Varga J, Uitto J, Jimenez SA. The cause and pathogenesis of the eosinophilia-myalgia syndrome. Ann Intern Med 1992;116(2):140–7.
16. Kilbourne EM, Philen RM, Kamb ML, Falk H. Tryptophan produced by Showa Denko and epidemic eosinophilia-myalgia syndrome. J Rheumatol Suppl 1996;46:81–8.
17. Bogaerts Y, Van Renterghem D, Vanvuchelen J, Praet M, Michielssen P, Blaton V, Willemot JP. Interstitial pneumonitis and pulmonary vasculitis in a patient taking an L-tryptophan preparation. Eur Respir J 1991;4(8):1033–6.

Tubocurarine

See also Neuromuscular blocking drugs

General Information

D-Tubocurarine is the standard non-depolarizing neuromuscular blocking agent against which all others of the group are compared. The molecule has one quaternary and one tertiary nitrogen, the latter being protonated at body pH, making it a bisquaternary entity. Its main action at the neuromuscular junction is to block the access of acetylcholine to the receptor recognition sites competitively; it may also block some ion channels, but only to a small extent and at very high concentrations.

Blockade of neuromuscular transmission by D-tubocurarine is easily reversed (if twitch height has recovered to at least 10%) by anticholinesterases. Sensitivity to D-tubocurarine and other non-depolarizing relaxants is highly variable, even in apparently healthy patients, so that the small doses given for precurarization can lead to appreciable paralysis (1–3). More commonly, residual blockade can be detected postoperatively (4,5), long after the expected recovery of neuromuscular transmission.

About 40–50% of a normal dose of D-tubocurarine is bound to plasma proteins, mostly gammaglobulins (about 25%). This binding is highly variable, giving a variable amount of non-bound drug available for neuromuscular blockade. Metabolism does not occur. Tubocurarine is eliminated principally via glomerular filtration (about 40–60% in 24 hours), but has an alternative pathway for excretion in the bile (normally only about 12% in 24 hours). The initial dose for healthy patients is 0.2–0.5 mg/kg, dependent on the anesthetic agents used and whether suxamethonium is given beforehand or not. Maintenance doses are about one-third of the initial dose and are required at approximately 30–40-minute intervals. Accumulation can occur and is more likely if large doses are given too frequently or if excretion is impaired. Smaller doses should be given if the patient has received D-tubocurarine within the previous 24 hours.

General adverse effects

A fall in blood pressure occurs almost always with D-tubocurarine. It is often mild, but may be marked, particularly if a large dose is given rapidly or if the patient is hypovolemic, or has a diminished cardiac reserve or capacity for vasoconstriction (as is not infrequently the case in old age, in diabetes, and in other diseases with sympathetic neuropathy), and is potentiated by other anesthetic agents such as halothane. Myasthenic patients or patients with other neuromuscular pathology are markedly sensitive to non-depolarizing relaxants.

Histamine-mediated reactions are common, leading to local wheal-and-flare effects near the injection site, frequent hypotension (mostly about a 20% fall), and occasionally bronchospasm.

Malignant hyperthermia has also been reported after D-tubocurarine.

Tumor-inducing effects have not been reported.

Drug resistance

Patients with burns require more D-tubocurarine (and higher plasma concentrations) for the same degree of blockade compared with non-burned patients (6). The mechanism is not known, but it appears not to be altered pharmacokinetics (7). The resistance to non-depolarizing neuromuscular blocking agents (SEDA-8, 136) appears to be influenced by the size of the body surface area burned and by the time which has elapsed since the injury (see Atracurium). In extensive burns dose requirements are increased approximately by a factor of 2–3.

Patients with upper motor neuron lesions such as hemiplegia (8–11) and possibly multiple sclerosis (SEDA-13, 105) (12) can be resistant to various non-depolarizing blockers. Lower motor neuron injury has so far only been reported to produce this phenomenon in rats (13) and dogs. Affected muscles in these conditions are paralysed to a lesser degree than unaffected muscles, and this has to be taken into account when siting the electrodes for monitoring a block and in assessing recovery therefrom. The mechanism is probably a quantitative and/or qualitative change in acetylcholine receptors. Resistance is seen too in patients taking certain drugs such as phenytoin, carbamazepine, and, disputedly, azathioprine.

In liver disease, increased amounts of D-tubocurarine may be required. In the past it has been suggested that this could be due to reduced synthesis of acetylcholinesterase, or to increased concentrations of gammaglobulins binding the relaxant (14), although this is disputed (15). Similar kinetic mechanisms to those suggested for pancuronium may be involved, but there are no studies on D-tubocurarine. In primary liver cancer in children, resistance to D-tubocurarine (and alcuronium) has been reported (SEDA-13, 104) (16).

Hyperkalemia tends to reduce the neuromuscular blocking effects of tubocurarine.

Organs and Systems

Cardiovascular

D-Tubocurarine commonly causes a fall in blood pressure, associated with a slight tachycardia and a reduction in total peripheral resistance; cardiac output is not affected. The frequency of hypotension is reported as being 20–90%. This wide range probably reflects the methods of measurement, the anesthetic agents used, and the general condition of the patients in the various studies, as well as the criteria for diagnosing hypotension. The magnitude of the fall in blood pressure is generally about 20%, and it occurs within 5 minutes of injection. Histamine release is considered to be the principal cause (17), but blockade of autonomic ganglia may also contribute. It has been suggested that prostacycline, released by histamine acting on H_1 receptors, is the final mediator; intravenous administration of aspirin or an H_1 receptor antagonist beforehand affords some protection (SEDA-15, 126) (18). Ganglion blockade may also contribute, particularly if high doses are used (19). Reduction in venous return secondary to muscle relaxation and alterations in intrathoracic and intra-abdominal pressures may also play a role. The fall in blood pressure can be greatly exaggerated in hypovolemic patients, in the elderly, and in others with reduced sympathetic tone. Tubocurarine should be used very cautiously in such patients or another relaxant should be chosen. Concurrent administration of agents known to cause circulatory depression aggravates the problem. The higher the halothane concentration, for example, the greater the fall in blood pressure after D-tubocurarine (20). Since the degree of hypotension seems to be linked to dose (17) and the rate of injection (21), it seems reasonable to use the smallest dose that produces adequate relaxation (under 0.5 mg/kg) and to inject it slowly (over at least 180 seconds) (SEDA-7, 141).

Respiratory

Tubocurarine can cause apnea. The muscles involved in protecting and maintaining the airway are more sensitive to D-tubocurarine than the muscles of ventilation (22,23) so that aspiration and airway obstruction are possible in the partially curarized patient at a time when spontaneous ventilation is adequate. Airway obstruction in the presence of vigorous respiratory efforts can eventually (and is rarely reported to) lead to negative pressure pulmonary edema (24,25). Hypoventilation can occur after doses as low as 1.5 mg in exceptionally sensitive patients. Postoperative hypoventilation, or apnea, is a danger in patients given certain antibiotics and antidysrhythmic drugs before or after apparently successful spontaneous reversal or antagonism of a non-depolarizing block.

Potentiation of undetected residual curarization can also occur postoperatively from respiratory acidosis.

Histamine release, common with D-tubocurarine, can cause bronchospasm. Tubocurarine is relatively contraindicated in asthmatic patients and in those with an allergic tendency.

Nervous system

Minute amounts of D-tubocurarine have been detected in cerebrospinal fluid (26). Although convulsions have been produced in animals by injection into the cerebrospinal fluid, and it has been suggested that exceptionally large doses can cause depression of medullary centers, there is insufficient information to draw any conclusions.

Pancuronium is reported to lower the MAC for halothane, but whether this is a central or peripheral action is not known.

Gastrointestinal

The motility of the gut may be reduced by tubocurarine, as a result of ganglion blockade.

Body temperature

Tubocurarine has been implicated as a trigger of malignant hyperthermia, particularly in combination with halothane (27), although doubts have been expressed (28). Increased muscular tone is not a feature with D-tubocurarine.

Second-Generation Effects

Pregnancy

Placental transfer of D-tubocurarine occurs (as with all relaxants) and low concentrations of the drug have been detected in umbilical blood. Under normal circumstances no untoward effects have been reported in neonates.

Paralysis occurred in a 28-week fetus, whose mother received D-tubocurarine for status epilepticus, and joint deformities possibly resulting from 4 weeks' maternal curarization during the first trimester have been reported (29).

Experiments in chick embryos have shown that D-tubocurarine can cause retardation of bone growth (30) and that malformations can be produced by in utero curarization (31). Long-term curarization during pregnancy is undesirable.

Susceptibility Factors

Genetic factors

Individual responses to these compounds differ (32–34). Racial differences and environmental factors can influence the response to relaxants and hence the extent of problems due to excessive activity. Patients in the USA reportedly require less D-tubocurarine than in the UK, and the West Indians need more. Difference in cholinesterase activities, perhaps brought about by more organophosphorus insecticides being used in one country than in another, or differences in protein-binding as a result of dietary factors, are possible explanations (35). Vecuronium has been reported to be approximately 30% more potent in Montreal than in Paris (36).

Age

In the elderly extreme falls in blood pressure can occur with D-tubocurarine (37).

Renal disease

In renal insufficiency the action of D-tubocurarine is increased (38) and prolonged (39).

The half-life in the complete absence of renal function is increased by 70% or more. The reduced ability of plasma proteins to bind the drug (40), if this indeed occurs, will result in a greater proportion of unbound D-tubocurarine and therefore increased potency.

Increased biliary excretion of D-tubocurarine occurs in renal insufficiency and compensates to a varying degree for reduced renal excretion (41). The slower rate of biliary (as opposed to renal) excretion will result in sharply increasing prolongation of neuromuscular blockade if large single doses are used or if multiple doses are given (42). A single small dose will result in little or no prolongation of effect, since redistribution will be mainly responsible for termination of the drug's effect. It has been suggested for several other non-depolarizing relaxants that the initial dose produces less effect in renal insufficiency (SEDA-13, 103).

The problem of accumulation may be marked in intensive care situations, where D-tubocurarine is used to maintain long-term paralysis (42). These patients may also have impaired renal and hepatic function, with protein and electrolyte imbalance. The timing of repeat injections of D-tubocurarine (and, indeed, all relaxant drugs) in such cases should be guided by monitoring of neuromuscular function (by response to single twitch, train-of-four, or tetanic stimulation, which is more sensitive but painful), or clinically by observing the return of muscle tone.

Other features of the patient

In hypovolemic patients, in patients with impaired sympathetic autonomic activity, and in patients operated on in the anti-Trendelenburg position, extreme falls in blood pressure can occur with D-tubocurarine. Hypotension is aggravated by the use of halothane in particular, and by other drugs that produce circulatory depression. In such cases, and in patients with hypertension, coronary artery disease, and arteriosclerosis, D-tubocurarine is better avoided.

Asthmatic and atopic individuals are at special risk from D-tubocurarine's histamine-releasing potential, and severe bronchospasm can result (43).

Greatly increased sensitivity occurs in myasthenia (44) and may even be seen in "premyasthenic" patients with no overt symptoms (45). Increased sensitivity has also been reported in amyotrophic lateral sclerosis (46), von Recklinghausen's disease (47), and ocular muscular dystrophy (48). Patients with Duchenne muscular dystrophy have prolonged block in the regional curare test (49), but other investigators have disputed whether an altered response to non-depolarizing relaxants occurs in this condition.

Patients with thyrotoxic myopathy, as with all forms of myopathy, are exceedingly sensitive to all non-depolarizing agents.

Drug–Drug Interactions

Antidysrhythmic drugs

Class I antidysrhythmic drugs, such as procainamide, lidocaine, propranolol, diphenylhydantoin (50), quinidine (51), and lidocaine (52) have all been claimed to enhance neuromuscular blockade by D-tubocurarine and other non-depolarizing agents. Bretylium (53) and disopyramide (54) are also reported to have their neuromuscular blocking activities potentiated by low concentrations of D-tubocurarine in animal experiments; neostigmine failed to reverse disopyramide-induced blockade (SEDA-13, 102) (55). The greatest hazard from these agents is that they can cause "recurarization" when given postoperatively. With bretylium this can occur several hours after its administration, as a result of its slow kinetics (53). Effects in man have still to be documented for bretylium, but "recurarization" 15 minutes after adequate reversal of vecuronium blockade with neostigmine has been described in a patient given disopyramide intravenously (SEDA-14, 116) (56).

Aprotinin

Reparalysis has been reported when aprotinin was used after operations during which suxamethonium had been given alone or in combination with normal doses of D-tubocurarine (57).

Azathioprine

Azathioprine reduces sensitivity to D-tubocurarine in experimental animals, possibly as a result of phosphodiesterase inhibition, increasing transmitter release (SEDA-4, 87) (58), (SEDA-13, 104).

Calcium channel blockers

Calcium channel blockers, such as verapamil and nifedipine, can potentiate neuromuscular blocking agents (59,60) and it has been suggested that in long-term use they can accumulate in muscle and make block-reversal difficult (61).

Corticosteroids

There have been several contradictory reports of possible interactions of tubocurarine with corticosteroids. In general, it seems that the long-term use of steroids can reduce sensitivity to non-depolarizing neuromuscular blocking agents, while acute administration can cause potentiation (62). Long-term steroid treatment may be associated with the development of a myasthenic syndrome in some patients, who will therefore be very sensitive to neuromuscular blocking agents.

Diuretics

Furosemide (40–80 mg) has been reported to enhance and prolong D-tubocurarine-induced block in anephric patients (63). In animals low doses potentiated D-tubocurarine (and suxamethonium) probably via presynaptic effects, while high doses (1–40 mg/kg in cats) reversed the neuromuscular actions of these relaxants (64). The effects of high doses were similar to those of theophylline, and phosphodiesterase inhibition leading to increased acetylcholine release was postulated as a possible mechanism for the antagonism.

Potassium and magnesium loss as a result of the use of diuretics can affect non-depolarizing relaxants.

Doxapram

Doxapram, used as a respiratory stimulant, increased partial D-tubocurarine and pancuronium neuromuscular blockade when used in high concentrations in rats (SEDA-14, 113) (65). There have been no reports in man so far.

Ganglion-blocking agents

Trimetaphan and hexamethonium can potentiate D-tubo-curarine-induced block, but clinical reports clearly showing this are lacking. Tubocurarine will increase their hypotensive effect. Neostigmine could theoretically facilitate the postulated end-plate ion channel block of trimetaphan (SEDA-13, 102) (66), which would complicate reversal of neuromuscular block.

Local anesthetics

Local anesthetics have diverse effects on the neuromuscular junction. In very large doses they produce paralysis on their own. When the recommended doses are used for local anesthesia, systemic absorption is small and interaction with relaxants is not to be expected. However, large doses injected intravascularly (accidentally, or therapeutically for dysrhythmias) can potentiate relaxants of both types (67,68).

Magnesium sulfate

Magnesium inhibits the release of acetylcholine and reduces the sensitivity of the postjunctional membrane. Thus, magnesium sulfate can cause neuromuscular transmission failure and enhance the effect of D-tubocurarine and other non-depolarizing neuromuscular blocking drugs (69). Not only have potentiation and prolongation of D-tubocurarine block been reported, but also respiratory depression when magnesium sulfate was given an hour after reversal of the relaxant. Presumably the muscle weakness resulted from potentiation of residual curarization. Whether the effects are additive or synergistic is disputed. Muscle relaxants must be used with caution and in reduced dosage in patients receiving magnesium sulfate. Reversal of the block may be difficult.

References

1. Rao TL, Jacobs HK. Pulmonary function following "pretreatment" dose of pancuronium in volunteers. Anesth Analg 1980;59(9):659–61.
2. Mayrhofer O. Die Wirksamheit von d-Tubocurarin zur Verhütung der Muskelschmerzen nach Succinylcholin. [The efficacy of d-tubocurarine in the prevention of muscle pains after succinylcholine.] Anaesthesist 1959;8:313.
3. Musich J, Walts LF. Pulmonary aspiration after a priming dose of vecuronium. Anesthesiology 1986;64(4):517–19.
4. Viby-Mogensen J, Jorgensen BC, Ording H. Residual curarization in the recovery room. Anesthesiology 1979;50(6):539–41.
5. Lennmarken C, Lofstrom JB. Partial curarization in the postoperative period. Acta Anaesthesiol Scand 1984;28(3):260–2.
6. Martyn JA, Szyfelbein SK, Ali HH, Matteo RS, Savarese JJ. Increased d-tubocurarine requirement following major thermal injury. Anesthesiology 1980;52(4):352–5.
7. Martyn JA, Matteo RS, Greenblatt DJ, Lebowitz PW, Savarese JJ. Pharmacokinetics of d-tubocurarine in patients with thermal injury. Anesth Analg 1982;61(3):241–6.
8. Shayevitz JR, Matteo RS. Decreased sensitivity to metocurine in patients with upper motoneuron disease. Anesth Analg 1985;64(8):767–72.
9. Moorthy SS, Hilgenberg JC. Resistance to non-depolarizing muscle relaxants in paretic upper extremities of patients with residual hemiplegia. Anesth Analg 1980;59(8):624–7.
10. Graham DH. Monitoring neuromuscular block may be unreliable in patients with upper-motor-neuron lesions. Anesthesiology 1980;52(1):74–5.
11. Laycock JR, Smith CE, Donati F, Bevan DR. Sensitivity of the adductor pollicis and diaphragm muscles to atracurium in a hemiplegic patient. Anesthesiology 1987;67(5):851–3.
12. Brett RS, Schmidt JH, Gage JS, Schartel SA, Poppers PJ. Measurement of acetylcholine receptor concentration in skeletal muscle from a patient with multiple sclerosis and resistance to atracurium. Anesthesiology 1987;66(6):837–9.
13. Hogue CW Jr, Itani MS, Martyn JA. Resistance to d-tubocurarine in lower motor neuron injury is related to increased acetylcholine receptors at the neuromuscular junction. Anesthesiology 1990;73(4):703–9.
14. Stovner J, Theodorsen L, Bjelke E. Sensitivity to tubocurarine and alcuronium with special reference to plasma protein pattern. Br J Anaesth 1971;43(4):385–91.
15. Duvaldestin P. Common disease states affecting the action of neuromuscular blocking drugs. In: Agoston S, Bowman WC, editors. Monographs in Anaesthesiology. Amsterdam: Elsevier Science Publishers BV, 1990;19:253.
16. Brown TC, Gregory M, Bell B, Campbell PC. Liver tumours and muscle relaxants. Electromyographic studies in children. Anaesthesia 1987;42(12):1284–6.
17. Moss J, Rosow CE, Savarese JJ, Philbin DM, Kniffen KJ. Role of histamine in the hypotensive action of d-tubocurarine in humans. Anesthesiology 1981;55(1):19–25.
18. Hatano Y, Arai T, Noda J, Komatsu K, Shinkura R, Nakajima Y, Sawada M, Mori K. Contribution of prostacyclin to D-tubocurarine-induced hypotension in humans. Anesthesiology 1990;72(1):28–32.
19. Marshall IG. Pharmacological effects of neuromuscular blocking agents: interaction with cholinoceptors other than nicotinic receptors of the neuromuscular junction. Anest Rianim 1986;27:19.
20. Munger WL, Miller RD, Stevens WC. The dependence of a d-tubocurarine-induced hypotension on alveolar concentration of halothane, dose of d-tubocurarine, and nitrous oxide. Anesthesiology 1974;40(5):442–8.
21. Stoelting RK, McCammon RL, Hilgenberg JC. Changes in blood pressure with varying rates of administration of d-tubocurarine. Anesth Analg 1980;59(9):697–9.
22. Pavlin EG, Holle RH, Schoene RB. Recovery of airway protection compared with ventilation in humans after paralysis with curare. Anesthesiology 1989;70(3):381–5.
23. Knill RL. D-tubocurarine and upper airway obstruction: a historical perspective. Anesthesiology 1989;71(3):480–1.
24. Warner LO, Martino JD, Davidson PJ, Beach TP. Negative pressure pulmonary oedema: a potential hazard

of muscle relaxants in awake infants. Can J Anaesth 1990;37(5):580–3.

25. Brown RE. Negative pressure pulmonary edema. In: Berry FA, editor. Anesthetic Management of Difficult and Routine Pediatric Patients. New York: Churchill Livingstone, 1986:169.

26. Matteo RS, Pua EK, Khambatta HJ, Spector S. Cerebrospinal fluid levels of d-tubocurarine in man. Ancsthesiology 1977;46(6):396–9.

27. Britt BA, Webb GE, LeDuc C. Malignant hyperthermia induced by curare. Can Anaesth Soc J 1974;21(4):371–5.

28. Gronert GA. Malignant hyperthermia. Anesthesiology 1980;53(5):395–423.

29. Older PO, Harris JM. Placental transfer of tubocurarine. Case report. Br J Anaesth 1968;40(6):459–63.

30. Ahmed W. The effect of relaxant drugs on the growth and development of bone and cartilage in the chick embryo. Ain Shams Med J 1970;21:679.

31. Drachman DB, Coulombre AJ. Experimental clubfoot and arthrogryposis multiplex congenita. Lancet 1962;2:523–6.

32. Azar I. The response of patients with neuromuscular disorders to muscle relaxants: a review. Anesthesiology 1984;61(2):173–87.

33. Martz DG, Schreibman DL, Matjasko MJ. Neurological diseases. In: Katz RL, Benumof JL, Kadis LB, editors. Anesthesia and Uncommon Diseases. 3rd ed. Philadelphia: W.B. Saunders, 1990:560.

34. Miller JD, Lee C. Muscle diseases. In: Katz RL, Benumof JL, Kadis LB, editors. Anesthesia and Uncommon Diseases. 3rd ed. Philadelphia: W.B. Saunders; 1990:590.

35. Stovner J. Clinical use of relaxants in Europe. In: Katz RL, editor. Muscle Relaxants. Amsterdam: Excerpta Medica, 1975:268.

36. Fiset P, Donati F, Balendran P, Meistelman C, Lira E, Bevan DR. Vecuronium is more potent in Montreal than in Paris. Can J Anaesth 1991;38(6):717–21.

37. McCullough LS, Reier CE, Delaunois AL, Gardier RW, Hamelberg W. The effects of d-tubocurarine on spontaneous postganglionic sympathetic activity and histamine release. Anesthesiology 1970;33(3):328–34.

38. Orko R, Heino A, Rosenberg PH, Alanen T. Dose-response of tubocurarine in patients with and without renal failure. Acta Anaesthesiol Scand 1984;28(4):452–6.

39. Miller RD, Matteo RS, Benet LZ, Sohn YJ. The pharmacokinetics of d-tubocurarine in man with and without renal failure. J Pharmacol Exp Ther 1977;202(1):1–7.

40. Miller RD, Eger EI 2nd. Early and late relative potencies of pancuronium and d-tubocurarine in man. Anesthesiology 1976;44(4):297–300.

41. Cohen EN, Brewer HW, Smith D. The metabolism and elimination of d-tubocurarine-H3. Anesthesiology 1967;28(2):309–17.

42. Riordan DD, Gilbertson AA. Prolonged curarization in a patient with renal failure. Case report. Br J Anaesth 1971;43(5):506–8.

43. Yeung ML, Ng LY, Koo AW. Severe bronchospasm in an asthmatic patient following alcuronium and D-tubocurarine. Anaesth Intensive Care 1979;7(1):62–4.

44. Foldes FF. Myasthenia gravis. In: Katz RL, editor. Muscle Relaxants. Amsterdam: Excerpta Medica, 1975:345.

45. Enoki T, Naito Y, Hirokawa Y, Nomura R, Hatano Y, Mori K. Marked sensitivity to pancuronium in a patient without clinical manifestations of myasthenia gravis. Anesth Analg 1989;69(6):840–2.

46. Rosenbaum KJ, Neigh JL, Strobel GE. Sensitivity to non-depolarizing muscle relaxants in amyotrophic lateral sclerosis: report of two cases. Anesthesiology 1971;35(6):638–41.

47. Baraka A. Myasthenic response to muscle relaxants in von Recklinghausen's disease. Br J Anaesth 1974;46(9):701–3.

48. Robertson JA. Ocular muscular dystrophy. A cause of curare sensitivity. Anaesthesia 1984;39(3):251–3.

49. Brown JC, Charlton JE. Study of sensitivity to curare in certain neurological disorders using a regional technique. J Neurol Neurosurg Psychiatry 1975;38(1):34–45.

50. Harrah MD, Way WL, Katzung BG. The interaction of d-tubocurarine with antiarrhythmic drugs. Anesthesiology 1970;33(4):406–10.

51. Miller RD, Way WL, Katzung BG. The potentiation of neuromuscular blocking agents by quinidine. Anesthesiology 1967;28(6):1036–41.

52. Katz RL, Gissen AJ. Effects of intravenous and intra-arterial procaine and lidocaine on neuromuscular transmission in man. Acta Anaesthesiol Scand Suppl 1969;36:103–13.

53. Welch GW, Waud BE. Effect of bretylium on neuromuscular transmission. Anesth Analg 1982;61(5):442–4.

54. Healy TE, O'Shea M, Massey J. Disopyramide and neuromuscular transmission. Br J Anaesth 1981;53(5):495–8.

55. Jones SV, Marshall IG. Non-competitive effects of disopyramide at the neuromuscular junction: evidence for endplate ion channel block. Br J Anaesth 1987;59(6):776–83.

56. Baurain M, Barvais L, d'Hollander A, Hennart D. Impairment of the antagonism of vecuronium-induced paralysis and intra-operative disopyramide administration. Anaesthesia 1989;44(1):34–6.

57. Chasapakis G, Dimas C. Possible interaction between muscle relaxants and the kallikrein-trypsin inactivator "Trasylol". Report of three cases. Br J Anaesth 1966;38(10):838–9.

58. Dretchen KL, Morgenroth VH 3rd, Standaert FG, Walts LF. Azathioprine: effects on neuromuscular transmission. Anesthesiology 1976;45(6):604–9.

59. Durant NN, Nguyen N, Katz RL. Potentiation of neuromuscular blockade by verapamil. Anesthesiology 1984;60(4):298–303.

60. Jones RM, Cashman JN, Casson WR, Broadbent MP. Verapamil potentiation of neuromuscular blockade: failure of reversal with neostigmine but prompt reversal with edrophonium. Anesth Analg 1985;64(10):1021–5.

61. Bikhazi GB, Leung I, Flores C, Mikati HM, Foldes FF. Potentiation of neuromuscular blocking agents by calcium channel blockers in rats. Anesth Analg 1988;67(1):1–8.

62. Maestrone E. Interaction of neuromuscular blocking agents in surgical patients. In: Agoston S, Bowman WC, editors. Monographs in Anaesthesiology. . Amsterdam: Elsevier Science Publishers BV, 1990;19:199.

63. Miller RD, Sohn YJ, Matteo RS. Enhancement of d-tuborcurarine neuromuscular blockade by diuretics in man. Anesthesiology 1976;45(4):442–5.

64. Scappaticci KA, Ham JA, Sohn YJ, Miller RD, Dretchen KL. Effects of furosemide on the neuromuscular junction. Anesthesiology 1982;57(5):381–8.

65. Pollard BJ, Randall NP, Pleuvry BJ. Doxapram and the neuromuscular junction. Br J Anaesth 1989;62(6):664–8.

66. Nakamura K, Hatano Y, Mori K. The site of action of trimethaphan-induced neuromuscular blockade in isolated rat and frog muscle. Acta Anaesthesiol Scand 1988;32(2):125–30.

67. Matsuo S, Rao DB, Chaudry I, Foldes FF. Interaction of muscle relaxants and local anesthetics at the neuromuscular junction. Anesth Analg 1978;57(5):580–7.

68. Telivuo L, Katz RL. The effects of modern intravenous local analgesics on respiration during partial neuromuscular block in man. Anaesthesia 1970;25(1):30–5.

69. Giesecke AH Jr, Morris RE, Dalton MD, Stephen CR. Of magnesium, muscle relaxants, toxemic parturients, and cats. Anesth Analg 1968;47(6):689–95.

Tumor necrosis factor alfa

General Information

Tumor necrosis factor alfa is naturally produced by activated macrophages and monocytes and has pleiotropic effects on normal and malignant cells. Unfortunately, the systemic administration of tumor necrosis factor alfa as a single agent gave disappointing results with severe adverse effects and no significant clinical antitumor effect (SED-13, 1110) (1,2). However, tumor necrosis factor alfa combined with interferon gamma, interleukin-2, or cytotoxic drugs produced positive clinical results, and these combinations reduced the maximum tolerated dose of tumor necrosis factor alfa two to four-fold.

Severe hypotension, thought to be nitrous oxide-mediated, is the main dose-limiting toxicity at all doses. Other frequent and sometimes dose-limiting adverse effects included fever, chills and rigors, myalgias, diarrhea, nausea or vomiting, and local reactions at the injection site. During combination therapy with tumor necrosis factor alfa, hyperbilirubinemia, neurotoxicity, severe febrile reactions, and hypotension were the most frequent complications (SED-13, 1110) (1–4). Transient liver dysfunction, oliguria, and raised creatinine concentrations are common.

Organs and Systems

Cardiovascular

Hypotension, perhaps nitrous oxide-mediated, is a dose-limiting adverse effect of tumor necrosis factor alfa (5).

Severe hypophosphatemia with myocardial dysfunction was noted in patients receiving tumor necrosis factor alfa by continuous hepatic arterial infusion (SEDA-17, 433).

Congestive cardiomyopathy has been attributed to tumor necrosis factor alfa in isolated patients (SED-13, 1110) (6).

Respiratory

A reversible reduction in pulmonary diffusing capacity (7) and pulmonary hemorrhage have been attributed to tumor necrosis factor alfa in isolated patients (SED-13, 1110) (8).

Nervous system

Tumor necrosis factor alfa is considered to be a major neurotoxic agent, and most patients who received large doses developed central nervous system symptoms, most commonly headache, lethargy, fatigue, confusion, disorientation, and reduced performance. Seizures, transient amnesia, aphasia, hallucinations, and diplopia sometimes occur (9).

Psychological, psychiatric

Evaluation of cognitive function in patients receiving tumor necrosis factor alfa alone or combined with interleukin-2 showed reversible attentional deficits, memory disorders, deficits in motor coordination and frontal lobe executive functions (9). There was reversible hypoperfusion in the frontal lobes.

Endocrine

Exacerbation of hypothyroidism was noted in one patient with chronic thyroiditis who received tumor necrosis factor alfa (10).

Metabolism

Metabolic effects of tumor necrosis factor alfa include a reduction in cholesterol and high-density lipoproteins, increases in triglycerides and very low-density lipoproteins, and hyperglycemia.

Hematologic

The hematological effects of tumor necrosis factor alfa mostly consist of dose-related thrombocytopenia and granulocytopenia, and decreased monocyte or lymphocyte counts (SED-13, 1111) (11,12). Septic episodes are sometimes associated with leukopenia. Coagulopathy with laboratory evidence of disseminated intravascular coagulopathy was found in 30% of patients and was sometimes associated with thromboembolic events (13). Other coagulation disorders include transient alterations in prothrombin time, and a rise in the plasma concentrations of von Willebrand factor was found in healthy volunteers (14).

Gastrointestinal

Hemorrhagic gastritis has been attributed to tumor necrosis factor alfa (15).

Immunologic

Anaphylactic-like reactions, dyspnea, or acute bronchospasm have been attributed to tumor necrosis factor alfa in patients also treated with interleukin-2 (16).

Drug Administration

Drug administration route

Local (intralesional, intra-arterial, or intraperitoneal) administration of tumor necrosis factor alfa may well prove to be a more promising and less toxic route of administration. Although mild adverse effects, namely fever, hypotension, and fatigue, were similar to those reported after intravenous administration, coagulation disorders, pulmonary, central nervous system, liver, and renal forms of toxicity were usually not observed (17).

The most interesting and encouraging experience has been obtained using hyperthermic isolated limb perfusion (HILP) of tumor necrosis factor alfa combined with cytostatic drugs (for example melphalan) in melanoma and sarcoma (18). Although systemic toxicity was moderate in this setting, there was still a risk of severe hemodynamic changes, with clinical features of septic shock and a direct nephrotoxic effect of tumor necrosis factor alfa (19,20). A mild neuropathy, marked by transient paresthesia, is also frequent (21). Other rare adverse effects included lung infiltrates, fever, neutropenia, thrombocytopenia, coagulation disorders, transient rise in transaminases and bilirubin, and an increased risk of more severe rhabdomyolysis (SED-13, 1111) (22).

References

1. Sidhu RS, Bollon AP. Tumor necrosis factor activities and cancer therapy—a perspective. Pharmacol Ther 1993;57(1):79–128.
2. Hieber U, Heim ME. Tumor necrosis factor for the treatment of malignancies. Oncology 1994;51(2):142–53.
3. Schiller JH, Witt PL, Storer B, Alberti D, Tombes MB, Arzoomanian R, Brown RR, Proctor RA, Voss SD, Spriggs DR, et al. Clinical and biologic effects of combination therapy with gamma-interferon and tumor necrosis factor. Cancer 1992;69(2):562–71.
4. Smith JW 2nd, Urba WJ, Clark JW, Longo DL, Farrell M, Creekmore SP, Conlon KC, Jaffe H, Steis RG. Phase I evaluation of recombinant tumor necrosis factor given in combination with recombinant interferon-gamma. J Immunother 1991;10(5):355–62.
5. Hanson DS, Leggette CT. Severe hypotension following inadvertent intravenous administration of interferon alfa-2a. Ann Pharmacother 1997;31(3):371–2.
6. Hegewisch S, Weh HJ, Hossfeld DK. TNF-induced cardiomyopathy. Lancet 1990;335(8684):294–5.
7. Kuei JH, Tashkin DP, Figlin RA. Pulmonary toxicity of recombinant human tumor necrosis factor. Chest 1989;96(2):334–8.
8. Schilling PJ, Murray JL, Markowitz AB. Novel tumor necrosis factor toxic effects. Pulmonary hemorrhage and severe hepatic dysfunction. Cancer 1992;69(1):256–60.
9. Meyers CA, Valentine AD, Wong FC, Leeds NE. Reversible neurotoxicity of interleukin-2 and tumor necrosis factor: correlation of SPECT with neuropsychological testing. J Neuropsychiatry Clin Neurosci 1994; 6(3):285–8.
10. Miyakoshi H, Ohsawa K, Yokoyama H, Nagai Y, Ieki Y, Bando YI, Kobayashi K. Exacerbation of hypothyroidism following tumor necrosis factor-alpha infusion. Intern Med 1992;31(2):200–3.
11. Mittelman A, Puccio C, Gafney E, Coombe N, Singh B, Wood D, Nadler P, Ahmed T, Arlin Z. A phase I pharmacokinetic study of recombinant human tumor necrosis factor administered by a 5-day continuous infusion. Invest New Drugs 1992;10(3):183–90.
12. Logan TF, Kaplan SS, Bryant JL, Ernstoff MS, Krause JR, Kirkwood JM. Granulocytopenia in cancer patients treated in a phase I trial with recombinant human tumor necrosis factor. J Immunother 1991;10(2):84–95.
13. Muggia FM, Brown TD, Goodman PJ, Macdonald JS, Hersh EM, Fleming TR, Leichman L. High incidence of coagulopathy in phase II studies of recombinant tumor necrosis factor in advanced pancreatic and gastric cancers. Anticancer Drugs 1992;3(3):211–17.
14. van der Poll T, van Deventer SJ, Pasterkamp G, van Mourik JA, Buller HR, ten Cate JW. Tumor necrosis factor induces von Willebrand factor release in healthy humans. Thromb Haemost 1992;67(6):623–6.
15. Krigel RL, Padavic-Shaller KA, Rudolph AA, Young JD, Weiner LM, Konrad M, Comis RL. Hemorrhagic gastritis as a new dose-limiting toxicity of recombinant tumor necrosis factor. J Natl Cancer Inst 1991;83(2):129–31.
16. Negrier MS, Pourreau CN, Palmer PA, Ranchere JY, Mercatello A, Viens P, Blaise D, Jasmin C, Misset JL, Franks CR, et al. Phase I trial of recombinant interleukin-2 followed by recombinant tumor necrosis factor in patients with metastatic cancer. J Immunother 1992;11(2):93–102.
17. Watanabe N, Yamauchi N, Maeda M, Neda H, Tsuji Y, Okamoto T, Tsuji N, Akiyama S, Sasaki H, Niitsu Y. Recombinant human tumor necrosis factor causes regression in patients with advanced malignances. Oncology 1994;51(4):360–5.
18. Eggermont AM, Schraffordt Koops H, Klausner JM, Kroon BB, Schlag PM, Lienard D, van Geel AN, Hoekstra HJ, Meller I, Nieweg OE, Kettelhack C, Ben-Ari G, Pector JC, Lejeune FJ. Isolated limb perfusion with tumor necrosis factor and melphalan for limb salvage in 186 patients with locally advanced soft tissue extremity sarcomas. The cumulative multicenter European experience. Ann Surg 1996;224(6):756–65.
19. Eggimann P, Chiolero R, Chassot PG, Lienard D, Gerain J, Lejeune F. Systemic and hemodynamic effects of recombinant tumor necrosis factor alpha in isolation perfusion of the limbs. Chest 1995;107(4):1074–82.
20. Zwaveling JH, Hoekstra HJ, Maring JK, v Ginkel RJ, Schraffordt Koops H, Smit AJ, Girbes AR. Renal function in cancer patients treated with hyperthermic isolated limb perfusion with recombinant tumor necrosis factor-alpha and melphalan. Nephron 1997;76(2):146–52.
21. Drory VE, Lev D, Groozman GB, Gutmann M, Klausner JM. Neurotoxicity of isolated limb perfusion with tumor necrosis factor. J Neurol Sci 1998;158(1):1–4.
22. Hohenberger P, Haier J, Schlag PM. Rhabdomyolysis and renal function impairment after isolated limb perfusion—comparison between the effects of perfusion with rhTNF alpha and a "triple-drug" regimen. Eur J Cancer 1997;33(4):596–601.

Tylosin

General Information

Tylosin is a polyketide lactone substituted with three deoxyhexose sugars. It is used as an antimicrobial growth promoter in animals. Acquired resistance has been observed in potentially human pathogenic strains isolated from animals (1). Of further concern is the fact that tylosin confers cross-resistance on erythromycin (2).

References

1. Butaye P, Devriese LA, Haesebrouck F. Phenotypic distinction in *Enterococcus faecium* and *Enterococcus faecalis* strains between susceptibility and resistance to growth-enhancing antibiotics. Antimicrob Agents Chemother 1999;43(10):2569–70.
2. Pedersen KB. Some growth promoters in animals do confer antimicrobial resistance in humans. BMJ 1999; 318(7190):1076.

Typhoid vaccine (including typhoid-paratyphoid vaccine)

See also Vaccines

General Information

The different typhoid vaccines commercially available for civilian use are:

- an oral live attenuated vaccine based on the Ty21a strain of *Salmonella typhi*;
- a parenteral heat-phenol-inactivated vaccine, containing either killed *Salmonella typhi* or killed *Salmonella typhi* and *Salmonella paratyphi* A, B organisms; this

preparation is no longer recommended by the WHO, although it is still produced in some countries;

- Vi capsular polysaccharide vaccine and vaccines based on auxotrophic mutants of Vi-positive and Vi-negative *Salmonella typhi* (SED-11, 687) (SEDA-12, 278) (SEDA-13, 284) (SEDA-14, 281).

Oral live vaccine

During volunteer studies and field trials using Ty21a vaccine, adverse reactions were rare and consisted of abdominal discomfort, nausea, vomiting, and rash or urticaria. Adverse reactions occurred with equal frequencies among groups receiving vaccine or placebo. There has been a report of a typhoid-fever-like syndrome after the use of Ty21a live oral vaccine (SEDA-15, 350).

Inactivated vaccine

Vaccines administered parenterally are not well tolerated. Severe local pain and/or swelling occurred in 6–40% of vaccinees; systemic reactions have been reported in 9–30% (headache), and in 14–29% (fever); 13–24% of vaccinees missed work or school due to adverse effects. More severe reactions (hypotension, shock) have been reported sporadically (1).

General adverse effects

There have been individual reports of fatal angio-immunoblastic lymphadenopathy, hemolytic uremic syndrome (after typhoid/paratyphoid/diphtheria vaccination), fatal hyperpyrexia (SED-11, 687), transverse myelitis (SEDA-10, 288), erythema nodosum (SEDA-11, 289) (SEDA-14, 281), and Reiter's syndrome (SEDA-15, 350).

The efficacy and safety of typhoid fever vaccine have been estimated in a meta-analysis of about 1.8 million vaccinees in efficacy trials and about 11 000 vaccinees in safety studies (2). The 3-year cumulative efficacy was 73% (65–80%) for two doses of whole cell vaccines, 51% (35–63%) for three doses of Ty21 live attenuated vaccine, and 55% (30–71%) for one dose of Vi vaccine. After immunization, fever occurred in 16% (12–21%) of whole cell vaccine recipients, 2% (0.7–5.3%) of Ty21a vaccine recipients, and 1.1% (0.1–12.3%) of Vi vaccine recipients (Table 1) (3).

A meta-analysis of studies of the efficacy and toxicity of typhoid fever vaccines (SEDA-23, 343) has been criticized as an interesting mathematical exercise but of little practical relevance (4). The meta-analysis had lumped together different parenteral whole-cell vaccines (alcohol-inactivated, formalin-inactivated, acetone-inactivated, and dried whole-cell vaccines), but the only

Table 1 Local and systemic reactions after the administration of typhoid fever vaccines

Study	Age (years)	Type of study	Number vaccinated	Fever (%)	Swelling (%)	Vomiting (%)	Diarrhea (%)	Missed school or work (%)
Ty21a vaccine								
Gilman et al.	Adults	Clinic	155	1	NA	3	10	ND
Murphy et al.	0.5–2	Clinic	18	11	NA	17	11	ND
Rahman et al.	3–78	Clinic	157	2	NA	0	1	ND
Cryz et al.	2–6	Clinic	317	<1	NA	1	<1	ND
Cryz et al.	16–56	Clinic	30	2	NA	0	20	ND
Pooled estimate (95% CI)				2.0 (0.7–5.3)		2.1 (0.6–7.8)	5.1 (1.7–15)	
Vi vaccine								
Levin et al.	ND	Clinic	21	24	ND	NA	NA	ND
Tacket et al.	20–24	Clinic	19	0	ND	NA	NA	0
Klugman et al.	5–15	Field	253	<1	4	NA	NA	ND
Cumberland et al.	18–22	Clinic	388	<1	1	NA	NA	ND
Mirza et al.	5–15	Field	435	0	8	NA	NA	ND
Pooled estimate (95% CI)				1.1 (0.1–1.2)	3.7 (1.3–9.6)			
Whole-cell vaccine (heat inactivated)								
YTC	5-50	Field	214	9	5	NA	NA	11
Ashcroft et al.	5–15	Field	193	13	61	NA	NA	14
YTC	NA	Field	66	29	ND	NA	NA	17
Hejfez et al.	7–18	Field	2621	30	19	NA	NA	ND
Hejfez et al.	ND	Field	3463	26	21	NA	NA	ND
Hejfez et al.	7–20	Field	2157	13	13	NA	NA	ND
Dimache et al.	16–18	Field	94	27	ND	NA	NA	ND
Dimache et al.	21	Clinic	113	1	ND	NA	NA	ND
Dimache	20	Field	100	34	ND	NA	NA	2
Cumberland et al.	18–22	Clinic	390	2	20	NA	NA	ND
Pooled estimate (95% CI)				16 (21–21)	20 (13–30)			10 (6–16)

For references, see (3)

YTC = Yugoslav Typhoid Commission

NA = Not applicable

ND = Not described in study

parenteral killed whole-cell vaccine that is available is the heat-inactivated phenol-preserved vaccine. The analysis should therefore have been limited to heat-phenolized vaccine. It was also mentioned that the quoted data on the occurrence of adverse reactions failed to include the largest clinical trial of Ty21a vaccine. Last but not least, the authors of the meta-analysis failed to relate the severity of reactions connected with the use of parenteral whole-cell vaccine. These adverse reactions, including high fever, malaise, and nausea, make the killed whole-cell vaccine among the most reactogenic vaccine ever licensed. In contrast, oral Ty21a and parenteral Vi vaccines are well tolerated.

Combined meningococcal and typhoid fever vaccine

A combined meningococcal and typhoid vaccine (Mérieux) was evaluated in 158 volunteers in a single-blind study (5). Comparing the effects with those in vaccinees receiving monocomponent vaccines or the combination vaccine, there was no significant difference in the reported frequency or duration of local and systemic reactions. However, vaccinees who received the monocomponent typhoid fever vaccine alone were less likely to complain of swelling or pain at the injection site.

Organs and Systems

Musculoskeletal

Two cases of arthritis temporally connected with the administration of oral typhoid vaccine have been reported (6).

- Arthritis of the knees, ankles, and hands occurred 8 weeks after immunization in a 27-year-old woman.
- Bilateral sacroiliitis was observed in a 66-year-old woman 1 day after she had completed the four-capsule series.

A rheumatologist evaluated both patients and felt that the diagnosis was reactive arthritis, in his opinion most probably vaccine-related. The two cases are the first reports of reactive arthritis following oral typhoid immunization. However, the time-courses (1 day, 8 weeks) make a causal relation doubtful.

References

1. Immunization Practices Advisory Committee (ACIP). Typhoid immunization. MMWR Recomm Rep 1990;39(RR-10):1–5.
2. Hodsagi M, Uhereczky G, Kiraly L, Pinter E. BCG dissemination in chronic granulomatous disease (CGD). Dev Biol Stand 1986;58(Pt A):339–46.
3. Engels EA, Falagas ME, Lau J, Bennish ML. Typhoid fever vaccines: a meta-analysis of studies on efficacy and toxicity. BMJ 1998;316(7125):110–16.
4. Clemens J, Hoffman S, Ivanoff B, Klugman K, Levine MM, Neira M, Pang T. Typhoid fever vaccines. Vaccine 1999;17(20–21):2476–8.
5. Khoo SH, St Clair Roberts J, Mandal BK. Safety and efficacy of combined meningococcal and typhoid vaccine. BMJ 1995;310(6984):908–9.
6. Adachi JA, D'Alessio FR, Ericsson CD. Reactive arthritis associated with typhoid vaccination in travelers: report of two cases with negative HLA-B27. J Travel Med 2000;7(1):35–6.

U

Ultrasound contrast agents

General Information

The ideal contrast agent for enhancing ultrasound images and Doppler signals would be non-toxic, injectable intravenously, capable of crossing the pulmonary capillary bed, stable for the duration of the ultrasound examination, and useful for both Doppler and grey scale enhancement.

The first generation of echo contrast agents comprised compounds made of air bubbles stabilized with human serum albumin or D-galactose, which pass through the lung capillaries and reach the left heart chambers. The second generation comprises agents made of stabilized microbubbles of gases of high molecular weight and low solubility in water, mainly fluorocarbons, which provide better resistance to pressure. The high molecular weight fluorocarbon gases have lower diffusivity and blood solubility and thus give better persistence of microbubbles in the circulation. These agents can actually be considered as blood pool agents. Other factors, such as the size and stability of the particles, play a major role in optimal examination. Microbubbles larger than 7 μm will not cross the pulmonary vasculature after intravenous administration and hence the mean size of the microbubbles should be 2–5 μm.

Non-thermal bioeffects can develop with ultrasound equipment with high acoustic input in the presence of ultrasound contrast agents with a high mechanical index. Mechanical index is defined as the maximal rarefactional acoustic pressure divided by the acoustic frequency. Ventricular extra beats have been reported in people subjected to strong ultrasound fields but not with diagnostic ultrasonography, which is generally considered safe and without adverse effects. However, new ultrasound machines can provide high acoustic pressures, and the maximum mechanical index currently allowed is 1.9 (1).

Albumin microspheres

Albunex is a suspension of air-filled human albumin microspheres. In an assessment of the safety of Albunex (Molecular Biosystem Inc USA, Nycomed, Oslo Norway) in imaging the left ventricle in 52 patients, there were no major or minor adverse events and no changes in vital signs (2).

Optison is a second-generation contrast agent based on sonicated human albumin (albumin microspheres containing the gas perfluoropropane). In 191 patients with chronic pulmonary disease and/or cardiomyopathy (aged 21–83 years) given intravenous Optison 0.2, 0.5, 3.0, and 5.0 ml, adverse effects were observed in 6.5% (3). The most frequent adverse events were transient alterations in taste (2.5% of patients), headache (2.0%), and a warm sensation/flushing (2.0%). The adverse events were similar to those reported with first-generation ultrasound contrast agents.

In 50 patients (mean age 59 years) in an intensive care unit who underwent echocardiography examination with intravenous Optison (dose 0.5–1.5 ml), there were no contrast-related adverse effects (4). Good quality echocardiography was obtained in all cases.

Albunex has been compared with Optison in 203 patients undergoing echocardiography (5). There were no clinically significant changes in physical examination, vital signs, or electrocardiography in either group. Adverse effects were few in each group and were most commonly related to flushing, warmth, or taste disturbance. Similar results have been reported from a comparison of Echogen (2% dodecafluoropentane emulsion) with Albunex (SEDA-22, 505) (5).

AIP10119 is a contrast agent that consists of heat-stabilized, air-filled, albumin microcapsules with a median diameter of 4 μm. It contains 1.5×10^8 microcapsules/ml after reconstitution with water for injection. It can be prepared in a formulation with a relatively high acoustic pressure (mechanical index 1.5). In a phase I study in healthy men (mean age 28 years) who received continuous infusions of 1 ml/minute of AIP10119 (mechanical index 1.5) for 10 minutes ($n = 6$) or 20 minutes ($n = 4$) there was a significant dose-dependent increase in the number of ventricular extra beats during end-systolic imaging but not during end-diastolic imaging (1). Nine volunteers received AIP10119 as a single infusion of 1 ml/minute for 25 minutes (mechanical index 1.1) followed by three rapid bolus injections of 1 ml at least 5 minutes apart, the infusion and the series of bolus injections being separated by at least 2 hours; there was no increase in the number of ventricular extra beats. The authors concluded that precautionary measures would include using formulations with a low mechanical index or end-diastolic imaging.

Galactose

The galactose-based ultrasound contrast agents include Echovist and Levovist. Levovist consists of microbubbles less than 8 μm in size. After injection it crosses the lung and enters the systemic circulation. The lack of any adverse effects has been reported in several studies and clinical trials (SEDA-20, 418).

There has been a meta-analysis of the use of Echovist in 986 patients in the assessment of fallopian tube patency. It was well tolerated, although there were adverse events in 47%. By far the most common adverse effect was abdominal pain during the examination (38%). This correlated with tubal patency and was most severe in patients with blockage of both fallopian tubes, presumably because of increased intraluminal pressure. The only other common adverse events were vasovagal reactions (2.8%) and nausea (1.5%), which may not have been directly related to contrast administration (SEDA-22, 505).

Levovist has been assessed in 5073 patients. In addition, spontaneous reporting of adverse events in 100 000 patients given injections of Levovist has been analysed (6). The incidence of adverse events (12%) was similar in the Levovist group and in the controls, who were given isotonic saline. The adverse events included sensations of pain, cold, and warmth during injection, abnormal taste sensations, headache, nausea, and vomiting. There were no serious adverse events. The overall adverse event rate in spontaneous reports was 0.02%. One patient developed bronchospasm, another had a generalized skin rash, and two other patients had urticaria. The other reported adverse events were not serious and may not have been caused by the contrast agent.

Intravesical Levovist has been used for voiding uroso-nography in 118 patients (aged 3 weeks to 16 years) (7). The diagnostic accuracy of the examination was high and no adverse effects were reported.

A phase-3 assessment of the accuracy of Levovist (SHU508A, Schering, Berlin) in investigating the portal system has been reported (8). It was injected into peripheral veins in 588 patients in concentrations of 200–400 mg/ml. During the 24 hours after the last injection, pain at the site of injection, vasodilatation, and paresthesia were the only adverse effects definitely related to the injection. There were 18 adverse events in 12 patients and the only severe reaction (fever) was not considered to have been related to Levovist.

There has been further confirmation of the safety of Levovist in a phase 3b clinical trial in 38 patients with hepatocellular carcinoma (9). There were only two minor reactions of nausea and vomiting.

Perfluorocarbons

NC100100

NC100100 (Nycomed, Oslo, Norway) is composed of stabilized perfluorocarbon microbubbles. In a randomized comparison of ^{99m}technetium sestamibi single-photon emission-computed tomography (SPECT) and NC100100 in the assessment of myocardial perfusion in 203 patients with myocardial infarction, NC100100 was well tolerated, with no serious adverse events or deaths (10). Similarly there were no clinically important changes in vital signs, laboratory parameters, or electrocardiography. NC100100 correctly identified the vast majority of normally perfused segments assessed by SPECT.

Octafluoropropane

Octafluoropropane gas encapsulated as microspheres in lipid shells (Definity) is given intravenously as an echocardiographic contrast agent. In a review of its diagnostic efficacy and safety, the authors concluded that it improves the diagnostic accuracy of echocardiographic examinations and has a good safety profile (11). Minor adverse effects were reported, such as headache, back pain, flushing, and nausea. There were no serious adverse effects. However, Definity should not be used in patients with intracardiac shunts or in pregnant or lactating women. It should also be used with caution in patients with severe liver or renal disease.

Perflenapent

Perflenapent emulsion (EchoGen) is an ultrasound contrast agent for echocardiography. It is a liquid-in-liquid emulsion of dodecafluoropentane in water, which becomes a dispersion of microbubbles after hypobaric activation. The microbubbles cross the lung capillary bed and persist in solution much longer than microbubbles of air or other gases of similar size, providing prolonged contrast enhancement. A review of 21 clinical studies involving 743 patients who received perflenapent emulsion and 151 patients who received placebo showed no clinically important abnormalities in laboratory tests, pulse oximetry, vital signs, or electrocardiography. There were adverse events in 6.7% of patients after perflenapent emulsion and 2.6% of patients after placebo. The most frequent adverse effects considered relevant to perflenapent emulsion were vasodilatation (2.8%) and taste disturbances (1.2%). Adverse events were generally mild to moderate, started within 10–20 minutes of contrast administration, and resolved spontaneously within 10–20 minutes. These reassuring findings are in keeping with safety reports about other ultrasound contrast agents (SEDA-22, 505).

A double-blind, placebo-controlled evaluation of perflenapent emulsion as a contrast agent for the liver, kidneys, and vasculature has been reported in 151 patients of whom 12 had adverse effects compared with nine who received placebo (12). Injection site pain, vasodilatation, rash, and rhinitis occurred more often with perflenapent than placebo.

The safety of perflenapent has been evaluated in multicenter phase II studies in 146 patients with congestive heart failure (NYHA class III or IV, mean age 68 years), of whom 99 received perflenapent and 47 received isotonic saline, and in 134 patients with severe chronic obstructive pulmonary disease (FEV_1 no more than 60% of predicted, mean age 65 years), of whom 91 received perflenapent and 43 received isotonic saline (13). Blood pressure, heart rate, respiratory rate, oxygen saturation, the electrocardiogram, FEV_1, complete serum biochemistry, hematology, and mental state were assessed. Adverse events were mild and required no treatment. There was no significant difference in the incidence of adverse reactions between those given perflenapent (15%) and those given placebo (11%). The most frequent adverse events with perflenapent were vasodilatation ($n = 8$), taste disturbance ($n = 6$), nausea ($n = 5$), and headache ($n = 3$).

Perflubron

Perflubron (perfluoro-octylbromide) is composed predominantly of carbon and fluorine, and the absence of protons results in a signal void wherever it is found. When it is given enterically the bowel is labeled as a signal void on the abdominal image.

The enteric use of perflubron has been studied and the authors concluded that it is relatively safe and effective. The main adverse effects were vomiting, which developed in 8% of patients, and a feeling of fullness reported in 5% of cases. Other adverse events involved complaints about the taste of the agent. There were no life-threatening or fatal events (SEDA-21, 484).

An intravenous infusion of an emulsion of perflubron as a hepatic and splenic enhancement agent during CT examination caused lower back pain and transient fever (SEDA-15, 505). This problem appeared to be due to the lipid emulsion and seems to have been overcome with more recent formulations.

Perflutren

Perflutren is an ultrasound agent that consists of perfluoropropane gas encapsulated in lipid microbubbles. It has been used in patients with suspected cardiac disease and suboptimal baseline echocardiography in doses of 5 µl/kg ($n = 85$) or 10 µl/kg ($n = 84$); 42 patients received isotonic saline (14). The magnitude of clinically useful opacification was not dose-dependent, but its duration was 81 seconds with 5 µl/kg and 99 seconds with 10 µl/kg. There were no clinically significant changes in physical examination, vital signs, electrocardiography, biochemistry, or hematology. Headache was the most frequent averse event, in nine patients who received perflutren and in three controls.

Simethicone-coated cellulose

Artefacts that arise from gas in the stomach and adjacent bowel often limit the diagnostic accuracy of abdominal ultrasound. Research to overcome this problem has focused on cellulose-based suspensions. An agent has been developed based on simethicone-coated cellulose—SonoRx (Bracco Diagnostics, Princeton, NJ), which displaces and disperses gas bubbles. In a phase 2 clinical study, 93 patients underwent upper abdominal sonography before and after a randomized dose of the contrast agent (200, 400, 600, 800, or 1000 ml) (15). Anatomical visualization was improved as follows: the stomach in 82% of patients, the duodenum in 63%, the pancreatic head and body in 61%, and the pancreatic tail in 67%. There were 14 adverse events in 11 patients and only five were considered to be related to the contrast agent. The main adverse effects were mild diarrhea and nausea.

Sulfur hexafluoride

Sono Vue (BR1) is an ultrasound contrast medium that consists of microbubbles containing sulfur hexafluoride gas stabilized by phospholipids. The diameter of each microbubble is 2.5 µm and there are about 0.5×10^9 microbubbles/ml. It is isotonic with human plasma, has the same viscosity as blood, and has minimal antigenic potential, since it contains no protein material.

The pharmacokinetics of Sono Vue have been studied in 12 healthy volunteers (aged 20–36 years, seven men), who received two intravenous doses of 0.03 and 0.3 ml/kg in random order (16). Sono Vue was rapidly cleared from the blood, with a half-life of 5–7 minutes. About 40–50% of the dose was eliminated in the expired air during the first minute after injection and 80–90% was eliminated by 11 minutes. Within 90 minutes, sulfur hexafluoride could no longer be detected in the expired air in most cases. There were no adverse effects.

The diagnostic efficacy and the safety of Sono Vue has been assessed in 218 patients with suspected coronary artery disease who underwent echocardiography (17). Each received intravenous Sono Vue 0.5, 1.0, 2.0, and 4.0 ml in random order at intervals of at least 5 minutes between injections. There were no clinically significant changes in physical examination, vital signs, or electrocardiography. There were no serious adverse effects, even in patients who had heart failure and a history of myocardial infarction. The non-serious adverse reactions were mild and transient and required no treatment. The most common adverse effects were headache (4%) and nausea (1.4%).

Assessment of vascularity can be useful in differentiating benign and malignant breast lesions using color Doppler examination. However, some neoplasms have low blood flow and Doppler may be suboptimal. In these cases, ultrasound contrast may be beneficial. In a phase II/III, multicenter, randomized study 220 patients

with breast lesions in different anatomical areas received intravenous Sono Vue 0.3, 0.6, 1.2, and 2.4 ml (18). Sono Vue improved the quality of Doppler blood flow information in both parenchymal and focal lesions. There were mild adverse events in two patients only; one complained of nausea and the other of discomfort. It is not clear whether these events were related to the contrast agent or not.

The safety of Sono Vue as an intravenous bolus injection of 0.3, 0.6, 1.2, or 2.4 ml in transcranial Doppler examination of the cerebral arteries has been investigated in 40 patients (mean age 64 years) (19). The interval between each dose was at least 10 minutes or until total disappearance of the contrast effect from the previous dose. Eight patients reported 12 adverse events. There were no serious adverse events and no patient withdrew because of an adverse event. The most common adverse events were pain at the injection site, headache, and a feeling of warmth; all were mild.

The safety of Sono Vue has been evaluated in 36 healthy volunteers who were given a single dose of isotonic saline or Sono Vue, 0.003, 0.01, 0.03, 0.06, 0.09, or 0.12 ml/kg and in 30 volunteers who were given cumulative doses of 0.15–0.6 ml/kg (20). The volunteers were aged 20–35 years. Another 12 subjects, patients with chronic obstructive airways disease, were given a single dose of Sono Vue 4 ml and placebo (isotonic saline 4 ml) in two sessions, separated by 48–72 hours. All adverse events were minor or mild and rapidly resolved. The adverse effects in the healthy volunteers were heat at the injection site, facial flushing, headache, and a tingling sensation in the hand (one patient each). There were no differences in the frequencies of adverse events in the different dosages groups or between Sono Vue and placebo. In the patient with chronic obstructive airways disease, vomiting and lethargy occurred in one patient each. There were no significant changes in respiratory function tests (FEV_1, FVC, forced mid-expiratory flow, and oxygen saturation).

The excellent safety and efficacy of Sono Vue at doses of 0.7, 1, 2, and 4 ml has been demonstrated in 138 patients (mean age 57 years) (21). There were mild adverse events, such as headache, nausea, paresthesia, and taste disturbance, but no severe adverse reactions.

References

1. van Der Wouw PA, Brauns AC, Bailey SE, Powers JE, Wilde AA. Premature ventricular contractions during triggered imaging with ultrasound contrast. J Am Soc Echocardiogr 2000;13(4):288–94.
2. Castini D, Gentile F, Ornaghi M, Mangiarotti E, Garbin M, Ravaglia R, Gioventu M, Mantero A, Corno R, Limido A, Morandi F, Fiorentini C, Pezzano A, Repetto S, Haider T, Morris H, Marelli C. Left ventricular opacification by intravenous contrast echocardiography. G Ital Cardiol 1999;29(6):620–9.
3. Ellahham S, Hausnerova E, Gottdiener J. Intravenous Optison (FS069) enhances pulmonary vein flow velocity signals: a multicenter study. Clin Cardiol 2000;23(2):91–5.
4. Daniel GK, Chawla MK, Sawada SG, Gradus-Pizlo I, Feigenbaum H, Segar DS. Echocardiographic imaging of technically difficult patients in the intensive care unit: use

of Optison in combination with fundamental and harmonic imaging. J Am Soc Echocardiogr 2001;14(9):917–20.

5. Cohen JL, Cheirif J, Segar DS, Gillam LD, Gottdiener JS, Hausnerova E, Bruns DE. Improved left ventricular endocardial border delineation and opacification with OPTISON (FS069), a new echocardiographic contrast agent. Results of a phase III Multicenter Trial. J Am Coll Cardiol 1998;32(3):746–52.

6. Schlief R, Alhassan A, Wiggins J, Schumann W, Niendorf HP. Safety of the galactose-based ultrasound contrast agent Levovist. Acad Radiol 2002;9(Suppl 1):S240–2.

7. Mentzel HJ, Vogt S, John U, Kaiser WA. Voiding urosonography with ultrasonography contrast medium in children. Pediatr Nephrol 2002;17(4):272–6.

8. Gebel M, Caselitz M, Bowen-Davies PE, Weber S. A multicenter, prospective, open label, randomized, controlled phase IIIb study of SH U 508 a (Levovist) for Doppler signal enhancement in the portal vascular system. Ultraschall Med 1998;19(4):148–56.

9. Khong PL, Chau MT, Fan ST, Leong LL. Ultrasound contrast agent Levovist in colour Doppler sonography of hepatocellular carcinoma in Chinese patients. Australas Radiol 1999;43(2):156–9.

10. Binder T, Assayag P, Baer F, Flachskampf F, Kamp O, Nienaber C, Nihoyannopoulos P, Pierard L, Steg G, Vanoverschelde JL, Van der Wouw P, Meland N, Marelli C, Lindvall K. NC100100, a new echo contrast agent for the assessment of myocardial perfusion—safety and comparison with technetium-99m sestamibi single-photon emission computed tomography in a randomized multicenter study. Clin Cardiol 1999;22(4):273–82.

11. Murthy TH, Weissman NJ. The advanced echocardiographic contrast agent Definity (perflutren lipid microspheres). Today's Ther Trends 2002;20:233–41.

12. Robbin ML, Eisenfeld AJ. Perflenapent emulsion: a US contrast agent for diagnostic radiology—multicenter, double-blind comparison with a placebo. EchoGen Contrast Ultrasound Study Group Radiology 1998;207(3):717–22

13. Kitzman DW, Wesley DJ. Safety assessment of perflenapent emulsion for echocardiographic contrast enhancement in patients with congestive heart failure or chronic obstructive pulmonary disease. Am Heart J 2000;139(6):1077–80.

14. Kitzman DW, Goldman ME, Gillam LD, Cohen JL, Aurigemma GP, Gottdiener JS. Efficacy and safety of the novel ultrasound contrast agent perflutren (Definity) in patients with suboptimal baseline left ventricular echocardiographic images. Am J Cardiol 2000;86(6):669–74.

15. Lev-Toaff AS, Langer JE, Rubin DL, Zelch JV, Chong WK, Barone AE, Goldberg BB. Safety and efficacy of a new oral contrast agent for sonography: a phase II trial. Am J Roentgenol 1999;173(2):431–6.

16. Morel DR, Schwieger I, Hohn L, Terrettaz J, Llull JB, Cornioley YA, Schneider M. Human pharmacokinetics and safety evaluation of SonoVue, a new contrast agent for ultrasound imaging. Invest Radiol 2000;35(1):80–5.

17. Senior R, Andersson O, Caidahl K, Carlens P, Herregods MC, Jenni R, Kenny A, Melcher A, Svedenhag J, Vanoverschelde JL, Wandt B, Widgren BR, Williams G, Guerret P, la Rosee K, Agati L, Bezante G. Enhanced left ventricular endocardial border delineation with an intravenous injection of SonoVue, a new echocardiographic contrast agent: A European multicenter study. Echocardiography 2000;17(8):705–11.

18. Madjar H, Prompeler HJ, Del Favero C, Hackeloer BJ, Llull JB. A new Doppler signal enhancing agent for flow assessment in breast lesions. Eur J Ultrasound 2000;12(2):123–30.

19. Kaps M, Legemate DA, Ries F, Ackerstaff RG, Markus H, Pezzoll C, Llull JB, Spinazzi A. SonoVue in transcranial Doppler investigations of the cerebral arteries. J Neuroimaging 2001;11(3):261–7.

20. Bokor D, Chambers JB, Rees PJ, Mant TG, Luzzani F, Spinazzi A. Clinical safety of SonoVue, a new contrast agent for ultrasound imaging, in healthy volunteers and in patients with chronic obstructive pulmonary disease. Invest Radiol 2001;36(2):104–9.

21. Nanda NC, Wistran DC, Karlsberg RP, Hack TC, Smith WB, Foley DA, Picard MH, Cotter B. Multicenter evaluation of SonoVue for improved endocardial border delineation. Echocardiography 2002;19(1):27–36.

Unoprostone

See also Prostaglandins

General Information

Unoprostone is a synthetic prostaglandin analogue of $PGF_{2\alpha}$ used in the treatment of glaucoma. Its mechanism of action is believed to be by enhancing uveoscleral outflow, like latanoprost.

Organs and Systems

Sensory systems

The use of unoprostone in the treatment of open-angle glaucoma and ocular hypertension has been reviewed (1). Most of the literature is in Japanese. The adverse effects of unoprostone are similar to those of latanoprost: conjunctival hyperemia, iris pigmentation, hypertrichosis and hyperpigmentation of eyelashes, and rarely systemic effects (1).

Reference

1. Eisenberg DL, Camras CB. A preliminary risk-benefit assessment of latanoprost and unoprostone in open-angle glaucoma and ocular hypertension. Drug Saf 1999;20(6):505–14.

Urticaceae

See also Herbal medicines

General Information

The genera in the family of Urticaceae (Table 1) include various types of nettle.

Urtica dioica

Urtica dioica (stinging nettle) has been used to treat rheumatism and benign prostatic hyperplasia.

Adverse effects
Gastrointestinal

A secondary source states that tea prepared from stinging nettle leaves can occasionally cause gastric irritation, skin reactions, edema, and oliguria, but primary references are not provided.

Table 1 The genera of Urticaceae

Boehmeria (false nettle)
Cypholophus (lopleaf)
Elatostema
Hesperocnide (stinging nettle)
Laportea (laportea)
Neraudia (ma'oloa)
Parietaria (pellitory)
Pilea (clearweed)
Pipturus (pipturus)
Pouzolzia (pouzolzia)
Rousselia (rousselia)
Soleirolia (soleirolia)
Touchardia (touchardia)
Urera (urera)
Urtica (nettle)

Skin

The blister-raising properties of topical stinging nettle extracts are well known; there is no definitive treatment (1).

A positive patch test reaction to *U. dioica* has been obtained in a patient who had developed edematous gingivostomatitis following the regular use of stinging nettle tea as a tonic; the patient also had positive reactions to chamomile (*Anthemis nobilis*) and its allergens (sesquiterpene lactones) (2).

References

1. Anderson BE, Miller CJ, Adams DR. Stinging nettle dermatitis. Am J Contact Dermat 2003;14(1):44–6.
2. Bossuyt L, Dooms-Goossens A. Contact sensitivity to nettles and camomile in "alternative" remedies. Contact Dermatitis 1994;31(2):131–2.

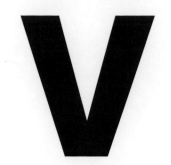

Vaccines

See also Individual agents

General Information

In the early days of vaccine development the majority of untoward effects after immunization were associated with faulty production, and the control of biological products as they exist today has been developed largely as a result of major accidents. For example, the Cutter incident in the USA in 1955, in which a batch of "inactivated" poliomyelitis vaccine containing live poliovirus was inadvertently released, had devastating consequences. The World Health Organization (WHO) subsequently took over the responsibility for international biological standardization. Currently, more than 50 WHO requirements for the manufacture and control of biological substances have been adopted and updated. As a result of the incorporation of WHO requirements, and their strict observance by manufacturers and control authorities, accidents due to faulty production of vaccines have become rare (SEDA-13, 271).

However, during the last two decades rapid increases in immunization coverage have been reported worldwide; globally, 5–10 billion injections are now given each year, mainly for treatment of illness but also for prophylactic purposes such as immunization. Unavoidably, the growth of WHO's Expanded Program on Immunization has sometimes resulted in extension of immunization work into areas of the developing world where logistic support and training programs have not been adequate. In such circumstances, avoidable faults have been made, involving variously improper or inadequate sterilization, incorrect doses and routes of vaccine administration, or substitution of drugs for diluents or vaccines (SEDA-15, 340). The use of unsterilized or improperly sterilized needles and syringes is particularly common in these regions and contributes largely to the spread of hepatitis B and C as well as to the spread of human immunodeficiency virus (HIV) and other blood-borne pathogens. The WHO recognizes this as a major public health problem and has initiated a program of activities to ensure safe injections (1).

In some highly developed countries that have had great success in reducing dangerous infectious diseases through immunization, there are controversial discussions regarding the benefits to harm balance of immunization. Because the incidence of vaccine-preventable diseases is reduced by increasing coverage with an efficacious vaccine, adverse events, both those caused by vaccines themselves (that is true adverse reactions) and those associated with immunization only by coincidence or as a result of faulty routines, become increasingly frequent. Not surprisingly, vaccine safety concerns have become increasingly prominent in successful immunization programs. Chronic illnesses recently claimed to be linked with immunizations include asthma, autism, diabetes, and multiple sclerosis. Given the current increasingly "anti-vaccine" environment that has developed in some countries, it is hard to imagine that the full potential of new vaccines will be harnessed. To avoid damage to current and future immunization programs considered as among the most successful and cost-effective public health interventions, we need to examine critically the factors that have influenced this change in public attitudes.

We have been relatively slow in appreciating the importance that the public now places on vaccine safety. In fact, much of our resource allocations still unfortunately reflect safety last rather than safety first. This reflects in part an unfortunate legacy, in which we have characterized this arena for years in narrow, negative terms of adverse events, instead of the more broad and positive terms of safety. Furthermore, it shows that we have not been as interested in preventing vaccine-induced illnesses as we are in vaccine-preventable diseases (2). Increasing interest in this problem can therefore be observed in many developed and developing countries, and international institutions and organizations, for example the World Health Organization (WHO), the United Nations Children's Fund (UNICEF), and vaccine manufacturers. The careful review of the current knowledge on adverse effects after immunization is a useful contribution to vaccine safety and helps to maintain confidence in immunization programs.

On the other hand, we must not forget that the ultimate goal of an immunization program is control of disease or even its regional elimination or worldwide eradication. A successful immunization program can lead to the eradication of disease and opens up the possibility of ultimately abandoning immunization (and with it the occurrence of adverse effects) completely. Smallpox eradication made it possible to stop smallpox immunization and poliomyelitis eradication, which is expected to be achieved within a few years, will mean the end of polio vaccine.

Surveillance of adverse events following immunization

Currently, in many highly developed countries in which the incidences of dangerous infectious diseases have been markedly reduced through immunization, there are controversial discussions about the balance of benefits and harms in immunization. Vaccine adverse events, both those caused by vaccines (that is true adverse reactions) and those associated with immunization only by coincidence, become more visible than the natural disease. Not surprisingly, vaccine safety concerns have become increasingly prominent in such successful immunization programs. Vaccines have been spuriously linked by various researchers to asthma, autism, diabetes, inflammatory bowel disease, multiple sclerosis, permanent brain damage, and sudden infant death syndrome (SIDS). Modern communication is providing even more penetrating ways of communicating messages on the subject through the World Wide Web. The result is a formidable challenge to immunization service providers. Neil Halsey, head of the Institute for Vaccine Safety at Johns Hopkins University, has summarized the features common to recent publications on vaccine adverse effects:

- a causal link is usually claimed with a disease or condition of unknown or unclear cause;
- the association is claimed by one investigator or a group of investigators;

- the association is not confirmed by peers or by subsequent research;
- the claims are made with no apparent concern for potential harm from public loss of confidence and refusal to immunize;
- findings of subsequent studies that fail to confirm the original claim never get the publicity given to the original finding, and so the public never gets a balanced view(2,3).

A critical examination (4) of a report (5) of several children whose chronic bowel and behavioral abnormalities were linked to measles, mumps, and rubella (MMR) immunization can be used as an example to underline Halsey's comments. Without effective and credible systems for the detection of vaccine-associated adverse events through pharmacovigilance, for distinguishing causal reactions from coincidental reactions by pharmacoepidemiological or other studies, and for risk communication, vaccine safety concerns may confuse the media and the public.

A concerted effort is needed to improve communications at all levels regarding the real risks associated with vaccines and immunization and helping to reassure the public of the overwhelming safety record of vaccines. The medical community is still preeminent as advice givers to the public on matters of immunization and should play the key role in improved communication (3,6).

The US Vaccine Adverse Events Reporting System (VAERS) has been described (SEDA-14, 919) and the pros and cons of the system have been discussed (7). About 1000 reports per month are submitted by manufacturers (39%), state health coordinators (34%), health care professionals (25%), and parents (2%). Manufacturers' reports are primarily based on information received from health care providers or the parents of vaccinees. As a passive reporting system, VAERS is subject to numerous well-known deficiencies, such as underreporting, incomplete and missing data, and recall bias. Resources are not adequate to allow follow-up for complete or accurate data in all cases. However, VAERS is useful to detect early warning signals and to generate hypotheses. For example, the information from a parent that her daughter had lost her hair after the second and third doses of hepatitis B vaccine initiated a study that found 59 similar cases, including three cases of positive rechallenge. As a result of this study, alopecia was added to the list of adverse reactions in the hepatitis B vaccine package insert. Individual case reports can also trigger a complete review of the VAERS database. For example, three reports of idiopathic thrombocytopenic purpura after measles-containing vaccine were received in a short period of time. The study of idiopathic thrombocytopenic purpura reported in the database found 54 other reports during the period 1990–95, including one case of positive rechallenge, which increased the likelihood that the association was causal.

Reports on adverse events after the administration of the two hepatitis B vaccines licensed in the US (Engerix-B and Recombivax HB) have been compared in two different surveillance systems: VAERS and Vaccine Safety Datalink (VSD) (8). VSD is a computerized record linkage system designed to allow more rigorous evaluation of causality of adverse events after immunization. Since 1989, VSD has actively maintained medical files on over 500 000 children, aged from birth to 6 years enrolled at four West-coast health maintenance organizations. Immunization records, medical diagnoses, and diseases from clinic, hospitalization, and emergency room visits are coded. Whereas VAERS found that the reporting rate for events after brand 1 vaccine was at least three times higher than the reporting rate after brand 2 vaccine, VSD found no difference between rates of hospitalization or emergency room visits in recipients of the two brands. The authors concluded that the results of the VAERS database are subject to the inherent limitations of a passive surveillance system. This study underlined the importance of using other analytical studies, such as VSD, to evaluate preliminary results obtained by VAERS.

Adverse events reported to the VAERS during the period 1991–2001 have been summarized and evaluated (9). The main results were as follows:

- During 1991–2001, annual reports of deaths constituted 1.4–2.3% of all reports, and reports of life-threatening illness constituted 1.4–2.8% of all reports.
- A clinical research team followed up all deaths reported to VAERS; most of these deaths were ultimately classified as SIDS; analysis of the age distribution and seasonality of infant deaths reported to VAERS showed that they matched the age distribution and seasonality of SIDS: both peaked at 2–4 months and during the winter; the reduction in the number of deaths reported to VAERS since 1992–93 parallels the overall reduction in the incidence of SIDS in the US population since the implementation of the "Back to sleep" campaign; the Food and Drug Administration (FDA) and the Institute of Medicine (IOM) reviewed 206 deaths reported to VAERS during 1990–91: only one death was believed to have resulted from a vaccine.
- Intussusception after rotavirus vaccine was described as an example to underline the value of passive surveillance systems as an indicator for carefully designed follow-up studies.
- An increase in the number of reports of Guillain–Barré syndrome after the receipt of influenza vaccine was noted in VAERS data by week 29 of the 1993–94 influenza season; the numbers of reports of Guillain–Barré syndrome increased from 23 during 1991-92 to 40 during 1992–93 and to 80 during 1993–94; a study of the VAERS signal showed that slightly more than one additional case of Guillain–Barré syndrome occurred per 1 million people immunized against influenza, a risk that is less than the risk from severe influenza, which can be prevented by the vaccine.
- A detailed review of VAERS reports received during the first 3 years after the licensure of the *Varicella* vaccine documented that the majority of reported adverse events were minor and serious adverse events were rare.

Terms and definitions used in surveillance programs of adverse events and adverse effects after immunization

Definitions are fundamental to the establishment of any functioning surveillance system. There must be different definitions for monitoring and evaluation. An international voluntary collaboration has been established to develop globally accepted standardized case definitions of adverse events following immunization (AEFI). The so-called Brighton Collaboration (initiated in 1999 during a vaccine meeting in Brighton, UK) took into consideration that there is a general lack of widely accepted and implemented case definitions, because only a limited set of case definitions elaborated by WHO has been available internationally. Working groups on fever, local reactions, intussusception, persistent crying, convulsion, and hypotonic-hyporesponsive episodes were already established. The website of the Brighton Collaboration contains information about the process and progress of the collaboration, the work statement for the working groups, a template format for draft definitions, and much more (10).

On behalf of the Brighton Collaboration, an electronic discussion on the wisdom of using the term "adverse event following immunization" (AEFI) has been undertaken during the year 2001. Concern has sometimes been expressed that the word "following" could imply causality. At least 10 alternative terms have been proposed and discussed. Finally, the term "adverse event possibly related to immunization" (AEPRI) received the majority of votes. However, there were many participants in the discussion who believed that the term AEFI should be kept because it is used in many countries as well as in guidelines issued by the WHO and UNICEF and because a change will create new confusion. It therefore seems that the term AEFI will not be replaced (11).

The Brighton Collaboration took into consideration the fact that there is a general lack of widely accepted and implemented case definitions in order to allow comparability between studies. Based on a network of more than 300 participants from 34 countries and collaborating with many national and international organizations, institutions, and manufacturers (for example WHO, FDA, CDC, GlaxoSmithKline), case definitions and guidelines have been developed for intussusception, fever, prolonged crying, seizure, hypotonic-hyporesponsive episodes, and local reactions, such as nodules, swelling, cellulitis, and abscesses. A Brighton Internet site has been created (10).

Monitoring

Data collection is the first step in surveillance. Terms and definitions developed for monitoring purposes should be useful both for practitioners and health workers. Monitoring definitions therefore have to cover a broad range. For monitoring purposes, the term "adverse event" has been introduced, defined as an untoward event temporally associated with immunization, which might or might not be caused by the vaccine or the immunization process. The term "adverse effect" does not seem useful for monitoring purposes, since it relates to an untoward effect after immunization that is linked to the vaccine (antigen or vaccine component) or to the immunization procedure. The term and its definition imply a distinct degree of causality. However, the term "suspected adverse effect" is acceptable.

Evaluation

Statistical analysis and expert evaluation of the collected data should be carried out centrally. Expert evaluation of reports should be based on precise evaluation definitions, taking into account current scientific knowledge. One classification of events is that concerning causality, for example certain, probable, possible, unlikely, unclassified (when no attempt to classify has been made), and unclassifiable events (for example due to lack of data) (12). Alternatively one can classify reports into those for which there is no evidence of a causal relation, those for which evidence is insufficient to indicate a causal relation, those for which the evidence does not indicate a causal relation, those for which the evidence is consistent with a causal relation, and finally those for which the evidence indicates a causal relation (13,14). An evaluated adverse event classified as either "certain" or "probable" or "consistent with a causal relation" or "indicating a causal relation" fulfils the criteria for the recognition of an adverse effect after immunization.

Following WHO's proposal to distinguish four types of adverse events after immunization, the evaluation should furthermore try to distinguish:

- vaccine-induced adverse events (for example BCG lymphadenitis, BCG osteitis, vaccine-associated poliomyelitis, allergic reactions);
- vaccine-precipitated events (for example a simple febrile seizure following DPT immunization in a predisposed child);
- programmatic errors (for example an abscess due to improper sterilization);
- coincidental events (15).

Most commonly, passive surveillance systems are used for the surveillance of adverse events after immunization. Spontaneous reports from health care providers on temporally related adverse events suspected of being caused by the vaccine or the immunization procedure are collected and evaluated. However, the significant degree of under-reporting, together with the non-specific nature of most adverse events reports, highlights the limitations of passive surveillance systems of adverse events after immunization. A critical evaluation of the limitations of the US Vaccine Adverse Event Reporting System (VAERS) (SED-13, 919) and its predecessor, the Monitoring System for Adverse Events Following Immunization (MSAEFI) (SEDA-13, 273) (SEDA-16, 320) has been made by Rosenthal and Chen (16,17). The authors concluded that reports to VAERS and MSAEFI are essentially non-controlled clinical case reports or case series, useful for generating hypotheses but not for testing them. Other controlled studies are therefore often necessary to evaluate hypotheses raised by passive surveillance system reports: whether a given adverse event can be caused by a specific vaccine and if so how commonly it occurs. However, if reporting is reasonably consistent, it may be possible to detect changes in trends of known common adverse events. In addition, passive surveillance remains a potentially cost-effective way of monitoring rare events that cannot be detected in small prelicensing trials.

Cohort studies of rare adverse events would be useful, but are generally not feasible, particularly for economic reasons. One promising alternative approach is the use of large linked databases. The databases appropriate for such studies are derived from defined populations, such as members of health maintenance organizations, universal health care systems, and Medicaid programs. Information on both exposure (immunization records) and outcome (for example diagnoses recording potential adverse events) is usually computerized for members of such populations. These databases can be linked for epidemiological studies assessing potential associations between immunization and outcomes. Large linked databases have already been used by various groups to examine the association between DTP vaccine and SIDS, DTP vaccine and neurological events, and MMR vaccine and seizures. The Centers for Disease Control and Prevention (CDC) in Atlanta use large linked databases (now called Vaccine Safety Datalink) in addition to VAERS Vaccine Safety Datalink, covering a defined cohort of approximately 500 000 children up to the age of 5 years (17–19).

An epidemiological and statistical method based on linkage of routinely available computerized hospital admission records with vaccination records has been described by Farrington (20). This active surveillance method has been used to assess the attributable risk of convulsions after DTP and MMR immunization and to investigate the relation between MMR vaccine and idiopathic thrombocytopenic purpura in children under 2 years of age in five districts in England.

Causality assessment of adverse events following immunization (AEFI)

Adverse events following immunization can be causally related to the inherent properties of the vaccine, linked to errors in administration, quality, storage, and transport of the vaccine (programmatic errors), but also occurring coincidentally after immunization. It is therefore necessary to investigate and evaluate AEFI, particularly those that are serious or unknown.

The most reliable way of determining the causality of an AEFI is by randomized comparisons of events in an immunized group with events in a non-immunized group. However, such trials can never be large enough to detect very rare events; postmarket surveillance is required to identify rare events. A Global Advisory Committee on Vaccine Safety, constituted by the WHO in 1999, has developed criteria for AEFI causality assessment. Criteria to be considered are consistency (the findings should be replicable), strengths of association (in an epidemiological sense), specificity, temporal relation, and biological plausibility (according to what is known about the natural history and biology of the disease). Not all these criteria need to be present to establish causality (21).

In Canada, an advisory committee on causality assessment (ACCA) has been established to evaluate serious individual adverse event reports collected through active surveillance of pediatric hospitals or a passive voluntary reporting system. The ACCA is composed of specialists in epidemiology, immunology, infectious diseases, microbiology, neurology, pathology, and pediatrics. A causality assessment form has been developed (including criteria similar to the WHO criteria described above). For final classification of the evaluated adverse events the causality assessment criteria of the WHO (see Table 1) are used. The great majority of reports collected through the surveillance system describe minor or well-known reactions (over 95%);

Table 1 WHO causality assessment criteria for adverse reactions to vaccines

Probability	Criteria
Very likely/ certain	Clinical event with a plausible time relationship to vaccine administration, and which cannot be explained by concurrent disease or other drugs or chemicals
Probable	Clinical event with a reasonable time relationship to vaccine administration, and is unlikely to be attributed to concurrent disease or other drugs or chemicals
Possible	Clinical event with a reasonable time relationship to vaccine administration, but which could also be explained by concurrent disease or other drugs or chemicals
Unlikely	Clinical event whose time relationship to vaccine administration makes a causal connection improbable, but which could plausibly be explained by underlying disease or other drugs or chemicals
Unrelated	Clinical event with an incompatible time relationship to vaccine administration, and which could be explained by underlying disease or other drugs or chemicals
Unclassifiable	Clinical event with insufficient information to permit assessment and identification of the cause

only the most serious and unusual adverse events after immunization requiring detailed review are submitted to ACCA. At each twice-yearly meeting of the ACCA 60–110 reports of severe and unusual reports are evaluated (22).

Surveillance systems in different countries and between-country collaboration

Some countries have long experience in monitoring adverse events after immunization, starting with smallpox vaccination.

Worldwide, under 10% of countries have implemented postlicensure surveillance systems. The withdrawal of rotavirus vaccine (Rotashield, Wyeth Laboratories) based on postmarketing surveillance data that showed an excess risk of intussusception after the use of the vaccine convincingly showed that such systems are essential components of vaccine program implementation. However, the event also showed the power of active surveillance systems. Active systems in Minnesota and the Northern California Kaiser Permanente Health Maintenance Organization have provided preliminary data that suggest an increased risk of intussusception after the administration of Rotashield. Further analysis of the data collected both from the passive US national AEFI reporting system (VAERS) and from various active postmarketing surveillance systems led to a decision to withdraw the vaccine from the market (23).

USA

Since March 21, 1988, health care providers and vaccine manufacturers have been required by law to report certain events following specific immunizations (SED-12, 792) to the US Department of Health and Human Services. Table 2 shows the updated table for reportable

Table 2 Reportable events after vaccination

Vaccine/toxoid	Event	Interval from vaccination
Tetanus in any combination; DTaP, DTP, DTP-HiB, DT, Td, TT	A. Anaphylaxis or anaphylactic shock B. Brachial neuritis C. Any sequel (including death) of the above events D. Events described in the manufacturers' package insert as contraindications to additional doses of the vaccine	7 days 28 days Not applicable See package insert
Pertussis in any combination; DTaP, DTP, DTP-HiB, P	A. Anaphylaxis or anaphylactic shock B. Encephalopathy (or encephalitis) C. Any sequel (including death) of the above events D. Events described in the manufacturers' package insert as contraindications to additional doses of the vaccine	7 days 7 days Not applicable See package insert
Measles, mumps, and rubella, in any combination; MMR, MR, M, R	A. Anaphylaxis or anaphylactic shock B. Encephalopathy (or encephalitis) C. Any sequel (including death) of the above events D. Events described in the manufacturers' package insert as contraindications to additional doses of the vaccine	7 days 15 days Not applicable See package insert
Rubella in any combination; MMR, MR, R	A. Chronic arthritis B. Any sequel (including death) of the above event C. Events described in the manufacturers' package insert as contraindications to additional doses of the vaccine	42 days No limit See package insert
Measles in any combination; MMR, MR, M	A. Thrombocytopenic purpura B. Vaccine-strain measles viral infection in an immunodeficient recipient C. Any sequel (including death) of the above events D. Events described in the manufacturers' package insert as contraindications to additional doses of the vaccine	7–30 days 6 months No limit See package insert
Oral polio (OPV)	A. Paralytic polio B. Vaccine-strain polio viral infection C. Any sequel (including death) of the above events D. Events described in the manufacturers' package insert as contraindications to additional doses of the vaccine	30 days/6 months 30 days/6 months Not applicable See package insert
Inactivated polio (IPV)	A. Anaphylaxis or anaphylactic shock B. Any sequel (including death) of the above events C. Events described in the manufacturers' package insert as contraindications to additional doses of the vaccine	7 days Not applicable See package insert
Hepatitis B	A. Anaphylaxis or anaphylactic shock B. Any sequel (including death) of the above events C. Events described in the manufacturers' package insert as contraindications to additional doses of the vaccine	7 days Not applicable See package insert
Hemophilus influenzae type b (conjugate)	A. Events described in the manufacturers' package insert as contraindications to additional doses of the vaccine	See package insert
Varicella	A. Events described in the manufacturers' package insert as contraindications to additional doses of the vaccine	See package insert
Rotavirus	A. Intussusception B. Any sequel (including death) of the above events C. Events described in the manufacturers' package insert as contraindications to additional doses of the vaccine	30 days Not applicable See package insert
Pneumococcal conjugate	A. Events described in the manufacturers' package insert as contraindications to additional doses of the vaccine	See package insert

events after vaccination, effective from August 26, 2002. The VAERS accepts all reports of suspected adverse events after the administration of any vaccine, including but not limited to those certain events required by law to be reported.

Canada

The reporting of vaccine-associated adverse events temporally associated with immunization by health-care providers is voluntary in Canada, except in the province of Ontario, which has specific mandatory requirements. However, there is no evidence of a higher reporting rate with the latter approach. This is partly explained by the fact that immunization in Ontario is usually provided by physicians, who have lower reporting rates than public-health nurses. In addition to its spontaneous voluntary reporting system, Canada also has an active surveillance system, IMPACT, for serious adverse events, vaccination failures, and selected infectious diseases. It involves a network of 11 pediatric centers across Canada. The results of the Canadian surveillance system have been reviewed (SEDA-16, 367) (SEDA-17, 363) (SEDA-21, 324) (SEDA-22, 333).

The Netherlands
A special committee of the Health Council of the Netherlands has been created (12), with the task of analysing, classifying, and interpreting the adverse effects which are reported to the National Institute of Health and Environmental Protection in Bilthoven (SEDA-12, 271) (SEDA-13, 278) (SEDA-14, 269) (SEDA-15, 341) (SEDA-16, 365) (SEDA-17, 363) (SEDA-18, 325).

New Zealand
Reported adverse events after immunization in New Zealand from 1990 to 1995 have been presented (24). Reactions at the injection site following adult teta-nus + diphtheria vaccine were the most commonly reported (68 reports per 100 000 immunizations). The authors concluded that the picture confirmed the overall safety of vaccines and the value of an adverse events monitoring system.

Spain
In Spain, reports on adverse events after immunization are collected through the Spanish Pharmacovigilance System by means of a yellow card. In children, the most commonly involved pharmaceutical groups were antibiotics, respiratory drugs, and vaccines. A review of reports received over 10 years (1982–91) has been provided (25). In the framework of the Global Training Network, a WHO initiative to improve the quality of vaccines and their use, a model for a simple national system for dealing with vaccine safety and emergencies as they arise has been elaborated. The authors have described the model and have outlined a training program designed to help develop such a system (26).

Other countries
There are other national surveillance programs on adverse events after immunization, for example in Denmark, Germany, Sweden, the UK, Hungary; developing countries such as India (SEDA-17, 363) and Brazil (SEDA-16, 367) have also already started to collect data on severe adverse events.

International surveillance programs
The Program on International Drug Monitoring of the WHO has participation from over 50 member states. In all member countries, national Drug Reaction Monitoring Centers collect reports from health professionals and pass them on for entry into the international database housed at the WHO Collaborating Center for International Drug Monitoring in Uppsala, Sweden. Currently, there are some 2.5 million reports on file, and each year about 200 000 new reports are added. The database generates signals of potentially severe drug toxicity and provides confirmation of signals generated in specific countries. The Center also acts as the guardian of the standardized terminology of adverse drug reactions in computerized

systems. Although vaccines are considered to be safe, the work of the Center underlines the importance of collecting information on the safety of vaccines to provide sound reference data in the event of a problem. Since vaccines are administered to healthy people, mostly children, the impact of a perceived problem can be enormous. Because of these considerations, many countries have already established specific programs for the monitoring of adverse events after immunization (27).

Clinical immunization safety assessment centers
The National Immunization Program of the Centers for Disease Control and Prevention (CDC), Atlanta, GA, USA, is trying to set up a network of Clinical Immunization Safety Assessment Centers (CISA). Based on standardized clinical evaluation protocols the centers will assist health care providers in evaluating patients who may have had an adverse reaction after immunization. Furthermore, the centers will evaluate newly hypothesized syndromes or events identified through the routine VAERS (28).

Guaranteeing vaccine quality
During the last 20–30 years, great progress has been achieved in both vaccine production technologies and testing technologies. In addition to sophisticated tests, vaccine regulation entails a number of procedures that ensure safety, including the characterization of starting material, cell banking, seed lot systems, principles of good manufacturing practices, independent release of vaccines on a lot-by-lot basis by national regulatory authorities, and enhanced premarketing and postmarketing surveillance for possible rare adverse events after immunization (29).

Perspectives on prelicensure trials
The withdrawal of tetravalent rhesus-based rotavirus vaccine from the market illustrates an important problem regarding prelicensure testing and its ability to identify rare vaccine-related adverse events. A sample size of 10 000 volunteers may provide excellent estimates of reactogenicity (local and systemic reactions) and efficacy but be inadequate as a denominator for ruling out rare adverse events. Table 3 shows how trial size determines the ability to detect frequent and rare events. Plans for future large prelicensure trials, for example for newly developed rotavirus vaccines, therefore include 10 000–60 000 volunteers. These large trials can be seen as a

Table 3 Sample size necessary to have 80% power to detect an increase in the risk of a rare event

Background rate (1:1 randomization)	Detectable relative risk	Total study population required
1:100	5	1443
1:100	2	5916
1:1000	5	14 428
1:1000	2	59 160
1:10 000	5	144 280
1:10 000	2	591 600

bridge between prelicensure and improved postlicensure surveillance (30,31).

Improving monitoring of vaccine safety through postlicensure studies
Gaps in current vaccine safety monitoring methods have been analysed and the needs for improvements outlined (32,33). The well-known limitations associated with prelicensure trials have led to the expectation that postlicensure studies would address safety issues better. To meet this expectation, steps that should be taken include bar-code labeling of vaccines to improve the accuracy and completeness of information about administered vaccines, establishing immunization registers to provide numerator data, developing generally agreed case definitions for adverse events following immunization (AEFI), to allow comparability between studies, to facilitate long-term follow-up, and to do linked database studies. Only by investing in vaccine safety infrastructure will the high expectations of postlicensure studies be met.

Passive surveillance and reported fatalities
The fatalities reported to the federally administered (US) VAERS have been examined (34). A total of 1266 deaths were reported to VAERS between July 1990 and June 1997. Table 4 shows the numbers of deaths by age (total sample 1199 individuals) and Table 5 shows the causes of death (total sample 1244 individuals).

Nearly half of the deaths were attributed to SIDS. Since 1992/93, the trend of decreasing numbers of reported deaths follows that observed for SIDS overall in the US general population following implementation of the "Back to Sleep" program. Therefore, the VAERS data support the findings of controlled studies that show that the association between infant immunization and SIDS is coincidental and not causal.

Adverse events after immunization—the need for improved research, surveillance, and communication
The success of vaccines is not only impressive and convincing but also makes immunization its own worst enemy. When a naturally occurring disease becomes less common, concerns about vaccine safety increase, particularly since no vaccine can be regarded as being completely safe, although some are very much safer than others. Progress in the development, manufacture, and control of modern vaccines has contributed to the safety of current vaccines. However, it is absolutely necessary to know what the true

Table 4 Deaths related in time to immunization reported to VAERS 1990–97, by age

Age (years)	Number (%)
Overall	1199 (100)
<1	808 (67)
1–4	117 (9.8)
5–9	18 (1.5)
10–17	17 (1.4)
18–45	43 (3.6)
46–64	55 (4.6)
≥65	141 (12)

Table 5 Causes of death related in time to immunization reported to VAERS 1990–97

Cause of death	Number (%)
Overall	1244 (100)
SIDS	592 (48)
Congenital	38 (3.1)
Infectious	164 (13)
Neoplastic	15 (1.2)
Other	261 (21)
Unknown	174 (14)

complications of immunization are, what the gaps in our current knowledge are, and when there is no evidence linking immunization and a suspected adverse effect.

Current knowledge about vaccine risks is incomplete, as was noted in extensive reviews in the early 1990s by the IOM in the USA (13,14). Two-thirds of the 76 vaccine-associated adverse events evaluated by the IOM had either no evidence or inadequate evidence to assess the causal role of the vaccine. Specifically, the reviews identified the following limitations:

- inadequate understanding of the biological mechanisms that underlie adverse events;
- insufficient or inconsistent information from case reports and case series;
- inadequate size or length of follow-up of many population-based epidemiological studies;
- limitations of existing surveillance systems to provide persuasive evidence of causation;
- few experimental studies published relative to the total number of epidemiological studies published.

A concerted effort is therefore needed to improve both research on and surveillance of the risks associated with immunization, as well as better communication aiming to reassure health-care providers, parents, and the public (including the media) about the steps taken to ensure vaccine safety and the overwhelming safety record of vaccines. The medical community still has preeminence as the purveyor of advice to the public on matters of immunization and should play a key role in improving communication. Nothing will strengthen our ability to communicate risk more than ensuring that there is adequate capacity and funding for vaccine safety infrastructure and research (2).

The response to a newly published adverse event associated with immunization must be rapid. First, if the reported association is correct, urgent re-evaluation of the immunization program is necessary. However, if the reported association is false, a credible countermessage must be sent, to minimize the negative impact on the immunization program (35).

The pros and cons of the (US) VAERS (SEDA-14, 919) have been critically reviewed (SEDA-23, 336) (36).

Among the many new developments in the communication of adverse events, the increasing role of the Internet should be mentioned. Many national bodies (for example the FDA, Rockville, Maryland, USA, www.fda.gov, or the CDC, Atlanta, Georgia, USA, www.vaers.org) and intergovernmental health authorities responsible for licensure of vaccines (for example the European Agency for the Evaluation of Medicinal Products (EMEA), www.eudra.org/emea.html), and/or vaccine safety (for example the World Health Organization, www.who.int/vaccines-diseases/safety/), as well as vaccine manufacturers (through postmarketing surveillance of their products, for example SmithKline Biologicals, www.worldwidevaccines.com), universities, and private organizations have also launched Websites providing information on vaccine safety and immunization risks.

National compensation programs for vaccine-related injuries

The need for some form of compensation when an individual is seriously injured by vaccination, particularly when the immunization has been compulsory or recommended by the health authority, has been accepted in many countries. Table 6 shows details of compensation programs in Canada (the province of Quebec), Denmark, France, Germany, Italy, Japan, New Zealand, Norway, Sweden, Switzerland, Taiwan, the UK, and the USA (37).

In the USA, the National Childhood Vaccine Injury Act of 1986 established the National Vaccine Injury Compensation Program as a federal no-fault compensation system for individuals who may have been injured by specific vaccines. This compensation program relies on a Vaccine Injury Table that lists the vaccines that are covered by the program, as well as injuries, disabilities, illnesses, and conditions (including death) for which compensation may be awarded. To better reflect current scientific knowledge about vaccine injuries, the Vaccine Injury Table was revised in 1995 and has been subsequently further modified. The latest modification, which became effective on December 1, 2004, is shown in Table 7. This revision took into account a review of the literature on specific adverse consequences of pertussis and rubella vaccines performed and published by the IOM (SED-12, 817) (SED-12, 825). In addition to the seven vaccines (diphtheria, pertussis, tetanus, measles, mumps, rubella, and poliomyelitis) included in the first Vaccine Injury Table, the 1997 revision includes hepatitis B, *Hemophilus influenzae* type b, and *Varicella* vaccines, as well as any future licensed vaccine recommended by the Advisory Committee on Immunization Practices (ACIP) for routine administration to children (38).

There are other compensation programs, for example in Japan, where the program covers damage caused by compulsory immunizations; provisions include medical allowance, care giver's allowance, disability pension, and a funeral grant; a national expert committee reviews applications.

Although not focusing primarily on vaccine-induced injury, attention should be paid to a contribution to the field of liability for drug-induced disease (39).

On December 1, 2004, the Secretary published a notice in the Federal Register announcing the addition of hepatitis A vaccines to the Vaccine Injury Table under Category XIV with an effective date of December 1, 2004.

The balance of benefits and harms in immunization

The risks of adverse effects after immunization against diphtheria, pertussis, tetanus, poliomyelitis, measles, and tuberculosis have been discussed in the framework of the WHO Expanded Program on Immunization and compared with the complication rate following natural disease (40). Table 8 presents a comparison of the estimated risks of adverse reactions after DTP immunization with the complication rates of natural whooping cough, while Table 9 shows a similar comparison for measles immunization and natural measles. The authors concluded that no vaccine is without adverse effects, but that the risks of serious complications from vaccines used in WHO's Expanded Program on Immunization are much lower than the risks from the natural disease.

Bioterrorism and prevention through immunization

Anthrax

Human anthrax is endemic in agricultural regions of the world where animal anthrax is common; sporadic cases occur in industrialized countries. Cutaneous, intestinal, and pulmonary anthrax can be distinguished clinically. Untreated cutaneous anthrax has a case fatality rate of 5–10%; death occurs only rarely in properly treated patients. Intestinal and pulmonary anthrax have much higher case fatality rates, even in properly treated patients. Transmission from person to person is very rare. Recently, anthrax has been considered a leading potential agent in bioterrorism. As was first demonstrated in 1979 at Sverdlovsk, USSR (an environmental accident in a biological weapon manufacturing facility), inhalational anthrax accounts for most of the cases and for all deaths following the use of anthrax as an aerosolized biological weapon (41).

In 2001, the first bioterrorist anthrax attack occurred in the USA. From 3 October 2001 to 21 November 2001, the CDC had received reports of 23 human cases of anthrax, 18 confirmed and five suspected. There were five deaths from pulmonary anthrax (42).

Three human vaccines against anthrax are currently available commercially (produced in the UK, the USA, and Russia). Two are inactivated cell-free products, whereas the Russian product contains a live attenuated vaccine. Current vaccine supplies are limited; however, even if enough vaccine were available, mass immunization would not be recommended. Immunization could be considered for essential service personnel and, following a terroristic attack, would be combined with an antibiotic to protect against residual retained spores. In 1970, an anthrax vaccine, derived from a sterile filtrate of an avirulent non-encapsulated strain of *Bacillus anthracis* and adsorbed on to aluminium hydroxide, was licensed by the FDA to protect people who might be exposed to anthrax. The ACIP has recommended immunization with this vaccine for people working with *B. anthracis* in the laboratory, those working with imported animal hides or furs in conditions that are inadequate to prevent exposure to anthrax spores, and military personnel deployed to areas with high risk for exposure. The vaccine was used to protect military personnel during the 1991 Gulf War.

Table 6 Vaccine injury compensation programs

	Denmark	France	Germany	Italy	Japan	New Zealand
Enacted	1972 (1978)	1964	1961	1992	1970 (1977)	1974
Administrative entity	National Social Security Office	Ministry of Solidarity, Health and Welfare	State (Länder) pension system (federal law guides outcome)	Ministry of Health	Ministry of Health and Welfare	Accident Rehabilitation and Compensation Insurance Corporation (semi-governmental)
Vaccines covered	Government-provided (free) (D, T, P, M, MR, polio, Hib, BCG)	Compulsory (HBV, D, T, polio, BCG, typhoid)	Recommended (most routine and specific use vaccines)	Compulsory (D, T, polio, HBV, typhoid)	Recommended (polio, D, P, M, R, JE, and others for control of epidemics)	All that are administered
Filing deadlines	1 year after onset of symptoms	4 years after injury stabilization	None (states may have limitations)	Injury: 3 years; Death: no limit	No limit	1 year (exceptions if claim is incomplete)
Compensatable injuries	Injuries with reasonable probability caused by vaccine	All damage directly attributable to vaccination	Injuries exceeding normal extent of reactions—aggravation of pre-existing	Death or injury resulting in permanent physical or mental impairment	Disability or death resulting from vaccination	Vaccine-related injury that is rare and severe
Process and decision-making	Notice must be filed within 1 year of symptoms	Choice of ministerial commission or administrative tribunal	Claims evaluated by pension office; 1971 law gives more flexibility on causation	Medical Hospital Board for eligibility; compensation based on category level of injury (8 levels)	Committee on Public Health decides eligibility and damages	Patient files claim form, reviewed by ACC Medical Misadventure Advisory Committee
Proof needed	Reasonable probability	Clear and convincing evidence	Probable cause	Not specified	Not specified	Balance of probabilities
Elements of compensation	Medical costs, lost wages, death benefits, non-economic damages	Medical costs, disability pensions, lost wages, death benefits, non-economic damages	Medical costs, disability pensions, lost wages, funeral costs, non-economic damages	Free medical care, medications, disability pension, death benefit	Medical costs, lost wages, disability pensions, death benefits	Medical costs, disability pensions, lost wages, death benefits
Funding source	National treasury	National treasury	General revenues of the state	National treasury	Treasury (50%), Municipal (25%), Prefecture (25%)	Employers, wage earners, auto licensing fees, government, investment income
Appeal rights	Yes	Yes	Yes	Yes	Yes	Yes
Litigation rights	Yes (with limits)	No	Yes (with limits)	Yes	Yes	No
Total number of claims filed to June 1999	55	51	4569	366	2982	211
Number compensated	5 (9%)	37 (73%)	1139 (25%)	260 (71%)	2720 (91%)	68 (32%)

Continued

Table 6 Continued

	Norway	Quebec	Sweden	Switzerland	Taiwan	UK	USA
Enacted	1995	1985	1978	1970	1988	1979	1988
Administrative entity	Ministry of Health and Social Affairs	Ministry of Health and Social Services	Pharmaceutical insurance (non-governmental)	State (Canton) (federal law guides outcome)	Department of Health	Department of Social Security	Department of Health and Human Services
Vaccines covered	Routine childhood (D, T, P, Hib, M, MR, polio, BCG)	Voluntary (none is compulsory) (D, T, P, MMR, BCG, HAV, HBV, typhoid)	All approved products marketed in Sweden	Recommended by cantons (D, T, P, HBV, Hib, M, MR, polio)	Compulsory (BCG, HBV, OPV, D, T, P, MMR, JE, D, T)	Routine childhood (D, T, P, M, MR, polio, BCG, Hib)	Routine childhood (D, T, P, MMR, polio, Hib, *Varicella*, HBV, rotavirus)
Filing deadlines	3 years after vaccination or death, or onset of chronic illness	3 years after being made first aware of injury	None (states may have limitations)	1 year after vaccination	Within 6 years of the later of immunization date or age	Injury: 3 years; Death: 2 years (new vaccination or conditions—8 years)	
Compensatable injuries	Not specified	Any serious permanent damage, whether physical or mental, including death	Those noted as adverse effects in FASS or in medical literature	Injury has to exceed a normal post-vaccination reaction	Table of compensatable injuries	Severe disability to extent of 80% or more as a result of immunization	Injuries listed on the Vaccine Injury Table or by proving causation or significant aggravation
Process and decision-making	Minister of Health decides eligibility	Claim reviewed by three-member Medical Evaluation Committee; final decision by Minister of Health	Claims manager with Zurich insurance company makes decision with medical consultations as needed	Health dept. reviews claim and seeks supporting information	Vaccine Injury Comfort Fund Working Group, Department of Health	Claim evaluated by medical officer; makes recommendation to Secretary of State for Social Security	DHHS reviews claim and makes recommendation US Court of Federal Claims makes decision
Proof needed	Balance of probabilities	Balance of probabilities	Strong probability of cause and effect	Not specified	Balance of probabilities	Balance of probabilities	Balance of probabilities

	Norway	Quebec	Sweden	Switzerland	Taiwan	UK	USA
Elements of compensation	No precedent (only award to date was a lump sum payment)	Unreimbursed medical costs, lost wages, rehabilitation, death benefits	Unreimbursed medical costs, lost wages, death benefits	Medical costs, lost wages, death benefits, non-economic damages	Medical costs, health care expenses, burial expenses	Lump sum of payment of statutory sum (40 000 pounds)	Unreimbursed past and future medical expenses, non-economic damage, attorneys' fees
Funding source	National treasury with contribution from manufacturer	National treasury	Manufacturers pay premiums into fund	General revenues of the states	Manufacturers and local society and community	Consolidated fund provided by Parliament	National treasury (pre-enactment); excise tax on covered immunization (postenactment)
Appeal rights	Yes	Yes	Yes	Yes	Yes	Yes	Yes
Litigation rights	Yes	Yes	No	Yes (with limits)	Yes	Yes (with limits)	Yes (with limits)
Total number of claims filed to June 1999	1	142	140	1	123	4012	5355
Number compensated	1 (100%)	17 (12%)	79 (56%)	1 (100%)	62 (50%)	890 (22%)	1390 (26%)

Table 7 National Childhood Vaccine Injury Act: Vaccine Injury Table

Vaccine	Illness, disability, injury, or condition covered	Time interval
I. Vaccines containing tetanus toxoid (for example DTaP, DTP-Hib, DT, Td, or TT)	A. Anaphylaxis B. Brachial neuritis C. Any acute complication or sequel (including death) of the above events	0–4 hours 2–28 days Not applicable
II. Pertussis antigen-containing vaccines (for example DTaP, DTP, P, DTP-Hib)	A. Anaphylaxis or anaphylactic shock B. Encephalopathy (or encephalitis) C. Any acute complication or sequel (including death) of the above events	0–4 hours 0–72 hours Not applicable
III. Vaccines containing measles, mumps, and rubella viruses in any combination (for example MMR, MR, M, R)	A. Anaphylaxis or anaphylactic shock B. Encephalopathy (or encephalitis) C. Any acute complication or sequel (including death) of the above events	0–4 hours 5–15 days Not applicable
IV. Vaccines containing rubella virus (for example MMR, MR, R)	A. Chronic arthritis B. Any acute complication or sequel (including death) of the above event	7–42 days Not applicable
V. Vaccines containing measles virus (for example MMR, MR, M)	A. Thrombocytopenic purpura B. Vaccine-strain measles viral infection in an immunodeficient recipient C. Any acute complication or sequel (including death) of the above events	7–30 days 0–6 months Not applicable
VI. Vaccines containing live oral polio virus (OPV)	A. Paralytic polio in a non-immunodeficient recipient in an immunodeficient recipient in a vaccine associated community case B. Vaccine-strain polio viral infection in a non-immunodeficient recipient in an immunodeficient recipient in a vaccine associated community case C. Any acute complication or sequela (including death) of the above events	 0–30 days 0–6 months Not applicable 0–30 days 0–6 months Not applicable Not applicable
VII. Vaccines containing polio inactivated virus (for example IPV)	A. Anaphylaxis or anaphylactic shock B. Any acute complication or sequela (including death) of the above event	0–4 hours Not applicable
VIII. Hepatitis B antigen-containing vaccines	A. Anaphylaxis or anaphylactic shock B. Any acute complication or sequel (including death) of the above event	0–4 hours Not applicable
IX. *Hemophilus influenzae* type b polysaccharide conjugate vaccines	No condition specified for compensation	Not applicable
X. Varicella vaccine	No condition specified for compensation	Not applicable
XI. Rotavirus vaccine	No condition specified for compensation	Not applicable
XII. Vaccines containing live, oral, rhesus-based rotavirus	A. Intussusception B. Any acute complication or sequel (including death) of the above event	0–30 days Not applicable
XIII. Pneumococcal conjugate vaccines	No condition specified for compensation	Not applicable
XIV. Any new vaccine recommended by the Centers for Disease Control and Prevention for routine administration to children, after publication of a notice of coverage by the Secretary of the HHS	No condition specified for compensation	Not applicable

Although it has a safety record based on clinical trials carried out in the 1950s and 1960s and on the experience of over 30 years of use by thousands of military personnel, woolworkers, and veterinarians (43,44), the debate over its safety has come to the forefront in recent years, including the hypothesis of an alleged link between anthrax vaccine and disease reported by military personnel after the 1991 Gulf War. As a result of this concern, Congress ordered an in-depth investigation into the safety of the anthrax vaccine. The IOM was asked to initiate a comprehensive study and to report on the safety and efficacy of the vaccine in an effort to answer the questions raised by Congress, the Department of Defense, and the public. Because of immediate concerns over anthrax vaccine safety issues, the IOM provided on 30 March 2000 a letter report to the Department of

Table 8 A comparison of the estimated risks of adverse reactions after DTP immunization with the complication rates of natural whooping cough

Adverse reaction	Whooping cough complication rates per 100 000 cases	DTP vaccine adverse reaction rates per 100 000 immunizations
Permanent brain damage	600–2000 (0.6–2.0%)	0.2–0.6
Death	100–400 (0.1–4.0%)	0.2
Encephalopathy/ encephalitis*	90–4000 (0.09–4.0%)	0.1–3.0
Convulsions	600–8000 (0.6–8.0%)	0.3–90
Shock		0.5–30

*Including seizures, focal neurological signs, coma, and Reye's syndrome

Defense, summarizing the Institute's literature review on the safety of anthrax vaccine, prepared by its Committee on Health Effects Associated with Exposures during the Gulf War (45). The committee evaluated primary peer-reviewed literature and did not draw conclusions from secondary literature. It considered that there have been only a few published peer-reviewed studies of the safety of the anthrax vaccine in humans, and only one published series of studies discussed the long-term follow-up of individuals who received multiple vaccines including the anthrax vaccine. The committee concluded that (a) published studies have reported no significant adverse effects of the vaccine, but the literature is limited to a few short-term studies and (b) in peer-reviewed publications there is inadequate/insufficient evidence to determine whether there is or is not an association between anthrax immunization and long-term adverse health outcomes. The committee considered the findings and conclusions as an early step in the complex process of understanding the vaccine's safety, which began with its licensure in 1970 and includes the 1985 FDA advisory panel's finding that categorized the anthrax vaccine as safe and effective. The committee included in its evaluation the results of the VAERS, and considered the VAERS data as being useful as a sentinel for adverse events but of limited value for assessing the rate of causality of adverse events. The VAERS data are as follows:

(a) From 1 January 1990 to 31 August 2000, 1544 adverse events after anthrax immunization (nearly 2 million doses administered) were reported to VAERS.

(b) The most frequently reported adverse events were local reactions (864 reports).

(c) Other reports included headache (239 reports), arthralgia (232 reports), weakness (215 reports), pruritus (212 reports), and a few other systemic reactions.

(d) There were 76 (5%) serious adverse events (death or life-threatening disease, hospitalization, permanent disability); based on autopsy results, one of two reported deaths was due to aplastic anemia and the other was due to coronary arteritis (46).

- A 34-year-old man reported mild tenderness at the injection site after the first dose of anthrax vaccine; after the second dose he felt sweaty and weak and was pale; 20 hours after the third dose he had a life-threatening anaphylactic reaction (dyspnea, sweating, pallor, and urticarial wheals on the face, arms, and torso). After intensive care measures all his symptoms and signs resolved (47).

In 1997 manufacturers in South Korea started to develop a new anthrax vaccine. However, it will take a few years more to put the vaccine to practical use (42).

Botulism

Worldwide, sporadic cases and limited outbreaks of botulism can occur when food and food products are prepared or preserved by improper methods that do not destroy the spores of *Clostridium botulinum* and permit the formation of botulinum toxin. In industrially developed countries, the case fatality rate of food-borne botulism is 5–10%. Person-to-person transmission of botulism is not known. Botulinum toxin is the most poisonous substance known and poses a major bioweapon threat. In addition to the clinical forms of natural botulism (food-borne, wound, and intestinal), there is a fourth, man-made form of inhalational botulism that results from aerosolized botulinum toxin.

A pentavalent botulinum toxoid (botulinum toxin in different antigenic types) has been used for more than 30 years in some countries to prevent the disease in laboratory workers and to protect troops against attack. Pre-exposure immunization for the general population is neither feasible nor desirable; the vaccine is ineffective for postexposure prophylaxis. Treatment of botulism consists of passive immunization and supportive care. Most licensed antitoxins contain antibodies against the most common toxin types A, B, and E. About 9% of recipients of equine antitoxin developed urticaria, serum sickness, or other hypersensitivity reactions. In 2% of recipients anaphylaxis occurred within 10 minutes of antitoxin

Table 9 A comparison of the estimated risks of adverse reactions after measles immunization with the complication rates of natural measles

Adverse reaction	Measles complication rates per 100 000 cases	Adverse reaction rates per 100 000 vaccines	Background illness rate per 100 000
Encephalopathy/encephalitis	50–400 (0.05–0.4%)	0.1	0.1–0.3
Subacute sclerosing panencephalitis	500–2000 (0.5–2.0%)	0.05–0.1	—
Pneumonia	3800–7300 (3.8–7.3%)	—	—
Convulsions	500–1000 (0.5–1.0%)	0.02–190	30
Death	10–10 000 (0.01–10%)	0.02–0.3	—

administration. Before administering antitoxin the patient should be screened for hypersensitivity (48).

Plague

The large plague pandemics (the Justinian plague in the 6th century and pandemics in the 14th–15th centuries and 19th century) killed millions of people worldwide and were feared as the Black Death, a term that was actually not introduced until Victorian times. There is evidence that all three plagues were caused by the same variant of the plague bacterium, *Yersinia pestis*, var Orientalis (49). Progress in hygiene, public health, and antibiotic therapy make future pandemics improbable.

Wild rodent plague still exists in many parts of the world, including areas of Africa, Latin America, Asia, South-Eastern Europe, and the Western half of the USA. Domestic pets, for example house cats and dogs, can bring infected wild rodent fleas into homes, and the bite of infected fleas can result in human disease. Bubonic, pulmonary, and septicemic plague are life-threatening diseases with very high case fatality rates in untreated patients and in patients in whom treatment is delayed. Pneumonic plague is highly communicable, particularly in overcrowded facilities.

The potential use of *Y. pestis*, the causative agent of plague, as a biological weapon is of great concern. A killed whole bacillus plague vaccine (limited data on reactogenicity; see SED-14, 1086) is no longer available in the USA. This killed vaccine was efficacious in preventing or ameliorating bubonic plague but was ineffective against primary pneumonic plague. A live plague vaccine is manufactured in Russia, but no data on its efficacy and safety are available. Recommendations for antibiotic therapy of plague are available (50).

Smallpox

The last natural case of smallpox occurred in 1977 in Somalia. Because of the success of worldwide co-ordinated efforts, particularly the use of smallpox vaccine, natural smallpox has been eradicated. In 1989, the WHO declared the global eradication of this dangerous and often deadly disease (the case fatality rate in non-immunized patients was 20–40%). During natural smallpox outbreaks the secondary attack rate in non-immunized contacts was about 50%.

The smallpox virus belongs to the limited number of organisms that could be used as a biological weapon, causing one of the most serious diseases. There is no causal treatment of smallpox available. Immunization is the most effective measure for pre-exposure prevention and postexposure infection control. However, there were severe complications associated with the use of the old vaccines: encephalitis (mainly in primary vaccines; sometimes fatal or causing permanent neurological sequelae), progressive vaccinia (in both primary and secondary vaccinees), eczema vaccinatum (in vaccinees with either active or healed eczema), and generalized vaccinia resulting from viremia.

With the global eradication of smallpox, smallpox immunization was stopped in all countries of the world, and complications of smallpox vaccination became largely of historical interest. However, recently, the threat of bioterrorism has made it necessary again to consider immunization strategies and the potential hazards of immunization. The old vaccine used for prevention of smallpox contained vaccinia virus strains grown on scarified calves. Some countries and manufacturers have retained limited stocks of vaccine, and the WHO has 500 000 doses. However, there is no reserve large enough to meet more than very limited potential emergency needs (51). Strategies for smallpox immunization in emergencies have been elaborated, focusing on priority immunization of individuals at greatest risk and immunization to contain outbreaks (52). However, the old smallpox vaccine hardly meets modern safety requirements. Therefore, the development and licensure of a modern tissue cell culture vaccine and the establishment of new vaccine production facilities is necessary. Various manufacturers have initiated such developments. A British biotechnology company announced its intention to begin clinical trials on immunogenicity and reactogenicity of a newly developed tissue culture smallpox vaccine in early 2002 (53).

Tularemia

Tularemia is a zoonotic bacterial disease that occurs in North America, China, Japan, parts of Europe, and parts of the former USSR. Various wild animals are the reservoir of the causative agent, *Francisella tularensis*, which is transmitted through the bite of arthropods, including ticks and mosquitoes, by eating insufficiently cooked meat, by drinking contaminated water, or by inhalation of dust from a contaminated environment. Clinically, an ulceroglandular type can be distinguished from an oropharyngeal type; inhalation of infectious material can be followed by pneumonia or septicemia, with a 30–60% case fatality rate in untreated patients. Person-to-person transmission of tularemia is not known.

Francisella tularensis is considered to be a dangerous potential biological weapon. Live tularemia vaccines have been developed and used in the USSR (to protect millions of persons in endemic areas) and the USA (as an investigational vaccine to protect laboratory workers). After the administration of the US vaccine, symptoms of ulceroglandular disease were considered milder; however, the vaccine did not protect all recipients against aerosol challenge with *F. tularensis*. The live vaccine is currently under review by the US Food and Drug Administration (FDA), and its future availability is undetermined. Taking into account the short incubation period of tularemia and incomplete protection through immunization with the current live vaccine, post-exposure immunization is not recommended. Treatment with antibiotics is recommended (54).

General adverse effects after immunization

The reports of the Institute of Medicine, National Academy of Sciences, Washington (on adverse events after pertussis and rubella immunization (SED-12, 817) (SED-12, 825) and on adverse events after immunization against tetanus, diphtheria, measles, mumps, poliomyelitis, *H. influenzae* type b, and hepatitis B (SEDA-18, 325) have provided useful reviews (13,14). The 1996 "Update on vaccine side effects, adverse reactions, contraindications, and precautions" elaborated and published by the US Advisory Committee on Immunization Practices includes summarized conclusions of evidence for possible associations between specific adverse effects and childhood vaccines (Table 10 and Table 11). The conclusions are based on the reports of the IOM mentioned above (55). The respective chapters of "Vaccines" (56) also provide useful information on adverse effects and immunization risks.

General risks of multiple immunizations

Some parents, particularly in industrialized countries, believe that infants get more vaccines than are good for them, and they fear that too many immunizations could overwhelm the infant's immune system. However, the actual number of antigens that children receive in the USA (the schedule includes 11 vaccines) or in some Western European countries (on average 9 vaccines) has declined when compared with immunization programs used during the 1960s or 1980s. Whereas smallpox vaccine contained about 200 proteins, the current routinely recommended vaccines for children in countries in which whole-cell pertussis vaccine was replaced by acellular pertussis vaccine (for example Austria, Germany, Japan, the Scandinavian countries, the USA) contain a total of 50–125 proteins and polysaccharides. The replacement of whole-cell pertussis vaccine by acellular pertussis vaccine reduced the content of immunogenic proteins and polysaccharides from about 3000 to a range of 2-5. (Table 12) (57).

If vaccines overwhelmed the immune system, smaller immune responses would be expected. However, the authors of many carefully designed studies have concluded that there is no evidence that adding vaccines to combination products increases the burden on the immune system. Young infants have a large capacity to respond to multiple vaccines, as well as to many other environmental challenges. Increased reactogenicity after the receipt of combination vaccines has not been a major issue. Combining antigens usually does not increase the risk of adverse effects, and can actually lead to an overall reduction in the numbers of adverse events (58) despite public concern (59).

The Safety Review Committee of the IOM has reviewed the evidence regarding multiple immunizations and immune dysfunction (60). The review did not support the hypothesis that an infant's immune system is inherently incapable of handling the number of antigens to which children in the USA are exposed during routine immunizations. The committee rejected a causal relation between multiple immunizations and increased risks of infections or type 1 diabetes mellitus. The evidence was inadequate to accept or reject a causal relation between multiple immunizations and allergic disease, particularly asthma.

Organs and Systems

Respiratory

There is a hypothesis that the seeds of immune system problems, perhaps including asthma, may be sown in the early weeks of life and activated later by immunization. However, studies have given inconsistent results. A randomized controlled trial showed no effect of pertussis vaccine on the risk of asthma (61), which was suggested by a cohort study (62). A British cohort study also showed no association between immunization and wheeze, but there was a lower risk of eczema (63). Data from the Christchurch Health and Development Study showed a link between immunization and asthma (64). However, the findings were based on only 23 children who had not received DTP or polio vaccine. There was no effect from measles vaccine. This is somewhat in contrast to data from Africa suggesting that measles may protect against asthma (SEDA-21, 323).

Nervous system

Guillain–Barré syndrome
Many drugs and vaccines are associated with Guillain–Barré syndrome. However, a cause-and-effect relation has generally not been established. The issue has been reviewed (SEDA-21, 323).

Haemophilus influenzae
Guillain–Barré syndrome has occasionally been reported after immunization with a conjugate vaccine against *H. influenzae* type b. In one case there were immunoglobulin antibodies against the *H. influenzae* type b polysaccharide (PRP) component of the vaccine, with a high titer of anti-PRP IgM antibody (65).

Hepatitis
Guillain–Barré syndrome has been reported after the administration of plasma-derived hepatitis B vaccines. In the 3 years between 1 June 1982 and 31 May 1985, an estimated 850 000 people received a new plasma derived hepatitis B vaccine (Heptavax-B, Merck Sharp and Dohme) and there were 41 reports of the following neurological adverse events: Bell's palsy ($n = 10$), Guillain–Barré syndrome ($n = 9$), convulsions ($n = 5$), lumbar radiculopathy ($n = 5$), optic neuritis ($n = 5$), transverse myelitis ($n = 4$), and brachial plexus neuropathy ($n = 3$) (66). Half occurred after the first of three doses. There were no deaths.

Guillain–Barré syndrome has also occasionally been reported after the administration of recombinant hepatitis B vaccines (67,68).

Influenza
Following the swine-flu immunization campaign in 1976/77 in the USA there was a significant increase in the incidence of Guillain–Barré syndrome in immunized versus non-immunized people, from 2.6 per million to 13.3 per million (69). Peak time of onset was 2–3 weeks after receiving the vaccine, and cases among vaccinees were less likely to have a history of antecedent infection than were cases in unvaccinated persons. Since 1977 the risk of influenza vaccine–induced syndrome appears to be the same as the risk in the non-immunized population.

Measles–mumps–rubella
Guillain–Barré syndrome has been reported to be associated with measles, mumps, and rubella immunization (70).

Table 10 Evidence for possible associations between specific adverse effects and childhood vaccines

Evidence	DT/Td/tetanus toxoid	Measles vaccine	Mumps vaccine	OPV/IPV	Hepatitis B vaccine	Hemophilus influenzae type b (Hib) vaccine
None available to establish a causal relation	None	None	Neuropathy Residual seizure disorder	Transverse myelitis (IPV) Thrombocytopenia (IPV)	None	None
Inadequate to accept or reject a causal relation	Residual seizure disorder other than infantile spasms Demyelinating diseases of the central nervous system Mononeuropathy Arthritis Erythema multiforme	Encephalopathy Subacute sclerosing panencephalitis Residual seizure disorder Sensorineural deafness (MMR) Optic neuritis Transverse myelitis Guillain–Barré syndrome Thrombocytopenia Insulin-dependent diabetes mellitus	Encephalopathy Aseptic meningitis Sensorineural deafness (MMR) Insulin-dependent diabetes mellitus Sterility Thrombocytopenia Anaphylaxis	Transverse myelitis (OPV) Guillain–Barré syndrome (IPV) Death from SIDS	Guillain–Barré syndrome Demyelinating diseases of the central nervous system Arthritis Death from SIDS	Guillain–Barré syndrome Transverse myelitis Thrombocytopenia Anaphylaxis Death from SIDS
Favored rejection of a causal relation	Encephalopathy Infantile spasms (DT only) Death from SIDS (DT only)	None	None	None	None	Early-onset Hib disease (conjugate vaccines)
Favored acceptance of a causal relation	Guillain–Barré syndrome Brachial neuritis	Anaphylaxis	None	Guillain–Barré syndrome (OPV)	None	Early-onset Hib disease in children aged 18 months whose first Hib vaccination was with unconjugated PRP vaccine
Established a causal relation	Anaphylaxis	Thrombocytopenia (MMR) Anaphylaxis (MMR) Death from measles infection	None	Poliomyelitis in recipient or contact (OPV) Death from polio infection	Anaphylaxis	None

See the original paper for extensive notes to this table.
OPV—oral poliovirus vaccine
IPV—inactivated poliovirus vaccine
DT—diphtheria and tetanus toxoids for pediatric use
Td—diphtheria and tetanus toxoids for adult use
SIDS—sudden infant death syndrome

Table 11 Evidence for possible associations between specific adverse effects and childhood vaccines (DTP and MMR)

Evidence	Adverse effect	DTP vaccine-RA 27/3 MMR
Strong evidence against a causal relation	Autism	None
Inadequate to accept or reject a causal relation	Aseptic meningitis	Radiculoneuritis and other neuropathies
	Chronic neurological damage	Thrombocytopenic purpura
	Erythema multiforme or other rash	
	Guillain–Barré syndrome	
	Hemolytic anemia	
	Type 1 diabetes	
	Learning disabilities and attention-deficit disorder	
	Peripheral mononeuropathy	
	Thrombocytopenia	
Favored rejection of a causal relation	Infantile spasms	None
	Hypsarrhythmia	
	Reye's syndrome	
	Sudden infant death syndrome	
Favored acceptance of a causal relation	Acute encephalopathy	Chronic arthritis
	Shock and unusual shock-like state	
Causal relation established	Anaphylaxis	Acute arthritis
	Protracted inconsolable crying	

DTP—diphtheria toxoid, tetanus toxoid, and pertussis vaccine
MMR—measles, mumps, and rubella vaccine

Table 12 Number of immunogenic pathogens/polysaccharides in vaccines over the past 100 years

1900		1960s		1980s		2000	
Vaccine	Proteins	Vaccine	Proteins	Vaccine	Proteins	Vaccine	Proteins/polysaccharides
Smallpox	~200	Smallpox	~200	Diphtheria	1	Diphtheria	1
—	—	Diphtheria	1	Tetanus	1	Tetanus	1
—	—	Tetanus	1	WC-pertussis	~3000	AC-pertussis	2–5
—	—	WC-pertussis	~3000	Poliomyelitis	15	Poliomyelitis	15
—	—	Poliomyelitis	15	Measles	10	Measles	10
—	—	—	—	Mumps	9	Mumps	9
—	—	—	—	Rubella	5	Rubella	5
—	—	—	—	—	—	H. influenzae	2
—	—	—	—	—	—	Hepatitis B	1
—	—	—	—	—	—	Varicella*	69
—	—	—	—	—	—	Pneumococcus*	8
Total		200		3200		3040	46–49 (Germany) 123–126 (USA)

Polio

Following a mass immunization campaign against poliomyelitis in Finland (1984/85), an analysis based on hospital records covering a population of 1.17 million and 6 years showed a significantly increased incidence of Guillain–Barré syndrome coinciding with the campaign (71).

In a retrospective analysis of the incidence of Guillain–Barré syndrome in Finland in 1981–86 by examination of medical records identified from the nationwide Hospital Discharge Register, based on a population of 5 million people, 247 patients fulfilled the accepted criteria of Guillain–Barré syndrome corresponding to a mean annual incidence of 0.82 per 100 000 (72). Monthly rates showed an increased incidence of Guillain–Barré syndrome in March 1985, a few weeks after the start of the nationwide oral poliovirus vaccine campaign and partly overlapping it. However, the increase had begun just before the onset of the campaign and may have been due to wild-type 3 poliovirus in the population immediately before the campaign and could have been due to that rather than the administration of the oral poliovirus vaccine.

Rabies

Guillain–Barré syndrome was a well-known complication in the era of brain tissue rabies vaccines, and there have been a few cases associated with the use of human diploid cell rabies vaccines (73,74).

Tetanus and diphtheria

Tetanus and diphtheria toxoid vaccines are reportedly associated with polyradiculitis, polyneuritis, and mononeuritis (75–77).

Immunization and multiple sclerosis (encephalitis disseminata)

The possible relation between immunization and an attack of encephalitis disseminata has been investigated in an analysis of 16 confirmed cases and 24 suspected cases in connection with the distribution of approximately 100 million doses of vaccines manufactured by Behringwerke (1980–89) (78). The data did not support an increased risk of initial manifestation of encephalitis disseminata or of renewed attacks in patients with pre-existing disease.

Studies of the role of influenza or influenza immunization in multiple sclerosis have been reviewed by Jeffery (79). He considers that in patients with multiple sclerosis and advanced disability influenza can constitute a life-threatening illness. Even in patients who have minimal disability, severe influenza can be followed by secondary bacterial infection. The risk of relapse after influenza may be as high as 33%, whereas the risk of relapse after influenza immunization appears to be negligible. The only exception to the general rule that influenza immunization is beneficial for patients with multiple sclerosis is in patients with rapidly evolving neurological deficits due to active disease, in whom immunization should be withheld pending treatment with high-dose glucocorticoids to suppress inflammation or stabilization through immunomodulatory treatment. In the absence of active disease, Jeffery strongly recommends influenza immunization for patients with multiple sclerosis. Regarding hepatitis B immunization and multiple sclerosis, Jeffery recommends hepatitis B immunization only for patients with multiple sclerosis at high risk of hepatitis B infection. If a high-risk patient has active multiple sclerosis, immunization should be withheld until the disease activity has been adequately treated. With regard to other immunizations, Jeffery has made similar recommendations: immunization should be postponed if a patient with multiple sclerosis shows disease activity.

Musculoskeletal

A child with fibrodysplasia ossificans progressiva developed permanent heterotopic ossification at the injection site after intramuscular DTP immunization (80). The authors considered that intramuscular injections in children with fibrodysplasia ossificans progressiva were potentially risky, but that subcutaneous injections could be carried out.

Immunologic

The questions of whether early childhood immunization affects the development of atopy and whether it causes allergic reactions have been reviewed (81). The authors concluded that immunization programs do not explain the increasing incidence of allergic diseases, but that

individual children may uncommonly develop an allergic reaction to a vaccine.

Non-sterile injection equipment can transmit HIV and other infectious agents, including hepatitis viruses. There is also a possibility of needle transmission from an HIV-infected person to a vaccinator. Data from the USA show that the risk of transmission of HIV through needle stick is very low, perhaps 20 times lower than in the case of hepatitis B, and in the order of one per 100 accidents. Furthermore, the types of injections given during immunization sessions do not as a rule cause bleeding. The risk of transmission is thus extremely low. No instances of immunization-related spread of HIV to other infants have been reported, and if proper sterilization of needles and syringes is performed and vaccines are administered correctly the risk of HIV transmission is zero (82). However, the use of unsterilized or improperly sterilized needles and syringes is common, particularly in many developing countries, and contributes largely to the spread of hepatitis B and C, as well to the spread of human immunodeficiency virus and other blood-borne pathogens. These risks are recognized by the WHO as major public health problems and led the Organization to initiate a broad program of activities to ensure safe injection techniques (1). The guidelines published by WHO and UNICEF in 1986/87 (83,84), which can be set out briefly as follows, are still valid. Essentially they state that:

(a) a single sterile needle and a single sterile syringe should be used with each injection;
(b) reusable needles and syringes are recommended for use in developing countries; they should be steam-sterilized between uses; boiling is an acceptable alternative procedure when steam sterilization is not available;
(c) disposable needles and syringes should only be used if an assurance can be obtained that they will be destroyed after a single use;
(d) disease transmission by use of jet injectors is theoretically possible and has been demonstrated in human beings in a single situation (SEDA-11, 296); until further studies clarify the risks of disease transmission with different types of injectors, their use should be restricted to special circumstances in which large numbers of persons need to be immunized within a short period of time.

Jet-gun-associated infections

The first outbreak of a disease in which a jet injector was implicated as the vehicle of transmission has been reported. Thirty-one attendees at a weight-reduction clinic in Southern California experienced hepatitis B after daily parenteral injections of human chorionic gonadotrophin given by jet injectors; transmission appeared to have resulted from the multiple repeated jet injections (85). WHO and UNICEF have stated in their "Guidelines for selecting injection equipment for the Expanded Program on Immunization" that the use of jet injectors should be restricted to circumstances in which reusable or disposable equipment is not feasible because of the large number of persons to be immunized within a short period of time (83).

A new type of needleless jet-injector (Mini-Imojet) administers liquid vaccines from a single-use, prefilled cartridge ("imule"), thereby avoiding the risk of cross-contamination. Administration of various vaccines by jet-injector has been compared with standard syringe technique. All the jet-administered vaccines were of equivalent or superior immunogenicity. The most common reactions were mild (minor bleeding, superficial papules, erythema, induration). The technical and safety advantages of the Mini-Imojet reinforce the potential use of this technique for mass immunization (86).

Mixed bacterial vaccines

Starting in the 1920s, very many different mixed bacterial vaccine products (including inactivated bacteria such as *Staphylococcus aureus*, *Streptococcus* species, *Streptococcus pneumoniae*, *Moraxella catarrhalis*, *Klebsiella pneumoniae*, *H. influenzae*) were marketed worldwide. Currently, there are still several products available in European countries, and one product in the USA. Most vaccines have been used for treatment of recurrent and chronic infections of the respiratory tract. The efficacy of these products is doubtful. Delayed hypersensitivity to bacterial products is common. Delayed reactions, sometimes associated with vague malaise or myalgia, can occur after the administration of maintenance doses for months. If delayed skin reactions are accompanied by any systemic symptoms, administration of the mixed vaccine should be drastically reduced or stopped (87).

Immunization and autoimmune disease

Autoimmunity is characterized by the development of one or several immune responses, directed against antigenic components of the host. The detection of antibodies against host antigens (autoantibodies) or autoreactive T cells does not indicate current or future disease, and autoimmunity does not always result in autoimmune disease. An autoimmune disease results from autoimmunity when autoantibodies or autoreactive T cells reach the corresponding antigen in a target organ and become pathogenic, or when autoantibodies form pathogenic immune complexes with antigens released from host cells. An autoimmune disease can be clinically silent for months or years before the destruction of the tissues involved leads to clinical symptoms, for example the appearance of type 1 diabetes following the autoimmune destruction of pancreatic islets.

As many as 5% of individuals in Europe and North America have some form of autoimmune disease. There is clear evidence that genetic predisposition is necessary for the development of some autoimmune diseases. In genetically predisposed individuals an infection can induce or trigger an autoimmune disease. Of the many potential environmental factors, infections are the most likely cause. The causal linkage between some infections and autoimmune diseases has raised the question as to whether autoimmune diseases might also be triggered by vaccines (88).

Autoimmune diseases include autoimmune thrombocytopenia, Graves' disease, hemolytic anemia, Hashimoto's thyroiditis, insulin-dependent diabetes mellitus (diabetes type 1), multiple sclerosis, myasthenia gravis, rheumatoid arthritis, systemic lupus erythematosus, dermatomyositis, and Reiter's syndrome (88–90).

The number of publications that include claims and counterclaims about the risk of autoimmune diseases after immunization is increasing. However, only in rare instances has evidence established a causal relation or favored acceptance of a causal relation:

(a) Rabies vaccine produced in rabbit nervous tissue caused acute disseminated encephalomyelitis in some immunized individuals (91).
(b) During the US swine flu immunization campaign (1976–77) immunized individuals had a much higher risk of Guillain–Barré syndrome than non-immunized individuals (relative risk 7.60); currently, the risk of Guillain–Barré syndrome after immunization (one additional case per million people immunized) is estimated to be substantially lower than the risk of severe influenza and its complications (92).
(c) Idiopathic thrombocytopenia can occur after MMR immunization (about one case in 30 000 immunized children); however, the risks of thrombocytopenia after natural measles or rubella are respectively five and 10 times higher (88,93).

For other potential association between vaccines and autoimmune diseases, the evidence favors rejection of a causal relation:

(a) hepatitis B vaccine and multiple sclerosis (SEDA-24, 374) (SEDA-25, 386);
(b) vaccines and diabetes mellitus (94,95);
(c) Lyme disease vaccine and a treatment-resistant form of autoimmune arthritis; however, owing to public misperception and the promotion of false concerns about its safety, the demand for Lyme disease vaccine did not reach a sustainable level and the manufacturer withdrew it (SEDA-24, 366) (SEDA-26, 357).

How to assess a potential link between a vaccine and an autoimmune condition

Careful epidemiological studies should be the basis of conclusions about an association between a specific vaccine and a particular autoimmune disease. Wraith and colleagues took into account WHO recommendations for the assessment of adverse events after immunization and established the following four basic principles that apply to autoimmune diseases:

1. consistency of findings in various studies;
2. strength (in an epidemiological sense);
3. specificity;
4. temporal relation (95).

Death

Sudden infant death syndrome and multiple immunizations

Current recommendations call for infants and very young children to receive multiple doses of vaccines during their first year of life, and since SIDS is the most frequent cause of death in highly developed countries during that early period of life, it is important to take into account concerns that multiple immunization might play a role in SIDS. SIDS is the diagnosis most commonly used to explain unexpected sudden death of uncertain cause occurring mainly in infancy at 2–7 months of life, sometimes later. By definition, the cause or causes of SIDS are unknown, but risk factors (for example maternal characteristics, prenatal factors, and postnatal conditions, including the infant's sleeping position) have been identified. The results of the most comprehensive analysis "Vaccinations and sudden unexpected death in infancy" have been provided by the Immunization Safety Review Committee of the IOM (96). The committee reviewed an extensive collection of material, primarily from published peer-reviewed scientific and medical literature. The causality conclusions of the committee were as follows:

(a) The evidence favors rejection of a causal relation between exposure to multiple vaccines and SIDS.
(b) The evidence favors acceptance of a causal relation between diphtheria toxoid and whole cell pertussis vaccine and death due to anaphylaxis in infants; however, anaphylaxis of infants following vaccination is very rare, and a fatal outcome is extremely rare.
(c) The committee has not recommended a policy review of the recommended (US) childhood immunization schedule on the basis of concerns about SIDS.

The committee also noted that there are studies that show that vaccinated infants are at a reduced risk of SIDS (96,97).

Susceptibility Factors

It is well known that immune deficiency can play a distinct role in the development of adverse effects after immunization, particularly in connection with the administration of live virus vaccines. The first such experience was with smallpox vaccine; people with immune defects had a markedly increased risk of complications, for example generalized vaccinia. Disseminated BCG infection is usually associated with severe abnormalities of cellular immunity. The risk of vaccine-associated poliomyelitis is increased in immunodeficient children. There have been several reports of adverse events or death after measles immunization in immunodeficient children. Based on these experiences, there is a general consensus that live vaccines should not be given to people with immune deficiency diseases or to those whose immune response is suppressed because of leukemia, lymphoma, generalized malignancy, or therapy with glucocorticoids, alkylating agents, antimetabolites, or radiation (SEDA-12, 268).

Various studies in both symptomatic and asymptomatic HIV-infected individuals have failed to show any special sensitivity to adverse effects after other immunizations, for example in children receiving live oral or inactivated polio vaccine, DPT or DT vaccine, or measles vaccine (98–101).

Recommendations by the US ACIP, WHO's Global Programme on Immunization, and the European Advisory Group on Expanded Program on Immunization have all been published in detail (SEDA-12, 270) (SEDA-13, 273). Based on the recommendations elaborated by WHO and ACIP, similar recommendations have been prepared in other countries. WHO recommends that non-immunized individuals with symptomatic HIV infection should not receive BCG, but should receive the other vaccines; whereas ACIP recommends that children with symptomatic HIV infection should not receive live virus or live bacterial vaccines. Taking into account the hazard of measles in children with AIDS and HIV-infection, ACIP additionally recommends measles vaccine for all (both symptomatic and asymptomatic) HIV-infected children.

Drug Administration

Drug additives

Thiomersal

Thiomersal (see the monograph on Mercury and mercurial salts) has been used as an additive to biologics and vaccinessince the 1930s because it is very effective in killing bacteria used in several vaccines and in preventing bacterial contamination, particularly in opened multidose containers. Some but not all vaccines contain thiomersal. Billions of children and adults have been immunized worldwide and there is no scientific data that thiomersal-containing products have caused problems of toxicity in humans. The main causes of concern with thiomersal are allergic reactions and the potential risk of neurotoxicity. The WHO has recommended a Permissible Total Weekly Intake (PTWI) of 200 µg for non-pregnant adults. Owing to the vulnerability of the developing brain, the PTWI for pregnant women and infants should be lower, but there is currently no international recommendation for maximum intake in infants. Considering the thiomersal content of some vaccines, intake of mercury in infants can exceed that which could be considered safe. The US Public Health Service, the American Academy of Pediatrics, and US vaccine manufacturers are in agreement that thiomersal should be eliminated from vaccine manufacture as soon as possible. Similar conclusions were reached in 1999 in a meeting attended by the European vaccine manufacturers, European regulatory agencies, and the FDA. Already, many new vaccines are thiomersal-free and the manufacturers are committed to the target of reducing as much as possible the thiomersal content in all vaccines. However, given that the known risks of not immunizing children far outweigh the unknown and much smaller risk of thiomersal, clinicians and parents are encouraged to continue immunizing all infants with the currently available vaccines despite their thiomersal content (102).

Questions and answers on thiomersal have been provided by the WHO, which has underlined the fact that the risk of adverse effects of thiomersal is theoretical, uncertain, and at most extremely small (103). However, the WHO aims to replace thiomersal with other preservatives in the long term. Combination vaccines can reduce the amount of mercury to an absolute minimum.

In 2001 the Immunization Safety Review Committee of the Institute of Medicine issued a report on thiomersal-containing vaccines and neurodevelopmental disorders (104). "The committee concluded that although the hypothesis that exposure to thiomersal-containing vaccines could be associated with neurodevelopmental disorders is not established and rests on indirect and incomplete information, primarily from analogies with methylmercury and levels of maximum mercury exposure from vaccines given in children, the hypothesis is biologically plausible. ... [However,] the evidence is inadequate to accept or reject a causal relationship between thiomersal exposure from childhood vaccines and the neurodevelopmental disorders of autism, attention deficit/hyperactivity disorder, and speech or language delay." Hypersensitivity to thiomersal is a contraindication to immunization (105).

Vaccine adjuvants

A vaccine adjuvant is defined as an agent that increases specific immune responses to an antigen (106). The only vaccine adjuvants currently licensed by the FDA are aluminum salts. All other adjuvants are considered experimental and must undergo special preclinical testing. Real and theoretical risks of vaccine adjuvants comprise various local acute or chronic inflammation with formation of abscesses and nodules; induction of hypersensitivity to the host's own tissues, producing autoimmune arthritis, amyloidosis, anterior uveitis; cross-reactions with human antigens, such as glomerular basement membranes or neurolemma, causing glomerulonephritis or meningoencephalomyelitis; sensitization to tuberculin or to other skin test antigens; carcinogenesis; pyogenesis; teratogenesis; abortion; and adverse pharmacological effects, such as hypoglycemia.

Drug contamination

Since the problem of bovine spongiform encephalitis (BSE) emerged in Europe around 1987, the WHO and ministries of health have been alert to the danger that BSE-contaminated materials might be used in biological products, including vaccines. Guidelines were created that ensured that when bovine materials were needed in a biological product, the materials were obtained from countries that were free from BSE. Bovine products are used in the production of certain vaccines, in creating seed lots, or in amplifying the seed lot into working lots. The material is generally calf serum, which, even if it came from an infected animal, is extremely unlikely to transmit the prions that cause the disease. An exceptional situation arose on 20 October 2000, when the UK withdrew one manufacturer's OPV because of the possibility that the vaccine had been manufactured using serum from calves that were from a BSE-infected country. Even though the risk was extremely remote, the health authorities decided to have the vaccine withdrawn. This particular product was not the main OPV used in the UK. To clarify the situation in the UK and to reassure countries throughout the world that there were no implications for OPV used in the eradication of poliomyelitis, the WHO issued the following position statement (107): "On 20 October 2000, Evans/Medeva Oral Polio Vaccine (OPV), which to the knowledge of the World Health Organization has only been used in the United Kingdom and Republic of Ireland, was recalled in the UK. This vaccine has never been used in the immunization campaigns that are ongoing as part of the Global Polio Eradication Initiative. The recall was prompted by evidence that the Evans/Medeva vaccine was manufactured in contravention of European Union guidelines, and was not based on any adverse events related to the vaccine. The specific concern is that fetal bovine calf serum (FCS) from the UK was used in the manufacture of the Evans/Medeva vaccine, at a time when there was a risk of bovine spongiform encephalopathy (BSE) in that country. WHO endorses the recall step as a precaution, even though FCS is removed in the manufacturing process of the vaccine and there is no evidence that FCS could transmit BSE. Due to this breach of EU guidelines and acting on a precautionary basis, the Health Departments in the UK have withdrawn remaining shelf stocks of the Evans/Medeva brand of polio vaccine, which had already ceased production. The World Health Organization imposes strict production and quality controls to ensure the safety and efficacy of OPV. WHO recommends that manufacturers use the safest source of materials from countries which have not reported indigenous BSE cases and have a compulsory BSE notification system, compulsory clinical and laboratory verification of suspected cases and a surveillance program. The Global Polio Eradication Initiative only distributes vaccine supplied by vaccine manufacturers who follow National Control Authorities' criteria provided by WHO."

Two advisory committees of the US FDA, the Transmissible Spongiform Encephalopathies Advisory Committee and the Vaccines and Related Biologicals Product Advisory Committee, said at a joint meeting on 3 August 2000 that vaccines made from bovine-derived materials from countries with a known or uncertain risk of BSE carry only an infinitesimal risk of new variant Creutzfeldt–Jakob disease, and that no change in US immunization practice is indicated (Evans G, personal communication, 3 August 2000).

References

1. Kane M. Unsafe injections. Bull World Health Organ 1998;76(1):99–100.
2. Chen R. Vaccine risks: real, perceived, and unknown. 4th European Conference on Vaccinology, March 17–19, 1999. Brighton, United Kingdom, 1999.
3. Clements CJ, Evans G, Dittman S, Reeler AV. Vaccine safety concerns everyone. Vaccine 1999;17(Suppl 3):S90–4.
4. Chen RT, DeStefano F. Vaccine adverse events: causal or coincidental? Lancet 1998;351(9103):611–12.
5. Wakefield AJ, Murch SH, Anthony A, Linnell J, Casson DM, Malik M, Berelowitz M, Dhillon AP, Thomson MA, Harvey P, Valentine A, Davies SE, Walker-Smith JA. Ileal-lymphoid-nodular hyperplasia, non-specific colitis, and pervasive developmental disorder in children. Lancet 1998;351(9103):637–41.
6. Jefferson T. Vaccination and its adverse effects: real or perceived. Society should think about means of linking exposure to potential long term effect. BMJ 1998;317(7152):159–60.
7. Varricchio F. The vaccine adverse event reporting system. J Toxicol Clin Toxicol 1998;36(7):765–8.
8. Niu MT, Rhodes P, Salive M, Lively T, Davis DM, Black S, Shinefield H, Chen RT, Ellenberg SS, Braun M, Donlon J,

Krueger C, Rastogi S, Varricchio F, Wise R, Haber P, Lloyd J, Terracciano G, Eltermann D, Gordon S, DeStefano F, Glasser J, Handler S, Kimsey D Jr, Swint E Jr, Fireman B Jr, Hiatt R Jr, Lewis N Jr, Lieu T Jr, the VAERS and VSD Working Group T Jr. Comparative safety of two recombinant hepatitis B vaccines in children: data from the Vaccine Adverse Event Reporting System (VAERS) and Vaccine Safety Datalink (VSD). J Clin Epidemiol 1998;51(6):503–10.

9. Surveillence for safety after immunization: Vaccine Adverse Event Reporting System (VAERS)-United States, 1991–2001. MMWR Morb Mortal Wkly Rep 2003;52(SS-1):1.

10. The Brighton Collaboration. http://brightoncollaboration.org, 27/12/2001.

11. The term AEFI — a debate. VACSAF-L@LIST.NIH.GOV (accessed July 2001).

12. Health Council of the Netherlands. Adverse reactions to vaccines used in the national vaccination programme in 1989. Report, Gezondheidsraad, The Hague, 1999.

13. Howson CP, Howe CJ, Fineberg HV, editors. Adverse effects of pertussis and rubella vaccines. A report of the Committee to Review the Adverse Consequences of Pertussis and Rubella Vaccines. Washington, DC: National Academy Press, 1991.

14. Stratton KR, Howe CJ, Johnson RB Jr, editors. Adverse effects associated with childhood vaccines. Washington, DC: National Academy of Sciences, 1994.

15. Centers for Disease Control (CDC). Vaccine Adverse Event Reporting System—United States. MMWR Morb Mortal Wkly Rep 1990;39(41):730–3.

16. Rosenthal S, Chen R. The reporting sensitivities of two passive surveillance systems for vaccine adverse events. Am J Public Health 1995;85(12):1706–9.

17. Chen RT, Rastogi SC, Mullen JR, Hayes SW, Cochi SL, Donlon JA, Wassilak SG. The Vaccine Adverse Event Reporting System (VAERS). Vaccine 1994;12(6):542–50.

18. Wassilak SG, Glasser JW, Chen RT, Hadler SC. Utility of large-linked databases in vaccine safety, particularly in distinguishing independent and synergistic effects. The Vaccine Safety Datalink Investigators. Ann NY Acad Sci 1995;754:377–82.

19. Chen RT, Glasser JW, Rhodes PH, Davis RL, Barlow WE, Thompson RS, Mullooly JP, Black SB, Shinefield HR, Vadheim CM, Marcy SM, Ward JI, Wise RP, Wassilak SG, Hadler SC, Swint E, Hardy JR, Payne T, Benson P, Draket J, Drew L, Mendius B, Ray P, Lewis N, Fireman BH, Jing J, Wulfsohn M, Lugg MM, Osborne P, Rastogi S, Patriarca P, Caserta V. Vaccine Safety Datalink project: a new tool for improving vaccine safety monitoring in the United States. The Vaccine Safety Datalink Team. Pediatrics 1997;99(6):765–73.

20. Farrington P, Pugh S, Colville A, Flower A, Nash J, Morgan-Capner P, Rush M, Miller E. A new method for active surveillance of adverse events from diphtheria/tetanus/pertussis and measles/mumps/rubella vaccines. Lancet 1995;345(8949):567–9.

21. Anonymous. Causality assessment of adverse events following immunization. Wkly Epidemiol Rec 2001; 76(12):85–9.

22. Collet JP, MacDonald N, Cashman N, Pless R, Halperin S, Landry M, Palkonyay L, Duclos P, Mootrey G, Ward B, LeSaux N, Caserta V. Monitoring signals for vaccine safety: the assessment of individual adverse event reports by an expert advisory committee. Advisory Committee on Causality Assessment. Bull World Health Organ 2000;78(2):178–85.

23. Delage G. Rotavirus vaccine withdrawal in the United States: the role of post-marketing surveillance. Can J Infect Dis 2000;11:10–12.

24. Mansoor O, Pillans PI. Vaccine adverse events reported in New Zealand 1990–5. NZ Med J 1997;110(1048):270–2.

25. Morales-Olivas FJ, Martinez-Mir I, Ferrer JM, Rubio E, Palop V. Adverse drug reactions in children reported by means of the yellow card in Spain. J Clin Epidemiol 2000;53(10):1076–80.

26. Mehta U, Milstien JB, Duclos P, Folb PI. Developing a national system for dealing with adverse events following immunization. Bull World Health Organ 2000; 78(2):170–7.

27. Adverse drug reaction monitoring: new issues. WHO Drug Inf 1997;11:1–4.

28. Announcing funding for clinical immunization safety assessment centers. www.cdc.gov/od/pgo/funding/01112.htm, 27/06/2001.

29. Dellepiane N, Griffiths E, Milstien JB. New challenges in assuring vaccine quality. Bull World Health Organ 2000;78(2):155–62.

30. Black S. Perspectives on the design and analysis of prelicensure trials: bridging the gap to postlicensure studies. Clin Infect Dis 2001;33(Suppl 4):S323–6.

31. Jacobson RM, Adegbenro A, Pankratz VS, Poland GA. Adverse events and vaccination—the lack of power and predictability of infrequent events in pre-licensure study. Vaccine 2001;19(17–19):2428–33.

32. Heijbel H, Jefferson T. Vaccine safety—improving monitoring. Vaccine 2001;19(17–19):2457–60.

33. Chen RT, Pool V, Takahashi H, Weniger BG, Patel B. Combination vaccines: postlicensure safety evaluation. Clin Infect Dis 2001;33(Suppl 4):S327–33.

34. Silvers LE, Ellenberg SS, Wise RP, Varricchio FE, Mootrey GT, Salive ME. The epidemiology of fatalities reported to the vaccine adverse event reporting system 1990–1997. Pharmacoepidemiol Drug Saf 2001;10(4): 279–85.

35. Duclos P, Ward BJ. Measles vaccines: a review of adverse events. Drug Saf 1998;19(6):435–54.

36. Singleton JA, Lloyd JC, Mootrey GT, Salive ME, Chen RT. An overview of the vaccine adverse event reporting system (VAERS) as a surveillance system. VAERS Working Group. Vaccine 1999;17(22):2908–17.

37. Evans G. Personal communication, 1999.

38. Red Book. Report of the Committee on Infectious Diseases, 24th ed. American Academy of Pediatrics, 1997:681–8.

39. Dukes MNG, Swartz B. Responsibility for Drug-induced Injury. Amsterdam: Elsevier, 1988.

40. Galazka AM, Lauer BA, Henderson RH, Keja J. Indications and contraindications for vaccines used in the Expanded Programme on Immunization. Bull World Health Organ 1984;62(3):357–66.

41. Inglesby TV, Henderson DA, Bartlett JG, Ascher MS, Eitzen E, Friedlander AM, Hauer J, McDade J, Osterholm MT, O'Toole T, Parker G, Perl TM, Russell PK, Tonat K. Anthrax as a biological weapon: medical and public health management. Working Group on Civilian Biodefense. JAMA 1999;281(18):1735–45.

42. Anonymous. South Korea: development of anthrax vaccine close to completion. The Korea Herald, 14/01/2000.

43. Snyder JW. The anthrax vaccine: a question of safety. Clin Microbiol Newslett 2001;23:51–4.

44. Pittman PR, Gibbs PH, Cannon TL, Friedlander AM. Anthrax vaccine: short-term safety experience in humans. Vaccine 2001;20(5–6):972–8.

45. Committee on Health Effects Associated with Exposures during the Gulf War. An assessment of the safety of the anthrax vaccine. A letter report. Washington, DC: Institute of Medicine. http://www.nap.edu/html/anthrax_vaccine, 02/10/2027.

46. Advisory Committee on Immunization Practices. Use of anthrax vaccine in the United States. MMWR Recomm Rep 2000;49(RR-15):1–20.

47. Swanson-Biearman B, Krenzelok EP. Delayed life-threatening reaction to anthrax vaccine. J Toxicol Clin Toxicol 2001;39(1):81–4.

48. Arnon SS, Schechter R, Inglesby TV, Henderson DA, Bartlett JG, Ascher MS, Eitzen E, Fine AD, Hauer J, Layton M, Lillibridge S, Osterholm MT, O'Toole T, Parker G, Perl TM, Russell PK, Swerdlow DL, Tonat K; Working Group on Civilian Biodefense. Botulinum toxin as a biological weapon: medical and public health management. JAMA 2001;285(8):1059–70.

49. Drancourt M, Roux V, Dang LV, Tran-Hung L, Castex D, Chenal-Francisque V, Ogata H, Fournier PE, Crubezy E, Raoult D. Genotyping, Orientalis-like *Yersinia pestis*, and plague pandemics. Emerg Infect Dis 2004;10(9):1585–92.

50. Inglesby TV, Dennis DT, Henderson DA, Bartlett JG, Ascher MS, Eitzen E, Fine AD, Friedlander AM, Hauer J, Koerner JF, Layton M, McDade J, Osterholm MT, O'Toole T, Parker G, Perl TM, Russell PK, Schoch-Spana M, Tonat K. Plague as a biological weapon: medical and public health management. Working Group on Civilian Biodefense. JAMA 2000;283(17):2281–90.

51. Henderson DA, Inglesby TV, Bartlett JG, Ascher MS, Eitzen E, Jahrling PB, Hauer J, Layton M, McDade J, Osterholm MT, O'Toole T, Parker G, Perl T, Russell PK, Tonat K. Smallpox as a biological weapon: medical and public health management. Working Group on Civilian Biodefense. JAMA 1999;281(22):2127–37.

52. Centers for Disease Control and Prevention (CDC). Interim smallpox response plan and guidelines (draft 2.0—21 November 2001). http://www.bt.cdc.gov/DocumentsApp/Smallpox?RPG/plan.

53. Reuters Medical News. New smallpox vaccine nears clinical trial. http://primarycare.medscape.com/reuters/prof/2001/09/09.21/20010920drgd002.html.

54. Dennis DT, Inglesby TV, Henderson DA, Bartlett JG, Ascher MS, Eitzen E, Fine AD, Friedlander AM, Hauer J, Layton M, Lillibridge SR, McDade JE, Osterholm MT, O'Toole T, Parker G, Perl TM, Russell PK, Tonat K; Working Group on Civilian Biodefense. Tularemia as a biological weapon: medical and public health management. JAMA 2001;285(21):2763–73.

55. Advisory Committee on Immunization Practices (ACIP). Update: vaccine side effects, adverse reactions, contraindications, and precautions. MMWR Recomm Rep 1996;45(RR-12):1–35.

56. Plotkin SA, Orenstein WA, editors. Vaccines. 3rd ed. Philadelphia: Saunders, 1999.

57. Offit PA, Quarles J, Gerber MA, Hackett CJ, Marcuse EK, Kollman TR, Gellin BG, Landry S. Addressing parents' concerns: do multiple vaccines overwhelm or weaken the infant's immune system? Pediatrics 2002;109(1):124–9.

58. Halsey NA. Safety of combination vaccines: perception versus reality. Pediatr Infect Dis J 2001;20(Suppl 11):S40–4.

59. Andreae MC, Freed GL, Katz SL. Safety concerns regarding combination vaccines: the experience in Japan. Vaccine 2004;22(29–30):3911–6.

60. Institute of Medicine (IOM) Report. Immunizations Safety Review. Multiple immunizations and immune dysfunction. http://www.cdc.gov/nip//vacsafe/concerns/gen/multiplevac_iom.htm, 28/10/2002.

61. Nilsson L, Kjellman NI, Storsaeter J, Gustafsson L, Olin P. Lack of association between pertussis vaccination and symptoms of asthma and allergy. JAMA 1996;275(10):760.

62. Odent MR, Culpin EE, Kimmel T. Pertussis vaccination and asthma: is there a link? JAMA 1994;272(8):592–3.

63. Butler NR, Golding J, editors. From birth to 5: a study of the health and behaviour of Britain's 5-year-olds. Oxford: Pergamon Press, 1986.

64. Kemp T, Pearce N, Fitzharris P, Crane J, Fergusson D, St George I, Wickens K, Beasley R. Is infant immunization a risk factor for childhood asthma or allergy? Epidemiology 1997;8(6):678–80.

65. Gervaix A, Caflisch M, Suter S, Haenggeli CA. Guillain–Barré syndrome following immunisation with *Haemophilus influenzae* type b conjugate vaccine. Eur J Pediatr 1993;152(7):613–14.

66. Shaw FE Jr, Graham DJ, Guess HA, Milstien JB, Johnson JM, Schatz GC, Hadler SC, Kuritsky JN, Hiner EE, Bregman DJ, et al. Postmarketing surveillance for neurologic adverse events reported after hepatitis B vaccination. Experience of the first three years. Am J Epidemiol 1988;127(2):337–52.

67. Sinsawaiwong S, Thampanitchawong P. Guillain–Barré syndrome following recombinant hepatitis B vaccine and literature review. J Med Assoc Thai 2000;83(9):1124–6.

68. Khamaisi M, Shoenfeld Y, Orbach H. Guillain–Barré syndrome following hepatitis B vaccination. Clin Exp Rheumatol 2004;22(6):767–70.

69. Marks JS, Halpin TJ. Guillain–Barré syndrome in recipients of A/New Jersey influenza vaccine. JAMA 1980;243(24):2490–4.

70. Morris K, Rylance G. Guillain–Barré syndrome after measles, mumps, and rubella vaccine. Lancet 1994;343(8888):60.

71. Kinnunen E, Farkkila M, Hovi T, Juntunen J, Weckstrom P. Incidence of Guillain–Barré syndrome during a nationwide oral poliovirus vaccine campaign. Neurology 1989;39(8):1034–6.

72. Kinnunen E, Junttila O, Haukka J, Hovi T. Nationwide oral poliovirus vaccination campaign and the incidence of Guillain–Barré syndrome. Am J Epidemiol 1998;147(1):69–73.

73. Knittel T, Ramadori G, Mayet WJ, Lohr H, Meyer zum Buschenfelde KH. Guillain–Barré syndrome and human diploid cell rabies vaccine. Lancet 1989;1(8650):1334–5.

74. Courrier A, Stenbach G, Simonnet P, Rumilly P, Lopez D, Coquillat G, Scherer C, Chopin J. Peripheral neuropathy following fetal bovine cell rabies vaccine. Lancet 1986;1(8492):1273.

75. Bakshi R, Graves MC. Guillain–Barré syndrome after combined tetanus–diphtheria toxoid vaccination. J Neurol Sci 1997;147(2):201–2.

76. Dieckhofer K, Scholl R, Wolf R. Neurologische Storungen nach Tetanusschutzimpfung. Ein kasuistischer Beitrag. [Neurologic disorders following tetanus vaccination. A case report.] Med Welt 1978;29(44):1710–2.

77. Hamati-Haddad A, Fenichel GM. Brachial neuritis following routine childhood immunization for diphtheria, tetanus, and pertussis (DTP): report of two cases and review of the literature. Pediatrics 1997;99(4):602–3.

78. Quast U, Herder C, Zwisler O. Vaccination of patients with encephalomyelitis disseminata. Vaccine 1991;9(4):228–30.

79. Jeffery DR. The use of vaccinations in patients with multiple sclerosis. Infect Med 2002;19:73–9.

80. Lanchoney TF, Cohen RB, Rocke DM, Zasloff MA, Kaplan FS. Permanent heterotopic ossification at the injection site after diphtheria–tetanus–pertussis immunizations in children who have fibrodysplasia ossificans progressiva. J Pediatr 1995;126(5 Pt 1):762–4.

81. Gruber C, Nilsson L, Bjorksten B. Do early childhood immunizations influence the development of atopy and

do they cause allergic reactions? Pediatr Allergy Immunol 2001;12(6):296–311.

82. La Force FM. Immunization of children infected with human immunodeficiency virus. WHO/EPI/GEN/86.6 Rev 1, Geneva, 1986.

83. Expanded Programme on Immunization. Immunization policy. WHO/EPI/GEN/86.7 Rev 1, Geneva, 1986.

84. Expanded Programme on Immunization. Joint WHO/UNICEF statement on immunization and AIDS. Wkly Epidemiol Rec 1987;62(9):53.

85. Shah RH, Mackey K, Wallace H, Yawata K, Roberto R, Meissinger J, Ascher M, Hagens S, Chin J. Centers for Disease Control (CDC). Hepatitis B associated with jet gun injection—California. MMWR Morb Mortal Wkly Rep 1986;35(23):373–6.

86. Parent du Chatelet I, Lang J, Schlumberger M, Vidor E, Soula G, Genet A, Standaert SM, Saliou P, Gueye A, Julien H, Lafaix C, Lemardeley P, Monnereau A, Spiegel A, Soke M, Varichon JP. Clinical immunogenicity and tolerance studies of liquid vaccines delivered by jet-injector and a new single-use cartridge (Imule): comparison with standard syringe injection. Imule Investigators Group. Vaccine 1997;15(4):449–58.

87. Grabenstein JD. A miscellany of obscure vaccines: adenovirus, anthrax, mixed bacteria, and staphylococcus. Hosp Pharm 1993;28:259–66.

88. Wraith DC, Goldman M, Lambert PH. Vaccination and autoimmune disease: what is the evidence? Lancet 2003;362(9396):1659–66. http://image.thelancet.com/extras/02art9340web.pdf.

89. Offit PA, Hackett CJ. Addressing parents' concerns: do vaccines cause allergic or autoimmune diseases? Pediatrics 2003;111(3):653–9.

90. Shoenfeld Y, Aron-Maor A. Vaccination and autoimmunity-vaccinosis: a dangerous liaison? J Autoimmun 2000;14(1):1–10.

91. Stuart G, Krikorian KS. The neuroparalytic accidents of anti-rabies treatment. Ann Trop Med Parasitol 1928;22:327–77.

92. Kilbourne ED, Arden NH. Inactivated influenza vaccines. In: Plotkin SA, Orenstein WA, editors. Vaccines. 3rd ed. Philadelphia: Saunders, 1999:542.

93. Miller E, Waight P, Farrington CP, Andrews N, Stowe J, Taylor B. Idiopathic thrombocytopenic purpura and MMR vaccine. Arch Dis Child 2001;84(3):227–9.

94. CDC. National Immunization program. Diabetes and vaccines. Questions and answers. http://www.cdc.gov/nip/vac-safe/concerns/diabetes/q&a.htm, 10/05/2003.

95. World Health Organization. Vaccines and Biologicals. Diabetes. http://www.who.int/vaccines-diseases/safety/infobank/diabetes.shtml, 29/11/2003.

96. Institute of Medicine (IOM) Report. Immunization Safety Review. Vaccinations and sudden unexpected death in infancy. The National Academies Press. http://www.nap.edu/nap-cgi, 20/06/2003.

97. Fleming PJ, Blair PS, Platt MW, Tripp J, Smith IJ, Golding J. The UK accelerated immunisation programme and sudden unexpected death in infancy: case-control study. BMJ 2001;322(7290):822.

98. Centers for Disease Control (CDC). Immunization of children infected with human T-lymphotropic virus type III/lymphadenopathy-associated virus. MMWR Morb Mortal Wkly Rep 1986;35(38):595–8, 603–6.

99. McLaughlin M, Thomas P, Onorato I, Rubinstein A, Oleske J, Nicholas S, Krasinski K, Guigli P, Orenstein W. Live virus vaccines in human immunodeficiency virus-infected children: a retrospective survey. Pediatrics 1988;82(2):229–33.

100. Gutfreund K, Cheatham-Speth D, Rossol S, Voth R, Clemens R, Hess G. The effect of vaccination against

hepatitis B on the CD4 cell account in anti-HIV positive man. In: Abstracts, V International Conference on AIDS, Montreal, 1989;5:435.

101. Buchbinder SP, Hessol N, Lifson A, O'Malley P, Barnhart I, Rutherford G, Hadler S. The interaction of HIV and hepatitis B vaccination in a cohort of homosexual and bisexual men. In: Abstracts, V International Conference on AIDS, Montreal, 1989;5:259.

102. Centers for Disease Control and Prevention (CDC). Thimerosal in vaccines: a joint statement of the American Academy of Pediatrics and the Public Health Service. MMWR Morb Mortal Wkly Rep 1999;48(26):563–5.

103. World Health Organization. Questions and answers on thiomersal. July 1999. http://www.who.int/vaccines-diseases/safety/hottop/thiomersal.htm, 15/11/2000.

104. Immunization Safety Review. Thimerosal-Containing Vaccines and Neurodevelopmental Disorders. Washington, DC: National Academy Press, 2001.

105. Advisory Committee on Immunization Practices (ACIP). Inactivated Japanese encephalitis virus vaccine. MMWR Recomm Rep 1993;42(RR-1):1–15.

106. Edelman R. An update on vaccine adjuvants in clinical trial. AIDS Res Hum Retroviruses 1992;8(8):1409–11.

107. World Health Organization. Bovine spongiform encephalitis and oral polio vaccine. Position statement. October 2000. http://www.who.int/vaccines-diseases/safety/hottop/bse.htm, 11/10/2000.

Vacuum devices

General Information

Vacuum tumescence constriction therapy is the use of an external device that creates a vacuum to cause penile erection, which is then maintained by a constriction band. It produces rigidity sufficient for intercourse in 91% of men, with satisfaction in 80%.

Adverse effects of this procedure have been reported (1): ecchymosis (37%), discomfort (28%), hematoma (10%), numbness (6.9%), penile skin irritation, and edema. Subcutaneous penile hematoma occurred in two patients using anticoagulants and penile gangrene occurred in one patient; all had worn the constriction band overnight (2). The current recommendation is to apply the constriction band for not more than 30 minutes.

- A 55-year-old African–American, tetraplegic after a motor vehicle accident in 1969, had been using an erection aid device for 4–5 years (3). He used the device, but forgot the constricting ring, which remained on overnight. The next morning his penis was markedly swollen and 2 days later he developed septicemia. He had a gangrenous penis and necrotizing fasciitis with a foul smelling discharge.

References

1. Witherington R. Vacuum constriction device for management of erectile impotence. J Urol 1989;141(2):320–2.

2. Rivas DA, Chancellor MB. Complications associated with the use of vacuum constriction devices for erectile

dysfunction in the spinal cord injured population. J Am Paraplegia Soc 1994;17(3):136–9.
3. Eltorai I, Mentory R, Laurente F. Gangrene of the penis in a tetraplegic due to the use of vacuum constriction device for erection. Sex Disabil 2000;18:105–14.

Vaginal tampons

General Information

A tampon is a pad made of cotton, cotton wool, sponge, or other materials, used in surgery for the control of hemorrhage or absorption of secretions. Vaginal tampons are widely used to absorb menstrual flow, and have been used to absorb disagreeable secretions in women with inflammatory diseases of the vagina or cervix and to administer drugs locally after operations (1). They have also been used to collect vaginal material for diagnostic purposes (2). Tampons containing miconazole have been used to treat vaginal candidiasis (3).

Toxic shock syndrome

Toxic shock syndrome is generally associated with the use by women of internal vaginal tampons, but does not occur solely in those circumstances. Two large clinical epidemiological studies (4,5) have contributed to an understanding of the conditions that lead to toxic shock syndrome. Of all patients with toxic shock syndrome, 95% were women; in 98% of cases it began during the menstrual period, and in 98% *Staphylococcus aureus* phage group 1 was isolated from the vaginal swab. In no case was the organism isolated from the blood. It is clear that shock was caused not by bacteremia but by an epidermal toxin. Only some 8% of healthy controls harbored *S. aureus* vaginally. The mortality rate of toxic shock syndrome is estimated to be 10–15% (6,7). Since contamination with staphylococci, vaginal and extravaginal, usually occurs without any clinical consequences, special attention has focused on the association with vaginal tampons. A particular brand (Rely) has been withdrawn from the market, but other brands have also been linked with the syndrome.

A number of surviving patients had several recurrences during subsequent menstrual periods (up to five), these events each being progressively less severe in their clinical course (8,9). Insertion of a contraceptive diaphragm can trigger the toxic shock syndrome, even at times other than during menstruation.

Pathogenesis

The pathogenesis of toxic shock syndrome is not well understood. The tampons are not contaminated, and they cannot be regarded as the direct cause of toxic shock syndrome; they are rather a trigger for the events that lead to the syndrome. A plausible explanation is that the toxin produced by *S. aureus* accumulates in the tampon and is absorbed either directly from the vagina or after reflux of menstrual blood through the fallopian tubes into the peritoneal cavity. In support of this, some cases have occurred in women who have left the tampon in situ for a long time (up to 3 days). It is unclear why the incidence of toxic shock syndrome has increased since 1978. Highly absorbent tampons may partly explain this, but that is not the only explanation. The toxic shock syndrome is likely to be the result of the coincidence of staphylococcus in the vagina and conditions favoring their growth or colonization, such as a tampon saturated with menstrual blood.

Incidence and susceptibility factors

The risk of toxic shock syndrome in association with vaginal tampons is small: 10–15 per 100 000 menstruating women per year. Poor hygiene (leaving tampons in situ for several days) is not the only cause; toxic shock syndrome has been described in women changing their tampons regularly. Women who have previously had febrile episodes during menstruation should use tampons with utmost restraint or abandon them in favour of external tampons.

Toxic shock syndrome has also been described in association with use of a vaginal contraceptive sponge; vaginal cultures grew *S. aureus* (10).

Women using contraception, either oral contraceptive pills or topical spermicides, appear to be at lower risk of developing toxic shock syndrome. A study of patients with toxic shock syndrome found only six spermicide users and eight oral contraception users, against 60 not using a contraceptive method (11). It has been suggested that an antibacterial effect of spermicidal ingredients prevents the intravaginal growth of *S. aureus*. The postulated protective action of oral contraceptives has been explained by reduced menstrual flow and duration, and an alteration in cervical mucus.

References

1. Geipel K. Scheidentampons in Klinik und Praxis. [The use of vaginal tampons in hospital and practice.] Fortschr Med 1976;94(18):1077–81.
2. Sturm PD, Connolly C, Khan N, Ebrahim S, Sturm AW. Vaginal tampons as specimen collection device for the molecular diagnosis of non-ulcerative sexually transmitted infections in antenatal clinic attendees. Int J STD AIDS 2004;15(2):94–8.
3. Balsdon MJ. Comparison of miconazole-coated tampons with clotrimazole vaginal tablets in the treatment of vaginal candidosis. Br J Vener Dis 1981;57(4):275–8.
4. Davis JP, Chesney PJ, Wand PJ, LaVenture M. Toxic-shock syndrome: epidemiologic features, recurrence, risk factors, and prevention. N Engl J Med 1980;303(25):1429–35.
5. Shands KN, Schmid GP, Dan BB, Blum D, Guidotti RJ, Hargrett NT, Anderson RL, Hill DL, Broome CV, Band JD, Fraser DW. Toxic-shock syndrome in menstruating women: association with tampon use and *Staphylococcus aureus* and clinical features in 52 cases. N Engl J Med 1980;303(25):1436–42.
6. Glasgow LA. Staphylococcal infection in the toxic-shock syndrome. N Engl J Med 1980;303(25):1473–5.
7. Anonymous. Toxic shock and tampons. BMJ 1980; 281(6249):1161–2.
8. Anonymous. Toxic shock and tampons. BMJ 1980; 281(6252):1426.

9. Lea S, Ellis-Pegler RB. Toxic shock and tampons. BMJ 1980;281(6255):1639.
10. Faich G, Pearson K, Fleming D, Sobel S, Anello C. Toxic shock syndrome and the vaginal contraceptive sponge. JAMA 1986;255(2):216–18.
11. Shelton JD, Higgins JE. Contraception and toxic-shock syndrome: a reanalysis. Contraception 1981; 24(6):631–4.

Valaciclovir

General Information

Valaciclovir is the L-valyl ester of aciclovir. After oral administration, it is rapidly and extensively converted to aciclovir by first-pass metabolism, resulting in plasma aciclovir concentrations previously only attainable with intravenous administration. Like aciclovir, valaciclovir is generally well tolerated. Compared with oral aciclovir, the systemic availability of aciclovir from oral valaciclovir is markedly improved.

Valaciclovir is highly active against *Herpes simplex* and *Herpes zoster*. It is also effective in suppressing recurrent episodes of genital herpes (1). Prophylactic administration of high doses of valaciclovir to prevent CMV disease was effective in patients with AIDS and in liver transplant recipients (2,3).

Observational studies

In a double-blind comparison of two regimens of valaciclovir 500 mg bd for recurrent genital herpes, a 5-day course ($n = 398$) and a 3-day course ($n = 402$), there were no significant differences in therapeutic outcome or adverse events between the two regimens (4). The most common adverse events were headache (10%), nausea (4%), diarrhea (3%), and fatigue (1.5%).

Comparative studies

The effects of aciclovir and valaciclovir for anogenital herpes have been studied in HIV-infected individuals in two controlled trials (5). In the first study, 1062 patients with CD4+ counts over 100×10^6/l received valaciclovir or aciclovir for 1 year and were assessed monthly. In the second study, 467 patients were treated episodically for at least 5 days with valaciclovir or aciclovir and were assessed daily. Valaciclovir was as effective as aciclovir for suppression and episodic treatment of herpesvirus infections. Hazard ratios for the time to recurrence with valaciclovir 500 mg bd and 1000 mg od compared with aciclovir were 0.73 (95% CI = 0.50, 1.06) and 1.31 (0.94, 1.82). Valaciclovir 1000 mg bd and aciclovir had similar effects on the duration of infective episodes (HR = 0.92; CI = 0.75, 1.14). The most common adverse events, which occurred at similar rates with all regimens, were diarrhea, headache, infections, rashes, nausea, rhinitis, pharyngitis, abdominal pain, fever, depression, and cough.

Placebo-controlled studies

In large, placebo-controlled comparisons of the efficacy of valaciclovir and aciclovir in treating or suppressing recurrent genital *Herpes simplex* infections in immunocompetent people, dosages up to 2 g/day were well tolerated, with safety profiles comparable to aciclovir (1,6). In a comparison of high-dose valaciclovir (8 g/day) with two doses of aciclovir (0.8 and 3.2 g/day) for prophylaxis of cytomegalovirus disease in patients with advanced human immunodeficiency virus infection, intention-to-treat analysis showed a trend toward earlier mortality in those who received valaciclovir. In those who actually received valaciclovir, survival was significantly shorter. In view of the unexplained trend toward earlier mortality, as well as higher frequencies of renal toxicity (see the section on Urinary tract) and premature treatment discontinuation, the authors concluded that the dose of valaciclovir was too high and that better tolerated doses, which maintain a protective effect on cytomegalovirus disease, need to be identified (2).

Organs and Systems

Nervous system

Valaciclovir is a prodrug of aciclovir and can therefore cause similar effects, as two cases of nervous system effects have demonstrated (7).

- A 65-year-old man was given valaciclovir 1 g bd for 36 hours and had reduced concentration and was incoherent. All investigations were normal or negative. He improved rapidly on withdrawal of valaciclovir.
- A 44-year-old man was given valaciclovir 1 g tds for 5 days and developed a fever, disorientation, confusion, ataxia, dysarthria, and photophobia. All investigations were normal or negative. He was given antimicrobial drugs, including aciclovir, but his symptoms did not improve until the aciclovir was withdrawn.

Elderly patients and people with chronic renal insufficiency are most susceptible to the neurotoxic effects of aciclovir: confusion, hallucinations, dizziness, irritability, ataxia, tremor, myoclonus, and seizures. The symptoms usually occur within 3 days of the start of therapy and resolve within 5 days after withdrawal. Plasma aciclovir concentrations do not correlate with symptoms. Lumbar puncture and CT scans of the head are essentially unremarkable. The most common electroencephalographic abnormality is diffuse generalized slowing of brain wave activity.

Psychological, psychiatric

At high doses (8 g/day) hallucinations and confusion were a significant concern (2,3), but similar symptoms have also occurred at lower doses and in patients with renal insufficiency.

- Ocular and auditory hallucinations have been reported in a 60-year-old female patient on CAPD (8).
- A 58-year-old man with chronic renal insufficiency, who was hemodialysed twice a week, was treated with valaciclovir (1 g tds) for *Herpes zoster* (9). Two days

later he became disoriented, dizzy, dysarthric, and experienced hallucinations. The serum aciclovir concentration was 21 µg/ml. Treatment was discontinued and he was treated with hemodialysis for 6 hours, resulting in marked clinical improvement. The next day his symptoms of dysarthria recurred, but immediately and completely resolved after a second hemodialysis.

Hematologic

In one study, high-dose valaciclovir was associated with an increased risk of a thrombotic microangiopathy-like syndrome, reported as thrombocytopenic purpura or hemolytic-uremic syndrome (2). This syndrome occurred in 14 of 523 patients who received valaciclovir and in only four of 704 patients who received aciclovir after a median of 54 (range 8–84) weeks of treatment. The precise relation to valaciclovir remains unclear, since eight of 14 patients who were treated with valaciclovir had stopped treatment at least 1 week before the onset of the syndrome. In addition, all patients with thrombotic microangiopathy-like syndromes had taken multiple concomitant medications, and most had other intercurrent illnesses, which could have explained the hematological and renal abnormalities. The authors concluded that additional data are required to understand the role of valaciclovir and other medications for thrombotic microangiopathy-like syndromes, which are recognized with increasing frequency in patients with advanced HIV disease.

Gastrointestinal

Nausea, vomiting, and abdominal pain were commonly reported in human volunteers, but only diarrhea was significantly associated with exposure (10).

Urinary tract

Aciclovir is excreted renally. High plasma concentrations of aciclovir can lead to precipitation in renal tubules, causing impaired renal function, which is generally reversible. Since oral valaciclovir can result in plasma aciclovir concentrations comparable to those attained with intravenous dosing, reversible impairment of renal function can also occur after prolonged use of high-dose valaciclovir. Indeed, in a study of high-dose valaciclovir for prevention of cytomegalovirus disease in HIV-infected people, there was an association between treatment with valaciclovir and moderate nephrotoxicity (serum creatinine more than 1.5 times the upper limit of normal; estimated creatinine clearance under 50 ml/minute) (2).

Second-Generation Effects

Fetotoxicity

In a phase I trial, valaciclovir administered in the third trimester of pregnancy was well tolerated (11).

Susceptibility Factors

Renal disease

Adverse effects of valaciclovir, the L-valyl ester of aciclovir, can be associated with increased drug concentrations when the dose is not adjusted for reduced renal function. For example, aseptic meningitis has been associated with valaciclovir in a patient with renal insufficiency (12).

- An 88-year-old man with renal insufficiency took valaciclovir 1000 mg tds. After the first dose, he became disoriented and incontinent. Valaciclovir was withdrawn, but the symptoms continued and progressed to drowsiness and nuchal rigidity. After an extensive work-up, aseptic meningitis was diagnosed.

Given the patient's age and renal dysfunction, it is likely that excessive valaciclovir accumulation was responsible for this presentation.

Drug–Drug Interactions

Cimetidine

In an open, single-dose study of the effects of probenecid and cimetidine on the pharmacokinetics of valaciclovir and its metabolite aciclovir in 12 healthy men, valaciclovir 1 g, valaciclovir plus probenecid 1 g, valaciclovir plus cimetidine 800 mg, and valaciclovir with a combination of probenecid and cimetidine were studied (13). At three subsequent administrations, drug regimens were alternated among groups so that each group received each regimen. Probenecid and cimetidine respectively increased the mean C_{max} of valaciclovir by 23 and 53% and its AUC by 22 and 73%. Probenecid and cimetidine also respectively increased the mean aciclovir C_{max} by 22 and 8% and its AUC by 48 and 27%. The combination had a greater effect than either drug alone. Neither cimetidine nor probenecid affected the absorption of valaciclovir.

Probenecid

In an open, single-dose study of the effects of probenecid and cimetidine on the pharmacokinetics of valaciclovir and its metabolite aciclovir in 12 healthy men, valaciclovir 1 g, valaciclovir plus probenecid 1 g, valaciclovir plus cimetidine 800 mg, and valaciclovir with a combination of probenecid and cimetidine were studied (13). At three subsequent administrations, drug regimens were alternated among groups so that each group received each regimen. Probenecid and cimetidine respectively increased the mean C_{max} of valaciclovir by 23 and 53% and its AUC by 22 and 73%. Probenecid and cimetidine also respectively increased the mean aciclovir C_{max} by 22 and 8% and its AUC by 48 and 27%. The combination had a greater effect than either drug alone. Neither cimetidine nor probenecid affected the absorption of valaciclovir.

References

1. Reitano M, Tyring S, Lang W, Thoming C, Worm AM, Borelli S, Chambers LO, Robinson JM, Corey L. Valaciclovir for the suppression of recurrent genital *Herpes*

simplex virus infection: a large-scale dose range-finding study. International Valaciclovir HSV Study Group. J Infect Dis 1998;178(3):603–10.

2. Feinberg JE, Hurwitz SCooper D, Sattler FR, MacGregor RR, Powderly W, Holland GN, Griffiths PD, Pollard RB, Youle M, Gill MJ, Holland FJ, Power ME, Owens S, Coakley D, Fry J, Jacobson MA. A randomized, double-blind trial of valaciclovir prophylaxis for cytomegalovirus disease in patients with advanced human immunodeficiency virus infection. AIDS Clinical Trials Group Protocol 204/ Glaxo Wellcome 123-014 International CMV Prophylaxis Study Group. J Infect Dis 1998;177(1):48–56.

3. Lowance D, Neumayer HH, Legendre CM, Squifflet JP, Kovarik J, Brennan PJ, Norman D, Mendez R, Keating MR, Coggon GL, Crisp A, Lee IC. Valacyclovir for the prevention of cytomegalovirus disease after renal transplantation. International Valacyclovir Cytomegalovirus Prophylaxis Transplantation Study Group. N Engl J Med 1999;340(19):1462–70.

4. Leone PA, Trottier S, Miller JM. Valacyclovir for episodic treatment of genital herpes: a shorter 3-day treatment course compared with 5-day treatment. Clin Infect Dis 2002;34(7):958–62.

5. Conant MA, Schacker TW, Murphy RL, Gold J, Crutchfield LT, Crooks RJ, Acebes LO, Aiuti F, Akil B, Anderson J, Melville RL, Ballesteros Martin J, Berry A, Weiner M, Black F, Anderson PL, Bockman W, Borelli S, Bradbeer CS, Braffman M, Brandon W, Clark R, Wisniewski T, Bruun JN, Burdge D, Caputo RM, Chateauvert M, LaLonde R, Chiodo F, et al; International Valaciclovir HSV Study Group. Valaciclovir versus aciclovir for *Herpes simplex* virus infection in HIV-infected individuals: two randomized trials. Int J STD AIDS 2002;13(1):12–21.

6. Tyring SK, Douglas JM Jr, Corey L, Spruance SL, Esmann J. A randomized, placebo-controlled comparison of oral valacyclovir and acyclovir in immunocompetent patients with recurrent genital herpes infections. The Valaciclovir International Study Group. Arch Dermatol 1998;134(2):185–91.

7. Tornero C, Sanchez P, Castejon P, Rull S. Regrassion de la lipomatosis multiple con la administration de indinavir. [Reversal of multiple lipomatosis after indinavir treatment.] Med Clin (Barc) 1999;113(7):278–9.

8. Izzedine H, Launay-Vacher V, Aymard G, Legrand M, Deray G. Pharmacokinetic of nevirapine in haemodialysis. Nephrol Dial Transplant 2001;16(1):192–3.

9. Linssen-Schuurmans CD, van Kan EJ, Feith GW, Uges DR. Neurotoxicity caused by valacyclovir in a patient on hemodialysis. Ther Drug Monit 1998;20(4):385–6.

10. Jacobson MA, Gallant J, Wang LH, Coakley D, Weller S, Gary D, Squires L, Smiley ML, Blum MR, Feinberg J. Phase I trial of valaciclovir, the L-valyl ester of acyclovir, in patients with advanced human immunodeficiency virus disease. Antimicrob Agents Chemother 1994;38(7):1534–40.

11. Kimberlin DF, Weller S, Whitley RJ, Andrews WW, Hauth JC, Lakeman F, Miller G. Pharmacokinetics of oral valacyclovir and acyclovir in late pregnancy. Am J Obstet Gynecol 1998;179(4):846–51.

12. Fobelo MJ, Corzo Delgado JE, Romero Alonso A, Gomez-Bellver MJ. Aseptic meningitis related to valacyclovir. Ann Pharmacother 2001;35(1):128–9.

13. De Bony F, Tod M, Bidault R, On NT, Posner J, Rolan P. Multiple interactions of cimetidine and probenecid with valaciclovir and its metabolite acyclovir. Antimicrob Agents Chemother 2002;46(2):458–63.

Valerianaceae

See also Herbal medicines

General Information

The family of Valerianaceae contains four genera:

1. *Centranthus* (centranthus)
2. *Plectritis* (seablush)
3. *Valeriana* (valerian)
4. *Valerianella* (cornsalad).

Valeriana species

Valeriana (all-heal, amantilla, heliotrope, valerian), 400–900 mg 30–60 minutes before bedtime, is a traditional herbal sleep remedy (1), but although it has subjective effects on sleep objective sleep measures have been inconsistently affected (2). The roots of members of the *Valeriana* (valerian) species contain valepotriates, which have alkylating properties. Valtrate/isovaltrate and dihydrovaltrate are mutagenic in bacterial test systems in the presence of a metabolic activator, and their degradation products baldrinal (from valtrate) and homobaldrinal (from isovaltrate) are mutagenic even without metabolic activation. These latter compounds also have direct genotoxic effects. As far as is known, decomposition of dihydrovaltrate does not yield baldrinals.

The amounts of valepotriates and baldrinals in valerian extracts depend on the botanical species: root extracts of *Valeriana officinalis* contain up to 0.9% of valepotriates, compared with 2–4% and 5–7% of valepotriates in root extracts of *Valeriana wallichii* and *Valeriana mexicana* respectively.

Another relevant variable is the dosage form: when a herbal tea is prepared by hot extraction from valerian root, up to 60% of the valepotriates remain in the root material and only 0.1% can be recovered from the tea. A freshly prepared tincture contains 11% of the valepotriates originally found in the root material. Storage at room temperature rapidly reduces this to 3.7% after 1 week and 0% after 3 weeks. In view of this rapid degradation, it is not surprising that commercially available tincture samples yield baldrinals.

Valerian-containing tablets and capsules provide up to 1 mg of baldrinals per piece.

Valepotriates are poorly absorbed from the gastrointestinal tract, but 2% is degraded in vivo to baldrinals after oral administration of valtrate/isovaltrate to mice. In other words, a tablet with 50 mg of valepotriates may add 1 mg of baldrinals to the amount of baldrinals, which are already present before ingestion. In contrast to the valepotriates, the degradation product homobaldrinal is absorbed fairly well after oral administration to mice. As much as 71% of the administered dose can be recovered from the urine in the form of baldrinal glucuronide. Since no unchanged homobaldrinal can be demonstrated in body fluids or liver samples after oral administration, the compound appears to undergo substantial first-pass metabolism. As this glucuronidation leads to loss of its mutagenic properties, the primary target organs that are at risk from valepotriates and baldrinals are the gastrointestinal tract and the liver (3). However, the toxicological significance of all these data is still unclear, since the carcinogenic potential of valerian formulations has not been evaluated.

Adverse effects
Liver

- A 13-year-old child with fulminant seronegative liver failure required liver transplantation (4). A liver biopsy showed non-specific necrosis of more than 90% of hepatocytes. Possible exogenous toxic factors were ruled out and it was thought that the most likely cause of the liver damage was self-medication with Euphytose, a herbal mixture of *V. officinalis*, *Ballota nigra*, *Crataegus oxyacantha*, *Passiflora incarnata*, and *Cola nitida*.

The authors suggested that of these medicinal plants valerian was the most likely to have caused the liver damage. However, it could just as easily have been due to one of the other constituents or some other cause entirely.

Drug withdrawal
Delirium has been attributed to valerian withdrawal (5).

- A 58-year-old man who had regularly taken excessive doses of valerian root extract for many years was given naloxone postoperatively and developed extreme tremulousness and worsening ventilation. His condition deteriorated and he became delirious. He was treated with midazolam, lorazepam, and finally reducing doses of clonazepam and made an uneventful recovery.

The authors suggested that the anxiolytic action of valerian is similar to that of benzodiazepines and that the patient had been suffering from a valerian withdrawal syndrome.

Drug overdose
In one case of overdose with about 20 times the recommended therapeutic dose, there were only mild symptoms, all of which resolved within 24 hours (6).

In 23 patients who took an overdose of "Sleep-Qik" (valerian dry extract 75 mg, mean dose 2.5 g, hyoscine hydrobromide 0.25 mg, and cyproheptadine hydrochloride 2 mg) the main problems were central nervous system depression and anticholinergic poisoning (7). There was no evidence of liver damage, subclinical, acute, or delayed. It is unlikely that valerian contributed to the adverse effects in these cases.

References

1. Hadley S, Petry JJ. Valerian. Am Fam Physician 2003;67(8):1755–8.
2. Pallesen S, Bjorvatn B, Nordhus IH, Skjerve A. Valeriana som sovemiddel. [Valerian as a sleeping aid?] Tidsskr Nor Laegeforen 2002;122(30):2857–9.
3. Dieckmann H. Untersuchungen zur Pharmakokinetik, Metabolismus und Toxikologie von Baldrinalen. Inaugural Dissertation, Free University, Berlin, 1988.
4. Bagheri H, Broue P, Lacroix I, Larrey D, Olives JP, Vaysse P, Ghisolfi J, Montastruc JL. Fulminant hepatic failure after herbal medicine ingestion in children. Therapie 1998;53(1):82–3.
5. Garges HP, Varia I, Doraiswamy PM. Cardiac complications and delirium associated with valerian root withdrawal. JAMA 1998;280(18):1566–7.
6. Willey LB, Mady SP, Cobaugh DJ, Wax PM. Valerian overdose: a case report. Vet Hum Toxicol 1995;37(4):364–5.
7. Chan TY, Tang CH, Critchley JA. Poisoning due to an over-the-counter hypnotic, Sleep-Qik (hyoscine, cyproheptadine, valerian). Postgrad Med J 1995;71(834):227–8.

Valproic acid

See also Antiepileptic drugs

General Information

Valproic acid is available as sodium, magnesium, and calcium salts, as the free acid, and as a coordination compound, valproate semisodium (divalproex sodium), which comprises the sodium salt of valproic acid and free valproic acid in a 1:1 molar ratio. All share the same active principle (valproic acid) and have virtually identical tolerability, although the formulation influences the incidence of gastrointestinal adverse effects. Valpromide (rINN) is a prodrug of valproate, to which it is converted with a half-life of less than 1 hour. Valnoctamide (rINN) is an isomer of valpromide.

The therapeutic uses of valproate in psychiatric conditions have been reviewed (1,2). The major adverse effects in one study of 150 patients were tremor (9.3%), gastrointestinal effects (8.9%), drowsiness (8.6%), hair loss (7.9%), weight gain (6.9%), weakness (6.9%), dizziness (4.1%), thrombocytopenia (2.9%), and headache (2.7%).

General adverse effects

Weight gain, gastrointestinal symptoms, hair loss, and tremor are relatively common adverse effects. Sedation, fatigue, dizziness, headache, ataxia, insomnia, and behavioral problems are less frequent than with other anticonvulsants. Hyperammonemia is relatively common, but it is often asymptomatic. Fatal liver failure has an incidence of up to 1:600 in young infants, but is extremely rare in adults. Uncommon effects include parkinsonism, encephalopathy, pseudoatrophy of the brain, pancreatitis, and disorders of hemostasis (especially thrombocytopenia).

Hypersusceptibility reactions
Hypersusceptibility reactions can affect any organ and system, but are very rare. Lupus-like syndrome has been reported.

Second-generation effects
Valproate can cause fetal malformations, particularly neural tube defects (2–3% risk).

Organs and Systems

Cardiovascular

Very rarely, valproate-induced carnitine deficiency adversely affects cardiac function (see Metabolism in this monograph).

Hypotension has been attributed to valproate (3).

- In an 11-year-old girl who was treated with intravenous valproate (30 mg/kg over 1 hour) for status epilepticus, the blood pressure fell from 130/80 mmHg to 70/55 mmHg after about 40 minutes of infusion. Her seizures stopped, but her blood pressure fluctuated for several hours between 90/60 mmHg and 60/30 mmHg, requiring intravenous fluids and pressor therapy. Endotracheal intubation was also performed and she eventually recovered.

In this case a relatively high dosage of valproate, concurrent *Varicella* infection, and previous use of benzodiazepines may have contributed.

In 775 patients who received intravenous phenytoin, valproate, or placebo, intravenous site reactions occurred in 18% of patients who received valproate (4). Most of the events (70%) occurred in the first intravenous site and all occurred in peripheral administration sites. When patients who received the drug by central line were excluded, the estimated incidence was 21%. There were fewer adverse events when phenytoin was given alone than when it was given together with valproate.

Respiratory

Respiratory failure and truncal weakness occurred in one patient given dosages up to 3200 mg/day, the association being proven by withdrawal and rechallenge (SEDA-18, 68).

Fatal pulmonary hemorrhage occurred during high-dose valproate monotherapy in a 30-year-old woman (5). It was accompanied by a low platelet count (15×10^9/l).

Nervous system

Tremor is seen in 15% of patients taking valproate (6), although its incidence can increase to over 60% at serum drug concentrations in a high range (80–150 µg/ml) (7); it is clinically reminiscent of essential tremor and responds to dosage reduction. Asterixis has been associated with intoxication by most anticonvulsants, but with valproate it can occur at therapeutic drug concentrations (SED-12, 133) (8).

Sedation, fatigue, dizziness, headache, ataxia, and insomnia are less frequent with valproate than with other anticonvulsants. However, encephalopathy, sometimes associated with hyperammonemia and/or liver failure, has been described on several occasions, with symptoms ranging from acute confusion to stupor and even deep coma (SEDA-18, 69) (9). The stupor tends to be associated with bilaterally synchronous high-voltage, slow-wave EEG activity. Psychiatric symptoms and increased seizure frequency can also occur. Although in some cases valproate-induced stupor can be associated with increased epileptiform activity, it appeared to be triggered by a cortical non-epileptic mechanism in six patients who developed negative myoclonus and stupor after taking valproate for a few days (SEDA-19, 74).

Rarely valproate causes a parkinsonian-like reaction (SEDA-18, 69) (SEDA-19, 74). Involuntary movements and twitching of the face and limbs have been also reported. Intermittent choreiform movements were observed in two girls and one man, all with pre-existing severe brain damage, after they had taken valproate for 27 years (SEDA-20, 68).

When a 25-year-old woman with a hypothalamic hamartoma was given valproate (up to 2500 mg/day) in addition to phenytoin and phenobarbital, she became increasingly somnolent and spike and wave activity in her electroencephalogram deteriorated to the point when she appeared to be in absence status (10). Her blood ammonia concentration was about three times the upper limit of the reference range. During wakefulness, electroencephalographic paroxysms increased with increasing plasma valproic acid concentrations and resolved (together with mental status changes and hyperammonemia) when valproate was withdrawn. The data are suggestive of a paradoxical effect of valproic acid on spike and wave activity, possibly related to the underlying pathology or hyperammonemia.

A most unusual adverse effect, uncontrollable laughter, was reported in two men aged 17 and 20 years (11). The laughter persisted for 4–6 hours after an intravenous injection of 800 mg valproate over 1 hour.

Valproate rarely causes severe mental deterioration and CT/MRI findings suggestive of cortical atrophy, reversible after withdrawal (SEDA-20, 67). Two possible additional cases have been reported in women with juvenile myoclonic epilepsy aged 22 and 46 years (12). In one case mental function and brain atrophy regressed over a few months after stopping valproate, while in the other cognitive function improved but CT/MRI abnormalities persisted. The authors suggested that valproate-induced pseudoatrophy of the brain may not be always fully reversible, especially when the interval between onset of the condition and diagnosis is prolonged (2 years in this case). However, the possibility exists that the persistent cortical atrophy had other causes in their patient.

Retrospective studies have suggested that anticonvulsants may be associated with peripheral nerve dysfunction. This has been studied prospectively in 81 patients (aged 13–67 years) without polyneuropathy who took sodium valproate ($n = 44$) or carbamazepine ($n = 37$) as monotherapy in standard daily doses (13). After 2 years one patient had clinical signs of polyneuropathy and six patients had symptoms of polyneuropathy, but electrophysiology did not show significant changes or trends. Only one patient had abnormal electrophysiological findings, which were only subclinical, and eight patients had abnormal values at two subsequent visits. There were no consistent patterns, and the data were unaffected when the drugs were examined separately or when patients were grouped according to whether or not they had symptoms of polyneuropathy. The authors concluded that previously untreated young to middle-aged patients who take valproic acid or carbamazepine for 2 years are not at risk of polyneuropathy.

Valproate can cause altered visual evoked potentials and brainstem evoked potentials (14). In 100 epileptic patients aged 8–18 years taking valproate in a modified-release formulation, interpeak latencies of I-III and III-V of brainstem evoked potentials were significantly delayed and N75/P100 and P100/N145 amplitudes in the visual evoked potentials were reduced.

Valproate toxicity has been reported to have caused a neurodegenerative condition that mimicked multisystem atrophy in a 67-year-old woman (15).

Valproate can occasionally cause aggravation of absence seizures in children (16). Eight patients with typical and myoclonic absence epilepsy and electroencephalography that showed generalized 3-Hz spike-and-wave had an increase in the frequency of absence seizures within days of valproate introduction. Dosage increments resulted in further aggravation. Serum concentrations of valproate were in the target range in all cases. All the children improved on valproate withdrawal; in five valproate was reintroduced, resulting in further seizure aggravation.

In one report of 36 adults chronically treated with valproate at a veterans' clinic, intellectual deterioration, sleep disorders, sexual dysfunction, personality changes, hearing difficulties, gait instability, tremor, parkinsonism, bradykinesia, abulia, and upper motor neuron signs were found in a large proportion, but selection bias was likely (17). The severity of symptoms and signs varied from minimal to a degree that could lead to diagnosis of Parkinson's disease or dementia. Improvement followed valproate withdrawal, and in two patients retested by CT scan cerebral atrophy regressed after drug withdrawal.

Psychological, psychiatric

Psychotic reactions had been reported to the WHO monitoring system on 16 occasions by 1993, and other occasional cases have been published (SED-13, 149) (18).

Behavioral problems are less frequent with valproate than with other anticonvulsants and include sedation, hyperactivity, irritability, and aggression (19).

There has been a randomized, double-blind, single crossover study of the effects of sodium valproate on cognitive performance and behavior in eight children with learning and behavioral problems associated with electroencephalographic epileptiform discharges but without clinical seizures (20). The children became more distractable, had increased delay in response time, and had lower memory scores while taking valproate. Their parents reported higher internalizing scores on the Child Behavior Checklists.

Although valproate has little effect on cognitive function compared with other anticonvulsants, it can occasionally cause reversible dementia, sometimes associated with MRI evidence of pseudoatrophy of the brain (SEDA-20, 67) (SEDA-21, 76). The presentation can be striking, with progressive motor and intellectual deterioration and apathy appearing shortly after the introduction of valproate, or sometimes after as long as 2 years. Many affected patients have relatively high serum drug concentrations (100–120 mg/l), other signs of toxicity, such as tremor and ataxia, and normal electroencephalographic background activity. The presentation differs from valproate-induced stupor, in which consciousness is impaired, and there may be clinical or electroencephalographic signs of increased seizure activity. In all cases, clinical and imaging signs improved rapidly after drug withdrawal. The incidence of this syndrome is probably very low, although there is concern about possible underdiagnosis.

Endocrine

The use of valproate in young women has been associated with an increased incidence of menstrual abnormalities (21), polycystic ovaries, and hyperandrogenism (SEDA-18, 69) (SEDA-20, 68). Of 22 valproate-treated women who underwent endocrine evaluation, 13 were obese and 11 had marked weight gain (mean 21 kg) after starting valproate (22). There were polycystic ovaries, hyperandrogenism, or both in 64%, but the clinical relevance of these findings remains uncertain.

The syndrome of polycystic ovaries and hyperandrogenism associated with weight gain and hyperinsulinemia was reversible in 16 women with valproate-related polycystic ovaries and/or hyperandrogenism who were switched to lamotrigine (23). While taking valproate, they had centripetal obesity with associated hyperinsulinism and unfavorable serum lipid profiles. After switching to lamotrigine, in the 12 patients available for follow-up at 1 year, body-mass index and fasting serum insulin and testosterone concentrations fell, whereas HDL cholesterol/total cholesterol ratios increased from 0.17 to 0.26. The total number of polycystic ovaries fell from 20 to 11 after 1 year of lamotrigine.

Pubertal growth arrest has been described in a 12-year-old girl who had taken valproate for 18 months (SED-13, 152) (24).

Among 45 valproate-treated girls aged 8–18 years, hyperandrogenism (serum testosterone concentrations more than two standard deviations above the mean for healthy controls) was seen in 38% of prepubertal girls, 36% of pubertal girls, and 57% of postpubertal girls (25). Obesity was more common in postpubertal valproate-treated girls than in controls. The authors concluded that valproate may cause hyperandrogenism in girls with epilepsy during the sensitive period of pubertal maturation.

There were increased serum androgen concentrations in 60% of those who took valproate (22).

The endocrine consequences of valproate or carbamazepine monotherapy have been evaluated in a cross-sectional study in two groups of women with epilepsy, who were treated for at least 2 years with valproate ($n = 52$) or carbamazepine monotherapy ($n = 53$) (26). Menstrual disturbances were reported by 29 of the women, 12 of those taking valproate and 17 of those taking carbamazepine. Polycystic ovaries were found in 28 patients, of whom 13 were taking valproate and 15 carbamazepine. Postprandial concentrations of insulin, C-peptide, and proinsulin were significantly higher with valproate than carbamazepine, but there were no differences in the fasting state. In conclusion, this study did not show an increase in the frequency of polycystic ovaries in valproate-treated women, although valproate does appear to increase glucose-stimulated pancreatic insulin secretion.

Metabolism

Valproate can cause hyperglycinemia and hyperglycinuria, sometimes with raised spinal fluid glycine concentrations (SED-12, 133). These changes are usually asymptomatic.

Chronic valproate treatment did not change serum concentrations of lipids, vitamin B12, or folic acid in 26 children with epilepsy (27).

Weight gain

Weight increase, sometimes associated with increased appetite, occurs in 8–60% of patients taking valproate (6) and may be unrelated to dose.

A randomized, double-blind study was conducted for 32 weeks to analyse weight change in patients taking lamotrigine ($n = 65$; mean age 35 years; target dosage 200 mg/day) and valproate ($n = 68$; mean age 30 years; target dosage 20 mg/kg/day) (28). Weight remained stable in the patients taking lamotrigine. However, there was significant weight gain in the patients taking valproate by the 10th week of treatment, and weight continued to increase throughout the study. After 32 weeks, mean weight gain was significantly higher in those taking valproate (5.8 kg) compared with lamotrigine (0.6 kg). Similar proportions of patients taking lamotrigine (29%) or valproate (26%) were seizure-free. The frequencies of adverse events were similar in the two groups.

The mechanisms involved have been assessed in 40 women with epilepsy evaluated before and after 1 year of therapy (29). At the end of follow-up, 15 patients were obese and had higher serum leptin and insulin concentrations than patients who did not gain weight. The rise in serum leptin is consistent with that observed in other types of obesity.

In a prospective cohort study of the role of insulin and leptin (a signal factor that regulates body weight and energy expenditure) in valproate-related obesity, 81 patients with epilepsy taking valproate and 51 healthy controls were analysed (30). Mean serum insulin concentrations were significantly higher in the valproate-treated patients than in the controls, despite similar body mass indexes. Furthermore, serum insulin concentrations were significantly higher both in lean men and lean women compared with lean controls of same sex and similar body mass indexes. This implies that the hyperinsulinemia seen in obese people taking valproate is not merely a consequence of insulin resistance induced by weight gain. Serum leptin concentrations did not differ between the valproate-treated patients and the controls. Thus, both obese and lean patients taking valproate have hyperinsulinemia, suggesting insulin resistance. This may be one of the factors that leads to weight gain during valproate treatment. Similar findings, that is increased insulin concentrations without changes in leptin concentrations, have also been published in three other reports from one center (26,31,32).

Hyperammonemia

Hyperammonemic encephalopathy has been attributed to valproate (33).

- A 61-year-old man with epilepsy had altered consciousness after his dose of valproate was increased because of poor seizure control. Electroencephalography showed triphasic waves and high-amplitude delta-wave activity with frontal predominance. Although serum aspartate transaminase and alanine transaminase were normal, the serum ammonium concentration was high at 960 ng/ml (reference range 30–470). Serum amino acid analysis showed multiple minor abnormalities. Valproate was withdrawn. He improved within 4 days and the electroencephalogram, serum ammonium concentration, and amino acid profile were normal by day 8.

In two other cases the addition of topiramate was thought to have precipitated valproate-induced hyperammonemic encephalopathy (34). Recovery occurred after withdrawal of valproate or topiramate. The authors suggested that topiramate may have contributed to the hyperammonemia by inhibiting carbonic anhydrase and cerebral glutamine synthetase.

Asymptomatic hyperammonemia, with ammonia concentrations as high as 140 mmol/l, has been found in up to over 50% of patients (35) and may be due to increased renal production or inhibition of nitrogen elimination, although carnitine deficiency, nutritional influences, metabolic abnormalities secondary to increased glycine or propionic acid concentrations, and multiple drug therapy may play a role (SED-13, 149) (35). In individual patients, the condition can be associated with severe symptoms (SEDA-20, 69). Deaths have occurred after the use of valproate in patients with ornithine transcarbamylase deficiency (SED-12, 133) (36), (SED-13, 149) (37). Additional evidence points to a need for caution in patients with any enzyme disorder: an 18-year-old woman with progressive dementia and spastic paraparesis became comatose with hyperammonemia when taking valproate; moderate hyperammonemia persisted for months after drug withdrawal, coma recurred without exposure to valproate, and congenital argininemia was diagnosed (38). Carnitine supplementation has been proposed in symptomatic hyperammonemia caused by valproate (see below).

Valproate-induced hyperammonemic encephalopathy has been reviewed (39). Proton magnetic resonance spectroscopy was performed in a patient with valproate-induced hyperammonemic encephalopathy; there was a significant fall in the choline and myoinositol resonances and an increase in glutamine in the hyperintense basal ganglia lesions (40). A similar pattern has been observed in other hyperammonemic encephalopathies, such as hepatic encephalopathy. In another study in seven patients with valproate-related hyperammonemia serum or cerebrospinal fluid glutamine concentrations were initially raised in most patients, sometimes in the absence of hyperammonemia (41).

Carnitine deficiency

Valproate is often associated with low carnitine concentrations and occasionally with true carnitine deficiency, especially in young children with neurological disabilities taking several anticonvulsants. The condition is usually asymptomatic, but it can occasionally cause significant toxicity (42).

- Life-threatening cardiac dysfunction in a 7-year-old boy required urgent carnitine supplementation (SEDA-17, 74).
- In one patient with acute valproate-associated encephalopathy associated with biochemical evidence of severe carnitine deficiency and a defect in valproate

metabolism, L-carnitine substitution corrected the biochemical abnormalities, but the patient died (SED-13, 150) (43).

- In another case, there was late-onset lipid storage myopathy, with secondary carnitine deficiency (SED-13, 150) (44).

While measurement of carnitine concentrations is advisable in patients with symptoms and signs suggestive of carnitine deficiency (SED-12, 133) (45), indiscriminate carnitine supplementation is unwarranted. A panel of pediatric neurologists recently recommended intravenous carnitine for valproate hepatotoxicity and for valproate overdose (SEDA-20, 69), whereas oral supplementation was suggested for patients with symptomatic valproate-associated hyperammonemia, multiple risk factors for valproate hepatotoxicity, and infants and young children receiving valproate (46). It was mentioned that carnitine might be deleterious in some disorders of long-chain fatty acid oxidation. Others have considered carnitine to be valuable in valproate-induced hyperammonemia, but have suggested reserving it for patients with subnormal blood carnitine concentrations or known risk factors for carnitine deficiency (47). In a double-blind trial in 47 children taking carbamazepine or valproate, carnitine (100 mg/kg/day for 4 weeks) was not more effective than placebo in improving subjective well-being (SEDA-19, 74).

Nutrition

Concentrations of plasma homocysteine, plasma pyridoxal 5'-phosphate (active vitamin B6), serum folate, erythrocyte folate, and serum vitamin B12 have been measured both fasting and after methionine in 60 epileptic patients (aged 14–18 years) and 63 sex- and age-matched controls before therapy and after 1 year of therapy with valproate or carbamazepine (48). After 1 year the patients who took valproate and carbamazepine had significantly increased plasma homocysteine concentrations compared with both baseline and control values and there was a significant fall in serum folate and plasma pyridoxal 5'-phosphate. Serum vitamin B12 and erythrocyte folate were unchanged.

The genetic determinants of this effect on homocysteine have been determined in 136 epileptic children taking carbamazepine or valproate as monotherapy (49). Nutritional determinants (folate and vitamins B6 and B12) and genetic determinants (MTHFR 677CT) of plasma homocysteine were studied in a random sample of 59 of those children. Total homocysteine concentrations were significantly increased and folate and vitamin B6 concentrations were significantly reduced. Carbamazepine lowered folate concentrations in association with hyperhomocysteinemia, which seemed to be related to the homozygous MTHFR 677CT mutation. Valproate, although also associated with hyperhomocysteinemia, only reduced vitamin B6 concentrations, independent of the MTHFR genotype.

In 15 patients who had a serious adverse reaction to valproate (including behavioral changes and emesis in six, raised aspartate transaminase in three, raised aspartate transaminase and pancreatitis in one, thombocytopenia in two, and unexpected death in two), erythrocyte glutathione peroxidase activity and plasma selenium and zinc concentrations were significantly reduced, whereas erythrocyte glutathione reductase activity was significantly raised

relative to matched healthy controls or patients with good tolerance of valproate (50). These findings may indicate a role for selenium-dependent antioxidant activity in individual susceptibility to the adverse effects of valproate.

Mineral balance

- Hyponatremia (serum sodium of 128 mmol/l) was discovered accidentally in a 50-year-old man during follow-up for Henoch-Schönlein nephritis (51). He was taking sodium valproate 2000 mg/day. Repeated water loads at different dosages of valproate confirmed that the ability to excrete water was dose-dependently reduced.

Fluid balance

Edema has been attributed to valproate.

- A 42-year-old man with bipolar disorder developed peripheral edema 14 days after starting treatment with valproate in a dosage of 1400 mg/day (52). Within 3 weeks he gained 11 kg in body weight, his legs were very swollen, and periorbital edema was present after a night's sleep. Blood chemistry and hematology tests were normal. The diagnosis was avid salt retention by the renal tubules, secondary to treatment with valproate, and recovery occurred when diuretics were given and valproate was substituted with lithium.
- An 18-year-old woman also developed leg edema while taking valproate 800 mg/day for epilepsy (53). Although she had taken valproate for 10 years without edema, the lack of alternative explanations and the disappearance of the condition after withdrawal suggested a drug-related effect. She also had dysmenorrhea, hirsutism, and obesity, which were thought to have been caused by valproate.

There have been eight other published cases of valproate-induced edema, plus two additional cases in whom edema developed when risperidone was added to valproate.

- Severe peripheral edema occurred in a 42-year-old man taking valproate 1.5 g/day and resolved on withdrawal (52).

The authors proposed that increased GABA activity had inhibited natriuresis by altering the action of nitric oxide in the kidneys or by inhibiting the central production of C-type natriuretic peptide.

Hematologic

Hematological abnormalities, mostly of little or no clinical significance, occur in about 30% of patients taking valproate (SEDA-18, 69).

Thrombocytopenia can be caused by autoimmune mechanisms (SED-13, 150) (54), tends to be related to high serum drug concentrations, and often responds to dosage reduction (SEDA-19, 74). Of 131 patients randomized to high plasma concentrations of valproic acid (80–150 µg/ml), 36 (27%) had at least one platelet count below 75×10^9/l, compared with only one patient in a group randomized to drug concentrations of 25–50 µg/ml (55).

As well as reducing platelet count or function valproate can impair procoagulatory thrombocytic functions as reflected by reduced platelet activation and an increased thrombin time (56). Valproate-induced platelet dysfunction may be related, at least in part and in some patients, to inhibition of the arachidonic acid cascade (57).

- There was a small reduction in platelet count (from 150 to $110 \times 10^9/l$) in association with gastrointestinal symptoms in a 45-year-old man when he took valproate 750 mg tds, but not when he took the same dose of divalproex, an enteric-coated formulation (58).
- A small reduction in platelet count (from 170 to $110 \times 10^9/l$) in a 37-year-old woman was associated with disproportionate perioperative bleeding (59). An antiplatelet antibody was also detected and the authors therefore proposed that valproate must also have caused reduced platelet aggregation.
- Small reductions in red cell, white cell, and platelet counts occurred in a 65-year-old man taking valproate; the changes were dose-related but did not merit the description of pancytopenia that the authors used in the title of their paper (60).

Bleeding complications occasionally occur. In an unusual case, thrombocytopenic purpura, anemia, and reticulocytosis occurred in a 3-month-old breast-fed infant whose mother was taking valproic acid 1200 mg/day. The serum valproic acid concentration in the infant was 6.6 μg/ml, and recovery occurred when breast-feeding was stopped (61).

Depressed fibrinogen concentrations have been reported (SED-12, 134) (62,63), but they are unlikely to be important, except perhaps in patients due to undergo surgery. However, two neonates from mothers who had taken valproate during pregnancy developed bleeding associated with fibrinogen depletion soon after birth, and one of them died from afibrinogenemia (SEDA-19, 75).

In one study there were marked reductions in von Willebrand factor and ristocetin co-factor in most valproate-treated children (SEDA-17, 74), leading to deranged hemostasis, although not always to a clinically important extent. In the event of bleeding or need for surgical procedures, a high-purity factor VIII concentrate (Haemate P) provided sufficient hemostasis in valproate-induced von Willebrand's disease, despite the fact that Haemate P is ineffective in the platelet type of the disease (64). Despite frequent changes in hemostasis and blood coagulation in patients taking valproate, bleeding complications during or after neurosurgery are uncommon (SEDA-21, 76).

Very rare effects include bone-marrow suppression associated with platelet autoantibodies and coagulopathy, transient leukopenia, lethal bone-marrow failure due to self-poisoning, reversible intravascular hemolysis, and pure red cell aplasia (SED-12, 134) (65–68).

A 5-year-old girl with acquired protein C deficiency had a stroke while taking valproate (69). The authors then measured protein C concentrations in 20 children taking valproate monotherapy and 20 children taking other anticonvulsants. There were significantly lower protein C concentrations in those taking valproate. Protein S and antithrombin III were not affected. Despite this, there is no known association between valproate therapy and a risk of thromboembolic disease, and the clinical relevance of this effect on protein C is not clear.

Gastrointestinal

Gastrointestinal symptoms, such as nausea, anorexia, vomiting, gastritis, and diarrhea, occur in 36% of patients (6), although over 20% may be affected at high dosages (7). Stomatitis, parotid gland enlargement, and gingival hyperplasia are exceedingly rare (SED-13, 151) (70–72).

In a retrospective survey, gastrointestinal adverse effects were less common in 150 patients taking valproate semisodium than in an equal number taking valproic acid (15 versus 29%), despite the fact that serum valproic acid concentrations were comparable in the two groups (73). Patients taking valproate semisodium were less likely to discontinue medication because of gastrointestinal adverse effects (4 versus 13%). The difference was ascribed to the enteric-coated formulation of valproate semisodium.

The suggestion that divalproex (valproate semisodium) causes fewer gastrointestinal adverse reactions than valproate (SEDA-23, 94) (58) has been challenged (74). In other cited studies divalproex was associated with a higher risk of gastrointestinal effects.

Liver

Liver abnormalities due to valproate range from transient dose-related asymptomatic rises in liver enzymes (in as many as 40% of patients) to rare and often fatal hepatic failure. Rises in liver enzymes up to three times normal may abate, even without a reduction in dosage, but the drug should be withdrawn if the rise in enzyme concentrations is greater.

At least 132 patients have died of liver failure (and/or pancreatitis) (75). The risk is highest (1:600) in children under 2 years of age with complex neurological disorders taking valproate as part of a multidrug regimen (46,76). In older patients the incidence is no more than 1:37 000 for monotherapy and 1:12 000 for multidrug therapy. Deaths beyond 20 years of age are exceedingly rare. Risk factors include mental retardation, congenital abnormalities, neurological disorders, familial hepatic disease, the addition of valproate within 3 months of liver dysfunction, and concomitant salicylate use. Fatal hepatotoxicity usually occurs within the first 3 months, although the proportion of patients who developed their first symptoms after 6 months has increased lately, possibly because of greater awareness of the problem and a reduced death rate, owing to rapid drug withdrawal (75). The presenting symptoms include nausea, vomiting, loss of appetite, reduced alertness, apathy, coma, fever, jaundice, hemorrhage, edema, and increased seizure frequency, including status epilepticus. The importance of fever and increased seizure frequency as diagnostic features may have been underestimated in the past.

A Reye-like syndrome, as yet only in children, has also been described. The mechanisms involved remain elusive, and possible roles of carnitine deficiency (46) and hepatotoxic metabolites (SED-13, 151) (77) have been discussed.

Knowledge of symptoms is more important than laboratory tests in early detection and prevention, although monitoring liver function during the first 6 months of therapy is recommended. There is some evidence that hepatotoxicity is related to carnitine deficiency, and retrospective data suggest that the outcome can be improved by early intravenous administration of carnitine (46).

- Valproate-induced fatal liver failure developed in a 29-year-old woman with Friedreich's disease (78). The first symptoms (apathy during febrile upper airways infection) occurred after 2 months of therapy at a dosage of 20 mg/kg. The drug was withdrawn 10 days later, when she had hepatic encephalopathy and a severe bleeding diathesis; supportive treatment was provided but she died after 4 weeks.

This was the third published case of fatal valproate liver toxicity in an adult with Friedreich's disease, suggesting that this condition is a predisposing factor. Although the risk of valproate hepatotoxicity in adults is much lower than in children, adults still represented over 15% of the cases known to the authors. Overall, a total of 26 other adults (age range 17–62 years) with fatal valproate-induced liver failure have been reported: of these, 3 were taking monotherapy and 12 had no underlying disease or a clearly non-metabolic and non-hepatic disease. The duration of treatment before the first symptoms varied between 6 days and 6 years.

Fatal hepatitis has been reported in a child taking valproate (79).

- An 8-year-old boy with complex partial seizures had taken valproate for more than 3 years. His sister developed uncomplicated hepatitis A, and 1 month later he became jaundiced, developed fulminant hepatic failure, quickly became encephalopathic, and died, despite withdrawal of valproate, aggressive supportive therapy, and treatment with carnitine. He had positive hepatitis A IgM; other causes for acute hepatitis were ruled out. Liver pathology showed distended hepatocytes with cholestasis and microvesicular changes.

The authors thought that valproate-induced hepatotoxicity may have exacerbated this child's infective hepatitis.

Hepatotoxicity due to valproate has been attributed to reactive hepatotoxic metabolites of valproate, which are normally detoxified by glutathione conjugation followed by mercapturic acid metabolism to their respective *N*-acetylcysteine conjugates (80).

The Alpers–Huttenlocher syndrome, progressive neuronal degeneration of childhood, which is associated with seizures and abnormal liver function tests, can lead a clinician to use valproate, which can then precipitate acute liver damage, as has been reported in five cases (81). In all cases liver transplantation for valproate-induced liver damage was then associated with worsening neurological function. In another case Alpers–Huttenlocher syndrome was misdiagnosed as valproate toxicity (82).

The association between valproate and raised transaminase activities has been studied in a retrospective review of the medical records of patients positive for hepatitis C virus (83). Of 214 patients 28 were taking valproate and 186 were not. The controls and those who had been hepatitis-positive for longer were significantly more likely to have worse hepatotoxicity. Valproate, either alone or in the presence of other potential hepatotoxins, was not associated with raised transaminases.

Pancreas

There have been over 50 published reports of acute pancreatitis associated with valproate (SEDA-18, 70) (84), including several confirmed by rechallenge. Deaths have occurred from hemorrhagic pancreatic necrosis; complications can include pleural and pericardial effusions, coagulopathy, pseudocyst, ascites, wound infection, and pneumonia (SED-13, 151) (85). Hepatotoxicity can co-exist. There is suggestive evidence that end-stage renal insufficiency (SEDA-22, 92) and mental retardation (84) can be predisposing factors.

In a study of intravenous valproate in status epilepticus, three of 19 patients (ages and dosages not specified) developed a rise in serum lipase activity above 4000 IU/ml within 1–3 weeks (86); one of these developed overt exudative pancreatitis. Based on these data, it may be prudent to monitor serum lipase when using intravenous valproate.

However, in a review of valproate-induced pancreatitis (87) the author discouraged routine checking of amylase activity in the absence of other clinical signs and symptoms.

Urinary tract

Enuresis in children can occasionally be a problem (88). There have been single cases of Fanconi syndrome (SED-13, 151) (89), and hematuria with acute renal insufficiency (SEDA-20, 69).

A child with developmental delay and epilepsy developed glycosuria about 16 months after starting to take valproic acid (90). Laboratory evaluation showed global defects in proximal tubule function, consistent with the De Toni–Debré–Fanconi syndrome. The authors reviewed the literature on this rare complication, which is reversible on valproate withdrawal.

Skin

Skin rashes are uncommon (2–4%), and photosensitivity and cutaneous vasculitis, if they occur at all, are exceedingly rare (SED-13, 152) (91,92).

Cutaneous pseudolymphoma has been attributed to valproate (93).

- A 41-year-old man presented with an erythematous papule, histologically mimicking a non-epidermotropic T cell lymphoma. Polymerase chain reaction in the skin biopsy showed monoclonal rearrangement of the T cell receptor gamma gene. Withdrawal of valproate was followed by regression of the lesion, but 5 months after substitution by carbamazepine, two further papules appeared, with similar histological features. Carbamazepine was withdrawn and the lesions disappeared without relapse over 4 years.

Hair

Hair loss and changes in hair texture or color are seen in 1–11% of patients (SED-12, 135) (6,94,95). Alopecia has been reported in 4% of patients with concentrations below 50 µg/ml and in 28% of patients with serum drug concentrations above 80 µg/ml (7).

Musculoskeletal

Accumulation of microvesicular lipid droplets between myofibrils adjacent to mitochondria was found in muscle biopsies from seven children taking valproate (SEDA-22, 92). Ultrastructural abnormalities in the mitochondria suggested that these could have resulted from impaired mitochondrial fatty acid oxidation.

Sexual function

- A 32-year-old man developed infertility and a low sperm count (under $50 \times 10^6/l$), with no motile sperm, less than 10% viability, and 100% with abnormal structure while taking valproate monotherapy for 5 years (96). Within 4 months of switching to felbamate, he and his wife conceived twin girls, and the sperm abnormalities were largely reversed.

These findings suggest that occasionally valproate can cause male infertility.

Reproductive system

Polycystic ovary syndrome (polycystic ovaries, hyperandrogenism, obesity, hirsutism, anovulatory cycles, and menstrual disorders) is more common in women with epilepsy. Valproate has been associated with alterations in reproductive hormonal function beginning in the first month of treatment. Serum androgen concentrations increase in patients taking valproate but the profile of hormonal changes is different in women and men (97). Animal studies have corroborated the adverse ovarian and endocrine effects of valproate (98). Four review articles have dealt with this reported adverse event, highlighting controversial views (99–102).

The estimated prevalence of polycystic ovary syndrome in patients with epilepsy is 13–25%, compared with 4–6% in the general population (99). Polycystic ovary syndrome has been described in women with epilepsy taking valproate, especially those who start treatment before 20 years of age (22,103), and the frequency is high: in a cross-sectional study of 22 women taking valproate monotherapy, 59% were obese and 64% had polycystic ovaries, hyperandrogenism, or both (22).

In a prospective study of polycystic ovary syndrome in 52 controls and 72 women with epilepsy (37 taking valproate monotherapy and 35 carbamazepine monotherapy), the frequency of polycystic ovaries, hyperandrogenism, or both was significantly higher in those taking valproate than in the controls (70 versus 19%) (104). They occurred in 20% of the patients taking carbamazepine. The obese women taking valproate who had polycystic ovaries or hyperandrogenism or both had hyperinsulinemia and associated unfavorable changes in serum lipid concentrations consistent with insulin resistance. In both obese and lean women, polycystic ovaries and related hyperandrogenism were similarly found. Most of the abnormalities were reversed when valproate was withdrawn (23).

Three women taking valproate developed hyperandrogenism and polycystic ovaries, associated in two cases with weight gain and menstrual disorders (105). Valproate was replaced by lamotrigine, and the serum testosterone concentrations fell in all three women, the polycystic changes disappeared from the ovaries in two,

and the two women who had gained weight and developed amenorrhea lost weight and started menstruating. In the light of this report others have clarified the distinction between polycystic ovary syndrome and polycystic ovary morphology, and have pointed out that it was not clear which of these valproate had actually caused (106,107). The report also contrasts with a report that polycystic ovary syndrome was identified in two of 19 patients taking no medications, four of 38 patients taking valproate or carbamazepine monotherapy, and one of 36 patients taking more than one antiepileptic drug, suggesting that polycystic ovary syndrome in women with focal epilepsy is not related to valproate or carbamazepine (108).

Although the association between polycystic ovary syndrome and valproate treatment appears to be established, current published studies are limited, owing to small sample sizes and diverse definitions of polycystic ovary syndrome. Thus, the true clinical relevance and frequency of the association needs further investigation in large, multicenter, prospective studies.

Women taking valproate should be asked about menstrual disorders. The presence of a menstrual disorder, hirsutism, or weight gain should trigger thorough evaluation and, if necessary, valproate withdrawal.

Immunologic

Hypersensitivity reactions to valproate are rare. Lupus-like syndrome has been reported occasionally with valproate (SEDA-19, 75) (SEDA-20, 69) and valpromide (109).

In vitro tests have shown that valproate can increase the viral burden in HIV-infected individuals by potentiating replication of the virus (110). In a retrospective review of 11 HIV-positive patients with behavioral disturbances taking valproate HIV-1 viral load did not increase in six of the nine patients who had measurements between the first week and 3.5 months after the start of valproate treatment; no follow-up was available for the other three (111). These data suggest that, contrary to in vitro data, HIV-1 viral load is not adversely affected by valproate in the presence of effective antiretroviral therapy.

Body temperature

Hypothermia related to valproate has been reported in a child (112). There have been five previously described cases in adults or elderly patients (113).

- A 2-year-old boy was admitted after a prolonged febrile seizure that stopped only after he was given several doses of benzodiazepines plus phenobarbital. A CT scan showed a right arachnoid cyst. He was given valproate 13 mg/kg/day and 2 days later developed hypothermia (33.8–34.5°C). He was lethargic and irritable. Valproate was withdrawn. His lethargy improved within 48 hours and the temperature slowly returned to normal over the course of 1 week.

Second-Generation Effects

Teratogenicity

The association of valproate with spina bifida, cardiac malformations, hypospadias, porencephaly, and other specified anomalies of the brain, anomalies of the face, coarctation of the aorta, and limb reduction defects has been found.

There has been a case-control study of the relation between prenatal exposure to valproate and the presence of limb deficiencies in newborn infants, using data from the Spanish Collaborative Study of Congenital Malformations (ECEMC) (114). Of 22 294 consecutive malformed infants (excluding genetic syndromes) and 21 937 control infants with specified data on anticonvulsants during gestation, 57 malformed infants and 10 control infants had been exposed to valproate during the first trimester of pregnancy. Of the malformed infants who had been exposed to valproate 21 had congenital limb defects of different types (including overlapping digits, talipes, clubfoot, clinodactyly, arachnodactyly, hip dislocation, and preaxial and postaxial polydactyly); three had limb deficiencies. After controlling for potential confounding factors there was an odds ratio of limb deficiencies of 6.2 (CI = 1.3, 30). The estimated risk for women taking valproate of having a baby with limb deficiencies was around 0.42%.

Fetotoxicity

Two neonates born of mothers who had taken valproate during pregnancy developed bleeding associated with fibrinogen depletion soon after birth, and one of them died from afibrinogenemia (SEDA-19, 75).

Of 17 infants born of mothers taking valproate, 12 had possible withdrawal effects (irritability, jitteriness, abnormal tone, seizures, feeding problems), which correlated with the dosage of valproate during the last trimester, and four of the affected children also had hypoglycemia (SEDA-18, 70).

Three cases of lung hypoplasia after prenatal exposure to valproate have been reported in two female siblings and an unrelated girl (115). The two siblings had no other malformations, whereas the third neonate had a number of major birth defects. All three died a few hours after birth. The possibility that lung hypoplasia was caused by valproate remains speculative.

Fetal valproate syndrome comprises a number of typical dysmorphic features and major organ system anomalies (116). In a case file review of 2220 children with craniosynostosis, detailed maternal health information was obtained in 1676 cases (117). Of these, 17 mothers had taken valproate monotherapy during pregnancy. All 17 children had trigonocephaly (caused by premature fusion of the metopic suture). Their IQs were 45–100 (mean 75). IQs were significantly higher in patients who underwent surgery before 6 months of age. This is the first study to have reported trigonocephaly associated with fetal valproate syndrome.

Five patients with fetal valproate syndrome and autism have been described (118).

Lactation

In an unusual case, thrombocytopenic purpura, anemia, and reticulocytosis occurred in a 3-month-old breast-fed infant whose mother was taking valproic acid 1200 mg/day. The serum valproic acid concentration in the infant

was 6.6 µg/ml; recovery occurred when breast-feeding was stopped (61).

Susceptibility Factors

Genetic factors

Deaths have occurred after the use of valproate in patients with ornithine transcarbamylase deficiency (SED-12, 133) (36) (SED-13, 149) (37). Additional evidence points to a need for caution in patients with any enzyme disorder.

- An 18-year-old woman with progressive dementia and spastic paraparesis became comatose with hyperammonemia when taking valproate; moderate hyperammonemia persisted for months after drug withdrawal, coma recurred without exposure to valproate, and congenital argininemia was diagnosed (38).

Carnitine supplementation has been proposed for the treatment of symptomatic hyperammonemia caused by valproate.

Since glutathione peroxidase deficiency could predispose to severe reactions such as pancreatic or hepatic failure in children, screening for such deficiency might prove useful (SEDA-17, 72).

Age

At least 132 patients have died of liver failure (and/or pancreatitis) (75). The risk is highest (1 : 600) in children under 2 years of age with complex neurological disorders taking valproate as part of a multidrug regimen (46,76). In older patients the incidence is no more than 1:37 000 for monotherapy and 1:12 000 for multidrug therapy. Deaths beyond 20 years of age are exceedingly rare.

Valproate should not be prescribed for children with metabolic defects possibly associated with Reye-like symptoms, including acyl CoA-dehydrogenase deficiency (SEDA-22, 92) (75). In patients under 2 years old and in children with psychomotor retardation metabolic screening should be performed before therapy, and the drug should be avoided whenever a metabolic defect is known or suspected.

Hepatic disease

Valproate should be avoided in patients with a personal or family history of liver disorders or pancreatic dysfunction (75,119).

Other features of the patient

At least 132 patients have died of liver failure (and/or pancreatitis) (75). Risk factors include mental retardation, congenital abnormalities, neurological disorders, a family history of hepatic disease, the addition of valproate within 3 months of liver dysfunction, and concomitant salicylate use.

- A 24-year-old man with demyelinating disease had fulminant progression of the disease after he experienced valproate-induced hyperammonemic encephalopathy (120).

Although the role of hyperammonemia is uncertain, this case raises concern for possible risks in using valproic acid in patients with fulminant demyelinating disease.

The importance of hypoalbuminemia as a risk factor in valproate toxicity has been emphasized (121).

- A 53-year-old woman had a heart transplantation and developed worsening cardiac function, possible rejection, and increased lethargy. Her dose of valproate had been adjusted based on the total serum valproate concentration, but hypoalbuminemia prompted the measurement of the unbound serum valproate concentration, which was high. When the dose of valproate was adjusted based on the unbound rather than the total serum concentration she eventually improved.

Non-linear protein binding of valproate can result in disproportionate increases in unbound drug; adverse effects can then result when dosage adjustments are based solely on measurement of total valproate serum concentrations in patients with hypoalbuminemia.

Drug Administration

Drug formulations

Extended-release (ER) divalproex (valproate semisodium) is not bioequivalent to delayed-release (DR) divalproex. In a randomized, crossover study in 36 healthy volunteers the bioequivalence of divalproex ER once a day and divalproex DR at 14% and 20% lower daily doses given twice a day were compared (122). The two formulations gave equivalent exposure (AUC) with lower peak and higher trough concentrations, that is less fluctuation during the dosage interval, with divalproex DR.

Drug administration route

The successful use of intravenous valproate in psychiatric practice has been described (123). The safety of rapid infusion of valproate has been studied in 20 patients with acute repetitive seizures, who received 20 mg/kg loading doses at rates of 33–555 mg/minute (124). Consciousness and respiratory function were not affected. There was no significant local irritation. Two patients with significant contributing factors developed hypotension and required vasopressors.

Drug overdose

- After a valproate overdose a 27-year-old man developed seizures, hypernatremia, respiratory failure, metabolic acidosis, liver failure, and bone marrow depression (125). His plasma valproic acid concentration was 1414 µg/ml. Treatment with hemodialysis was effective in enhancing valproic acid clearance, while hemoperfusion was relatively less effective, because of saturation of the column. Overall, the half-life of the drug was reduced from over 20 hours before treatment to less than 3 hours during hemodialysis/hemoperfusion; drug removal was probably favored by saturation of drug binding to plasma proteins, which resulted in a low unbound fraction (32% at the start of treatment). He was comatose for 5 days but recovered fully thereafter.

A beneficial effect of high-flux hemodialysis without hemoperfusion has been described in valproate overdose (126).

- A 25-year-old white woman took an unknown amount of valproic acid, became comatose, and developed hypotension and lactic acidosis. Her valproic acid concentrations rose to over 8400 µmol/l. High-flux hemodialysis was performed for 4 hours; the calculated half-life during the procedure was 2.7 hours, compared with a posthemodialysis value of 23 hours, suggesting that high-flux hemodialysis had increased the clearance rate of valproic acid. Her hemodynamic status and mental function improved in conjunction with the acute reduction in valproic acid concentrations.

Three patients who took overdoses of valpromide presented with no symptoms or only moderate ones and serum valproate concentrations below or within the usual target range; in two cases more than 3 hours after ingestion (127). However, there was marked deterioration more than 10 hours after ingestion, when serum valproate concentrations were in the toxic range.

Drug–Drug Interactions

General

An encephalopathy leading to stupor is occasionally observed after valproate is added to other anticonvulsants.

Valproate has no enzyme-inducing properties and does not interact with oral contraceptives.

Carbamazepine

In patients taking carbamazepine, valproate slightly increases the serum concentration of the active metabolite carbamazepine-10,11-epoxide, by inhibiting epoxide hydrolase and perhaps also by inhibiting the glucuronidation of carbamazepine-10,11-trans-diol (128).

Valpromide is a more potent inhibitor than valproate of carbamazepine epoxide hydrolase in vitro (129) and in six healthy volunteers it caused a marked rise in carbamazepine-10,11-epoxide, prolonging the half-life of carbamazepine-10,11-epoxide from 6.4 to 21 hours and reducing its clearance three-fold, suggesting that valpromide inhibits epoxide hydrolase in the liver in vivo as well as in vitro, despite the fact that it is rapidly converted in vivo to valproate (130).

In 12 adults with epilepsy taking carbamazepine, valpromide produced a larger increase in plasma concentrations of carbamazepine-10,11-epoxide than valproate (131).

In healthy subjects valnoctamide 200 mg tds for 8 days prolonged the half-life of carbamazepine-10,11-epoxide from 7 to 20 hours and reduced its oral clearance fourfold, suggesting that valnoctamide, like its isomer valpromide, is a potent inhibitor of carbamazepine epoxide hydrolase (130).

Clozapine

Chronic valproate (600–1500 mg/day) has been associated with a slight increase in plasma clozapine concentrations and a slight fall in norclozapine concentrations (132). These changes are unlikely to be clinically significant.

Lamotrigine

Valproate inhibits the metabolism of lamotrigine (133).

Levodopa

Valproate caused a fall in growth hormone concentrations at varying times after the administration of levodopa (134).

Panipenem–betamipron

- The intravenous administration of panipenem + betamipron in a 22-year-old man and in two young girls resulted in a marked and rapid fall in the serum concentrations of valproic acid to 0–40% of the pretreatment concentration (135). In two patients, the effect was associated with epileptic seizures. Serum valproic acid began to rise again within 2 hours of stopping the antibiotic.

Although the mechanism of this interaction is unknown, animal studies suggest that suppression of the enterohepatic circulation of valproic acid may have been involved (136).

Phenobarbital

Valproate inhibits the metabolism of phenobarbital (137).

Phenytoin

Serum phenytoin concentrations can be increased or reduced by valproate (138): since valproic acid displaces phenytoin from plasma proteins, therapeutic and toxic effects of phenytoin occur at total phenytoin concentrations lower than usual.

Risperidone

Steady-state plasma concentrations of risperidone and 9-hydroxyrisperidone have been measured in 23 patients taking risperidone alone and in 10 co-medicated with sodium valproate (139). Valproate had no effect on the kinetics of risperidone.

Salicylates

Simultaneous use of salicylates and valproate should be avoided (140).

Sertraline

- In a 34-year-old man with bipolar depression treated with valproate, the addition of sertraline (100 mg/day) was associated with signs of valproate intoxication and an increase in serum valproic acid concentration from 378 to 1127 µmol/l (141). The serum valproic acid concentration returned to baseline after sertraline withdrawal.

Inhibition of valproic acid metabolism was a probable cause for this interaction.

Tricyclic antidepressants

In 10 patients taking amitriptyline 125 mg/day, for 20 days valpromide increased amitriptyline and nortriptyline plasma concentrations from 71 to 106 ng/ml for amitriptyline, and from 61 to 101 ng/ml for nortriptyline (142).

Zidovudine

At a concentration of 100 µg/ml, valproic acid inhibits the glucuronidation of zidovudine in human liver microsomes by 50% (143). This observation explains the previously reported effect of valproate to increase plasma zidovudine concentrations in HIV-infected patients.

Diagnosis of Adverse Drug Reactions

The tentative target range for plasma concentrations is 350–700 µmol/l (50–100 µg/ml).

References

1. Lennkh C, Simhandl C. Current aspects of valproate in bipolar disorder. Int Clin Psychopharmacol 2000;15(1):1–11.
2. Davis LL, Ryan W, Adinoff B, Petty F. Comprehensive review of the psychiatric uses of valproate. J Clin Psychopharmacol 2000;20(1 Suppl. 1):S1–17.
3. White JR, Santos CS. Intravenous valproate associated with significant hypotension in the treatment of status epilepticus. J Child Neurol 1999;14(12):822–3.
4. Anderson GD, Lin Y, Temkin NR, Fischer JH, Winn HR. Incidence of intravenous site reactions in neurotrauma patients receiving valproate or phenytoin. Ann Pharmacother 2000;34(6):697–702.
5. Sleiman C, Raffy O, Roue C, Mal H. Fatal pulmonary hemorrhage during high-dose valproate monotherapy. Chest 2000;117(2):613.
6. Davis R, Peters DH, McTavish D. Valproic acid. A reappraisal of its pharmacological properties and clinical efficacy in epilepsy. Drugs 1994;47(2):332–72.
7. Beydoun A, Sackellares JC, Shu V. Safety and efficacy of divalproex sodium monotherapy in partial epilepsy: a double-blind, concentration-response design clinical trial. Depakote Monotherapy for Partial Seizures Study Group. Neurology 1997;48(1):182–8.
8. Bodensteiner JB, Morris HH, Golden GS. Asterixis associated with sodium valproate. Neurology 1981;31(2):194–5.
9. Duarte J, Macias S, Coria F, Fernandez E, Claveria LE. Valproate-induced coma: case report and literature review. Ann Pharmacother 1993;27(5):582–3.
10. Stecker MM, Kita M. Paradoxical response to valproic acid in a patient with a hypothalamic hamartoma. Ann Pharmacother 1998;32(11):1168–72.
11. Jacob PC, Chand RP. Pathological laughter following intravenous sodium valproate. Can J Neurol Sci 1998;25(3):252–3.
12. La Fiore LA, Jorge CL, Yacubian EMT. Reversible pseudoatrophy of the brain caused by valproate treatment: How reversible is it? Epilepsia 1999;40(Suppl. 2):129–30.
13. Bogliun G, Di Viesti P, Monticelli LM, Beghi E, Zarrelli M, Simone P, Airoldi L, Frattola L. Anticonvulsants and peripheral nerve function results of prospective monitoring in patients with newly diagnosed epilepsy. Clin Drug Invest 2000;20:173–80.
14. Zgorzalewicz M, Galas-Zgorzalewicz B. Visual and auditory evoked potentials during long-term vigabatrin treatment in children and adolescents with epilepsy. Clin Neurophysiol 2000;111(12):2150–4.
15. Shill HA, Fife TD. Valproic acid toxicity mimicking multiple system atrophy. Neurology 2000;55(12):1936–7.
16. Lerman-Sagie T, Watemberg N, Kramer U, Shahar E, Lerman P. Absence seizures aggravated by valproic acid. Epilepsia 2001;42(7):941–3.

17. Armon C, Shin C, Miller P, Carwile S, Brown E, Edinger JD, Paul RG. Reversible parkinsonism and cognitive impairment with chronic valproate use. Neurology 1996;47(3):626–35.

18. Chadwick DW, Cumming WJ, Livingstone I, Cartlidge NE. Acute intoxication with sodium valproate. Ann Neurol 1979;6(6):552–3.

19. American Academy of Pediatrics. Committee on Drugs. Behavioral and cognitive effects of anticonvulsant therapy. Pediatrics 1985;76(4):644–7.

20. Ronen GM, Richards JE, Cunningham C, Secord M, Rosenbloom D. Can sodium valproate improve learning in children with epileptiform bursts but without clinical seizures? Dev Med Child Neurol 2000;42(11):751–5.

21. Margraf JW, Dreifuss FE. Amenorrhea following initiation of therapy with valproic acid. Neurology 1981;31:159.

22. Isojarvi JI, Laatikainen TJ, Knip M, Pakarinen AJ, Juntunen KT, Myllyla VV. Obesity and endocrine disorders in women taking valproate for epilepsy. Ann Neurol 1996;39(5):579–84.

23. Isojarvi JI, Rattya J, Myllyla VV, Knip M, Koivunen R, Pakarinen AJ, Tekay A, Tapanainen JS. Valproate, lamotrigine, and insulin-mediated risks in women with epilepsy. Ann Neurol 1998;43(4):446–51.

24. Cook JS, Bale JF Jr, Hoffman RP. Pubertal arrest associated with valproic acid therapy. Pediatr Neurol 1992;8(3):229–31.

25. Vainionpaa LK, Rattya J, Knip M, Tapanainen JS, Pakarinen AJ, Lanning P, Tekay A, Myllyla VV, Isojarvi JI. Valproate-induced hyperandrogenism during pubertal maturation in girls with epilepsy. Ann Neurol 1999;45(4):444–50.

26. Luef G, Abraham I, Haslinger M, Trinka E, Seppi K, Unterberger I, Alge A, Windisch J, Lechleitner M, Bauer G. Polycystic ovaries, obesity and insulin resistance in women with epilepsy. A comparative study of carbamazepine and valproic acid in 105 women. J Neurol 2002;249(7):835–41.

27. Geda G, Caksen H, Icagasioglu D. Serum lipids, vitamin B12 and folic acid levels in children receiving long-term valproate therapy. Acta Neurol Belg 2002;102(3):122–6.

28. Biton V, Mirza W, Montouris G, Vuong A, Hammer AE, Barrett PS. Weight change associated with valproate and lamotrigine monotherapy in patients with epilepsy. Neurology 2001;56(2):172–7.

29. Verrotti A, Basciani F, Morresi S, de Martino M, Morgese G, Chiarelli F. Serum leptin changes in epileptic patients who gain weight after therapy with valproic acid. Neurology 1999;53(1):230–2.

30. Pylvanen V, Knip M, Pakarinen A, Kotila M, Turkka J, Isojarvi JI. Serum insulin and leptin levels in valproate-associated obesity. Epilepsia 2002;43(5):514–17.

31. Luef G, Abraham I, Hoppichler F, Trinka E, Unterberger I, Bauer G, Lechleitner M. Increase in postprandial serum insulin levels in epileptic patients with valproic acid therapy. Metabolism 2002;51(10):1274–8.

32. Luef G, Abraham I, Trinka E, Alge A, Windisch J, Daxenbichler G, Unterberger I, Seppi K, Lechleitner M, Kramer G, Bauer G. Hyperandrogenism, postprandial hyperinsulinism and the risk of PCOS in a cross sectional study of women with epilepsy treated with valproate. Epilepsy Res 2002;48(1–2):91–102.

33. Kifune A, Kubota F, Shibata N, Akata T, Kikuchi S. Valproic acid-induced hyperammonemic encephalopathy with triphasic waves. Epilepsia 2000;41(7):909–12.

34. Hamer HM, Knake S, Schomburg U, Rosenow F. Valproate-induced hyperammonemic encephalopathy in the presence of topiramate. Neurology 2000;54(1):230–2.

35. Murphy JV, Marquardt K. Asymptomatic hyperammonemia in patients receiving valproic acid. Arch Neurol 1982;39(9):591–2.

36. Kay JD, Hilton-Jones D, Hyman N. Valproate toxicity and ornithine carbamoyltransferase deficiency. Lancet 1986;2(8518):1283–4.

37. Hjelm M, de Silva LV, Seakins JW, Oberholzer VG, Rolles CJ. Evidence of inherited urea cycle defect in a case of fatal valproate toxicity. BMJ (Clin Res Ed) 1986;292(6512):23–4.

38. Christmann R. Valproate-induced coma in a patient with urea cycle enzyme deficiency. Epilepsia 1990;31:228.

39. Verrotti A, Trotta D, Morgese G, Chiarelli F. Valproate-induced hyperammonemic encephalopathy. Metab Brain Dis 2002;17(4):367–73.

40. Ziyeh S, Thiel T, Spreer J, Klisch J, Schumacher M. Valproate-induced encephalopathy: assessment with MR imaging and ^{1}H MR spectroscopy. Epilepsia 2002;43(9):1101–5.

41. Vossler DG, Wilensky AJ, Cawthon DF, Kraemer DL, Ojemann LM, Caylor LM, Morgan JD. Serum and CSF glutamine levels in valproate-related hyperammonemic encephalopathy. Epilepsia 2002;43(2):154–9.

42. Coulter DL. Carnitine, valproate, and toxicity. J Child Neurol 1991;6(1):7–14.

43. Murakami K, Sugimoto T, Nishida N, Kobayashi Y, Kuhara T, Matsumoto I. Abnormal metabolism of carnitine and valproate in a case of acute encephalopathy during chronic valproate therapy. Brain Dev 1992;14(3):178–81.

44. Papadimitriou A, Servidei S. Late onset lipid storage myopathy due to multiple acyl CoA dehydrogenase deficiency triggered by valproate. Neuromuscul Disord 1991;1(4):247–52.

45. Gram L. Valproate. In: Dam M, Gram L, editors. Comprehensive Epileptology. New York: Raven Press, 1990:537.

46. De Vivo DC, Bohan TP, Coulter DL, Dreifuss FE, Greenwood RS, Nordli DR Jr, Shields WD, Stafstrom CE, Tein I. L-carnitine supplementation in childhood epilepsy: current perspectives. Epilepsia 1998;39(11):1216–25.

47. Coulter DL. Carnitine deficiency in epilepsy: Risk factors and treatment. J Child Neurol 1995;10(Suppl. 2):S32–9.

48. Verrotti A, Pascarella R, Trotta D, Giuva T, Morgese G, Chiarelli F. Hyperhomocysteinemia in children treated with sodium valproate and carbamazepine. Epilepsy Res 2000;41(3):253–7.

49. Vilaseca MA, Monros E, Artuch R, Colome C, Farre C, Valls C, Cardo E, Pineda M. Anti-epileptic drug treatment in children: hyperhomocysteinaemia, B-vitamins and the 677C→T mutation of the methylenetetrahydrofolate reductase gene. Eur J Paediatr Neurol 2000;4(6):269–77.

50. Graf WD, Oleinik OE, Glauser TA, Maertens P, Eder DN, Pippenger CE. Altered antioxidant enzyme activities in children with a serious adverse experience related to valproic acid therapy. Neuropediatrics 1998;29(4):195–201.

51. Branten AJ, Wetzels JF, Weber AM, Koene RA. Hyponatremia due to sodium valproate. Ann Neurol 1998;43(2):265–7.

52. Haviv YS, Kuper A. Severe peripheral oedema associated with valproic acid. Clin Drug Invest 2000;19:385–7.

53. Basel-Vanagaite L, Zeharia A, Amir J, Mimouni M. Edema associated with valproate therapy. Ann Pharmacother 1999;33(12):1370–1.

54. Bentsen KD, Gram L, Veje A. Serum thyroid hormones and blood folic acid during monotherapy with carbamazepine or valproate. A controlled study. Acta Neurol Scand 1983;67(4):235–41.

55. Carney P, Nasreddine W, Drury I, Varma N, Payne T, Shu V, Beydoun A. Relation between thrombocytopenia and valproate dose. Epilepsia 1997;38(Suppl. 8):102.

56. Zeller JA, Schlesinger S, Runge U, Kessler C. Influence of valproate monotherapy on platelet activation and hematologic values. Epilepsia 1999;40(2):186–9.

57. Kis B, Szupera Z, Mezei Z, Gecse A, Telegdy G, Vecsei L. Valproate treatment and platelet function: the role of arachidonate metabolites. Epilepsia 1999;40(3):307–10.

58. Levine J, Chengappa KN, Parepally H. Side effect profile of enteric-coated divalproex sodium versus valproic acid. J Clin Psychiatry 2000;61(9):680–1.

59. Proulle V, Masnou P, Cartron J, Kaplan C, Ajzenberg N, Tchernia G, Dreyfus M. GPIaIIa as a candidate target for anti-platelet autoantibody occurring during valproate therapy and associated with peroperative bleeding. Thromb Haemost 2000;83(1):175–6.

60. Oluboka OJ, Haslam D, Gardner DM. Pancytopenia and valproic acid: a dose-related association. J Am Geriatr Soc 2000;48(3):349–50.

61. Stahl MM, Neiderud J, Vinge E. Thrombocytopenic purpura and anemia in a breast-fed infant whose mother was treated with valproic acid. J Pediatr 1997;130(6):100–1.

62. Von Czettritz G, Windorfer A, Steinhoff U. Nebenwirkungen bei Valproinat-Therapie. Med Klin (Munich) 1983;78:305.

63. Loiseau P. Sodium valproate, platelet dysfunction, and bleeding. Epilepsia 1981;22(2):141–6.

64. Kreuz W, Mentzer D, Becker S, Scharrer I, Kornhuber B. Haemate P in children with von Willebrand's disease. Haemostasis 1994;24(5):304–10.

65. Smith FR, Boots M. Sodium valproate and bone marrow suppression. Ann Neurol 1980;8(2):197–9.

66. Coulter DL, Wu H, Allen RJ. Valproic acid therapy in childhood epilepsy. JAMA 1980;244(8):785–8.

67. Boillot A, Bourgeois F, Barale F, Lenys R, Daoudal P, Delacour JL. Atteinte médulaire mortelle au cours d'une intoxication aiguë volontaire para dipropylacétate de sodium. [Fatal bone marrow involvement voluntary acute poisoning with sodium dipropylacetate.] Nouv Presse Med 1981;10(24):2038.

68. Hirose Y, Konda S. Depakene-induced intravascular hemolysis and pure red cell aplasia. Nippon Ketsueki Gakkai Zasshi 1984;47(6):1366–70.

69. Gruppo R, Degrauw A, Fogelson H, Glauser T, Balasa V, Gartside P. Protein C deficiency related to valproic acid therapy: a possible association with childhood stroke. J Pediatr 2000;137(5):714–18.

70. Syrjanen SM, Syrjanen KJ. Hyperplastic gingivitis in a child receiving sodium valproate treatment. Proc Finn Dent Soc 1979;75(5–6):95–8.

71. Reisser C, Maier H. Sialadendose durch Valproat-dauermedikation. [Sialadenosis caused long-term Valproate medication.] Laryngorhinootologie 1991;70(7):384–6.

72. Behari M. Gingival hyperplasia due to sodium valproate. J Neurol Neurosurg Psychiatry 1991;54(3):279–80.

73. Zarate CA Jr, Tohen M, Narendran R, Tomassini EC, McDonald J, Sederer M, Madrid AR. The adverse effect profile and efficacy of divalproex sodium compared with valproic acid: a pharmacoepidemiology study. J Clin Psychiatry 1999;60(4):232–6.

74. Wagner PG, Welton SR, Hammond CM. Gastrointestinal adverse effects with divalproex sodium and valproic acid. J Clin Psychiatry 2000;61(4):302–3.

75. Konig SA, Siemes H, Blaker F, Boenigk E, Gross-Selbeck G, Hanefeld F, Haas N, Kohler B, Koelfen W, Korinthenberg R, et al. Severe hepatotoxicity during valproate therapy: an update and report of eight new fatalities. Epilepsia 1994;35(5):1005–15.

76. Bryant AE 3rd, Dreifuss FE. Valproic acid hepatic fatalities. III. U.S. experience since 1986. Neurology 1996;46(2):465–9.

77. Baille TA, Rettenmaier AW. Valproate—biotransformation. In: Levy R, Mattson R, Meldrum B, Penry JK, Dreifuss FE, editors. Antiepileptic Drugs. 3rd ed. New York: Raven Press, 1989:601.

78. Konig SA, Schenk M, Sick C, Holm E, Heubner C, Weiss A, Konig I, Hehlmann R. Fatal liver failure associated with valproate therapy in a patient with Friedreich's disease: review of valproate hepatotoxicity in adults. Epilepsia 1999;40(7):1036–40.

79. Fayad M, Choueiri R, Mikati M. Fatality from hepatitis A in a child taking valproate. J Child Neurol 2000;15(2):135–6.

80. Gopaul SV, Farrell K, Abbott FS. Identification and characterization of N-acetylcysteine conjugates of valproic acid in humans and animals. Drug Metab Dispos 2000;28(7):823–32.

81. Thomson MA, Lynch S, Strong R, Shepherd RW, Marsh W. Orthotopic liver transplantation with poor neurologic outcome in valproate-associated liver failure: a need for critical risk-benefit appraisal in the use of valproate. Transplant Proc 2000;32(1):200–3.

82. Delarue A, Paut O, Guys JM, Montfort MF, Lethel V, Roquelaure B, Pellissier JF, Sarles J, Camboulives J. Inappropriate liver transplantation in a child with Alpers–Huttenlocher syndrome misdiagnosed as valproate-induced acute liver failure. Pediatr Transplant 2000;4(1):67–71.

83. Lott RS, Helmboldt KM, Madaras-Kelly KJ. Retrospective evaluation of the effect of valproate therapy on transaminase elevations in patients with hepatitis C. Pharmacotherapy 2001;21(11):1345–51.

84. Buzan RD, Firestone D, Thomas M, Dubovsky SL. Valproate-associated pancreatitis and cholecystitis in six mentally retarded adults. J Clin Psychiatry 1995;56(11):529–32.

85. Ng JY, Disney AP, Jones TE, Purdie G. Acute pancreatitis and sodium valproate. Med J Aust 1982;2(8):362.

86. Grosse P, Rusch L, Schmitz B. Pancreatitis complicating treatment with intravenous valproate: three case reports. Epilepsia 1999;40(Suppl. 2):267.

87. Pellock JM, Wilder BJ, Deaton R, Sommerville KW. Acute pancreatitis coincident with valproate use: a critical review. Epilepsia 2002;43(11):1421–4.

88. Choonara IA. Sodium valproate and enuresis. Lancet 1985;1(8440):1276.

89. Lenoir GR, Perignon JL, Gubler MC, Broyer M. Valproic acid: a possible cause of proximal tubular renal syndrome. J Pediatr 1981;98(3):503–4.

90. Zaki EL, Springate JE. Renal injury from valproic acid: case report and literature review. Pediatr Neurol 2002;27(4):318–19.

91. Kinnell HG. Heated reaction to valproate. Hosp Doctor 1984;C4(23):4.

92. Kamper AM, Valentijn RM, Strickler BH, Purcell PM. Cutaneous vasculitis induced by sodium valproate. Lancet 1991;337(8739):497–8.

93. Cogrel O, Beylot-Barry M, Vergier B, Dubus P, Doutre MS, Merlio JP, Beylot C. Sodium valproate-induced cutaneous pseudolymphoma followed by recurrence with carbamazepine. Br J Dermatol 2001;144(6):1235–8.

94. Jeavons PM, Clark JE, Harding GF. Valproate and curly hair. Lancet 1977;1(8007):359.

95. Herranz JL, Arteaga R, Armijo JA. Change in hair colour induced by valproic acid. Dev Med Child Neurol 1981;23(3):386–7.

96. Yerby MS, McCoy GB. Male infertility: possible association with valproate exposure. Epilepsia 1999;40(4):520–1.

97. Rattya J, Pakarinen AJ, Knip M, Repo-Outakoski M, Myllyla VV, Isojarvi JI. Early hormonal changes during valproate or carbamazepine treatment: a 3-month study. Neurology 2001;57(3):440–4.

98. Roste LS, Tauboll E, Berner A, Isojarvi JI, Gjerstad L. Valproate, but not lamotrigine, induces ovarian morphological changes in Wistar rats. Exp Toxicol Pathol 2001;52(6):545–52.

99. Herzog AG, Schachter SC. Valproate and the polycystic ovarian syndrome: final thoughts. Epilepsia 2001;42(3):311–15.

100. Isojarvi JI, Tauboll E, Tapanainen JS, Pakarinen AJ, Laatikainen TJ, Knip M, Myllyla VV. On the association between valproate and polycystic ovary syndrome: a response and an alternative view. Epilepsia 2001; 42(3):305–10.

101. Genton P, Bauer J, Duncan S, Taylor AE, Balen AH, Eberle A, Pedersen B, Salas-Puig X, Sauer MV. On the association between valproate and polycystic ovary syndrome. Epilepsia 2001;42(3):295–304.

102. Duncan S. Polycystic ovarian syndrome in women with epilepsy: a review. Epilepsia 2001;42(Suppl. 3):60–5.

103. Isojarvi JI, Laatikainen TJ, Pakarinen AJ, Juntunen KT, Myllyla VV. Polycystic ovaries and hyperandrogenism in women taking valproate for epilepsy. N Engl J Med 1993;329(19):1383–8.

104. Isojarvi JI, Tauboll E, Pakarinen AJ, van Parys J, Rattya J, Harbo HF, Dale PO, Fauser BC, Gjerstad L, Koivunen R, Knip M, Tapanainen JS. Altered ovarian function and cardiovascular risk factors in valproate-treated women. Am J Med 2001;111(4):290–6.

105. Isojarvi JI, Tapanainen JS. Valproate, hyperandrogenism, and polycystic ovaries: a report of 3 cases. Arch Neurol 2000;57(7):1064–8.

106. Reuber M, Goulding PJ. Valproate, polycystic ovary syndrome and the need for a prospective study. Seizure 2000;9(3):235–6.

107. Betts T. Editorial comment. Seizure 2000;9:236.

108. Bauer J, Jarre A, Klingmuller D, Elger CE. Polycystic ovary syndrome in patients with focal epilepsy: a study in 93 women. Epilepsy Res 2000;41(2):163–7.

109. Bonnet F, Morlat P, De Witte S, Combe C, Beylot J. Lupus-like syndrome and vasculitis induced by valpromide. J Rheumatol 2003;30(1):208–9.

110. Jennings HR, Romanelli F. The use of valproic acid in HIV-positive patients. Ann Pharmacother 1999;33(10): 1113–16.

111. Maggi JD, Halman MH. The effect of divalproex sodium on viral load: a retrospective review of HIV-positive patients with manic syndromes. Can J Psychiatry 2001;46(4):359–62.

112. Nagarajan L, Johnston K, Williams S. Hypothermia and thermoregulatory derangements induced by valproic acid. Neurology 2001;56(1):139.

113. Zachariah SB, Zachariah A, Ananda R, Stewart JT. Hypothermia and thermoregulatory derangements induced by valproic acid. Neurology 2000;55(1):150–1.

114. Rodriguez-Pinilla E, Arroyo I, Fondevilla J, Garcia MJ, Martinez-Frias ML. Prenatal exposure to valproic acid during pregnancy and limb deficiencies: a case-control study. Am J Med Genet 2000;90(5):376–81.

115. Janas MS, Arroe M, Hansen SH, Graem N. Lung hypoplasia—a possible teratogenic effect of valproate. Case report. APMIS 1998;106(2):300–4.

116. Kozma C. Valproic acid embryopathy: report of two siblings with further expansion of the phenotypic abnormalities and a review of the literature. Am J Med Genet 2001;98(2):168–75.

117. Lajeunie E, Barcik U, Thorne JA, Ghouzzi VE, Bourgeois M, Renier D. Craniosynostosis and fetal exposure to sodium valproate. J Neurosurg 2001;95(5):778–82.

118. Williams G, King J, Cunningham M, Stephan M, Kerr B, Hersh JH. Fetal valproate syndrome and autism: additional evidence of an association. Dev Med Child Neurol 2001;43(3):202–6.

119. Levin TL, Berdon WE, Seigle RR, Nash MA. Valproic-acid-associated pancreatitis and hepatic toxicity in children with endstage renal disease. Pediatr Radiol 1997;27(2):192–3.

120. Blindauer KA, Harrington G, Morris GL 3rd, Ho KC. Fulminant progression of demyelinating disease after valproate-induced encephalopathy. Neurology 1998;51(1): 292–5.

121. Haroldson JA, Kramer LE, Wolff DL, Lake KD. Elevated free fractions of valproic acid in a heart transplant patient with hypoalbuminemia. Ann Pharmacother 2000;34(2):183–7.

122. Dutta S, Zhang Y, Selness DS, Lee LL, Williams LA, Sommerville KW. Comparison of the bioavailability of unequal doses of divalproex sodium extended-release formulation relative to the delayed-release formulation in healthy volunteers. Epilepsy Res 2002;49(1):1–10.

123. Norton JW, Quarles E. Intravenous valproate in neuropsychiatry. Pharmacotherapy 2000;20(1):88–92.

124. Limdi NA, Faught E. The safety of rapid valproic acid infusion. Epilepsia 2000;41(10):1342–5.

125. Franssen EJ, van Essen GG, Portman AT, de Jong J, Go G, Stegeman CA, Uges DR. Valproic acid toxicokinetics: serial hemodialysis and hemoperfusion. Ther Drug Monit 1999;21(3):289–92.

126. Kane SL, Constantiner M, Staubus AE, Meinecke CD, Sedor JR. High-flux hemodialysis without hemoperfusion is effective in acute valproic acid overdose. Ann Pharmacother 2000;34(10):1146–51.

127. Payen C, Frantz P, Martin O, Parant F, Moulsma M, Pulce C, Descotes J. Delayed toxicity following acute ingestion of valpromide. Hum Exp Toxicol 2004;23(3):145–8.

128. Bernus I, Dickinson RG, Hooper WD, Eadie MJ. The mechanism of the carbamazepine–valproate interaction in humans. Br J Clin Pharmacol 1997;44(1):21–7.

129. Kerr BM, Rettie AE, Eddy AC, Loiseau P, Guyot M, Wilensky AJ, Levy RH. Inhibition of human liver microsomal epoxide hydrolase by valproate and valpromide: in vitro/in vivo correlation. Clin Pharmacol Ther 1989;46(1):82–93.

130. Pisani F, Fazio A, Artesi C, Oteri G, Spina E, Tomson T, Perucca E. Impairment of carbamazepine-10, 11-epoxide elimination by valnoctamide, a valpromide isomer, in healthy subjects. Br J Clin Pharmacol 1992;34(1):85–7.

131. Pisani F, Fazio A, Oteri G, Spina E, Perucca E, Bertilsson L. Effect of valpromide on the pharmacokinetics of carbamazepine-10, 11-epoxide. Br J Clin Pharmacol 1988;25(5):611–13.

132. Facciola G, Avenoso A, Scordo MG, Madia AG, Ventimiglia A, Perucca E, Spina E. Small effects of valproic acid on the plasma concentrations of clozapine and its major metabolites in patients with schizophrenic or affective disorders. Ther Drug Monit 1999;21(3):341–5.

133. Goa KL, Ross SR, Chrisp P. Lamotrigine. A review of its pharmacological properties and clinical efficacy in epilepsy. Drugs 1993;46(1):152–76.

134. Franceschi M, Perego L, Cavagnini F, Cattaneo AG, Invitti C, Caviezel F, Strambi LF, Smirne S. Effects of long-term antiepileptic therapy on the hypothalamic–pituitary axis in man. Epilepsia 1984;25(1):46–52.

135. Yamagata T, Momoi MY, Murai K, Ikematsu K, Suwa K, Sakamoto K, Fujimura A. Panipenem–betamipron and

decreases in serum valproic acid concentration. Ther Drug Monit 1998;20(4):396–400.

136. Kojima S, Nadai M, Kitaichi K, Wang L, Nabeshima T, Hasegawa T. Possible mechanism by which the carbapenem antibiotic panipenem decreases the concentration of valproic acid in plasma in rats. Antimicrob Agents Chemother 1998;42(12):3136–40.

137. Schmidt D, Seldon L. Adverse Effects of Antiepileptic Drugs. New York: Raven Press, 1982.

138. Bruni J, Wilder BJ, Willmore LJ, Barbour B. Valproic acid and plasma levels of phenytoin. Neurology 1979;29(6):904–5.

139. Spina E, Avenoso A, Facciola G, Salemi M, Scordo MG, Giacobello T, Madia AG, Perucca E. Plasma concentrations of risperidone and 9-hydroxyrisperidone: effect of comedication with carbamazepine or valproate. Ther Drug Monit 2000;22(4):481–5.

140. Dreifuss FE, Langer DH, Moline KA, Maxwell JE. Valproic acid hepatic fatalities. II. US experience since 1984. Neurology 1989;39(2 Pt 1):201–7.

141. Berigan T, Harazin J. A sertraline/valproic acid drug interaction. Int J Psychiatry Clin Pract 1999;3:287–8.

142. Bertschy G, Vandel S, Jounet JM, Allers G. Interaction valpromide-amitriptyline. Augmentation de la biodisponibilité de l'amitriptyline et de la nortriptyline par le valpromide. [Valpromide–amitriptyline interaction. Increase in the bioavailability of amitriptyline and nortriptyline caused by valpromide.] Encephale 1990;16(1):43–5

143. Trapnell CB, Klecker RW, Jamis-Dow C, Collins JM. Glucuronidation of 3'-azido-3'-deoxythymidine (zidovudine) by human liver microsomes: relevance to clinical pharmacokinetic interactions with atovaquone, fluconazole, methadone, and valproic acid. Antimicrob Agents Chemother 1998;42(7):1592–6.

Valsartan

See also Angiotensin II receptor antagonists

General Information

Valsartan is a highly selective antagonist at angiotensin II type 1 (AT$_1$) receptors (1). It has a half-life of about 8 hours, and is metabolized to a negligible extent. Most of its clearance is via the feces.

In 1378 patients with mild to moderate hypertension valsartan 80 mg/day has been compared with losartan 50 mg/day and placebo for 8 weeks (2). This study confirmed the excellent tolerance profile, not different from placebo, of both angiotensin II receptor antagonists.

References

1. Thurmann PA. Valsartan: a novel angiotensin type 1 receptor antagonist. Expert Opin Pharmacother 2000;1(2):337–50.

2. Hedner T, Oparil S, Rasmussen K, Rapelli A, Gatlin M, Kobi P, Sullivan J, Oddou-Stock P. A comparison of the angiotensin II antagonists valsartan and losartan in the treatment of essential hypertension. Am J Hypertens 1999;12(4 Pt 1):414–17.

Vancomycin

General Information

Vancomycin is a narrow-spectrum glycopeptide antibiotic with potent antistaphylococcal activity. It was developed in the early 1950s. Early formulations contained substantial impurities, which were presumably responsible for some adverse reactions (1). When rapid infusion rates are avoided, vancomycin is rarely associated with serious toxicity. Reviews have suggested that the potential for vancomycin to cause significant ototoxicity or nephrotoxicity has been exaggerated (2,3). Improved manufacturing has resulted in a purer product and fewer toxic effects, but vancomycin is still associated with potentially serious adverse reactions (4).

Vancomycin inhibits bacterial cell wall synthesis and is bactericidal during cell division at therapeutic concentrations. Bacterial resistance to vancomycin has not been an issue during the first decades of its use. More recently, vancomycin-resistant enterococci have been recovered with increasing frequency from hospitalized patients. In some institutions, multidrug-resistant and vancomycin-resistant enterococci have become important nosocomial pathogens, difficult to treat. Vancomycin-resistant enterococcal bacteremia is associated with a poor prognosis. Judicious use of vancomycin and broad-spectrum antibiotics is recommended, and strict infection control measures must be implemented to prevent nosocomial transmission of these organisms (5).

Vancomycin is particularly useful in infections caused by meticillin-resistant or penicillinase-producing staphylococci and diphtheroids, as well as in the prophylaxis of bacterial endocarditis and in the treatment of antibiotic-associated colitis. Sufficient fecal concentrations can be achieved with oral therapy. It is poorly absorbed from the gastrointestinal tract and painful when injected intramuscularly. It diffuses moderately well into bone tissue (6).

Lactoferrin, a protein contained in tears, increases the activity of vancomycin against biofilms of strains of *Staphylococcus epidermidis* and may be therapeutically helpful in the treatment of infections such as endophthalmitis associated with intraocular lenses (7).

Observational studies

In a prospective, observational study of 742 consecutive patients (390 men; mean age 51 years, range 17–86), the incidence, outcomes, and predictive factors of vancomycin-associated toxic effects in general oncology practice were assessed (8). In all, 47% had hematological malignancies, and of the patients with solid tumors, primary urogenital (12%) and breast (10%) tumors were most common. In 72% vancomycin was given in a dosage of 2 g/day, 16% received a prophylactic dose of 1 g/day, and 12% had another regimen not specified. Phlebitis occurred in 3%, predominantly those with recently inserted central venous catheters. All responded promptly to local therapy, and withdrawal of the catheter or vancomycin was never required. Skin rashes occurred in 11%. However, all but four patients concomitantly received a beta-lactam antibiotic. None of the rashes required withdrawal, although the beta-lactam antibiotic was often withdrawn. There was clinical evidence of ototoxicity in 6% of the patients who received other ototoxic drugs and only 3% of patients who were not receiving other ototoxic drugs. There was nephrotoxicity in 17%. Logistic regression was used to derive a model of risk of nephrotoxicity. Factors associated with an increased risk of nephrotoxicity included administration of other mild to moderate nephrotoxic agents or APACHE II scores over 40. Raised serum vancomycin concentrations did not reliably predict subsequent nephrotoxicity. The derived model was prospectively tested in a validation set of 359 patients. Sensitivity of the Nephrotoxicity Risk Index for any nephrotoxicity was 71% and for serious nephrotoxicity 100%. Specificity for any nephrotoxicity was 90% and for serious nephrotoxicity 81%. A main limitation of the study was the lack of patients who received only vancomycin. The concomitant administration of other agents may therefore have confounded the results.

The adverse effects of once-daily or twice-daily vancomycin were not significantly different in 121 hospitalized patients (9). Nephrotoxicity developed in 11 and 7.7% of the patients respectively; hearing loss in 3.2 and 16%; phlebitis in 14 and 23%; and red man syndrome in 14 and 9.6%.

Comparative studies

In a prospective, randomized trial in 34 drug abusers a short course of a combination of a glycopeptide (vancomycin or teicoplanin) with gentamicin was significantly less effective in right-sided endocarditis caused by *Staphylococcus aureus* than a combination of cloxacillin and gentamicin (10).

Use in non-infective conditions

Many parents of children with regressive-onset autism have noted antecedent antibiotic exposure followed by chronic diarrhea. In a subgroup of children, disruption of indigenous gut flora might promote colonization by one or more neurotoxin-producing bacteria, contributing at least in part to their autistic symptoms. In 11 children with regressive-onset autism who had broad-spectrum antimicrobial exposure followed by chronic persistent diarrhea, oral vancomycin resulted in short-term improvement; however, these gains had largely waned at follow-up (11).

Red man syndrome

A unique and peculiar adverse reaction related to the rapid infusion of large doses is the so-called red neck or red man syndrome. It is the most common adverse reaction to vancomycin, characterized by fever, chills, paresthesia, and erythema at the base of the neck and the upper back, and can be followed by a hypotensive episode (12). It is not a true allergic reaction. It seems to be due to vancomycin-induced release of histamine and possibly other vasoactive substances without the involvement of preformed antibodies (13,14). In rat peritoneal mast cells vancomycin provoked histamine release dose-dependently; fosfomycin inhibited this effect (15).

Antihistamines (H_1 receptor antagonists) prevent anaphylactoid reactions to vancomycin (16). The recommended method of administration is by intravenous infusion of a solution of 0.25–0.5% over 60 minutes, and patients have to be monitored closely. A possible red man syndrome has also been associated with systemic absorption of oral vancomycin in a patient with normal renal function (17).

In a prospective, randomized, double-blind, placebo-controlled study in 30 patients who required vancomycin chemoprophylaxis before elective arthroplasty, oral pretreatment with either a histamine H_1 receptor antagonist (diphenhydramine 1 mg/kg) or a histamine H_2 receptor antagonist (cimetidine 4 mg/kg) significantly reduced the histamine-related adverse effects of rapid vancomycin infusion (18).

It has been stressed that near-fatal red man syndrome can also occur after slow administration of vancomycin (19).

- An 83-year-old white man became distressed and had nausea and facial flushing after 10 minutes of a slow infusion of vancomycin (1 g scheduled over 2 hours). Despite interruption, he developed suffocating respiratory distress requiring intubation and mechanical ventilation. Uncharacteristic of anaphylactoid reactions, he became severely hypertensive. Subsequently, his condition rapidly normalized. During the acute event, there was an increase in serum troponin concentration.
- A 45-year-old man developed hypotension, bradycardia, a change in consciousness, and an erythematous macular rash 10 minutes after the slow infusion of 0.1% vancomycin (20). After appropriate management, he recovered well and was discharged on the following day.

In 50 patients, in whom vancomycin 15 mg/kg was continuously infused at a constant rate over 30 minutes, the occurrence of pruritus suggested that systemic vascular resistance was falling, exposing the patient to a risk of hypotension (21). Therapy with a beta-blocker appeared to confer protection against this hemodynamic effect.

Pretreatment with H_1 and H_2 receptor antagonists (diphenhydramine 1 mg/kg and cimetidine 4 mg/kg) intravenously serially over 3 minutes starting 10 minutes before the infusion of vancomycin permitted rapid vancomycin administration (1 g over 10 minutes) in 17 of 19 patients compared with eight of 19 patients treated with placebo in a prospective, randomized, double-blind, placebo-controlled study of patients undergoing elective arthroplasty (22). Hypotension occurred in 2 versus 12 of the patients, and 12 versus 19 of the patients had a rash. Serum histamine concentrations were raised after vancomycin administration in both groups.

Possible synergism between vancomycin and narcotics in the induction of red man syndrome due to histamine release has been suggested in a 19-year-old women treated with fentanyl and vancomycin during orthopedic surgery (23). Evidence from an animal study has suggested that the risk can also be enhanced by the co-administration of muscle relaxants, resulting in enhanced release of histamine (24).

Pharmacoeconomics

The pharmacoeconomic impact of adverse effects of antimicrobial drugs is enormous. Antibacterial drug reactions account for about 25% of adverse drug reactions. The adverse effects profile of an antimicrobial agent can contribute significantly to its overall direct costs (monitoring costs, prolonged hospitalization due to complications or treatment failures) and indirect costs (quality of life, loss of productivity, time spent by families and patients receiving medical care). In one study an adverse event in a hospitalized patient was associated on average with an excess of 1.9 days in the length of stay, extra costs of $US2262 (1990–93 values), and an almost two-fold increase in the risk of death. In the outpatient setting, adverse drug reactions result in 2–6% of hospitalizations, and most of them were thought to be avoidable if appropriate interventions had been taken. In a review, economic aspects of antibacterial therapy with vancomycin have been summarized and critically evaluated (25).

In a randomized, prospective, cost-effectiveness study both teicoplanin and vancomycin were assessed as second-line therapy in 66 neutropenic patients after the failure of empirical treatment with a combination of piperacillin + tazobactam and amikacin (26). The primary success of second-line therapy was equivalent, and the direct total costs were similar. Acquisition costs per dose were in favor of vancomycin, but costs derived from administering vancomycin and serum concentration monitoring led to similar costs for both regimens. With the exception of the red man syndrome, which occurred in 10% of vancomycin-treated patients but none of the teicoplanin-treated patients, toxicity (renal, liver, and ear toxicity, diarrhea, phlebitis) was also similar.

In a retrospective cost analysis, the records of 527 patients with acute leukemia were studied (27). They had been treated in a multicenter, randomized trial for febrile neutropenia with ceftazidime and amikacin plus either teicoplanin (6 mg/kg in a single dose; $n = 275$) or vancomycin (30 mg/kg/day in 2 doses; $n = 252$). Clinical responses were equivalent. Again the higher acquisition costs for teicoplanin were counterbalanced by the lower incidence of adverse events and easier administration, resulting in overall similar costs for both regimens. A total of 8% of patients treated with vancomycin reported adverse events compared with 3.2% of patients treated with teicoplanin. Rashes occurred in 6.0 versus 1.4% respectively. Nephrotoxicity, ototoxicity, fever, and hypotension occurred in very few patients.

Organs and Systems

Cardiovascular

Vancomycin can cause phlebitis if infused peripherally (28,29).

Nervous system

It is still controversial whether vancomycin can cause ototoxicity when given alone. However, vancomycin can augment the ototoxicity of aminoglycosides (30). Tinnitus and dizziness have been noted, resolving on withdrawal (31). Hearing loss can be transient or permanent. If vancomycin is combined with aminoglycosides, toxicity may be additive (32).

Sensory systems

Eyes

In 118 consecutive patients undergoing cataract surgery, the use of supplementary prophylactic vancomycin in the irrigating solution during extracapsular lens extraction was significantly associated with an increased incidence of angiographic and clinical cystoid macular edema (33).

Ears

The risk of ototoxicity has been assessed in a prospective study in 16 patients on continuous ambulatory peritoneal dialysis treated with two infusions of vancomycin (30 mg/kg) in 2 liters of peritoneal dialysate administered at 6-day intervals for episodes of peritonitis (34). Patients who were too ill to respond appropriately, those with pre-existing sensorineural hearing loss, those with a narrow auditory canal, those with a discharging ear or perforated tympanic membrane, and those receiving concurrent ototoxic drugs were excluded. The authors found no evidence of ototoxicity (pure-tone audiometry, electronystagmography, and clinical assessment), even with repeated courses of vancomycin. Average serum concentrations were in the target range. No adverse effects were recorded, except for a transient generalized pruritus in one patient after the start of infusion.

In a prospective multicenter study in 152 children with peritoneal dialysis-associated peritonitis one patient with vancomycin intoxication had a 20–30 dB increase in hearing threshold (35).

Hearing loss due to vancomycin toxicity has been treated by hemoperfusion and hemodialysis (36).

- A 14-month-old girl with chronic renal insufficiency due to renal dysplasia was empirically treated with ceftazidime and vancomycin for fever. Her calculated creatinine clearance was 10 ml/minute/1.73 m². She erroneously received vancomycin 1.5 g in 3 doses 6 hours apart. Her serum creatinine concentration increased and her vancomycin concentrations remained markedly high (338 mg/l 5 hours after the third dose). The half-life of vancomycin was 145 hours. Hearing loss developed. Continued charcoal hemoperfusion and hemodialysis were used to treat the disorder. Thrombocytopenia was noted as significant consequence of hemoperfusion. The patient did not fully recover her previous renal function and became dialysis dependent. The audiogram normalized by 6 months.

Metabolism

Lactic acidosis occurred in a 56-year-old woman who was given intravenous vancomycin 1 g bd for 10 days (37).

Hematologic

Hemophagocytosis after vancomycin and teicoplanin occurred in a 45-year-old woman (38).

Treatment with vancomycin can rarely cause reversible pancytopenia (39).

- Neutropenia occurred in a 48-year-old man 16 days after the start of vancomycin therapy (40). Vancomycin was withdrawn and he was given a granulocyte-colony stimulating factor. He was then rechallenged with a single dose of vancomycin 1 g. His white blood cell count fell to 600×10^9/l but returned to normal with continued granulocyte-colony stimulating factor therapy.

- A 43-year-old white woman was given vancomycin for a suspected methicillin-resistant *S. aureus* infection (41). On day 10 she developed a fever, chills, and a disseminated lacy macular rash. Vancomycin was withdrawn but reinstituted 48 hours later. Another 24 hours later, she again developed a fever, chills, and a confluent erythematous rash. Sepsis developed, and ceftazidime was added. There was thrombocytopenia (118×10^9/l), and a fall in the white blood count (from 7.6 to 3.5×10^9/l) and hemoglobin (from 13.8 to 12.2 g/dl). One day later the leukocyte count was 2.6×10^9/l and the hemoglobin fell to 10 g/dl. Both drugs were withdrawn. The rash disappeared, the temperature returned to normal, and the blood cell counts completely recovered 4 days later.

- An 87-year-old white woman was treated with vancomycin for an abscess due to methicillin-resistant *S. epidermidis* (42). On day 30, her white blood cell count fell to 0.5×10^9/l after a total dose of 55 g of vancomycin. Vancomycin was withdrawn, and the white blood cell count returned to normal within 5 days. After 6 weeks vancomycin was reintroduced, and the white blood cell count fell to 0.325×10^9/l after a total dose of 14 g of vancomycin on day 9, but resolved rapidly after vancomycin was withdrawn.

Leukocytes

Vancomycin-induced neutropenia occurs in about 2% of treated patients, and complete recovery takes place in 2–5 days after withdrawal (43,44). It occurs after prolonged treatment with high doses in patients with normal renal function (for example more than 20 days of more than 15–20 mg/kg) or in the prolonged presence of high serum concentrations in patients with severe renal insufficiency (45). After withdrawal of vancomycin, neutropenia disappeared promptly. The bone marrow seemed to be unaffected. Other cases of agranulocytosis related to vancomycin therapy have been reported (46–48).

Neutropenia normally recovers after drug withdrawal, and the neutrophil count can recover when vancomycin is replaced by teicoplanin (49).

- A 35-year-old man was given vancomycin (1.5 g bd) for a wound infection with a coagulase-negative staphylococcus, a peptostreptococcus, and a coryneform Gram-positive bacillus. On day 37 hi white blood cell count was 2.8×10^9/l (baseline 5.2) with a low neutrophil count (0.5×10^9/l). Vancomycin was withdrawn and 2 days later he was given teicoplanin 400 mg/day, by which time the cell count had increased to 3.5×10^9/l, neutrophils 0.9×10^9/l. On day 45, the total white cell count was 4.9×10^9/l, neutrophils 2.3×10^9/l. Teicoplanin was continued for 1 month, and the white cell count remained normal.

A direct toxic effect of vancomycin and/or an immune-mediated mechanism (antineutrophil antibodies, sensitized lymphocytes) have been discussed.

- A typical case of vancomycin-induced neutropenia has been reported in a 39-year-old woman with sickle cell SS disease treated with vancomycin for methicillin-resistant coagulase-negative staphylococcal bacteremia (50). However, in addition to neutropenia, the clinical course was defined by a febrile period characteristic of drug fever, with delayed onset and resolution 48 hours after vancomycin was withdrawn. In this case, fluconazole and cefazoline were also administered, but their contribution to neutropenia was judged unlikely (negative rechallenge with fluconazole, withdrawal of cefazoline after less than 5 days of therapy).

Platelets

Thrombocytopenia is a rare adverse effect of vancomycin and may be associated with the presence of vancomycin-dependent antiplatelet IgG antibodies. Reports of drug-induced thrombocytopenia have been systematically reviewed (51). Among the 98 different drugs described in 561 articles the following antibiotics were found with level I (definite) evidence: co-trimoxazole, rifampicin, vancomycin, sulfisoxazole, cefalothin, piperacillin, methicillin, novobiocin. Drugs with level II (probable) evidence were oxytetracycline and ampicillin.

- Vancomycin-associated thrombocytopenia has been reported in a 72-year-old woman who was treated with gentamicin and vancomycin for infectious endocarditis due to *Clostridium pseudodiphtheriticum* (52). On the 4th day of treatment, the platelet count fell and reached a nadir of 14×10^{12}/l on day 7. Two days after withdrawal of vancomycin (day 8) the platelet count began to rise and reached 150×10^{12}/l within 5 days. Vancomycin-dependent antiplatelet IgG antibodies were not detected 10 days after vancomycin.

- Thrombocytopenia also developed in a 72-year-old man who was treated with vancomycin for staphylococcal sepsis after treatment with gemcitabine for metastatic pancreatic cancer (53). On day 12 thrombocytopenia developed, reached a nadir on day 18 (13×10^{12}/l), and did not respond to platelet transfusions. Bone-marrow megakaryocytes were adequate. Platelet-associated IgG and IgM were increased. Vancomycin was withdrawn on day 28, with prompt recovery of the platelet count to 136×10^{12}/l in 10 days.

Vancomycin was associated with subsequent thrombocytopenia in a retrospective study that included 193 patients in a surgical trauma intensive care unit (54).

Patients undergoing allogeneic hemopoietic stem cell transplantation always require platelet transfusions, but the increase in platelet count is often less than expected. The factors responsible for poor responses to platelet transfusions in this clinical setting are largely unknown. In a prospective study in 87 consecutive transplanted children univariate analysis showed that concomitant therapy with vancomycin is significantly associated with a lower post-transfusion corrected increment in platelet count (55).

Gastrointestinal

Antibiotic-associated diarrhea can develop with any antibacterial agent. Vancomycin has been implicated as a rare cause of diarrhea associated with *Clostridium difficile* (56), despite the fact that vancomycin is often used to treat it.

- Diarrhea developed in a 60-year-old man on chronic hemodialysis after 20 doses of parenteral vancomycin (250 mg at each dialysis) (57). Although culture for *C. difficile* was not performed, latex agglutination was positive for *C. difficile* toxin.

A few other cases of antibiotic-associated diarrhea with vancomycin have been described in association with *C. difficile*. This paradoxical association, although very uncommon, should be considered in patients who develop diarrhea during vancomycin therapy.

Urinary tract

Of 69 neonates (including 8 with peak vancomycin concentrations over 40 µg/ml) with culture-proven *S. aureus* or coagulase-negative staphylococcal septicemia who received vancomycin for more than 3 days, 6 had a doubling of serum creatinine concentration during vancomycin treatment, and all were in the group with peak serum vancomycin concentrations under 40 µg/ml (58).

Nephrotoxicity of vancomycin is often mild and reversible after withdrawal. It occurs in 6–17% of courses (59). Higher frequencies of nephrotoxicity were reported when vancomycin was used in combination with an aminoglycoside, which is consistent with toxicological data obtained in rats (60). Nevertheless, evidence of synergistic toxicity between vancomycin and aminoglycosides is controversial (2,31,59). Endotoxins seem to potentiate the nephrotoxic effect of vancomycin, at least in rats (61).

Acute interstitial nephritis has been reported in a patient receiving vancomycin (62).

- A 64-year-old white man was treated with intravenous cloxacillin 2 g 4-hourly for a *S. aureus* sternal wound infection and osteomyelitis. On day 14, cloxacillin was discontinued because of a fall in renal function. Urinalysis was positive for occasional red blood cells and hyaline casts, but there were no eosinophils. He was given intravenous vancomycin 1.5 g 36-hourly. Renal function gradually improved and the dosing regimen was adjusted to 1.5 g/day. Predose vancomycin serum concentrations were 11.0 and 6.3 mg/l on days 23 and 30 respectively. On day 32, oral ciprofloxacin 500 mg bd was added for suspected sepsis (catheter tip cultures grew *Klebsiella pneumoniae*, although blood cultures were negative). Other medications were enteric-coated aspirin, warfarin, acebutolol, and digoxin. The next day, a progressing maculopapular rash developed and the patient continued to have a fever. Acute interstitial nephritis was confirmed by kidney biopsy. Hemodialysis was required, and he was treated with prednisone and made a gradual recovery. Four months later, he was treated with vancomycin for a relapse of the sternal infection. His eosinophil count rose and peaked at 18%, and there were eosinophils in the urine.

The authors found four other published cases of vancomycin-induced acute interstitial nephritis.

There was a fall in residual renal function during episodes of peritonitis in a prospective multicenter study in 152 children with peritoneal dialysis-associated peritonitis (35). The study evaluated the efficacy, safety, and clinical acceptance of combination treatment, including a glycopeptide (teicoplanin or vancomycin) and ceftazidime, each given either intermittently or continuously. Irreversible anuria developed in 19% of the patients with residual diuresis. In patients who retained residual renal function, there was a strong trend toward a decreased residual glomerular filtration rate (−11%). There was no difference with respect to the type of glycopeptide or the mode of use. Aminoglycosides were used concomitantly in only 12 patients and did not seem to affect the evolution of residual renal function. Underdosing/non-adherence or overdosing occurred in 8.2% of continuously treated versus 4.9% of intermittently treated patients. Intermittent and continuous intraperitoneal treatment with glycopeptides and ceftazidime were equally efficacious and safe when measured by objective clinical criteria.

In children with febrile neutropenia and Gram-positive bacteremia associated with antineoplastic drug therapy, teicoplanin was significantly less nephrotoxic than vancomycin (63).

The effect of co-administration of fosfomycin on glycopeptide antibiotic-induced nephrotoxicity for 3 days has been investigated in rats (64). Fosfomycin reduced glycopeptide antibiotic-induced nephrotoxicity, as shown by reduced urinary excretion of *N*-acetyl-beta-D-glucosaminidase and fewer histological signs of nephrotoxicity in those treated with a combination of glycopeptide and fosfomycin compared with a glycopeptide alone. In addition, the higher the dose of fosfomycin, the more it reduced urinary *N*-acetyl-beta-D-glucosaminidase activity, suggesting that the role of fosfomycin in alleviating nephrotoxicity is dose-dependent. There was significantly less accumulation of teicoplanin and vancomycin in the renal cortex of rats treated with glycopeptide antibiotics plus fosfomycin compared with the glycopeptide antibiotics alone.

Skin

Epidermolysis bullosa acquisita occurred in a 73-year-old man after a course of vancomycin for 15 days (65).

A fixed drug eruption after the fifth dose of vancomycin 1 g occurred in a 45-year-old white woman (66).

Vancomycin reportedly caused a severe delayed skin reaction with allergic cross-reactivity between vancomycin and teicoplanin requiring steroid therapy (67).

- A 68-year-old woman who was being treated with vancomycin for *S. epidermidis* bacteremia developed pruritus and a generalized maculopapular skin rash after 2 weeks. After a short course of prednisolone, she was given teicoplanin and developed general malaise, fever, conjunctival injection, an extensive rash, and later blisters on the legs, again requiring treatment with steroids.

Erythema multiforme

Erythema multiforme has been attributed to vancomycin (67).

- A 70-year-old woman given vancomycin postoperatively developed fever on day 5 and vancomycin was withdrawn. She then developed a generalized urticarial rash with oral and vaginal erosive lesions on day 6, requiring treatment with steroids and antihistamines. The diagnosis was confirmed by skin biopsy.

Vancomycin can cause the severe forms of erythema multiforme, both Stevens–Johnson syndrome (involvement of 10–30% of the skin surface) (68) and toxic epidermal necrolysis (more than 30% of the skin surface involved); both conditions include mucosal involvement.

- A 53-year-old white woman with liver cirrhosis took vancomycin (1 g bd) for sepsis due to methicillin-resistant *S. aureus* and a catheter-associated infection due to *Enterococcus faecalis*, developed oral and vaginal mucositis and conjunctivitis followed by a maculopapular rash (69). The diagnosis was confirmed by skin biopsy. Vancomycin was replaced by teicoplanin and corticosteroids; the symptoms disappeared within 7 days.
- A 36-year-old white woman with relapsing acute myeloid leukemia took ceftazidime (2 g tds) and aciclovir for febrile neutropenia and *Herpes labialis*. She developed an itchy rash and treatment was changed to imipenem (500 mg qds for 5 days), vancomycin (1 g bd for 3 days), and gentamicin (2 mg/kg for 3 days); chemotherapy included idarubicin, cytarabine, etoposide, ondansetron, and dexamethasone for 3 days. Within a few days the rash developed into blisters and erosions, affecting more than 80% of the skin. The diagnosis was confirmed histologically, and she subsequently died from shock (70).

Linear IgA bullous disease

Linear IgA bullous disease is an autoimmune subepidermal disorder, characterized by a linear deposition of IgA along the blister base, with a predominantly neutrophilic dermal infiltrate. Most often idiopathic, a subset of linear IgA bullous disease is induced by drugs, and intravenous vancomycin is the best-documented drug that triggers it (71). The diagnosis can be confirmed by direct immunofluorescence (72,73). In some cases the blisters resolve only after withdrawal of therapy and in others glucocorticoid therapy is required.

In a review of 17 cases the features were: mean age 65 years; 11 men/6 women; eruption latency 1–15 days; normal trough concentrations (when reported); cutaneous manifestations included bullous, urticarial, erythematous, and targetoid erythema multiforme-like lesions favoring the trunk, extremities, palms, and soles, and sparing the head and neck; six patients had mucosal involvement (74). The gold standard for diagnosis is direct immunofluorescence of the perilesional skin. Circulating antibasement membrane zone antibodies were identified only in a minority of patients. Therapies included drug withdrawal, prednisone, and dapsone. No spontaneous recurrences were reported.

Linear immunoglobulin A bullous disease has been reported in a 69-year-old white woman treated with vancomycin and ciprofloxacin, in a 53-year-old white man with septic shock, and in other cases in which both vancomycin and *Varicella zoster* infection were present as triggers (75–78).

- An 87-year-old white woman treated with vancomycin and phenytoin and a 65-year-old white man with renal insufficiency developed linear immunoglobulin A bullous disease (79,80).
- A 72-year-old woman developed a bullous eruption on her palms, soles, and conjunctivae a day after receiving vancomycin (intravenously and via a cecostomy tube) for staphylococcal sepsis (81). Immunofluorescence of the skin biopsy showed linear IgA deposition along the basement membrane. The lesions cleared over the next 2 weeks after withdrawal of vancomycin.
- A blistering eruption developed in the skin and buccal mucosa of a 79-year-old man after 8 days of vancomycin therapy for an infected leg ulcer (82). Biopsy showed linear IgA deposition along the basement membrane. The lesions cleared spontaneously within two days of withdrawal.
- After 7 days of antibiotic therapy with intravenous vancomycin, gentamicin, and ticarcillin + clavulanate for *Pseudomonas aeruginosa* and *S. aureus* sepsis, confluent erythematous-based vesicobullae developed in a 65-year-old woman with subarachnoid hemorrhage secondary to a ruptured aneurysm (72). Other medications included ranitidine, glyceryl trinitrate, nimodipine, ferrous sulfate, and phenytoin.
- On the tenth day of antibiotic therapy with vancomycin, imipenem, and gentamicin for an infected enterocutaneous fistula, widespread bullae developed in a 60-year-old woman (72).
- In a 71-year-old woman with pneumonia, vesicles and bullae developed on the eighth day of antibiotic therapy that consisted of one dose of intravenous vancomycin followed by a course of nafcillin (73).
- A 52-year-old woman was given vancomycin 1 g intravenously bd and within 12 hours developed a generalized pruritic maculopapular rash (83). Over the next few days, the lesions progressively worsened and transformed into hemorrhagic and non-hemorrhagic vesicles and bullae. Mucosal surfaces, palms, and soles were spared. The skin lesions completely healed without scarring within 2 weeks of vancomycin withdrawal. There was no recurrence 5 months later.

Sexual function

- Prostatitis due to vancomycin-resistant enterococci has been reported in a 42-year-old liver transplant recipient (84). The organism, *Enterococcus faecium*, was resistant to vancomycin, ampicillin, ciprofloxacin, and doxycycline. Treatment with a combination of rifampicin and nitrofurantoin for 6 weeks resulted in a long-lasting cure.
- Priapism has been reported in a 37-year-old man with a 30-year history of severe diabetes mellitus after two doses of vancomycin 1 g intravenously for treatment of methicillin-resistant *S. aureus* bursitis (85).

The authors noted that an interaction between vancomycin and other medications (cefazolin, aztreonam, ciclosporin, prednisone, mycophenolate mofetil, and co-trimoxazole) could not be ruled out.

Immunologic

Allergic reactions with vancomycin, such as rashes, chills, fever, and eosinophilia, can occur in up to 5% of patients. Severe anaphylactic reactions are rare. Alpha-tryptase is only detected in the blood during systemic anaphylactic reactions, having been released by degranulation from activated mast cells. Plasma tryptase activities were unchanged, independent of increased histamine concentrations, antihistamine pretreatment, and clinical symptoms of anaphylactoid reaction in 40 patients receiving vancomycin (1 g over 10 minutes) before elective arthroplasty (86). The authors conclude that plasma tryptase activities can be used to distinguish chemical from immunological reactions.

Vancomycin anaphylaxis is a major management problem in patients with methicillin-resistant *S. aureus* sepsis. However, desensitization in patients with previous anaphylaxis is possible (87).

- An anaphylactic reaction occurred in a 77-year-old woman 5 minutes after the start of a vancomycin infusion, when she had received only 40 mg (88). She became unconscious and had a severe cardiovascular collapse, from which she was resuscitated with intravenous ephedrine and adrenaline.
- A 47-year-old white woman with end-stage renal disease had had anaphylactoid shock after vancomycin 1 g intravenously infused over 1.5 hours and gentamicin 90 mg 3 years before, despite premedication with diphenhydramine (89). She was treated with doubling doses of vancomycin every 30 minutes for methicillin-resistant *S. epidermidis*. She had no reaction.

The authors of the second report could not exclude that the previous anaphylactoid reaction had not been due to gentamicin, as no specific testing was done. Although successful vancomycin desensitization has been described, this would be the first time in a patient with a history of anaphylactoid reaction.

In some patients the clinical presentation of red man syndrome is identical to that of acute IgE-mediated anaphylaxis. Vancomycin desensitization should therefore be considered for severe red man syndrome reactions that do not respond to premedication and a slower rate of infusion, and in anaphylactic reactions to vancomycin when substitution of another antibiotic is not feasible. Rapid desensitization is preferred, as it is effective in the majority of patients and enables administration of vancomycin within 24 hours. In patients who fail rapid desensitization, a slow desensitization protocol may be tried (90).

Vasculitic rashes have been described rarely. Two case reports have suggested that there may be cross-reactivity between vancomycin and teicoplanin with respect to biopsy-proven leukocytoclastic vasculitis (91). In both cases, vancomycin-induced vasculitis improved after drug withdrawal. Teicoplanin was started and the rash reappeared several days later. In one case the rash faded after teicoplanin had been withdrawn. In the other, teicoplanin was continued, but the rash improved after prednisolone was given.

Long-Term Effects

Drug resistance

The increasing rate of antimicrobial drug resistance has been a matter of great concern and is the most serious unwanted effect of these drugs. However, in spite of the fact that the problem is now very well recognized (SEDA-25, 279), it continues to grow.

History

Most antimicrobial drugs are natural products, that is they are produced by micro-organisms such as bacteria or fungi, often found in the soil. In fact, they can be looked upon as nature's regulatory principle for microbial society. Resistance to antimicrobial drugs is therefore a natural phenomenon. Before the introduction of penicillin in the 1940s, resistance to antimicrobial drugs was not a clinical problem. At that time, the large majority of commensal and infectious bacteria associated with infections in man were susceptible.

Over the last six decades, however, increased use of antimicrobial drugs, not only in human medicine, but in other areas, such as veterinary medicine, agriculture, and fish farming, has had an enormous impact on the microbial society. Nearly everywhere, the numbers of susceptible strains have reduced and resistant strains or variants have increased in numbers. It has been repeatedly reported that the susceptibility profile of bacteria in any human compartment, such as the skin, intestine, and respiratory tract, is very different from what it was in the pre-antibiotic era, and even 15 years ago. The same trend is reported from hospitals and homes. Multidrug resistance, that is resistance to several antimicrobial drugs, is commonly found in bacteria that cause infections as well as in commensal organisms.

A few decades ago, it was a common opinion that various compartments in nature have their own flora. As an example, it was claimed that you could use antimicrobial drugs relatively freely in fish farming without increasing the burden of resistance in humans. Now we have learned the lesson. Micro-organisms circulate everywhere, and there is a continuous exchange of strains between all compartments in nature (humans, animals, birds, fish, etc.). Even if a bacterial species is host-specific, the genetic material that codes for resistance is not. In fact, antibiotics have shown that bacteria have great genetic adaptability, in terms of their ability to exchange genetic traits among genera and species which are evolutionarily millions of years apart. Antibiotic resistance genes on plasmids and transposons flow to and from nearly all types of bacteria. Sometimes they leave the plasmid and jump into bacterial chromosomes; sometimes they jump back again.

However, this knowledge is not being heeded everywhere. Small doses of antimicrobial drugs as "growth promoters" are still commonly used, even in countries in which the health authorities should be aware of the problems. It is easy to blame developing countries for using antimicrobial drugs as growth promoters, or for selling antimicrobial drugs over the counter without prescription, but it took the European Community many years before it started to look into the problem of using antimicrobial drugs as growth promoters. The history of cross-resistance between avoparcin and vancomycin may have provided important background for this alteration in attitude.

Avoparcin and vancomycin are glycopeptide antibiotics, large molecules that are produced by a variety of environmental micro-organisms, which may therefore contain genes that code for antimicrobial drug resistance. Both of these drugs are mostly active against Gram-positive bacteria, such as enterococci and staphylococci. In Europe, avoparcin was allowed to be used as an animal food additive in many countries, while the use of vancomycin was limited to humans. Nobody bothered about the possibility of cross-resistance between avoparcin and vancomycin until 10 years ago. After the emergence of vancomycin-resistant enterococci and after more than 2 years of hard lobbying by several groups, avoparcin was withdrawn from the market in the European Community. However, in the meantime, vancomycin-resistant enterococci had become widespread in many European countries.

Instead of focusing on the development of resistance to a specific antimicrobial drug in a specific species, we should focus on the microbial community as a single entity or a "metagenome". Any use of any microbial agent might cause resistance to develop in one or more microbial species. When such genes have first become established, they may float around and be picked up by other species. This approach to the development and spread of resistance can, and should, be applied to the microbial flora in all mammals, as well as in the environment. The consequence of this approach is that we should, every time we prescribe an antimicrobial drug, try to find a drug that hits nothing but the pathogen in the infected organ(s). Of course, this can be difficult and sometimes even close to impossible. But that should not stop us from trying. For example, in nearly all cases, a third-generation cephalosporin for acute pharyngitis caused by Group A streptococci, or of a fluoroquinolone for acute cystitis, are not the best alternatives.

Ecology

In our struggle for prudent use of antimicrobial drugs, the so-called eco-shadow concept represents a challenging way of following alterations in mammalian and environmental ecosystems produced by exposure of these systems to antibiotics (92). In brief, an eco-shadow (ecological shadow) can be defined as any alteration in any ecosystem following exposure of the system to an antimicrobial drug (or any compound that influences the system). The alterations can be of variable length and may involve a variable number of species and functions, including the development and spread of resistance. When possible, the sum of all the alterations caused by an antibiotic can be included in an "eco-shadow index." A large eco-shadow or high eco-shadow index indicates a high tendency to the development of microbial resistance.

At present, it seems that Europe has taken the lead in the fight against antimicrobial drug resistance. At the Fourth European Conference on Antibiotic Resistance, organized by the European Commission and held in Rome in November 2003, it was strongly emphasized that only a multidisciplinary approach, involving all stakeholders—physicians, researchers, industry, politicians,

and patients—can overcome the problem of increasing resistance. It is to be hoped that this problem will be established as a major objective for the forthcoming European Centre for Disease Prevention and Control.

Reports of organisms that are resistant to vancomycin

The first case of methicillin-resistant *S. aureus* with intermediate resistance to vancomycin was documented in May 1996. Additional cases have been described in the USA:

- a 59-year-old man with diabetes mellitus and chronic renal insufficiency suffering from peritonitis;
- a 66-year-old man with diabetes who developed a septicemia after 18 weeks of vancomycin treatment for recurrent methicillin-resistant *S. aureus* bacteremia;
- a 79-year-old man with diabetes and chronic renal insufficiency, who developed intermediate vancomycin-resistance after a 6-week therapy with vancomycin for MRSA bloodstream infection.

In the last case the strain was identical to eight MRSA isolates obtained from hospitals in the New York City metropolitan area, and all eight isolates, but not control isolates, could be transformed in vitro to develop intermediate resistance to vancomycin. Both the presence of glycopeptides and environmental factors, as demonstrated by increased resistance of *S. aureus* to antibiotics in the presence of prosthetic material in animals, can exert selective pressure to develop new resistance mechanisms (93–95).

There are reports of vancomycin-dependent enterococci that grow only in the presence of vancomycin and are best treated by withdrawal of the compound (96).

Vancomycin/glycopeptide intermediately resistant and methicillin-resistant *S. aureus* have been described in Japan, Europe, the Far East, and the USA. Some vancomycin-susceptible strains of *S. aureus* contain subpopulations with intermediate resistance to vancomycin (heterogeneous strains), and these may escape laboratory detection (93,94,97–99).

Numerous risk factors have been identified for infection with vancomycin-resistant enterococci. In one study the severity of mucositis in cancer patients was significantly associated with vancomycin-resistant enterococci (100). Previous vancomycin therapy was also believed to be a risk factor. However, a meta-analysis concluded that the reported strong association between vancomycin treatment and hospital-acquired vancomycin-resistant enterococci results from selection bias, confounding by duration of hospitalization, and publication bias (101).

Glycopeptide resistance in a cluster of three clinical isolates of vancomycin-resistant *Enterococcus faecium* was due to vanD, which was located on the chromosome and was not transferable to other enterococci. These isolates were indistinguishable but differed from the strain in which vanD-mediated resistance has been reported previously (102). A type of acquired glycopeptide resistance, named vanE, has been characterized in *E. faecalis* BM 4405. It results in low-level resistance of vancomycin but susceptibility to teicoplanin (103). Defects in penicillin-binding protein 4 result in a distorted peptidoglycan composition of the cell of vancomycin-resistant and teicoplanin-resistant laboratory mutants of *S. aureus* and are suggested to be part of the mechanism of glycopeptide resistance in these microbes (104).

Vancomycin-dependent enterococci growing only in the presence of vancomycin are best treated by withdrawing vancomycin (96). However, vancomycin-independent revertants can rapidly emerge in vitro, endangering the cure of patients treated by interruption of vancomycin only (105).

In a study of antibiotic resistance in enterococci from raw meat, there was a high prevalence of glycopeptide-resistant strains (106). Resistance to vancomycin was significantly associated with resistance to teicoplanin, erythromycin, tetracycline, and chloramphenicol.

The prevalence of vancomycin-resistant enterococci (VRE) has been investigated in 49 laboratories from 27 European countries, which collected 4208 clinical isolates; 18 vanA and 5 vanB isolates of VRE were identified (107). The prevalence of vanA VRE was highest in the UK (2.7%), while the prevalence of vanB VRE was highest in Slovenia (2%). Most vanA and vanB vancomycin-resistant enterococci were identified as *E. fecium*. A total of 71 isolates containing the vanC gene were identified. The prevalence of vanC VRE was highest in Latvia and Turkey, where rates were 14 and 12% respectively. Two-thirds of these isolates were identified as *Enterococcus gallinarum* and one-third as *Enterococcus casseliflavus*.

In 155 methicillin-resistant strains of *S. aureus* isolated from patients in Thailand, one-point population analysis identified three methicillin-resistant strains, which contained subpopulations of cells with reduced susceptibility to vancomycin (108).

Susceptibility Factors

Renal disease

Vancomycin is eliminated almost exclusively by renal excretion. In oliguria 1 g can produce therapeutic plasma concentrations for 10–14 days. Hemodialysis fails to remove vancomycin from the body to any significant extent. If renal function is compromised, even oral therapy with vancomycin can lead to high and potentially toxic serum and CSF drug concentrations (109).

Drug Administration

Drug contamination

Vancomycin underwent spontaneous chemical modification when kept at room temperature at neutral pH in aqueous solutions containing traces of formaldehyde or acetaldehyde (110). In vitro studies on two different strains of bacteria showed that the resulting compounds had reduced antibacterial activity.

Drug administration route

In a multicenter, prospective, randomized comparison of continuous infusion of vancomycin (targeted serum plateau concentrations of 20–25 µg/ml) and intermittent infusions of vancomycin (targeted serum trough concentrations of 10–15 µg/ml) in 119 critically ill patients, microbiological and clinical outcomes and safety were similar (111). Continuous infusion of vancomycin produced the target concentration faster, and fewer samples were required for monitoring. Serum creatinine concentrations and creatinine clearance increased non-significantly from baseline to the end of treatment in the two groups. There was nephrotoxicity in 21 patients (10 of whom received the continuous infusion). Vancomycin given concomitantly with other antibiotics was associated with a significant increase in the serum creatinine concentration, but not when it was given alone. Dialysis was required for three of those who were given intermittent infusions and six of those who were given continuous infusions. Red man syndrome was reported in one patient who was given an intermittent infusion, and phlebitis and fever in two patients who were given continuous infusions.

Drug overdose

- Accidental 10-fold vancomycin overdose in a 6-month-old girl resulted in flushing and a transient rise in serum creatinine concentration, but she recovered completely without specific therapeutic intervention (112).
- Two preterm twins, born in the 35th week of gestation, accidentally received an overdose of vancomycin as an intravenous bolus injection (113). Both were treated from the day of birth with piperacillin (100 mg/kg/day) and cefotaxime (100 mg/kg/day) for congenital pneumonia. On the 6th day of antibiotic therapy, vancomycin (38 and 35 mg/kg respectively) was given over 1 minute. A few minutes later the twins developed flushed faces and trunks and peripheral cyanosis. Other findings were a prolonged capillary refill time, apnea and hypoxemia, bradycardia (40–60/minute), a fall in systolic blood pressure of 10 mmHg, and metabolic acidosis (pH 7.29 and 7.24 and base excess −10.5 and −10.9 respectively). Metabolic acidosis and the red man syndrome disappeared after 30 minutes. Serum vancomycin concentrations were 32 and 34.5 µg/ml respectively 9 hours after administration. Fundoscopy and repeated otoacoustic emissions were normal. There was minimal reduction in creatinine clearance. Tubular proteinuria, paralleled by increased activity of *N*-acetyl-beta-D-glucosaminidase in the urine, resolved completely within 1 week.
- Hemodialysis with high-efficiency dialysis membranes resulted in a removal of plasma vancomycin of about 60% (calculated half-life 2 hours) in two children with initial plasma vancomycin concentrations of 238 µg/ml and 182 µg/ml (114).
- In a 6-day-old neonate with a solitary hypodysplastic kidney, suspected sepsis, and acute renal insufficiency, venovenous hemodiafiltration with a high-flux membrane was successfully used to treat a 10-fold overdose of vancomycin (115).

Multiple-dose activated charcoal does not increase the elimination of vancomycin and is therefore not recommended for detoxification of acute poisoning (116).

Drug–Drug Interactions

Aminoglycoside antibiotics

Vancomycin is more nephrotoxic than teicoplanin when it is combined with aminoglycosides (117).

Beta lactam antibiotics

Vancomycin and ceftazidime are incompatible in vitro because of precipitation due to the alkaline pH of vancomycin relative to ceftazidime. This phenomenon was encountered in two cases of post-traumatic endophthalmitis (118). Immediately on local administration of the antibiotics, which were injected using different needles and syringes for each drug, dense yellow-white precipitates were observed along the needle tract in the vitreous cavity. During follow-up the vitreous opacities gradually disappeared over a period of 2 months, with complete resolution.

Co-administration of imipenem + cilastatin may reduce the nephrotoxicity of vancomycin, as suggested by a study in rats (119).

Dexamethasone

Intravitreal application of dexamethasone may reduce the elimination of intravitreal vancomycin and may enhance this therapy, as suggested by an in vivo study in rabbits (120).

Dobutamine

In critically ill patients, co-administration with dobutamine can enhance vancomycin clearance by increasing cardiac output and renal blood flow and by interacting with the renal anion transport system, increasing glomerular filtration rate and renal tubular secretion (121).

Dopamine

In critically ill patients, co-administration with dopamine can enhance vancomycin clearance by increasing cardiac output and renal blood flow and by interacting with the renal anion transport system, increasing glomerular filtration rate and renal tubular secretion (121).

Fosfomycin

Co-administration of fosfomycin may reduce the nephrotoxicity of vancomycin, as suggested by a study in rats (119).

Furosemide

Preterm infants often receive theophylline for apnea of prematurity and furosemide to improve dynamic lung compliance and to reduce total pulmonary resistance. In 10 preterm infants receiving furosemide plus theophylline, vancomycin was introduced according to the generally recommended dosing schedules but failed to achieve anticipated therapeutic concentrations (122). In nine infants the addition of furosemide to vancomycin plus theophylline resulted in a fall in serum vancomycin concentrations to subtherapeutic within 24 hours, and only in one did vancomycin concentrations remain within the target range. The addition of furosemide reduced the serum creatinine concentration by 24% (range 12–43). These data suggest that furosemide enhances the excretion of vancomycin, and an acute and transient increase in glomerular filtration rate and creatinine clearance may be the explanation.

Gelatin

Vancomycin is incompatible with gelatin-containing fluids, resulting in precipitation (123).

Levofloxacin

Changes in pharmacokinetics were studied in male Wistar rats when intravenous vancomycin 100 mg/kg and levofloxacin 20 mg/kg were administered together (124). There was an increase in the AUC and half-life of vancomycin. There was also an increase in the AUC and a delay in the t_{max} of levofloxacin, but no effect on C_{max}; these data suggested delayed absorption of levofloxacin. Concomitant administration had no effect on the correlation between serum and hepatic tissue concentrations of levofloxacin, but it markedly reduced the correlation between the serum and renal tissue concentrations of vancomycin. Vancomycin increased serum creatinine concentrations 8 hours after administration. However, there was no difference in animals who received monotherapy compared with animals who received combined therapy. The authors suggested the cautious use of a combination of levofloxacin and vancomycin and advised monitoring blood concentrations of vancomycin in such cases.

Neuromuscular blocking drugs

Some authors stress the fact that vancomycin can interact with anesthetic drugs, particularly muscle relaxants. In the reported cases anaphylactoid reactions were seen, with intense erythema and marked permeability changes (125).

Monitoring Therapy

There is evidence that predose concentrations of teicoplanin are related to clinical outcome; the evidence is less conclusive for vancomycin. Predose concentrations can be linked to some toxic effects (nephrotoxicity for vancomycin and thrombocytopenia to teicoplanin) (SEDA23.26.77) (126,127). Monitoring of serum concentrations has therefore been advocated to reduce potential nephrotoxicity and ototoxicity due to interpatient variability in vancomycin pharmacokinetics. However, routine monitoring is probably unnecessary in most patients (3,128). Clinical settings in which monitoring is wise include combination therapies with an aminoglycoside and treatment of patients with poor or unstable renal function (2). Vancomycin-induced nephrotoxicity is clearly related to drug plasma concentrations: trough vancomycin concentrations over 15 µg/ml were associated with significantly more nephrotoxicity (129).

In a prospective study to determine if standardized vancomycin doses could produce adequate serum concentrations in 25 full-term neonates with sepsis 13 had adequate peak vancomycin serum concentrations (20–40 mg/ml) and one had a peak concentration with a risk of ototoxicity (over 40 µg/ml) (130). Only 12 had adequate trough concentrations (5–10 mg/ml) and 7 had a risk of nephrotoxicity (over 10 µg/ml). There was no significant difference between peak or trough concentrations and good or bad clinical outcomes.

Intravenous vancomycin 30–40 mg/kg/day, divided every 6 hours, was given to167 infants and children without cancer and 42 cancer patients aged 3 months to 17.5

years with normal serum creatinine concentrations and without evidence of renal dysfunction (131). In 93% of the children without cancer, peak serum vancomycin concentrations were in an adequate target range (8–55 µg/ml). However, 10% of the children with cancers had peak serum vancomycin concentrations below 10 µg/ml, and 21% had trough concentrations less than 5 µg/ml; an increased dosage was required to achieve adequate peak concentrations. There were no treatment failures. The authors suggested the following guidelines:

- the serum creatinine concentration should be measured within 24 hours of beginning therapy, to verify normal renal function, and weekly thereafter to detect an eventual reduction in creatinine clearance;
- an increase of serum creatinine of more than 44 µmol/l (0.5 mg/dl) over baseline should be followed by monitoring serum vancomycin concentrations;
- peak and trough vancomycin serum concentrations measurements are not necessary in children without cancer receiving 40 mg/kg/day or less who have normal renal function and do not receive other potentially nephrotoxic drugs; this approach should be individualized, based on factors such as degree of illness, poor clinical response, or persistent positive cultures;
- monitoring should be considered for patients with cancer, neonates, those receiving concurrent nephrotoxic drugs, patients with renal insufficiency, and for dosages over 40 mg/kg/day.

Fluorescence polarization immunoassay determination of serum vancomycin concentrations can result in falsely high vancomycin concentrations in excess of 30–80% in patients with renal dysfunction. This is due to the formation of a non-toxic, non-microbiologically active pseudometabolite, the vancomycin crystalline degradation product (132). A report on a 48-year-old man underlies the significance of resulting underdosing and eventually suboptimal clinical response (133).

Managing Adverse Effects

Vancomycin clearance is minimally altered by hemodialysis using standard cuprophane membranes. However, it is significantly increased using a high-flux polysulfone membrane.

- A 17-year-old anuric woman with end-stage renal insufficiency received a massive overdose of vancomycin (40 mg/kg/day for 8 days) and was treated three times with high-flux hemodiafiltration with a polysulfone membrane (134). The vancomycin concentration fell from 101 to 17 mg/l at the end of the procedure. There were no adverse effects of either vancomycin or hemodiafiltration.
- In a 46-year-old African-American woman with sickle-cell disease there was clinically significant removal of vancomycin during a plasma exchange transfusion (135).

References

1. Griffith RS. Introduction to vancomycin. Rev Infect Dis 1981;3(Suppl):S200–4.
2. Moellering RC Jr. Monitoring serum vancomycin levels: climbing the mountain because it is there? Clin Infect Dis 1994;18(4):544–6.
3. Cantu TG, Yamanaka-Yuen NA, Lietman PS. Serum vancomycin concentrations: reappraisal of their clinical value. Clin Infect Dis 1994;18(4):533–43.
4. Anderson JL, Muhlestein JB, Carlquist J, Allen A, Trehan S, Nielson C, Hall S, Brady J, Egger M, Horne B, Lim T. Randomized secondary prevention trial of azithromycin in patients with coronary artery disease and serological evidence for *Chlamydia pneumoniae* infection: The Azithromycin in Coronary Artery Disease: Elimination of Myocardial Infection with Chlamydia (ACADEMIC) study. Circulation 1999;99(12):1540–7.
5. Hospital Infection Control Practices Advisory Committee (HICPAC). Recommendations for preventing the spread of vancomycin resistance. Am J Infect Control 1995;23(2):87–94.
6. Boselli E, Allaouchiche B. Diffusion osseuse des antibiotiques. [Diffusion in bone tissue of antibiotics.] Presse Méd 1999;28(40):2265–76.
7. Leitch EC, Willcox MD. Lactoferrin increases the susceptibility of *S. epidermidis* biofilms to lysozyme and vancomycin. Curr Eye Res 1999;19(1):12–19.
8. Elting LS, Rubenstein EB, Kurtin D, Rolston KV, Fangtang J, Martin CG, Raad II, Whimbey EE, Manzullo E, Bodey GP. Mississippi mud in the 1990s: risks and outcomes of vancomycin-associated toxicity in general oncology practice. Cancer 1998;83(12):2597–607.
9. Cohen E, Dadashev A, Drucker M, Samra Z, Rubinstein E, Garty M. Once-daily versus twice-daily intravenous administration of vancomycin for infections in hospitalized patients. J Antimicrob Chemother 2002;49(1):155–60.
10. Fortun J, Navas E, Martinez-Beltran J, Perez-Molina J, Martin-Davila P, Guerrero A, Moreno S. Short-course therapy for right-side endocarditis due to Staphylococcus aureus in drug abusers: cloxacillin versus glycopeptides in combination with gentamicin. Clin Infect Dis 2001;33(1):120–5.
11. Sandler RH, Finegold SM, Bolte ER, Buchanan CP, Maxwell AP, Vaisanen ML, Nelson MN, Wexler HM. Short-term benefit from oral vancomycin treatment of regressive-onset autism. J Child Neurol 2000;15(7):429–35.
12. Newfield P, Roizen MF. Hazards of rapid administration of vancomycin. Ann Intern Med 1979;91(4):581.
13. Davis RL, Smith AL, Koup JR. The "red man's syndrome" and slow infusion of vancomycin. Ann Intern Med 1986;104(2):285–6.
14. Healy DP, Sahai JV, Fuller SH, Polk RE. Vancomycin-induced histamine release and "red man syndrome": comparison of 1- and 2-hour infusions. Antimicrob Agents Chemother 1990;34(4):550–4.
15. Toyoguchi T, Ebihara M, Ojima F, Hosoya J, Shoji T, Nakagawa Y. Histamine release induced by antimicrobial agents and effects of antimicrobial agents on vancomycin-induced histamine release from rat peritoneal mast cells. J Pharm Pharmacol 2000;52(3):327–31.
16. Polk RE. Anaphylactoid reactions to glycopeptide antibiotics. J Antimicrob Chemother 1991;27(Suppl B):17–29.
17. Bergeron L, Boucher FD. Possible red-man syndrome associated with systemic absorption of oral vancomycin in a child with normal renal function. Ann Pharmacother 1994;28(5):581–4.
18. Renz CL, Thurn JD, Finn HA, Lynch JP, Moss J. Oral antihistamines reduce the side effects from rapid vancomycin infusion. Anesth Analg 1998;87(3):681–5.
19. Johnson JR, Burke MS, Mahowald ML, Ytterberg SR. Life-threatening reaction to vancomycin given for noninfectious fever. Ann Pharmacother 1999;33(10):1043–5.
20. Hui YL, Yu CC, Ng YT, Lau WM, Hsieh JR, Chung PC. Red Man's syndrome following administration of vancomycin in a patient under spinal anesthesia—a case report. Acta Anaesthesiol Sin 2002;40(3):149–51.

21. Bertolissi M, Bassi F, Cecotti R, Capelli C, Giordano F. Pruritus: a useful sign for predicting the haemodynamic changes that occur following administration of vancomycin. Crit Care 2002;6(3):234–9.

22. Renz CL, Thurn JD, Finn HA, Lynch JP, Moss J. Antihistamine prophylaxis permits rapid vancomycin infusion. Crit Care Med 1999;27(9):1732–7.

23. Aissaoui M, Mathelier-Fusade P, Leynadier F. Le syndrome vancomycine/narcotiques. [The vancomycin/narcotic syndrome.] Presse Méd 1999;28(39):2152.

24. Shuto H, Sueyasu M, Otsuki S, Hara T, Tsuruta Y, Kataoka Y, Oishi R. Potentiation of vancomycin-induced histamine release by muscle relaxants and morphine in rats. Antimicrob Agents Chemother 1999;43(12):2881–4.

25. Beringer PM, Wong-Beringer A, Rho JP. Economic aspects of antibacterial adverse effects. Pharmacoeconomics 1998;13(1 Pt 1):35–49.

26. Vazquez L, Encinas MP, Morin LS, Vilches P, Gutierrez N, Garcia-Sanz R, Caballero D, Hurle AD. Randomized prospective study comparing cost-effectiveness of teicoplanin and vancomycin as second-line empiric therapy for infection in neutropenic patients. Haematologica 1999;84(3):231–6.

27. Bucaneve G, Menichetti F, Del Favero A. Cost analysis of 2 empiric antibacterial regimens containing glycopeptides for the treatment of febrile neutropenia in patients with acute leukaemia. Pharmacoeconomics 1999;15(1):85–95.

28. Garrelts JC, Smith DF Jr, Ast D, LaRocca J, Peterie JD. Phlebitis associated with vancomycin therapy. Clin Pharm 1988;7(10):720–1.

29. Hadaway L, Chamallas SN. Vancomycin: new perspectives on an old drug. J Infus Nurs 2003;26(5):278–84.

30. Brummett RE. Ototoxicity of vancomycin and analogues. Otolaryngol Clin North Am 1993;26(5):821–8.

31. Mellor JA, Kingdom J, Cafferkey M, Keane CT. Vancomycin toxicity: a prospective study. J Antimicrob Chemother 1985;15(6):773–80.

32. Cook FV, Farrar WE Jr. Vancomycin revisited. Ann Intern Med 1978;88(6):813–18.

33. Axer-Siegel R, Stiebel-Kalish H, Rosenblatt I, Strassmann E, Yassur Y, Weinberger D. Cystoid macular edema after cataract surgery with intraocular vancomycin. Ophthalmology 1999;106(9):1660–4.

34. Gendeh BS, Gibb AG, Aziz NS, Kong N, Zahir ZM. Vancomycin administration in continuous ambulatory peritoneal dialysis: the risk of ototoxicity. Otolaryngol Head Neck Surg 1998;118(4):551–8.

35. Schaefer F, Klaus G, Muller-Wiefel DE, Mehls O. Intermittent versus continuous intraperitoneal glycopeptide/ceftazidime treatment in children with peritoneal dialysis-associated peritonitis. The Mid-European Pediatric Peritoneal Dialysis Study Group (MEPPS). J Am Soc Nephrol 1999;10(1):136–45.

36. Panzarino VM, Feldstein TJ, Kashtan CE. Charcoal hemoperfusion in a child with vancomycin overdose and chronic renal failure. Pediatr Nephrol 1998;12(1):63–4.

37. Gavazzi C, Stacchiotti S, Cavalletti R, Lodi R. Confusion after antibiotics. Lancet 2001;357(9266):1410.

38. Lambotte O, Costedoat-Chalumeau N, Amoura Z, Piette JC, Cacoub P. Drug-induced hemophagocytosis. Am J Med 2002;112(7):592–3.

39. Rocha JL, Kondo W, Baptista MI, Da Cunha CA, Martins LT. Uncommon vancomycin-induced side effects. Braz J Infect Dis 2002;6(4):196–200.

40. Schwartz MD. Vancomycin-induced neutropenia in a patient positive for an antineutrophil antibody. Pharmacotherapy 2002;22(6):783–8.

41. Shahar A, Berner Y, Levi S. Fever, rash, and pancytopenia following vancomycin rechallenge in the presence of ceftazidime. Ann Pharmacother 2000;34(2):263–4.

42. Petit N, Rohrbach P, Mathieu P, Cronier B. Neutropénie a la vancomycine confirmée par une épreuve de réintroduction positive. Med Mal Infect 2000;20:665–6.

43. Weitzman SA, Stossel TP. Drug-induced immunological neutropenia. Lancet 1978;1(8073):1068–72.

44. Henry K, Steinberg I, Crossley KB. Vancomycin-induced neutropenia during treatment of osteomyelitis in an outpatient. Drug Intell Clin Pharm 1986;20(10):783–5.

45. Eich G, Neftel KA. Hämatologische Nebenwirkungen der antiinfektiösen Therapie. Infection 1991;19:S1–35.

46. Adrouny A, Meguerditchian S, Koo CH, Gadallah M, Rasgon S, Idroos M, Oppenheimer E, Glowalla M. Agranulocytosis related to vancomycin therapy. Am J Med 1986;81(6):1059–61.

47. West BC. Vancomycin-induced neutropenia. South Med J 1981;74(10):1255–6.

48. Koo KB, Bachand RL, Chow AW. Vancomycin-induced neutropenia. Drug Intell Clin Pharm 1986;20(10):780–2.

49. Sanche SE, Dust WN, Shevchuk YM. Vancomycin-induced neutropenia resolves after substitution with teicoplanin. Clin Infect Dis 2000;31(3):824–5.

50. Smith PF, Taylor CT. Vancomycin-induced neutropenia associated with fever: similarities between two immune-mediated drug reactions. Pharmacotherapy 1999;19(2):240–4.

51. George JN, Raskob GE, Shah SR, Rizvi MA, Hamilton SA, Osborne S, Vondracek T. Drug-induced thrombocytopenia: a systematic review of published case reports. Ann Intern Med 1998;129(11):886–90.

52. Kuruppu JC, Le TP, Tuazon CU. Vancomycin-associated thrombocytopenia: case report and review of the literature. Am J Hematol 1999;60(3):249–50.

53. Govindarajan R, Baxter D, Wilson C, Zent C. Vancomycin-induced thrombocytopenia. Am J Hematol 1999;62(2):122–3.

54. Cawley MJ, Wittbrodt ET, Boyce EG, Skaar DJ. Potential risk factors associated with thrombocytopenia in a surgical intensive care unit. Pharmacotherapy 1999;19(1):108–13.

55. Balduini CL, Salvaneschi L, Klersy C, Noris P, Mazzucco M, Rizzuto F, Giorgiani G, Perotti C, Stroppa P, Pumpo MD, Nobili B, Locatelli F. Factors influencing post-transfusional platelet increment in pediatric patients given hematopoietic stem cell transplantation. Leukemia 2001;15(12):1885–91.

56. Hurley BW, Nguyen CC. The spectrum of pseudomembranous enterocolitis and antibiotic-associated diarrhea. Arch Intern Med 2002;162(19):2177–84.

57. Schenfeld LA, Pote HH Jr. Diarrhea associated with parenteral vancomycin therapy. Clin Infect Dis 1995;20(6):1578–9.

58. Bhatt-Mehta V, Schumacher RE, Faix RG, Leady M, Brenner T. Lack of vancomycin-associated nephrotoxicity in newborn infants: a case-control study. Pediatrics 1999;103(4):e48.

59. Downs NJ, Neihart RE, Dolezal JM, Hodges GR. Mild nephrotoxicity associated with vancomycin use. Arch Intern Med 1989;149(8):1777–81.

60. Wold JS, Turnipseed SA. Toxicology of vancomycin in laboratory animals. Rev Infect Dis 1981;3(Suppl):S224–9.

61. Ngeleka M, Auclair P, Tardif D, Beauchamp D, Bergeron MG. Intrarenal distribution of vancomycin in endotoxemic rats. Antimicrob Agents Chemother 1989;33(9):1575–9.

62. Wai AO, Lo AM, Abdo A, Marra F. Vancomycin-induced acute interstitial nephritis. Ann Pharmacother 1998;32(11):1160–4.

63. Sidi V, Roilides E, Bibashi E, Gompakis N, Tsakiri A, Koliouskas D. Comparison of efficacy and safety of teicoplanin and vancomycin in children with antineoplastic therapy-associated febrile neutropenia and Gram-positive bacteremia. J Chemother 2000;12(4):326–31.

64. Yoshiyama Y, Yazaki T, Wong PC, Beauchamp D, Kanke M. The effect of fosfomycin on glycopeptide antibiotic-induced nephrotoxicity in rats. J Infect Chemother 2001;7(4):243–6.

65. Delbaldo C, Chen M, Friedli A, Prins C, Desmeules J, Saurat JH, Woodley DT, Borradori L. Drug-induced epidermolysis bullosa acquisita with antibodies to type VII collagen. J Am Acad Dermatol 2002;46(Suppl 5):S161–4.

66. Joshi PP, Ahmed N. Fixed drug eruption with vancomycin. Ann Pharmacother 2002;36(6):1104.

67. Padial MA, Barranco P, Lopez-Serrano C. Erythema multiforme to vancomycin. Allergy 2000;55(12):1201.

68. Packer J, Olshan AR, Schwarts AB. Prolonged allergic reaction to vancomycin in endstage renal disease. Dialysis Transplant 1987;16:87.

69. Santaeugenia S, Pedro Botet ML, Sabat M, Sopena N, Sadria M. Sindrome de Stevens–Johnson asociado a vancomicina. [Stevens–Johnson syndrome associated with vancomycin.] Rev Esp Quimioter 2000;13(4):425–6.

70. Thestrup-Pedersen K, Hainau B, Al'Eisa A, Al'Fadley A, Hamadah I. Fatal toxic epidermal necrolysis associated with ceftazidine and vancomycin therapy: a report of two cases. Acta Dermatol Venereol 2000;80(4):316–17.

71. Danielsen AG, Thomsen K. Vancomycin-induced linear IgA bullous disease. Br J Dermatol 1999;141(4):756–7.

72. Nousari HC, Costarangos C, Anhalt GJ. Vancomycin-associated linear IgA bullous dermatosis. Ann Intern Med 1998;129(6):507–8.

73. Bernstein EF, Schuster M. Linear IgA bullous dermatosis associated with vancomycin. Ann Intern Med 1998;129(6):508–9.

74. Nousari HC, Kimyai-Asadi A, Caeiro JP, Anhalt GJ. Clinical, demographic, and immunohistologic features of vancomycin-induced linear IgA bullous disease of the skin. Report of 2 cases and review of the literature. Medicine (Baltimore) 1999;78(1):1–8.

75. Wiadrowski TP, Reid CM. Drug-induced linear IgA bullous disease following antibiotics. Australas J Dermatol 2001;42(3):196–9.

76. Chang A, Camisa C, Ormsby A. Intertriginous bullae in a 53-year-old man. Arch Dermatol 2001;137(6):815–20.

77. Palmer RA, Ogg G, Allen J, Banerjee A, Ryatt KS, Ratnavel R, Wojnarowska F. Vancomycin-induced linear IgA disease with autoantibodies to BP180 and LAD285. Br J Dermatol 2001;145(5):816–20.

78. Ahkami R, Thomas I. Linear IgA bullous dermatosis associated with vancomycin and disseminated varicella-zoster infection. Cutis 2001;67(5):423–6.

79. Mofid MZ, Costarangos C, Bernstein B, Wong L, Munster A, Nousari HC. Drug-induced linear immunoglobulin A bullous disease that clinically mimics toxic epidermal necrolysis. J Burn Care Rehabil 2000;21(3):246–7.

80. Klein PA, Callen JP. Drug-induced linear IgA bullous dermatosis after vancomycin discontinuance in a patient with renal insufficiency. J Am Acad Dermatol 2000;42(2 Pt 2):316–23.

81. Richards SS, Hall S, Yokel B, Whitmore SE. A bullous eruption in an elderly woman. Vancomycin-associated linear IgA dermatosis (LAD). Arch Dermatol 1995;131(12):1447–51.

82. Geissmann C, Beylot-Barry M, Doutre MS, Beylot C. Drug-induced linear IgA bullous dermatosis. J Am Acad Dermatol 1995;32(2 Pt 1):296.

83. Neughebauer BI, Negron G, Pelton S, Plunkett RW, Beutner EH, Magnussen R. Bullous skin disease: an unusual allergic reaction to vancomycin. Am J Med Sci 2002;323(5):273–8.

84. Taylor SE, Paterson DL, Yu VL. Treatment options for chronic prostatitis due to vancomycin-resistant *Enterococcus faecium*. Eur J Clin Microbiol Infect Dis 1998;17(11):798–800.

85. Czachor JS, Garzaro P, Miller JR. Vancomycin and priapism. N Engl J Med 1998;338(23):1701.

86. Renz CL, Laroche D, Thurn JD, Finn HA, Lynch JP, Thisted R, Moss J. Tryptase levels are not increased during vancomycin-induced anaphylactoid reactions. Anesthesiology 1998;89(3):620–5.

87. Chopra N, Oppenheimer J, Derimanov GS, Fine PL. Vancomycin anaphylaxis and successful desensitization in a patient with end stage renal disease on hemodialysis by maintaining steady antibiotic levels. Ann Allergy Asthma Immunol 2000;84(6):633–5.

88. Duffy BL. Vancomycin reaction during spinal anaesthesia. Anaesth Intensive Care 2002;30(3):364–6.

89. Sorensen SJ, Wise SL, al-Tawfiq JA, Robb JL, Cushing HE. Successful vancomycin desensitization in a patient with end-stage renal disease and anaphylactic shock to vancomycin. Ann Pharmacother 1998;32(10):1020–3.

90. Wazny LD, Daghigh B. Desensitization protocols for vancomycin hypersensitivity. Ann Pharmacother 2001;35(11):1458–64.

91. Marshall C, Street A, Galbraith K. Glycopeptide-induced vasculitis—cross-reactivity between vancomycin and teicoplanin. J Infect 1998;37(1):82–3.

92. Midtvedt T. The ECO-SHADOW concept—a new way of following environmental impacts of antimicrobials. Heidelberg, New York: Springer-Verlag, 2001:230–6.

93. Smith TL, Pearson ML, Wilcox KR, Cruz C, Lancaster MV, Robinson-Dunn B, Tenover FC, Zervos MJ, Band JD, White E, Jarvis WR, Arduino MJ, Carr JH, Clark N, Hill B, McAllister S, Miller JM, Jennings G. Emergence of vancomycin resistance in *Staphylococcus aureus*. Glycopeptide-Intermediate Staphylococcus Aureus Working Group. N Engl J Med 1999;340(7):493–501.

94. Sieradzki K, Roberts RB, Haber SW, Tomasz A. The development of vancomycin resistance in a patient with methicillin-resistant *Staphylococcus aureus* infection. N Engl J Med 1999;340(7):517–23.

95. Waldvogel FA. New resistance in *Staphylococcus aureus*. N Engl J Med 1999;340(7):556–7.

96. Majumdar A, Lipkin GW, Eliott TS, Wheeler DC. Vancomycin-dependent enterococci in a uraemic patient with sclerosing peritonitis. Nephrol Dial Transplant 1999;14(3):765–7.

97. Bierbaum G, Fuchs K, Lenz W, Szekat C, Sahl HG. Presence of *Staphylococcus aureus* with reduced susceptibility to vancomycin in Germany. Eur J Clin Microbiol Infect Dis 1999;18(10):691–6.

98. Endtz HP, van den Braak N, Verbrugh HA, van Belkum A. Vancomycin resistance: status quo and quo vadis. Eur J Clin Microbiol Infect Dis 1999;18(10):683–90.

99. Perl TM. The threat of vancomycin resistance. Am J Med 1999;106(5A):S26–37.

100. Kuehnert MJ, Jernigan JA, Pullen AL, Rimland D, Jarvis WR. Association between mucositis severity and vancomycin-resistant enterococcal bloodstream infection in hospitalized cancer patients. Infect Control Hosp Epidemiol 1999;20(10):660–3.

101. Carmeli Y, Samore MH, Huskins C. The association between antecedent vancomycin treatment and hospital-acquired vancomycin-resistant enterococci: a meta-analysis. Arch Intern Med 1999;159(20):2461–8.

102. Ostrowsky BE, Clark NC, Thauvin-Eliopoulos C, Venkataraman L, Samore MH, Tenover FC, Eliopoulos GM, Moellering RC Jr, Gold HS. A cluster of VanD vancomycin-resistant *Enterococcus faecium*: molecular characterization and clinical epidemiology. J Infect Dis 1999;180(4):1177–85.

103. Fines M, Perichon B, Reynolds P, Sahm DF, Courvalin P. VanE, a new type of acquired glycopeptide resistance in Enterococcus faecalis BM4405. Antimicrob Agents Chemother 1999;43(9):2161–4.

104. Sieradzki K, Pinho MG, Tomasz A. Inactivated pbp4 in highly glycopeptide-resistant laboratory mutants of *Staphylococcus aureus*. J Biol Chem 1999;274(27):18942–6.

105. Van Bambeke F, Chauvel M, Reynolds PE, Fraimow HS, Courvalin P. Vancomycin-dependent *Enterococcus faecalis* clinical isolates and revertant mutants. Antimicrob Agents Chemother 1999;43(1):41–7.

106. Pavia M, Nobile CG, Salpietro L, Angelillo IF. Vancomycin resistance and antibiotic susceptibility of enterococci in raw meat. J Food Prot 2000;63(7):912–15.

107. Schouten MA, Hoogkamp-Korstanje JA, Meis JF, Voss A; European VRE Study Group. Prevalence of vancomycin-resistant enterococci in Europe. Eur J Clin Microbiol Infect Dis 2000;19(11):816–22.

108. Trakulsomboon S, Danchaivijitr S, Rongrungruang Y, Dhiraputra C, Susaemgrat W, Ito T, Hiramatsu K. First report of methicillin-resistant *Staphylococcus aureus* with reduced susceptibility to vancomycin in Thailand. J Clin Microbiol 2001;39(2):591–5.

109. Thompson CM Jr, Long SS, Gilligan PH, Prebis JW. Absorption of oral vancomycin—possible associated toxicity. Int J Pediatr Nephrol 1983;4(1):1–4.

110. Heck AJ, Bonnici PJ, Breukink E, Morris D, Wills M. Modification and inhibition of vancomycin group antibiotics by formaldehyde and acetaldehyde. Chemistry 2001;7(4):910–16.

111. Wysocki M, Delatour F, Faurisson F, Rauss A, Pean Y, Misset B, Thomas F, Timsit JF, Similowski T, Mentec H, Mier L, Dreyfuss D. Continuous versus intermittent infusion of vancomycin in severe staphylococcal infections: prospective multicenter randomized study. Antimicrob Agents Chemother 2001;45(9):2460–7.

112. Balen RM, Betts T, Ensom MHH. Vancomycin overdose in 6-month-old girl. Can J Hosp Pharm 2000;53:32–5.

113. Muller D, Hufnagel M, Suttorp M. Accidental overdose of vancomycin in preterm twins. Pediatr Infect Dis J 1999;18(8):744–5.

114. Bunchman TE, Valentini RP, Gardner J, Mottes T, Kudelka T, Maxvold NJ. Treatment of vancomycin overdose using high-efficiency dialysis membranes. Pediatr Nephrol 1999;13(9):773–4.

115. Goebel J, Ananth M, Lewy JE. Hemodiafiltration for vancomycin overdose in a neonate with end-stage renal failure. Pediatr Nephrol 1999;13(5):423–5.

116. American Academy of Clinical Toxicology; European Association of Poisons Centres and Clinical Toxicologists. Position statement and practice guidelines on the use of multi-dose activated charcoal in the treatment of acute poisoning. J Toxicol Clin Toxicol 1999;37(6):731–51.

117. Paganini H, Marin M. Caracteristicas farmacocineticas y espectro antimicrobiano de la teicoplanina. [Pharmacokinetic characteristics and antimicrobial spectrum of teicoplanin.] Medicina (B Aires) 2002;62(Suppl 2):52–5.

118. Lifshitz T, Lapid-Gortzak R, Finkelman Y, Klemperer I. Vancomycin and ceftazidime incompatibility upon intravitreal injection. Br J Ophthalmol 2000;84(1):117–18.

119. Nakamura T, Kokuryo T, Hashimoto Y, Inui KI. Effects of fosfomycin and imipenem-cilastatin on the nephrotoxicity of vancomycin and cisplatin in rats. J Pharm Pharmacol 1999;51(2):227–32.

120. Park SS, Vallar RV, Hong CH, von Gunten S, Ruoff K, D'Amico DJ. Intravitreal dexamethasone effect on intravitreal vancomycin elimination in endophthalmitis. Arch Ophthalmol 1999;117(8):1058–62.

121. Pea F, Porreca L, Baraldo M, Furlanut M. High vancomycin dosage regimens required by intensive care unit patients cotreated with drugs to improve haemodynamics following cardiac surgical procedures. J Antimicrob Chemother 2000;45(3):329–35.

122. Yeung MY, Smyth JP. Concurrent frusemide–theophylline dosing reduces serum vancomycin concentrations in preterm infants. Aust J Hosp Pharm 1999;29:269–72.

123. Ng HP, Koh KF, Tham LS. Vancomycin causes dangerous precipitation when infused with gelatin fluid. Anaesthesia 2000;55(10):1039–40.

124. Mori H, Nakajima T, Nakayama A, Yamori M, Izushi F, Gomita Y. Interaction between levofloxacin and vancomycin in rats—study of serum and organ levels. Chemotherapy 1998;44(3):181–9.

125. Symons NL, Hobbes AF, Leaver HK. Anaphylactoid reactions to vancomycin during anaesthesia: two clinical reports. Can Anaesth Soc J 1985;32(2):178–81.

126. Wilson AP. Comparative safety of teicoplanin and vancomycin. Int J Antimicrob Agents 1998;10(2):143–52.

127. MacGowan AP. Pharmacodynamics, pharmacokinetics, and therapeutic drug monitoring of glycopeptides. Ther Drug Monit 1998;20(5):473–7.

128. Freeman CD, Quintiliani R, Nightingale CH. Vancomycin therapeutic drug monitoring: is it necessary? Ann Pharmacother 1993;27(5):594–8.

129. Launay-Vacher V, Izzedine H, Mercadal L, Deray G. Clinical review: use of vancomycin in haemodialysis patients. Crit Care 2002;6(4):313–16.

130. Machado JK, Feferbaum R, Diniz EM, Okay TS, Ceccon ME, Costa Vaz FA. Monitoring the treatment of sepsis with vancomycin in term newborn infants. Rev Hosp Clin Fac Med Sao Paulo 2001;56(1):17–24.

131. Thomas MP, Steele RW. Monitoring serum vancomycin concentrations in children: is it necessary? Pediatr Infect Dis J 1998;17(4):351–3.

132. Smith PF, Morse GD. Accuracy of measured vancomycin serum concentrations in patients with end-stage renal disease. Ann Pharmacother 1999;33(12):1329–35.

133. Kim JS, Perkins RJ, Briceland LL, Tobin EH. Clinical significance of falsely elevated vancomycin concentrations in end-stage renal disease. Ann Pharmacother 1999;33(1):116–18.

134. Akil IO, Mir S. Hemodiafiltration for vancomycin overdose in a patient with end-stage renal failure. Pediatr Nephrol 2001;16(12):1019–21.

135. Foral MA, Heineman SM. Vancomycin removal during a plasma exchange transfusion. Ann Pharmacother 2001;35(11):1400–2.

Varicella vaccine

See also Vaccines

General Information

A live attenuated *Varicella* vaccine was developed in 1973 by Takahashi using the Oka strain, which was isolated from a boy with chickenpox and named after the boy. Several producers use this live vaccine strain, for example Biken Institute, Merck, Sharp & Dohme, and SmithKline Beecham. Whereas the first Oka strain vaccines needed to be stored at −20°C, subsequent reformulation of the vaccine provided a shelf-life of up to 2 years at +2°C, with immunogenicity and safety comparable to other Oka strain *Varicella* vaccines (1). The safety and efficacy of *Varicella* vaccine have been critically reviewed (2).

Non-infective uses

In an experimental model of multiple sclerosis, repeated high doses of antigen (myelin basic protein) deleted both the clinical and pathological manifestations of the disease. The effects of *Varicella* vaccine on 50 patients with chronic progressive multiple sclerosis have therefore been studied (3). The patients were immunized with *Varicella* vaccine and followed for 1 year. All were seropositive for *Varicella* before immunization and all had rises in *Varicella* antibodies after being given the vaccine. There was improvement in 14 patients, 4 became worse, and 29 were unchanged. Four patients developed mild chickenpox after immunization. No other untoward adverse effects occurred.

General adverse effects

There have been many clinical trials to assess the immunogenicity and safety of *Varicella* vaccine, in both healthy and immunocompromised individuals (SEDA-12, 285) (SEDA-13, 290) (SEDA-14, 285) (SEDA-15, 289) (SEDA-17, 379). The vaccine was safe and immunogenic. The reports of different investigators were similar. Mild local reactions at the injection site were the most commonly reported adverse effects, occurring in about 10% after the first and second dose. Vaccine-associated rashes about 1 month after the first dose were reported in about 6% of vaccinees, sore throat in 8%, and fever over 37.8°C in 2%. Rash and fever after the second dose of vaccine were reported by less than 1% of vaccinees. Maculopapular or papulovesicular rashes occurred much more often in vaccinees with suspended chemotherapy (42%) (4,5).

Oka strain *Varicella* vaccine (Merck) has been evaluated in immunocompromised children with leukemia in remission (6,7). Most children had chemotherapy stopped 1 week before and 1 week after immunization; glucocorticoids were also stopped for 3 weeks (from 1 week before to 2 weeks after immunization). *Varicella* vaccine was safe, immunogenic, and effective in leukemic children at risk of serious disease or death from chickenpox. The major adverse effect was a mild rash in 50% of the children within 1 month of immunization, about 40% of whom were treated with aciclovir. A mild form of *Varicella* developed in 14% of immunized children exposed to *Varicella* (household contacts). The vaccine protected completely against severe *Varicella*. Leukemic vaccinees were less likely to develop zoster than were comparable children with leukemia who had wild type *Varicella*.

Between 1987 and 1993, *Varicella* vaccine developed by the Biken Institute was given to 1.39 million individuals in Japan and 1.93 million individuals in South Korea. Adverse effects occurred in 6.9% of vaccinees. Despite more than 100 well-documented contacts with *Varicella* patients, only 2% of those immunized developed breakthrough *Varicella*, with very mild clinical features (8).

In 1995, live virus *Varicella* vaccine (Oka strain) was licensed in the USA. Of the 6574 reported adverse events 4% (67.5 per 100 000 doses) after immunization were serious, while the majority were minor reactions, such as rash, redness, or injection site pain (9). About 10% of immunized children developed mild chickenpox. A total 193 vaccinees reported neurological symptoms, including Bell's palsy, convulsions, and demyelinating syndromes; febrile seizures accounted for half of the cases of convulsions. There were 14 deaths, but a role for the vaccine was not proven.

Organs and Systems

Hematologic

Acute thrombocytopenic purpura developed 3 weeks after *Varicella* immunization (10).

Skin

Extensive *Varicella* vaccine-associated rashes occurred in four leukemic children; there was a relation between rash and glucocorticoid treatment (11).

Immunologic

In one case a hypersensitivity vasculitis developed 2 weeks after *Varicella* immunization (12).

Infection risk

Spread of infection to the siblings of immunized leukemic children has been observed. Between 18 and 36 days after the receipt of *Varicella* vaccine 2–10% of exposed children developed mild *Varicella* and/or seroconversion to *Varicella* virus.

Transmission of the *Varicella* vaccine virus from a toddler (with a history of allergic diathesis) to his pregnant mother has been reported and discussed (SEDA-22, 354).

Complicated wild *Varicella* in immunized individuals has been reported (13); among the two cases the first reported case of *Varicella* meningitis occurring in a child with documented immunization and seroconversion (14).

Cases of zoster both in healthy and in immunosuppressed persons have been reported (15–17).

A 19-month-old girl was immunized against *Varicella* at 15 months of age and later developed zoster infection (18). Viral cultures from various lesions isolated *Varicella zoster* virus. The Oka vaccine strain was revealed by polymerase chain reaction.

There have been three case reports of suspected reactivation of *Varicella zoster* through hepatitis A vaccine, influenza vaccine, and simultaneous administration of rabies and Japanese encephalitis vaccine (19).

- A 53-year-old woman without signs of immunodeficiency developed zoster in the left T10 dermatome 14 days after influenza immunization. The rash resolved without sequelae. Five months later she received another injection of influenza vaccine and 12 days later developed zoster in the left T1 dermatome. Recovery was prolonged.
- An 80-year-old woman with carcinoma developed long-lasting left thoracic zoster 6 days after influenza

immunization. Influenza vaccination before and after the event had no adverse effect.

- A 27-year-old man developed zoster in the second and third branches of the trigeminal nerve 1 day after immunization against rabies and Japanese encephalitis.

Zoster in childhood is unusual and probably even less common after *Varicella* immunization.

- A 6-year-old boy developed a zoster infection (with a vesicular rash in a left second thoracic dermatome pattern on his back extending to the back of his left arm) 15 days after the receipt of *Varicella* vaccine (Oka strain) (20). Molecular biological analysis of the virus isolated from the vesicles showed a pattern consistent with wild-type *Varicella zoster* virus.

The authors felt that this case mandated a careful review of all cases of zoster after *Varicella* immunization. Zoster induced by *Varicella* immunization could have implications for the use of immunization to prevent zoster in the elderly, a population with almost uniform *Varicella zoster* latent virus and at higher risk of zoster.

Susceptibility Factors

Age

In 29 children aged 1–12 years with chronic liver disease who received one dose of *Varicella* vaccine, seroconversion rates at 8 weeks after immunization were 100% (21). The geometric mean titers tended to relate to the severity of liver disease. Local and systemic reactions did not differ from reactions reported in healthy children.

- A 5-year-old boy developed zoster-like vesicular lesions 4 years after *Varicella* immunization. Virological examination showed *Herpes simplex* virus type 1, and so the vesicular lesions could not be attributed to the *Varicella zoster* virus vaccine strain, demonstrating the difficulty in confirming causality between time-related events (22).

Other features of the patient

To determine the safety and immunogenicity of *Varicella* immunization in HIV-infected children, 41 children (aged 1–8 years) who were asymptomatic or mildly affected (according to CDC stages) received two doses of live attenuated *Varicella* vaccine 12 weeks apart (23). Two months after the second dose, 60% of the recipients had anti-*Varicella* antibody in their serum. A minority of recipients developed mild local or systemic reactions. The immunization had no effect on the clinical stage of HIV infection or the HIV RNA plasma load.

Live virus vaccines, such as *Varicella*, are contraindicated in pregnancy.

Drug–Drug Interactions

Other vaccines

Reaction rates were not increased if the administration of *Varicella* vaccine was combined with other vaccines, for example MMR vaccine (SEDA-15, 358).

References

1. Tan AY, Connett CJ, Connett GJ, Quek SC, Yap HK, Meurice F, Lee BW. Use of a reformulated Oka strain varicella vaccine (SmithKline Beecham Biologicals/Oka) in healthy children. Eur J Pediatr 1996;155(8):706–11.
2. Skull SA, Wang EE. Varicella vaccination—a critical review of the evidence. Arch Dis Child 2001;85(2):83–90.
3. Ross RT, Nicolle LE, Cheang M. The *Varicella zoster* virus: a pilot trial of a potential therapeutic agent in multiple sclerosis. J Clin Epidemiol 1997;50(1):63–8.
4. Gershon AA, Steinberg SP, LaRussa P, Ferrara A, Hammerschlag M, Gelb L. Immunization of healthy adults with live attenuated *Varicella* vaccine. J Infect Dis 1988;158(1):132–7.
5. Gershon AA, Steinberg SP, Gelb L. Live attenuated *Varicella* vaccine use in immunocompromised children and adults. Pediatrics 1986;78(4 Pt 2):757–62.
6. Gershon AA, LaRussa P, Steinberg S. The *Varicella* vaccine. Clinical trials in immunocompromised individuals. Infect Dis Clin North Am 1996;10(3):583–94.
7. LaRussa P, Steinberg S, Gershon AA. *Varicella* vaccine for immunocompromised children: results of collaborative studies in the United States and Canada. J Infect Dis 1996;174(Suppl 3):S320–3.
8. Asano Y. *Varicella* vaccine: the Japanese experience. J Infect Dis 1996;174(Suppl 3):S310–13.
9. Wise RP, Salive ME, Braun MM, Mootrey GT, Seward JF, Rider LG, Krause PR. Postlicensure safety surveillance for *Varicella* vaccine. JAMA 2000;284(10):1271–9.
10. Lee SY, Komp DM, Andiman W. Thrombocytopenic purpura following *Varicella-zoster* vaccination. Am J Pediatr Hematol Oncol 1986;8(1):78–80.
11. Lydick E, Kuter BJ, Zajac BA, Guess HA. Association of steroid therapy with vaccine-associated rashes in children with acute lymphocytic leukaemia who received Oka/Merck *Varicella* vaccine. NIAID Varicella Vaccine Collaborative Study Group. Vaccine 1989;7(6):549–53.
12. Fraunfelder FW, Rosenbaum JT. Drug-induced uveitis. Incidence, prevention and treatment. Drug Saf 1997;17(3):197–207.
13. Pillai JJ, Gaughan WJ, Watson B, Sivalingam JJ, Murphey SA. Renal involvement in association with post-vaccination *Varicella*. Clin Infect Dis 1993;17(6):1079–80.
14. Naruse H, Miwata H, Ozaki T, Asano Y, Namazue J, Yamanishi K. *Varicella* infection complicated with meningitis after immunization. Acta Paediatr Jpn 1993;35(4):345–7.
15. Plotkin SA, Starr SE, Connor K, Morton D. Zoster in normal children after *Varicella* vaccine. J Infect Dis 1989;159(5):1000–1.
16. Hammerschlag MR, Gershon AA, Steinberg SP, Clarke L, Gelb LD. Herpes zoster in an adult recipient of live attenuated *Varicella* vaccine. J Infect Dis 1989;160(3):535–7.
17. Magrath DI. Prospective vaccines for national immunization programmes. In: Proceedings, 3rd Meeting of National Programme Managers on Expanded Programme on Immunization, St Vincent, Italy, 22–25 May 1990. ICP/EPI 023/31, 1990.
18. Liang MG, Heidelberg KA, Jacobson RM, McEvoy MT. Herpes zoster after *Varicella* immunization. J Am Acad Dermatol 1998;38(5 Pt 1):761–3.
19. Walter R, Hartmann K, Fleisch F, Reinhart WH, Kuhn M. Reactivation of herpesvirus infections after vaccinations? Lancet 1999;353(9155):810.
20. Kohl S, Rapp J, La Russa P, Gershon AA, Steinberg SP. Natural *Varicella-zoster* virus reactivation shortly after varicella immunization in a child. Pediatr Infect Dis J 1999;18(12):1112–13.

21. Nithichaiyo C, Chongsrisawat V, Hutagalung Y, Bock HL, Poovorawa Y. Immunogenicity and adverse effects of live attenuated *Varicella* vaccine (Oka-strain) in children with chronic liver disease. Asian Pac J Allergy Immunol 2001;19(2):101–5.
22. Takayama N, Takayama M, Takita J. *Herpes simplex* mimicking *Herpes zoster* in a child immunized with *Varicella* vaccine. Pediatr Infect Dis J 2001;20(2):226–8.
23. Levin MJ, Gershon AA, Weinberg A, Blanchard S, Nowak B, Palumbo P, Chan CY; AIDS Clinical Trials Group 265 Team. Immunization of HIV-infected children with *Varicella* vaccine. J Pediatr 2001; 139(2):305–10.

Vasopressin and analogues

See also Individual agents

General Information

Vasopressin, a hypothalamic octapeptide that is secreted by the neurohypophysis, has both antidiuretic and vasoconstrictor properties. Its short half-life (about 10 minutes) necessitates continuous intravenous infusion or frequent nasal application.

Because its vasoconstrictor effects limit the use of the native hormone, analogues with greater or lesser affinity for vasopressin V_2 receptors and more selective antidiuretic effects have been developed:

- argipressin (8-arginine vasopressin)
- desmopressin (*N*-deamino-8-D-arginine vasopressin, DDAVP); desmopressin is covered in a separate monograph
- felypressin (2-phenylalanine, 8-lysine vasopressin)
- lypressin (8-lysine vasopressin; pig vasopressin)
- ornipressin (8-onithine vasopressin)
- terlipressin (triglycyl-lysine vasopressin).

Vasopressin receptor antagonists, such as relcovaptan (an antagonist at V_{1a} receptors), lixivaptan and tolvaptan (V_2), and conivaptan (mixed V_{1a}/V_2), are also under development (1).

Desmopressin has little vasoconstrictor effect but has potent antidiuretic action, through renal vasopressin V_2 receptors, and at high doses hemostatic properties, by increasing concentrations of factor VIII and von Willebrand factor in the blood.

Ornipressin is a selective agonist at vasopressin V_1 receptors and has weaker antidiuretic activity than the native hormone.

Terlipressin, a long-acting vasopressin analogue, is metabolized to the active drug lysine vasopressin. The use of terlipressin to treat acute variceal bleeding has been reviewed (2,3).

Although vasopressin and its analogues have been used in the acute management of bleeding esophageal varices, they do not reduce mortality (2,3) and the rate of adverse effects is higher than with octreotide (3).

Uterine and abdominal cramps, nausea, and an urge to defecate have been reported in vasopressin-treated patients.

Organs and Systems

Cardiovascular

Dose-related adverse effects of vasopressin include skin pallor, hypertension, cardiac dysrhythmias, and myocardial ischemia or infarction; treatment has to be stopped in 20–30% of patients because of these effects (3).

Intestinal and peripheral vasoconstriction can follow prolonged infusion, resulting in gangrene of intestinal segments or of skin, fingers, or limbs. This has been fatal in several cases, and vasopressin should be withdrawn if skin necrosis occurs (SEDA-13, 1310) (4).

Of 10 patients with hepatorenal syndrome one had to be withdrawn 2 hours after receiving 12 units of ornipressin (6 IU/hour) because of a ventricular tachydysrhythmia, and an infusion of dopamine 2–3 micrograms/kg/minute was started (5).

Terlipressin has similar, but less pronounced, systemic hemodynamic effects to vasopressin, including increases in mean arterial pressure and reduced heart rate (6). Of 105 patients who had continuous terlipressin infusions for variceal bleeding in a multicenter study, lower limb ischemia developed in two and cardiac ischemia in one (7).

Of 86 cirrhotic patients treated with terlipressin 10 developed a tachycardia, four developed atrial fibrillation, and one developed ventricular tachycardia. Four patients in the same study developed hypertension (8). In another study, tachycardia occurred in 23% of patients randomized to pitressin for acute variceal bleeding and 8% developed transient hypertension (9).

Myocardial ischemia has been associated with terlipressin (10).

- A 61-year-old man with coronary artery stenosis became hypotensive during elective surgery, refractory to ephedrine (cumulative dose of 36 mg over 45 minutes). Immediately after terlipressin 1 mg, he developed hypertension and bradycardia, with evidence of myocardial ischemia.

One of 21 patients with hepatorenal syndrome developed finger ischemia on the fourth day of intermittent intravenous terlipressin and recovered after terlipressin was stopped (11).

Respiratory

An elderly patient (over 70 years old) with cirrhosis and hepatorenal syndrome developed severe bronchospasm and died after intravenous terlipressin administration; the mechanism was not determined (12).

Electrolyte balance

Profound hyponatremia due to reduced free water clearance is a predictable dose-related effect of vasopressin (13). This is a particular risk in patients who are unconscious or who have disturbed thirst sensation (SEDA-22, 487).

Of 105 patients who had continuous infusions of terlipressin for variceal bleeding in a multicenter study, four developed hyponatremia, severe in one case (7).

High-dose terlipressin (1 mg intravenously every 4 hours for 5 days) was associated with severe hyponatremia and loss of consciousness in one of 45 cirrhotic patients in a randomized trial (8). Of course, cirrhosis itself is associated with hyponatremia.

Hematologic

Mild lymphangitis was reported in one of 105 patients in a multicenter study of the effects of terlipressin (7).

Gastrointestinal

Tongue ischemia and ischemic colitis have been described after 4–9 days of treatment with ornipressin 6 IU/hour combined with plasma volume expansion (14).

Skin

Skin necrosis is often reported after vasopressin therapy. In a retrospective study, two of five patients treated with a continuous infusion of terlipressin developed skin necrosis at the infusion site and a third developed scrotal necrosis (12).

- A 46-year-old woman with septic shock had a peripheral venous infusion of vasopressin 0.04 U/minute in addition to dobutamine, via the subclavian vein; extravasation of vasopressin to local soft tissue resulted in ischemic skin necrosis (15).

Purpuric skin necrosis, due to local vasoconstriction, has been reported in 19 patients within a few days of starting vasopressin infusion (16).

Bullous necrosis developed within 48 hours of starting an infusion of terlipressin in a 44-year-old man (17). There have been only four previous reports of skin necrosis.

Musculoskeletal

Rhabdomyolysis has been attributed to terlipressin (18).

- A 36-year-old man with nephrotic syndrome was given an infusion of terlipressin (an intravenous bolus of 2 mg followed by 2 mg over 24 hours) to treat diffuse gastric bleeding, and 12 hours later developed acute pain and livedo reticularis in both legs. High plasma concentrations of myoglobin and creatine kinase confirmed the diagnosis of toxic rhabdomyolysis, thought to be due to the vasoconstrictor action of terlipressin. He made a gradual recovery over the next few weeks after terlipressin was withdrawn.

Pre-existing blood vessel disease due to amyloidosis may have contributed to the outcome in this patient.

References

1. Serradeil-Le Gal C, Wagnon J, Valette G, Garcia G, Pascal M, Maffrand JP, Le Fur G. Nonpeptide vasopressin receptor antagonists: development of selective and orally active V1a, V2 and V1b receptor ligands. Prog Brain Res 2002;139:197–210.
2. Avgerinos A. Approach to the management of bleeding esophageal varices: role of somatostatin. Digestion 1998;59(Suppl 1):1–22.
3. Burroughs AK, Planas R, Svoboda P. Optimizing emergency care of upper gastrointestinal bleeding in cirrhotic patients. Scand J Gastroenterol Suppl 1998;226:14–24.
4. Moreno-Sanchez D, Casis B, Martin A, Ortiz P, Castellano G, Munoz MT, Vanaclocha F, Solis-Herruzo JA. Rhabdomyolysis and cutaneous necrosis following intravenous vasopressin infusion. Gastroenterology 1991;101(2):529–32.
5. Gulberg V, Bilzer M, Gerbes AL. Long-term therapy and retreatment of hepatorenal syndrome type 1 with ornipressin and dopamine. Hepatology 1999;30(4):870–5.
6. Romero G, Kravetz D, Argonz J, Bildozola M, Suarez A, Terg R. Terlipressin is more effective in decreasing variceal pressure than portal pressure in cirrhotic patients. J Hepatol 2000;32(3):419–25.
7. Escorsell A, Ruiz del Arbol L, Planas R, Albillos A, Banares R, Cales P, Pateron D, Bernard B, Vinel JP, Bosch J. Multicenter randomized controlled trial of terlipressin versus sclerotherapy in the treatment of acute variceal bleeding: the TEST study. Hepatology 2000; 32(3):471–6.
8. Bruha R, Marecek Z, Spicak J, Hulek P, Lata J, Petrtyl J, Urbanek P, Taimr P, Volfova M, Dite P. Double-blind randomized, comparative multicenter study of the effect of terlipressin in the treatment of acute esophageal variceal and/or hypertensive gastropathy bleeding. Hepatogastroenterology 2002;49(46):1161–6.
9. Zhang HB, Wong BC, Zhou XM, Guo XG, Zhao SJ, Wang JH, Wu KC, Ding J, Lam SK, Fan DM. Effects of somatostatin, octreotide and pitressin plus nitroglycerine on systemic and portal haemodynamics in the control of acute variceal bleeding. Int J Clin Pract 2002; 56(6):447–51.
10. Medel J, Boccara G, Van de Steen E, Bertrand M, Godet G, Coriat P. Terlipressin for treating intraoperative hypotension: can it unmask myocardial ischemia? Anesth Analg 2001;93(1):53–5.
11. Ortega R, Gines P, Uriz J, Cardenas A, Calahorra B, De Las Heras D, Guevara M, Bataller R, Jimenez W, Arroyo V, Rodes J. Terlipressin therapy with and without albumin for patients with hepatorenal syndrome: results of a prospective, nonrandomized study. Hepatology 2002; 36(4 Pt 1):941–8.
12. Halimi C, Bonnard P, Bernard B, Mathurin P, Mofredj A, di Martino V, Demontis R, Henry-Biabaud E, Fievet P, Opolon P, Poynard T, Cadranel JF. Effect of terlipressin (Glypressin) on hepatorenal syndrome in cirrhotic patients: results of a multicentre pilot study. Eur J Gastroenterol Hepatol 2002; 14(2):153–8.
13. Robson WL, Norgaard JP, Leung AK. Hyponatremia in patients with nocturnal enuresis treated with DDAVP. Eur J Pediatr 1996;155(11):959–62.
14. Crowther CA, Hiller JE, Haslam RR, Robinson JS. Australian Collaborative Trial of Antenatal Thyrotropin-Releasing Hormone: adverse effects at 12-month follow-up. ACTOBAT Study Group. Pediatrics 1997; 99(3):311–17.
15. Kahn JM, Kress JP, Hall JB. Skin necrosis after extravasation of low-dose vasopressin administered for septic shock. Crit Care Med 2002;30(8):1899–901.
16. Lemlich G, Di Grandi S, Szaniawski WK. Cutaneous reaction to vasopressin. Cutis 1996;57(5):330–2.
17. Tomassini E, Guiot P, Poussel JF, De Cubber J, Schnitzler B. Bullous disease following intravenous terlipressin infusion. Reanim Urgences 2000;9:313–14.
18. Rolla D, Cannella G, Ravetti JL. Toxic rhabdomyolysis induced by terlipressin infusion in a uraemic patient suffering from AA-type amyloidosis. Nephron 1999; 83(2):167–8.

Vecuronium bromide

See also Neuromuscular blocking drugs

General Information

Vecuronium is a monoquaternary analogue of pancuronium, with a similar speed of onset, a duration of action of 15–30 minutes, rapid spontaneous recovery, and virtually no cumulative effects (1). Being monoquaternary, it is more lipophilic than pancuronium. About 30% is bound to plasma proteins. It is deacetylated in the liver, the principal metabolite being 3-desacetylvecuronium, which is believed to have about 50% of the neuromuscular blocking potency of the parent drug in man; small amounts of 17-desacetyl-vecuronium and 3,17-didesacetylvecuronium are also formed. In balanced anesthesia vecuronium is slightly more potent than pancuronium, but during halothane anesthesia it has been reported to be 1.4 times as potent as the latter. Suitable doses during balanced anesthesia are similar to those for pancuronium; potentiation by volatile agents (2) allows these doses to be reduced, after equilibration has occurred between the volatile agent and the tissues, by 25 or 45% when halothane or enflurane are used (3,4). In another study, after 1 hour of constant 90% neuromuscular blockade under nitrous oxide (60%), isoflurane (1.2% end-tidal), or enflurane (1.2% end-tidal) anesthesia the vecuronium infusion requirements were reduced by as much as 70% (compared with the nitrous oxide/fentanyl group) (SEDA-13, 105) (5).

In animals, histamine release, cholinesterase inhibition, and autonomic effects are minimal and occur only at concentrations of vecuronium considerably greater than those required for neuromuscular block (6–9). Interactions with antimicrobial drugs, analgesics, and anesthetic agents were similar to those known for other non-depolarizing relaxants, apart from a possible potentiating effect by metronidazole (6). These animal findings have been confirmed in man by the relative paucity of reported adverse effects. In man, the intradermal injection of vecuronium produces a considerably smaller local histamine reaction than d-tubocurarine, metocurine, pancuronium, or atracurium do (10,11) and plasma histamine is not raised in the clinical dose range (12,13). Nevertheless, minor skin reactions have been reported (14,15), as well as hypotension (16) and severe anaphylactoid reactions with circulatory collapse (17,18) and bronchospasm (19,20). Cross-sensitivity with pancuronium may occur (SEDA-10, 111).

Organs and Systems

Cardiovascular

The expected cardiovascular stability of vecuronium has been confirmed in man (2,21–23). Even doses as large as 0.28 mg/kg in patients undergoing coronary artery bypass grafting produced negligible effects (24). Bradycardia is the only cardiovascular adverse effect reported, and this is seen in association with opioids such as fentanyl (25) and sufentanil (SEDA-11, 125) (26) or other drugs that are themselves capable of producing bradycardia. The lack of vagolytic and sympathomimetic activity of vecuronium

means that it does not counteract the bradycardia or the hypotensive effects of other drugs or surgical manipulations. It is an ideal relaxant for patients with pheochromocytoma (27).

Musculoskeletal

Masseter muscle rigidity is a rare but potentially dangerous adverse effect of suxamethonium and can prevent successful airway management. Furthermore, it can be the first sign of malignant hyperthermia and rhabdomyolysis. Non-depolarizing neuromuscular blocking agents are thought to be safe with regard to masseter muscle rigidity. However, masseter muscle rigidity not associated with the use of suxamethonium can also complicate airway management (28).

- A 42-year-old woman had anesthesia induced with propofol 200 mg, vecuronium 8 mg, and mask ventilation with oxygen, nitrous oxide, and 2% isoflurane. Laryngoscopy proved impossible because of spasm of the masseter muscles, and the airway was secured by blind nasal intubation. There was no evidence of rigidity of other muscle groups. Body temperature and end-tidal carbon dioxide concentration remained in the reference ranges. Masseter muscle rigidity persisted throughout the operation and resolved during recovery from anesthesia after neostigmine 2.5 mg had been given.

The authors suggested that in this case the phenomenon had been caused by vecuronium. Masseter muscle rigidity persisted during anesthesia and resolved during recovery from anesthesia after neostigmine had been given and isoflurane inhalation had been stopped. If vecuronium caused muscle rigidity in this case it was probably not mediated by effects on acetylcholine receptors, but rather by an interaction of vecuronium with ion channels (sodium, potassium, and/or calcium), but it is hard to imagine how this effect could have been antagonized by a cholinesterase inhibitor. It therefore seems likely that the masseter muscle rigidity was rather caused by isoflurane, which would explain why the symptoms improved after withdrawal of isoflurane. There have been previous reports of masseter muscle rigidity associated with non-depolarizing neuromuscular blocking agents (SEDA-21, 144) (29,30). The mechanism is unclear. One wonders how muscle specimens from these patients might react to exposure to an inhalational anesthetic during in vitro contracture testing. Regarding the link between masseter muscle rigidity and malignant hyperthermia, muscle biopsy would not be inappropriate in patients who have masseter muscle rigidity severe enough to prevent mouth opening and conventional orotracheal intubation.

Second-Generation Effects

Fetotoxicity

There is placental transfer of vecuronium, but no effects have been detected in the newborn (the feto-maternal concentration ratio is about 10% less than for pancuronium (31). Postpartum, vecuronium has been reported to have an appreciably longer duration of action (SEDA-13, 105) (32,33) when given in a dose of 0.1 mg/kg.

Susceptibility Factors

Age

Spontaneous recovery of neuromuscular function after a bolus dose of vecuronium (0.1 mg/kg) was significantly prolonged in elderly patients compared with younger adults (SEDA-17, 153). The elimination half-life was significantly prolonged (125 versus 78 minutes) and the plasma clearance reduced (2.5 versus 5.6 ml/kg/minute) in the elderly versus the younger patients.

Renal disease

About 25–30% of an injected dose of vecuronium is excreted in the urine in normal patients, mostly as unchanged drug. Renal dysfunction has been reported as having no significant effect on the duration of action of vecuronium (SEDA-11, 125) (34–36). Nevertheless, slight resistance to the neuromuscular blocking effect of an initial dose (ED_{50} increased by 20%) and a small reduction (of 23%) in infusion requirements to maintain a 90% block after 1 hour of relaxation have been described in end-stage renal insufficiency (SEDA-13, 103) (37). These findings are in line with those for other non-depolarizing agents, with the exception of atracurium; the changes, however, are minor compared with the older relaxants, as is to be expected from the kinetics of vecuronium. There is a slight tendency for the action of vecuronium to be prolonged in renal insufficiency, and monitoring of neuromuscular transmission is advisable if several doses are to be given.

Hepatic disease

In liver disease (cirrhosis and cholestasis), the plasma clearance of vecuronium is reduced, its half-life is increased, and its duration of action is prolonged (SEDA-10, 112) (38,39). Rapid uptake in the liver appears to be an important factor in its plasma clearance and in determining its relatively short duration of action; it is estimated that about 40% of the injected drug is excreted via the bile (40). Prolongation of the action of large single doses and accumulation after repeated doses are therefore to be expected in liver disease.

Drug–Drug Interactions

Azathioprine

In humans with renal insufficiency, azathioprine 3 mg/kg produced a negligible and transient reduction in neuromuscular blockade maintained by infusion of vecuronium (37).

Carbamazepine

Resistance to vecuronium has been described in patients taking carbamazepine (41).

Ciclosporin

Ciclosporin can cause considerable prolongation of the neuromuscular paralysis induced by vecuronium (42),

causing difficulties with reversal (SEDA-14, 116) (43). Potentiation of vecuronium in cats has also been described (SEDA-12, 188) (44).

Disopyramide

Disopyramide has also been associated with impairment of neostigmine antagonism of vecuronium-induced neuromuscular blockade (45).

- A 63-year-old man was given vecuronium 70 µg/kg followed by increments of 20 µg/kg, and three intravenous doses of disopyramide 10 mg for supraventricular extra beats, followed by an infusion of 25 mg/hour. Paralysis was reversed using atropine 0.75 mg and neostigmine 2.5 mg. The twitch height returned to normal and the train-of-four was above 85%, but the responses to tetanic stimulation at 100 and 50 Hz remained severely depressed (10 and 45% respectively). The plasma concentration of disopyramide was 5.1 µg/ml.

Phenytoin

Acute administration of phenytoin (10 mg/kg intravenously) has been reported to enhance slightly, but statistically significantly, steady blockade maintained by an infusion of vecuronium (SEDA-15, 124) (46). This is in contrast to reports of resistance to non-depolarizing neuromuscular blocking agents, including vecuronium, associated with long-term phenytoin (SEDA-13, 104) (47).

Testosterone

Testosterone enanthate, given over 10 years to produce virilization, has been claimed to have been responsible for a case of marked resistance to vecuronium (SEDA-14, 116) (48).

References

1. Miller RD, Rupp SM, Fisher DM, Cronnelly R, Fahey MR, Sohn YJ. Clinical pharmacology of vecuronium and atracurium. Anesthesiology 1984;61(4):444–53.
2. Mirakhur RK, Ferres CJ, Clarke RS, Bali IM, Dundee JW. Clinical evaluation of Org NC 45. Br J Anaesth 1983;55(2):119–24.
3. Foldes FF, Bencini A, Newton D. Influence of halothane and enflurane on the neuromuscular effects of ORG NC 45 in man. Br J Anaesth 1980;52(Suppl 1):S64–5.
4. Ording H, Viby-Mogensen J. Dose response curves for Org NC 45 and pancuronium. Acta Anaesthesiol Scand 1981;25(Suppl 72):73.
5. Cannon JE, Fahey MR, Castagnoli KP, Furuta T, Canfell PC, Sharma M, Miller RD. Continuous infusion of vecuronium: the effect of anesthetic agents. Anesthesiology 1987;67(4):503–6.
6. McIndewar IC, Marshall RJ. Interactions between the neuromuscular blocking drug Org NC 45 and some anaesthetic, analgesic and antimicrobial agents. Br J Anaesth 1981;53(8):785–92.
7. Son SL, Waud BE, Waud DR. A comparison of the neuromuscular blocking and vagolytic effects of ORG NC45 and pancuronium. Anesthesiology 1981;55(1):12–18.
8. Durant NN, Marshall IG, Savage DS, Nelson DJ, Sleigh T, Carlyle IC. The neuromuscular and autonomic blocking activities of pancuronium, Org NC 45, and other

pancuronium analogues, in the cat. J Pharm Pharmacol 1979;31(12):831–6.

9. Marshall RJ, McGrath JC, Miller RD, Docherty JR, Lamar JC. Comparison of the cardiovascular actions of ORG NC 45 with those produced by other non-depolarizing neuromuscular blocking agents in experimental animals. Br J Anaesth 1980;52(Suppl 1):S21–32.

10. Booij LH, Krieg N, Crul JF. Intradermal histamine releasing effect caused by Org-NC 45. A comparison with pancuronium, metocurine and d-tubocurarine Acta Anaesthesiol Scand 1980;24(5):393–4.

11. Robertson EN, Booij LH, Fragen RJ, Crul JF. Intradermal histamine release by 3 muscle relaxants. Acta Anaesthesiol Scand 1983;27(3):203–5.

12. Basta SJ, Savarese JJ, Ali HH, et al. Vecuronium does not alter serum histamine within the clinical dose range. Anesthesiology 1983;59:A273.

13. Goudsouzian NG, Young ET, Moss J, Liu LM. Histamine release during the administration of atracurium or vecuronium in children. Br J Anaesth 1986;58(11):1229–33.

14. Clayton DG, Watkins J. Histamine release with vecuronium. Anaesthesia 1984;39(11):1143–4.

15. Spence AG, Barnetson RS. Reaction to vecuronium bromide. Lancet 1985;1(8435):979–80.

16. Lavery GG, Hewitt AJ, Kenny NT. Possible histamine release after vecuronium. Anaesthesia 1985;40(4):389–90.

17. Thacker MA, Boon von Ochssee D. Anaphylactoid reaction to vecuronium. Anaesth Intensive Care 1988;16(1):129–30.

18. Treuren BC, Buckley DH. Anaphylactoid reaction to vecuronium. Br J Anaesth 1990;64(1):125–6.

19. Conil C, Bornet JL, Jean-Noel M, Conil JM, Brouchet A. Choc anaphylactique au pancuronium et au vécuronium. [Anaphylactic shock caused by pancuronium and vecuronium.] Ann Fr Anesth Reanim 1985;4(2):241–3.

20. Holt AW, Vedig AE. Anaphylaxis following vecuronium. Anaesth Intensive Care 1988;16(3):378–9.

21. Barnes PK, Smith GB, White WD, Tennant R. Comparison of the effects of Org NC 45 and pancuronium bromide on heart rate and arterial pressure in anaesthetized man. Br J Anaesth 1982;54(4):435–9.

22. Gregoretti SM, Sohn YJ, Sia RL. Heart rate and blood pressure changes after ORG NC45 (vecuronium) and pancuronium during halothane and enflurane anesthesia. Anesthesiology 1982;56(5):392–5.

23. Lienhart A, Desnault H, Guggiari M, et al. Vecuronium bromide: dose response curve and haemodynamic effects in anaesthetized man. In: Agoston S, editor. Clinical Experiences with Norcuron. Amsterdam: Excerpta Medica, 1982:46.

24. Morris RB, Cahalan MK, Miller RD, Wilkinson PL, Quasha AL, Robinson SL. The cardiovascular effects of vecuronium (ORG NC45) and pancuronium in patients undergoing coronary artery bypass grafting. Anesthesiology 1983;58(5):438–40.

25. Salmenpera M, Peltola K, Takkunen O, Heinonen J. Cardiovascular effects of pancuronium and vecuronium during high-dose fentanyl anesthesia. Anesth Analg 1983;62(12):1059–64.

26. Starr NJ, Sethna DH, Estafanous FG. Bradycardia and asystole following the rapid administration of sufentanil with vecuronium. Anesthesiology 1986;64(4):521–3.

27. Gencarelli PJ, Roizen MF, Miller RD, Joyce J, Hunt TK, Tyrrell JB. ORG NC45 (Norcuron) and pheochromocytoma: a report of three cases. Anesthesiology 1981;55(6):690–3.

28. Jenkins JG. Masseter muscle rigidity after vecuronium. Eur J Anaesthesiol 1999;16(2):137–9.

29. Polta TA, Hanisch EC Jr, Nasser JG, Ramsborg GC, Roelofs RI. Masseter spasm after pancuronium. Anesth Analg 1980;59(7):509–11.

30. Albrecht A, Wedel DJ, Gronert GA. Masseter muscle rigidity and nondepolarizing neuromuscular blocking agents. Mayo Clin Proc 1997;72(4):329–32.

31. Demetriou M, Depoix JP, Diakite B, Fromentin M, Duvaldestin P. Placental transfer of org nc 45 in women undergoing Caesarean section. Br J Anaesth 1982;54(6):643–5.

32. Hawkins JL, Adenwala J, Camp C, Joyce TH 3rd. The effect of H2-receptor antagonist premedication on the duration of vecuronium-induced neuromuscular blockade in postpartum patients. Anesthesiology 1989;71(2):175–7.

33. Camp CE, Tessem J, Adenwala J, Joyce TH 3rd. Vecuronium and prolonged neuromuscular blockade in postpartum patients. Anesthesiology 1987;67(6):1006–8.

34. Fahey MR, Morris RB, Miller RD, Nguyen TL, Upton RA. Pharmacokinetics of Org NC45 (Norcuron) in patients with and without renal failure. Br J Anaesth 1981;53(10):1049–53.

35. Bencini AF, Scaf AH, Sohn YJ, Meistelman C, Lienhart A, Kersten UW, Schwarz S, Agoston S. Disposition and urinary excretion of vecuronium bromide in anesthetized patients with normal renal function or renal failure. Anesth Analg 1986;65(3):245–51.

36. Bevan DR, Donati F, Gyasi H, Williams A. Vecuronium in renal failure. Can Anaesth Soc J 1984;31(5):491–6.

37. Gramstad L. Atracurium, vecuronium and pancuronium in end-stage renal failure. Dose-response properties and interactions with azathioprine. Br J Anaesth 1987;59(8):995–1003.

38. Lebrault C, Berger JL, D'Hollander AA, Gomeni R, Henzel D, Duvaldestin P. Pharmacokinetics and pharmacodynamics of vecuronium (ORG NC 45) in patients with cirrhosis. Anesthesiology 1985;62(5):601–5.

39. Lebrault C, Duvaldestin P, Henzel D, Chauvin M, Guesnon P. Pharmacokinetics and pharmacodynamics of vecuronium in patients with cholestasis. Br J Anaesth 1986;58(9):983–7.

40. Bencini AF, Scaf AH, Sohn YJ, Kersten-Kleef UW, Agoston S. Hepatobiliary disposition of vecuronium bromide in man. Br J Anaesth 1986;58(9):988–95.

41. Ebrahim Z, Bulkley R, Roth S. Carbamazepine therapy and neuromuscular blockade with atracurium and vecuronium. Anesth Analg 1988;67:555.

42. Crosby E, Robblee JA. Cyclosporine–pancuronium interaction in a patient with a renal allograft. Can J Anaesth 1988;35(3 Pt 1):300–2.

43. Wood GG. Cyclosporine-vecuronium interaction. Can J Anaesth 1989;36(3 Pt 1):358.

44. Gramstad L, Gjerlow JA, Hysing ES, Rugstad HE. Interaction of cyclosporin and its solvent, Cremophor, with atracurium and vecuronium. Studies in the cat. Br J Anaesth 1986;58(10):1149–55.

45. Baurain M, Barvais L, d'Hollander A, Hennart D. Impairment of the antagonism of vecuronium-induced paralysis and intra-operative disopyramide administration. Anaesthesia 1989;44(1):34–6.

46. Gray HS, Slater RM, Pollard BJ. The effect of acutely administered phenytoin on vecuronium-induced neuromuscular blockade. Anaesthesia 1989;44(5):379–81.

47. Ornstein E, Matteo RS, Schwartz AE, Silverberg PA, Young WL, Diaz J. The effect of phenytoin on the magnitude and duration of neuromuscular block following atracurium or vecuronium. Anesthesiology 1987;67(2):191–6.

48. Reddy P, Guzman A, Robalino J, Shevde K. Resistance to muscle relaxants in a patient receiving prolonged testosterone therapy. Anesthesiology 1989;70(5):871–3.

Venlafaxine

See also Antidepressants, second-generation

General Information

Venlafaxine inhibits the re-uptake of both serotonin and noradrenaline. Trials have shown efficacy comparable to that of tricyclic antidepressants, and it may be particularly effective in refractory depression (1)(2).

Reported adverse effects were nausea, somnolence, dry mouth, insomnia, dizziness, constipation, weakness, nervousness, and sweating. Other adverse effects include nervousness, weight loss, and a dose-dependent increase in blood pressure.

Because of its serotonin-potentiating effect, venlafaxine can cause a serotonin syndrome when combined with monoamine oxidase (MAO) inhibitors (SEDA-20, 9) (SEDA-21, 13).

Adverse sexual effects are reported in a frequency similar to that of SSRIs (SEDA-20, 9).

Withdrawal reactions have been reported in several cases after abrupt discontinuation (SEDA-21, 13) (3)(4).

Preliminary data suggest that venlafaxine is safer in acute overdose than tricyclic antidepressants but more dangerous than SSRIs. Seizures have been reported in several cases of overdose (5–7).

Organs and Systems

Cardiovascular

A meta-analysis of the effect of venlafaxine on blood pressure in patients studied in randomized placebo-controlled trials of venlafaxine, imipramine, and placebo showed that at the end of the acute phase (6 weeks) the incidence of a sustained rise in supine diastolic blood pressure (over 90 mmHg) was significantly higher in both active treatment groups: venlafaxine 4.8% (135/2817), imipramine 4.7% (15/319), and placebo 2.1% (13/605) (8). The effect of venlafaxine in causing a rise in diastolic blood pressure appeared to be dose related, with an incidence of 1.7% in patients taking under 100 mg/day and 9.1% in those taking over 300 mg/day.

These data confirm that venlafaxine, particularly in higher dosages, can significantly increase blood pressure. At high doses, venlafaxine inhibits the re-uptake of noradrenaline as well as that of serotonin, which probably accounts for the pressor effect.

In physically healthy subjects venlafaxine has a generally benign cardiovascular profile, although hypotension and dose-related hypertension have been reported (SEDA-23, 20).

Venlafaxine is often used in high doses in patients with treatment-resistant depression. If there is continuing failure to respond, electroconvulsive therapy might be used, often in combination with venlafaxine. A 73-year-old woman taking venlafaxine (112.5 mg/day) had sustained hypertension for several hours after her first treatment (9). However, electroconvulsive therapy can cause transient hypertension, and the patient had essential hypertension controlled by bendroflumethiazide. It is therefore possible that the reaction might have occurred had she not been taking venlafaxine. Nevertheless, the fact that venlafaxine can cause hypertension when used as sole treatment suggests that blood pressure should be monitored carefully in patients receiving electroconvulsive therapy and venlafaxine together, particularly if there is a history or current evidence of hypertension.

Venlafaxine has not been studied systematically in patients with cardiovascular disease, although there are reports that older patients can have clinically significant disturbances of cardiac rhythm (10).

- A 69-year-old woman with stable angina and mild single-vessel coronary artery disease developed acute myocardial ischemia within a week of starting venlafaxine (75 mg/day).

Taken together with the information that the authors cited in their review, the current data suggest that venlafaxine should be used with caution in patients with established cardiovascular disease.

Nervous system

Antidepressant drugs, such as tricyclic antidepressants and SSRIs, suppress rapid eye movement (REM) sleep, the period of sleep during which dreaming occurs. Despite this, antidepressant treatment is sometimes associated with recurrent nightmares. Venlafaxine also suppresses REM sleep and was associated with nightmares in a 35-year-old woman with body image disturbance; the nightmares remitted when the venlafaxinc was withdrawn (11). The authors speculated that indirect activation of 5-HT$_2$ receptors might have played a causal role, because 5-HT$_2$ receptor antagonists, such as nefazodone, can be helpful in the treatment of nightmares, for example in patients with post-traumatic stress disorder.

Sensory systems

Tricyclic antidepressants predispose to acute angle closure glaucoma, probably through an anticholinergic action. However, acute angle closure has also been reported with SSRIs, suggesting that all serotonin-potentiating drugs can cause glaucoma (SEDA-21, 13) (SEDA-23, 17).

- Acute angle closure glaucoma has been reported in a 45-year-old woman taking venlafaxine (75 mg/day) and chlorpromazine (150 mg/day) (12). She had previously taken low-dose dosulepin (75 mg/day), chlorpromazine, and SSRIs without ophthalmic problems.

Chlorpromazine has mild anticholinergic properties and may have contributed to the angle closure in this case. She also had hypermetropia which is an another risk factor for glaucoma. However, this case supports the view that potent blockade of serotonin re-uptake can cause glaucoma in predisposed subjects.

Psychological, psychiatric

The use of antidepressants in patients with documented bipolar illness is often associated with a risk of manic illness (13).

- A 63-year-old man with a long history of bipolar illness and alcohol dependence took nefazodone 400 mg/day for 8 months, with no relief of a depressive episode. He was also taking valproate 1500 mg/day as a mood stabilizer, aspirin 81 mg/day, ranitidine 300 mg/day, and docusate calcium 240 mg/day. Nefazodone was tapered over 4 days and venlafaxine begun in a dosage of 37.5 mg/day and gradually increased to 150 mg/day over 3 weeks. Venlafaxine led to improvement in depressive symptoms, but 6 days after the dose reached 150 mg/day he became agitated, verbally and physically threatening, grandiose, and sexually disinhibited. He also had paranoid thinking and appeared to be hallucinating. The venlafaxine was withdrawn but the manic symptoms persisted and eventually required increases in the dosages of valproate and antipsychotic drugs.

This report illustrates the difficulty of treating depression in bipolar disorder with antidepressants. The presence of a mood stabilizer did not prevent the manic episode that emerged during venlafaxine treatment, and it is in any case difficult to know whether the mania was in fact due to the venlafaxine or instead represented a spontaneous mood swing.

Electrolyte balance

It is well established that SSRIs can cause hyponatremia. Similar cases have now been reported with venlafaxine.

- A 90-year-old woman had a depressive disorder in addition to other medical problems, including congestive cardiac failure, seizures, dementia, and osteoporosis (14). She was also taking phenobarbital 120 mg/day, enalapril 40 mg/day, furosemide 80 mg/day, calcium carbonate 1300 mg/day, and nortriptyline 50 mg at night. She was given additional paroxetine 20 mg/day, but there was no clinical response and she was changed to venlafaxine, increasing to 75 mg/day. Two months later her sodium concentration had fallen to 130 mmol/l and the furosemide was withdrawn. However, 4 months later the sodium concentration had fallen to 124 mmol/l. The venlafaxine was then withdrawn and the sodium normalized within a week and remained within the reference range for the following year.

This was a complex case, because of the multiple medical problems and treatments. However, it has been reported that since the launch of venlafaxine in Australia in 1996, the Adverse Drug Reactions Advisory Committee there has received 15 reports of hyponatremia, suggesting that the association is real (15).

Liver

Raised liver enzymes have been rarely found in patients taking venlafaxine, and it appears that hepatitis may also be rare adverse effect (16).

- A 44-year-old woman developed weakness with abnormal liver function tests (aspartate transaminase 661 IU/l) about 6 months after starting to take venlafaxine 150 mg/day. Biopsy showed confluent necrosis in zone 3, with unaffected portal tracts. No other cause for the hepatitis could be found. The clinical

and biochemical features resolved within 12 weeks of withdrawal of venlafaxine.

Hair

SSRIs can cause occasional, idiosyncratic hair loss in some patients (SEDA-19, 10), and this has also been attributed to venlafaxine (17).

- A 50-year-old woman took venlafaxine 75 mg/day for depression, and the dosage was increased to 150 mg/day after 2 weeks. After 4 weeks she noted increased hair loss when brushing or washing her hair. After 3 months she stopped taking venlafaxine and 1 month later her hair loss stopped completely. However, 10 months later she had another depressive episode and was again successfully treated with venlafaxine. Once again she noted excessive hair loss. She was subsequently treated with sertraline 50 mg/day, which helped her depression without causing hair loss.

The fact that sertraline did not cause hair loss in this patient suggests that the mechanism was not related to blockade of serotonin re-uptake.

Sexual function

Antidepressant drugs can rarely cause priapism. The agent most often implicated has been trazodone, perhaps because of its α_1-adrenoceptor antagonist properties. In general venlafaxine has an inhibitory effect on sexual function, but perhaps, like SSRIs, it can rarely cause priapism (18).

- A 16-year-old youth taking venlafaxine (150 mg/day) had several episodes of prolonged erections, which persisted for several hours after intercourse. The episodes remitted after the venlafaxine was withdrawn.

Pain on ejaculation is also a rare adverse effect of tricyclic antidepressants and SSRIs and has been reported with venlafaxine (19).

- Painful ejaculation occurred in a 59-year-old man taking venlafaxine 150 mg/day. It remitted when the venlafaxine was withdrawn and did not recur when citalopram 40 mg/day was used instead.

Long-Term Effects

Drug withdrawal

Both SSRIs and venlafaxine can cause troublesome withdrawal symptoms (SEDA-22, 12) (SEDA-22, 17). Because venlafaxine blocks the re-uptake of both serotonin and noradrenaline the mechanism of venlafaxine-induced abstinence symptoms is not clear.

- A 72-year-old woman taking venlafaxine 150 mg/day for depression was abruptly switched to the noradrenaline re-uptake inhibitor maprotiline 75 mg/day; 1 day later she developed agitation, sweating, nausea, vomiting, tinnitus, and insomnia (20). These symptoms continued for another week, but disappeared on the second day of sertraline treatment 50 mg/day.

The symptoms experienced by this patient were typical of venlafaxine and SSRI withdrawal (although they could also be experienced after sudden withdrawal of tricyclic antidepressants). The fact that they were relieved by a serotonin but not a noradrenaline re-uptake inhibitor suggests that venlafaxine-induced withdrawal symptoms are mediated by serotonergic mechanisms.

Drug Administration

Drug overdose

Venlafaxine is generally regarded as being reasonably safe in overdose relative to conventional tricyclic antidepressants.

However, it has been associated with occasional reports of cardiac conduction disturbances at both therapeutic doses and in overdose (SEDA-24, 19).

Deaths have been described after venlafaxine overdose, but in combination with other agents and alcohol. However, there have been two fatal cases of overdosage in which venlafaxine was the only agent detected postmortem (21). It therefore appears that venlafaxine can occasionally prove fatal in overdosage, probably through cardiac conduction abnormalities and seizures (21,22). It is possible that poor metabolizers may be especially liable to develop toxic effects.

- A 44-year-old woman took an overdose of venlafaxine 3 g. An electrocardiogram showed sinus rhythm and incomplete right bundle branch block (23). She was monitored in an intensive care unit and 10 hours later a further electrocardiogram showed atrial fibrillation with a wide QRS complex. Both of these abnormalities resolved with sodium bicarbonate (100 ml of a 1 M solution). No further conduction disturbances were noted over the following days.

The authors suggested that the effect of venlafaxine on cardiac conduction is mediated by its ability to block the fast inward sodium current in cardiac myocytes. This might promote membrane stabilizing effects in a similar way to tricyclic antidepressants. They recommended that the management of venlafaxine overdose should include cardiac monitoring.

Drug–Drug Interactions

Caffeine

Venlafaxine 150 mg/day did not alter the disposition of caffeine, a probe of CYP1A2 activity (24). This suggests that at therapeutic doses venlafaxine, in contrast to fluvoxamine (SEDA-22, 13), does not inhibit CYP1A2.

Dexamfetamine

Psychostimulants, such as dexamfetamine, are being increasingly prescribed for patients who meet the criteria for adult attention deficit disorder. Many such patients also have co-morbid major depression.

- A 32-year-old man taking dexamfetamine 15 mg/day developed the serotonin syndrome, with shivering, sweating, myoclonus, and pyrexia, following the

addition of venlafaxine 150 mg/day (25). Venlafaxine and dexamfetamine were withdrawn, and he was given the serotonin receptor antagonist, cyproheptadine (32 mg over 3 hours). His symptoms remitted a few hours later and he subsequently restarted dexamfetamine without incident. A later trial of citalopram, while he was still taking dexamfetamine, also led to symptoms of serotonin toxicity.

The combination of stimulants and SSRIs is not uncommon in clinical practice, but reports of serotonin toxicity are unusual, perhaps because drugs such as dexamfetamine and methylphenidate predominantly release dopamine and noradrenaline rather than serotonin. However, psychostimulants do cause some degree of serotonin release, which might have been sufficient to cause serotonin toxicity in this case.

Fluoxetine

Four depressed patients (age range 21–73 years) had anticholinergic adverse effects when venlafaxine 37.5 mg/day was added to fluoxetine 20 mg/day (26). Venlafaxine does not have direct anticholinergic effects, but could cause them indirectly as a result of its ability to increase noradrenergic neurotransmission. This effect would be expected only at much higher doses of venlafaxine than those used here, which led the author to suggest that in the presence of CYP2D6 inhibition by fluoxetine, venlafaxine concentrations could have been substantially higher than expected.

Imipramine

In six healthy men, venlafaxine (150 mg/day for 10 days) produced an increase of 28% in the systemic availability of a single dose of imipramine (100 mg); the availability of the active metabolite of imipramine, desipramine, was also increased (27). These data suggest that venlafaxine inhibits CYP2D6; the effects appear to be modest relative to those of fluoxetine and are similar to those produced by sertraline.

Monoamine oxidase inhibitors

There have been previous reports of serotonin toxicity when venlafaxine was combined with therapeutic doses of conventional MAO inhibitors (SEDA 20, 21). The serotonin syndrome has been reported in four patients who were switched from the MAO inhibitor phenelzine to venlafaxine (28). In two of the subjects, the 14-day washout period recommended when switching from phenelzine to other antidepressant drugs had elapsed.

- A 25-year-old woman had been taking phenelzine 45 mg/day for refractory migraine and tension headache, but suffered intolerable adverse effects (weight gain, edema, and insomnia). Phenelzine was withdrawn and 15 days elapsed before she took a single dose of venlafaxine 37.5 mg. Within 1 hour she developed agitation, twitching, shakiness, sweating, and generalized erythema with hyperthermia (38°C). Her symptoms resolved within 3 hours with no sequelae.

These cases suggest that even after the recommended 2-week washout from MAO inhibitors, venlafaxine can provoke serotonin toxicity in some patients. In principle it should be possible to switch from one conventional MAO inhibitor to another without a washout period. However, there have been reports that patients who switched from phenelzine to tranylcypromine had hypertensive reactions, with disastrous consequences (29). Whenever possible, a 2-week washout period when switching MAO inhibitors or when introducing serotonin re-uptake inhibitors seems advisable.

Quinidine

Venlafaxine is metabolized by CYP2D6. In healthy volunteers the oral clearance of venlafaxine (37.5 mg/day for 2 days) was fourfold less in poor metabolizers ($n = 6$) than extensive metabolizers ($n = 8$) (30). Administration of the CYP2D6 inhibitor quinidine, 200 mg/day for 2 days, to the extensive metabolizers reduced the oral clearance of venlafaxine to the level seen in poor metabolizers. Quinidine had no effect on venlafaxine clearance in subjects who were poor metabolizers before treatment. The authors suggested that poor metabolizers may be at particular risk of venlafaxine toxicity, as could subjects who take inhibitors of CYP2D6.

Risperidone

Unlike SSRIs, venlafaxine only weakly inhibits CYP2D6. Venlafaxine (up to 150 mg/day for 10 days) modestly but significantly increased the plasma AUC of a single dose of risperidone (1 mg) in 38 healthy volunteers in an open longitudinal design, but did not affect its active metabolite, 9-hydroxyrisperidone (31). The authors suggested that their study had shown a small potentiating effect of venlafaxine on risperidone availability, probably through weak inhibition by venlafaxine of CYP2D6. Venlafaxine is therefore less likely to increase risperidone concentrations than are fluoxetine and paroxetine.

Trifluoperazine

Drugs that potentiate the function of serotonin, such as venlafaxine, can produce pharmacodynamic interactions with dopamine receptor antagonists, perhaps because serotonin pathways can inhibit dopamine neurotransmission.

- A 44-year-old man with major depression had been taking the antipsychotic drug trifluoperazine (3 mg/day) for anxiety for several years (32). He was given venlafaxine 75 mg/day, and 12 hours after the first dose developed anxiety and malaise. He was sweating and had tremor and rigidity. His blood pressure fluctuated and his creatine phosphokinase activity was raised at 11 320 IU/l. A diagnosis of neuroleptic malignant syndrome was made and he was given dantrolene and bromocriptine. His symptoms settled within 24 hours and trifluoperazine was reintroduced uneventfully.

This case suggests that venlafaxine can rarely increase the risk of neuroleptic malignant syndrome in patients taking a dopamine receptor antagonist. However, this combination of drugs is often used, and it is not clear why only very few patients appear to be susceptible to this reaction, and then only on some occasions.

References

1. Nemeroff CB. Evolutionary trends in the pharmacotherapeutic management of depression. J Clin Psychiatry 1994;55(Suppl):3–15.
2. Montgomery SA. Venlafaxine: a new dimension in antidepressant pharmacotherapy. J Clin Psychiatry 1993;54(3):119–26.
3. Dallal A, Chouinard G. Withdrawal and rebound symptoms associated with abrupt discontinuation of venlafaxine. J Clin Psychopharmacol 1998;18(4):343–4.
4. Parker G, Blennerhassett J. Withdrawal reactions associated with venlafaxine. Aust NZ J Psychiatry 1998;32(2):291–4.
5. White CM, Gailey RA, Levin GM, Smith T. Seizure resulting from a venlafaxine overdose. Ann Pharmacother 1997;31(2):178–80.
6. Zhalkovsky B, Walker D, Bourgeois JA. Seizure activity and enzyme elevations after venlafaxine overdose. J Clin Psychopharmacol 1997;17(6):490–1.
7. Leaf EV, Peano C, Leikin JB, Hanashiro PK. Seizures, ventricular tachycardia, and rhabdomyolysis as a result of ingestion of venlafaxine and lamotrigine. Ann Emerg Med 1997;30(5):704–8.
8. Thase ME. Effects of venlafaxine on blood pressure: a meta-analysis of original data from 3744 depressed patients. J Clin Psychiatry 1998;59(10):502–8.
9. West S, Hewitt J. Prolonged hypertension: a case report of a potential interaction between electroconvulsive therapy and venlafaxine. Int J Psychiatr Clin Pract 1999;3:55–7.
10. Reznik I, Rosen Y, Rosen B. An acute ischaemic event associated with the use of venlafaxine: a case report and proposed pathophysiological mechanisms. J Psychopharmacol 1999;13(2):193–5.
11. Zullino DF, Riquier F. Venlafaxine and vivid dreaming. J Clin Psychiatry 2000;61(8):600.
12. Ng B, Sanbrook GM, Malouf AJ, Agarwal SA. Venlafaxine and bilateral acute angle closure glaucoma. Med J Aust 2002;176(5):241.
13. Stoner SC, Williams RJ, Worrel J, Ramlatchman L. Possible venlafaxine-induced mania. J Clin Psychopharmacol 1999;19(2):184–5.
14. Masood GR, Karki SD, Patterson WR. Hyponatremia with venlafaxine. Ann Pharmacother 1998;32(1):49–51.
15. Boyd IW, Karki SD, Masood GR. Comment: hyponatremia with venlafaxine. Ann Pharmacother 1998;32(9):981–2.
16. Horsmans Y, De Clercq M, Sempoux C. Venlafaxine-associated hepatitis. Ann Intern Med 1999;130(11):944.
17. Pitchot W, Ansseau M. Venlafaxine-induced hair loss. Am J Psychiatry 2001;158(7):159–60.
18. Samuel RZ, Horrigan JP, Barnhill LJ. Priapism associated with venlafaxine use. J Am Acad Child Adolesc Psychiatry 2000;39(1):16–17.
19. Michael A. Venlafaxine-induced painful ejaculation. Br J Psychiatry 2000;177:282.
20. Luckhaus C, Jacob C. Venlafaxine withdrawal syndrome not prevented by maprotiline, but resolved by sertraline. Int J Neuropsychopharmacol 2001;4(1):43–4.
21. Jaffe PD, Batziris HP, van der Hoeven P, DeSilva D, McIntyre IM. A study involving venlafaxine overdoses: comparison of fatal and therapeutic concentrations in postmortem specimens. J Forensic Sci 1999;44(1):193–6.
22. Blythe D, Hackett LP. Cardiovascular and neurological toxicity of venlafaxine. Hum Exp Toxicol 1999;18(5):309–13.
23. Combes A, Peytavin G, Theron D. Conduction disturbances associated with venlafaxine. Ann Intern Med 2001;134(2):166–7.
24. Amchin J, Zarycranski W, Taylor KP, Albano D, Klockowski PM. Effect of venlafaxine on CYP1A2-dependent

pharmacokinetics and metabolism of caffeine. J Clin Pharmacol 1999;39(3):252–9.

25. Prior FH, Isbister GK, Dawson AH, Whyte IM. Serotonin toxicity with therapeutic doses of dexamphetamine and venlafaxine. Med J Aust 2002;176(5):240–1.

26. Benazzi F. Venlafaxine–fluoxetine interaction. J Clin Psychopharmacol 1999;19(1):96–8.

27. Albers LJ, Reist C, Vu RL, Fujimoto K, Ozdemir V, Helmeste D, Poland R, Tang SW. Effect of venlafaxine on imipramine metabolism. Psychiatry Res 2000;96(3):235–43.

28. Diamond S, Pepper BJ, Diamond ML, Freitag FG, Urban GJ, Erdemoglu AK. Serotonin syndrome induced by transitioning from phenelzine to venlafaxine: four patient reports. Neurology 1998;51(1):274–6.

29. Mattes JA. Stroke resulting from a rapid switch from phenelzine to tranylcypromine. J Clin Psychiatry 1998;59(7):382.

30. Lessard E, Yessine MA, Hamelin BA, O'Hara G, LeBlanc J, Turgeon J. Influence of CYP2D6 activity on the disposition and cardiovascular toxicity of the antidepressant agent venlafaxine in humans. Pharmacogenetics 1999;9(4):435–43.

31. Amchin J, Zarycranski W, Taylor KP, Albano D, Klockowski PM. Effect of venlafaxine on the pharmacokinetics of risperidone. J Clin Pharmacol 1999;39(3):297–309.

32. Nimmagadda SR, Ryan DH, Atkin SL. Neuroleptic malignant syndrome after venlafaxine. Lancet 2000; 355(9200):289–90.

Verapamil

See also Calcium channel blockers

General Information

Verapamil is a phenylalkylamine calcium channel blocker, with actions mainly on the heart.

Organs and Systems

Cardiovascular

Heart failure

Verapamil can cause cardiac failure, because it has a potent negative inotropic effect and causes increased capillary filtration pressure by vasodilatation (1). There are also reports of drug-induced acute right heart failure in patients with pulmonary hypertension due to valvular heart and chronic pulmonary obstructive airways diseases (2).

- A 16-year-old boy who took long-term verapamil after a Mustard operation for transposition of the great arteries developed severe congestive heart failure, which did not respond to diuretics. Systemic vascular resistance was increased by 75% and pulmonary vascular resistance by 150%; the cardiac index was reduced from 3.0 to 1.8 l/minute/m^2. Ejection fraction and atrial pressure were unchanged and neurohormonal causes were excluded. The heart failure resolved after withdrawal of verapamil.

Cardiogenic shock after the ingestion of verapamil has been reported, in one case with a small dose (3).

- A 78-year-old woman with a history of biventricular heart failure developed cardiogenic shock after she took a single tablet of verapamil 80 mg. She was resuscitated with artificial ventilation, dobutamine, noradrenaline, and calcium gluconate. Toxicological analysis showed an unexpectedly high plasma verapamil concentration, which was attributed to liver failure.

In patients with advanced heart failure a single oral therapeutic dose of verapamil may have a severe toxic effect.

Cardiac dysrhythmias

Relatively harmless and asymptomatic disturbances of heart rhythm are common during treatment with verapamil. For example, Wenckebach phenomenon (Mobitz type I second-degree atrioventricular block), sinus bradycardia and junctional escape, and accelerated junctional rhythm have been seen during the treatment of angina pectoris (4). In the DAVIT II study (5), 23 of 878 patients who took verapamil and seven of 897 who took placebo in a survival study after myocardial infarction developed second- or third-degree AV block. It has been suggested that the extent of PR prolongation may be proportional to the pharmacological effect of verapamil in patients with sinus rhythm (6). Patients with diseased conduction systems can develop atrioventricular block, sinoatrial block, sinus arrest, or sinus bradycardia with verapamil (7).

Severe cardiac conduction disturbances have been reported in patients with chronic renal insufficiency taking verapamil, mainly related to modified-release formulations.

- A serious bradydysrhythmia with complete atrioventricular block occurred after some months of conventional verapamil at normal doses and dose-adjusted digoxin in a 72-year-old woman with chronic renal insufficiency of unknown cause; the atrioventricular block resolved after 2 hours of hemodialysis (8).

Problems can also occur in patients with aberrant conduction pathways; for example, verapamil caused an increased ventricular response in patients with Wolff–Parkinson–White syndrome associated with atrial fibrillation (9–11). The danger lies in provocation of ventricular fibrillation from advanced anterograde conduction in accessory pathways (12).

Nervous system

Myoclonic dystonia has been described in a 70-year-old man who took verapamil for supraventricular tachycardia for 10 months; the abnormal movements disappeared within 3 weeks of substituting diltiazem, but rechallenge was not attempted (13).

Myoclonic seizures have been attributed to verapamil (14).

- An 18-month-old girl with supraventricular tachycardia was given intravenous verapamil 0.2 mg/kg, which was discontinued after half the dose had been given, because she developed irregular, repetitive, jerky movements in both upper and lower limbs which lasted for 2 minutes. As the supraventricular tachycardia had not responded, second and third doses of 0.2 mg/kg were given intravenously under diazepam cover, but similar myoclonic seizures occurred again. There were no predisposing factors.

Fasciculation occurred when a patient with background peripheral neuropathy was given verapamil (SEDA-16, 197).

Feelings of "painful coldness and numbness" in the legs, in the absence of a neurological deficit, have been reported with verapamil (15); the symptoms disappeared with drug withdrawal and recurred with rechallenge.

Endocrine

There was a significant rise in serum alkaline phosphatase of skeletal origin in a group of patients taking verapamil for hypertension. It was associated with a slight increase in parathyroid hormone, indicating involvement of bone metabolism, although there was no change in the urinary excretion of calcium, phosphate, or potassium. It has yet to be shown whether verapamil causes osteopenia in man, as it does in animals (SEDA-16, 197).

Verapamil-induced hyperprolactinemia has been reported in a 74-year-old man, who presented with impotence and who was subsequently found to have a benign 6 mm pituitary microadenoma (16). The withdrawal of verapamil was associated with the normalization of serum prolactin concentrations.

The mechanism for this adverse effect is unclear and has not been reported with other calcium channel blockers.

Hair

Increased hair growth has been associated with modified-release verapamil (SEDA-17, 238).

Musculoskeletal

Arthralgia has been associated with verapamil (17).

- A 28-year-old man with migraine and vascular pain of the face was given verapamil 480 mg/day when sumatriptan did not control the pain. Verapamil was withdrawn after 1 month and reintroduced in a dosage of 960 mg/day after a new episode of pain. He then developed arthralgia in the right hand and arm, which disappeared after withdrawal and recurred after rechallenge.

Susceptibility Factors

In therapeutic doses, verapamil has a negative dromotropic effect, reflected in plasma concentration-dependent prolongation of the PR interval and AV nodal block. PR interval prolongation is detectable even after small single doses. The effects of rheumatoid arthritis on the pharmacokinetics and pharmacodynamics of verapamil have been studied in eight patients and eight age- and sex-matched healthy volunteers (18). Verapamil and norverapamil concentrations were substantially increased in the patients with rheumatoid arthritis, accompanied by significantly less dromotropic activity. Regardless of the mechanism involved in the altered pharmacokinetics of verapamil, the rise in drug concentrations was accompanied by a significant reduction in dromotropic activity.

Therefore, administration of verapamil to patients with rheumatoid arthritis may require close attention to prevent therapeutic failure.

Drug Administration

Drug overdose

Verapamil poisoning can cause cardiac toxicity with cardiogenic shock, conduction abnormalities (including life-threatening dysrhythmias), hypotension, and death.

- A 15-year-old woman survived a total of 65 minutes cardiac arrest after taking 7200 mg of verapamil and 240 mg of paroxetine, which potentiates verapamil toxicity (19). Despite the length of cardiopulmonary resuscitation, with evidence of subsequent myocardial damage and renal impairment, she was discharged 17 days after admission, having made a full recovery, without evidence of neurological impairment.

The authors considered that the lack of neurological damage may have been related to the possible neuroprotective effect of a large dose of verapamil.

- A 28-year-old man developed rhabdomyolysis and acute renal insufficiency 10 hours after taking four capsules containing verapamil 180 mg plus trandolapril 2 mg. He survived with gastric lavage and activated charcoal 70 g. By 4 hours after admission he was awake and complained of diffuse muscle cramps and myalgia. Creatinine and creatine kinase reached 565 µmol/l (6.7 mg/dl) and 10 700 U/l respectively. After 6 days the laboratory tests were all within the reference ranges.

The authors suggested that rhabdomyolysis should be considered in patients with myalgia and muscle cramps taking verapamil plus trandolapril, and that routine serum creatinine kinase should be checked (20).

Non-cardiogenic pulmonary edema has been reported after the ingestion of a large quantity of verapamil (21).

- Two 19-year-old-girls developed pulmonary edema after taking massive overdoses of verapamil (6000 mg and 7200 mg). In each case a chest X-ray showed diffuse bilateral patchy infiltration. Left ventricular size and function was normal on transthoracic echocardiography. They were both treated successfully with mechanical ventilatory support.

Several mechanisms may be involved in non-cardiogenic pulmonary edema subsequent to verapamil intoxication, including leaky capillary syndrome attributable to inhibition of prostacyclin, a cellular membrane protector. Prolonged hypotension and a shock-like state may also contribute. The authors recommended pressor/inotropic therapy and mechanical ventilation as therapy.

Different therapeutic approaches have been described in suicide attempts with verapamil.

- Enoximone has been used to treat cardiogenic shock in a case of self-poisoning with verapamil 2.4 g in a 40-year-old woman; treatment with calcium and noradrenaline had been unsuccessful (22).

- A 41-year-old man who had taken 4800–6400 mg of verapamil presented 5 hours later and had a cardiac arrest; cardiopulmonary resuscitation was started and he underwent percutaneous cardiopulmonary by-pass, to maintain adequate tissue perfusion and sufficient cerebral oxygen supply until the drug concentration was reduced and restoration of spontaneous circulation was achieved (23).
- Severe poisoning with modified-release verapamil was associated with respiratory failure in a 27-year-old man, who presented 2 hours after taking 24 g, one of the largest reported overdoses (24). He survived after receiving 4 days of partial liquid ventilation as a part of his medical management.
- A 61-year-old woman developed profound hypotension, bradycardia, oliguria, and multifocal myoclonus after verapamil overdose. Her serum verapamil concentration was 800 ng/ml (1760 nmol/l) (usual target range 50–200 ng/ml, 110–440 nmol/l). She was treated with supportive care, vasopressin, dopamine, and calcium gluconate. After about 60 hours the myoclonus and hemodynamic compromise resolved completely (25).
- Two patients took 2400 mg and 9600 mg of verapamil, resulting in life-threatening hypotension and bradycardia, needing cardiac pacing and resuscitation (26). Gastric lavage was not carried out in the first patient, owing to clouded consciousness. Both patients underwent plasmapheresis within 4 hours of ingestion, with dramatic improvement. However, the first patient died 38 hours after admission with multiorgan failure, probably because of the long period of cardiogenic shock. The second patient survived without infirmity, despite the higher verapamil dose.

The authors of the last report emphasized the role of vigorous gastrointestinal lavage with repeated administration of activated charcoal to reduce gastrointestinal absorption of the drug.

Drug–Drug Interactions

ACE inhibitor

The addition of low doses of verapamil to ACE inhibitor therapy reversed ACE inhibitor-induced increases in creatinine concentrations in eight elderly hypertensive patients (27). During an average of 25 weeks, ACE inhibitors significantly reduced blood pressure, but serum creatinine concentrations rose. During an average of 10 weeks, the addition of verapamil did not reduce the blood pressure further, but the serum creatinine concentrations were normalized. Verapamil appears to have a beneficial effect, through dilatation of constricted afferent and efferent arterioles and reduction of the mesangial cell contraction induced by endothelin-1, factors that have been implicated in the increase in intraglomerular pressure and proteinuria due to ACE inhibitors.

Calcium adipinate and calciferol

Treatment of osteoporosis with calcium adipinate and calciferol counteracts the antidysrhythmic effect of verapamil (28).

Ciclosporin

Calcium channel blockers are given to transplant patients for their protective effect against ciclosporin-induced nephrotoxicity. Verapamil has been particularly preferred, as it causes a significant increase in plasma ciclosporin concentrations and also seems to have a direct immunosuppressive action. However, in a study in 152 kidney transplant recipients, verapamil increased the incidence of postoperative infections (29). The patients, all of whom were taking ciclosporin, were assigned either to verapamil 240 mg/day or to no verapamil; during a postoperative period of 2–14 months, the incidence of infections was 22% (17/77) of those given verapamil compared with 5% (4/75) of the others. However, since the study was not randomized, it is not possible to draw reliable conclusions.

Dofetilide

By increasing its rate of absorption, verapamil produced transient rises in peak plasma concentrations of dofetilide in 12 young healthy male volunteers (30). During combination treatment at steady state there was a significant, albeit modest, increase in the mean C_{max} and AUC of dofetilide. These changes were associated with corresponding short-lived increases in its pharmacodynamic effect, as measured by changes in the QT_c interval. These two drugs should not be administered concurrently.

Grape fruit juice

The interaction with grapefruit juice observed with several calcium channel blockers, including felodipine, nifedipine, and nisoldipine, has not been confirmed with verapamil. A single dose of grapefruit juice had no effect on the pharmacokinetics of verapamil in 10 hypertensive patients taking chronic verapamil (31).

Macrolide antibiotics

Verapamil is both a substrate and an inhibitor of CYP3A4, which is inhibited by clarithromycin and erythromycin. Giving these macrolide antibiotics during verapamil therapy is likely to reduce the first-pass metabolism of verapamil, increase its systemic availability, and impair its elimination. In patients taking this combination, verapamil should be started in a low dosage and its hemodynamic effects should be monitored closely.

Clarithromycin

- A 53-year-old woman had periods of dizziness and episodes of fainting when she stood up 24 hours after having been given clarithromycin for an acute exacerbation of chronic obstructive pulmonary disease and verapamil for atrial fibrillation (32). One day later she developed severe hypotension and bradycardia (32). Since her symptoms matched those of severe verapamil overdosage, the drug was withdrawn and her condition improved within two days.
- A 77-year-old hypertensive woman receiving both verapamil and propranolol for hypertrophic cardiomyopathy and paroxysmal atrial fibrillation developed symptomatic bradycardia within 2–4 days of initiation of both

erythromycin or clarithromycin on two separate occasions, for pneumonia and sinusitis respectively (33).

Erythromycin

- A 79-year-old white woman developed extreme fatigue and dizziness (34). Her heart rate was 40/minute and her blood pressure 80/40 mmHg. An electrocardiogram showed complete atrioventricular block, an escape rhythm at 50/minute, and QT_c interval prolongation to 583 milliseconds. This event was attributed to concomitant treatment with verapamil 480 mg/day and erythromycin 2000 mg/day, which had been prescribed 1 week before admission.

This is the first report of complete AV block and prolongation of the QT interval after co-administration of erythromycin and verapamil, both of which are principally metabolized by CYP3A4. Both drugs are potent inhibitors of CYP3A4 and P-glycoprotein, which may be the basis of this interaction.

The effects of a combination of erythromycin and verapamil on the pharmacokinetics of a single dose of simvastatin have been studied in a randomized, double-blind, cross-over study in 12 healthy volunteers simultaneously taking the three drugs. Both erythromycin and verapamil interacted with simvastatin, producing significant increases in the serum concentrations of simvastatin and its active metabolite simvastatin acid. The mean C_{max} of active simvastatin acid was increased about five-fold and the AUC_{0-24} four-fold by erythromycin; verapamil increased the C_{max} of simvastatin acid 3.4-fold and the AUC_{0-24} 2.8-fold. There was a substantial interindividual variation in the extent of these interactions. Concomitant use of erythromycin, verapamil, and simvastatin should be avoided (35).

Rifampicin

Rifampicin reduces the systemic availability of verapamil, presumably by enzyme induction in the liver (36).

References

1. Buchhorn R, Motz R, Bursch J. Hemodynamic and neurohormonal causes of a severe verapamil induced cardiac decompensation in a child after mustard operation. Herz Kreisl 2000;32:74–7.
2. Shimoni A, Maor-Kendler Y, Neuman Y. Verapamil-induced acute right heart failure. Am Heart J 1996;132(1 Pt 1):193–4.
3. Stajer D, Bervar M, Horvat M. Cardiogenic shock following a single therapeutic oral dose of verapamil. Int J Clin Pract 2001;55(1):69–70.
4. Pine MB, Citron PD, Bailly DJ, Butman S, Plasencia GO, Landa DW, Wong RK. Verapamil versus placebo in relieving stable angina pectoris. Circulation 1982;65(1):17–22.
5. Held PH, Yusuf S, Furberg CD. Calcium channel blockers in acute myocardial infarction and unstable angina: an overview. BMJ 1989;299(6709):1187–92.
6. Dominic JA, Bourne DW, Tan TG, Kirsten EB, McAllister RG Jr. The pharmacology of verapamil. III. Pharmacokinetics in normal subjects after intravenous drug administration. J Cardiovasc Pharmacol 1981;3(1):25–38.
7. Opie LH. Drugs and the heart. III. Calcium antagonists. Lancet 1980;1(8172):806–10.
8. Martin-Gago J, Pascual J, Rodriguez-Palomares JR, Marcen R, Teruel JL, Liano F, Ortuno J. Complete atrioventricular blockade secondary to conventional-release verapamil in a patient on hemodialysis. Nephron 1999;83(1):89–90.
9. Harper R, Whitford E, Middlebrook K, et al. Verapamil in patients with Wolff–Parkinson–White syndrome—a potential hazard? NZ J Med 1981;11:456.
10. Strasberg B, Sagie A, Rechavia E, Katz A, Ovsyscher IA, Sclarovsky S, Agmon J. Deleterious effects of intravenous verapamil in Wolff–Parkinson–White patients and atrial fibrillation. Cardiovasc Drugs Ther 1989;2(6):801–6.
11. Garratt C, Antoniou A, Ward D, Camm AJ. Misuse of verapamil in pre-excited atrial fibrillation. Lancet 1989;1(8634):367–9.
12. Jacob AS, Nielsen DH, Gianelly RE. Fatal ventricular fibrillation following verapamil in Wolff–Parkinson–White syndrome with atrial fibrillation. Ann Emerg Med 1985;14(2):159–60.
13. Hicks CB, Abraham K. Verapamil and myoclonic dystonia. Ann Intern Med 1985;103(1):154.
14. Maiteh M, Daoud AS. Myoclonic seizure following intravenous verapamil injection: case report and review of the literature. Ann Trop Paediatr 2001;21(3):271–2.
15. Kumana CR, Mahon WA. Bizarre perceptual disorder of extremities in patients taking verapamil. Lancet 1981;1(8233):1324–5.
16. Dombrowski RC, Romeo JH, Aron DC. Verapamil-induced hyperprolactinemia complicated by a pituitary incidentaloma. Ann Pharmacother 1995;29(10):999–1001.
17. Nicolas X, Bellard S, Zagnoli F. Arthralgies induites par de fortes doses de vérapamil. [Arthralgia induced by large doses of verapamil.] Presse Méd 2001;30(25 Pt 1):1256–7.
18. Mayo PR, Skeith K, Russell AS, Jamali F. Decreased dromotropic response to verapamil despite pronounced increased drug concentration in rheumatoid arthritis. Br J Clin Pharmacol 2000;50(6):605–13.
19. Evans JS, Oram MP. Neurological recovery after prolonged verapamil-induced cardiac arrest. Anaesth Intensive Care 1999;27(6):653–5.
20. Gokel Y, Paydas S, Duru M. High-dose verapamil–trandolapril induced rhabdomyolysis and acute renal failure. Am J Emerg Med 2000;18(6):738–9.
21. Sami Karti S, Ulusoy H, Yandi M, Gunduz A, Kosucu M, Erol K, Ratip S. Non-cardiogenic pulmonary oedema in the course of verapamil intoxication. Emerg Med J 2002;19(5):458–9.
22. Link A, Hammer B, Weisgerber K, Bohm M. Therapie der Verapamil-Intoxikation mit Noradrenalin und dem Phosphodiesterasehemmer Enoximon. [Therapy of verapamil poisoning with noradrenaline and the phosphodiesterase inhibitor enoximone.] Dtsch Med Wochenschr 2002;127(39):2006–8.
23. Holzer M, Sterz F, Schoerkhuber W, Behringer W, Domanovits H, Weinmar D, Weinstabl C, Stimpfl T. Successful resuscitation of a verapamil-intoxicated patient with percutaneous cardiopulmonary bypass. Crit Care Med 1999;27(12):2818–23.
24. Szekely LA, Thompson BT, Woolf A. Use of partial liquid ventilation to manage pulmonary complications of acute verapamil-sustained release poisoning. J Toxicol Clin Toxicol 1999;37(4):475–9.
25. Vadlamudi L, Wijdicks EF. Multifocal myoclonus due to verapamil overdose. Neurology 2002;58(6):984.
26. Kuhlmann U, Schoenemann H, Muller TF, Keuchel M, Lange H. Plasmapheresis in fatal overdose with verapamil. Intensive Care Med 1999;25(12):1473.
27. Bitar R, Flores O, Reverte M, Lopez-Novoa JM, Macias JF. Beneficial effect of verapamil added to chronic ACE

inhibitor treatment on renal function in hypertensive elderly patients. Int Urol Nephrol 2000;32(2):165–9.

28. Bar-Or D, Gasiel Y. Calcium and calciferol antagonise effect of verapamil in atrial fibrillation. BMJ (Clin Res Ed) 1981;282(6276):1585–6.

29. Nanni G, Panocchia N, Tacchino R, Foco M, Piccioni E, Castagneto M. Increased incidence of infection in verapamil-treated kidney transplant recipients. Transplant Proc 2000;32(3):551–3.

30. Johnson BF, Cheng SL, Venitz J. Transient kinetic and dynamic interactions between verapamil and dofetilide, a class III antiarrhythmic. J Clin Pharmacol 2001;41(11):1248–56.

31. Zaidenstein R, Dishi V, Gips M, Soback S, Cohen N, Weissgarten J, Blatt A, Golik A. The effect of grapefruit juice on the pharmacokinetics of orally administered verapamil. Eur J Clin Pharmacol 1998;54(4):337–40.

32. Kaeser YA, Brunner F, Drewe J, Haefeli WE. Severe hypotension and bradycardia associated with verapamil and clarithromycin. Am J Health Syst Pharm 1998; 55(22):2417–18.

33. Steenbergen JA, Stauffer VL. Potential macrolide interaction with verapamil. Ann Pharmacother 1998;32(3):387–8.

34. Goldschmidt N, Azaz-Livshits T, Gotsman, Nir-Paz R, Ben-Yehuda A, Muszkat M. Compound cardiac toxicity of oral erythromycin and verapamil. Ann Pharmacother 2001; 35(11):1396–9.

35. Kantola T, Kivisto KT, Neuvonen PJ. Erythromycin and verapamil considerably increase serum simvastatin and simvastatin acid concentrations. Clin Pharmacol Ther 1998;64(2):177–82.

36. Barbarash RA, Bauman JL, Fischer JH, Kondos GT, Batenhorst RL. Near-total reduction in verapamil bioavailability by rifampin. Electrocardiographic correlates. Chest 1988;94(5):954–9.

Verbenaceae

See also Herbal medicines

General Information

The genera in the family of Verbenaceae (Table 1) include mangrove and vervain.

Vitex agnus-castus

Vitex agnus-castus (chaste tree, hemp tree, monk's pepper) is a plant with estrogen-like activities, used for a variety of gynecological problems, particularly on the European continent, particularly premenstrual symptoms (1).

Adverse effects

Vitex agnus-castus can cause ovarian hyperstimulation and increase the risk of miscarriage.

- A woman took *V. agnus-castus* during an unstimulated cycle while undergoing in vitro fertilization (2). She had considerable derangements of gonadotrophin and ovarian hormone concentrations.

Table 1 The genera of Verbenaceae

Aegiphila (spiritweed)
Aloysia (bee brush)
Avicennia (mangrove)
Bouchea (bouchea)
Callicarpa (beauty berry)
Caryopteris (caryopteris)
Citharexylum (fiddlewood)
Clerodendrum (glory bower)
Congea (congea)
Cornutia (cornutia)
Duranta (duranta)
Faradaya
Glandularia (mock vervain)
Gmelina (gmelina)
Holmskioldia (holmskioldia)
Lantana (lantana)
Lippia (lippia)
Nashia (nashia)
Petitia (petitia)
Petrea (petrea)
Phryma (phryma)
Phyla (fog fruit)
Premna (premna)
Priva (priva)
Stachytarpheta (porterweed)
Stylodon (stylodon)
Tamonea (tamonea)
Tectona (tectona)
Tetraclea (tetraclea)
Verbena (vervain)
Vitex (chaste tree)

References

1. Wuttke W, Jarry H, Christoffel V, Spengler B, Seidlova-Wuttke D. Chaste tree (*Vitex agnus-castus*)—pharmacology and clinical indications. Phytomedicine 2003;10(4):348–57.

2. Cahill DJ, Fox R, Wardle PG, Harlow CR. Multiple follicular development associated with herbal medicine. Hum Reprod 1994;9(8):1469–70.

Vesnarinone

See also Phosphodiesterase type III, selective inhibitors of

General Information

Vesnarinone is an inhibitor of phosphodiesterase type III, and has a positive inotropic effect. Although vesnarinone was originally developed for the treatment of cardiac failure, its action on tumor cells has prompted its use in the treatment of cancer. In 26 patients who received combinations of vesnarinone and gemcitabine there was no pharmacokinetic interaction between the two drugs (1). Although there were cases of neutropenia and thrombocytopenia, those effects could have occurred with gemcitabine alone and could not necessarily be attributed to vesnarinone. Other adverse effects of the combination included nausea and vomiting, anorexia and fatigue, diarrhea, headache, and fever. There were no cases of QT interval prolongation or ventricular dysrhythmias. There were rises in hepatic transaminase activities in up to 25% of cases. Again it was not possible to distinguish between adverse effects of gemcitabine and vesnarinone.

Organs and Systems

Hematologic

Vesnarinone causes reversible neutropenia in up to 2.5% of patients (2,3). In 3833 patients with heart failure of Class III or IV and a left ventricular ejection fraction of 30% or less despite optimal treatment, followed for 286 days, there was dose-dependent agranulocytosis, in 0.2% of those taking vesnarinone 30 mg/day and 1.2% of those taking 60 mg/day (3).

Gastrointestinal

In 3833 patients with heart failure of Class III or IV and a left ventricular ejection fraction of 30% or less despite optimal treatment, followed for 286 days, there was a slight increase in the risk of diarrhea, which occurred in 17% of those taking 60 mg/day compared with 12% of those taking placebo and 14.5% of those taking 30 mg/day (3).

Death

Vesnarinone has been reported to reduce mortality at low doses and to increase it at high doses (SEDA-18, 199) (2,4). In 3833 patients with heart failure of Class III or IV and a left ventricular ejection fraction of 30% or less despite optimal treatment, followed for 286 days, vesnarinone 60 mg/day was associated with significantly more deaths and a shorter duration of survival (3). The increased death rate was due to an increase in sudden deaths, presumably because of cardiac dysrhythmias. There were similar trends in patients who took 30 mg/day, but the changes were not significant. In contrast to the increased mortality with vesnarinone there was a short-term increase in quality of life, which occurred during the first 16 weeks but was not maintained at 6 months. Probably the increased mortality due to vesnarinone outweighs the improvement in quality of life.

References

1. Patnaik A, Rowinsky EK, Tammara BK, Hidalgo M, Drengler RL, Garner AM, Siu LL, Hammond LA, Felton SA, Mallikaarjun S, Von Hoff DD, Eckhardt SG. Phase I and pharmacokinetic study of the differentiating agent vesnarinone in combination with gemcitabine in patients with advanced cancer. J Clin Oncol 2000;18(23):3974–85.
2. Feldman AM, Bristow MR, Parmley WW, Carson PE, Pepine CJ, Gilbert EM, Strobeck JE, Hendrix GH, Powers ER, Bain RP, et al. Effects of vesnarinone on morbidity and mortality in patients with heart failure. Vesnarinone Study Group. N Engl J Med 1993;329(3):149–55.
3. Cohn JN, Goldstein SO, Greenberg BH, Lorell BH, Bourge RC, Jaski BE, Gottlieb SO, McGrew F 3rd, DeMets DL, White BG. A dose-dependent increase in mortality with vesnarinone among patients with severe heart

failure. Vesnarinone Trial Investigators. N Engl J Med 1998;339(25):1810–16.
4. Feldman AM, Baughman KL, Lee WK, Gottlieb SH, Weiss JL, Becker LC, Strobeck JE. Usefulness of OPC-8212, a quinolinone derivative, for chronic congestive heart failure in patients with ischemic heart disease or idiopathic dilated cardiomyopathy. Am J Cardiol 1991;68(11):1203–10.

Vidarabine

General Information

Intravenous vidarabine is effective in the treatment of kerato-uveitis in animals and man, and has been used intravenously to treat herpetic eye infections in man (1). It has also been used as an ointment for treating superficial keratitis that does not respond to idoxuridine, but it penetrates the eye poorly (2). It is no longer used because of unacceptable toxicity and inferior activity compared with newer drugs for *Herpes simplex* and *Varicella zoster*. Its rapid inactivation and poor solubility are practical disadvantages.

Long-Term Effects

Mutagenicity

Vidarabine is oncogenic and mutagenic in animals (3).

References

1. Kaufman HE. Systemic therapy of ocular herpes. Int Ophthalmol Clin 1975;15(4):163–9.
2. Colin J. L'adenine-arabinoside en ophtalmologie. [Arabinosyladenine in ophthalmology.] J Fr Ophtalmol 1981;4(6–7):525–30.
3. Chang TW, Snydman DR. Antiviral agents: action and clinical use. Drugs 1979;18(5):354–76.

Vigabatrin

See also Antiepileptic drugs

General Information

Vigabatrin is used mainly in the treatment of refractory partial seizures and infantile spasms. Weight gain and mostly transient sedation are its most common adverse effects, but visual field defects are the main cause for concern and severely restrict its use.

In a placebo-controlled add-on comparison of three dosages of vigabatrin (1, 3, and 6 g/day) in 174 patients with partial epilepsy, fatigue, drowsiness, and dizziness were the most common treatment-related adverse events, especially at the highest dosage (1). The incidence of severe events was 2.2% in the placebo group and 8.7, 11, and 16% with 1, 3, and 6 g/day respectively. The proportion of patients who withdrew owing to adverse events was 2.2% in the placebo group and 6.5, 11, and 18% with 1, 3, and 6 g/day respectively. Four vigabatrin patients (three of whom were taking 6 g/day) had a reduction in erythrocyte counts to $3.4–3.5 \times 10^9/l$. Symptoms suggestive of retinal toxicity were not reported, but the duration of treatment was short (18 weeks) and there was no formal ophthalmological testing. Overall, efficacy and safety data from this trial suggested that 3 g/day gave optimal results. Although higher dosages may provide additional benefit in selected patients, the occurrence of retinal toxicity (see below) warrants caution about the use of high doses.

Vigabatrin has been studied in an open 1-year extension of a randomized, double-blind, placebo-controlled Canadian trial in 97 adults with resistant partial epilepsy (2). There was a mean weight gain of 3.7 kg by the end of the study. Treatment was discontinued in 12% because of adverse effects. Neurological/psychiatric adverse effects were the most common reason for withdrawal, including three behavioral reactions attributed to the drug.

In a single-blind, randomized trial of vigabatrin for 2 weeks in children with newly diagnosed infantile spasms the children were randomly assigned to low-dose vigabatrin (18–36 mg/kg/day) or high-dose vigabatrin (100–148 mg/kg/day) (3). The time to response was evaluated during the first 3 months, and safety was evaluated during the entire study. Eight of 75 children who took low-dose vigabatrin and 24 of 67 who took high-dose vigabatrin responded. The time to response was significantly shorter in those who took high-dose vigabatrin and in those with tuberous sclerosis. The most common treatment-related adverse events were sedation (42/167), insomnia (15/167), and irritability (15/167). There were no dose-related adverse events, and adverse event rates were similar in the low-dose and high-dose groups. Only nine patients withdrew because of adverse events.

Vigabatrin efficacy and tolerability have been evaluated for a mean of 16 months in children in a retrospective study of 73 patients (mean age 87 months) (4). In 16% of the children vigabatrin was given as monotherapy and patients with either partial or generalized seizures were included. Vigabatrin was highly effective in 30 children (over 90% seizure reduction) and partially effective in 4 (50–90% seizure frequency reduction). There were adverse effects in 24%, the commonest being irritability, aggression, opposition/defiance, self-injurious behaviors, and deterioration in behavioral control. There was seizure deterioration in 7% of the children; worsening of myoclonic seizures was most common. Visual field testing by perimetry was possible in only 12 of the children; 2 had visual field constriction.

Organs and Systems

Nervous system

Central nervous system adverse events are mostly mild and transient and consist especially of drowsiness and fatigue. Other effects include irritability, nervousness, dizziness, headache, confusion, and depression. In a double-blind add-on trial at dosages of 2 or 3 g/day, drowsiness, diplopia, ataxia, and visual abnormalities were the only adverse effects that increased with dosage (5).

In a randomized open comparison of carbamazepine and vigabatrin in newly diagnosed epilepsy (6), patients randomized to vigabatrin reported less frequent drowsiness (44 versus 62%) and dizziness (7 versus 20%), and more frequent myoclonic jerks (14 versus 2%) and visual scintillae (16 versus 0%).

Like other GABAergic drugs, vigabatrin can aggravate absence seizures and may precipitate absence status in patients with generalized epilepsies. Occasionally, absence seizures are also precipitated in patients with partial epilepsy, as in a 28-year old man who developed de novo absence status 4 days after the dosage of vigabatrin was increased to 2 g/day (7).

Vigabatrin produces intramyelinic edema (neuronal vacuolization) in rats, mice, and dogs, but probably not in non-human primates (8). These findings have been reassessed on the background of clinical safety data, to determine the potential for a similar effect in man (8). In animals intramyelinic edema correlates with changes in multimodality-evoked potentials and MRI, but many studies in patients treated with vigabatrin in dosages of 1–6 g/day for up to 12 years have failed to provide evidence for similar changes in humans. Histological examinations of autopsy brain tissue from 24 patients exposed to vigabatrin for 0.6 months to 9.6 years also failed to show any evidence of astrocytosis or axonal changes similar to those associated with vigabatrin-induced microvacuolization. These findings do not provide any support to the hypothesis that intramyelinic edema occurs in patients treated with vigabatrin.

Acute encephalopathy has previously been attributed to vigabatrin in adults. There has also been a case in a child (9).

- A 6-month-old girl with infantile Alexander disease with hydrocephalus developed apathy, somnolence, and stupor, with slowing of background encephalographic activity, 3 days after starting vigabatrin, which was withdrawn. During the next 2 days her symptoms abated and after 10 days her electroencephalogram normalized.

Vigabatrin can exacerbate myoclonic and absence seizures and occasionally other seizure types, especially in children with generalized epilepsies. After the administration of vigabatrin, seizures worsened in all of four children with Angelman syndrome (10), and generalized seizures occurred for the first time in a boy with succinic semialdehyde dehydrogenase deficiency (SEDA-21, 77). De novo myoclonic jerks and precipitation of status epilepticus have also been reported (SEDA-20, 70).

There have been several reports of acute encephalopathy (SEDA-18, 71) and occasional cases of akathisia, hyperkinesia, and dyskinesias. Toxicology studies in mice, rats, and dogs showed dose-related intramyelinic edema, with microvacuoles in the white matter of the brain, but there is no evidence that these have clinical relevance (SEDA-21, 77).

Sensory systems

Vigabatrin causes a variety of changes in visual function, including reductions in visual field, visual acuity, color vision, and electroretinographic and electro-oculographic amplitudes (11–16).

Visual field defects

DoTS classification (BMJ 2003;327:1222–5)
   Dose-relation: collateral
   Time-course: long-term
   Susceptibility factors: male sex

Severe symptomatic visual field constriction, affecting mostly the peripheral fields and without loss of visual acuity, was first reported in 1997 in three patients who had taken vigabatrin for 2–3 years (17), and reports continue to appear (18–24). Electrophysiological investigations suggested damage to the outer retina, and there was no recovery for up to 12 months after withdrawal. Over 50 other cases of visual field defects (including asymptomatic cases) were published thereafter, and 28 were known to the manufacturer before the initial publication (SEDA-21, 78) (SEDA-22, 92).

Features

Visual field loss due to vigabatrin has been studied in 18 patients taking long-term treatment (0.5–9.5 years) and five controls (25). Of the 18 patients taking vigabatrin, there were mild visual field defects in six right eyes and eight left eyes, and severe defects in nine right eyes and eight left eyes. Most of the defects were peripheral constriction with nasal predominance.

Even patients with relatively severe constriction can partly compensate through adjustments in eye movements. Because the disorder develops insidiously, these patients may remain unaware of their condition, even though their visual impairment puts them at risk in special circumstances, such as driving a car.

The safety of continuing vigabatrin therapy in adults who have taken prolonged treatment (over 2 years) has been assessed by serially monitoring changes in visual function over 1 year of continued therapy (26). Fifteen patients who continued to take vigabatrin had visual function testing (visual acuity, color vision, and kinetic and static perimetry) every 3 months for 1 year. Nine had normal visual fields and six had visual field constriction. During follow-up, they showed no worsening of visual acuity, color vision, or visual field constriction, beyond that measured in the initial test. This study showed that mild changes in visual function after long-term vigabatrin generally remain stable with continued treatment. However, patient consistency was variable and repeated testing was necessary in some cases to assess the reliability of the apparent worsening or improvement experienced by some patients.

Frequency

Visual field defects have been commonly reported in patients taking vigabatrin (10–30%) (27,28), although if asymptomatic cases are included, the incidence may be as high as 40% (29) or even 60% (30). In an observational cohort study the prevalence was relatively low, at 0.8% of 7228 patients (31); however, this result was challenged as a probable underestimate, because of the use of a questionnaire to elicit the diagnosis (12–14). These different rates have probably been related to the diverse methods of patient inclusion and visual field testing.

In a prospective study in patients evaluated for epilepsy surgery, absolute concentric contraction of the visual field of 10–30 degrees was found in 20 (17%) of 118 patients who had ever taken vigabatrin, compared with none of 39 patients who had never taken vigabatrin (27). Men were more frequently affected than women (21 versus 6%), and the degree of visual field loss was more severe in patients who had taken vigabatrin for more than 2 years. None of the affected patients complained spontaneously of visual field loss.

Expert review of 25 cases of visual field defects reported to the manufacturer suggested that in 13 of the patients the visual field loss could not be assigned to an alternative known cause and had to be ascribed to vigabatrin (11). In an open extension study in Japan, 29 of 99 patients treated with vigabatrin for 2.7–6.7 years had visual field defects attributed to vigabatrin (11).

Among 57 patients aged 19–73 years treated with vigabatrin as add-on or as monotherapy for 2–14 years, there were mildly abnormal or severely abnormal fields in 14 and 8 patients respectively (32). Two patients with severe field abnormalities were symptomatic.

Of 20 consecutive patients treated with vigabatrin 12 had visual field constriction, severe in four and symptomatic in two (33). Visual field defects were more common in patients who were also taking valproate. Although most reports concerned adults, children may also be affected (34).

In a randomized monotherapy trial in newly diagnosed epilepsy, seven of 32 patients who were still taking vigabatrin after 3–9 years had concentrically constricted visual fields, and the defect was rated as severe in two (35). Of the seven patients with field defects, five had reduced oscillatory potentials and two also had abnormal a and b waves in rod and cone electroretinography. In contrast, none of the 20 patients who were still taking carbamazepine had abnormal visual fields. There is also preliminary evidence that a pre-existing visual field defect increases susceptibility to vigabatrin-induced visual field constriction.

In a double-blind, randomized study in patients with partial epilepsy three of 32 patients taking vigabatrin had abnormal visual perimetry after the end of the study (36).

In a retrospective study in 158 patients with partial epilepsy visual field defects were detected in 21 (13%); 13 patients had concentric visual field constriction without subjective spontaneous manifestations. Of these 13 patients, 9 were taking vigabatrin (37).

The efficacy and adverse effects of steroids and vigabatrin in children with infantile spasms have been reviewed (38). The authors found a high rate of visual field defects and concluded that although vigabatrin is efficacious it does not seem to be more effective than steroids or corticotrophin, and that the benefits of vigabatrin do not justify the associated risks of possible irreversible visual changes.

The prevalence of visual field constriction associated with vigabatrin has been evaluated in 91 children aged 5.6–18 years (39). There were visual field defects in 17, but there was wide intrasubject variation between successive test sessions, and children often performed better in later test sessions, making evaluation difficult.

Pathophysiology
Electroretinographic findings in affected patients are consistent with reduced inner retinal cone response (40,41), but interpretation of the results has been disputed (42,43).

Visual fields have been studied in eight patients with vigabatrin-attributed visual field loss; six were no longer taking vigabatrin (44). Seven patients had marked visual field constriction with some sparing of the temporal visual field; the eighth had concentric constriction. Two patients had subnormal Arden electro-oculography indices; one patient had an abnormally delayed photopic b wave; five patients had delayed 30-Hz flicker b waves; and seven patients had delayed oscillatory potentials. Multifocal electroretinography confirmed that the effects occurred at the retinal level.

Visual fields, visual evoked potentials, and electroretinography have been assessed in 24 children treated with vigabatrin; 13 had at least one abnormal study (45). There was visual field constriction in 11 of 17 patients who had perimetry; five of 15 patients who underwent visual evoked potential testing and four of 11 who underwent electroretinography had abnormal examinations. Abnormal visual evoked potentials and electroretinography were mostly found in children who also had visual field constriction. Of five patients who were taking vigabatrin alone, three had abnormalities; however, all the other patients were taking other antiepileptic drugs and additive effects could not be ruled out.

The retinal electrophysiological markers associated with vigabatrin-attributed visual field loss have been distinguished from those associated with current vigabatrin therapy in 8 previous and 18 current vigabatrin users (46). They underwent electro-oculography, electroretinography, and automated static threshold perimetry and 22 healthy subjects underwent electroretinography. Of 26 patients exposed to vigabatrin, 18 had visual field loss; none taking other antiepileptic drugs had this type of visual field abnormality. The presence and severity of the visual field loss were significantly associated with the latency (implicit time) and amplitude of the electroretinographic cone function. The amplitude of the cone flicker response was the strongest predictor of visual field loss. The electro-oculogram, the photopic and scotopic electroretinogram, and the latency of the electroretinographic second oscillatory potential were not significantly related to the presence of visual field loss. Vigabatrin was significantly associated with the photopic amplitude, the scotopic a-wave latency, and the latency of the second oscillatory potential.

The pathological features of visual field constriction have been described in a patient taking vigabatrin (47).

- A 41-year-old man who had taken vigabatrin for 2 years in doses of 3–6 g/day developed bilateral concentric visual field defects, with greater loss in the nasal fields. Vigabatrin was withdrawn. Later he had a cardiopulmonary arrest and died. At postmortem there was peripheral retinal atrophy with loss of ganglion cells, severe in the peripheral retina and less severe in the maculae.

There was loss of nerve fibers in the optic nerves, chiasm, and tracts. There was no evidence of intramyelin edema.

These findings suggest that vigabatrin may be directly associated with direct retinal injury (to the ganglion cells). The degree of cell loss suggested that the visual field loss was irreversible.

Mechanism
The mechanism responsible for the development of the visual field defects is unknown. However, they may be related to accumulation of GABA in the retina. In rats treated either with vigabatrin or tiagabine, vigabatrin reduced the activity of GABA transaminase and increased GABA concentrations in the brain, but these effects were more pronounced in the retina, in which vigabatrin concentrations are as much as five-fold higher than in the brain (48). On the other hand, tiagabine concentrations are considerably lower in the retina than in the brain. Tiagabine has not been associated with visual field defects.

Vigabatrin-induced inhibition of ornithine transaminase has been suggested as an alternative mechanism (49).

Diagnosis
Visual field defects are difficult to detect by simple clinical examination, even in patients with severe constriction at perimetric assessment. Visual field testing should be done before treatment and at regular intervals thereafter. Patients should be questioned about visual disturbances and referred to an ophthalmologist if relevant symptoms are recognized.

Potential correlations between visual field defects and the results of ophthalmological tests have been assessed. The use of the electroretinogram as a marker for vigabatrin-induced visual field alterations has been questioned (42), and the suggestion has been made that the electroretinographic changes described in some patients on vigabatrin may be due to a physiological effect of GABA not necessarily related to retinal toxicity (43). Of 20 consecutive patients 14 had a reduced light/dark ratio (Arden ratio) in the standard electro-oculogram and 10 had absent oscillatory potentials in the electroretinogram (33). Overall, 17 patients had abnormal electro-oculography, electroretinography, or both, although only 12 had constricted visual fields at perimetric testing.

The value of electroretinography and electro-oculography in the early diagnosis of vigabatrin-associated visual field defects has been assessed in 30 patients with temporal lobe epilepsy (50,51). The patients were stratified into three groups: (A) concentric contraction of the visual field associated with vigabatrin ($n = 15$), (B) normal visual field with vigabatrin use ($n = 11$), and (C) normal visual field without vigabatrin ($n = 4$). There were abnormal electrophysiological results in 50% of the patients in group A. The electro-oculographic Arden ratio was lowered in 57%. The amount of visual field loss and the total dose of vigabatrin used correlated only weakly with the results of electroretinography and electro-oculography. These results suggest that ocular electrophysiology is not a good method for detecting patients at risk of vigabatrin-related visual field defects. Regular visual field examination remains the cornerstone in screening. This has been confirmed by a retrospective, comparative case series in which the degree of electroretinal dysfunction was analysed using electroretinography in 40 patients taking vigabatrin, 24 as monotherapy (52). There was no statistically significant relation between the frequency of electrodiagnostic abnormalities and the duration of use or the total cumulative dosage of vigabatrin.

Dose-relation
Visual function has been studied in 21 epileptic patients taking vigabatrin and compared with visual function in 11 similar epileptic patients who had never taken it, in order to investigate whether the severity of visual field defect is related to the dose of vigabatrin and to consider other factors that may correlate with severity (53). Nine of 20 patients taking vigabatrin complained of blurring of vision compared with two of 11 controls. Four patients taking vigabatrin described flickering lights compared with one control. None had a posterior vitreous detachment. Three of 30 eyes of patients taking vigabatrin had distant visual acuity of 6/12 or worse compared with three of 22 controls, and five of 30 had near visual acuity worse than N6 compared with one of 22 controls. A mean of 1.73 Ishihara plates were misread by patients taking vigabatrin compared with 0.18 in the controls. There was a significant correlation between the severity of visual field defect and the total dose of vigabatrin.

In a cohort study of 99 patients taking vigabatrin, the prevalence of visual field defects increased significantly with increasing total vigabatrin dose. The prevalence ranged from four of 51 patients who had been exposed to 1 g/day or less to six of 8 patients taking a total dose of 3–5 g/day (28).

Time-course
The longer the duration of vigabatrin treatment and the higher the dose the greater the probability of field defects (28,30,51).

In a reference cohort of 42 patients exposed to other antiepileptic drugs without vigabatrin, 7 had visual field defects, but in all of them this could be ascribed to a known cause (11). The prevalence of visual field loss ascribed to the drug did not differ between patients treated for less than 4 years and those treated for more than 4 years (32 versus 28%), suggesting that the disorder is unlikely to increase with continuous treatment beyond 4 years. Visual field loss occurred in 17 of 45 men (38%) versus 12 of 54 women (22%), indicating that men have a two-fold increase in risk. Age, body weight, daily or cumulative vigabatrin dose, and concomitant antiepileptic drugs did not predict the occurrence of visual field loss. The appearance in the central field out to 30° eccentricity was typically that of a localized bilateral binasal loss, particularly with static threshold perimetry, extending in an annulus over the horizontal midline, together with a relative sparing of the temporal field. In severe cases, there was a concentric appearance. All cases except one were asymptomatic. The authors concluded that the visual field defect induced by vigabatrin is unique in pattern and profound in terms of frequency of occurrence and location and severity of the loss.

Susceptibility factors
Concentric visual field loss found in the presurgical evaluation of patients with drug-resistant temporal lobe epilepsy taking vigabatrin has been studied and related to potential susceptibility factors in 157 consecutive patients with drug-resistant temporal lobe epilepsy (27). There was absolute concentric contraction of the visual field of 10–30 degrees presurgically in 20 of 118 patients who had ever used vigabatrin and in none of 39 who had not. Men were significantly more often affected than women (15 of 72 versus 5 of 85). The degree of visual field loss correlated with the duration of vigabatrin medication. There was no correlation of visual field contraction with a history of meningitis as potential cause of the epilepsy, duration of the epilepsy, status epilepticus in the medical history, or histological abnormality of the brain tissue removed. Ophthalmological examination of the patients with concentric contraction showed no abnormalities. None of the patients with concentric contraction complained spontaneously of their visual field loss.

The long-term retinal effects of vigabatrin in children are unknown, and visual field testing is usually impossible. Recent evidence has suggested that a short course of vigabatrin (6 months) in children with infantile spasms may be sufficient (54) and minimizes the potential for visual adverse effects.

Reversibility
Vigabatrin-induced visual field loss is generally considered to be irreversible (28,51), although partial reversibility has been described in some cases.

Long-term changes in the concentric contraction of the visual field have been studied in 27 patients with temporal lobe epilepsy taking vigabatrin (55). Concentric contraction of the visual field did not change in 16 patients who stopped taking vigabatrin before the first examination but there was slight but significant worsening of visual field loss in 11 patients who continued taking vigabatrin. The authors concluded that vigabatrin-associated visual field loss is not reversible and that progression can occur when vigabatrin is continued.

The reversibility of visual function loss from vigabatrin has been studied in 13 patients who had discontinued the drug up to a year before because of lack of efficacy or reductions in visual field (56). Although electroretinographic cone implicit time improved, most of the patients did not have improvement in either clinical measures of visual function (that is visual acuity, color vision, visual fields) or in electroretinographic amplitudes. However, several patients who had minimal visual field loss while taking vigabatrin had substantial recovery of the electroretinographic amplitudes. There was no association between recovery of function and either duration of treatment or cumulative dosage. Multifocal electroretinography showed a diffuse loss of function that was not isolated to the periphery.

In contrast, in another study there was partial reversibility of visual field constriction and retinal function after withdrawal in two patients (57).

Of 30 children with epilepsy (14 boys and 16 girls, aged 4–20 years) taking vigabatrin for infantile spasms and simple and complex partial epilepsy, who had never complained of ophthalmologic disturbances, 4 had visual field constriction in the nasal hemifield (58). In one child, visual abnormalities were stable even 10 months after vigabatrin withdrawal, while in another there was improvement 5 months after withdrawal.

- Although in a 10-year-old girl a severe visual field defect was said to have reversed after withdrawal (59), repeat confirmatory testing was not performed before the withdrawal of vigabatrin and the pattern of constriction was suggestive of an artefact related to inadequate compliance with the testing procedure (J Wild, personal communication, 1999).

However, other preliminary reports have suggested that reversibility of the visual field defects may in fact occur following early withdrawal (57,60).

Of 12 vigabatrin-treated patients with visual field defects re-examined 2–10 years after vigabatrin withdrawal, all still had visual field defects (28). In five cases there was apparent worsening. Exceptional cases of reversible visual field defects have been reported in children (61). However, perimetry assessment in children is burdened with multiple methodological problems that usually preclude reliable results.

In a study in 60 adults with partial epilepsy, progression or reversibility of vigabatrin-associated visual field defects were examined (51). The patients had taken vigabatrin for 7 months to 14 years as monotherapy or add-on therapy and were examined with repeated kinetic Goldmann perimetry. A follow-up examination was performed after 4–38 months in 55 patients. There was vigabatrin-associated visual field constriction in 40%, and in 13% the defect was severe. During follow-up after withdrawal of vigabatrin, there was no significant recovery of visual fields in any patient. Conversely, there was no progression in those who continued therapy.

Effects of other antiepileptic drugs and interaction with vigabatrin
Other antiepileptic drugs can also alter visual evoked potentials and brainstem evoked potentials. Visual field defects associated with various antiepileptic drugs (carbamazepine, diazepam, gabapentin, phenytoin, tiagabine, and vigabatrin) have been reviewed (37).

In 100 epileptic patients aged 8–18 years taking carbamazepine or valproate in modified-release formulations either alone or with added vigabatrin interpeak latencies of I-III and III-V of brainstem evoked potentials were significantly delayed and N75/P100 and P100/N145 amplitudes in the visual evoked potentials were reduced (62). However, the addition of vigabatrin did not worsen the effects caused by the other two drugs alone.

Retinal dysfunction
Retinal dysfunction has been retrospectively assessed in 29 children taking vigabatrin 25–114 mg/kg/day for 6.5 years (63). Ophthalmic examination was performed before treatment and every 6 months thereafter. Four children developed eye changes (retinal pigmentation, hypopigmented retinal spots, vascular sheathing, and optic atrophy). Visual evoked potentials were abnormal in 16. Electroretinography and electro-oculography were not performed.

Color vision defects
There was abnormal color perception in 32% of 32 patients taking vigabatrin monotherapy; in four cases there was an abnormality in the blue-yellow axis (64). In the same patients there was a positive correlation between visual contrast sensitivity and the size of the visual field; macular photo-stress and glare tests were equal in both groups and did not differ from normal values; there was no effect on glare sensitivity (65).

Changes in color vision have been investigated in healthy volunteers who took a single oral dose of either vigabatrin or carbamazepine in a single-blind, placebo-controlled, randomized trial (66). All underwent color visual-evoked potential testing and color perimetry at baseline and after taking placebo, vigabatrin (2000 mg), or carbamazepine (400 mg). Carbamazepine caused mild overall impairment of the chromatic and achromatic systems. Vigabatrin caused selective blue impairment, consistent with GABAergic inhibition in the retina. The relation of this change in color perception to visual field defects, if any, is unknown.

Psychological, psychiatric

Although abnormal behavior, psychosis, and depression occur with increased frequency (around 2–4% or even higher) in patients with refractory epilepsy, the risk is increased during treatment with vigabatrin or on its abrupt withdrawal (SEDA-18, 71) (SEDA-19, 76) (SEDA-20, 70) (SEDA-21, 77) (67). The risk depends on the patient's characteristics, the dosage, and the rate of dose escalation. In the manufacturer's safety database, the incidence of psychosis was reported as being 1.1% or 0.64% based on postmarketing Prescription Event Monitoring (68). However, in adults with refractory partial epilepsy, severe behavioral or mood disturbances can be anticipated in 26% of treated cases (SEDA-18, 72), although higher figures have also been presented (SEDA-20, 70). In one study depression occurred with a frequency of about 9% with vigabatrin and 1% with placebo (5).

Psychiatric complications occur in both children and adults. While there is some evidence that a positive psychiatric history may increase the risk (and may represent a relative contraindication), behavioral and mood disturbances can occur in patients who had no similar episodes in the past. A retrospective survey of 50 patients with vigabatrin-associated psychosis ($n = 28$) or depression ($n = 22$) suggested that psychosis tends to occur in patients with more severe epilepsy and may be related to a right-sided EEG focus or suppression of seizures (64% of patients were free of seizures). On the other hand, patients with depression tended to have a past history of depressive illness and to have had little or no change in seizure frequency (69). To minimize risks, vigabatrin should be introduced in low dosages and increased slowly, and it should not be withdrawn abruptly. Psychiatric symptoms usually remit with drug withdrawal, although if treatment needs to be continued, neuroleptic medication may be useful.

That vigabatrin can cause psychosis and depression has been confirmed in an analysis of data from double-blind, controlled, add-on trials (70). Compared with placebo, vigabatrin-exposed patients had a significantly higher incidence of events coded as depression (12 versus 3.5%) and psychosis (2.5 versus 0.3%). Although these events occurred during the first 3 months, most of the studies lasted 12–18 weeks and therefore definite conclusions could not be reached about timing.

Metabolism

Weight gain occurs in as many as 40% of patients during the first 6 months of therapy.

Mouth and teeth

Gingival overgrowth occurred in a 29-year-old man who had taken vigabatrin for 5 years for partial epileptic seizures (71).

Liver

Liver toxicity, if it occurs, is exceedingly rare. Fatal acute hepatic failure was described in a 3-year-old boy (SEDA-21, 78).

Pancreas

Pancreatitis occurred in a patient whose polytherapy included vigabatrin (SEDA-20, 58), but cause and effect was uncertain.

Skin

Skin reactions to vigabatrin are very rare. One case of erythema multiforme was complicated by concomitant multiple pathology, and cause and effect was dubious (SEDA-20, 71).

Susceptibility Factors

Renal disease

Acute encephalopathy with stupor and generalized slow wave electroencephalographic activity developed in three men with mild renal insufficiency aged 24–74 years within 1–3 days of starting vigabatrin (1–2 g/day) or increasing the dosage (from 2 to 3 g/day) (72). The symptoms subsided rapidly after drug withdrawal or dose reduction. Special caution is recommended when vigabatrin is used in patients with impaired renal function.

Drug Administration

Drug overdose

Doses of vigabatrin up to 10 g have been taken without serious effects. Toxic manifestations include vertigo, tremor, sedation, coma, myoclonic jerks, and psychosis. Gastric lavage within 1–2 hours is recommended after doses in excess of 12 g in adults and 2 g in children (SEDA-22, 85). The development of discontinuous partial complex status epilepticus in a patient with partial epilepsy who had taken a 20 g overdose 6 days earlier was considered to be a possible effect of withdrawal (SEDA-22, 85).

- After an overdose of vigabatrin 45 g, a 17-year-old girl developed a behavioral disorder (73). A CT scan of the

brain was normal but an electroencephalogram showed abnormal delta waves.

Drug–Drug Interactions

Carbamazepine

One report suggesting that carbamazepine reduces serum vigabatrin concentrations (SEDA-21, 80) requires confirmation.

Although vigabatrin is not metabolized by liver enzymes it increased serum carbamazepine concentrations by at least 10% in 66 epileptic patients aged 10–66 years with focal seizure onset with or without secondary generalization (74).

Ethinylestradiol

Vigabatrin does not produce enzyme induction and did not generally alter the kinetics of ethinylestradiol and levonorgestrel, although two women had an approximate 50% reduction in ethinylestradiol concentrations during vigabatrin treatment (SEDA-21, 80).

Phenytoin

Vigabatrin can reduce serum phenytoin concentrations by about one-third, but this interaction is inconsistent.

Interference with Diagnostic Tests

General

Vigabatrin can produce an abnormal urinary amino acid pattern, which can be diagnostically confusing (SEDA-16, 74). It increases plasma and urinary alpha-aminoadipic acid concentrations, possibly complicating the diagnosis of alpha-aminoadipicaciduria (SEDA-20, 71).

Vigabatrin inhibits alanine transferase, and the resulting underestimation of enzyme activity could mask evidence of hepatic disease (SEDA-20, 70).

References

1. Dean C, Mosier M, Penry K. Dose-Response Study of Vigabatrin as add-on therapy in patients with uncontrolled complex partial seizures. Epilepsia 1999;40(1):74–82.
2. Guberman A, Bruni J. Long-term open multicentre, add-on trial of vigabatrin in adult resistant partial epilepsy.The Canadian Vigabatrin Study Group. Seizure 2000;9(2):112–18.
3. Elterman RD, Shields WD, Mansfield KA, Nakagawa J. US Infantile Spasms Vigabatrin Study Group. Randomized trial of vigabatrin in patients with infantile spasms. Neurology 2001;57(8):1416–21.
4. Prasad AN, Penney S, Buckley DJ. The role of vigabatrin in childhood seizure disorders: results from a clinical audit. Epilepsia 2001;42(1):54–61.
5. Beran RG, Berkovic SF, Buchanan N, Danta G, Mackenzie R, Schapel G, Sheean G, Vajda F. A double-blind, placebo-controlled crossover study of vigabatrin 2 g/day and 3 g/day in uncontrolled partial seizures. Seizure 1996;5(4):259–65.
6. Kalviainen R, Aikia M, Saukkonen AM, Mervaala E, Riekkinen PJ Sr. Vigabatrin vs carbamazepine

monotherapy in patients with newly diagnosed epilepsy. A randomized, controlled study. Arch Neurol 1995;52(10):989–96.

7. Cocito L, Primavera A, Panayiotopoulos CP, Agathonikou A, Sharoqi IA, Parker APJ. Vigabatrin aggravates absences and absence status. Neurology 1998;51(5):1519–20.

8. Cohen JA, Fisher RS, Brigell MG, Peyster RG, Sze G. The potential for vigabatrin-induced intramyelinic edema in humans. Epilepsia 2000;41(2):148–57.

9. Haas-Lude K, Wolff M, Riethmuller J, Niemann G, Krageloh-Mann I. Acute encephalopathy associated with vigabatrin in a six-month-old girl. Epilepsia 2000; 41(5):628–30.

10. Kuenzle C, Steinlin M, Wohlrab G, Boltshauser E, Schmitt B. Adverse effects of vigabatrin in Angelman syndrome. Epilepsia 1998;39(11):1213–15.

11. Wild JM, Martinez C, Reinshagen G, Harding GF. Characteristics of a unique visual field defect attributed to vigabatrin. Epilepsia 1999;40(12):1784–94.

12. Comaish IF, Gorman C, Galloway NR. Visual field defect associated with vigabatrin. Many more patients may be affected than were found in study. BMJ 2000;320(7246):1403.

13. Manuchehri K. Visual field defect associated with vigabatrin. Method of estimating prevalence was inappropriate. BMJ 2000;320(7246):1403–4.

14. Midelfart A. Visual field defect associated with vigabatrin. Means of selecting patients was misleading. BMJ 2000;320(7246):1404.

15. Spence SJ, Sankar R. Visual field defects and other ophthalmological disturbances associated with vigabatrin. Drug Saf 2001;24(5):385–404.

16. Kalviainen R, Nousiainen I. Visual field defects with vigabatrin: epidemiology and therapeutic implications. CNS Drugs 2001;15(3):217–30.

17. Eke T, Talbot JF, Lawden MC. Severe persistent visual field constriction associated with vigabatrin. BMJ 1997;314(7075):180–1.

18. Schmitz B, Schmidt T, Jokiel B, Pfeiffer S, Tiel-Wilck K, Ruther K. Visual field constriction in epilepsy patients treated with vigabatrin and other antiepileptic drugs: a prospective study. J Neurol 2002;249(4):469–75.

19. Schmidt T, Ruther K, Jokiel B, Pfeiffer S, Tiel-Wilck K, Schmitz B. Is visual field constriction in epilepsy patients treated with vigabatrin reversible? J Neurol 2002;249(8):1066–71.

20. Newman WD, Tocher K, Acheson JF. Vigabatrin associated visual field loss: a clinical audit to study prevalence, drug history and effects of drug withdrawal. Eye 2002;16(5):567–71.

21. Jensen H, Sjo O, Uldall P, Gram L. Vigabatrin and retinal changes. Doc Ophthalmol 2002;104(2):171–80.

22. Hilton EJ, Cubbidge RP, Hosking SL, Betts T, Comaish IF. Patients treated with vigabatrin exhibit central visual function loss. Epilepsia 2002;43(11):1351–9.

23. Besch D, Kurtenbach A, Apfelstedt-Sylla E, Sadowski B, Dennig D, Asenbauer C, Zrenner E, Schiefer U. Visual field constriction and electrophysiological changes associated with vigabatrin. Doc Ophthalmol 2002;104(2):151–70.

24. Arndt CF, Salle M, Derambure PH, Defoort-Dhellemmes S, Hache JC. The effect on vision of associated treatments in patients taking vigabatrin: carbamazepine versus valproate. Epilepsia 2002;43(8):812–17.

25. Midelfart A, Midelfart E, Brodtkorb E. Visual field defects in patients taking vigabatrin. Acta Ophthalmol Scand 2000;78(5):580–4.

26. Paul SR, Krauss GL, Miller NR, Medura MT, Miller TA, Johnson MA. Visual function is stable in patients who continue long-term vigabatrin therapy: implications for clinical decision making. Epilepsia 2001;42(4):525–30.

27. Hardus P, Verduin WM, Postma G, Stilma JS, Berendschot TT, van Veelen CW. Concentric contraction of the visual field in patients with temporal lobe epilepsy and its association with the use of vigabatrin medication. Epilepsia 2000;41(5):581–7.

28. Malmgren K, Ben-Menachem E, Frisen L. Vigabatrin visual toxicity: evolution and dose dependence. Epilepsia 2001;42(5):609–15.

29. Nousiainen I, Mantyjarvi M, Kalviainen R. No reversion in vigabatrin-associated visual field defects. Neurology 2001;57(10):1916–17.

30. Toggweiler S, Wieser HG. Concentric visual field restriction under vigabatrin therapy: extent depends on the duration of drug intake. Seizure 2001;10(6):420–3.

31. Wilton LV, Stephens MD, Mann RD. Visual field defect associated with vigabatrin: observational cohort study. BMJ 1999;319(7218):1165–6.

32. Nousiainen I, Kalviainen R, Mantiyarvi M, Riekkinen PJ. Prevalence of concentric visual field constriction in adult epilepsy patients with vigabatrin treatment. Neurology 1999;52(Suppl. 2):A235–6.

33. Arndt CF, Derambure P, Defoort-Dhellemmes S, Hache JC. Outer retinal dysfunction in patients treated with vigabatrin. Neurology 1999;52(6):1201–5.

34. Vanhatalo S, Paakkonen L, Nousiainen I. Visual field constriction in children treated with vigabatrin. Neurology 1999;52(8):1713–14.

35. Kalviainen R, Nousianen I, Nikoskelainen A, Partanen J, Partanen K, Mantijarvi M, Riekkinen PJ. Visual field defects associated with initial vigabatrin monotherapy as compared with initial carbamazepine monotherapy. Epilepsia 1998;39(Suppl. 2):5.

36. Lindberger M, Alenius M, Frisen L, Johannessen SI, Larsson S, Malmgren K, Tomson T. Gabapentin versus vigabatrin as first add-on for patients with partial seizures that failed to respond to monotherapy: a randomized, double-blind, dose titration study. GREAT Study Investigators Group.Gabapentin Refractory Epilepsy Add-on Treatment. Epilepsia 2000;41(10):1289–95.

37. Stefan H, Bernatik J, Knorr HLJ. Visual field constriction and antiepileptic drug treatment. Neurol Psychiatry Brain Res 2000;7:185–90.

38. Riikonen RS. Steroids or vigabatrin in the treatment of infantile spasms? Pediatr Neurol 2000;23(5):403–8.

39. Vanhatalo S, Nousiainen I, Eriksson K, Rantala H, Vainionpaa L, Mustonen K, Aarimaa T, Alen R, Aine MR, Byring R, Hirvasniemi A, Nuutila A, Walden T, Ritanen-Mohammed UM, Karttunen-Lewandowski P, Pohjola LM, Kaksonen S, Jurvelin P, Granstrom ML. Visual field constriction in 91 Finnish children treated with vigabatrin. Epilepsia 2002;43(7):748–56.

40. Krauss GL, Johnson MA, Miller NR. Vigabatrin-associated retinal cone system dysfunction: electroretinogram and ophthalmologic findings. Neurology 1998;50(3):614–18.

41. Krauss GL, Johnson MA, Miller NR. Vigabatrin-associated retinal cone system dysfunction. Neurology 1998;51:1779–81.

42. Beck RW. Vigabatrin-associated retinal cone system dysfunction. Neurology 1998;51(6):1778–9.

43. Brigell MG. Vigabatrin-associated retinal cone system dysfunction. Neurology 1998;51(6):1779–81.

44. Harding GF, Wild JM, Robertson KA, Lawden MC, Betts TA, Barber C, Barnes PM. Electro-oculography, electroretinography, visual evoked potentials, and multifocal electroretinography in patients with vigabatrin-attributed visual field constriction. Epilepsia 2000; 41(11):1420–31.

45. Gross-Tsur V, Banin E, Shahar E, Shalev RS, Lahat E. Visual impairment in children with epilepsy treated with vigabatrin. Ann Neurol 2000;48(1):60–4.

46. Harding GF, Wild JM, Robertson KA, Rietbrock S, Martinez C. Separating the retinal electrophysiologic effects of vigabatrin: treatment versus field loss. Neurology 2000;55(3):347–52.

47. Ravindran J, Blumbergs P, Crompton J, Pietris G, Waddy H. Visual field loss associated with vigabatrin: pathological correlations. J Neurol Neurosurg Psychiatry 2001;70(6):787–9.

48. Sills GJ, Patsalos PN, Butler E, Forrest G, Ratnaraj N, Brodie MJ. Visual field constriction: accumulation of vigabatrin but not tiagabine in the retina. Neurology 2001;57(2):196–200.

49. Roubertie A, Bellet H, Echenne B. Vigabatrin-associated retinal cone system dysfunction. Neurology 1998;51(6):1779–81.

50. Hardus P, Verduin WM, Berendschot TT, Kamermans M, Postma G, Stilma JS, van Veelen CW. The value of electrophysiology results in patients with epilepsy and vigabatrin associated visual field loss. Acta Ophthalmol Scand 2001;79(2):169–74.

51. Hardus P, Verduin WM, Engelsman M, Edelbroek PM, Segers JP, Berendschot TT, Stilma JS. Visual field loss associated with vigabatrin: quantification and relation to dosage. Epilepsia 2001;42(2):262–7.

52. Coupland SG, Zackon DH, Leonard BC, Ross TM. Vigabatrin effect on inner retinal function. Ophthalmology 2001;108(8):1493–6.

53. Manuchehri K, Goodman S, Siviter L, Nightingale S. A controlled study of vigabatrin and visual abnormalities. Br J Ophthalmol 2000;84(5):499–505.

54. Nabbout R, Melki I, Gerbaka B, Dulac O, Akatcherian C. Infantile spasms in Down syndrome: good response to a short course of vigabatrin. Epilepsia 2001;42(12):1580–3.

55. Hardus P, Verduin WM, Postma G, Stilma JS, Berendschot TT, van Veelen CW. Long term changes in the visual fields of patients with temporal lobe epilepsy using vigabatrin. Br J Ophthalmol 2000;84(7):788–90.

56. Johnson MA, Krauss GL, Miller NR, Medura M, Paul SR. Visual function loss from vigabatrin: effect of stopping the drug. Neurology 2000;55(1):40–5.

57. Krakow K, Polizzi G, Riordan-Eva P, Holder G, MacLeod WN, Fish DR. Recovery of visual field constriction following discontinuation of vigabatrin. Seizure 2000;9(4):287–90.

58. Iannetti P, Spalice A, Perla FM, Conicella E, Raucci U, Bizzarri B. Visual field constriction in children with epilepsy on vigabatrin treatment. Pediatrics 2000;106(4):838–42.

59. Versino M, Veggiotti P. Reversibility of vigabatrin-induced visual-field defect. Lancet 1999;354(9177):486.

60. Kramer G, Ried S, Landau K, Harding GFA. Vigabatrin: reversibility of severe concentric visual field defects after early detection and drug withdrawal—a case report. Epilepsia 2000;41(Suppl Florence):144.

61. Vanhatalo S, Alen R, Riikonen R, Rantala H, Aine MR, Mustonen K, Nousiainen I. Reversed visual field constrictions in children after vigabatrin withdrawal—true retinal recovery or improved test performance only? Seizure 2001;10(7):508–11.

62. Zgorzalewicz M, Galas-Zgorzalewicz B. Visual and auditory evoked potentials during long-term vigabatrin treatment in children and adolescents with epilepsy. Clin Neurophysiol 2000;111(12):2150–4.

63. Koul R, Chacko A, Ganesh A, Bulusu S, Al Riyami K. Vigabatrin associated retinal dysfunction in children with epilepsy. Arch Dis Child 2001;85(6):469–73.

64. Nousiainen I, Kalviainen R, Mantyjarvi M. Contrast and glare sensitivity in epilepsy patients treated with vigabatrin or carbamazepine monotherapy compared with healthy volunteers. Br J Ophthalmol 2000;84(6):622–5.

65. Miyaoka T, Seno H, Itoga M, Horiguchi J. Reversible pitch perception deficit caused by carbamazepine. Clin Neuropharmacol 2000;23(4):219–21.

66. Mecarelli O, Rinalduzzi S, Accornero N. Changes in color vision after a single dose of vigabatrin or carbamazepine in healthy volunteers. Clin Neuropharmacol 2001;24(1):23–6.

67. Ferrie CD, Robinson RO, Panayiotopoulos CP. Psychotic and severe behavioural reactions with vigabatrin: a review. Acta Neurol Scand 1996;93(1):1–8.

68. Levinson D, Mumford J. Vigabatrin and psychosis. Epilepsia 1995;36(Suppl. 4):32.

69. Guberman A, Andermann F, McLachlan R, Savard G, Manchanda R. The Vigabatrin Behavioral Effects Study Group. Severe behavioral/psychiatric reactions on vigabatrin: a Canadian study. Epilepsia 1996;37(Suppl. 5):170.

70. Levinson DF, Devinsky O. Psychiatric adverse events during vigabatrin therapy. Neurology 1999;53(7):1503–11.

71. Mesa FL, Lopez C, Gonzalez MA, Del-Moral R, O'Valle FJ. Clinical and histopathological description of a new case of vigabatrin-induced gingival overgrowth. Med Oral 2000;5(2):133–7.

72. Ifergane G, Masalha R, Zigulinski R, Merkin L, Wirguin I, Herishanu YO. Acute encephalopathy associated with vigabatrin monotherapy in patients with mild renal failure. Neurology 1998;51(1):314–15.

73. Mouton P, Defer GL. Troubles comportmentaux par intoxication aiguë au vigabatrin. [Behavior disorders due to acute vigabatrin intoxication.] Rev Neurol (Paris) 2000;156(2):184–6.

74. Jedrzejczak J, Dlawichowska E, Owczarek K, Majkowski J. Effect of vigabatrin addition on carbamazepine blood serum levels in patients with epilepsy. Epilepsy Res 2000;39(2):115–20.

Viloxazine

See also Antidepressants, second-generation

General Information

Viloxazine, a bicyclic compound, is related structurally (but not pharmacologically) to the beta-adrenoceptor antagonists. In animal tests, its profile shows properties of both the imipramine-like compounds (reversal of reserpine-induced hypothermia) and amphetamine (stimulation of the electroencephalogram). A review of animal and clinical data confirmed the impression that viloxazine has efficacy comparable to that of imipramine but with a different adverse effects profile (1). There is a reduced frequency of anticholinergic and sedative effects and a tendency to lose rather than to gain weight. However, viloxazine has some limiting adverse effects of its own. These include nausea, vomiting, and gastrointestinal distress, which may be reduced by the use of an enteric-coated formulation (2,3). Viloxazine has also been implicated in migraine, even in patients with no previous history (4).

Organs and Systems

Cardiovascular

Although hypotension and tachycardia can occur, an extensive review of its animal and clinical pharmacology suggested that viloxazine is relatively free of direct cardiotoxic effects (1). In a controlled comparison of doxepin and viloxazine (150–450 mg/day), one patient taking viloxazine developed chest pain after 26 days; an electrocardiogram confirmed changes compatible with ischemia but there were no progressive electrocardiographic or enzyme changes, and the patient recovered fully after being dropped from the study (5).

Nervous system

Viloxazine has previously been reported to lack epileptogenic properties (SEDA-10, 52). In a review of eight patients (six reported to the UK Committee on Safety of Medicines and two in Japan) it was concluded that there was a possible causal connection with seizures in only two cases, and that such an association was inconsistent with the results of animal studies and with a worldwide review of clinical trials (6). The reviewers concluded that if there is a risk of inducing epilepsy with viloxazine, it is probably only one-tenth that of tricyclic compounds.

Drug Administration

Drug overdose

It has been claimed that viloxazine is relatively free of cardiotoxic effects and therefore safe in patients who take an overdose. Indeed, 12 cases of overdose have been reported, with complete recovery and no electrocardiographic changes (SEDA-1, 9). In an authoritative review it was concluded that although coma, hypotension, and loss of tendon reflexes have been reported, serious complications do not develop in most cases (7).

Drug–Drug Interactions

Carbamazepine

In seven patients with epilepsy taking carbamazepine the addition of viloxazine 300 mg/day resulted in a pronounced increase in plasma carbamazepine concentrations (8.1–12.1 ng/ml), with symptoms of intoxication (dizziness, fatigue, ataxia, and drowsiness), resolving on withdrawal of viloxazine (8). The mechanism was unclear, but serum concentrations of phenytoin in two patients were unchanged.

References

1. Pinder RM, Brogden RN, Speight TM, Avery GS. Viloxazine: a review of its pharmacological properties and therapeutic efficacy in depressive illness. Drugs 1977;13(6):401–21.
2. Pichot P, Guelfi J, Dreyfus JF. A controlled multicentre therapeutic trial of viloxazine. J Int Med Res 1975;3:80.
3. Ichimaru I. Evaluation of Vivalan: additional studies (Japan). J Int Med Res 1975;3:97.
4. Barnes TR, Kidger T, Greenwood DT. Viloxazine and migraine. Lancet 1979;2(8156–8157):1368.
5. Pinder RM, Brogden RN, Speight TM, Avery GS. Doxepin up-to-date: a review of its pharmacological properties and therapeutic efficacy with particular reference to depression. Drugs 1977;13(3):161–218.
6. Edwards JG, Glen-Bott M. Does viloxazine have epileptogenic properties? J Neurol Neurosurg Psychiatry 1984; 47(9):960–4.
7. Crome P. Antidepressant overdosage. Drugs 1982;23(6):431–61.
8. Pisani F, Narbone MC, Fazio A, Crisafulli P, Primerano G, D'Agostino AA, Oteri G, Di Perri R. Effect of viloxazine on serum carbamazepine levels in epileptic patients. Epilepsia 1984;25(4):482–5.

Vinca alkaloids

See also Cytostatic and immunosuppressant drugs

General Information

From among nearly 30 different alkaloids that have been isolated from the periwinkle *Catharanthus roseus* (Apocynaceae), vincristine and vinblastine have been assessed to have the highest antitumor activity. Both have a large dimeric asymmetric structure composed of a dihydroindole nucleus (vindoline ring) and an indole nucleus, linked by a carbon–carbon bond. In contrast, the derivatives vindesine (deacetyl vinblastine amide sulfate (DVAS)) and vinorelbine are semisynthetic (1–3). Finally, vinflunine, the latest semisynthetic vinca alkaloid, is a fluorinated derivative that is still under clinical investigation and has a different inhibitory action than other vinca alkaloids. Preliminary results suggest that this congener may be less toxic on the peripheral and autonomic nervous systems (4).

Vincristine (rINN)

Vincristine is part of many chemotherapeutic regimens, based on its lack of myelosuppressive toxicity. It is used, for example, in the treatment of acute lymphocytic leukemia (ALL), acute myeloid leukemia (AML), lymphomas, neuroblastoma, brain tumors, and Wilms' tumor. The generally recommended dose in adults is 1.4 mg/m^2/week intravenously (5). Some clinicians have recommended an absolute upper limit of 2 mg, but this limitation is still a matter of debate (6). The usual pediatric dosage is 1.5–2 mg/m^2, but for children weighing 10 kg or less or who have a body surface area less than 1 m^2, the manufacturers recommend that treatment should be begun at 0.05 mg/kg once a week (5).

Vinblastine (rINN)

Vinblastine is used in combination with other cytotoxic agents for the treatment of disseminated Hodgkin's disease stages III and IV, non-Hodgkin's lymphoma, histiocytic lymphoma, and advanced carcinoma of the testis. It has also been used for the treatment of bladder cancer, melanoma, and renal cell cancer. The usual adult dosage is 3–6 mg/m^2 intravenously for the treatment of testicular germ cell tumors and Hodgkin's disease (1,2).

Vindesine (rINN)

Vindesine (DVAS) was the first semi-synthetic vinca alkaloid derivative introduced into clinical oncology. It differs solely from vinblastine in the nature of the substituted functional group attached to the vindoline ring. Vindesine has been most extensively studied in the treatment of non-small cell lung cancers. A randomized study has shown that vindesine (3 mg/m^2 intravenously) was substantially better than vincristine (1.4 mg/m^2 intravenously) both given weekly for 4 weeks, then every 2 weeks for 1 month, then monthly. However, another study showed that vindesine may be inferior to the structurally related vinorelbine in the treatment of advanced non-small cell lung cancers with overall response rates of 9 and 29%, respectively. Vindesine has also been used in patients with advanced malignant melanomas. Potential indications that have been studied with vindesine include head and neck cancer, ALL, lymphomas, and breast cancer. However, its precise role and clinically relevant advantages to other available vinca alkaloids needs further investigation (7–10).

Vinorelbine (rINN)

Vinorelbine has become a pivotal agent for treating adjuvant non-small cell lung cancer (stages IB-III) and the palliative treatment of non-small cell lung cancer (stages IIIB and IV), often in combination with drugs like cisplatin. In addition, vinorelbine plays an important part in the treatment of advanced and metastatic breast cancer. Its role in the treatment of advanced cervical cancer is still under investigation. The usual intravenous dosage is 20–30 mg/m^2 (vinorelbine base) given once a week. In contrast to the other congeners, vinorelbine can also be taken orally based on its absolute systemic availability of about 44% after administration as a capsule. Oral dosages of 60 and 80 mg/m^2 have been said to be pharmacokinetically and clinically equivalent to intravenous dosages of 25 and 30 mg/m^2 respectively (2,11).

Mechanism of action

All four vinca alkaloids block mitosis with metaphase arrest. Their antitumor activity is based on their high binding affinity to intracellular tubulin, which is the protein subunit of the spindle microtubules. The binding constants of vincristine, vinblastine, and vindesine for tubulin are 8, 6, and 3.3 nmol/l respectively (9,10). The formation of complexes between the vinca alkaloids and tubulin prevents the polymerization of the tubulin subunits to microtubules, which results in depolymerization of microtubules and inhibition of microtubule assembly. Based on the fact that microtubule assemblies also play a pivotal role in the movement of neurotransmitter substances along neuronal axons, vinca alkaloids can cause neurotoxicity, particularly at higher concentrations (9,10).

Pharmacokinetics

After intravenous administration, plasma concentrations of vinca alkaloids fall triphasically, with an initial rapid phase. All four congeners are extensively distributed into peripheral compartments, but passage across the blood–brain barrier is limited (11,12). In addition to tissue binding, vinca alkaloids bind to blood constituents like human platelets and lymphocytes. Binding to plasma proteins has been estimated to be from about 80% to more than 90%, with an unbound fraction of about 0.10–0.20. Binding to whole blood is usually higher than in serum, which reflects substantial binding to platelets (11,12).

All four congeners are extensively metabolized in the liver and excreted in the bile (13). Their metabolic biotransformation is primarily mediated by CYP3A. Deacetylvinorelbine, the primary metabolite of vinorelbine, has remarkable antitumor activity; however, the amounts detected in blood after conventional doses of vinorelbine are very low, which suggests that this metabolite does not contribute significantly to the overall antitumor activity of vinorelbine (14,15). Based on the pivotal role of CYP3A isozymes during the catabolism of vinca alkaloids, care is warranted when using concomitant drugs that inhibit these isozymes (16,17).

The half-lives of vinblastine, vindesine, and vinorelbine are all about 24 hours; vincristine has a much longer half-life of about 3.5 days (5). Because biliary and fecal drug excretion is of major quantitative importance during the elimination of vinca alkaloids, patients with impaired hepatic clearance and increased bilirubin concentrations may need dosage modification in order to avoid critical drug accumulation. CYP3A4 activity measurement (for example by the monoethylglycinexylidide test) might be the most appropriate method to estimate individual capacity to metabolize drugs like vinorelbine; however, such methods have not yet been routinely established in most cancer centers. Empirically, it is prudent to reduce doses by about 50% in patients with liver volume replacement by tumor that exceeds 75% (18).

Vinorelbine is the only vinca congener that can also be used orally. Its oral availability averages 43% and is not affected by food (19). The interpatient variability in blood concentrations is in the same range as after intravenous administration (15).

General adverse effects

The most important adverse effects of vinca alkaloids include nervous system disorders, hematological effects, and gastrointestinal discomfort. Respiratory and cardiovascular adverse effects have to be particularly considered during combination chemotherapy. All the vinca alkaloids are tissue irritants, and extravasation without any adequate supportive management can result in severe local ulceration (1,2,5,8,20).

Vinca alkaloids are primarily metabolized by CYP3A4, inducers, inhibitors of which can significantly change their pharmacokinetics (16,17,21).

Organs and Systems

Cardiovascular

Vinca alkaloid-associated myocardial infarction, angina pectoris, and transient electrocardiographic changes related to coronary ischemia are limited to case reports (22–24). In addition, patients with these adverse effects received combination cancer chemotherapy, containing drugs such as bleomycin and cisplatin, which both have been suggested to cause cardiovascular adverse effects.

- A 64-year-old Japanese man developed chest pain with concomitant lateral ST segment depression after treatment with intravenous cisplatin 70 mg/m^2, vincristine 1.2 mg/m^2, and bleomycin 12 U/m^2. There was no history of predisposing factors and the symptoms disappeared quickly with glyceryl trinitrate. During the following cycle, containing cisplatin and verapamil as an antianginal agent, chest pain did not reoccur (23).
- A 46-year-old man developed a Q-wave inferior and a right ventricular myocardial infarct with postinfarction angina after the third cycle of vincristine + doxorubicin for multiple myeloma. The patient had no risk factors for ischemic heart disease, except for a positive smoking history, nor for hyperviscosity (24).

There is some evidence that both vincristine and doxorubicin are more often associated with ischemic heart disease than other cancer chemotherapeutic agents. Whether drug-induced platelet activation, altered clotting, or endovascular damage are responsible for vascular toxicity is still unclear. The risk of ischemic heart disease must therefore be kept in mind when patients receive a combination of doxorubicin and vincristine, especially when potential risk factors have been identified. Whether the structural similarity between vinca alkaloids and ergot alkaloids, which are vasospastic, is relevant is highly speculative.

After administration of vinorelbine, chest pain occurs in up to 5% of patients. However, subsequent analysis showed that most patients had underlying cardiovascular disease or a tumor in the chest, making interpretation difficult (2,20). Three patients developed acute cardiopulmonary toxicity after vinorelbine therapy (25). The symptoms mimicked acute cardiac ischemia, but with no electrocardiographic changes or raised cardiac enzymes. In two patients, tachypnea, râles, wheezing, and severe dyspnea responded to inhaled salbutamol. One patient developed pulmonary edema and bilateral pleural effusions, which contained no malignant cells when drained.

Venous discomfort and venous chemical phlebitis have been reported with vinorelbine 30 mg/m^2, with an incidence of up to 31% (26,27). The risk is increased in obesity (27). Pain along the vein occurred in five of 43 patients receiving vinorelbine 30 mg/m^2/week; none developed extravasation, but their symptoms were very similar (28). A similar rate of toxicity, 4.5%, has been reported in a review of the use of vinorelbine in 321 patients with breast cancer (29).

Respiratory

Acute shortness of breath and bronchospasm have been reported after the administration of vinca alkaloids, for example vinblastine and vindesine (30–34). The respiratory effects, including abrupt onset of progressive dyspnea, non-productive cough, pleuritic chest pain, profound wheezing, and diffuse basal crackles, were more common when mitomycin was used concomitantly. The onset of symptoms can be rapid (for example a few minutes to 1–5 hours after administration) or subacute (for example up to 2 weeks). If patients have pre-existing pulmonary dysfunction, intensified treatment, including glucocorticoids, may be indicated. Most case reports with vinca alkaloid-associated pulmonary toxicity included vinblastine, usually in combination with other known pneumotoxic agents, or thoracic irradiation. Patients receiving combination chemotherapy including vinca alkaloids should be monitored carefully for pulmonary symptoms. The underlying mechanism of vinca alkaloid pulmonary toxicity is unclear, but may involve a hypersensitivity reaction.

Nervous system

The most commonly reported dose-limiting toxic effect of vinca alkaloids is a mixed sensorimotor polyneuropathy (35). Vincristine has been associated with highest incidence, followed by vindesine and vinblastine; vinorelbine causes less neurotoxicity than the other congeners (2,5,8,36). The neurotoxic effects of vinca alkaloids are reversible (5).

The vinca alkaloids may have synergistic effects on the nervous system. Amongst 17 patients with metastatic breast cancer given the four-drug combination, vincristine + vinblastine + doxorubicin + cyclosphosphamide, there was a high incidence of acute neurotoxicity at half the usual therapeutic dose of vincristine and vinblastine (37).

Nerve palsies
Cranial nerve palsies can occur with the vinca alkaloids (38–42).

There have been several reports of isolated vincristine-induced recurrent laryngeal nerve paralysis (38,43–47).

Peripheral neuropathy
The features of vinca alkaloid-induced polyneuropathy include early loss of tendon reflexes at the ankles and distal paresthesia, followed by loss of touch, pain, and vibration sensations. Other symptoms include headache, malaise, weakness, dizziness, severe face and jaw pain, and vocal cord paralysis. The first symptoms usually occur a few days after drug administration (36). Gastrointestinal discomfort, particularly constipation, abdominal pain, and adynamic ileus, can occur through an autonomic neuropathy (5,48).

Higher drug concentrations during monotherapy (possibly related to impaired drug excretion in patients with hepatic dysfunction) or prolonged periods of treatment are important predisposing factors for more severe forms of neurotoxicity. The same is true of concomitant use of potent CYP3A inhibitors, such as erythromycin, itraconazole, or quinupristin/dalfopristin, which can increase plasma vinca alkaloid drug concentrations (5).

Of 22 patients given vindesine 2 mg/m^2 on 2 consecutive days weekly, four developed a peripheral neuropathy with paresthesia, and five developed muscle weakness with loss of deep tendon reflexes (49). Neuropathies were pronounced at sites of pre-existing nerve damage. If a tumor had previously damaged peripheral nerves, or if a chordotomy had been performed, the paresthesia that developed at that site was often painful. Neurotoxicity was reversible, and the longest interval to full recovery was 3 months.

In 40 patients, orofacial pain developed as a manifestation of neuropathy about 3 days after vincristine administration, lasting for a mean duration of 2 days. Half of the patients were affected in the first week, and pain was commonest in young patients and in smokers (50).

With vinorelbine, incidence rates of 1.3% for peripheral neuropathies (mainly loss of deep tendon reflexes) and 4.1% for autonomic neuropathies (manifested by constipation) have been reported from a European overview of 321 patients (29).

The pathogenesis of vincristine-induced neuropathy has not been fully elucidated, but very probably altered axoplasmic transport processes are of major importance, since neurons treated with vincristine lose portions of their axonal microtubules (35). There is marked interindividual variability in sensitivity to this toxic effect, partially based on different predisposing factors, for example diabetes mellitus, pretreatment with other potentially neurotoxic agents (such as cisplatin and taxanes), or familial disorders (such as Charcot–Marie–Tooth syndrome) (37,51,52).

Several drugs have been proposed to be neuroprotective, including folinic acid, vitamin B_1, vitamin B_6, glutamic acid, Org 2766, insulin-like growth factor (IGF-1), and nerve growth factor. However, most drugs have been studied in experimental systems and there are only a few case reports suggesting clinical benefit. In contrast, folinic acid, vitamins B_1, B_{16}, and B_{12}, which were promising in experimental systems, failed to provide protection from vincristine-induced neuropathy in clinical studies. In the case of L-glutamic acid, which can be given orally, there was some neuroprotective activity; however, more information is needed to exclude any impairment of vincristine-induced antineoplastic activity, when both agents are used together on the same day (5).

The ACTH analogue Org 2766 was studied in a randomized, double-blind, placebo-controlled trial as a neuroprotective agent in patients receiving vincristine (53). In spite of positive results, the study design was later criticized because of a significantly higher number of younger patients in the Org 2766 group. In addition, there are contradictory results on the potential effect of Org 2766 on the overall antineoplastic activity of vincristine.

In a prospective, double-blind, placebo-controlled study, concurrent oral administration of 500 mg glutamic acid tds with vincristine reduced the incidence of subjective and objective signs of vincristine neurotoxicity (54). There were no differences in constipation, weakness, or loss of knee reflexes. There were no severe gastrointestinal adverse effects.

During recent years, more attention has been paid to nerve growth factor as a neuroprotective agent, since it may induce microtubule assembly, especially during neurite outgrowth. For instance, patients with a sensory neuropathy related to the use of cancer chemotherapy including paclitaxel, vincristine, or cisplatin had a significant reduction in plasma nerve growth factor concentrations (5). Acetyl-L -carnitine has been considered for neuroprotection because it increases nerve growth factor

expression. However, as in the case of L-glutamine or Org 2766, more information is needed to evaluate any potential effect on vincristine antitumor efficacy.

Pre-existing neurological disease can predispose to severe vincristine neuropathy (55). For example, Charcot–Marie–Tooth disease is regarded as a contraindication to the use of vincristine (56). There have been four cases of vincristine-induced neuropathy in Charcot–Marie–Tooth disease; one was fatal, and in the other three there was severe quadriplegia, which resolved. A predisposition to vincristine neuropathy has been described in a patient with pre-existing Friedreich's ataxia (56). When vincristine 0.625 mg/m^2/week was given to 264 patients for a maximum of 10 weeks, the incidence of grade 3/4 neuropathy rate was 7%, suggesting that dose intensity rather than total dose may be important for determining the severity of this toxic effect. The rate of grade 1–4 neuropathy was 56% (57).

Finally, the aminothiol amifostine has been proposed to be effective in preventing vincristine-induced neurotoxicity; however, clinical data are still lacking to assess its role as a neuroprotective agent in terms of vinca alkaloids (5).

Myeloencephalopathy

Central nervous system toxicity is unusual with vinca alkaloids, because they do not readily cross the blood–brain barrier. However, fatal myeloencephalopathy can occur a few hours after accidental intrathecal drug administration (58,59), with severe bilateral leg pain, and over the next 36 hours progressive leg weakness, urinary retention, meningism, fever, and somnolence. Other effects include absence of deep tendon and gag reflexes and disappearance of rectal tone. In spite of high-dose folinic acid rescue, patients became comatose, for example by the fourth day after injection, with loss of brain stem function a few days later.

Seizures

Seizures associated with intravenous use of vinca alkaloids are very rare (60–62). Some cases may have been due to SIADH-associated hyponatremia. Other forms include tumor-related effects, nervous system infections, or cerebral hemorrhage, which often make direct causal relations between drug exposure and nervous system adverse effects very difficult.

- An 8-year-old girl with leukemia had tonic-clonic convulsions and life-threatening encephalopathy after intravenous vincristine. After the second dose (1.5 mg/m^2 in combination with prednisone) she developed seizures and bilateral translucencies in the CT scan. When vincristine was withdrawn in subsequent cycles, the symptoms disappeared (61).

Four of 350 patients without a history of seizures developed generalized seizures 5–6 days after the first, second, and eleventh doses of intravenous vincristine. However, seizures did not recur in later cycles. It is difficult to implicate vincristine as a cause of these adverse effects (62). Tonic-clonic seizures were only reported in four patients 7 days after vindesine administration. All patients had pre-existing cerebral deposits of melanoma, possibly mimicking nervous system adverse effects (8).

Sensory systems

Eyes

Reversible visual damage has been attributed to vincristine.

- An 18-year-old man with lymphocytic leukemia became completely blind for 6 months after a fifth 10-day cycle of therapy with vincristine 2 mg intravenously followed by cyclophosphamide 600 mg orally for 5 days with prednisolone 100 mg orally for 5 days (63).
- A 15-year-old girl developed bilateral optic atrophy after treatment with weekly vincristine, posterior craniectomy, and whole neuraxis radiation therapy (64). Withdrawal resulted in recovery of visual function.

In 50 patients, ptosis and diplopia related to vincristine occurred in 16 (64). The exact pathomechanism of this adverse effect has not been elucidated.

Studies on monkeys have demonstrated visual loss and optic atrophy with intravitreous injection of vincristine. Clinical reports of postvincristine optic atrophy are rare. Most are irreversible, progressing to permanent blindness. There is commonly coexistent peripheral or cranial neuropathy (65). It is possible that certain patients are predisposed to vincristine-induced optic atrophy. Optic neuropathy after a single small dose of vincristine has been reported in a single case; the dose of vincristine was small (1275 mg), and the latent period before onset of visual loss was brief (6–8 weeks) (66). Previously reported cases have had multiple injections of vincristine and the latent period was longer than 3 months.

Ears

Vinca alkaloids can have ototoxic effects, such as tinnitus and transient hearing loss. In addition, vestibular disorders can cause dizziness, nystagmus, and vertigo (67,68).

- A 29-year-old man with recurrent Hodgkin's disease was treated with the ABVD regimen (doxorubicin, bleomycin, vinblastine, and dacarbazine) (69). He complained of tinnitus after each treatment cycle, with an onset of about 6 hours and a duration of 7–10 days. These symptoms interfered with reading, watching television, and general concentration. Based on audiography before and several hours after several cycles, there was evidence of mild sensorineural hearing loss in the high-decibel range 48 and 72 hours after drug administration. Six months after the completion of cancer chemotherapy, there was still some mild high-frequency sensorineural hearing loss in the left ear.

The authors concluded that vinblastine may have been responsible, because the other agents have not yet been associated with ototoxicity and because vincristine can cause ototoxicity too. The mechanism of this adverse effect is unclear but it may involve vinca alkaloid-associated damage to the eighth cranial nerve. This means that care should be taken when vinca alkaloids are used together with platinum compounds, especially cisplatin.

Endocrine

A rare but well-known adverse effect of vinca alkaloids, including vinorelbine, is the syndrome of inappropriate secretion of antidiuretic hormone (SIADH) (70–72). The diagnosis is usually based on clinical and laboratory findings. There are falls in plasma sodium (below 120 mmol/l), chloride (below 90 mmol/l), and osmolality (below 230 mosm/kg). Further features include lethargy, anorexia, nausea, listlessness, and rarely coma, particularly when serum sodium falls below 110 mmol/l. Treatment is based on withdrawal of the causative agent and the administration of 0.9% saline and potassium (for example 40 mmol/l) at an infusion rate of 200 ml/hour. Further treatment strategies include demeclocycline (for example 300 mg bd), which can be continued for the duration of further vinca alkaloid-containing cycles. In one case demeclocycline prevented SIADH during further courses of vinorelbine (72).

Asian patients have been proposed to be at higher risk of SIADH during treatment with vincristine. Between 1983 and 1999, 76 cases of hyponatremia and/or SIADH related to the use of vincristine were reported to the global adverse event database of Eli Lilly and Company. The average age of the patients was 36 years (range 2 weeks to 86 years) and 62% were male. Most of the patients had received vincristine for leukemia or lymphomas. Of the 76 reports, 39 included background information on race: 35 patients were Asian, three were Caucasian, and one was black. The authors concluded that there may be a correlation between race and vinca alkaloid-associated SIADH/hyponatremia; however, the reasons are still unclear (73).

Hematologic

The most frequent adverse effect of vinblastine, vindesine, and vinorelbine is hematological toxicity (1,2,5,7,8). Leukopenia, particularly neutropenia, occurs more often than thrombocytopenia or anemia. The nadir in the leukocyte count after vinblastine occurs 4–10 days after administration, with recovery within another 7–14 days. Blood counts should generally be measured weekly and before the administration of each dose, in order to avoid severe forms of myelosuppression, neutropenic fever, or infections (20).

Oral vinorelbine is also associated with neutropenia. In one small study in patients with breast cancer treated with 50–160 mg/week, the incidence of grade 3–4 neutropenia was 32% (14). The incidence of severe neutropenia is higher with vinorelbine than the other vinca alkaloids. However, mean recovery (about 9 days) appears to be somewhat shorter with vinorelbine than with compounds vinblastine and vindesine (average 14–21 days) (1,2).

Gastrointestinal

Constipation is common when vinca alkaloids cause an autonomic neuropathy. Laxatives such as lactulose or polyethylene glycol-containing solutions can prevent adynamic subileus during treatment courses containing vinca alkaloids (48,74).

In contrast to constipation, nausea and vomiting are neither frequent nor dose-limiting adverse effects of vinca alkaloids. The regular use of antiemetics, such as 5-HT$_3$ receptor antagonists in combination with dexamethasone, is not recommended. However, oral vinorelbine has been associated with more severe forms of nausea and vomiting, with a frequency that is higher than after intravenous administration; in these patients and in particular those with predisposing factors for nausea and vomiting, metoclopramide and 5-HT$_3$ receptor antagonists are justified (75).

Skin

Vinca alkaloids are potential vesicants (76–78) and accidental drug extravasation can cause severe soft tissue ulceration. The initial symptoms include marked pain, erythema, and local swelling for several hours up to a day; later effects include blisters and severe painful skin ulcers, several days and 3 weeks after extravasation respectively. The lesions usually heal very slowly and sometimes require surgical intervention. Because vinca alkaloid extravasation can have severe effects, the use of antidotes is highly recommended when extravasation is suspected. In addition, venous irritation can be worsened if the vinca alkaloid is infused over at least 20–30 minutes rather than 6–10 minutes.

Among several antidotes for the treatment of vinca alkaloid extravasation, hyaluronidase is the most effective (79). Seven patients with extravasation of vincristine, vinblastine, or vinorelbine received hyaluronidase 250 units diluted in 6 ml of 0.9% saline, through the indwelling needle or, when the needle had been already removed, as six subcutaneous injections around the extravasation site. None developed skin necrosis. Local mild skin warming in order to produce local vasodilatation may have an additional beneficial effect, but should be avoided when simultaneous extravasation of a vinca alkaloid and an anthracycline is suspected, because local warming can worsen the anthracycline-associated local reaction, whereas local cooling, which is generally beneficial in anthracycline-related extravasation alone, can worsen skin necrosis due to vinca alkaloids (76).

Hair

Vinca alkaloids are associated with a low incidence of alopecia. In about 10% of patients, there can be gradual thinning of hair, but very few patients develop total hair loss (1,5,7).

Reproductive system

Based on comparative studies of the relative gonadal toxicity of several antineoplastic agents in experimental models and humans, the vinca alkaloids vinblastine and vincristine have negligible potency for killing stem cells. Permanent recovery of sperm counts and preserved ovarian function, depending on the patient's age at the time of

treatment and the total cumulative dose, can be expected after treatment with vinca alkaloids (80–82).

Body temperature

Nine of 31 Japanese children receiving maintenance vincristine chemotherapy for either leukemia or lymphoma developed a fever over 38°C (83). An allergic mechanism was proposed. Concurrent glucocorticoids as part of the regimen appeared to be protective. Younger children were at greater risk. Peak temperatures occurred within 24 hours of vincristine administration. The pyrexia lasted from 6 hours to 4 days and the condition was self-limiting.

Long-Term Effects

Drug tolerance

Resistance to vinca alkaloids can be mediated by glycoprotein B, a transmembrane pump that is part of the multidrug resistance (MDR) phenotype (5).

Mutagenicity

Vinca alkaloids are less mutagenic than other cytotoxic agents like the N-Lost derivatives or bleomycin. Positive or negative results in mutagenicity tests depend on the test system used. For instance, vinorelbine significantly increased the frequencies of micronuclei in binucleate lymphocytes (84). In Chinese hamster ovary cells vinorelbine arrested cells at the first metaphase and caused an increase in abnormal anaphases, containing chiefly lagging chromosomes and multipolar spindles (85). These results suggest that vinorelbine does not directly damage DNA, but acts on spindle microtubules, altering chromosome movement and causing aneuploidy. However, it has no mutagenic effects in the Ames test.

Tumorigenicity

In the International Agency for Research and Treatment of Cancer (IARC), the vinca alkaloids were classified in group 3, which means that they cannot yet be classified in group 1 (proven human carcinogens), 2A (probably carcinogenic), or 2B (possibly carcinogenic) (86,87).

Second-Generation Effects

Teratogenicity

There is evidence that vinca alkaloids are teratogenic. Vinblastine caused malformations after first trimester administration (88–90). However, since vinca alkaloids are often combined with other cytotoxic drugs, it is difficult to relate any teratogenic effect to the vinca alkaloid alone (88). In mice and rabbits, vinblastine was embryotoxic and fetotoxic (89). However, it is unclear whether vinca alkaloids can cross the placenta because of their high molecular weights (about 1000 g/mol).

- Two pregnant women with breast cancer received two or three courses of intravenous vinorelbine 20–30 mg/m^2 and fluorouracil 500–750 mg/m^2 at 24, 28, and 29 weeks of gestation; there were no adverse effects in the two newborns (90). A third patient also had epirubicin and cyclophosphamide and her infant, who had been exposed to the four-drug regimen, developed transient anemia at 21 days of age which resolved spontaneously. All three infants were developing normally at 2–3 years of age.

According to the FDA classification, the potential therapeutic benefits of vinca alkaloids have to be outweighed with the potential teratogenic risks (FDA classification D). All women of childbearing potential should be advised to avoid becoming pregnant while receiving cytotoxic cancer chemotherapy (80).

Drug Administration

Drug administration route

In seven patients (median age 7 years), limb and jaw muscle pain, starting at days 3–5 of an intravenous infusion of vincristine and requiring opiate analgesia, was the most pronounced adverse effect (68).

Guidance on the safe administration of intrathecal chemotherapy has been issued in the UK (91), following a case in which vincristine was fatally injected into the cerebrospinal fluid (92).

Drug–Drug Interactions

Asparaginase

Asparaginase and vincristine should not be used together on the same day, since simultaneous administration can cause increased vincristine toxicity. It has been suggested that this is due to a deleterious effect of asparaginase on hepatic function, reducing the metabolism of vincristine (5).

Carbamazepine

In a small pharmacokinetic study the clearance of vincristine was 65% greater than in patients who were not taking carbamazepine and the half-life and AUC of vincristine were reduced by 35 and 43% respectively (93).

Erythromycin

Toward the end of a phase I study of vinblastine plus oral ciclosporin to reverse multidrug resistance, three patients also received erythromycin to raise their ciclosporin concentrations; all developed severe toxicity consistent with a much higher dose of vinblastine than was actually given (94).

Itraconazole

The concomitant use of itraconazole with vincristine increased the incidence of neurotoxicity in children and adults with ALL (95,96).

- A 19-year-old woman developed severe abdominal pain and constipation 28 days after starting to take itraconazole as antifungal prophylaxis when receiving vincristine

for ALL. She had hypertension, marked abdominal distension and tenderness, and absent bowel sounds. Withdrawal of itraconazole resulted in resolution of symptoms and vincristine was continued (96).

- A 72-year-old patient developed painful oral mucositis and constipation 3 days after being given vinorelbine and itraconazole (97). Further complications included neutropenia and hypoxia and he died.

Concomitant use of itraconazole 2.5 mg/kg/day and vincristine in five children receiving vincristine resulted in hypertension, paralytic ileus, and SIADH (95).

Phenytoin

In a small pharmacokinetic study, the clearance of vincristine was 65% greater than in patients who were not taking phenytoin and the half-life and AUC of vincristine were reduced by 35 and 43% respectively (93).

References

1. Zhou XJ, Rahmani R. Preclinical and clinical pharmacology of vinca alkaloids. Drugs 1992;44(Suppl 4):1–16.
2. Budman DR. New vinca alkaloids and related compounds. Semin Oncol 1992;19(6):639–45.
3. Malawista SE, Sato H, Bensch KG. Vinblastine and griseofulvin reversibly disrupt the living mitotic spindle. Science 1968;160(829):770–2.
4. Kruczynski A, Hill BT. Vinflunine, the latest vinca alkaloid in clinical development. A review of its preclinical anticancer properties. Crit Rev Oncol Hematol 2001;40(2):159–73.
5. Gidding CE, Kellie SJ, Kamps WA, de Graaf SS. Vincristine revisited. Crit Rev Oncol Hematol 1999;29(3):267–87.
6. McCune JS, Lindley C. Appropriateness of maximum-dose guidelines for vincristine. Am J Health Syst Pharm 1997;54(15):1755–8.
7. Cersosimo RJ, Bromer R, Licciardello JT, Hong WK. Pharmacology, clinical efficacy and adverse effects of vindesine sulfate, a new vinca alkaloid. Pharmacotherapy 1983;3(5):259–74.
8. Summerhayes M. Vindesine: ten years in the pharmacy. EHP 1996;2:214–21.
9. Jordan MA, Himes RH, Wilson L. Comparison of the effects of vinblastine, vincristine, vindesine, and vinepidine on microtubule dynamics and cell proliferation in vitro. Cancer Res 1985;45(6):2741–7.
10. Singer WD, Himes RH. Cellular uptake and tubulin binding properties of four vinca alkaloids. Biochem Pharmacol 1992;43(3):545–51.
11. Rahmani R, Gueritte F, Martin M, Just S, Cano JP, Barbet J. Comparative pharmacokinetics of antitumor vinca alkaloids: intravenous bolus injections of Navelbine and related alkaloids to cancer patients and rats. Cancer Chemother Pharmacol 1986;16(3):223–8.
12. Nelson RL, Dyke RW, Root MA. Comparative pharmacokinetics of vindesine, vincristine and vinblastine in patients with cancer. Cancer Treat Rev 1980;7(Suppl 1):17–24.
13. Jackson DV Jr, Castle MC, Bender RA. Biliary excretion of vincristine. Clin Pharmacol Ther 1978;24(1):101–7.
14. Deporte-Fety R, Simon N, Fumoleau P, Campone M, Kerbrat P, Bonneterre J, Fargeot P, Urien S. Population pharmacokinetics of short intravenous vinorelbine infusions in patients with metastatic breast cancer. Cancer Chemother Pharmacol 2004;53(3):233–8.

15. Variol P, Nguyen L, Tranchand B, Puozzo C. A simultaneous oral/intravenous population pharmacokinetic model for vinorelbine. Eur J Clin Pharmacol 2002;58(7):467–76.

16. Zhou-Pan XR, Seree E, Zhou XJ, Placidi M, Maurel P, Barra Y, Rahmani R. Involvement of human liver cytochrome P450 3A in vinblastine metabolism: drug interactions. Cancer Res 1993;53(21):5121–6.

17. Kajita J, Kuwabara T, Kobayashi H, Kobayashi S. CYP3A4 is mainly responsibile for the metabolism of a new vinca alkaloid, vinorelbine, in human liver microsomes. Drug Metab Dispos 2000;28(9):1121–7.

18. Robieux I, Sorio R, Borsatti E, Cannizzaro R, Vitali V, Aita P, Freschi A, Galligioni E, Monfardini S. Pharmacokinetics of vinorelbine in patients with liver metastases. Clin Pharmacol Ther 1996;59(1):32–40.

19. Rowinsky EK, Lucas VS, Hsieh AL, Wargin WA, Hohneker JA, Lubejko B, Sartorius SE, Donehower RC. The effects of food and divided dosing on the bioavailability of oral vinorelbine. Cancer Chemother Pharmacol 1996;39(1–2):9–16.

20. Furuse K, Kubota K, Kawahara M, Takada M, Kimura I, Fujii M, Ohta M, Hasegawa K, Yoshida K, Nakajima S, Ogura T, Niitani H. Phase II study of vinorelbine in heavily previously treated small cell lung cancer. Japan Lung Cancer Vinorelbine Study Group. Oncology 1996;53(2):169–72.

21. Chan JD. Pharmacokinetic drug interactions of vinca alkaloids: summary of case reports. Pharmacotherapy 1998;18(6):1304–7.

22. Cargill RI, Boyter AC, Lipworth BJ. Reversible myocardial ischaemia following vincristine containing chemotherapy. Respir Med 1994;88(9):709–10.

23. Dixon A, Nakamura JM, Oishi N, Wachi DH, Fukuyama O. Angina pectoris and therapy with cisplatin, vincristine, and bleomycin. Ann Intern Med 1989;111(4):342–3.

24. Calvo-Romero JM, Fernandez-Soria-Pantoja R, Arrebola-Garcia JD, Gil-Cubero M. Ischemic heart disease associated with vincristine and doxorubicin chemotherapy. Ann Pharmacother 2001;35(11):1403–5.

25. Karminsky N, Merimsky O, Kovner F, Inbar M. Vinorelbine-related acute cardiopulmonary toxicity. Cancer Chemother Pharmacol 1999;43(2):180–2.

26. Feun LG, Savaraj N, Hurley J, Marini A, Lai S. A clinical trial of intravenous vinorelbine tartrate plus tamoxifen in the treatment of patients with advanced malignant melanoma. Cancer 2000;88(3):584–8.

27. Yoh K, Niho S, Goto K, Ohmatsu H, Kubota K, Kakinuma R, Nishiwaki Y. High body mass index correlates with increased risk of venous irritation by vinorelbine infusion. Jpn J Clin Oncol 2004;34(4):206–9.

28. Frasci G, Comella G, Comella P, Salzano F, Cremone L, Della Volpe N, Imbriani A, Persico G. Mitoxantrone plus vinorelbine with granulocyte-colony stimulating factor (G-CSF) support in advanced breast cancer patients. A dose and schedule finding study. Breast Cancer Res Treat 1995;35(2):147–56.

29. Fumoleau P, Delozier T, Extra JM, Canobbio L, Delgado FM, Hurteloup P. Vinorelbine (Navelbine) in the treatment of breast cancer: the European experience. Semin Oncol 1995;22(2 Suppl 5):22–8.

30. Luedke D, McLaughlin TT, Daughaday C, Luedke S, Harrison B, Reed G, Martello O. Mitomycin C and vindesine associated pulmonary toxicity with variable clinical expression. Cancer 1985;55(3):542–5.

31. Kris MG, Pablo D, Gralla RJ, Burke MT, Prestifilippo J, Lewin D. Dyspnea following vinblastine or vindesine administration in patients receiving mitomycin plus vinca alkaloid combination therapy. Cancer Treat Rep 1984;68(7–8):1029–31.

32. Konits PH, Aisner J, Sutherland JC, Wiernik PH. Possible pulmonary toxicity secondary to vinblastine. Cancer 1982;50(12):2771–4.

33. Ballen KK, Weiss ST. Fatal acute respiratory failure following vinblastine and mitomycin administration for breast cancer. Am J Med Sci 1988;295(6):558–60.

34. Hoelzer KL, Harrison BR, Luedke SW, Luedke DW. Vinblastine-associated pulmonary toxicity in patients receiving combination therapy with mitomycin and cisplatin. Drug Intell Clin Pharm 1986;20(4):287–9.

35. Legha SS. Vincristine neurotoxicity. Pathophysiology and management. Med Toxicol 1986;1(6):421–7.

36. Chauncey TR, Showel JL, Fox JH. Vincristine neurotoxicity. JAMA 1985;254(4):507.

37. Stewart DJ, Maroun JA, Lefebvre B, Heringer R. Neurotoxicity and efficacy of combined vinca alkaloids in breast cancer. Cancer Treat Rep 1986;70(5):571–3.

38. Manelis G, Aderka D, Manelis J, Horn I. [Recurrent laryngeal nerve palsy and dysphagia for liquids due to vincristine.] Harefuah 1976;91(3–4):84–5.

39. Toker E, Yenice O, Ogut MS. Isolated abducens nerve palsy induced by vincristine therapy. J AAPOS 2004;8(1):69–71.

40. Lash SC, Williams CP, Marsh CS, Critchley C, Hodgkins PR, Mackie EJ. Acute sixth-nerve palsy after vincristine therapy. J AAPOS 2004;8(1):67–8.

41. Fujishita M, Tamura A, Yamada M, Uemura Y, Niiya K, Yoshimoto S, Kubonishi I, Taguchi H, Yoshino T, Ohtsuki Y, et al. [Quadriplegia and cranial nerve palsy during treatment by vincristine in blastic crisis of chronic myelocytic leukemia: report of an autopsy case.] Rinsho Ketsueki 1986;27(8):1437–42.

42. Mahajan SL, Ikeda Y, Myers TJ, Baldini MG. Acute acoustic nerve palsy associated with vincristine therapy. Cancer 1981;47(10):2404–6.

43. Annino DJ Jr, MacArthur CJ, Friedman EM. Vincristine-induced recurrent laryngeal nerve paralysis. Laryngoscope 1992;102(11):1260–2.

44. Nunez E, Solano D, Arreita A, Franco-Vicario R, Miguel F. Paralisis recurrencial inducida por vincristina. [Vincristine-induced recurrent laryngeal nerve paralysis.] Rev Clin Esp 1992;190(4):214–15.

45. Tobias JD, Bozeman PM. Vincristine-induced recurrent laryngeal nerve paralysis in children. Intensive Care Med 1991;17(5):304–5.

46. Delaney P. Vincristine-induced laryngeal nerve paralysis. Neurology 1982;32(11):1285–8.

47. Whittaker JA, Griffith IP. Recurrent laryngeal nerve paralysis in patients receiving vincristine and vinblastine. BMJ 1977;1(6071):1251–2.

48. Raphaelson MI, Stevens JC, Newman RP. Vincristine neuropathy with bowel and bladder atony, mimicking spinal cord compression. Cancer Treat Rep 1983;67(6):604–5.

49. Rhomberg WU. Vindesine for recurrent and metastatic cancer of the uterine cervix: a phase II study. Cancer Treat Rep 1986;70(12):1455–7.

50. McCarthy GM, Skillings JR. Jaw and other orofacial pain in patients receiving vincristine for the treatment of cancer. Oral Surg Oral Med Oral Pathol 1992;74(3):299–304.

51. Parimoo D, Jeffers S, Muggia FM. Severe neurotoxicity from vinorelbine–paclitaxel combinations. J Natl Cancer Inst 1996;88(15):1079–80.

52. Hogan-Dann CM, Fellmeth WG, McGuire SA, Kiley VA. Polyneuropathy following vincristine therapy in two patients with Charcot–Marie–Tooth syndrome. JAMA 1984;252(20):2862–3.

53. van Kooten B, van Diemen HA, Groenhout KM, Huijgens PC, Ossenkoppele GJ, Nauta JJ, Heimans JJ. A pilot study on the influence of a corticotropin (4–9)

analogue on vinca alkaloid-induced neuropathy. Arch Neurol 1992;49(10):1027–31.

54. Jackson DV, Wells HB, Atkins JN, Zekan PJ, White DR, Richards F 2nd, Cruz JM, Muss HB. Amelioration of vincristine neurotoxicity by glutamic acid. Am J Med 1988;84(6):1016–22.

55. Thoumie P, Diverrez JR, Guidet B. Polynevrite aiguë a la vincristine préscrite pour un cancer du sein chez une patiente atteinte de maladie de Friedreich. Sem Hop Paris 1989;65:30.

56. Griffiths JD, Stark RJ, Ding JC, Cooper IA. Vincristine neurotoxicity in Charcot-Marie-Tooth syndrome. Med J Aust 1985;143(7):305–6.

57. Budd GT, Green S, O'Bryan RM, Martino S, Abeloff MD, Rinehart JJ, Hahn R, Harris J, Tormey D, O'Sullivan J, et al. Short-course FAC-M versus 1 year of CMFVP in node-positive, hormone receptor-negative breast cancer: an intergroup study. J Clin Oncol 1995;13(4):831–9.

58. Zaragoza MR, Ritchey ML, Walter A. Neurourologic consequences of accidental intrathecal vincristine: a case report. Med Pediatr Oncol 1995;24(1):61–2.

59. Dettmeyer R, Driever F, Becker A, Wiestler OD, Madea B. Fatal myeloencephalopathy due to accidental intrathecal vincristin administration: a report of two cases. Forensic Sci Int 2001;122(1):60–4.

60. Johnson FL, Bernstein ID, Hartmann JR, Chard RL Jr. Seizures associated with vincristine sulfate therapy. J Pediatr 1973;82(4):699–702.

61. Hurwitz RL, Mahoney DH Jr, Armstrong DL, Browder TM. Reversible encephalopathy and seizures as a result of conventional vincristine administration. Med Pediatr Oncol 1988;16(3):216–19.

62. Murphy JA, Ross LM, Gibson BE. Vincristine toxicity in five children with acute lymphoblastic leukaemia. Lancet 1995;346(8972):443.

63. Awidi AS. Blindness and vincristine. Ann Intern Med 1980;93(5):781.

64. Shurin SB, Rekate HL, Annable W. Optic atrophy induced by vincristine. Pediatrics 1982;70(2):288–91.

65. Pinkerton CR, McDermott B, Philip T, Biron P, Ardiet C, Vandenberg H, Brunat-Mentigny M. Continuous vincristine infusion as part of a high dose chemoradiotherapy regimen: drug kinetics and toxicity. Cancer Chemother Pharmacol 1988;22(3):271–4.

66. Teichmann KD, Dabbagh N. Severe visual loss after a single dose of vincristine in a patient with spinal cord astrocytoma. J Ocul Pharmacol 1988;4(2):117–21.

67. Schweitzer VG. Ototoxicity of chemotherapeutic agents. Otolaryngol Clin North Am 1993;26(5):759–89.

68. Lugassy G, Shapira A. A prospective cohort study of the effect of vincristine on audition. Anticancer Drugs 1996;7(5):525–6.

69. Moss PE, Hickman S, Harrison BR. Ototoxicity associated with vinblastine. Ann Pharmacother 1999;33(4):423–5.

70. Cutting HO. Inappropriate secretion of antidiuretic hormone secondary to vincristine therapy. Am J Med 1971;51(2):269–71.

71. Stahel RA, Oelz O. Syndrome of inappropriate ADH secretion secondary to vinblastine. Cancer Chemother Pharmacol 1982;8(2):253–4.

72. Garrett CA, Simpson TA Jr. Syndrome of inappropriate antidiuretic hormone associated with vinorelbine therapy. Ann Pharmacother 1998;32(12):1306–9.

73. Hammond IW, Ferguson JA, Kwong K, Muniz E, Delisle F. Hyponatremia and syndrome of inappropriate anti-diuretic hormone reported with the use of vincristine: an over-representation of Asians? Pharmacoepidemiol Drug Saf 2002;11(3):229–34.

74. Tomomasa T, Miyazawa R, Kato M, Hoshino M, Tabata M, Kaneko H, Suzuki M, Kobayashi T, Morikawa A. Prolonged gastrointestinal dysmotility in a patient with hemophagocytic lymphohistiocytosis treated with vincristine. Dig Dis Sci 1999;44(9):1755–7.

75. Jassem J, Ramlau R, Karnicka-Mlodkowska H, Krawczyk K, Krzakowski M, Zatloukal P, Lemarie E, Hartmann W, Novakova L, O'Brien M, Depierr A. A multicenter randomized phase II study of oral vs. intravenous vinorelbine in advanced non-small-cell lung cancer patients. Ann Oncol 2001;12(10):1375–81.

76. Dorr RT. Managing extravasation of vesicant chemotherapy drugs. In: Lipp HP, editor. Anticancer Drug Toxicity; Prevention, Management and Clinical Pharmacokinetics. New York–Basel: Marcel Dekker Inc, 1999:279–318.

77. Bellone JD. Treatment of vincristine extravasation. JAMA 1981;245(4):343.

78. Rittenberg CN, Gralla RJ, Rehmeyer TA. Assessing and managing venous irritation associated with vinorelbine tartrate (Navelbine) Oncol Nurs Forum 1995;22(4):707–10.

79. Bertelli G, Dini D, Forno GB, Gozza A, Silvestro S, Venturini M, Rosso R, Pronzato P. Hyaluronidase as an antidote to extravasation of vinca alkaloids: clinical results. J Cancer Res Clin Oncol 1994;120(8):505–6.

80. Lamont EB, Schilsky RL. Gonadal toxicity and teratogenicity after cytotoxic chemotherapy. In: Lipp HP, editor. Anticancer Drug Toxicity. Prevention, Management and Clinical Pharmacokinetics. New York–Basel: Marcel Dekker Inc, 1999:491–523.

81. Meistrich ML. Effects of chemotherapy and radiotherapy on spermatogenesis. Eur Urol 1993;23(1):136–42.

82. Rautonen J, Koskimies AI, Siimes MA. Vincristine is associated with the risk of azoospermia in adult male survivors of childhood malignancies. Eur J Cancer 1992;28A(11):1837–41.

83. Ishii E, Hara T, Mizuno Y, Ueda K. [Vincristine-induced fever in children with leukaemia and lymphoma.] Saishin Igaku 1988;6:1341.

84. Gonzalez-Cid M, Cuello MT, Larripa I. Comparison of the aneugenic effect of vinorelbine and vincristine in cultured human lymphocytes. Mutagenesis 1999;14(1):63–6.

85. Gonzalez-Cid M, Cuello MT, Larripa I. Mitotic arrest and anaphase aberrations induced by vinorelbine in hamster cells in vitro. Anticancer Drugs 1997;8(5):529–32.

86. Bokemeyer C, Kollmannsberger C. Secondary malignancies. In: Lipp HP, editor. Anticancer Drug Toxicity. Prevention, Management and Clinical Pharmacokinetics. New York-Basel: Marcel Dekker Inc, 1999:525–47.

87. Boivin JF. Second cancers and other late side effects of cancer treatment. A review. Cancer 1990;65(Suppl 3):770–5.

88. Lacher MJ. Use of vinblastine sulfate to treat Hodgkin's disease during pregnancy. Ann Intern Med 1964;61:113–15.

89. Product information. Navelbine. Glaxo Wellcome, 1999.

90. Cuvier C, Espie M, Extra JM, Marty M. Vinorelbine in pregnancy. Eur J Cancer 1997;33(1):168–9.

91. Toft B. Toft Report. External enquiry into the adverse incident that occurred at Queen's Medical Centre, Nottingham, 4 March, 2001. London: Department of Health;. 2001.

92. NHS Executive. National guidance on the safe administration of intrathecal chemotherapy. HSC 2000:022.

93. Villikka K, Kivisto KT, Maenpaa H, Joensuu H, Neuvonen PJ. Cytochrome P450-inducing antiepileptics increase the clearance of vincristine in patients with brain tumors. Clin Pharmacol Ther 1999;66(6):589–93.

94. Tobe SW, Siu LL, Jamal SA, Skorecki KL, Murphy GF, Warner E. Vinblastine and erythromycin: an unrecognized

serious drug interaction. Cancer Chemother Pharmacol 1995;35(3):188–90.

95. Bohme A, Ganser A, Hoelzer D. Aggravation of vincristine-induced neurotoxicity by itraconazole in the treatment of adult ALL. Ann Hematol 1995;71(6):311–12.
96. Gillies J, Hung KA, Fitzsimons E, Soutar R. Severe vincristine toxicity in combination with itraconazole. Clin Lab Haematol 1998;20(2):123–4.
97. Bosque E. Possible drug interaction between itraconazole and vinorelbine tartrate leading to death after one dose of chemotherapy. Ann Intern Med 2001;134(5):427.

Vincamine

General Information

Vincamine is an alkaloid extracted from the plant *Vinca minor*. Ethyl apovincaminate is a related synthetic ethyl ester of vincaminic acid. These drugs have spasmolytic effects similar to those of reserpine, but also have metabolic effects, including, in high doses, inhibition of phosphodiesterase. Although increased cerebral blood flow has been reported after the intravenous administration of vincamine, there have been no reliable studies of blood flow after oral medication. Improvement in scores on some psychometric tests have been obtained in some patients with cerebrovascular disease, but no clear-cut practical benefit has been demonstrated.

Organs and Systems

Cardiovascular

Commercial formulations obtained from the alkaloids in *Vinca minor* may not be free from adverse effects. Ventricular dysrhythmias have been observed, but only after intramuscular or intravenous administration, and they seem to reflect a direct effect on myocardial cells. Hypokalemia and a prolonged QT interval seem to be predisposing factors. Vincamine should therefore be avoided in patients with a prolonged QT interval (SEDA-2, 183) (SEDA-5, 206) (SEDA-5, 207) (SEDA-7, 228).

Psychological, psychiatric

Vincamine has minor psychoactive effects (1).

Reference

1. Crispi G, Di Lorenzo RS, Gentile A, Florino A, Pannone B, Sciorio G. Azione psicoattiva della vincamina in un gruppo di soggetti affetti da "sindrome depressiva recidivante". Nota preventiva. [Psychoactive effect of vincamine in a group of subjects affected by recurrent depressive syndrome. Preliminary note.] Minerva Med 1975;66(70):3683–5.

Vinegar

General Information

Vinegar was used topically in a Turkish neonate with suspected sepsis (1). The child was treated with antibiotics and his grandmother decided in addition to rub his upper thorax, back, and arms with vinegar. As a result the child developed chemical burns on the treated areas. Fortunately he made a full recovery after the grandmother stopped the treatment.

Reference

1. Korkmaz A, Sahiner U, Yurdakok M. Chemical burn caused by topical vinegar application in a newborn infant. Pediatr Dermatol 2000;17(1):34–6.

Viscaceae

See also Herbal medicines

General Information

The family of Viscaceae contains four genera of mistletoe:

1. *Arceuthobium* (dwarf mistletoe)
2. *Korthalsella* (korthal mistletoe)
3. *Phoradendron* (American mistletoe)
4. *Viscum* (mistletoe).

Phoradendron flavescens

In 14 cases of accidental exposure to *Phoradendron flavescens* (*Phoradendron serotinum*, American mistletoe) there were no symptoms, but there was one death from intentional ingestion of an unknown amount of an elixir brewed from the berries (1). In 92 patients aged 4 months to 42 years (median 2 years), 14 were symptomatic, 11 related to mistletoe exposure. All the symptomatic cases had onset of symptoms within 6 hours. The symptoms included gastrointestinal upsets (*n* = 6), mild drowsiness (*n* = 2), eye irritation (*n* = 1), ataxia (*n* = 1), and seizures (*n* = 1). Treatment included gastrointestinal decontamination in 54 patients, ocular irrigation in one, and an intravenous benzodiazepine in one; decontamination did not affect the outcome. The amount ingested ranged from one berry or leaf to more than 20 berries or five leaves. Eight of ten patients who had taken at least five berries were symptom-free. Of 11 patients who took only leaves (range 1–5 leaves), three had gastrointestinal upsets. There were no cardiovascular effects in any case.

Viscum album

The stems and leaves of *Viscum album* (all heal, bird lime, devil's fuge, golden bough, mistletoe) contain alkaloids, viscotoxins, and lectins. While the toxicity of the alkaloids remains to be assessed, the viscotoxins and lectins have been found to be very poisonous in animals when given parenterally. Mistletoe is a widely used alternative treatment for cancer, without convincing evidence of efficacy (2).

Adverse effects

Liver

Mistletoe is sometimes assumed to have hepatotoxic potential, based on a case report of hepatitis due to an herbal combination product claimed to have had mistletoe as one of its ingredients (3). However, the allegation that mistletoe was the probable cause of the illness has been rightly criticized, inter alia because the botanical material was not authenticated. The incriminated product also contained skullcap, which is hepatotoxic.

Immunologic

Parenteral administration of *V. album* can cause serious allergic reactions (4), and anaphylactic reactions have been described (5).

Tumorigenicity

- A 73-year-old man with a 5-year history of centrocytic non-Hodgkin's lymphoma presented with subcutaneous nodules in the abdominal wall at the sites where he had previously received subcutaneous injections of mistletoe (6). The nodules turned out to be infiltrations by the centrocytic lymphoma. The patient died 6 weeks later of bilateral pneumonia. The authors hypothesized that mistletoe has a growth-promoting action on lymphoma cells, mediated by high local concentrations of interleukin-6 liberated from the skin by mistletoe lectins.

References

1. Spiller HA, Willias DB, Gorman SE, Sanftleban J. Retrospective study of mistletoe ingestion. J Toxicol Clin Toxicol 1996;34(4):405–8.
2. Kleijnen J, Knipschild P. Mistletoe treatment for cancer. Review of controlled trials in humans. Phytomedicine 1994;1:255–60.
3. Harvey J, Colin-Jones DG. Mistletoe hepatitis. BMJ (Clin Res Ed) 1981;282(6259):186–7.
4. Pichler WJ, Angeli R. Allergie auf Mistelextrakt. [An allergy to mistletoe extract.] Dtsch Med Wochenschr 1991;116(35):1333–4.
5. Hutt N, Kopferschmitt-Kubler M, Cabalion J, Purohit A, Alt M, Pauli G. Anaphylactic reactions after therapeutic injection of mistletoe (*Viscum album* L.). Allergol Immunopathol (Madr) 2001;29(5):201–3.
6. Hagenah W, Dorges I, Gafumbegete E, Wagner T. Subkutane Manifestationen eines zentrozytischen Non-Hodgkin-Lymphoms an Injektionsstellen eines Mistelpräparats. [Subcutaneous manifestations of a centrocytic non-Hodgkin lymphoma at the injection site of a mistletoe preparation.] Dtsch Med Wochenschr 1998; 123(34–35):1001–4.

Vitamin A: Carotenoids

See also Vitamins *and* Vitamin A: Retinoids

General Information

The carotenoids are a class of hydrocarbons (carotenes) and their oxygenated derivatives (xanthophylls) that consist of eight isoprenoid units joined in such a manner that the arrangement of the units is reversed at the center of the molecule, so that the two central methyl groups are in a 1,6-positional relationship and the remaining non-terminal methyl groups are in a 1,5-positional relationship. Their nomenclature has been standardized by IUPAC [http://www.chem.qmul.ac.uk/iupac/carot/], and their formal names are all based on the term "carotene."

Vitamin A is a family of fat-soluble vitamins, of which retinol is the most active form. Beta-carotene is a provitamin carotenoid that is converted to retinol more efficiently than other provitamin carotenoids. Other provitamin carotenoids include alpha-carotene and (trivial names) b-cryptoxanthin, lycopene, lutein, and zeaxanthin; they are widely available in foods.

Canthaxanthin is an orange carotenoid that occurs naturally in fruits, vegetables, mushrooms, shellfish, algae, and other forms of marine life. It has been approved by the US Food and Drug Administration as a food coloring agent and has been promoted as a skin-tanning agent in oral formulations that supply larger amounts than would be normally consumed as a food additive. Unlike other carotenoids, canthaxanthin is not a precursor of vitamin A, and therefore does not carry the risk of hypervitaminosis A. Retinopathy, due to deposition of canthaxanthin, causes gold-yellow deposits around the macula. Canthaxanthin-associated aplastic anemia has been reported (1).

Vitamin A activity can be expressed either as international units IU (1 IU equaling 0.3 micrograms of all-*trans*-retinol or 0.6 micrograms of all-*trans*-beta-carotene) or, more correctly, in retinol equivalents (RE) where 1 RE equals 1 microgram of all-*trans*-retinol, 6 micrograms of all-*trans*-beta-carotene or 12 micrograms of other provitamin A carotenoids. Table 1 gives the activities of different forms of vitamin A in RE and IU.

The Average Requirement for vitamin A is 500 and 400 micrograms RE/day for adult men and women respectively, the Population Reference Intake 700 and 600 micrograms RE/day, and the Lowest Threshold Intake 300 and 250 micrograms RE/day. While a slightly higher Population Reference Intake is advised in pregnancy and lactation (700 and 950 micrograms RE/day respectively), concern about the possible teratogenic effect of vitamin A has led many European health authorities to advise pregnant women against taking vitamin A

Table 1 Relative activities of different forms of vitamin A

Vitamin A	Activity in RE	Activity in IU
Retinol (1 mg)	1000	3330
Retinyl acetate (1 mg)	870	2900
Retinyl palmitate (1 mg)	550	1830

supplements (2). However, much higher doses (over 60 000 micrograms RE/day or 200 000 IU/day) are routinely distributed at half-yearly intervals to children in populations deemed to be suffering from vitamin A deficiency, mainly in developing countries. Toxicity is occasionally observed during these massive-dose prophylactic programs (3), and their safety has sometimes been called into question (4,5). One study has suggested that high-dose vitamin A supplements cause modest adverse effects in children recovering from pneumonia (6).

Chronic toxic reactions are generally more frequent than acute toxic reactions, which are uncommon at dosages below 30 000 micrograms RE/day (7). Supplements that contain 8000 micrograms RE (25 000 IU) or more of vitamin A per capsule are available as over-the-counter formulations in many countries (8). The "Nutrient and Energy Intakes for the European Community" (9) advises against single doses over 120 000 micrograms RE, and regular doses over 9000 micrograms RE/day in men and 7500 micrograms RE/day in women.

The recommended daily allowance of vitamin A for children up to 12 years of age is 1500–4500 IU. Toxic reactions occur when retinol-binding proteins in the plasma are saturated with vitamin A. Excess vitamin A is bound to plasma lipoproteins, and in this form it causes toxic effects when it comes into contact with cells (10). Acute vitamin A intoxication can occur after ingestion of 500 000 IU in adults and proportionately less in children. Chronic intoxication is more common, and in children it can occur even with doses as small as 1500 IU/kg/day. The problem is under-recognized in children, and cases often present as diagnostic dilemmas.

The reference range for serum concentrations of vitamin A is 300–1500 IU/l (0.5–2.8 µmol/l) (11).

General adverse effects

Acute intoxication has been observed after ingestion of vitamin A-rich liver from the polar bear, halibut, or shark, or after the use of fish oil supplements used to lower plasma lipids. In adults, toxic doses have been in the range of one or more million units of vitamin A, but in children as low as 10 000 micrograms RE, or even in a few children under 650 micrograms RE/day (12). Symptoms occur at 6–24 hours after ingestion and include acute drowsiness, irritability, vertigo, headache, delirium and convulsions, intolerance of food, and diarrhea (SEDA-8, 344).

Long-term administration of 3000 micrograms RE/day (10 000 IU/day) can cause chronic hypervitaminosis A, and at greatest risk in this regard are those with impaired liver function (12,13). The risk further increases with low body weight, protein malnutrition, renal disease, hyperlipoproteinemia, high alcohol consumption, and ascorbic acid deficiency (7). Because of the multisystem manifestations of hypervitaminosis A, the symptoms are often misjudged and the diagnosis delayed. The main symptoms of chronic intoxication include malaise, intracranial hypertension, chronic headache, vertigo, nystagmus, photophobia, hyperkeratosis, gastrointestinal complaints,

changes in the skin and mucous membranes, tenderness and pain in the bone and joints, and fever.

Chronic intoxication with vitamin A has been reported to cause variously hypercalcemia, hyperglycaemia, increased alkaline phosphatase, hypoproteinemia, hypoprothrombinemia, increased sulfobromphthalein retention, raised serum transaminases, low serum ascorbic acid, reduced protein content of the cerebrospinal fluid, raised urinary hydroxyproline, and hypercalciuria (SED-8, 800) (14). It is not always clear, however, whether these deviations are a cause or an effect of hypervitaminosis A.

In some patients, adverse effects, especially disturbed liver function, become evident only when irreversible damage, for example liver cirrhosis or fibrosis with portal hypertension, is already present. It seems that the total cumulative intake of vitamin A, rather than the level of dosage, may be the critical factor for damage to the liver (15); this might hold true also for other adverse effects. A review found dosage ranges in reported cases of adverse events over the last 50 years to range from 650 to 20 000 micrograms RE/kg/day, and duration of administration to range from 41 to 3600 days, with an exponential relation between dose and duration with regard to symptoms of hypervitaminosis A (7). To avoid toxic reactions, the authors recommended, as a rule of thumb, that the daily dose (NB: in IU/kg) multiplied by the duration (in days) should not exceed one million.

Allergic reactions do not occur, but increased serum IgM concentrations were reported in patients with severe liver disease after prolonged administration of vitamin A (15).

Tumor-inducing effects of vitamin A have so far been suggested only with regard to prostatic cancer, especially in those 70 years of age and over (SEDA-13, 346).

Organs and Systems

Nervous system

Acute poisoning with vitamin A produces symptoms such as drowsiness, sluggishness, irritability, an irresistible desire to sleep, severe headache, and papilledema. In some cases papilledema is the only symptom (SEDA-11, 333) (16,17). In young children, raised intracranial pressure with bulging of the fontanelle, papilledema, and diplopia have been observed (SED-8, 799, 801) (SEDA-15, 411) (18).

In 50% of chronic vitamin A intoxications intracranial hypertension occurs, sometimes together with skin and hair changes, musculoskeletal pain, and fatigue (19). Benign intracranial hypertension (pseudotumor cerebri), vertigo, and papilledema have appeared after the intake of 3500–7000 micrograms RE/day of vitamin A for 2 years; in young children even a few months of treatment may precipitate these conditions (20) and symptoms can occur at low doses (even in a few children as low as 650 micrograms RE/kg/day) (12). Nystagmus, diplopia, photophobia, palsy of the ocular muscles, retinal hemorrhage, and protrusio bulbi (SED-8, 801) (21) have all been reported with vitamin A, and are an effect of raised intracranial pressure.

- A 15-year-old girl developed headache, vertigo, nausea, and epistaxis, diplopia, and reduced visual acuity (22). She had taken Arovit corresponding to vitamin A 200 000 IU/day for 6 months for acne. Ophthalmoscopy showed bilateral papilledema and minor bilateral abducens paresis. She had hypercalcemia (3.24 mmol/l) and a reduced parathyroid hormone concentration, a mild anemia (10.5 g/dl), and thrombocytopenia (112×10^9/l). Lumbar puncture showed a pressure of 62 cm H_2O with otherwise normal liquor. Her serum vitamin A concentration was 1.5 micrograms/ml (reference range 0.3–0.7 micrograms/ml).

Pseudotumor cerebri due to hypervitaminosis A is a serious complication, which can cause permanent visual impairment. Patients who take retinoids require proper surveillance. Raised serum concentrations of retinoids can persist for weeks after withdrawal.

Hypervitaminosis A can be a frequently overlooked cause of chronic headache (23). The precise cause of this, and of increased intracranial pressure in hypervitaminosis A, is controversial and unclear (24).

Psychological, psychiatric

Daily doses of 1 000 000 µg RE of vitamin A can cause acute symptomatic psychosis, with striking disturbances in the electroencephalogram and pathological changes in the cerebrospinal fluid (25). After withdrawal of vitamin A and administration of low doses of neuroleptic drugs the psychotic symptoms disappeared within a week.

Neuropsychiatric changes were reported to be the earliest dose-limiting symptomatic toxicity in patients with cancer taking high doses of retinol (26).

Metabolism

People with severe hypertriglyceridemia associated with Type V hyperlipoproteinemia may be at increased risk of hypervitaminosis A, even with moderate degrees of vitamin A supplementation (27). Long-term vitamin A administration is associated with an increase in serum cholesterol and serum triglyceride concentrations (28) and consequently might be linked with atherosclerosis (SEDA-8, 345) (29,30).

Mineral balance

Vitamin A toxicity in an adult woman resulted in hypercalcemia with renal insufficiency (31).

- An 86-year-old woman developed anorexia, thirst, and nocturia. During the previous 7 months her weight had fallen by 11 kg. She was taking domperidone and 1–6 vitamin tablets daily, each of which contained retinol palmitate 600 IU and colecalciferol 200 IU. She had hypercalcemia (serum calcium 3.34 mmol/l) and renal insufficiency (serum creatinine 333 µmol/l). Other causes of hypercalcemia were excluded.

In chronic vitamin A ingestion, risk factors for vitamin A toxicity are age, body weight, and renal insufficiency. The hypercalcemia caused by chronic vitamin A ingestion is explained by upregulation of osteoclasts by retinol metabolites.

Fluid balance

Edema and ascites are sometimes seen in chronic intoxication (SEDA-8, 799) (32,33).

Hematologic

High doses of vitamin A reduce the stability of the lipoprotein boundary layer of the erythrocytes, which can lead to hemolysis and anemia (34). Neutropenia, leukocytosis, thrombocytopenia, aplastic anemia, and increased sedimentation rate have also been reported after high doses of vitamin A (35–38).

Vitamin A toxicity appears to occur only when the amount of vitamin A exceeds the binding capability of the retinol binding protein. Hypervitaminosis A can cause severe anemia and thrombocytopenia, resulting from retinol-dependent bone marrow cell growth inhibition (39).

- A 3-month-old boy who was given Arovit (an aqueous solution of vitamin A palmitate, Roche, Italy), corresponding to vitamin A 62 000 IU/day for 80 days, developed signs of retinol intoxication (severe normochromic normocytic anemia, hemoglobin 5.9 g/dl, leukocyte count 6.2×10^9/l with lymphocytes 74%, neutrophils 17%, eosinophils 3%, and monocytes 6%, platelet count 20×10^9/l). The blood film showed anisopoikilocytosis. He had increased concentrations of unbound retinol, with high concentrations of retinyl esters and a raised retinol:retinol binding protein ratio. Vitamin A was withdrawn and 15 days later his hemoglobin rose to 7.5 g/dl and the platelet count to 105×10^9/l. The reticulocyte count increased from 8 to 300×10^9/l. The bone marrow showed normal populations of erythroid and myeloid cells and megakaryocytes. The retinyl esters fell by about 80% after 3 months.

These are the first findings to suggest that infant hypervitaminosis A can cause severe anemia and thrombocytopenia, probably due to the direct effect of vitamin A on the growth of all bone marrow cells. Investigation of the effect of retinol on the growth of the pluripotent hemopoietic cell line K-562 and on bone marrow mesenchymal stem cells showed strong inhibition of cell proliferation at concentrations similar to those found in vivo. Subsequent biochemical analysis of the cell cycle suggested that the effect was mediated by upregulation of the cyclin-dependent kinase-inhibitors $p21^{Cip1}$ and $p27^{Kip1}$.

Mouth and teeth

Dryness and scaling of the lips, gingivitis, and bleeding from the gums are common symptoms of acute vitamin A intoxication (32,35).

Gastrointestinal

Nausea, vomiting, and anorexia are common symptoms of acute vitamin A intoxication (34).

Liver

Enlargement of the liver, spleen, and lymph nodes in adults taking vitamin A were first reported many years ago (34–36).

The hepatotoxic effects of vitamin A have been reported after consumption of doses of about 100 000 IU/day for periods ranging from weeks to months, as well as after daily supplementation with 25 000 IU for a couple of years, accompanied by an increase in plasma vitamin A concentration to 10 times normal in users of health foods. The smallest daily supplement of vitamin A reported to be associated with liver cirrhosis is 25 000 IU taken for 6 years (15).

Liver biopsies have been performed in some patients with chronic vitamin A intoxication. Perisinusoidal fibrosis and massive accumulation of lipid-storing cells were found. Impairment of blood flow by perisinusoidal fibrosis probably resulted in secondary alterations in hepatocytes, including cellular atrophy and formation of cytoplasmic bullae. Histological examination also showed central vein sclerosis and focal congestion associated with perisinusoidal storage. The vitamin A concentration in the liver was increased (40–42).

For the diagnosis of hypervitaminosis A, plasma concentrations and retinol-binding protein may be misleading. Cases have been reported of hepatic fibrosis, secondary to chronic ingestion of massive doses of vitamin A, where plasma concentrations of vitamin A and retinol-binding protein at the time of diagnosis were within the reference range (43).

Long-term observation of 41 patients with varying forms of liver disease, all caused by prolonged vitamin A consumption, has given further insight into the range of histological lesions and the prognosis of liver disease related to hypervitaminosis A (15). Clinical examination showed hepatomegaly in 18 of the patients, splenomegaly in 13, signs of chronic hepatic disease in 12, ascites in 9, and icterus in 8. Repeat liver biopsies in three patients 3–6 years after diagnosis showed progression from steatosis or fibrosis to fully developed micronodular cirrhosis in all cases, showing that the liver damage can be irreversible. Nine patients died during follow-up, six of terminal liver failure. However, plasma retinol concentrations were above the reference range in only about 40%.

Liver damage due to vitamin A is not always irreversible; one patient, after prolonged intake of excessive amounts of vitamin A for treatment of psoriasis (90 000 micrograms RE/day), had not only reversible chronic intoxication, but reversible portal hypertension and deranged liver function tests without any histological signs of cirrhosis (44). In a similar case, portal hypertension disappeared after 6 months on a low vitamin A diet. The fact that there was no reduction in Ito cells either in size or number suggests that lipid venous obstruction is unlikely to be the only mechanism responsible for portal hypertension in vitamin A-induced liver disease (45).

Even moderate doses of vitamin A, when taken over a prolonged period of time, can cause significant hepatocellular injury, as seen in three family members with symptoms and biochemical evidence of hepatitis, who had taken 7000–15 000 micrograms/day RE (20 000–45 000 IU/day) for 7–10 years (46). A similar case involved a 45-year-old woman who had taken an over-the-counter supplement over 6 years, and developed severe and fatal liver damage (47).

Clinical presentations, changes in liver function tests, and liver morphology have previously been examined in 41 consecutive patients with vitamin A hepatotoxicity (15). The cause of liver disease was suspected at initial interview in only 13 instances, and there was histological evidence of fat-storage hyperplasia with fluorescent vacuoles in the other cases. Cirrhosis was found in 17 cases, mild chronic hepatitis in 10, non-cirrhotic portal hypertension in 5, and "increased storage" alone in 9. During a mean follow-up period of 4.6 years, six patients died of causes related to the liver disease. Precise appraisal of drug consumption was obtained in 29 cases. Among them the total cumulative intake was the highest in patients with cirrhosis (423 MIU) and significantly lower in those with non-cirrhotic liver disease (89 MIU). The smallest continuous daily consumption leading to cirrhosis was 25 000 IU for 6 years, whereas higher doses (greater than or equal to 100 000 IU/day) taken for 2.5 years resulted in similar histological changes.

Liver fibrosis induced by beta-carotene therapy for pigmentary retinopathy has been reported (48).

- A 66-year-old woman with a pigmentary retinopathy that had been treated for 30 years with antocyanosides combined with beta-carotene (total dose 165 g) developed anicteric cholestasis. Liver biopsy showed pronounced portal fibrosis with normal bile ducts and no evidence of portal inflammation. The usual causes of chronic hepatic diseases were excluded. The serum concentration of vitamin A was 0.43 (reference range: 0.5–0.8) mg/ml. After withdrawal of beta-carotene and administration of ursodeoxycholic acid for 6 months the cholestasis resolved.

Another feature of vitamin A hepatotoxicity, namely respiratory symptoms caused by hepatic hydrothorax, associated with excessive vitamin A consumption has been reported (49).

- A 52-year-old woman, who had taken multivitamin supplements daily for 17 years and vitamin A whenever she had a cold, became progressively breathless, with 18 kg weight loss, increasing abdominal girth, increasing fatigue, leg weakness and pain, worsening chronic diarrhea, and intermittent nose bleeds. Her total vitamin A intake over 17 years had been at least 63 MIU (average 10 273 IU/day) and in the previous year she had taken at least 98 MIU (270 000 IU/day). When she noted pruritus, epistaxis, hair loss, and nail degeneration, she reduced her vitamin A intake to 66 000–150 000 IU/day. She was thin with alopecia, dry skin, and dystrophic nails, and was in mild respiratory distress with reduced breath sounds throughout the right lung and mild expiratory wheezes at the apices. There was no hepatomegaly or splenomegaly, but her liver was tender. Her serum vitamin A concentration was within the reference range. She had marked ascites, a pleural effusion, and partial collapse of the right lung. Liver biopsy showed changes consistent with vitamin A hepatotoxicity, namely prominent aggregates of hypertrophied perisinusoidal hepatic stellate cells, focal pericellular fibrosis, and mild perivenular fibrosis.

Urinary tract

In chronic intoxication, polyuria, increased frequency of micturition, urinary incontinence, enuresis, and acute renal insufficiency due to tubular necrosis can occur (SED-11, 800).

Patients with renal dysfunction are known to have raised circulating vitamin A concentrations. In chronic dialysis patients, the concentration can rise steadily. The significantly increased osmotic fragility of erythrocytes observed in hemodialysed patients also seems to be related to high vitamin A concentrations. However, the similarity between uremic symptoms and those of vitamin A excess may explain why hypervitaminosis A in uremic patients is rarely reported as being associated with clinical toxicity (SEDA-12, 327).

Skin

In acute intoxication, peeling of the entire skin can occur as a delayed symptom (50). Among the early and most commonly reported symptoms of chronic vitamin A intoxication are erythema, pruritus, hyperkeratosis, and dryness, hemorrhages, and fissures of the lips. A yellow to yellow-orange discoloration of the skin, reduced tolerance to sunlight, changes in pigmentation, hair loss, and brittle nails have been observed (34,36,51–53).

Musculoskeletal

Excessive doses of vitamin A lead to accelerated resorption of trabecular and cortical bone because of increased osteoclastic activity. A raised alkaline phosphatase, increased urinary hydroxyproline concentrations, and hypercalciuria correlate with these findings (54). One study suggested that high dietary intake of retinol might be associated with osteoporosis (55).

Pain in the bones and joints is a common symptom in patients taking vitamin A. Bone tenderness often occurs without other bone symptoms, but possible complications include elevation of the periosteum, hyperostosis, and in children premature closure of the epiphyses of the long bones, causing growth arrest (54,56).

- There were skeletal deformities involving the lower limbs and the spine in a 15-month-old girl who had received a total dose of 3.5 million micrograms RE (10.5 million IU) of vitamin A during the previous few months (57).
- Skeletal signs were seen in a nursing infant who was given 35 drops of a vitamin formulation five times a day during the first month of life, corresponding to vitamin A 8000 micrograms RE/day, plus vitamin D 5000 IU/day, vitamin E 15 mg/day, and vitamin C 250 mg/day. Other symptoms included hydrocephalus, cutaneous effects, and hepatic signs (58).
- A fatal case of hypervitaminosis A involved a premature neonate who died after having ingested 30 000 micrograms RE/day (90 000 IU/day), that is 60 times the recommended intake of vitamin A, for 11 days. On autopsy the skeleton showed marked alterations of endochondral bone formation. There was also evidence of accelerated resorption of bone, hypercalcemia, and metastatic calcification of the skin, soft tissues, and organs (59).

These three cases illustrate a common misunderstanding with regard to vitamins found among medical and nonmedical people alike: vitamins are believed to be innocuous substances, and since a little of them is good for you,

Table 2 Toxic doses of vitamin A

Exposure	Population	Country or region	Retinol equivalents (micrograms)
Toxic concentrations	Adults	Nordic	7500
	Adults	Australia	20 000
	Pregnant woman	Australia	10 000
	Pregnant woman	USA	5000–10 000
Chronic intoxication[a]	Children		758/kg
	Adults		15 000–30 000
Acute intoxication[b]	Children		22 500–30 000
	Adults		300 000–600 000

[a] Defined as repeated and prolonged intake of high doses
[b] Defined as intake of single (or multiple) very high doses

much must be even better. Table 2 puts this misconception into perspective (60).

Reproductive system

The effects of all-*trans*-retinoic acid on the male reproductive system include gynecomastia, discomfort, potency disorders, reduced fertility, and ejaculatory failure (61). The incidence is reported to be very high, but exact figures do not seem to be available.

Immunologic

Large doses of vitamin A in children in poor socioeconomic conditions have often for logistic reasons been combined with other health-care interventions, such as immunization. A randomized, case-control study of 336 infants receiving either 33 000 micrograms RE/day (100 000 IU) of vitamin A or placebo simultaneously with measles vaccine showed a lower seroconversion to measles in the vitamin A group (62).

Long-Term Effects

Tumorigenicity

Negative outcomes in several supplementation trials of beta-carotene, especially the results of the Finnish Alpha-Tocopherol Beta-Carotene (ATBC) Cancer Prevention Study (63) (SEDA-20, 363), have again revived discussion about the carcinogenic potential of beta-carotene. The ATBC trial showed that there was a statistically significant increase in the incidence of lung cancer in heavy smokers who took beta-carotene.

Problems concerning the interactions of cigarette smoking, cancer, and carotenoids have been reviewed (64).

Over several decades, evidence has accumulated that a diet rich in fruit and vegetables is associated with a lower risk of cardiovascular disease and various forms of cancer, principally cancer of the lung and stomach, but also esophageal, oral, breast, and prostate cancer (65,66). It is possible that this effect is in part due to their beta-carotene content.

Beta-carotene and other micronutrients have been claimed to counteract oxidative processes that participate in various stages of carcinogenesis, and increased consumption of fruit and vegetables rich in carotenoids lowered urinary indices of oxidized lipids and DNA in healthy subjects (67). Although beta-carotene and other carotenoids are excellent in vitro quenchers of singulett oxygen and beta-carotene, and may also protect lipids from radical-initiated peroxidation under certain conditions, evidence for antioxidant properties of beta-carotene in vivo is much less compelling (68). Assessment of the antioxidant benefit of beta-carotene is especially complicated by the fact that carcinogenesis is a very complex multistage process, in which oxidative pathways play variable and incompletely understood roles. While a few early supplementation trials suggested a beneficial role of beta-carotene (66), many other studies did not show such an effect. The proposed beneficial properties of carotenoids appear to be consistent with findings that cigarette smokers generally have subnormal serum concentrations of various carotenoids and other micronutrients, such as vitamin C, supposed to be caused by the increased oxidative stress associated with smoking and its attendant activation of the inflammatory and immune systems. On the other hand, the low concentrations in smokers could also result from lower intake of these micronutrients. Lower concentrations of carotenoids and other micronutrients are also observed in passive smokers (69,70).

The constituents of cigarette smoke can degrade beta-carotene (71,72), but the conclusion that smoking causes increased carotenoid metabolism demands the demonstration of raised carotenoid oxidation products. Moreover, the consistent observation of subnormal carotenoid concentrations but unchanged alpha-tocopherol concentrations (70) suggests that factors other than oxidative stress contribute to the relative carotenoid deficiency.

The assumption that remedying the carotenoid deficit would minimize the risks of cancer and heart disease associated with passive smoking has not been supported by several large randomized supplemention trials. In two major trials there was an increased incidence of cancer with beta-carotene supplementation in both smokers and asbestos workers. Of course, both high-risk groups might already have been in the early stages of cancer development at the start of the studies (63,64).

These surprising findings have raised an interesting apparent paradox: how can supplementation with beta-carotene, a presumed antioxidant and possible chemo-protective agent, enhance cancer formation, even though this is thought to involve oxidative processes? In some experimental systems carotenoids have pro-oxidant properties at high concentrations, but these are not reached in vivo (69,70). Another mechanism is an increase or alteration in carotenoid metabolism in high-risk groups, resulting in the formation of metabolites or oxidation products that could be procarcinogenic (for instance by interfering with retinoid signaling pathways, by promoting DNA damage, or by inducing cytochrome P450 enzymes that might promote carcinogen activation) (66,73). Such induction of cytochrome P450 enzymes might also enhance the catabolism of retinoic acid, which plays an important role in lung epithelial proliferation and differentiation. Down-regulation of the retinoic acid receptor, RARb, by beta-carotene supplementation has been shown in recent studies in ferrets (73). RARb may act as a tumor suppressor gene. Moreover, lung expression of the proto-oncogenes c-jun and c-fos was increased in animals exposed to cigarette smoke and also receiving beta-carotene supplements (73).

In general, the negative outcomes of several supplementation trials and the lack of proof that carotenoids form the primary beneficial component of fruit and vegetables should serve as a warning against unregulated supplementation with these individual micronutrients, especially in view of the potential carcinogenic effect of carotenoids.

The carcinogenic effect of beta-carotene has recently been found to be reduced by vitamin E (74), suggesting that, rather than individual micronutrient supplementation, combinations of various such substances might be more advantageous.

Second-Generation Effects

Pregnancy

The benefits and safety of maternal and infant vitamin A supplementation administered with each of the three diphtheria-tetanus-pertussis (DPT) and poliomyelitis immunizations and with a fourth dose of measles immunization have been assessed in a randomized, double-blind, placebo-controlled study in 9424 mother–infant pairs from Ghana, India, and Peru (75). Vitamin A 200 000 IU was given to 4716 mothers and 25 000 IU to their infants with each of the first three doses of DPT/poliomyelitis immunization at 6, 10, and 14 weeks. Placebo was given to 4708 mothers and their infants. At 9 months, with measles immunization infants in the vitamin A group were given a further dose of 25 000 IU and those in the placebo group received 100 000 IU. At 6 months there was a small reduction in vitamin A deficiency in the vitamin A group compared with controls; this effect was no longer apparent at 9 months. There were no significant differences in mortality throughout the study. Adverse effects were a bulging fontanelle (in under 1% of the infants) and vomiting. Among the infants without a bulging fontanelle before the start of the study, more of the vitamin A recipients than placebo recipients had a bulging fontanelle within 48 hours of the dose at 6, 10, and 14 weeks. After the fourth dose at 9 months, a bulging fontanelle was more common among the controls than among the infants given vitamin A. However, after each dose under 1% of the infants in either group had a bulging fontanelle. Of the 62 infants in the vitamin A group who had a bulging fontanelle reported at 24 hours after a dose, the bulging had resolved within 48 hours in 445 (73%). Among the controls, in whom almost all the instances of bulging were reported with the 100 000 IU dose, 25 of 42 had resolution of bulging within 48 hours. Under 3% of mothers in each group reported a bulging fontanelle after each dose. Vomiting occurred only within 48 hours after administration of the fourth dose in 167

(4.9%) infants in the vitamin A group versus 236 (6.5%) in the control group. There were no significant differences in convulsions or raised temperature at any dose.

Teratogenicity

Although the retinoids are markedly teratogenic, vitamin A is less so. In animals vitamin A excess can be teratogenic, as can vitamin A deficiency. In humans several cases of teratogenicity associated with vitamin A have been observed (76–78), and high incidences of spontaneous abortions and birth defects have been observed in women who have taken therapeutic doses of isotretinoin (13-*cis*-retinoic acid) during the first trimester of pregnancy. Recommendations about dosages of vitamin A in pregnant women have been issued by several institutions (2), including the Teratology Society (8) and the American College of Obstetricians and Gynecologists (79). The Health Protection Branch of Health and Welfare Canada accepted the recommendation that the use of retinoic acid for acne be regarded as contraindicated in women during pregnancy and in those of childbearing age (80).

A study in Hungary of 1203 births to women who had taken a supplement containing 2000 micrograms RE (6000 IU)/day, compared with 1510 who had taken placebo, did not show any evidence of teratogenic effect (81). The lower limit of supplementation recommended varied between 1600 and 3300 micrograms RE (5000 and 10 000 IU) of vitamin A per day (SEDA-14, 330).

However, vitamin A may be harmful at even lower doses than had previously been appreciated, the prevalence of cranial neural crest tissue defects being 3.5 times higher when dietary and supplemental consumption of preformed vitamin A, taken together, exceeded 5000 micrograms RE (15 000 IU) than when it was 1600 (5000 IU) or less (82). For supplements considered alone, the prevalence of such defects was 4.8 times higher in the group consuming over 3300 micrograms RE (10 000 IU) than in the group consuming under 1600 micrograms RE (5000 IU). The risk seemed to start rising when consumption passed a threshold of about 3300 micrograms (10 000 IU).

The minimum human teratogenic daily dose of vitamin A is estimated to be 25 000–50 000 IU, and one report has suggested that it may be as little as 10 000 IU (82). The National Research Council's Committee on Dietary Allowance advocates a recommended daily allowance (RDA) of 800 retinol equivalents/day for non-pregnant women of childbearing age and pregnant women. The RDA is equivalent to 2700 IU of vitamin A obtained from a supplement as retinol or 4800 micrograms of beta-carotene. The committee of the American College of Obstetricians and Gynecologists recommends supplementation with 5000 IU/day as the maximum intake before and during pregnancy. This is well below the probable minimum human teratogenic dose. Prenatal multivitamin formulations in common use contain 5000 IU or less vitamin A, but vitamin tablets containing 25 000 IU or more of vitamin A are available as over-the-counter formulations. Pregnant women or those planning to become pregnant should be cautioned about the potential teratogenicity of high doses of vitamin A supplements. Warnings on labels were recommended as early as 1987 (8).

A summary of some cases of birth defects associated with high maternal intake of vitamin A is given in Table 3 (12).

To get further information about the teratogenicity of high doses of vitamin A, the European Network of the Teratology Information Services (ENTIS) prospectively evaluated data from 423 pregnancies exposed during the first 9 weeks of gestation to 10 000 IU/day or more (83). The presence of major structural malformations, excluding chromosomal and genetic diseases, was evaluated in 311 infants exposed to a median daily dose of vitamin A of 50 000 (range 10 000–300 000) IU/day. Three infants had a major malformation: pulmonary stenosis, stenotic anus with fistula, and bilateral inguinal hernia. There were no congenital malformations among 120 infants exposed to more than 50 000 IU/day. When the birth prevalence rate of major malformations in the study group was compared with two internal control groups of infants exposed to "high" doses of vitamin A later in pregnancy, and non-teratogenic doses, the respective rate ratios were 0.28 (CI = 0.06, 1.23) and 0.50

Table 3 Some cases of birth defects associated with high material intake of vitamin A

Maternal intake	Duration	Symptoms	Other conditions
Reports of individual cases			
~500 000 IU	Single dose, 2nd month	Preauricular appendices, epibulbar dermatoid (eye malfunctions similar to Goldenhar's syndrome)	Dose caused acute toxicity in the pregnant woman
150 000 IU	Periconceptual 2 to +3 months	Facial dysmorphism, pterygium colli, distended abdomen, absence of external genitalia and of anal and urethral openings, polycystic kidneys, dysmorphism of lumbar spine	Fetus aborted at 20 week because of spinal abnormality and polycystic kidney
25 000 IU	0–13 weeks	Unilateral ureteral duplication with one ureter ending in the vagina, hydronephrosis, hydroureters	
50 000 IU	14th week to term		
Reports of multiple cases			
18 000–100 000 IU	Before and throughout pregnancy	Abnormalities of the head, face, ears, eyes, mouth, lips, jaws, heart, and urinary system; other defects	Cases reported by physicians to the FDA; cases reported to the State Birth Defects Registry

(CI = 0.14, 1.76). There was no evidence for an increased risk of major malformations, associated with high vitamin A doses during organogenesis.

The incidence of the acute adverse effects of an oral dose of vitamin A 400 000 IU given to a newly delivered mother and a oral dose of 50 000 IU given at the same time to her baby has been assessed in a randomized, double-blind, placebo-controlled study, with follow-up 1 or 2 days after dosing in 839 mothers and babies, of whom 788 were assessed (84). The incidence of reported adverse effects was low. Only two mothers in each group spontaneously reported bulging fontanelles in their babies. One of these babies (in the placebo group) was reported to have been vomiting. The rates of bulging fontanelles were 1.5% and 1.0% in the treatment and control groups respectively (OR 1.48; CI = 0.35, 7.19) Only one baby (in the vitamin A group) of the 11 who had bulging fontanelles was symptomatic (with vomiting, possibly due to raised intracranial pressure). Maternal symptoms did not differ between the groups. Other reported symptoms in the vitamin A group ($n = 398$) compared with the controls ($n = 390$) were vomiting (6 versus 4.8%) and irritability (7.5 versus 5.4%). From these results it can be concluded that these large doses of vitamin A are well tolerated by newly delivered mothers and babies.

Susceptibility Factors

Age

Young children seem to be particularly at risk of vitamin A toxicity. Symptoms of chronic intoxication are seen with intakes of 800–16 000 micrograms/kg RE (2500–50 000 IU/kg) (21). Children with restricted protein intake may have reduced tolerance to vitamin A.

The National Prophylaxis Program for Prevention of Blindness due to Vitamin A Deficiency has been implemented in India since the 1970s and covers all children aged 9 months to 3 years (85). Children aged 9–12 months received a single dose of 100 000 IU and those aged 1–3 years received 200 000 IU every 6 months. According to the Assam State Government, 700 children of 3.2 million who were given vitamin A became ill and more than 15 children died. Whether all these cases were a direct consequence of high-dose vitamin A is being investigated. One of the possible reasons is overdose of vitamin A, because of use of a new 5 ml measuring cup, which was used instead of the traditional 2 ml spoon.

Hepatic disease

At special risk of vitamin A toxicity are those whose liver function is compromised by drugs, viral hepatitis, or protein-energy malnutrition (12). Elderly people may also be at increased risk for similar reasons but also from different causes. In addition to protein deficiency, alcohol intake and co-existing liver and renal disease may be present (86).

In alcoholics vitamin A supplementation, which might be a useful therapeutic measure, is complicated by the hepatotoxicity of large doses of the vitamin and the fact that chronic alcohol consumption results in an enhanced susceptibility to this effect (87).

Drug Administration

Drug formulations

The effects of variations in pharmaceutical formulation on plasma concentrations of vitamin A have only been partly documented. Vitamin A in aqueous dispersion results in higher plasma concentrations than in oily formulations (88).

Drug administration route

Vitamin A added to infusions can be absorbed by the plastic containers often used (89).

Drug overdose

Two children with vitamin A toxicity have been reported (90).

- A 2-year-old girl developed anorexia, lethargy, and bilateral leg pain and refused to walk. She had been unwell for the previous 3 weeks. She was lethargic and irritable and had tenderness over both tibial surfaces and an erythematous rash over her back and both elbows. She had a raised calcium concentration (3.05 mmol/l), a serum phosphate concentration in the reference range, and a raised serum vitamin A concentration (3.9 µmol/l; reference range 1.3–2.9 µmol/l). A skull X-ray showed widening of the coronal suture, and a leg X-ray showed abnormal metaphyseal densities at the knees and ankles. Radionuclide bone scans showed increased uptake in both anterior tibiae, anteriorly in multiple ribs close to the costochondral junctions, in the distal right ulnar shaft, and in the distal left femoral shaft. Her parents had given her a vitamin supplement containing 9000 IU/ml vitamin A 3 ml/day for several months. On withdrawal of the vitamin supplement her symptoms resolved over 2 weeks.
- A 4-year old boy presented with a 4-day history of bilateral leg pain and refusal to walk. He had tenderness over both tibial surfaces, generalized skin exfoliation, and reduced visual acuity in both eyes. Symmetrical bone scan changes (increased uptake throughout each ulna and tibia and foci in the 10th and 11th ribs and 11th thoracic vertebra), together with benign intracranial pressure, suggested vitamin A toxicity. His dermatologist had prescribed oral etretinate, but his parents had withdrawn it after consulting a naturopath. He was then given numerous medications, including vitamin A, D, and E supplements, calcium, and magnesium. After withdrawal of all vitamin supplements his condition steadily improved, except for visual acuity, which was unchanged.

These two cases clearly underline the importance of a detailed drug history, including the use of complementary medicines.

Drug–Drug Interactions

Ethanol

Ethanol and retinol are converted to their corresponding aldehydes by isozymes of alcohol dehydrogenase and other dehydrogenases. The pathways of retinol metabolism have been described in hepatic microsomes, partly involving cytochrome P450 isozymes, which can also metabolize various drugs. Multiple interactions of retinol, ethanol, and other drugs can therefore occur (91).

It is not therefore surprising that prolonged use of alcohol, drugs, or both not only results in reduced dietary intake of retinoids and carotenoids, but also accelerates the breakdown of retinol, through cross-induction of degradative enzymes. There is also competition between ethanol and retinoic acid precursors. Depletion of retinol and retinoic acid precursors is associated with hepatic and extrahepatic pathology, including carcinogenesis and fetal defects. Unfortunately, correction of vitamin A deficiency by supplementation is complicated by the intrinsic hepatotoxicity of retinol, which is potentiated by concomitant alcohol consumption. Furthermore, the precursor of vitamin A, beta-carotene, interacts with ethanol, interfering with the conversion of beta-carotin to retinol, while the combination of beta-carotene with ethanol results in hepatotoxicity.

In smokers who also consume alcohol, beta-carotene supplementation promotes pulmonary cancer and possibly cardiovascular complications.

It was already known in 1987 that foods that provide large amounts of retinol increase the risk of cancer of the esophagus (92,93), and in an epidemiological study the increased risk of cancer associated with the use of cigarettes and alcohol was enhanced by the ingestion of foods containing retinol (94).

The effect of alcohol abuse, one of the most common aggravating factors in vitamin A toxicity, has been elucidated. Vitamin A toxicity was potentiated in patients who took 10 000 IU/day for sexual dysfunction, and this effect was attributed to excess alcohol consumption (95). In animals, potentiation of vitamin A toxicity by ethanol resulted in striking hepatic inflammation and necrosis accompanied by a rise in serum glutamate dehydrogenase and aspartate transaminase (96).

Alcohol may also act indirectly by causing liver disease, which in turn can affect the capacity of the liver to export vitamin A, thereby enhancing its local toxicity. In alcoholics the carrying capacity of retinol binding protein was increased, even in those with low serum retinol concentrations (97). In such cases, caution in the amount of vitamin A used for therapy is recommended. Similarly, diets that are severely deficient in protein can affect the capacity of the liver to export vitamin A and enhance its hepatotoxicity.

In contrast to retinoids, carotenoids were considered non-toxic, even when taken chronically in large amounts, until recently, when it was found that ethanol interacts with carotenoids, interfering with their conversion to retinol. In baboons, the consumption of ethanol together with beta-carotene resulted in more striking hepatic injury than consumption of either compound alone (98). This interaction occurred at a total dose of 7.2–10.8 mg of beta-carotene per Joule of diet. This dose is common in people who take supplements and is the same order of magnitude used in the Beta-Carotene and Retinol Efficacy Trial (CARET) (30 mg/day) (99) and in another study (20 mg/day for 12 weeks) (100). The amount of alcohol given to the baboons was equivalent to that taken by an average alcoholic. The well-known toxicity

of ethanol was potentiated by large amounts of beta-carotene, and the concomitant administration of both beta-carotene and alcohol resulted in striking liver lesions, characterized by increased activity of plasma liver enzymes, an inflammatory response, and striking autophagic vacuoles and alterations in the endoplasmic reticulum and mitochondria (101).

Besides its hepatotoxic effects, beta-carotene supplementation can also cause cardiovascular complications in smokers and potentiate carcinogenicity. The Alpha-Tocopherol, Beta-Carotene and Cancer Prevention Study (ATBC) (72) and CARET (99) showed that supplementation of beta-carotene in smokers increased the incidence of death from coronary artery disease. Recent results suggest that beta-carotene participates as a pro-oxidant in the oxidative degradation of LDL, and that raised LDL concentrations may cancel the protective effect of alpha-tocopherol (102).

The two trials also showed that beta-carotene supplementation increased the incidence of pulmonary cancer in smokers. Because heavy smokers are commonly heavy drinkers it was supposed that alcohol might have contributed to the increased incidence of lung cancer. Subsequent analysis showed that there was indeed a relation between the incidence of pulmonary cancer and the amount of alcohol consumed.

As detrimental effects result from deficiency as well as an excess of retinoids and carotenoids, and since both have similar adverse effects in terms of fibrosis, carcinogenesis, and possibly embryotoxicity, therapeutic measures must pay attention to the narrow therapeutic window, especially in drinkers, in whom alcohol narrows the therapeutic window even further by promoting the depletion of retinoids and by potentiating their toxicity (91).

Liquid paraffin

Liquid paraffin used as a laxative can reduce the absorption of vitamin A and other fat-soluble vitamins (D, E, and K) (103).

Oral contraceptives

Earlier studies suggested that oral contraceptives could lead to an increase in plasma concentrations of vitamin A (104), the inference being that increased vitamin A concentrations might have a negative effect on conception, and that this might provide an explanation for the reduced fertility sometimes seen during the period immediately following withdrawal of contraceptive steroids. More recent work has not supported this theory.

References

1. Bluhm R, Branch R, Johnston P, Stein R. Aplastic anemia associated with canthaxanthin ingested for "tanning" purposes. JAMA 1990;264(9):1141–2.
2. Committee On Medical Aspects of Food Policy. Dietary Reference Values for Food Energy and Nutrients for the United Kingdom (1991). Report of the Panel on Dietary Reference Values. Report on Health and Social Subjects No. 41, Department of Health. London: Her Majesty's Stationery Office, 1991.

3. McLaren DS. Vitamin A deficiency and toxicity. Washington, DC: Nutrition Review, 1984:203.

4. Abdeljaber MH, Monto AS, Tilden RL, Schork MA, Tarwotjo I. The impact of vitamin A supplementation on morbidity: a randomized community intervention trial. Am J Public Health 1991;81(12):1654–6.

5. Herrera MG, Nestel P, el Amin A, Fawzi WW, Mohamed KA, Weld L. Vitamin A supplementation and child survival. Lancet 1992;340(8814):267–71.

6. Stephensen CB, Franchi LM, Hernandez H, Campos M, Gilman RH, Alvarez JO. Adverse effects of high-dose vitamin A supplements in children hospitalized with pneumonia. Pediatrics 1998;101(5):E3.

7. Meyers DG, Maloley PA, Weeks D. Safety of antioxidant vitamins. Arch Intern Med 1996;156(9):925–35.

8. Teratology Society position paper: recommendations for vitamin A use during pregnancy. Teratology 1987;35(2):269–75.

9. Scientific Committee for Food. Nutrient and energy intakes for the European Community. Directorate-General Industry, Commission of the European Communities. Luxembourg, 1993.

10. Bendich A, Langseth L. Safety of vitamin A. Am J Clin Nutr 1989;49(2):358–71.

11. Flores H, Azevedo MN, Campos FA, Barreto-Lins MC, Cavalcanti AA, Salzano AC, Varela RM, Underwood BA. Serum vitamin A distribution curve for children aged 2–6 y known to have adequate vitamin A status: a reference population. Am J Clin Nutr 1991;54(4):707–11.

12. Hathcock JN, Hattan DG, Jenkins MY, McDonald JT, Sundaresan PR, Wilkening VL. Evaluation of vitamin A toxicity. Am J Clin Nutr 1990;52(2):183–202.

13. Theiler R, Wirth HP, Flury R, Hanck A, Michel BA. Chronische Vitamin-A - Intoxikation mit muskulo-skelettalen Beschwerder und morphologischen Veranderungen der Leber: eine Fallbeschreibung. [Chronic vitamin A poisoning with musculoskeletal symptoms and morphological changes of the liver: a case report.] Schweiz Med Wochenschr 1993;123(51–52):2405–12.

14. Muntaner P, Rodriguez C, Arnau JM. Fever associated with chronic retinol therapy. Lancet 1990;335(8705):1588–9.

15. Geubel AP, De Galocsy C, Alves N, Rahier J, Dive C. Liver damage caused by therapeutic vitamin A administration: estimate of dose-related toxicity in 41 cases. Gastroenterology 1991;100(6):1701–9.

16. Marcus DF, Turgeon P, Aaberg TM, Wiznia RA, Wetzig PC, Bovino JA. Optic disk findings in hypervitaminosis A. Ann Ophthalmol 1985;17(7):397–402.

17. Hawkins TE, Burlon DT. Vitamin A intoxication. J Am Osteopath Assoc 1974;73(5):371–5.

18. de Francisco A, Chakraborty J, Chowdhury HR, Yunus M, Baqui AH, Siddique AK, Sack RB. Acute toxicity of vitamin A given with vaccines in infancy. Lancet 1993;342(8870):526–7.

19. Lombaert A, Carton H. Benign intracranial hypertension due to A-hypervitaminosis in adults and adolescents. Eur Neurol 1976;14(5):340–50.

20. Bauernfeind JC. Vitamin A-Application Technology: A Report of the International Vitamin A Consultative Group. Washington, DC: The Nutrition Foundation, 1980.

21. Morrice G Jr, Havener WH, Kapetansky F. Vitamin A intoxication as a cause of pseudotumor cerebri. JAMA 1960;173:1802–5.

22. Meyer-Heim A, Landau K, Boltshauser E. Aknetherapie mit Folgen—Pseudotumor cerebri durch Hypervitaminose A. [Treatment of acne with consequences—pseudotumor cerebri due to hypervitaminosis A.] Schweiz Rundsch Med Prax 2002;91(1–2):23–6.

23. Friedland S, Burde RM. Chronic headaches due to vitamin A abuse. J Neuroophthalmol 1996;16(1):72.

24. Marti TJ, Rusinol E, Santana JM, et al. Papiledema per ingesta excessiva de vitamina A: a proposit d'un cas. Bull Soc Catalana Pediatr 1985;45:193.

25. Haupt R. Akute symptomatische Psychose bei Vitamin A-Intoxikation. [Acute symptomatic psychosis in vitamin A intoxication.] Nervenarzt 1977;48(2):91–5.

26. Goodman GE, Alberts DS, Earnst DL, Meyskens FL. Phase I trial of retinol in cancer patients. J Clin Oncol 1983;1(6):394–9.

27. Ellis JK, Russell RM, Makrauer FL, Schaefer EJ. Increased risk for vitamin A toxicity in severe hypertriglyceridemia. Ann Intern Med 1986;105(6):877–9.

28. Pastorino U, Chiesa G, Infante M, Soresi E, Clerici M, Valente M, Belloni PA, Ravasi G. Safety of high-dose vitamin A. Randomized trial on lung cancer chemoprevention. Oncology 1991;48(2):131–7.

29. Gerber LE, Erdman JW Jr. Changes in lipid metabolism during retinoid administration. J Am Acad Dermatol 1982;6(4 Pt 2 Suppl):664–74.

30. Warrell RP Jr, de The H, Wang ZY, Degos L. Acute promyelocytic leukemia. N Engl J Med 1993;329(3):177–89.

31. Beijer C, Planken EV. Hypercalciemie door chronisch vitamine-A-gebruik bij een bejaarde patiente met nierinsufficientie. [Hypercalcemia due to chronic vitamin A use by an elderly patient with renal insufficiency.] Ned Tijdschr Geneeskd 2001;145(2):90–3.

32. Teo ST, Newth J, Pascoe BJ. Chronic vitamin A intoxication. Med J Aust 1973;2(7):324–6.

33. Mendoza FS, Johnson E, Kerner JA, Tune BM, Shochat SJ. Vitamin A intoxication presenting with ascites and a normal vitamin A level. West J Med 1988;148(1):88–90.

34. Leicht E, Strunz J, von Seebach HB, Meiser RJ, Mausle E. Akute Vitamin-A-Intoxikation mit hämolytischer Anämie, Hyperkalzämie und toxischer Hepatose. [Acute vitamin A intoxication with hemolytic anemia, hypercalcemia and toxic hepatosis.] Med Klin 1973;68(2):54–9.

35. Muenter MD, Perry HO, Ludwig J. Chronic vitamin A intoxication in adults. Hepatic, neurologic and dermatologic complications. Am J Med 1971;50(1):129–36.

36. Goeckenjan G, Goertz G, Pottgen W, Grabensee B, Herms W. Lebensbedrohliche Komplikationen der hochdosierten Vitamin-A Behandlung bei Psoriasis. [Life threatening complications in the treatment of psoriasis using large doses of vitamin A.] Dtsch Med Wochenschr 1972;97(38):1424–9.

37. Hatake K, Ohtsuki T, Uwai M, Takahashi H, Izumi T, Yoshida M, Kanai N, Saito K, Harigaya K, Miura Y. Tretinoin induces bone marrow collagenous fibrosis in acute promyelocytic leukaemia: new adverse, but reversible effect. Br J Haematol 1996;93(3):646–9.

38. Shimamoto Y, Suga K, Yamaguchi M, Kuriyama K, Tomonaga M. Prophylaxis of symptoms of hyperhistaminemia after the treatment of acute promyelocytic leukemia with all-trans retinoic acid. Acta Haematol 1994;92(2):109–12.

39. Perrotta S, Nobili B, Rossi F, Criscuolo M, Iolascon A, Di Pinto D, Passaro I, Cennamo L, Oliva A, Della Ragione F. Infant hypervitaminosis A causes severe anemia and thrombocytopenia: evidence of a retinol-dependent bone marrow cell growth inhibition. Blood 2002;99(6):2017–22.

40. Reuter H. Vitamine Chemie und Klinik. Stuttgart: Hippokrates Verlag, 1970.

41. Fleischmann R, Schlote W, Schomerus H, Wolburg H, Castrillon-Oberndorfer WL, Hoensch H. Kleinknotige Leberzirrhose mit ausgepragter portaler Hypertension als Folga einer Vitamin-A - intoxikation bei Psoriasis-Behandlung. [Small-nodular liver cirrhosis with marked portal hypertension due to vitamin A intoxication resulting from

psoriasis treatment.] Dtsch Med Wochenschr 1977; 102(45):1637–40.

42. Frokiaer E, Hertel L. Langvarig A-vitaminindtagelse og levercirrhose. [Prolonged intake of vitamin A and cirrhosis of the liver.] Ugeskr Laeger 1981;143(32):2038.

43. Sarles J, Scheiner C, Sarran M, Giraud F. Hepatic hypervitaminosis A: a familial observation. J Pediatr Gastroenterol Nutr 1990;10(1):71–6.

44. Kistler HJ, Pluer S, Dickenmann W, Pirozynski W. Portale Hypertonie ohne Leberzirrhose bei chronischer Vitamin-A-Intoxikation. [Portal hypertension without liver cirrhosis in chronic vitamin A intoxication.] Schweiz Med Wochenschr 1977;107(24):825–32.

45. Noseda A, Adler M, Ketelbant P, Baran D, Winand J. Massive vitamin A intoxication with ascites and pleural effusion. J Clin Gastroenterol 1985;7(4):344–9.

46. Minuk GY, Kelly JK, Hwang WS. Vitamin A hepatotoxicity in multiple family members. Hepatology 1988;8(2):272–5.

47. Kowalski TE, Falestiny M, Furth E, Malet PF. Vitamin A hepatotoxicity: a cautionary note regarding 25,000 IU supplements. Am J Med 1994;97(6):523–8.

48. Graffin B, Genty I, Cretel E, Jean R, Durand JM. Beta-carotene-induced hepatic fibrosis. Dig Dis Sci 2002;47(4):793.

49. Miksad R, de Ledinghen V, McDougall C, Fiel I, Rosenberg H. Hepatic hydrothorax associated with vitamin a toxicity. J Clin Gastroenterol 2002;34(3):275–9.

50. Nater JP, Doeglas HM. Halibut liver poisoning in 11 fishermen. Acta Dermatol Venereol 1970;50(2):109–13.

51. Wisse Smit J, Pott Hofstede D. Vitamine-A-intoxicatie bij volwassenen. [Vitamin A poisoning in adults.] Ned Tijdschr Geneeskd 1966;110(1):10–11.

52. Bartlett BH. An open evaluation of retinoic acid in acne. Australas J Dermatol 1972;13(3):132–9.

53. Linden V. Ketchup og hyperkarotenose. [Tomato-ketchup and hypercarotenosis.] Tidsskr Nor Laegeforen 1974; 94(13):855–6.

54. Frame B, Jackson CE, Reynolds WA, Umphrey JE. Hypercalcemia and skeletal effects in chronic hypervitaminosis A. Ann Intern Med 1974;80(1):44–8.

55. Melhus H, Michaelsson K, Kindmark A, Bergstrom R, Holmberg L, Mallmin H, Wolk A, Ljunghall S. Excessive dietary intake of vitamin A is associated with reduced bone mineral density and increased risk for hip fracture. Ann Intern Med 1998;129(10):770–8.

56. Bartolozzi G, Bernini G. Chronic hypervitaminosis A. Helv Paediatr Acta 1979;25:301.

57. Ruby LK, Mital MA. Skeletal deformities following chronic hypervitaminosis A: a case report. J Bone Joint Surg Am 1974;56(6):1283–7.

58. Gottrand F, Leclerc F, Chenaud M, Vallee L, Gaudier B. Une cause rare d'hydrocéphalie du nourrisson: l'intoxication chronique par la vitamine A. [A rare cause of hydrocephalus in an infant: chronic vitamin A poisoning.] Arch Fr Pediatr 1986;43(7):501–2.

59. Bush ME, Dahms BB. Fatal hypervitaminosis A in a neonate. Arch Pathol Lab Med 1984;108(10):838–42.

60. Noirfalise A. La vitamin A est-elle dangereuse? [Is vitamin A dangerous?] Rev Med Liege 1991;46(9):461–4.

61. Coleman R, MacDonald D. Effects of isotretinoin on male reproductive system. Lancet 1994;344(8916):198.

62. Semba RD, Munasir Z, Beeler J, Akib A, Muhilal, Audet S, Sommer A. Reduced seroconversion to measles in infants given vitamin A with measles vaccination. Lancet 1995;345(8961):1330–2.

63. The Alpha-Tocopherol, Beta Carotene Cancer Prevention Study Group. The effect of vitamin E and beta carotene on the incidence of lung cancer and other cancers in male smokers. N Engl J Med 1994;330(15):1029–35.

64. van der Vliet A. Cigarettes, cancer, and carotenoids: a continuing, unresolved antioxidant paradox. Am J Clin Nutr 2000;72(6):1421–3.

65. Block G, Patterson B, Subar A. Fruit, vegetables, and cancer prevention: a review of the epidemiological evidence. Nutr Cancer 1992;18(1):1–29.

66. Pryor WA, Stahl W, Rock CL. Beta carotene: from biochemistry to clinical trials. Nutr Rev 2000;58(2 Pt 1):39–53.

67. Thompson HJ, Heimendinger J, Haegele A, Sedlacek SM, Gillette C, O'Neill C, Wolfe P, Conry C. Effect of increased vegetable and fruit consumption on markers of oxidative cellular damage. Carcinogenesis 1999;20(12):2261–6.

68. Krinsky NI. The antioxidant and biological properties of the carotenoids. Ann NY Acad Sci 1998;854:443–7.

69. Cross CE, Traber M, Eiserich J, van der Vliet A. Micronutrient antioxidants and smoking. Br Med Bull 1999;55(3):691–704.

70. Alberg AJ, Chen JC, Zhao H, Hoffman SC, Comstock GW, Helzlsouer KJ. Household exposure to passive cigarette smoking and serum micronutrient concentrations. Am J Clin Nutr 2000;72(6):1576–82.

71. Handelman GJ, Packer L, Cross CE. Destruction of tocopherols, carotenoids, and retinol in human plasma by cigarette smoke. Am J Clin Nutr 1996;63(4):559–65.

72. Baker DL, Krol ES, Jacobsen N, Liebler DC. Reactions of beta-carotene with cigarette smoke oxidants. Identification of carotenoid oxidation products and evaluation of the prooxidant/antioxidant effect. Chem Res Toxicol 1999; 12(6):535–43.

73. Wang XD, Russell RM. Procarcinogenic and anti-carcinogenic effects of beta-carotene. Nutr Rev 1999;57(9 Pt 1):263–72.

74. Perocco P, Mazzullo M, Broccoli M, Rocchi P, Ferreri AM, Paolini M. Inhibitory activity of vitamin E and alpha-naphthoflavone on beta-carotene-enhanced transformation of BALB/c 3T3 cells by benzo(a)pyrene and cigarette-smoke condensate. Mutat Res 2000;465(1–2):151–8.

75. Arthur P, Bahl P, Bhan MK, Kirkwood BR, Martines J, Moulton LH, Panny ME, Ram M, Ram M, Underwood B. Randomised trial to assess benefits and safety of vitamin A supplementation linked to immunisation in early infancy. Lancet 1998;352:1257–63.

76. Rosa FW, Wilk AL, Kelsey FO. Teratogen update: vitamin A congeners. Teratology 1986;33(3):355–64.

77. Stange L, Carlstrom K, Eriksson M. Hypervitaminosis a in early human pregnancy and malformations of the central nervous system. Acta Obstet Gynecol Scand 1978; 57(3):289–91.

78. Nishimura H, Tanimura T. Clinical Aspects of the Teratogenicity of Drugs. Amsterdam, Oxford: Excerpta Medica, 1976:251.

79. ACOG Committee Opinion: Committee on Obstetrics. Maternal and fetal medicine, vitamin A supplementation during pregnancy. Intern J Gynecol Obstet 1993;40(2):175.

80. Danby FW. Retinoic acid in acne therapy. Can Med Assoc J 1978;119(8):854,856.

81. Dudas I, Czeizel AE. Use of 6,000 IU vitamin A during early pregnancy without teratogenic effect. Teratology 1992;45(4):335–6.

82. Rothman KJ, Moore LL, Singer MR, Nguyen US, Mannino S, Milunsky A. Teratogenicity of high vitamin A intake. N Engl J Med 1995;333(21):1369–73.

83. Mastroiacovo P, Mazzone T, Addis A, Elephant E, Carlier P, Vial T, Garbis H, Robert E, Bonati M, Ornoy A, Finardi A, Schaffer C, Caramelli L, Rodriguez-Pinilla E, Clementi M. High vitamin A intake in early pregnancy and major malformations: a multicenter prospective controlled study. Teratology 1999;59(1):7–11.

84. Iliff PJ, Humphrey JH, Mahomva AI, Zvandasara P, Bonduelle M, Malaba L, Nathoo KJ. Tolerance of large doses of vitamin A given to mothers and their babies shortly after delivery. Nutr Res 1999;19:1437–46.

85. Kapil U. Deaths in Assam during vitamin A pulse distribution: the needle of suspicion is on the new measuring cup. Indian Pediatr 2002;39(1):114–15.

86. Ward BJ. Retinol (vitamin A) supplements in the elderly. Drugs Aging 1996;9(1):48–59.

87. Lieber CS. Interaction of ethanol with drugs and vitamin therapy. Ration Drug Ther 1985;19(11):1–7.

88. Bauernfeind JC. The safe use of vitamin A: a report of the International Vitamin A Consultative Group. Washington DC: Nutrition Foundation, 1980.

89. Anonymous. Drug interactions with medical plastics. Drug Intell Clin Pharm 1983;17(10):726–31.

90. Coghlan D, Cranswick NE. Complementary medicine and vitamin A toxicity in children. Med J Aust 2001; 175(4):223–4.

91. Leo MA, Lieber CS. Alcohol, vitamin A, and beta-carotene: adverse interactions, including hepatotoxicity and carcinogenicity. Am J Clin Nutr 1999;69(6):1071–85.

92. Tuyns AJ, Riboli E, Doornbos G, Pequignot G. Diet and esophageal cancer in Calvados (France). Nutr Cancer 1987;9(2–3):81–92.

93. Decarli A, Liati P, Negri E, Franceschi S, La Vecchia C. Vitamin A and other dietary factors in the etiology of esophageal cancer. Nutr Cancer 1987;10(1–2):29–37.

94. Graham S, Marshall J, Haughey B, Brasure J, Freudenheim J, Zielezny M, Wilkinson G, Nolan J. Nutritional epidemiology of cancer of the esophagus. Am J Epidemiol 1990;131(3):454–67.

95. Worner TM, Gordon GG, Leo MA, Lieber CS. Vitamin A treatment of sexual dysfunction in male alcoholics. Am J Clin Nutr 1988;48(6):1431–5.

96. Leo MA, Lieber CS. Hepatic fibrosis after long-term administration of ethanol and moderate vitamin A supplementation in the rat. Hepatology 1983;3(1):1–11.

97. Chapman KM, Prabhudesai M, Erdman JW Jr. Vitamin A status of alcoholics upon admission and after two weeks of hospitalization. J Am Coll Nutr 1993;12(1):77–83.

98. Leo MA, Kim C, Lowe N, Lieber CS. Interaction of ethanol with beta-carotene: delayed blood clearance and enhanced hepatotoxicity. Hepatology 1992;15(5):883–91.

99. Omenn GS, Goodman GE, Thornquist MD, Balmes J, Cullen MR, Glass A, Keogh JP, Meyskens FL, Valanis B, Williams JH, Barnhart S, Hammar S. Effects of a combination of beta carotene and vitamin A on lung cancer and cardiovascular disease. N Engl J Med 1996;334(18):1150–5.

100. Rust P, Eichler I, Renner S, Elmadfa I. Effects of long-term oral beta-carotene supplementation on lipid peroxidation in patients with cystic fibrosis. Int J Vitam Nutr Res 1998;68(2):83–7.

101. Leo MA, Aleynik SI, Aleynik MK, Lieber CS. beta-Carotene beadlets potentiate hepatotoxicity of alcohol. Am J Clin Nutr 1997;66(6):1461–9.

102. Bowen HT, Omaye ST. Oxidative changes associated with beta-carotene and alpha-tocopherol enrichment of human low-density lipoproteins. J Am Coll Nutr 1998; 17(2):171–9.

103. Tarjan R, Kramer M. The effect of liquid paraffin on the utilization of carotene and vitamin A. Int Z Vitaminforsch 1963;33:304–10.

104. Wien EM, Ojo OA. Serum vitamin A, carotene and cholesterol levels in Nigerian women using various types of contraceptives. Nutr Rep Int 1982;25(4):687.

Vitamin A: Retinoids

See also Vitamins *and* Vitamin A: Carotenoids

General Information

Vitamin A (retinol) is a key regulator of epithelial cell proliferation and differentiation. Aberrations in these processes are a feature of many skin diseases, and dermatologists have therefore long taken an interest in vitamin A as a therapeutic agent. However, marginal efficacy and unacceptable adverse effects (Table 1) have minimized the usefulness of vitamin A itself. Therefore, derivatives of vitamin A (retinoids) have been developed.

Tretinoin

Tretinoin (*all-trans*-retinoic acid), a natural metabolite of vitamin A, was the first vitamin A analogue to be used orally, with some success, but its general therapeutic ratio did not differ markedly from that of vitamin A itself.

Tretinoin cream is used extensively for the treatment of acne and photodamaged skin, and local irritant dermatitis is common. With normal use, absorption is minimal and systemic adverse effects are therefore not expected.

Topical tretinoin has also been used as an ophthalmic ointment 0.01% in the treatment of squamous metaplasia associated with dry eyes. In 161 patients with either keratoconjunctivitis sicca or conjunctival cicatricial diseases (Stevens–Johnson syndrome, inactive pemphigoid, radiation-induced dry eye, drug-induced pseudopemphigoid, and toxic epidermal necrolysis) there were no beneficial effects in the former, but significant reversal of conjunctival keratinization in the temporal bulbar site in the latter (1). Adverse effects were limited to blepharoconjunctivitis and resolved on withdrawal.

Tretinoin has been evaluated in 26 patients with histologically confirmed adenocarcinoma of the prostate and manifestations of progressive metastatic disease (2). They received a single oral dose of tretinoin 45 mg/m^2/day for 7 days followed by no treatment for 7 days before starting to take tretinoin again. Toxicity was mostly mild. There was cheilosis in eleven patients and vomiting in one. In eight patients there were transient rises in serum

Table 1 Clinical effects of chronic hypervitaminosis A, in order of decreasing frequency (3,4)

Scaling of skin, erythema, pruritus, altered hair growth
Dry mucous membranes, cheilitis, angular stomatitis, gingivitis, glossitis
Pain and tenderness of the bones, restricted movement
Occipital headache
Hyperirritability, sleep disturbances
Papillary edema, diplopia
Anorexia, weight loss
Hepatomegaly, sometimes with splenomegaly
Peripheral edema
Fatigue, lassitude, occasionally somnolence
Hemorrhages, epistaxis, increased menstrual bleeding

triglyceride concentrations up to three times normal, returning to normal within 3–6 weeks, despite continuation of tretinoin. One patient had a severe headache with vomiting on day 1 and required a 30% dosage reduction. No patient withdrew because of toxicity.

Fatal adverse effects have been reported in patients given tretinoin for acute promyelocytic leukemia (5). Of 82 patients with acute promyelocytic leukemia, 35 developed leukocytosis and 22 had fatal adverse effects (15 with the retinoic acid syndrome and 7 with intracranial bleeding). Leukocytosis was a risk factor for fatal adverse effects. The authors suggested that the combination of tretinoin with low-dose harringtonine can reduce the incidence of leukocytosis-related intracranial bleeding and glucocorticoids can reduce mortality from the retinoic acid syndrome.

In another study of 413 patients with acute promyelocytic leukemia treated with tretinoin plus daunorubicin, the retinoic acid syndrome occurred in 64 cases, of which 5 were fatal (6).

Tretinoin 70, 110, 150, 190, or 230 mg/m^2/day has been given to 26 patients with advanced potentially hormone-responsive breast cancer taking tamoxifen 20 mg/day (7). At all doses headaches, nausea, skin changes, and bone pain occurred. The headaches were most severe during the first week of treatment, peaking at the end of the first week. They were sometimes associated with nausea and occasionally with vomiting, although there was no other evidence of raised cerebrospinal fluid pressure. Headaches and nausea tended to subside during the weeks when tretinoin was not given and recurred during the weeks of tretinoin reintroduction, although their severity tended to wane with subsequent cycles of treatment. Similarly, skin reactions, such as erythema and desquamation, were dose-related and were most severe during the initial cycles of treatment. Bone pain occurred intermittently. There was life-threatening hypercalcemia in one patient, but it was felt to be due to disease progression. The dose of 230 mg/m^2/day produced unacceptable headache and skin toxicity, but doses of up to 190 mg/m^2/day were tolerable.

A dry scaling skin rash and cheilitis were the most common adverse effects in 14 patients with prostate cancer treated with tretinoin and 20 patients treated with a combination of *cis*-retinoic acid and interferon α-2a (8). There was anorexia and significant weight loss in under 10% of the patients, but one patient discontinued treatment because of persistent fatigue and anorexia. Hematological toxic effects included leukopenia, neutropenia, anemia, and thrombocytopenia. Two patients with mild urinary hesitancy had acute urinary outlet obstruction within 1 week of starting *cis*-retinoic acid plus interferon. There were mild rises in hepatic transaminases and serum triglycerides in over half of the patients. Most triglyceride concentrations were below 2.3 (reference range 0.6–1.9) mmol/l, but one patient had an extreme rise of triglycerides to 3280 mg/dl. Sensory and mood changes were mild and occurred mostly in those given *cis*-retinoic acid plus interferon. Headaches were the most common neurological abnormality with tretinoin. Pulmonary adverse effects were

dyspnea and a non-fatal pulmonary embolism in one patient treated with tretinoin. Other adverse effects included constipation, fever, nausea, vomiting, diarrhea, fatigue, and stomatitis.

In 21 patients with squamous cell carcinomas of the head and neck randomized to tretinoin 45, 50, or 150 mg/m^2 either once daily or as divided doses every 8 hours for 1 year, severe adverse effects included headache in five patients, hypertriglyceridemia in six, mucositis in two, and hyperbilirubinemia, raised alkaline phosphatase, colitis, raised lipase, xerostomia, eczema, and arthritis in one patient each (9). The dose had to be reduced in seven of eight patients with severe toxicity at 90 mg/m^2/day. Three of nine patients taking 45 mg/m^2/day required dose reductions. The plasma AUC of tretinoin did not correlate with the severity or frequency of adverse effects. From these results it can be concluded that 15 mg/m^2/day every 8 hours is a tolerable dose for 1 year in patients with squamous cell carcinomas of the head and neck.

The adverse effects of tretinoin 50 mg/m^2/day for 3 months have been studied in 20 patients with emphysema in a randomized, double-blind, placebo-controlled trial (10). The treatment was well tolerated and associated with only mild adverse effects, including skin changes, such as dry skin and cracking lips in 15 (1 placebo), transient headache in 13 (1), hyperlipidemia in 11 (5), pruritus in 6 (2), muscle/bone pain in 6 (0), generalized fatigue in 6 (2), raised transaminases in 5 (1), a sensation of clogged ears in 3 (2), nausea in 2 (0), hair loss in 2 (0), and blurred vision in 1 (1).

Etretinate and isotretinoin

Since the beginning of the 1980s two synthetic retinoids, etretinate (the ethyl ester of trimethoxymethylphenyl retinoic acid; Tigason; Tegison) and isotretinoin (13-*cis*-retinoic acid; Acutane; Roaccutane), have been successfully administered for a variety of skin disorders, all of which involve disordered epidermal or epithelial cell growth and differentiation as prominent pathogenic features, for example psoriasis, ichthyosis, Darier's disease, lichen planus, and pityriasis rubra pilaris. Isotretinoin has been of great value in the treatment of cystic acne and acne conglobata, with no serious long-term adverse effects (11,12). It has also been used for milder forms of acne (13,14).

Acitretin

In 1990, etretinate (Tigason) was replaced by acitretin (Neo-Tigason), an aromatic retinoid, a carboxylic acid metabolite of etretinate (15). It is effective in pustular psoriasis and psoriatic palmoplantar keratoderma and in combination with PUVA or topical therapy (calcipotriol or glucocorticoids) in the treatment of other forms of psoriasis. It has also been used to treat disorders of keratinization (ichthyosis, palmoplantar keratoderma, Darier's disease) and severe cutaneous forms of lichen planus. It prevents new skin carcinomas in patients with xeroderma pigmentosum and those who are immunosuppressed. The main advantage of acitretin is its short half-life of 50 hours, compared with over 80 days for etretinate (16).

Adapalene

Topical retinoids and similar drugs, including tretinoin, adapalene, and tazaroten, are the most commonly used topical drugs for acne (17). Adapalene is a synthetic poly-aromatic retinoid and is formulated in a water-based gel (1.0%, Galderma Labs Inc, San Antonio, TX). In a double-blind, multicenter, parallel-group, randomized study the efficacy and adverse effects of 0.1% adapalene gel and 0.1% tretinoin gel in a microsphere formulation were compared over 12 weeks (18). The two drugs had similar effects on the resolution of acne lesions, but tretinoin was significantly more effective in reducing the number of comedones. There were no statistically significant differences between tretinoin and adapalene in the incidences of erythema, burning/stinging, or itching. Most patients had at least one sign of cutaneous irritation over the course of the study (tretinoin 95%, adapalene 91%). The most common adverse effect was erythema (tretinoin 83%, adapalene 66%), followed by peeling (80% and 66%), dryness (67% and 65%), burning/stinging (45% and 36%), and itching (37% and 35%). There were significant differences in the incidence of cutaneous effects in favor of adapalene for dryness at week 8 (tretinoin 34%, adapalene 18%) and week 10 (29% and 12%), and for peeling at week 3 (56% and 39%), week 6 (46% and 26%), week 8 (45% and 17%), and week 10 (35% and 17%). There were no serious adverse events in either group.

In another comparison of the efficacy and adverse effects of adapalene gel 1% or 0.025% tretinoin gel in 150 Chinese patients, similar effects were observed (19). In both groups skin irritation was mild, but it was more pronounced with tretinoin. Burning was the most common unwanted effect in those who used tretinoin compared with adapalene (34 versus 11%). There was dryness of the skin in 34% of those who used tretinoin and in 22% of those who used adapalene. The respective frequencies of scaling were 26 and 15%, and of erythema 26 and 2.7%. Pruritus was the only adverse effect experienced exclusively by those who used adapalene, and it occurred in under 4%. Overall, 46% of those who used tretinoin had some form of irritation, compared with 32% of those who used adapalene.

General adverse effects

Although the various retinoids have similar toxicity profiles, they differ in the extent to which they affect various body systems. Cutaneous and mucous membrane symptoms (up to 70%) are by far the most prominent adverse effects; patients who use isotretinoin have a 50% incidence of conjunctivitis and irritation of the eyes. Musculoskeletal symptoms occur in up to 15% of users. Hypersensitivity reactions are rare and consist of occasional drug rashes. The occurrence of sarcomas in patients treated with isotretinoin may well be a chance finding (SEDA-21, 164); retinoids may prevent or even cure certain malignancies (20). All the retinoids are strongly teratogenic (21–23).

The incidence and time-course of adverse events during a 4-month course of oral isotretinoin (1 mg/kg) for severe acne have been studied prospectively in 189 patients (24). Most of the adverse events were most

Table 2 Features of tretinoin toxicity in 22 patients

Organ system	N (%)	Symptoms	N (%)
Tretinoin-related toxicity	12 (55)	Retinoic acid syndrome	3 (14)
Cardiovascular	5 (23)	Pericardial effusion	1 (5)
		Weight gain	5 (23)
		Arterial hypotension	2 (9)
Respiratory	3 (14)	Adult respiratory distress syndrome	2 (9)
		Pleural effusion	1 (5)
		Pulmonary infiltrates	1 (5)
Nervous system	6 (27)	Headache	6 (27)
		Raised intracranial pressure	1 (5)
Liver and metabolism	12 (55)	Raised transaminases	6 (27)
		Raised bilirubin	1 (5)
		Raised triglycerides	2 (9)
Hematologic	4 (18)	Leukocytosis	4 (18)
Skin and musculoskeletal	4 (18)	Dry skin	1 (5)
		Itching	1 (5)
		Joint/bone/muscle pain	3 (14)
		Osteonecrosis	1 (5)

often reported during the first 3 months of treatment. However, only a few patients were seen every month as scheduled and only 50 of 189 filled in the questionnaire at 4 months.

In a retrospective study, 22 children taking tretinoin (median age 9.3 years, range 1.8–16.3) for a median of 38 (6–138) days were compared with 22 taking conventional therapy (median age 12.3 years, range: 3.2–16.7) (25). Overall, 12 of 22 patients had symptoms associated with tretinoin (Table 2). Three developed the retinoic acid syndrome.

Retinoic acid syndrome

The retinoic acid syndrome is a generalized severe capillary leakage syndrome with leukocyte activation, which results in weight gain, pulmonary infiltrates or pleural effusions with acute respiratory distress, and fever without infection. It occurs in up to 25% of patients. Postmortem reports of patients who have died from this syndrome have shown infiltration of maturing myeloid cells and edema in the lungs (26). The myeloid cells are considered to release various types of cytokines responsible for symptoms such as fever, weight gain, and heart failure. Improvement can be obtained by glucocorticoid treatment, which suppresses the effects of cytokines. Chest CT provides an accurate assessment of the size, number, and distribution of pulmonary opacities associated with the syndrome, as has been demonstrated anecdotally (27).

Of 69 patients with acute promyelocytic leukemia treated with tretinoin for 5 years, 15 developed retinoic acid syndrome (28). The following features were found on chest radiographs: an increased cardiothoracic ratio, an increased pedicle width, pulmonary congestion in 13, pleural effusion in 11, ground-glass opacities, septal lines, and peribronchial cuffing in 9, consolidation and nodules in 7, and an air bronchogram in 5. Three patients had pulmonary hemorrhages and bilateral, diffuse, poorly delineated nodules and ground-glass opacities on radiography. Lung infiltrates cleared completely within 8 days after administration of prednisolone.

- A 69-year-old man developed dyspnea, hypoxia, and heart failure 4 days after starting to take tretinoin 70 mg/day. His highest white blood cell count was $72 \times 10^9/l$. A plain chest X-ray showed two pulmonary opacities, increased attenuation in the left lower lobe, and bilateral pleural effusions, but a chest CT also showed multiple irregular-shaped opacities localized in the centrilobular and subpleural regions. He improved over 10 days with prednisolone (total dose 5750 mg) and daunorubicin (total dose 360 mg).

The retinoic acid syndrome, its incidence and clinical course, has been investigated in 167 patients taking tretinoin as induction and maintenance therapy for acute promyelocytic leukemia (29). The syndrome did not occur during maintenance therapy. During induction it occurred in 44 patients (26%) at a median of 11 (range 2–47) days. The major manifestations included respiratory distress (84%), fever (81%), pulmonary edema (54%), pulmonary infiltrates (52%), pleural or pericardial effusions (36%), hypotension (18%), bone pain (14%), headache (14%), congestive heart failure (11%), and acute renal insufficiency (11%). The median white blood cell count was $1.45 \times 10^9/l$ at diagnosis and $31 \times 10^9/l$ (range $6.8–72 \times 10^9/l$) at the time the syndrome developed. Tretinoin was continued in eight of the 44 patients, with subsequent resolution in 7. It was withdrawn in 36 patients and then reintroduced in 19, after which the syndrome recurred in 3, with one death attributable to reintroduction of the drug. Ten of these 36 patients received chemotherapy without further tretinoin, and 8 achieved complete remission. Of seven patients in whom tretinoin was not reintroduced and who were not given chemotherapy, five achieved complete remission and two died. Two deaths were definitely attributable to the syndrome.

In 63 patients with acute promyelocytic leukemia taking tretinoin (60 mg/day) the rates of leukocytosis, intracranial hypertension, and retinoic acid syndrome were 57%, 9.5%, and 3.2% respectively; the death rate was 11% (30). The authors suggested that progressive leukocytosis during tretinoin therapy should be an indication for chemotherapy (for example, with homoharringtonine); if the white cell count exceeds $10 \times 10^9/l$ before treatment, the patient should be given homoharringtonine only; if it is below $5.0 \times 10^9/l$ homoharringtonine plus tretinoin should be used.

A syndrome similar to that of the retinoic acid syndrome occurred after 10 days of tretinoin therapy in a patient with a relapse of acute myeloblastic leukemia (31).

- A 75-year-old woman whose acute myeloblastic leukemia relapsed was treated with one dose of intravenous idarubicin (10 mg/m²), cytarabine 20 mg subcutaneously for 10 days, and oral tretinoin 45 mg/m²/day.

Ten days later she developed a persistent fever. A chest X-ray and a CT scan showed bilateral pleural effusions and interstitial infiltrates, but no pulmonary embolus. Tretinoin was withdrawn and she was given intravenous dexamethasone 10 mg every 12 hours. Her fever disappeared within 24 hours and her respiratory distress gradually improved during the next 24–48 hours. A chest X-ray 7 days later showed total resolution.

The incidence, clinical features, and outcome of retinoic acid syndrome have been analysed in 413 cases of newly diagnosed acute promyelocytic leukemia (26). Patients under 65 years old with a white blood cell count below $5 \times 10^9/l$ were initially randomized to tretinoin followed by chemotherapy or to tretinoin with chemotherapy started on day 3. In patients with white cell counts over $5 \times 10^9/l$ chemotherapy was rapidly added if the white cell count was greater than 6, 10, and $15 \times 10^9/l$ by days 5, 10, and 15 of tretinoin treatment. The retinoic acid syndrome occurred during induction treatment in 64 of 413 patients (15%). Clinical signs developed after a median of 7 (range 0–35) days. In two cases they were present before the start of treatment; in 11 they occurred on recovery from the phase of aplasia due to the addition of chemotherapy. Respiratory distress (98% of patients), fever (81%), pulmonary infiltrates (81%), weight gain (50%), pleural effusion (47%), renal failure (39%), pericardial effusion (19%), cardiac failure (17%), and hypertension (12%) were the main clinical signs. Mechanical ventilation was required in 13 patients and dialysis in 2. A total of 55 patients (86%) who experienced the retinoic acid syndrome achieved complete remission, compared with 94% of patients who had no retinoic acid syndrome, and nine died of the syndrome. None of the patients with complete remission who received tretinoin for maintenance had recurrence of the syndrome. The syndrome was associated with a lower event-free survival and survival at 2 years.

Retinoic acid syndrome has been reported in a patient who developed diffuse alveolar hemorrhage while being treated with tretinoin for acute promyelocytic leukemia (32).

- An 18-year-old woman developed promyelocytic leukemia and was given tretinoin and dexamethasone. At 15 days she developed significant hemoptysis and respiratory failure, requiring mechanical ventilation. Her temperature was 39.1°C and she had disseminated intravascular coagulation. A lung biopsy showed diffuse interstitial neutrophilic infiltration, interstitial fibrinoid necrosis, and diffuse alveolar hemorrhage; pulmonary capillaritis was diagnosed. She was given intravenous methylprednisolone 1 g/day for 3 days followed by a tapering dose of oral prednisolone. She subsequently completed a full 45-day course of tretinoin.

Organs and Systems

Cardiovascular

An increased risk of thrombotic events, especially coronary thrombosis, has been reported in elderly patients taking retinoids (33). Two patients with acute promyelocytic leukemia developed thrombus in the right ventricle during induction treatment with tretinoin plus idarubicin (34).

- A 51-year-old man with acute promyelocytic leukemia suddenly developed hypoxemia, pulmonary infiltrates, and arterial hypotension, without fever or thoracic pain on day 11 of tretinoin treatment. He was pancytopenic, his coagulation parameters were normal, and cardiological examination was normal. High-dose dexamethasone (10 mg bd) was started, with prompt resolution of the clinical and radiological signs. Eight days later echocardiography showed a 3 cm non-homogeneous mass in the right ventricle. He was given subcutaneous low molecular weight heparin and the thrombus started to get smaller after 17 days. Oral anticoagulant therapy was started, and there was a further reduction of the size of the thrombus over the following year.
- A 32-year-old woman with acute promyelocytic leukemia developed severe retinoic acid syndrome after 3 days, with respiratory failure, fever, and bilateral lung infiltrates. Withdrawal of tretinoin and treatment with dexamethasone and antibiotics rapidly ameliorated the syndrome, and on day 10 tretinoin was restarted. However, routine echocardiography showed a 3 cm pedunculated mass in the right ventricle. There was consistent and stable reduction of the mass after 1 year of oral anticoagulant therapy.

Respiratory

The manufacturers have on record in the USA several pulmonary adverse effects during isotretinoin therapy, including worsening of asthma (SEDA-21, 162), recurrent pneumothorax, pleural effusion, interstitial fibrosis, pulmonary granuloma, and deterioration in lung function tests. Exercise-induced asthma (35) may be caused by a significant reduction in the forced expiratory flow rate (36) and a drying effect of isotretinoin on the mucous membranes of the respiratory tract (37).

Respiratory distress has been attributed to tretinoin.

- A 56-year-old woman with acute promyelocytic leukemia developed a fever of unknown origin, weight gain of 5 kg, and respiratory distress 9 days after the start of treatment with tretinoin 45 mg/m^2 (38). Her white cell count rose to 21×10^9/l despite treatment with cytosine arabinoside and idarubicin. A chest X-ray showed bilateral alveolar opacities. She recovered fully after 5 days of treatment with dexamethasone 10 mg bd.
- A 24-year-old woman with acute promyelocytic leukemia took tretinoin, and 2 days later developed dyspnea and general aching (39). Her total leukocyte count was 5.04×10^9/l, her PaO$_2$ was 42.5 mmHg, and a chest X-ray showed bilateral parenchymal infiltration consistent with respiratory distress syndrome. She recovered within 3 days of treatment with low-dose cytarabine and glucocorticoids, without withdrawal of the retinoic acid.

Although the retinoic acid syndrome involves the lungs, pulmonary hemorrhage has only rarely been reported. Two patients with acute promyelocytic leukemia developed severe lung hemorrhage during the first 3 weeks of treatment with tretinoin, shortly after the administration of chemotherapy (40).

- A 36-year-old man with acute promyelocytic leukemia was given tretinoin 45 mg/m^2/day, daunorubicin, and cytarabine. A week later his platelet count fell to 10×10^9/l, and the next day he developed dyspnea, hemoptysis, and fever. A chest X-ray showed diffuse bilateral patchy pulmonary infiltrates. Tretinoin was withdrawn, but despite high doses of glucocorticoids and blood products, hemoptysis and respiratory failure continued for 6 weeks, when he improved.
- A 59-year-old man with acute promyelocytic leukemia was given tretinoin 45 mg/m^2/day and chemotherapy. On day 6, his fibrinogen concentration fell to 940 mg/l and he developed a fever (39°C), dyspnea, and hypotension. A chest X-ray showed a right pleural effusion. Tretinoin was withdrawn and he was given dexamethasone. However, he deteriorated and developed hemoptysis. Despite glucocorticoids and blood products his pulmonary bleeding continued unabated. On day 29 he developed Gram-negative sepsis and died.

Eosinophilic pleural effusion has been attributed to isotretinoin (3).

Pneumonia has also been reported as a possible adverse effect (SEDA-20, 155) (36).

Nervous system

Nervous system disturbances include fatigue, lassitude, vertigo, sweating, hypesthesia, paresthesia, dizziness, fever, amnesia, delirium, flu-like symptoms, somnolence, pseudotumor cerebri, hyperirritability, sleep disturbance, lethargy, depression (41), and psychological changes. There was a direct correlation between intracranial hypertension and the use of isotretinoin in a retrospective study of spontaneous reports (42).

- An 8-year-old girl with acute promyelocytic leukemia was given cytarabine, etoposide, idarubicin, and tretinoin 25 mg/m^2/day (43). Five days later she developed fever, pleural effusions, and ascites, but the symptoms resolved spontaneously. On day 65 (cumulative dose of tretinoin 1.6 g/m^2) she had nausea and vomiting, severe headache, and diplopia. There was paralysis of the left trochlear nerve bilateral papilledema. A cranial MRI scan was normal. The intracranial pressure was not measured. Tretinoin was withdrawn and she was given glucocorticoids, mannitol, acetazolamide, and pethidine. Her symptoms resolved within 2 days.

A case of multiple mononeuropathies has been attributed to tretinoin (44). The neurological symptoms resembled atypical pseudotumor cerebri with focal neurological signs.

- A 23-year-old woman with acute promyelocytic leukemia was given tretinoin (45 mg/m^2/day) together with daunorubicin and cytarabine. She had a slight headache after the administration of tretinoin. On the 17th day an acute subdural hematoma required operation. Her headache persisted and she complained of diplopia, and burning pain and contact dysesthesia of the back of the left hand and the right foot, with accompanying weakness on day 21. Electrophysiology showed reduced conduction velocity and amplitude in the right peroneal nerve. She also had a right abducens nerve palsy and visual disturbance. There was no papilledema. MRI scan of the brain was normal. On day 51 tretinoin was discontinued. Her symptoms of peripheral neuropathy and the electrophysiological findings gradually improved as did her headache and dry skin, despite continued chemotherapy. The right abducens nerve palsy partly resolved.

The relation between isotretinoin and seizures is still unclear (SEDA-18, 169).

The possible negative effects of short-term oral acitretin 1 mg/kg/day on peripheral nerve function have been assessed in a small prospective study in 13 patients (45). Patients with conditions related to peripheral neuropathy were excluded. There was a fall in the mean amplitude of the sensory action potential of the superficial peroneal nerve after 1 and 3 months of therapy. There was a significant change in one or more neurophysiological parameters in three of 13 patients after 1 month and in nine of 13 patients after 3 months. None of the patients had detectable neurological abnormalities at any time during therapy. Acitretin was withdrawn, and after 6 months three patients gradually improved. Further studies are needed to determine whether neurophysiological evaluation should be routine during treatment with oral retinoids. Peripheral neuropathy has rarely been observed (SEDA-17, 183).

Sensory systems

Eyes

Ocular findings are among the more frequent adverse effects in patients taking isotretinoin (46,47), the most common being blepharoconjunctivitis, which also occurs in those who use tretinoin ophthalmic ointment (1).

Ocular adverse effects secondary to isotretinoin are generally benign in nature and reversible on reduction or withdrawal of therapy. However, papilledema necessitates withdrawal. Corneal opacities should be monitored closely. Although they do not usually interfere with vision, prudence dictates withdrawal of isotretinoin or reduction of the dosage when corneal opacities develop (48). Several cases of cataract have been (unconvincingly) ascribed to isotretinoin (SEDA-19, 157). Etretinate and isotretinoin have caused photophobia and reduced night vision (SEDA-17, 183), and possibly ectropion (SEDA-16, 152).

Corneal opacities after treatment with oral isotretinoin generally disappear after withdrawal. However, in one case they were persistent (49).

- A 39-year-old woman developed corneal opacities while taking oral isotretinoin 1 mg/kg for 6 months. The opacities persisted for at least 6 years after discontinuation of the drug. She had worn soft hydrophilic contact lenses for 10 years before, but without signs of corneal opacity 1 month before treatment was started.

Xerophthalmia, carrying a high risk of blindness, requires the immediate administration of massive doses of vitamin A. An infant who received intramuscular vitamin A for xerophthalmia secondary to cystic fibrosis developed an acute sixth nerve palsy (50).

- A 5-month-old boy with cystic fibrosis and xerophthalmia was given intramuscular vitamin A 50 000 IU (water-miscible retinyl palmitate). After the first dose prominent bulging of the fontanelle developed, but the infant remained alert and was feeding well. Two days later another dose of 50 000 IU was given in two divided doses over 2 days. These doses were well tolerated, with gradual improvement of the bulging fontanelle over 1 week. Five days later, a complete abduction deficit of the left eye developed, in keeping with an acute sixth nerve palsy. There were no other signs of raised intracranial pressure. The sixth nerve palsy resolved fully over the next 2 months. There were no other neurological sequelae. After discharge the infant continued to take oral vitamin A supplements.

In one study, 236 cases of adverse ocular reactions possibly associated with isotretinoin were evaluated (Table 3) (48).

Ears

Unilateral earache has been reported in two patients (SEDA-9, 134). Excessive cerumen production and otitis externa have also been reported.

Taste and smell

Taste and smell can be altered by isotretinoin (SEDA-16, 153) and loss of taste has been attributed to it (SEDA-21, 163).

Table 3 Adverse ocular effects associated with isotretinoin exposure in 236 patients (51)

Adverse effects	No. of patients
Eyelids	
Blepharoconjunctivitis or meibomianitis (52)	88
Photodermatitis	6
Cornea	
Corneal opacities	12
Dry eyes	47
Contact lens intolerance	19
Optic nerve	
Papilledema or pseudotumor cerebri	18
Optic neuritis	3
Congenital abnormalities	
Microphthalmos	5
Orbital hypertelorism	2
Optic nerve hypoplasia	4
Cortical blindness	1
Others	
Blurred vision	39
Myopia	5
Impaired night vision and dark adaptation (SEDA-10, 25)	3
Ocular inflammation (uveitis, scleritis, retinitis, ophthalmitis, iritis)	7

Psychological, psychiatric

In 1998 depression, psychosis, and suicidal ideation, suicide attempts, and suicide were added to the product label of isotretinoin. Since then the FDA has received increasing number of reports of these problems (53). From the time that isotretinoin was marketed in 1982 up to May 2000 the FDA received 37 reports of patients taking isotretinoin who committed suicide, 110 reports of patients who were hospitalized for depression, suicidal ideation, or suicide attempts, and 284 reports of patients with depression who did not need hospitalization (54). In 62% of the suicide cases a psychiatric history or possible contributing factors were identified, and 69% of patients hospitalized for depression had either a previous psychiatric history of possible contributing factors. Drug withdrawal led to improvement in about one-third of the patients, while in 29% depression persisted after withdrawal. In 24 cases dechallenge and rechallenge were positive. However, since this was a series of spontaneous reports, and since there are no good data on the incidence of depression and suicide among adolescents with acne, a causal relation cannot be concluded.

A change in dreaming pattern has been reported in two patients, occurring within 2–3 weeks after the start of treatment with isotretinoin 40 mg/day for cystic acne (55). One patient also reported increased irritability and bouts of depression. In both patients all the symptoms abated after 4–5 weeks without a change in isotretinoin dosage.

Endocrine

Small reductions in indices of thyroid function have been observed in patients taking etretinate (56). Thyrotoxicosis may have been triggered by isotretinoin in one patient (SEDA-12, 136).

Metabolism

Alterations in lipid metabolism are common and include increases in serum triglyceride and cholesterol concentrations, sometimes persisting after withdrawal of the therapy, and reductions in high-density lipoprotein cholesterol. The incidence of raised serum lipids during therapy with oral isotretinoin 1 mg/kg/day for acne has been reviewed retrospectively in 876 patients, of whom 54 had raised serum cholesterol concentrations (over 5.2 mmol/l) and 45 had triglyceride concentrations above 2.26 mmol/l (57).

Symptoms of hyperlipidemia and the metabolic syndrome have been investigated in a cross-sectional study in young adults who had used isotretinoin for acne for at least 4 weeks (mean dosage 0.56 mg/kg). Those in whom triglyceride concentrations increased by at least 1.0 mmol/l during therapy were termed hyper-responders ($n = 102$), and those in whom triglyceride concentrations changed by 0.1 mmol/l or less were termed non-responders ($n = 100$) (58). Despite similar pretreatment body weights and plasma lipid concentrations, 4 years after completion of isotretinoin therapy the hyper-responders were more likely to have hypertriglyceridemia (OR = 4.8; 95% CI = 1.6, 14), hypercholesterolemia (OR = 9.1; CI = 1.9, 43), truncal obesity (OR = 11.0; CI = 2.0, 59), and hyperinsulinemia (OR = 3.0,

CI = 1.6, 5.7) than non-responders. In addition, more hyper-responders had at least one parent with hypertriglyceridemia. Genotypes containing apoE ε2 and apoE ε4 alleles were over-represented among hyper-responders. Although a comparison of hyper-responders with non-responders may lead to overestimation of the risk, these data suggest that those who develop hyperlipidemia while taking isotretinoin are those who are already at risk of hyperlipidemia and the metabolic syndrome.

The consequences of hypertriglyceridemia are not well understood, but there may be an increased risk of cardiovascular disease and pancreatitis (SEDA-13, 123). Patients with an increased tendency to develop hypertriglyceridemia include those with diabetes mellitus, obesity, increased alcohol intake, and a positive family history. With a short course (16 weeks) of isotretinoin it is sufficient to ensure there is no hyperlipidemia before the start of therapy, and to determine the triglyceride response to therapy on one occasion after 4 weeks (59).

Mineral balance

Hypercalcemia has been reported as an adverse effect of systemic retinoid therapy (60).

- A 12-year-old girl with neuroblastoma and normal renal function developed severe hypercalcemia while receiving isotretinoin 160 mg/m²/day (61). Her hypercalcemia resolved with hydration, diuretic therapy, and temporary withdrawal of isotretinoin. Despite a dosage reduction to 80 mg/m²/day, severe hypercalcemia recurred during the next treatment cycle. Further treatment with isotretinoin was made tolerable by shortening the duration of the remaining cycles.
- An 11-year-old boy with acute promyelocytic leukemia was given *all-trans*-retinoic acid 47 mg/m²/day (62). On day 10 he developed headache and nausea. The dose was reduced to 39 mg/m²/day and he was given glycerol, but his symptoms of pseudotumor cerebri continued. Cranial CT showed neither space-occupying lesions nor brain edema. On day 25, hypercalcemia (3.2 mmol/l) was observed. In spite of conventional therapy the serum calcium concentration continued to rise to 4.0 mmol/l. Tretinoin was withdrawn on day 33. Within 1 week his symptoms resolved. On the second day of a second phase of *all-trans*-retinoic acid therapy, he again developed nausea and headache and the serum calcium concentration gradually increased to 3.3 mmol/l by day 7. Raised concentrations of type 1 cross-linked *N*-telopeptide and deoxypyridinoline suggested increased bone resorption. A bisphosphonate (pamidronate 30 mg) was administered intravenously; the calcium normalized within 2 days and the nausea and headache resolved.

Fluid balance

Generalized edema has been attributed to etretinate (63).

Hematologic

Altered blood clotting due to hypoprothrombinemia, raised erythrocyte sedimentation rate (64), altered red cell count (64), reduced white cell count (64), thrombocytopenia (SEDA-12, 136), and eosinophilia (SEDA-13, 122) have all been observed incidentally (SEDA-17, 184).

Of 31 patients with acute promyelocytic leukemia (15 men and 16 women, median age 43 years) 4 received tretinoin 45 mg/m^2/day and intravenous tranexamic acid 1–2 g for 6 days, 9 received tretinoin, daunorubicin, and cytarabine followed by thioguanine, 15 received chemotherapy, tretinoin, and tranexamic acid, 2 received chemotherapy and trancxamic acid, and 1 received chemotherapy only (65). Three of the four patients who received tretinoin plus tranexamic acid had sudden and rapid deterioration in their condition, leading to early death. At postmortem there were widespread microvascular thromboses in unusual sites (for example the brain and kidneys). The rapid progression to multiorgan failure and the widespread nature of the microthrombi suggests the need for caution in the simultaneous use of tretinoin and tranexamic acid.

Thrombosis during induction treatment with tretinoin, aprotinin, and chemotherapy has been described (66).

Transient polycythemia has been reported during treatment with isotretinoin for severe nodular acne (67).

- A 53-year-old man's hematocrit increased from 0.46 to 0.51 after he had taken isotretinoin for 11 months (180 mg/day for 3 months, 80 mg/day for 6 months, then 20 mg/day). No secondary causes of polycythemia were found and the hematocrit fell to 0.48 3 months after withdrawal of isotretinoin.

The reference range for hematocrit in men is 0.41–0.49, and so the clinical relevance of this observation is unclear.

Attacks of paroxysmal nocturnal hemoglobinuria may possibly be provoked by isotretinoin (SEDA-19, 156).

Extramedullary relapse of acute promyelocytic leukemia, which is rare after chemotherapy alone, was more common after tretinoin, but it is not clear whether it truly increases the risk of extramedullary recurrence and what the risk factors are. In a retrospective analysis of the incidence of extramedullary relapse in patients after prior treatment with tretinoin and in patients previously treated with chemotherapy alone (68) three of the 13 patients who received tretinoin had extramedullary involvement compared with none of the 11 patients previously treated with chemotherapy alone (RR = 2.1; CI = 1.34, 3.29). The retinoic acid syndrome during prior induction treatment was significantly associated with extramedullary relapse (three of five patients with the retinoic acid syndrome versus none of eight without the syndrome (RR = 5.0; CI = 1.4, 17)). Thus, tretinoin may predispose patients with acute promyelocytic leukemia to extramedullary involvement at relapse and the retinoic acid syndrome is a risk factor.

Gastrointestinal

The gastrointestinal adverse effects of retinoids include anorexia, nausea, vomiting, weight loss, stomach pain, thirst, splenomegaly, and acute esophagitis (SEDA-21, 162). Proctosigmoiditis has been reported (SEDA-13, 123).

- Ulcerative colitis occurred in a 17-year-old boy shortly after he had completed a 5-month course of isotretinoin

(dose not stated) for acne (69). There was no family history of inflammatory bowel disease.

Although three other cases of inflammatory bowel disease during isotretinoin therapy have been reported (70–72), there have also been reports of the safe use of isotretinoin in patents with a history of inflammatory bowel disease (that is without exacerbation of the inflammatory bowel disease) (70,73,74). Since retinoids are being increasingly used to treat moderately severe acne, larger studies are needed to elucidate the relation between retinoid use and inflammatory bowel disease.

Vasculitis and necrosis of the ileum developed in a patient with acute promyelocytic leukemia treated with *all-trans*-retinoic acid (75).

- A 29-year-old woman with acute promyelocytic leukemia was given tretinoin 45 mg/m^2. On day 20 she developed pain in both hands, wrists, feet, and ankles, with erythema and edema. On day 24 her fever increased to over 38°C and the white blood cell count was 10.9 × 10^9/l. She was given dexamethasone (8 mg intravenously on three consecutive days) and all her symptoms quickly resolved, but on day 37 she developed a low-grade fever and polyarthralgia, which persisted. On day 42 she had a profuse bloody stool and her abdominal pain worsened and spread all over the abdomen. At emergency operation there was segmental necrosis in several parts of the ileum, with inflammation invading the serosa. Histology of the ileum showed a leukocytoclastic vasculitis. After operation tretinoin was withdrawn and she had no fever, edema, arthralgia, or abdominal pain thereafter.

Liver

Hepatomegaly is an adverse effect of retinol and tretinoin. Transient slight rises in liver enzymes, notably aspartate transaminase, alanine transaminase, and alkaline phosphatase, are common, but some cases of hepatotoxicity due to etretinate and acitretin (SEDA-20, 154) have also been reported (76), as has cholestatic jaundice due to etretinate (77). Etretinate may have played a role in a case of liver failure leading to death (76).

The incidence of raised liver enzymes during therapy with oral isotretinoin 1 mg/kg/day for acne has been retrospectively reviewed in 876 patients (57). Liver enzymes (aspartate transaminase, alanine transaminase, and γ-glutamyl transferase) were transiently raised in a minority of patients (number not stated).

Acute liver damage has been attributed to tretinoin (78).

- A 40-year-old man with acute promyelocytic leukemia was given tretinoin 45 mg/m^2/day and intravenous daunorubicin. After 3 weeks his alkaline phosphatase rose to 370 (reference range 82–198) U/l, the gamma-glutamyltranspeptidase to 198 (reference range 7–43) U/l, and the direct bilirubin to 39 (reference range below 10) μmol/l. He had painful hepatomegaly without splenomegaly. Abdominal Doppler ultrasound ruled out biliary tract injury. Percutaneous liver biopsy showed intracellular cholestasis with preservation of hepatic architecture. He was given dexamethasone and tretinoin was withdrawn. After 3 days the symptoms and hepatomegaly abated.

Pancreas

Acute pancreatitis is a rare but serious adverse effect of tretinoin. Three cases associated with isotretinoin-induced hyperglyceridemia have previously been described and two cases associated with tretinoin (79,80).

- A 48-year-old man received tretinoin (45 mg/m^2/day) followed 9 days later by combination chemotherapy for 5 days (81). On day 15 he developed acute epigastric and upper left quadrant pain. He had raised serum lipase (1312 IU/l; reference range 27–208), amylase (509 IU/l; 30–110), and triglycerides (7.77 mmol/l; 0.45–1.82). Abdominal CT showed mild trabeculation of the peripancreatic adipose tissue, but no lithiasis or dilatation of the biliary ducts. Acute pancreatitis caused by hypertriglyceridemia was diagnosed and he was given supportive treatment plus fenofibrate (200 mg/day), without withdrawal of tretinoin. His lipase, amylase, and triglycerides normalized over 10 days.

Urinary tract

Impaired renal function has rarely been caused by isotretinoin (82) and etretinate (83). Abnormalities in urinary proteins, inflammation of the urethral meatus, and nephrolithiasis have rarely occurred. Urethritis may occur more often than has been realized (SEDA-21, 162) (84).

Nephrotic syndrome developed after 4 months treatment with isotretinoin 40 mg/day (85). No other causes were found and the symptoms disappeared within some months with appropriate treatment.

During tretinoin therapy, some patients with retinoic acid syndrome or with a hypercoagulable state develop acute renal insufficiency, usually accompanied by dysfunction of other organs. A patient with acute promyelocytic leukemia developed renal insufficiency alone during tretinoin treatment (86).

- A 72-year-old Japanese man with acute promyelocytic leukemia was given tretinoin 48 mg/m^2 plus idarubicin. On day 17 oliguria occurred and tretinoin was withdrawn on day 20 when the serum creatinine concentration rose to 619 µmol/l (7.0 mg/dl). There were no signs or symptoms of retinoic acid syndrome. A needle biopsy of the left kidney on day 38, when the serum creatinine concentration was 212 µmol/l (2.4 mg/dl), showed granulomatous tubulointerstitial nephritis. The glomeruli were mostly intact and there were no fibrin thrombi or leukemic cell infiltration. After one course of consolidation therapy he was discharged with a normal serum creatinine concentration.

Two cases of bone-marrow transplant nephropathy that developed coincident with retinoid therapy have been reported (87).

- A 3-year-old boy with a neuroblastoma was given cisplatin, adriamycin, and cyclophosphamide for five induction cycles and radiation to sites of residual bony metastases 1 month before autologous bone-marrow transplant, which resulted in an absolute neutrophil count of 500 $\times$ 10^6/l on day 9 and a self-sustaining platelet count over 50 $\times$ 10^{12}/l on day 72. He was randomized to receive retinoids 80 mg/m^2 bd by mouth, beginning on day 100 after bone-marrow transplant. Before beginning *cis*-retinoic acid, his highest serum creatinine concentration was 44 µmol/l on day 8. When *cis*-retinoic acid was begun, his hemoglobin was 9.8 g/dl and his platelet count 97 $\times$ 10^{12}/l. At the end of the second 2-week cycle of retinoic acid he developed a severe headache and diastolic hypertension (BP 120/108 mmHg), a blood urea nitrogen concentration of 4 mmol/l, serum creatinine of 133 µmol/l, hemoglobin of 5.8 g/dl, and platelet count of 57 $\times$ 10^{12}/l. Urinalysis showed erythrocytes and protein. Renal biopsy showed mesangiolysis, wide capillary loops, focal intimal thickening, and vacuolization of glomerular and tubular cells. His hematuria and proteinuria persisted for 4 weeks, and his blood urea nitrogen and serum creatinine gradually improved, as did the hypertension.

- A 5-year-old boy with a neuroblastoma was treated in the same way. On day 105 after bone-marrow transplantation he developed hypertension (BP 140/92 mmHg), hematuria, proteinuria, and a raised serum creatinine. His hemoglobin and platelet count fell. His urine contained protein 800 mg/l, a few hyaline casts, and 25–30 erythrocytes per high-power field. When nephritis developed, *cis*-retinoid acid was withdrawn. He gradually improved, and his urine cleared of casts, erythrocytes, and protein within 4 weeks.

Skin

Adverse effects of oral retinoids on the skin are common (up to 70%). The symptoms and signs are listed in Table 4. Three cases of scrotal ulceration during *all-trans*-retinoic acid therapy for a microgranular variant of acute promyelocytic leukemia (88,89), together with eight other reported cases (90–92), suggest that this adverse effect is specific for tretinoin. The incidence has been estimated at 12% (88). The pathogenesis is unknown, but it has been suggested to be a manifestation of the retinoic acid syndrome (88). Improvement after the withdrawal of tretinoin and the administration of glucocorticoids supports this assumption. However, activation of neutrophils by superoxide production may also be involved.

Acute febrile neutrophilic dermatosis (Sweet's syndrome) can occur in patients with acute promyelocytic leukemia given a retinoid. Sweet's syndrome is characterized by five cardinal features: fever, neutrophilia, multiple raised painful asymmetric erythematous cutaneous plaques, dermal infiltrates consisting of mature neutrophils, and a rapid response to glucocorticoid therapy. In up to 10–20% of cases it precedes or coincides with a diagnosis of malignancy, most commonly acute myelogenous leukemia. In cases associated with tretinoin the symptoms come on at 7–34 days and the skin lesions are seen on the face, limbs, and back.

- A 58-year-old woman was given tretinoin 45 mg/m^2/day for acute promyelocytic leukemia and after 9 days she developed symptoms of upper respiratory tract infection and fever (38.2°C) (96). The next day

Table 4 The adverse effects of oral retinoids on the skin and hair

Acne fulminans (SEDA-11, 137)
Angular stomatitis
Balanitis (rare)
Blepharoconjunctivitis
Bullous pemphigoid (SEDA-17, 184)
Cheilitis
Cystic and comedonal acne (SEDA-15, 142)
Dissemination of *Herpes simplex*
Dry mucous membranes
Epistaxis
Eruptive xanthomas (one report)
Erythema multiforme (SEDA-14, 124)
Erythema nodosum (SEDA-21, 163)
Erythroderma
Excess granulation tissue (SEDA-9, 134)
Facial cellulitis (*Staphylococcus aureus*)
Facial dermatitis
Facial erythema
Follicular eczema
Generalized edema
Gingivitis, bleeding gums
Glossitis
Hair curly, possibly due to the combination of isotretinoin +
    azathioprine (SEDA-21, 163)
Hair discoloration (SEDA-19, 157)
Hair growth disturbed
Hair loss
Hair thinning
Hair "unruly" (SEDA-11, 136)
Hirsutism
Hyperhidrosis
Hyperpigmentation
Hypopigmentation
Irritant dermatitis
Melasma (SEDA-21, 163)
Mucosal erosions
Mycosis fungoides-like dermatitis (SEDA-10, 125)
Nail deformities (softening, fragility, Beau's lines, onycholysis,
    onychomadesis, onchoschizia, paronychia, curly
    fingernails) (37)
Nail growth reduced
Nasal carriage of *Staphylococcus aureus* (SEDA-12, 131)
Nummular eczema (SEDA-12, 136)
Osteoma cutis exacerbation
Papulopustular palmoplantar eruptions
Pemphigus vulgaris (SEDA-20, 155)
Petechiae
Photoallergy (SEDA-17, 184)
Phototoxicity (SEDA-17, 184)
Pityriasis rosea-like dermatitis
Polyarteritis nodosa (93)
Porokeratosis exacerbation (SEDA-16, 152)
Prurigo nodularis (SEDA-12, 131)
Pruritus
Pseudoporphyria (SEDA-17, 184)
Psoriasis as a Koebner phenomenon (SEDA-13, 123)
Pyogenic granuloma
Rosacea-like eruption
Ruptured striae atrophicae
Sarcoid-like granulomas (SEDA-19, 157)
Scaling of the skin
Scalp folliculitis
Skin fragility and erosions (SEDA-22, 168)

Skin odor abnormal
Skin sticky
Thyroglossal cyst (SEDA-20, 155)
Toxic epidermal necrolysis
Vasculitis (94,95)
Vulvitis
Wound healing delayed
Xeroderma

multiple erythematous and painful cutaneous plaques appeared on her limbs. Her white cell count was 5.71×10^9/l. A skin biopsy showed a normal epidermis with subepidermal edema and dense diffuse perivascular aggregates composed of granulocytes and scattered eosinophils, compatible with Sweet's syndrome. Prednisolone 20 mg/day had no effect, but after 2 days treatment with cytarabine and daunorubicin the rash started to fade and gradually disappeared. Remission was achieved after one course and *all-trans*-retinoic acid was subsequently renewed without complications.

- A 39-year-old man with acute promyelocytic leukemia was given tretinoin 45 mg/m² (97). His leukocyte count rose to 34.3×10^9/l on day 11. On day 18 he developed rigors, mild dyspnea, and a fever (39°C). He had exquisite pain in the right posterior tibial muscle and had several 2-mm erythematous papular and pustular lesions on his limbs and trunk. He was given a cephalosporin and developed painful bilateral nodules in the quadriceps, posterior tibial, and right biceps muscles. An MRI scan showed focal areas of increased T2 signals in the quadriceps muscles bilaterally, in most of the left sartorius and soleus muscles, and in all the compartments of the right leg. There was thickening of the adjacent fascia with subcutaneous edema. Tretinoin was withdrawn and he was given dexamethasone 16 mg/day. The cutaneous lesions improved dramatically and tretinoin 45 mg/m² was restarted. The symptoms did not recur.

- A 35-year-old woman with acute promyelocytic leukemia was given tretinoin 45 mg/m²/day. On day 9 she became febrile (39.5°C) and had a sore throat with pharyngeal erythema and tender lymphadenopathy. The fever persisted despite cephalosporins, vancomycin, and antibiotics for anaerobic cover. On day 20 she developed severe bilateral anterior leg pain and both anterior tibial muscles were tender. Creatine kinase activity was 348 (reference range 38–176) U/l. Tretinoin was withdrawn and she was given intravenous dexamethasone 10 mg/day. Her fever resolved, her pain abated, and her leg muscles felt softer and less tender. Tretinoin was reintroduced and her symptoms returned.

- A 46-year-old man with promyelocytic leukemia was given tretinoin 45 mg/m² plus daunorubicin 60 mg/m²/day for 3 days and cytarabine 200 mg/m²/day by continuous infusion for 7 days (98). He became febrile on day 3 and was given cefotaxime and vancomycin. On day 6 he developed non-pruritic, erythematous, violaceous vesicles on the limbs and upper trunk. His temperature rose to 40°C and he gained 4.5 kg, which was attributed to a mild retinoic acid syndrome. Skin biopsy showed infiltration by neutrophilic granulocytes and marked edema in the dermis, without vasculitis or evidence of leukemic cells, fungi, or herpesvirus. Hepatic enzymes were moderately increased. The clinical presentation and histopathological findings were consistent with Sweet's syndrome. Tretinoin was withdrawn and he was given dexamethasone 40 mg/day for 10 days and then tapering doses of prednisone. He improved, and tretinoin was reintroduced without recurrence.

With topical application of tretinoin, special care should be taken when other drugs are given simultaneously. Dramatic photosensitivity has been associated with the combination of fluorouracil, prochlorperazine, and topical tretinoin (99).

- A 52-year-old woman with a colonic cancer was treated with chemotherapy after surgical resection. She had been applying topical tretinoin (Renova; Ortho Pharmac, Raritan N) cream 0.05% nightly to her face for about 5 years. During that time she had applied a sunscreen while outdoors and had tolerated tretinoin without incident. Her daily oral multivitamin supplement contained 5000 IU of retinol equivalents. About 3 days after her last dose of chemotherapy (leucovorin, fluorouracil, prochlorperazine) she exposed her face to the sun for about 1 hour after applying her usual sunscreen. Shortly afterwards the skin on her face became erythematous and worsened over several days. Her eyes became edematous, itchy, and painful. Within a week the skin on her face had completely desquamated. She stopped using tretinoin. The reaction began to improve and she was pain-free within 1 week. Her appearance returned to normal after about 10 days. During a second cycle of chemotherapy she received the same drugs as during the first, except tretinoin, and reported no significant change in sun exposure or sunscreen application. She tolerated subsequent cycles without adverse skin effects. After completing her monthly chemotherapy cycles, she resumed topical tretinoin without adverse effects.

Leukemia cutis is very rare in acute myelocytic leukemia. Cutaneous relapse in acute promyelocytic leukemia has been reported during a period of complete hematological remission after treatment with tretinoin (100).

- A 51-year-old man with acute promyelocytic leukemia was given induction chemotherapy and tretinoin 45 mg/m^2. After 1 month he developed discrete erythematous papules, although marrow biopsy suggested hematological remission. The papules were disseminated on all his limbs, trunk, and scalp, and were scattered, discrete, and 2–3 mm in diameter. Biopsy showed a moderate perivascular infiltration of medium to large atypical cells, mainly in the upper dermis, suggesting infiltrating promyelocytes. The clinical, histological, and histochemical findings were compatible with leukemia cutis. One week later, a bone-marrow biopsy still showed hematological remission.

Musculoskeletal

Musculoskeletal symptoms occur in 15% of patients who take isotretinoin. These are usually mild and consist of

pain, tenderness, and muscle stiffness. Creatine kinase activity can rise, especially in individuals engaging in strenuous physical activity (SEDA-10, 124). Clinical and subclinical muscle damage has been reported from etretinate, acitretin, and isotretinoin (SEDA-21, 162, 163).

Skeletal abnormalities associated with retinoid therapy include Achilles tendonitis (SEDA-17, 185), acute arthritis (SEDA-18, 168) (101), bridging of vertebral bodies, diffuse idiopathic skeletal hyperostosis (DISH), disc narrowing, nasal bone osteophytosis, osteoma cutis, hyperostosis, extraspinal calcifications, costochondritis, enthesiopathy, ossification of tendons and ligamentous insertions, ossification of the posterior longitudinal ligament, periosteal thickening, premature epiphyseal closure, reduced bone density/osteoporosis (102), skeletal aches and pains, slender long bones, and Tietze's syndrome.

Stiff man syndrome has been described 10 days after the start of oral isotretinoin treatment (1 mg/kg/day) and resolved completely within 2 weeks of withdrawal (103). There were no motor or sensory nerve conduction abnormalities. There were no conditions known to be associated with stiff man syndrome, either at the time or during 5 years of follow up.

Adult onset Still's disease occurred after 3 months of oral isotretinoin (104). No other causes were found and the symptoms disappeared with appropriate treatment within some months.

Reproductive system

Breast discharge has been reported (105). Menstrual disturbances occur, and may be under-reported (SEDA-13, 121, 123). Vaginal bleeding in a 64-year-old woman was convincingly ascribed to the daily use of tretinoin cream 0.05% to her face, suggesting a systemic effect (SEDA-16, 159).

Adverse effects of isotretinoin affecting the male reproductive system reported to the manufacturer include gynecomastia, local inflammation/discomfort, potency disorders, reduced fertility, and ejaculatory failure (SEDA-18, 168) (106).

Immunologic

Hypersensitivity reactions to retinoids are rare and consist of occasional drug rashes.

- Immunomodulatory effects of isotretinoin in the treatment of facial acne (40 mg/day for 4 weeks) were blamed for a recurrence of pulmonary alveolar proteinosis in a 16-year-old girl, in whom it had been in spontaneous remission for 2 years (107).

Although the time-course of this effect was suggestive, it should be borne in mind that about 25% of patients with this disease have exacerbations without a clear cause.

Body temperature

An increase in the frequency of attacks of familial Mediterranean fever has been reported after the start of systemic therapy with isotretinoin for nodulocystic acne (108).

- A 32-year-old man with familial Mediterranean fever had one or two attacks per year while taking colchicine twice daily for 10 years. During the first month after starting to take isotretinoin 50 mg/day he had three typical attacks, increasing to one attack a week after dosage increments to 60 mg/day and later 80 mg/day. Isotretinoin was withdrawn and he had no further attacks of familial Mediterranean fever during the following 10 months. Rechallenge was not performed.

Long-Term Effects

Mutagenicity

The reported occurrence of sarcomas in some patients treated with isotretinoin may be a chance finding (SEDA-21, 164); retinoids may prevent or even cure certain malignancies (20).

Second-Generation Effects

Teratogenicity

Retinoids are strongly teratogenic (21). Pregnancy should be ruled out and an effective form of contraception must be used for at least 1 month before starting therapy, during therapy, and for at least 1 month (isotretinoin) or 2 years (acitretin) after therapy is stopped. Retinoid-induced teratogenicity has been reviewed (22,23).

There are few data about the safety of topical retinoids during pregnancy. The risk of teratogenicity of topical tretinoin, if any, appears to be minimal (SEDA-18, 164) (109). However, there is a case report (110).

- A baby was born missing its right ear and external auditory canal. At 20 months an MRI scan of the brain showed focal atrophy and encephalomalacia of the right parieto-occipital lobe. His mother had used topical tretinoin (Retin A 0.025%) on her face and a large surface of the back before conception and during the first 2–3 months of pregnancy. His father had used oral isotretinoin before conception.

This type of ear abnormality is a typical feature of retinoic acid embryopathy. Given the pattern of malformations in this child, the authors thought that maternal use of topical tretinoin had been responsible. Three other cases of fetal malformations after topical tretinoin use have been reported (111–113).

Multiple congenital anomalies occurred after exposure to isotretinoin in the first trimester (114).

- A neonate whose mother had taken isotretinoin 40 mg/day during the first 2 months of pregnancy had absent auricles, tachypnea, and feeding difficulties. There were signs of heart failure, and echocardiography showed a large subpulmonary ventricular septal defect (Taussig–Bing malformation) and a secundum atrial septal defect. Both great arteries originated from the anterior right ventricle, and there was tricuspid insufficiency. A cranial CT scan showed atresia of the external ear canal, tympanic membrane, middle ear, and antrum. Other ear structures were normal. The child died at home.

Previously published information on outcomes after maternal exposure to topical tretinoin has been limited to three case reports (111–113). A fourth case has been reported (110).

- A boy, born at 41 weeks weighing 4090 g, had no right auricle or external auditory canal. Before conception and during the first months of pregnancy his mother had used topical tretinoin (Retin A 0.025%) on her face and a large area of her back. She had also used vitamins during pregnancy. His father had used oral isotretinoin before conception. At 16 months the baby was babbling. Optokinetic response was diminished and there was no oculovestibular response. At 20 months he was non-verbal and had poor receptive language, compatible with cognitive impairment. A cranial CT scan showed calcification of the right posterior hemisphere and MRI showed reduction in the volume of the right cerebral hemisphere, an infarct in the deep basal ganglia, focal atrophy, and encephalomalacia of the right parieto-occipital lobe. MRA showed marked attenuation of the posterior cerebral artery with poor declination of the more distal cortical, temporal, and occipital branches. A PET scan showed severe hypometabolism of the right posterior parietal, occipital, and temporal lobes, right basal ganglia, and thalamus, and mild hypometabolism of the left cerebellum.

Susceptibility Factors

Renal disease

The concentration of vitamin A is raised in chronic renal insufficiency, because reduced filtration of low molecular proteins results in increased concentrations of retinol binding protein. A retrospective evaluation of 18 liver biopsies in 71 patients on hemodialysis taking therapeutic doses of vitamin A showed hyperplasia of stellate cells in 7, but no evidence of fibrosis (115).

In a patient with renal insufficiency, stellate cell hyperplasia was accompanied by fibrosis (116).

- A 51-year-old man, with a 9-year history of renal insufficiency and an alcohol intake of 4 U/week, underwent transplant nephrectomy. At surgery, ascites and liver cirrhosis were noted. A needle biopsy of the liver 1 month later showed nodular regenerative hyperplasia but no cirrhosis. There were subendothelial vacuolated cells, suggestive of modified stellate cells, and there was adjacent focal perisinusoidal fibrosis. His medications included one multivitamin/mineral supplement per day containing vitamin A 4000 IU. His vitamin A concentration was 1045 (reference range 490–720) ng/ml. Viral and antibody studies were negative.

Drug Administration

Drug formulations

A novel intravenous liposomal formulation of tretinoin (Atragen®, Aronex Pharmaceuticals Inc, The Woodlands, TX), which provides a reliable dose for patients who are unable to swallow or absorb medications, has been evaluated in 69 patients with acute promyelocytic leukemia (117). Liposomal tretinoin (90 mg/m^2) was given every other day until complete remission or a maximum of 56 days. Treatment after complete remission was liposomal tretinoin with or without chemotherapy. Adverse effects (grade 1–2 according to the NCI common toxicity criteria) were the retinoic acid syndrome in 18 patients (grade 3/4 in 10), leukocytosis ($n = 36$), headache ($n = 46$), dry skin ($n = 23$), hypertriglyceridemia ($n = 23$), fever ($n = 18$), nausea ($n = 13$), stomatitis ($n = 11$), vomiting ($n = 10$), cheilitis ($n = 9$), exfoliative dermatitis ($n = 9$), rash ($n = 8$), myalgia ($n = 8$), liver enzyme abnormalities ($n = 7$), bone pain ($n = 6$), arthralgia ($n = 5$), raised LDH activity ($n = 4$), pseudotumor cerebri ($n = 4$; with severe headache, papilledema, increased CSF pressure, and absence of structural cranial lesions by CT or MRI scanning), hypercholesterolemia ($n = 4$), chills ($n = 4$), pruritus ($n = 3$), and diarrhea ($n = 2$).

Drug overdose

The possible symptoms and signs of overdosage are essentially the same as in hypervitaminosis A (see Table 1). The toxicity of overdosage appears to be low, and symptoms are restricted to headache and mucocutaneous adverse effects (118).

Drug–Drug Interactions

Alcohol

Concomitant intake of alcohol induces the transformation of acitretin to etretinate, which has a much longer half-life (84–168 days) (119).

Carbamazepine

No increase in seizure susceptibility was noted in a number of epileptic patients taking concomitant phenytoin, sodium valproate, or carbamazepine. However, it is recommended that carbamazepine concentrations be measured during therapy (12).

Tetracycline

Concurrent use of tetracycline has been considered contraindicated because of the risk of benign intracranial hypertension. However, although either compound alone can provoke this rare adverse effect, there is no evidence of any additive effect (12).

References

1. Soong HK, Martin NF, Wagoner MD, Alfonso E, Mandelbaum SH, Laibson PR, Smith RE, Udell I. Topical retinoid therapy for squamous metaplasia of various ocular surface disorders. A multicenter, placebo-controlled double-masked study. Ophthalmology 1988;95(10):1442–6.
2. Culine S, Kramar A, Droz JP, Theodore C. Phase II study of all-trans retinoic acid administered intermittently for hormone refractory prostate cancer. J Urol 1999;161(1):173–5.
3. Bunker CB, Sheron N, Maurice PD, Kocjan G, Johnson NM, Dowd PM. Isotretinoin and eosinophilic pleural effusion. Lancet 1989;1(8635):435–6.
4. Miller JA, Munro DD. Topical corticosteroids: clinical pharmacology and therapeutic use. Drugs 1980;19(2):119–34.
5. Junjie Y, Zhaoping H, Minfei P. Fatal side-effects of all-trans retinoic acid in the treatment of acute promyelocytic leukemia. Bull Hum Med Univ 1999;24:293–5.
6. Fenaux P, Chastang C, Chevret S, Sanz M, Dombret H, Archimbaud E, Fey M, Rayon C, Huguet F, Sotto JJ, Gardin C, Makhoul PC, Travade P, Solary E, Fegueux N, Bordessoule D, Miguel JS, Link H, Desablens B, Stamatoullas A, Deconinck E, Maloisel F, Castaigne S, Preudhomme C, Degos L. A randomized comparison of all transretinoic acid (ATRA) followed by chemotherapy and ATRA plus chemotherapy and the role of maintenance therapy in newly diagnosed acute promyelocytic leukemia. The European APL Group. Blood 1999;94(4):1192–200.
7. Budd GT, Adamson PC, Gupta M, Homayoun P, Sandstrom SK, Murphy RF, McLain D, Tuason L, Peereboom D, Bukowski RM, Ganapathi R. Phase I/II trial of all-trans retinoic acid and tamoxifen in patients with advanced breast cancer. Clin Cancer Res 1998;4(3):635–42.
8. Kelly WK, Osman I, Reuter VE, Curley T, Heston WD, Nanus DM, Scher HI. The development of biologic end points in patients treated with differentiation agents: an experience of retinoids in prostate cancer. Clin Cancer Res 2000;6(3):838–46.
9. Park SH, Gray WC, Hernandez I, Jacobs M, Ord RA, Sutharalingam M, Smith RG, Van Echo DA, Wu S, Conley BA. Phase I trial of all-trans retinoic acid in patients with treated head and neck squamous carcinoma. Clin Cancer Res 2000;6(3):847–54.
10. Mao JT, Goldin JG, Dermand J, Ibrahim G, Brown MS, Emerick A, McNitt-Gray MF, Gjertson DW, Estrada F, Tashkin DP, Roth MD. A pilot study of all-trans-retinoic acid for the treatment of human emphysema. Am J Respir Crit Care Med 2002;165(5):718–23.
11. Goulden V, Layton AM, Cunliffe WJ. Long-term safety of isotretinoin as a treatment for acne vulgaris. Br J Dermatol 1994;131(3):360–3.
12. Meigel WN. How safe is oral isotretinoin? Dermatology 1997;195(Suppl 1):22–8.
13. Cunliffe WJ, van de Kerkhof PC, Caputo R, Cavicchini S, Cooper A, Fyrand OL, Gollnick H, Layton AM, Leyden JJ, Mascaro JM, Ortonne JP, Shalita A. Roaccutane treatment guidelines: results of an international survey. Dermatology 1997;194(4):351–7.
14. Cunliffe WJ, Stables A. Optimum use of isotretinoin. J Cutan Med Surg 1996;1(Suppl):2–20.
15. Berbis P. Acitretine. [Acitretine.] Ann Dermatol Venereol 2001;128(6–7):737–45.
16. Pilkington T, Brogden RN. Acitretin. A review of its pharmacology and therapeutic use. Drugs 1992;43(4):597–627.
17. Leyden JJ. Therapy for acne vulgaris. N Engl J Med 1997;336(16):1156–62.
18. Nyirady J, Grossman RM, Nighland M, Berger RS, Jorizzo JL, Kim YH, Martin AG, Pandya AG, Schulz KK, Strauss JS. A comparative trial of two retinoids commonly used in the treatment of acne vulgaris. J Dermatolog Treat 2001;12(3):149–57.
19. Tu P, Li GQ, Zhu XJ, Zheng J, Wong WZ. A comparison of adapalene gel 0.1% vs. tretinoin gel 0.025% in the

treatment of acne vulgaris in China. J Eur Acad Dermatol Venereol 2001;15(Suppl 3):31–6.

20. Peck GL. Therapy and prevention of skin cancer. In: Saurat JH, editor. Retinoids. Basel: S. Karger, 1985;345.

21. Dai WS, LaBraico JM, Stern RS. Epidemiology of isotretinoin exposure during pregnancy. J Am Acad Dermatol 1992;26(4):599–606.

22. Teelmann K. Retinoids: toxicology and teratogenicity to date. Pharmacol Ther 1989;40(1):29–43.

23. Chan A, Hanna M, Abbott M, Keane RJ. Oral retinoids and pregnancy. Med J Aust 1996;165(3):164–7.

24. Hull PR, Demkiw-Bartel C. Isotretinoin use in acne: prospective evaluation of adverse events. J Cutan Med Surg 2000;4(2):66–70.

25. Mann G, Reinhardt D, Ritter J, Hermann J, Schmitt K, Gadner H, Creutzig U. Treatment with all-trans retinoic acid in acute promyelocytic leukemia reduces early deaths in children. Ann Hematol 2001;80(7):417–22.

26. De Botton S, Dombret H, Sanz M, Miguel JS, Caillot D, Zittoun R, Gardembas M, Stamatoulas A, Conde E, Guerci A, Gardin C, Geiser K, Makhoul DC, Reman O, de la Serna J, Lefrere F, Chomienne C, Chastang C, Degos L, Fenaux P. Incidence, clinical features, and outcome of all trans-retinoic acid syndrome in 413 cases of newly diagnosed acute promyelocytic leukemia. The European APL Group. Blood 1998;92(8):2712–18.

27. Amano Y, Tajika K, Mizuki T, Amano M, Dan K, Kumazaki T. All-trans retinoic acid syndrome: chest CT assessment. Eur Radiol 2001;11(8):1516–17.

28. Jung JI, Choi JE, Hahn ST, Min CK, Kim CC, Park SH. Radiologic features of all-trans-retinoic acid syndrome. Am J Roentgenol 2002;178(2):475–80.

29. Tallman MS, Andersen JW, Schiffer CA, Appelbaum FR, Feusner JH, Ogden A, Shepherd L, Rowe JM, Francois C, Larson RS, Wiernik PH. Clinical description of 44 patients with acute promyelocytic leukemia who developed the retinoic acid syndrome. Blood 2000;95(1):90–5.

30. Han ZP, Lu HB, Shen ZS. [Severe side effects of the treatment of acute promyelocytic leukemia with all-trans retinoic acid.] Hunan Yi Ke Da Xue Xue Bao 2000;25(3):283–4.

31. Lehmann S, Paul C. The retinoic acid syndrome in non-M3 acute myeloid leukaemia: a case report. Br J Haematol 2000;108(1):198–9.

32. Nicolls MR, Terada LS, Tuder RM, Prindiville SA, Schwarz MI. Diffuse alveolar hemorrhage with underlying pulmonary capillaritis in the retinoic acid syndrome. Am J Respir Crit Care Med 1998;158(4):1302–5.

33. Mandelli F, Diverio D, Avvisati G, Luciano A, Barbui T, Bernasconi C, Broccia G, Cerri R, Falda M, Fioritoni G, Leoni F, Liso V, Petti MC, Rodeghiero F, Saglio G, Vegna ML, Visani G, Jehn U, Willemze R, Muus P, Pelicci PG, Biondi A, Lo Coco F. Molecular remission in PML/RAR alpha-positive acute promyelocytic leukemia by combined all-trans retinoic acid and idarubicin (AIDA) therapy. Gruppo Italiano-Malattie Ematologiche Maligne dell'Adulto and Associazione Italiana di Ematologia ed Oncologia Pediatrica Cooperative Groups. Blood 1997;90(3):1014–21.

34. Torromeo C, Latagliata R, Avvisati G, Petti MC, Mandelli F. Intraventricular thrombosis during all-trans retinoic acid treatment in acute promyelocytic leukemia. Leukemia 2001;15(8):1311–13.

35. Fisher DA. Exercise-induced bronchoconstriction related to isotretinoin therapy. J Am Acad Dermatol 1985; 13(3):524.

36. Bunker CB, Tomlinson MC, Johnson NM, Dowd PM. Isotretinoin and the lung. Br J Dermatol 1991;125(Suppl 38):29.

37. Sabroe RA, Staughton RC, Bunker CB. Bronchospasm induced by isotretinoin. BMJ 1996;312(7035):886.

38. van de Loosdrecht AA, van Imhoff GW. Images in clinical medicine. All-trans-retinoic acid related pulmonary syndrome in acute promyelocytic leukemia. Neth J Med 1999;54(3):131–2.

39. Kim C, Ki Ko W, Hyun Kwon S, Myung Kang S, Nyun Kim C, Gyoo Yang D, Kyu Kim S, Chang J, Kyu Kim S, Young Lee W, Ik Yang W. A case of acute respiratory distress syndrome induced by all-trans-retinoic acid. Tuberc Respir Dis 2000;49:93–8.

40. Raanani P, Segal E, Levi I, Bercowicz M, Berkenstat H, Avigdor A, Perel A, Ben-Bassat I. Diffuse alveolar hemorrhage in acute promyelocytic leukemia patients treated with ATRA—a manifestation of the basic disease or the treatment. Leuk Lymphoma 2000; 37(5–6):605–10.

41. Byrne A, Hnatko G. Depression associated with isotretinoin therapy. Can J Psychiatry 1995;40(9):567.

42. Fraunfelder FW, Fraunfelder FT, Corbett JJ. Isotretinoin-associated intracranial hypertension. Ophthalmology 2004;111(6):1248–50.

43. Schroeter T, Lanvers C, Herding H, Suttorp M. Pseudotumor cerebri induced by all-trans-retinoic acid in a child treated for acute promyelocytic leukemia. Med Pediatr Oncol 2000;34(4):284–6.

44. Yamaji S, Kanamori H, Mishima A, Fujisawa S, Motomura S, Mohri H. All-trans retinoic acid-induced multiple mononeuropathies. Am J Hematol 1999;60(4):311.

45. Chroni E, Georgiou S, Monastirli A, Paschalis C, Tsambaos D. Effects of short-term oral acitretin therapy on peripheral nerve function: a prospective neurological and neurophysiological study. Acta Dermatol Venereol 2001;81(6):423–5.

46. Lebowitz MA, Berson DS. Ocular effects of oral retinoids. J Am Acad Dermatol 1988;19(1 Pt 2):209–11.

47. Gold JA, Shupack JL, Nemec MA. Ocular side effects of the retinoids. Int J Dermatol 1989;28(4):218–25.

48. Fraunfelder FT, LaBraico JM, Meyer SM. Adverse ocular reactions possibly associated with isotretinoin. Am J Ophthalmol 1985;100(4):534–7.

49. Ellies P, Dighiero P, Legeais JM, Pouliquen YJ, Renard G. Persistent corneal opacity after oral isotretinoin therapy for acne. Cornea 2000;19(2):238–9.

50. Ng EW, Congdon NG, Sommer A. Acute sixth nerve palsy in vitamin A treatment of xerophthalmia. Br J Ophthalmol 2000;84(8):931–2.

51. Parry MF, Rha CK. Pseudomembranous colitis caused by topical clindamycin phosphate. Arch Dermatol 1986;122(5):583–4.

52. Wester RC, Maibach HI. In vivo percutaneous absorption. In: Marzulli FN, Maibach HI, editors. Dermatotoxicology. 2nd ed. Washington: Hemisphere Publishing Corporation, 1983:131.

53. Wysowski DK, Pitts M, Beitz J. An analysis of reports of depression and suicide in patients treated with isotretinoin. J Am Acad Dermatol 2001;45(4):515–19.

54. Wysowski DK, Pitts M, Beitz J. Depression and suicide in patients treated with isotretinoin. N Engl J Med 2001;344(6):460.

55. Gupta MA, Gupta AK. Isotretinoin use and reports of sustained dreaming. Br J Dermatol 2001;144(4):919–20.

56. Fontan B, Bonafe JL, Moatti JP. Toxic effects of the aromatic retinoid etretinate. Arch Dermatol 1983;119(3):187–8.

57. Alcalay J, Landau M, Zucker A. Analysis of laboratory data in acne patients treated with isotretinoin: is there really a need to perform routine laboratory tests? J Dermatol Treat 2001;12(1):9–12.

58. Rodondi N, Darioli R, Ramelet AA, Hohl D, Lenain V, Perdrix J, Wietlisbach V, Riesen WF, Walther T, Medinger L, Nicod P, Desvergne B, Mooser V. High risk for hyperlipidemia and the metabolic syndrome after an episode of hypertriglyceridemia during 13-cis retinoic acid therapy for acne: a pharmacogenetic study. Ann Intern Med 2002;136(8):582–9.

59. Barth JH, Macdonald-Hull SP, Mark J, Jones RG, Cunliffe WJ. Isotretinoin therapy for acne vulgaris: a re-evaluation of the need for measurements of plasma lipids and liver function tests. Br J Dermatol 1993;129(6):704–7.

60. Suzumiya J, Asahara F, Katakami H, Kimuran N, Hisano S, Okumura M, Ohno R. Hypercalcaemia caused by all-trans retinoic acid treatment of acute promyelocytic leukaemia: case report. Eur J Haematol 1994;53(2):126–7.

61. Belden TL, Ragucci DP. Hypercalcemia induced by 13-cis-retinoic acid in a patient with neuroblastoma. Pharmacotherapy 2002;22(5):645–8.

62. Sakamoto O, Yoshinari M, Rikiishi T, Fujiwara I, Imaizumi M, Tsuchiya S, Iinuma K. Hypercalcemia due to all-trans retinoic acid therapy for acute promyelocytic leukemia: a case report of effective treatment with bis-phosphonate. Pediatr Int 2001;43(6):688–90.

63. Allan S, Christmas T. Severe edema associated with etretinate. J Am Acad Dermatol 1988;19(1 Pt 1):140.

64. Windhorst DB, Nigra T. General clinical toxicology of oral retinoids. J Am Acad Dermatol 1982;6(4 Pt 2 Suppl):675–82.

65. Brown JE, Olujohungbe A, Chang J, Ryder WD, Morganstern GR, Chopra R, Scarffe JH. All-trans retinoic acid (ATRA) and tranexamic acid: a potentially fatal combination in acute promyelocytic leukaemia. Br J Haematol 2000;110(4):1010–12.

66. Kocak U, Gursel T, Ozturk G, Kantarci S. Thrombosis during all-trans-retinoic acid therapy in a child with acute promyelocytic leukemia and factor VQ 506 mutation. Pediatr Hematol Oncol 2000;17(2):177–80.

67. Cakmakci A, Yilmaz AS, Akbulut S, Gul U, Ozyilkan E. Polycythemia in a patient treated with isotretinoin. Ann Pharmacother 2001;35(7–8):964–5.

68. Ko BS, Tang JL, Chen YC, Yao M, Wang CH, Shen MC, Tien HF. Extramedullary relapse after all-trans retinoic acid treatment in acute promyelocytic leukemia—the occurrence of retinoic acid syndrome is a risk factor. Leukemia 1999;13(9):1406–8.

69. Reniers DE, Howard JM. Isotretinoin-induced inflammatory bowel disease in an adolescent. Ann Pharmacother 2001;35(10):1214–16.

70. Godfrey KM, James MP. Treatment of severe acne with isotretinoin in patients with inflammatory bowel disease. Br J Dermatol 1990;123(5):653–5.

71. Martin P, Manley PN, Depew WT, Blakeman JM. Isotretinoin-associated proctosigmoiditis. Gastroenterology 1987;93(3):606–9.

72. Brodin MB. Inflammatory bowel disease and isotretinoin. J Am Acad Dermatol 1986;14(5 Pt 1):843.

73. Schleicher SM. Oral isotretinoin and inflammatory bowel disease. J Am Acad Dermatol 1985;13(5 Pt 1):834–5.

74. Rosen T, Unkefer RP. Treatment of pyoderma faciale with isotretinoin in a patient with ulcerative colitis. Cutis 1999;64(2):107–9.

75. Yamada K, Sugimoto K, Matsumoto T, Narumi K, Oshimi K. All-trans retinoic acid-induced vasculitis and hemonecrosis of the ileum in a patient with acute promyelocytic leukemia. Leukemia 1999;13(4):647–8.

76. Sanchez MR, Ross B, Rotterdam H, Salik J, Brodie R, Freedberg IM. Retinoid hepatitis. J Am Acad Dermatol 1993;28(5 Pt 2):853–8.

77. Gavish D, Katz M, Gottehrer N, Israeli A, Lijovetzky G, Holubar K. Cholestatic jaundice, an unusual side effect of etretinate. J Am Acad Dermatol 1985;13(4):669–70.

78. Perea G, Salar A, Altes A, Brunet S, Sierra J. Acute hepatomegaly with severe liver toxicity due to all-trans-retinoic acid. Haematologica 2000;85(5):551–2.

79. Izumi T, Hatake K, Miura Y. Acute promyelocytic leukemia. N Engl J Med 1994;330(2):141.

80. Yutsudo Y, Imoto S, Ozuru R, Kajimoto K, Itoi H, Koizumi T, Nishimura R, Nakagawa T. Acute pancreatitis after all-trans retinoic acid therapy. Ann Hematol 1997;74(6):295–6.

81. Abou Chacra L, Ghosn M, Ghayad E, Honein K. A case of pancreatitis associated with all-trans-retinoic acid therapy in acute promyelocytic leukemia. Hematol J 2001;2(6):406–7.

82. Pavese P, Kuentz F, Belleville C, Rouge PE, Elsener M. Renal impairment induced by isotretinoin. Nephrol Dial Transplant 1997;12(6):1299.

83. Cribier B, Welsch M, Heid E. Renal impairment probably induced by etretinate. Dermatology 1992;185(4):266–8.

84. Kellock DJ, Parslew R, Mendelsohn SS, O'Mahony CP. Non-specific urethritis—possible association with isotretinoin therapy. Int J STD AIDS 1996;7(2):135–6.

85. van Oers JA, de Leeuw J, van Bommel EF. Nephrotic syndrome associated with isotretinoin. Nephrol Dial Transplant 2000;15(6):923–4.

86. Tomita N, Kanamori H, Fujita H, Maruta A, Naitoh A, Nakamura S, Ota Y, Nozue N, Kihara M, Ishigatsubo Y. Granulomatous tubulointerstitial nephritis induced by all-trans retinoic acid. Anticancer Drugs 2001;12(8):677–80.

87. Turman MA, Hammond S, Grovas A, Rauck AM. Possible association of retinoic acid with bone marrow transplant nephropathy. Pediatr Nephrol 1999;13(9):755–8.

88. Charles KS, Kanaa M, Winfield DA, Reilly JT. Scrotal ulceration during all-trans retinoic (ATRA) therapy for acute promyelocytic leukaemia. Clin Lab Haematol 2000;22(3):171–4.

89. Esser AC, Nossa R, Shoji T, Sapadin AN. All-trans-retinoic acid-induced scrotal ulcerations in a patient with acute promyelocytic leukemia. J Am Acad Dermatol 2000;43(2 Pt 1):316–17.

90. Sun GL. [Treatment of acute promyelocytic leukemia (APL) with all-trans retinoic acid (ATRA): a report of five-year experience.] Zhonghua Zhong Liu Za Zhi 1993;15(2):125–9.

91. Tajima K, Sagae M, Yahagi A, Akiba J, Suzuki K, Hayashi T, Satoh S. [Scrotum exfoliative dermatitis with ulcers associated with treatment of acute promyelocytic leukemia with all-trans retinoic acid.] Rinsho Ketsueki 1998;39(1):48–52.

92. Mori A, Tamura S, Katsuno T, Nishimura Y, Itoh T, Saheki K, Takatsuka H, Wada H, Fujimori Y, Okamoto T, Takemoto Y, Kakishita E. Scrotal ulcer occurring in patients with acute promyelocytic leukemia during treatment with all-trans retinoic acid Oncol Rep 1999;6(1):55–8.

93. Newman JM, Rindler JM, Bergfeld WF, Brydon JK. Stevens–Johnson syndrome associated with topical nitrogen mustard therapy. J Am Acad Dermatol 1997;36(1):112–14.

94. Reynolds P, Fawcett H, Waldram R, Prouse P. Delayed onset of vasculitis following isotretinoin. Lancet 1989;2(8673):1216.

95. Silverman AK, Ellis CN, Voorhees JJ. Hypervitaminosis A syndrome: a paradigm of retinoid side effects. J Am Acad Dermatol 1987;16(5 Pt 1):1027–39.

96. Levi I, Raanani P, Shalmon B, Schiby-Brilliant R, Ben-Bassat I. Acute neutrophilic dermatosis induced by all-trans-retinoic acid treatment for acute promyelocytic leukemia. Leuk Lymphoma 1999; 34(3–4):401–4.

97. van Der Vliet HJ, Roberson AE, Hogan MC, Morales CE, Crader SC, Letendre L, Pruthi RK. All-trans-retinoic acid-induced myositis: a description of two patients. Am J Hematol 2000;63(2):94–8.

98. Astudillo L, Loche F, Reynish W, Rigal-Huguet F, Lamant L, Pris J. Sweet's syndrome associated with retinoic acid syndrome in a patient with promyelocytic leukemia. Ann Hematol 2002;81(2):111–14.

99. Birner AM, Meyer LP. Photosensitivity associated with fluorouracil, prochlorperazine, and topical tretinoin. Pharmacotherapy 2001;21(2):258–60.

100. Chang SE, Huh J, Choi JH, Sung KJ, Moon KC, Koh JK. Cutaneous relapse in acute promyelocytic leukaemia following treatment with all-trans retinoic acid. Br J Dermatol 1999;141(3):586–7.

101. Hughes RA. Arthritis precipitated by isotretinoin treatment for acne vulgaris. J Rheumatol 1993;20(7):1241–2.

102. DiGiovanna JJ, Sollitto RB, Abangan DL, Steinberg SM, Reynolds JC. Osteoporosis is a toxic effect of long-term etretinate therapy. Arch Dermatol 1995;131(11):1263–7.

103. Chroni E, Sakkis T, Georgiou S, Monastirli A, Pasmatzi E, Paschalis C, Tsambaos D. Stiff-person syndrome associated with oral isotretinoin treatment. Neuromuscul Disord 2002;12(9):886–8.

104. Leibovitch I, Amital H, Levy Y, Langevitz P, Shoenfeld Y. Isotretinoin-induced adult onset Still's disease. Clin Exp Rheumatol 2000;18(5):616–18.

105. Larsen GK. Iatrogenic breast discharge with isotretinoin. Arch Dermatol 1985;121(4):450–1.

106. Coleman R, MacDonald D. Effects of isotretinoin on male reproductive system. Lancet 1994;344(8916):198.

107. Khurshid I, Seymour JF, Nakata K, Downie GH. Recurrent manifestations of idiopathic pulmonary alveolar proteinosis after isotretinoin (Accutane) treatment. Chest 2001;120(Suppl):335.

108. Alli N, Toy GG. Familial Mediterranean fever: attacks during isotretinoin treatment. J Am Acad Dermatol 2002;47(6):967.

109. Jick SS, Terris BZ, Jick H. First trimester topical tretinoin and congenital disorders. Lancet 1993; 341(8854):1181–2.

110. Selcen D, Seidman S, Nigro MA. Otocerebral anomalies associated with topical tretinoin use. Brain Dev 2000; 22(4):218–20.

111. Camera G, Pregliasco P. Ear malformation in baby born to mother using tretinoin cream. Lancet 1992; 339(8794):687.

112. Lipson AH, Collins F, Webster WS. Multiple congenital defects associated with maternal use of topical tretinoin. Lancet 1993;341(8856):1352–3.

113. Navarre-Belhassen C, Blanchet P, Hillaire-Buys D, Sarda P, Blayac JP. Multiple congenital malformations associated with topical tretinoin. Ann Pharmacother 1998;32(4):505–6.

114. Ceviz N, Ozkan B, Eren S, Ors R, Olgunturk R. A case of isotretinoin embryopathy with bilateral anotia and Taussig–Bing malformation. Turk J Pediatr 2000; 42(3):239–41.

115. Vannucchi MT, Vannucchi H, Humphreys M. Serum levels of vitamin A and retinol binding protein in chronic renal patients treated by continuous ambulatorial peritoneal dialysis. Int J Vitam Nutr Res 1992;62(2):107–12.

116. Doyle S, Conlon P, Royston D. Vitamin A induced stellate cell hyperplasia and fibrosis in renal failure. Histopathology 2000;36(1):90–1.

117. Douer D, Estey E, Santillana S, Bennett JM, Lopez-Bernstein G, Boehm K, Williams T. Treatment of newly diagnosed and relapsed acute promyelocytic leukemia with intravenous liposomal all-trans retinoic acid. Blood 2001;97(1):73–80.

118. Aubin S, Lorette G, Muller C, Vaillant L. Massive isotretinoin intoxication. Clin Exp Dermatol 1995; 20(4):348–50.

119. Larsen FG, Jakobsen P, Knudsen J, Weismann K, Kragballe K, Nielsen-Kudsk F. Conversion of acitretin to etretinate in psoriatic patients is influenced by ethanol. J Invest Dermatol 1993;100(5):623–7.

Vitamin B$_{12}$ (cobalamins)

See also Vitamins

General Information

Vitamin B$_{12}$ is a mixture of cobalamins. Dietary vitamin B$_{12}$ is converted to the active forms, methylcobalamin (mecobalamin) and adenosylcobalamin. The Average Requirement of total cobalamins in adults is 1.0 microgram/day and the Population Reference Intake is 1.4 micrograms/day. The Lowest Threshold Intake is 0.6 micrograms/day. Hydroxocobalamin (rINN; vitamin B$_{12a}$) and cyanocobalamin (rINN) have been used therapeutically.

All the cobalamins have the same pattern of adverse reactions. The adverse effects of high doses of cobalamins include urticaria, eczematous and exanthematous skin lesions, and anaphylactic reactions (SEDA-4, 265), but it is not clear whether the reactions are caused by the drug itself, a preservative, or possibly by contaminants. High oral or parenteral doses of vitamin B$_6$ and especially hydroxocobalamin are also on rare occasions suspected to induce acne which is, however, always benign (SEDA-5, 347) (1). Several cases of vitamin B$_{12}$-induced folliculitis and acneiform eruptions have been described, in one case in connection with a patient receiving total parenteral nutrition (2).

Organs and Systems

Cardiovascular

Syncope was induced by intramuscular injection of hydroxocobalamin in a paraplegic patient (3).

- An 81-year-old man had been a prisoner of war 58 years before and had been fed mainly rice. At that time he had developed complete loss of power and sensation in the right leg, weakness in the left leg, and weakness and impaired sensation in the right arm; he had become almost blind and deaf in both ears. When he was given vitamin B tablets his sight became almost normal within 1 month, but recovery of motor power was slower. In 1945 he returned home and was given injections of vitamin B_{12} on and off without adverse effects. In 1997 he had a serum vitamin B_{12} concentration of 91 ng/l (reference range 223–1132), a normal folate concentration, a hemoglobin of 15.7 g/dl, and an MCV of 95 fl. He was given intramuscular vitamin B_{12} 1 mg every 4–6 weeks. In 1998 he fainted about 10 minutes after an injection of vitamin B_{12}. His blood pressure was 60/30 mmHg. Soon after the next injection the patient fainted again and developed red patches and blisters over his arms, chest, and legs. Oral vitamin B_{12} without intrinsic factor resulted in 3.47% excretion in 24 hours. Vitamin B_{12} with intrinsic factor led to a urinary excretion of 1.49%. No reactions to oral vitamin B_{12} were reported.

Hematologic

A mild form of polycythemia with peripheral vascular thrombosis has been described in patients with pernicious anemia treated with high doses of vitamin B_{12} (4).

Immunologic

Allergy to vitamin B_{12} injection is infrequent, but can be serious. Positive results of basophil histamine release assay and skin testing suggest an IgE-mediated mechanism (5). Severe hypersensitivity to cyanocobalamin or hydroxocobalamin has been reported in patients who took the other cobalamin without further allergic reactions (6).

- A 45-year-old woman with pernicious anemia was given intramuscular hydroxocobalamin and developed mild generalized pruritus (7). Subsequent monthly injections of hydroxocobalamin 1 mg were followed by incrementally worsening pruritus and then frank urticaria. The last of nine injections was followed by urticaria, bronchospasm, and oropharyngeal angioedema, which responded to adrenaline. She underwent skin prick and intradermal testing with hydroxocobalamin and cyanocobalamin. Wheal-and-flare reactions occurred after injection of hydroxocobalamin, suggesting an IgE-mediated response. There was no reaction to cyanocobalamin. She subsequently had a reaction to subcutaneous cyanocobalamin 0.1 ml (100 micrograms) and then intramuscular cyanocobalamin 0.5 ml (500 micrograms). Her macrocytic anemia resolved with monthly cyanocobalamin. After 1 year she had an episode of delayed urticaria after a routine injection of cyanocobalamin. Skin prick and intradermal tests were again negative with cyanocobalamin, but there were wheal-and-flare reactions to hydroxocobalamin. She then tolerated monthly intramuscular cyanocobalamin for over 12 months.
- A 42-year-old woman who had received monthly intramuscular cyanocobalamin for 4 years developed Quincke's edema. She was given hydroxocobalamin instead, each injection being preceded by 4 mg of dexamethasone. After 13 years of this treatment she had not had any allergic reactions.
- A 35-year-old woman who had received monthly intramuscular hydroxocobalamin for 6 years developed anaphylactic shock immediately after a dose. Later she was given cyanocobalamin with terfenadine 120 mg/day for 2 days before each injection. After 3 years she had not had any allergic reactions.

Skin prick and intradermal tests, with increasing concentrations of hydroxocobalamin and cyanocobalamin, and histamine release tests on blood basophils with hydroxocobalamin and cyanocobalamin were negative in the second and third patients.

One way of dealing with vitamin B_{12} allergy is to use the alternative compound after skin testing to exclude cross-reactivity. If cross-reactivity occurs, desensitization may be considered. Alternatively, oral B_{12} can be used.

References

1. Dupre A, Albarel N, Bonafe JL, et al. Acnes induites par la vitamine B12. Rev Med Toulouse 1975;11:391.
2. Gallastegui C, Cardona D, Pujol R, Garcia B, Bonal J, Andreu A. Vitamin B12-induced folliculitis. DICP 1989;23(12):1033–4.
3. Vaidyanathan S, Soni BM, Oo T, Watt JW, Sett P, Singh G. Syncope following intramuscular injection of hydroxocobalamin in a paraplegic patient: indication for oral administration of cyanocobalamin in spinal cord injury patients. Spinal Cord 1999;37(2):147–9.
4. Klemetti L. Is the vitamin B12 treatment of pernicious anaemia a predisposing factor for thrombosis in aged patients? Acta Med Scand 1964;176:121–2.
5. de Blay F, Sager MF, Hirth C, Alt M, Chamouard P, Baumann R, Pauli G. IGE-mediated reaction to hydroxocobalamin injection in patient with pernicious anaemia. Lancet 1992;339(8808):1535–6.
6. Tordjman R, Genereau T, Guinnepain MT, Weyer A, Lortholary O, Royer I, Casassus P, Guillevin L. Reintroduction of vitamin B12 in 2 patients with prior B12-induced anaphylaxis. Eur J Haematol 1998;60(4):269–70.
7. Heyworth-Smith D, Hogan PG. Allergy to hydroxycobalamin, with tolerance of cyanocobalamin. Med J Aust 2002;177(3):162–3.

Vitamin D analogues

See also Vitamins

General Information

The group of D vitamins includes the following naturally occurring compounds:

- lumisterol (vitamin D_1)
- ergocalciferol (calciferol or vitamin D_2)
- colecalciferol (vitamin D_3)

- dihydrotachysterol (vitamin D_4)
- 25-hydroxycolecalciferol (calcifediol)
- 1α,25-dihydroxycolecalciferol (calcitriol)
- 24,25-dihydroxycolecalciferol.

Ergocalciferol is derived from ergosterol in the diet. Colecalciferol is derived from endogenous cholesterol. Both are also synthesized in the skin. Colecalciferol and ergocalciferol are converted in the liver by hydroxylation to calcifediol, which is weakly active. Calcifediol is activated in the kidneys by further hydroxylation to alfacalcidol, which is highly active, and calcitriol, which is weakly active. Calcitriol is deactivated by further hydroxylation in the kidney to 1α,24,25-trihydroxycolecalciferol.

Synthetic derivatives of vitamin D include:

- 1α-hydroxycolecalciferol (alfacalcidol)
- 19-nor-1,25-dihydroxycalciferol (paracalcitol) (1)
- 1α-hydroxycalciferol (doxercalciferol).

Of these alfacalcidol has been the most widely used. It is hydroxylated in the liver to calcitriol, thus bypassing the kidney. Unlike calcitriol, which acts in the small intestine to stimulate absorption, doxercalciferol remains inactive until it reaches the liver, where it undergoes transformation to active vitamin D (2). As a result, doxercalciferol minimizes the risk of hypercalcemia by 67–80%. The manufacturers claim that doxercalciferol is as potent as calcitriol in lowering parathyroid hormone concentrations.

Dietary intake and synthesis of vitamin D in the skin under the influence of ultraviolet light complement one another. In practice, the Population Reference Intake for adults is 5–10 micrograms/day and for infants and children 10–25 micrograms/day. Colecalciferol 1 microgram = vitamin D 40 IU.

The reference ranges for serum concentrations are [http://europa.eu.int/comm/food/fs/sc/scf/]:

- calcifediol 130–150 nmol/l
- calcitriol 50–145 pmol/l
- 24,25-dihydroxycolecalciferol 2–10 nmol/l.

Alfacalcidol and calcitriol have some advantages over calciferol, but their high potency involves a risk of hypercalcemia even after small dosage increments, because of increased intestinal calcium absorption. Because of this, constant vigilance is required to prevent hypercalcemia, especially in patients with chronic renal insufficiency and associated renal osteodystrophy.

Comparative studies

The efficacy of intravenous paricalcitol and calcitriol and the risks of hypercalcemia and hyperphosphatemia have been studied in an international, randomized, double-blind comparison in 38 patients in dialysis units (3). The end points were a reduction of at least 50% in baseline parathyroid hormone concentration and the occurrence of hypercalcemia and hyperphosphatemia. Paricalcitol was started at a dose of 0.04 micrograms/kg and increased in 0.04 micrograms/kg increments every 4 weeks to a maximum allowable dose of 0.24 micrograms/kg or until

there was at least a 50% fall in serum parathyroid hormone concentration. Calcitriol was started at a dose of 0.01 micrograms/kg and increased in 0.01 micrograms/kg increments every 4 weeks to a maximum allowable dose of 0.06 micrograms/kg or until there was at least a 50% fall in serum parathyroid hormone concentration. Mean baseline serum parathyroid hormone, calcium, and phosphorus concentrations were similar. Reductions in parathyroid hormone occurred more rapidly with paricalcitol than with calcitriol, but there were no differences in serum calcium concentrations throughout the study between the groups. However, the respective percentages of subjects who had severe hyperphosphatemia (serum phosphorus over 0.84 mmol/l) after 8, 16, and 20 weeks were about 18, 16, and 14% in 19 patients treated with calcitriol and 6.8, 8.6, and 9.8% in 19 patients treated with paricalcitol. The results of this study suggest that paricalcitol reduces parathyroid hormone concentrations more rapidly than calcitriol does, with fewer episodes of hyperphosphatemia.

Placebo-controlled studies

In two placebo-controlled trials, 90% of dialysis patients with moderate to severe secondary hyperparathyroidism who received doxercalciferol for 16–24 weeks had about a 70% reduction in parathyroid hormone concentrations. The most frequently reported adverse effects include edema, headache, and malaise.

General adverse effects

Vitamin D intoxication is characterized by hypercalcemia and hypercalciuria as a result both of excessive gastrointestinal calcium absorption and of enhanced mobilization of calcium from bone (SEDA-8, 804) (4–6). Unintentional intoxication can result from the addition of vitamin D to food, especially to milk and milk products, for prevention of vitamin D deficiency. The established dosage for prophylaxis of vitamin D deficient rickets, 400 IU (10 micrograms), is commonly regarded as safe. The large vitamin D doses used in hypoparathyroidism, renal osteodystrophy, vitamin D-resistant rickets, and osteomalacia can predispose to intoxication. Close clinical and biochemical monitoring of patients taking vitamin D or vitamin D analogues is necessary, since intoxication can occur independent of dose and the period over which the drug has been taken.

The initial symptoms of hypervitaminosis D include weakness, fatigue, lassitude, headache, nausea, vomiting, and diarrhea. Renal function can be impaired at an early stage, with polyuria, polydipsia, nocturia, reduced urinary concentrating ability, and proteinuria.

The characteristic features of chronic intoxication are deposition of calcium salts in various tissues. A follow-up study of 24 children with vitamin D intoxication (13 900–200 000 IU/day) for up to 13 years showed that 23% of the patients had permanent damage. The severity of renal, neurological, and digestive symptoms was related to the daily dose, but the final consequences depended on the duration of overdosage (7). Vitamin D intoxication has also been seen after so-called "Stoss" prophylaxis in children, that is the use of single very high doses of vitamin D, and it has therefore been suggested that this procedure should be avoided (8).

It has been postulated that it is calcifediol that is the main factor involved in vitamin D intoxication (9). The serum concentration of this metabolite can remain high for several months after ingestion of excessive amounts, at least in infants (SEDA-12, 329) (10).

In elderly people, the amount of body fat is usually increased and total body fluid is reduced. These changes affect drug distribution and should be considered when administering lipophilic substances such as vitamin D, which can have a higher relative distribution volume, a longer half-life, increased accumulation, and prolongation of the pharmacological effect. Reduced dosages of vitamin D should therefore be considered in older patients (11).

Allergic reactions to vitamin D are rare and tumor-inducing effects are not reported.

Organs and Systems

Cardiovascular

Some individuals develop hypertension in response to vitamin D, which in some of them may be directly related to hypercalcemia and which may be reversible when renal function is normalized (12). Metastatic calcification is observed in various tissues (13), but arterial calcification is the most usual. In some patients undergoing dialysis, calcification of the blood vessels has been so extensive that cannulation could not be performed (14).

Respiratory

Calcification of the lung from vitamin D is rare, but has been reported in an infant after ingestion of toxic doses (15).

Nervous system

There have been very occasional reports of mental disturbances, including depression (16), cerebellar ataxia, peripheral facial paresis, apathy, lack of interest, and (in cases of acute poisoning) even stupor (SEDA-8, 804) (17–19). Mental changes can occur before the appearance of any somatic symptoms. There may be a correlation between the seriousness of hypervitaminosis D and the extent of electroencephalographic changes (20–22).

Sensory systems

Band keratopathy has been reported in patients taking vitamin D (23), as have calcium deposits in the cornea and the conjunctiva (24).

Tympanic membrane calcification can lead to severe, irreversible conductive deafness (25).

Mineral balance

Hypercalcemia
A single high dose of vitamin D can usually be given without ill effects, even though some workers have described subsequent characteristic changes in the concentrations of phosphorus and calcium in the blood

(SEDA-8, 804) (5,26,27). However, long-term administration, especially with intoxication, is characterized by hypercalcemia and hypercalciuria as a result both of excessive gastrointestinal calcium absorption and of enhanced mobilization of calcium from bone (SEDA-9, 637) (4–6). Hypercalcemia is not necessarily accompanied by clinical symptoms and disappears within 48 hours when the drug is withdrawn. In patients with hypoparathyroidism or chronic renal insufficiency, the rate of reversal of hypercalcemia after stopping treatment with the vitamin D analogues is slower than in healthy subjects. In these diseases, frequent control of blood biochemistry is recommended during treatment with vitamin D analogues (28).

In a comparative study the efficacy and adverse effects of calcitriol and ergocalciferol were investigated in 18 children with chronic renal insufficiency and histological evidence of renal osteodystrophy. Whereas therapeutic effects were similar with ergocalciferol and calcitriol, hypercalcemia was more common in the calcitriol-treated patients (11 episodes following calcitriol therapy and three episodes following ergocalciferol therapy) (29).

Calcitriol + calcium carbonate has been compared with calcium carbonate alone over 12 months in a prospective, randomized trial in 15 patients with secondary hyperparathyroidism (30). Calcitriol 2 micrograms was given after each dialysis; the dose of calcium carbonate was adjusted as needed to maintain calcium and phosphate concentrations at 2.4–2.6 and 1.0–1.5 mmol/l respectively. During the first 6 months, one patient taking calcitriol had an asymptomatic episode of hypercalcemia (2.8 mmol/l), which resolved on reduction of the dose of calcitriol to 1 microgram. In the control group two patients had asymptomatic episodes of hypercalcemia (each 2.9 mmol/l) during the first 6 months. There were two episodes of asymptomatic hypercalcemia (3.2 and 2.9 mmol/l) in two patients taking calcitriol during the last 6 months of the study, requiring a reduction in dose to 0.5 micrograms in one patient. There was one episode of hypercalcemia (2.8 mmol/l) in the control group during the last 6 months of the study.

Two cases of hypercalcemia following the administration of vitamin D analogues in end-stage renal insufficiency have been reported (31).

- A 10-year-old boy with terminal renal insufficiency and secondary hyperparathyroidism was treated with calcitriol (0.5 mg/day; 0.02 mg/kg). His serum calcium rose to 3.05 mmol/l with a parathyroid hormone concentration of 51 pg/ml (reference range 15–65 pg/ml; the target range is 2–4 times higher). Calcitriol was withdrawn, hemodialysis was performed, and oral calcium acetate 2 g/day was administered as a phosphate binder. His calcium returned to normal after 4 months.
- A 12-year-old girl with terminal renal insufficiency was given alfacalcidol (0.5 mg/day; 0.02 micrograms/kg) and calcium carbonate (1 g/day) and developed calcification of the papillary muscles, of the ventricular septum, and of the atrioventricular valves, with sinus bradycardia and heart block that required a cardiac pacemaker. Her serum calcium was 2.7 mmol/l, phosphate 3.14 mmol/l, and parathyroid hormone 23 pg/ml. Calcidiol and calcium carbonate

were withdrawn and hemodialysis was continued. She was given Sevelamer hydrochloride 4 g/day as a phosphate-binder and then several months later calcium acetate 5.2 g/day. After a further 4 months her laboratory values were near the upper limit of the reference ranges.

Because of its potent effects on parathyroid hormone, intestinal calcium absorption, and bone calcium mobilization, calcitriol can cause hypercalcemia, often precluding its use in therapeutic doses (32). Hyperphosphatemia is also a persistent problem in patients on chronic hemodialysis and can be aggravated by therapeutic doses of calcitriol. The use of large doses of calcium carbonate or acetate to control phosphate absorption can increase the risk of hypercalcemia from calcitriol (33).

Severe vitamin D intoxication with spontaneously reversible anemia and bisphosphonate-responsive hypercalcemia has been reported (34).

- A 31-year-old woman developed diffuse musculoskeletal pain. She had been taking calcium and dihydrotachysterol up to 4 mg/day for 6 months for hypoparathyroidism after subtotal thyroid resection. She had severe hypercalcemia (4.1 mmol/l), no detectable intact parathyroid hormone, renal insufficiency (serum creatinine 486 μmol/l), and a normochromic anemia (6.6 g/dl). Rehydration and forced diuresis initially improved renal function and reduced the serum calcium concentration, but the calcium concentration after 4 weeks was still 3.0 mmol/l and it did not normalize until she was given a single intravenous dose of pamidronate 15 mg.

Severe hypercalcemia in a child receiving vitamin D was associated with hyperlipidemia (35).

- An 11-month-old girl developed polyuria, polydipsia, and vomiting. She had been given vitamin D 400 IU/day for just 1 month. A misdiagnosis of rickets was made, and 1 month before admission she was given bolus vitamin D 600 000 IU in two doses 15 days apart. Her serum calcium concentration was 5.5 mmol/l; total cholesterol, high density lipoprotein cholesterol, very low density lipoprotein cholesterol, low density lipoprotein cholesterol, and triglyceride concentrations were respectively: 6.37 mmol/l, 0.77 mmol/l, 1.37 mmol/l, 4.1 mmol/l, and 3.0 mmol/l. After 16 days of therapy with intravenous fluids, furosemide, glucocorticoids, calcitonin, magnesium sulfate, and phosphorus, her serum calcium concentration fell below 3 mmol/l. Her hyperlipidemia resolved gradually.

Ectopic calcification

The prevalence and etiology of ectopic calcification due to alfacalcidol and associated susceptibility factors have been examined in 60 patients with systemic lupus erythematosus (13). The prevalence of ectopic calcification was 40%. Localization of calcification was in peripheral arteries (6.7%), in periarticular areas (33%), and in other soft tissues (17%). The incidence of lupus nephritis and nephrotic syndrome were significantly higher in those with ectopic calcification. Total protein concentrations (70 g/l) in patients with ectopic calcification were significantly lower than in patients without calcification (75 g/l).

Significantly more of the patient with ectopic calcification had received alfacalcidol (63 versus 19%). The authors concluded that alfacalcidol therapy and lupus nephritis increase the risk of ectopic calcification in patients with systemic lupus erythematosus.

Hypomagnesemia

Primary infantile hypomagnesemia is an uncommon cause of neonatal hypocalcemic seizures, but it is an important condition to recognize, because magnesium supplementation corrects the magnesium deficit, reverses the hypocalcemia due to hypoparathyroidism, and prevents further seizures (36). There is evidence of genetic heterogeneity, but the number of gene loci is not known and phenotypic classification is still evolving. Several reports have described primary infantile hypomagnesemia in children of unaffected Arab parents (37,38). One of the first reported patients, now an affected adult, used calcitriol as an alternative to the parenteral magnesium injections that had been part of his life for more than 20 years and developed hypomagnesemia (39).

- A 22-year-old man, first reported at 4 months of age and currently free of neurological deficits, had had intermittent and chronic diarrhea due to large oral doses of magnesium for hypomagnesemic tetany. On the hypothesis that modest hypercalcemia might prevent the tetany, he was given calcitriol 5 micrograms/day for 5 days. Despite the resultant increase in serum calcium concentration, he developed tetany and a fall in serum magnesium concentration from 0.63 to 0.39 mmol/l (reference range over 0.65 mmol/l). The calcitriol was withdrawn, and 33% of his usual oral magnesium supplement was given by continuous nasogastric infusion; the serum magnesium concentration rose to 0.60 mmol/l.

Mouth and teeth

High doses of vitamin D can affect dental development. In one case, caused by incorrectly fortified milk, there was dental hypoplasia and focal pulp calcification (40).

Pancreas

In patients with pancreatitis associated with hypercalcemia of unclear origin, vitamin D poisoning can be responsible, especially when episodes are recurrent (41). Metastatic calcification of the pancreatic ducts has also been reported (42,43).

Urinary tract

Daily doses of more than 40 micrograms of vitamin D can cause calcium deposition in the kidneys. Renal damage is largely due to this. Tubular function is impaired first, glomerular function later (44,45). Medullary nephrocalcinosis can develop as a result of therapy with high doses of vitamin D combined with calcium; this is mainly seen in infants and schoolchildren. Ultrasound screening of children treated with high doses of vitamin D and calcium is therefore recommended (46). Early high-dosage prophylaxis or treatment can cause nephrocalcinosis and hypercalciuria in children (47,48).

There is controversy about whether the long-term use of C1-hydroxylated vitamin D analogues in non-dialysed patients with chronic renal insufficiency is associated with an impairment of glomerular filtration rate (SEDA-9, 639) (49). Treatment with these drugs should be restricted to patients with severe renal osteodystrophy. A proper dose should be administered in order to avoid a deleterious effect on renal function. Serum calcium and creatinine concentrations should be monitored carefully. The treatment should be withdrawn if hypercalcemia develops.

A comparison between treatment of postmenopausal osteoporosis with calcitriol together with etidronate or calcitonin showed no improvement in spinal bone mineral density, but rather a high rate of adverse events indicating nephrotoxicity (50).

There have been increasing numbers of reports of nephrocalcinosis diagnosed by renal ultrasound in patients with X-linked hypophosphatemia treated with vitamin D and phosphate, and a study of a small group of treated and untreated patients pointed to an association between this therapy and nephrocalcinosis (51).

In a French analysis of 22 510 urinary calculi performed by infrared spectroscopy, drug-induced urolithiasis was divided into two categories: first, stones with drugs physically embedded ($n = 238$; 1.0%), notably indinavir monohydrate ($n = 126$; 53%), followed by triamterene ($n = 43$; 18%), sulfonamides ($n = 29$; 12%), and amorphous silica ($n = 24$; 10%); secondly, metabolic nephrolithiasis induced by drugs ($n = 140$; 0.6%), involving mainly calcium/vitamin D supplementation ($n = 56$; 40%) and carbonic anhydrase inhibitors ($n = 33$; 24%) (52). Drug-induced stones are responsible for about 1.6% of all calculi in France. Physical analysis and a thorough drug history are important elements in the diagnosis.

Skin

The efficacy, safety, and tolerability of twice-daily calcitriol ointment 3 micrograms/g ($n = 60$) has been investigated and compared with 0.25–2% dithranol cream (once daily for 30 minutes; $n = 54$) in an 8-week prospective, randomized, open, parallel-group trial in 114 patients with plaque psoriasis (53). Skin irritation was reported by three patients who used calcitriol and by 39% of those who used dithranol. Three patients who used calcitriol and four who used dithranol reported adverse effects on the skin (pruritus, erythema, rash, dry skin, eczema). One patient with 75% skin involvement used 3.38 mg of calcitriol over 56 days (about 140 g of ointment per week without any effect on serum calcium).

Vitamin D_3 has been reported to cause hyper-reactivity of skin with pseudoxanthoma elasticum (39).

- A 68-year-old woman with pseudoxanthoma elasticum was given oral vitamin D_3 0.25 micrograms/day. After 2 weeks she developed new yellow papules on pre-existing plaques on the neck and abdomen, without itching or pain. Biopsy showed a thicker epidermis and more abundant calcium deposition than in a biopsy before treatment. Electron microscopy showed electron-dense deposits between the degenerated elastic fibers, which had been surrounded by normal collagen fibers

before treatment. After treatment with vitamin D_3 there were lucent areas that suggested unusual mineralization in association with electron-dense deposits. Serum concentrations of calcium were within the reference range throughout.

Musculoskeletal

In children with chronic renal insufficiency, secondary hyperparathyroidism has been treated with intermittent calcitriol therapy. There is some reason to believe that growth is negatively influenced by this therapy, possibly due to the direct inhibitory effects of calcitriol on chondrocyte activity (54).

Of 19 chronic hemodialysis patients taking a combination of alfacalcidol and calcitriol for 12 months, six had increased bone resorption, six had reduced bone resorption, and seven had no change. Histologically documented aggravation of hyperparathyroidism was associated with a statistically significant increase in plasma concentrations of phosphate and parathyroid hormone. The administration of vitamin D analogues may therefore be either beneficial or noxious depending on whether or not induced hyperphosphatemia is adequately prevented (55).

A child with X-linked hypophosphatemic rickets developed vitamin D intoxication during treatment with alfacalcidol and phosphorus. Besides the usual findings in this condition he had precocious synostosis of the skull, with signs of raised intracranial pressure. In view of earlier reports of coincidence of craniostenosis and X-linked hypophosphatemic rickets the authors pointed to the possibility that intoxication with alfacalcidol was the precipitating factor. In addition, hypersensitivity to alfacalcidol was found 2 months after the end of treatment, with normal concentrations of calcitriol (56).

In severe hypervitaminosis D signs of hypomineralization and demineralization of the long bones and calcification of the soft tissues can be seen radiologically. Some cases of hypervitaminosis D with hypercalcemia and acute renal insufficiency have been reported in patients with osteoporosis or osteomalacia who have taken pharmacological doses of vitamin D for extended periods of time. This suggests that such therapy should be avoided. Vitamin D for prophylaxis or treatment of osteoporosis has no benefits greater than those from calcium alone or calcium with estrogens and fluoride (SEDA-14, 332) (57).

Second-Generation Effects

Teratogenicity

High doses of vitamin D during pregnancy, possibly together with genetic factors, can precipitate a severe form of idiopathic hypercalcemia and a clinical abnormality in the offspring, comprising valvular stenosis of the aorta, peculiar facies, mental retardation, and abnormal tooth formation. However, such abnormalities can also occur in the absence of hypervitaminosis D, and the doses needed to treat hypoparathyroidism in pregnancy, for example 100 000 IU/day, have been well tolerated (58,59).

- A 28-year-old woman with hereditary insensitivity to calcitriol took oral calcitriol in doses of 17–36 micrograms/day (usual dose for hypocalcemia 0.25–1.0 micrograms/day) during pregnancy (60). Her serum calcitriol concentration was extraordinarily high throughout gestation. At delivery, the calcium concentration was 2.40 mmol/l in maternal serum and 2.52 mmol/l in cord serum. The concentration of total calcitriol in cord serum was high (470 pg/ml; normal mean for placental venous serum 19 pg/ml); mostly derived from transplacental passage of maternal calcitriol and not from fetoplacental biosynthesis. The child had mild hypercalcemia in the first 2 days of life, showing that the calcitriol measured in the cord serum was active in vivo. The child had no somatic features of the syndrome of elfin facies and supravalvular aortic stenosis.

This case demonstrates that high serum vitamin D concentrations need not be teratogenic, although the maternal metabolite can enter the fetal circulation.

Susceptibility Factors

Age

Neonates with subcutaneous fat necrosis can have transient hypersensitivity to vitamin D (61). There is a relation between the syndrome known as infantile idiopathic hypercalcemia and vitamin D intake and/or vitamin D metabolism (26).

Renal disease

There is increased sensitivity to vitamin D in patients who are undergoing renal dialysis and who have an abnormal calcium/phosphorus ratio. Patients on continuous ambulatory peritoneal dialysis (CAPD) who develop secondary hyperparathyroidism may already have low bone turnover or adynamic bone lesions, and if treated indiscriminately with calcitriol their low bone turnover can get worse (62).

Other features of the patient

There is increased sensitivity to vitamin D in sarcoidosis (63).

Drug Administration

Drug formulations

Calcium combined with colecalciferol in one tablet (Orocal) has been compared with calcium administered in a sachet (Ostram) plus colecalciferol as a separate tablet (Devaron) in 119 elderly women (64). Three patients taking the combined formulation withdrew because of adverse effects (all gastrointestinal disturbances), but none of those taking the separate tablets. Of those taking the combined tablet ($n = 59$) 43 and 39 patients had adverse effects at 6 and 12 months respectively, compared with 46 and 41 of the 60 patients taking separate tablets. For the most part, patients complained

of arthralgia and gastrointestinal complaints. None of the patients had symptomatic calcium nephrolithiasis.

Drug overdose

Fortification of margarine and dairy products with vitamin D is mandatory in some countries, and permitted in others. Infant formula and liquid milk are commonly fortified with vitamin D, and two studies have shown that fortification can be vastly in excess of what is stated on the label (65,66). In one case this was detected when hypervitaminosis D was found in the population. In one case hypercalcemia occurred after prolonged feeding with a premature formula that was higher than normal in vitamin D (67).

Vitamin D intoxication occurred in a 7-week-old infant after an overdose of calcitriol (68).

- A 7-week-old boy lost weight, became dehydrated and apathetic, and developed muscular hypotonia and mild leukocyturia. His serum calcium was 4.1 mmol/l, his urine calcium 3.1 mmol/l, and his serum phosphate 51 micrograms/ml. He had been given vitamin D 200 000 U/day for 30 days in error, instead of the usual 500 U/day. Parathyroid hormone was unmeasurably low. The serum concentration of calcitriol on day 1 was 61 pg/ml (reference range 20–135), and the serum concentrations of calcifediol were 980, 2660, and 8280 ng/l (reference range 100–620) on days 8, 20, and 34 respectively. He was treated with a calcium-free diet, prednisolone, phenobarbital, fluids, and furosemide for 8 weeks. His nephrocalcinosis persisted and after 8 months a large area of suppurative, aseptic, subcutaneous necrosis in the left upper leg perforated. At 2 years of age he was well.

As routine prophylaxis with vitamin D is not entirely safe, because of errors of prescription or dispensing, and because of its narrow therapeutic range one should remember that the daily requirements of 100–400 U are usually met by the fortification of formula milk with 40 U/100 g alone. When an infant is breastfed the mother should ensure that her diet is adequate in vitamin D.

A case of accidental ingestion of a veterinary vitamin D concentrate (colecalciferol in peanut oil; 2 million IU/g) as a cooking oil sheds some light on the mechanism of pathogenesis in hypercalcemia in vitamin D toxicity. Serum concentrations of calcifediol in nine of the cases were 8–15 times greater than the upper limit of the reference range, while total calcitriol concentrations were increased in only three patients. The percentage of unbound calcitriol was increased in all patients, as was the total calcitriol concentration. Increased unbound calcitriol concentrations might play a role in the pathogenesis of hypercalcemia in vitamin D toxicity (69).

Hypercalcemia has been associated with the ingestion of an over-the-counter vitamin D supplement (70).

- A 42-year-old man who for 2 years had taken a supplement containing vitamin D_2 had a serum calcium concentration of 3.75 mmol/l and a serum calcifediol concentration of 487 ng/ml (reference range 9–47). He had normal concentrations of calcitriol, parathyroid hormone, angiotensin-converting enzyme, and thyroid hormone, and had normal bone marrow, radiography, and CT of the chest, neck, and abdomen. Vitamin D_2

was withdrawn and he was rehydrated. He was advised to wear sunscreen at all times when outdoors. Three months after discharge the results of all blood tests were in the reference ranges, including serum concentrations of calcium and calcifediol.

Examination of three lots of the over-the-counter formulations the patient had used showed mean vitamin D contents of 1.3, 13, and 22 mg/g of powder. The patient had taken 3 g/day, or 156 000–2 604 000 IU/day of vitamin D_2, which is about 80–1300 times the recommended safe upper limit of 2000 IU/day.

Drug–Drug Interactions

Anabolic steroids

The combined effects of vitamin D, calcium, and anabolic steroids in the treatment of senile osteoporosis have been investigated (71). Neither methandienone nor vitamin D_3 alone but only the two together seemed to increase coronary morbidity and mortality, and possibly in women only. Simultaneous use of these two drugs should be avoided.

Calcium carbonate

Symptomatic reversible hypercalcemia was seen in two elderly patients taking apparently safe amounts of vitamin D and thiazide diuretics. Their unusual susceptibility to this effect resulted from an interaction with calcium carbonate which had been taken simultaneously. In the presence of other predisposing factors, hypercalcemia can develop in patients taking calcium carbonate 5–10 g/day (72,73).

Enzyme inducers

Anticonvulsants (barbiturates and phenytoin) and other drugs that induce liver enzymes (such as rifampicin) can accelerate the hepatic catabolism of vitamin D and can lead to reduced serum concentrations of calcifediol and osteomalacia. Prophylactic vitamin D treatment of patients taking long-term enzyme inducers can be helpful and should be given at least in cases of anticonvulsant-drug-induced osteomalacia (74,75).

References

1. Goldenberg MM. Paricalcitol, a new agent for the management of secondary hyperparathyroidism in patients undergoing chronic renal dialysis. Clin Ther 1999;21(3):432–41.
2. Portyansky E. New vitamin D analogue arrives for hyperparathyroid patients. Drug Topics 1999;143:16.
3. Sprague SM, Lerma E, McCormmick D, Abraham M, Batlle D. Suppression of parathyroid hormone secretion in hemodialysis patients: comparison of paricalcitol with calcitriol. Am J Kidney Dis 2001;38(5 Suppl 5):S51–6.
4. Roe DA. Nutrient toxicity with excessive intake. NY St J Med 1966;66:869.
5. Fournier A, Pauli A, Cousin J, Barry M, Paoli M, Lefebvre F. Hypercalcémie iatrogène. [Iatrogenic hypercalcemia.] J Sci Med Lille 1967;85(5):319–26.
6. Najjar SS, Yazigi A. Abuse of vitamin D: a report on 15 cases of vitamin D poisoning. J Med Liban 1972;25(1):113–22.
7. Navarro M, Acevedo C, Espinosa L, Pena A, Picazo ML, Larrauri M. Intoxicacion por vitamina D3 y secuelas irreversibles. [Vitamin D3 poisoning and irreversible sequela.] An Esp Pediatr 1985;22(2):99–106.
8. Hoppe B, Gnehm HE, Wopmann M, Neuhaus T, Willi U, Leumann E. Vitamin-D-Intoxikation beim Saugling: eine vermeidbare Ursache von Hypercalciurie und Nephrocalcinose. [Vitamin D poisoning in infants: a preventable cause of hypercalciuria and nephrocalcinosis.] Schweiz Med Wochenschr 1992;122(8):257–62.
9. Saggese G, Baroncelli GI, Bertelloni S. Intossicazione da vitamina D. [Vitamin D poisoning. Physiopathological aspects.] Minerva Pediatr 1986;38(22):1057–60.
10. Misselwitz J, Hesse V. Hypercalzämie nach Vitamin-D Stossprophylaxe. [Hypercalcemia following prophylactic vitamin D administration.] Kinderarztl Prax 1986;54(8):431–8.
11. Schutz RM. Aspekte der Pharmakotherapie im Alter. [Aspects of pharmacotherapy in old age.] Dtsch Med Wochenschr 1993;118(45):1652–4.
12. Blum M, Kirsten M, Worth MH Jr. Reversible hypertension. Caused by the hypercalcemia of hyperparathyroidism, vitamin D toxicity, and calcium infusion. JAMA 1977;237(3):262–3.
13. Okada J, Nomura M, Shirataka M, Kondo H. Prevalence of soft tissue calcifications in patients with SLE and effects of alfacarcidol. Lupus 1999;8(6):456–61.
14. Tsuchihashi K, Takizawa H, Torii T, Ikeda R, Nakahara N, Yuda S, Kobayashi N, Nakata T, Ura N, Shimamoto K. Hypoparathyroidism potentiates cardiovascular complications through disturbed calcium metabolism: possible risk of vitamin D(3) analogue administration in dialysis patients with end-stage renal disease. Nephron 2000;84(1):13–20.
15. Bartolozzi G, Calzolari C, Pela I, Terni M, Cappelli E, Biagini R. Calcificazioni polmonari in corso di intossicazione de vitamina D in un bambino. [Pulmonary calcification in vitamin D poisoning in an infant.] Pediatr Med Chir 1988;10(5):541–2.
16. Anderson DC, Cooper AF, Naylor GJ. Vitamin D intoxication, with hypernatraemia, potassium and water depletion, and mental depression. BMJ 1968;4(633):744–6.
17. Dolmierski R. Zaburzenia psychiczne wywolane hiperwitaminoza D. [Mental disorders caused by hypervitaminosis D.] Neurol Neurochir Psychiatr Pol 1965;15(6):859–62.
18. Dent CE. Dangers of vitamin-D intoxication. BMJ 1964;5386:834.
19. Gegick CG, Danowski TS, De Luca HF, Holick MF. Idiosyncratic reaction to 25-hydroxylated Vitamin D3. Ann Intern Med 1974;80(3):416–17.
20. Bagchi BK, Robinson WD, Bauer JM. Electro encephalographic changes in a case of vitamin D intoxication Med Bull (Ann Arbor) 1957;23(12):439–45.
21. Deluca G, Zecchini A. Il tracciato elletroencefalografico nell'intossicazione da vitamina D. [The electroencephalographic tracing in vitamin D intoxication.] Minerva Pediatr 1964;16:1276–9.
22. Lynch HT, Lemon HM, Henn MJ, Ellingson RJ, Grissom RL. Vitamin D-intoxicated patient with hypoparathyroidism; hypercalcemia, acute cerebellar ataxia, and EEG changes: magnesium sulfate therapy. Arch Intern Med 1964;114:375–80.
23. Gifford ES Jr, Maguire EF. Band keratopathy in vitamin D intoxication; report of a case. AMA Arch Ophthalmol 1954;52(1):106–7.
24. Severin M, Bulla M. Hornhautablagerung bei Kindern mit Dialysebehandlung unter einer Therapie mit Vitamin D3 und 1,25 Dihydroxy-Cholecalciferol. [Corneal deposits in children

on dialysis and treatment with vitamin D3 and 1,25 DHCC.] Klin Monatsbl Augenheilkd 1979;175(5):670–6.

25. Cohen HN, Fogelman I, Boyle IT, Doig JA. Deafness due to hypervitaminosis D. Lancet 1979;1(8123):985.

26. Fraser D. The relation between infantile hypercalcemia and vitamin D—public health implications in North America. Pediatrics 1967;40(6):1050–61.

27. Verhaegen H. Lésions gastriques dans l'hypercalcémie iatrogène. [Gastric lesions in iatrogenic hypercalcemia.] Acta Gastroenterol Belg 1966;29(5):529–34.

28. Chan JC, Young RB, Alon U, Mamunes P. Hypercalcemia in children with disorders of calcium and phosphate metabolism during long-term treatment with 1,25-dihydroxy-vitamin-D3. Pediatrics 1983;72(2):225–33.

29. Hodson EM, Evans RA, Dunstan CR, Hills E, Wong SY, Rosenberg AR, Roy LP. Treatment of childhood renal osteodystrophy with calcitriol or ergocalciferol. Clin Nephrol 1985;24(4):192–200.

30. Delmez JA, Kelber J, Norwood KY, Giles KS, Slatopolsky E. A controlled trial of the early treatment of secondary hyperparathyroidism with calcitriol in hemodialysis patients. Clin Nephrol 2000;54(4):301–8.

31. Bosch B, Plank C, Rascher W, Dötsch J. Hyperkalzämie als Folge einer hoch dosierten Vitamin-D-Therapie bei terminaler Niereninsuffizienz. Monatsschr Kinderheilk 2002;150:1508–12.

32. Slatopolsky E, Brown AJ. Vitamin D analogues for the treatment of secondary hyperparathyroidism Blood Purif 2002;20(1):109–12.

33. Meyrier A, Marsac J, Richet G. The influence of a high calcium carbonate intake on bone disease in patients undergoing hemodialysis. Kidney Int 1973;4(2):146–53.

34. Blind E, Fassnacht M, Korber C, Korber-Hafner N, Reiners C, Allolio B. Schwere vitamin-D(dihydrotachysterol)-Intoxikation mit spontan reversibler Anämie und bisphosphonat-responsiver Hyperkalziämie. [Severe vitamin D(dihydrotachysterol)-intoxication with temporary anemia and hypercalcemia responsive to bisphosphonates.] Dtsch Med Wochenschr 2001;126(12):T21–4.

35. Evliyaoglu O, Berberoglu M, Ocal G, Adiyaman P, Aycan Z. Severe hypercalcemia of an infant due to vitamin D toxicity associated with hypercholesterolemia. J Pediatr Endocrinol Metab 2001;14(7):915–19.

36. Cole DEC, Carpenter TO, Goltzman D. Calcium homeostasis and disorders of bone and mineral metabolism. In: Collu R, Ducharna JR, Guyda HJ, editors. Pediatric Eudocrinology. 2nd ed. New York: Raven Press, 1989:509–80.

37. Abdulrazzaq YM, Smigura FC, Wettrell G. Primary infantile hypomagnesaemia; report of two cases and review of literature. Eur J Pediatr 1989;148(5):459–61.

38. Dudin KI, Teebi AS. Primary hypomagnesaemia. A case report and literature review. Eur J Pediatr 1987;146(3):303–5.

39. Hamamoto Y, Nagai K, Yasui H, Muto M. Hyperreactivity of pseudoxanthoma elasticum-affected dermis to vitamin D3. J Am Acad Dermatol 2000;42(4):685–7.

40. Giunta JL. Dental changes in hypervitaminosis D. Oral Surg Oral Med Oral Pathol Oral Radiol Endod 1998;85(4):410–13.

41. Waele BD, Smitz J, Willems G. Recurrent pancreatitis secondary to hypercalcemia following vitamin D poisoning. Pancreas 1989;4(3):378–80.

42. Leeson PM, Fourman P. Increased sensitivity to vitamin D after vitamin-D poisoning. Lancet 1966;1(118):2.

43. Leeson PM, Fourman P. Acute pancreatitis from vitamin-D poisoning in a patient with parathyroid deficiency. Lancet 1966;1:1185.

44. Barrucand D, Mayer G, Mollet E. Néphropathie hypercalcémique après traitement d'un hypoparathyroidisme primitif. Ann Méd Nancy 1968;7(1311).

45. Pereda JM, Arnal P, Cavanilles JM, Gonzalez Miranda F, Facal JL. Intoxicación por vitamina D con nefrocalcinosis radiológicamente visible. [Vitamin D intoxication with radiologically visible nephrocalcinosis.] Rev Clin Esp 1968;110(1):61–4.

46. Guckel C, Benz-Bohm G, Roth B. Die nephrokalzinose in Kindesalter. Sonographische Befunde und Differentialdiagnostik. [Nephrocalcinosis in childhood. Sonographic findings and differential diagnosis.] Rofo 1989;151(3):301–5.

47. Misselwitz J, Hesse V, Markestad T. Nephrocalcinosis, hypercalciuria and elevated serum levels of 1,25-dihydroxy-vitamin D in children. Possible link to vitamin D toxicity. Acta Paediatr Scand 1990;79(6–7):637–43.

48. Weber G, Cazzuffi MA, Frisone F, de Angelis M, Pasolini D, Tomaselli V, Chiumello G. Nephrocalcinosis in children and adolescents: sonographic evaluation during long-term treatment with 1,25-dihydroxycholecalciferol. Child Nephrol Urol 1988–89;9(5):273–6.

49. Kanis JA, Cundy T, Naik R. 1alpha-hydroxy derivatives of vitamin D3 and renal function. Lancet 1978;2(8084):316–17.

50. Gurlek A, Bayraktar M, Gedik O. Comparison of calcitriol treatment with etidronate–calcitriol and calcitonin–calcitriol combinations in Turkish women with postmenopausal osteoporosis: a prospective study. Calcif Tissue Int 1997;61(1):39–43.

51. Taylor A, Sherman NH, Norman ME. Nephrocalcinosis in X-linked hypophosphatemia: effect of treatment versus disease. Pediatr Nephrol 1995;9(2):173–5.

52. Cohen-Solal F, Abdelmoula J, Hoarau MP, Jungers P, Lacour B, Daudon M. Les lithiases urinaires d'origine medicamenteuse. [Urinary lithiasis of medical origin.] Therapie 2001;56(6):743–50.

53. Hutchinson PE, Marks R, White J. The efficacy, safety and tolerance of calcitriol 3 microg/g ointment in the treatment of plaque psoriasis: a comparison with short-contact dithranol. Dermatology 2000;201(2):139–45.

54. Kuizon BD, Salusky IB. Intermittent calcitriol therapy and growth in children with chronic renal failure. Miner Electrolyte Metab 1998;24(4):290–5.

55. Coevoet B, Sebert JL, DeGueris J, et al. Adverse effect of vitamin D metabolites on osteitis fibrosa in patients on chronic hemodialysis: critical role of induced hyperphosphatemia. Miner Electrolyte Metab 1979;2:217.

56. Carlsen NL, Krasilnikoff PA, Eiken M. Premature cranial synostosis in X-linked hypophosphatemic rickets: possible precipitation by 1-alpha-OH-cholecalciferol intoxication. Acta Paediatr Scand 1984;73(1):149–54.

57. Schwartzman MS, Franck WA. Vitamin D toxicity complicating the treatment of senile, postmenopausal, and glucocorticoid-induced osteoporosis. Four case reports and a critical commentary on the use of vitamin D in these disorders. Am J Med 1987;82(2):224–30.

58. Ruby LK, Mital MA. Skeletal deformities following chronic hypervitaminosis A; a case report. J Bone Joint Surg Am 1974;56(6):1283–7.

59. Nishimura H, Tanimura T. Clinical Aspects of the Teratogenicity of Drugs. Amsterdam, Oxford: Excerpta Medica, 1976:251.

60. Marx SJ, Swart EG Jr, Hamstra AJ, DeLuca HF. Normal intrauterine development of the fetus of a woman receiving extraordinarily high doses of 1,25-dihydroxyvitamin D3. J Clin Endocrinol Metab 1980;51(5):1138–42.

61. Wehinger H. Spätrachitis nach Vitamin-D-Überempfindlichkeit bei Adiponekrosis subcutanea in der Neugeborenenperiode. [Vitamin D deficiency rickets after vitamin D hypersensitivity with subcutaneous fat necrosis in the newborn period.] Z Kinderheilkd 1969;107(1):42–52.

62. Delmez JA. Calcitriol and secondary hyperparathyroidism in continuous ambulatory peritoneal dialysis patients. Perit Dial Int 1993;13(2):95–7.

63. Bell NH, Bartter FC. Studies of 47-Ca metabolism in sarcoidosis: evidence for increased sensitivity of bone to vitamin D. Acta Endocrinol (Copenh) 1967;54(1):173–80.

64. Deroisy R, Collette J, Chevallier T, Breuil V, Reginster JY. Effects of two 1-year calcium and vitamin D3 treatments on bone remodeling markers and femoral bone density in elderly women. Curr Ther Res Clin Exp 1998;59:850–62.

65. Jacobus CH, Holick MF, Shao Q, Chen TC, Holm IA, Kolodny JM, Fuleihan GE, Seely EW. Hypervitaminosis D associated with drinking milk. N Engl J Med 1992;326(18):1173–7.

66. Holick MF, Shao Q, Liu WW, Chen TC. The vitamin D content of fortified milk and infant formula. N Engl J Med 1992;326(18):1178–81.

67. Nako Y, Fukushima N, Tomomasa T, Nagashima K, Kuroume T. Hypervitaminosis D after prolonged feeding with a premature formula. Pediatrics 1993;92(6):862–4.

68. v Muhlendahl KE, Nawracala J. Vitamin D intoxication. Eur J Pediatr 1999;158(3):266.

69. Pettifor JM, Bikle DD, Cavaleros M, Zachen D, Kamdar MC, Ross FP. Serum levels of free 1,25-dihydroxy-vitamin D in vitamin D toxicity. Ann Intern Med 1995;122(7):511–13.

70. Koutkia P, Chen TC, Holick MF. Vitamin D intoxication associated with an over-the-counter supplement. N Engl J Med 2001;345(1):66–7.

71. Inkovaara J, Gothoni G, Halttula R, Heikinheimo R, Tokola O. Calcium, vitamin D and anabolic steroid in treatment of aged bones: double-blind placebo-controlled long-term clinical trial. Age Ageing 1983;12(2):124–30.

72. Crowe M, Wollner L, Griffiths RA. Hypercalcaemia following vitamin D and thiazide therapy in the elderly. Practitioner 1984;228(1389):312–13.

73. Drinka PJ, Nolten WE. Hazards of treating osteoporosis and hypertension concurrently with calcium, vitamin D, and distal diuretics. J Am Geriatr Soc 1984;32(5):405–7.

74. Hahn TJ. Drug-induced disorders of vitamin D and mineral metabolism. Clin Endocrinol Metab 1980;9(1):107–27.

75. Krause KH, Bohn T, Schmidt-Gayk H, Prager P, Ritz E. Zur prophylaktischen Gabe von Vitamin D2 und D3 bei Anfallskranken. [Prophylactic treatment of epileptic patients with vitamin D2 and D3. Results of a comparative study of 86 patients.] Nervenarzt 1978;49(3):174–80.

Vitamin E

See also Vitamins

General Information

Vitamin E is a family of compounds that include several different isomers of tocopherols and tocotrienols, of which the most important is thought to be alpha-tocopherol, the form of vitamin E that has mostly been used in clinical trials (1). The actions of the different isoforms have not been fully elucidated.

It was suggested many years ago that vitamin E could be useful in patients with peripheral arterial disease, but the evidence is meager and incomplete. Nowadays, vitamin E is expected to have a role in the prevention of atherosclerosis, through inhibition of oxidation of low-density lipoprotein. The hypothesis that oxidative modification of low-density lipoprotein contributes to the progression of atherosclerosis is supported by an impressive amount of in vitro and animal data. Some epidemiological studies have associated high dietary intake or high serum concentrations of alpha-tocopherol with a reduced risk of cardiovascular events. Large intervention studies with clinical endpoints have tested the hypothesis that daily supplementation with a high dose of alpha-tocopherol reduces ischemic vascular events. In over 2000 patients there was a substantial reduction in non-fatal myocardial infarction, but not in cardiovascular deaths (2). Daily administration of 400 and 800 IU of vitamin E was well tolerated, and only 11 patients stopped treatment because of diarrhea, dyspepsia, or a rash. Withdrawals due to adverse effects were equally distributed between the placebo group and the two treatment groups.

Since vitamin E requirements depend on dietary polyunsaturated fatty acids, which vary considerably between individuals, it has not been seen as expedient to establish a single Population Reference Intake value.

General adverse effects

Several reviews of the adverse effects of vitamin E have been published (3,4), especially relating to premature infants (5), in whom high doses have been associated with infectious complications and fatal hepatic failure. In adults, thrombophlebitis, thromboembolism, pulmonary embolism, hypertension, fatigue, gynecomastia, and breast tumors have been described as particularly serious effects of vitamin E, but there is little evidence about their frequency. Diarrhea and abdominal pain can occur. For some of these effects there seems to be a dose relation. A dose of 800 mg/day for 30 days had no reported adverse effects in healthy elderly subjects (6). Table 1 shows reported adverse effects related to dosage in a review of about 50 publications on vitamin E (7).

Organs and Systems

Cardiovascular

Vitamin E 300 mg/day can increase serum cholesterol by an average of 1.9 mmol/l (74 mg/100 ml) (8). It is therefore advisable to use vitamin E with caution in patients with a family history of heart disease. Some studies have shown that vitamin E can prevent atherosclerosis and serious adverse events were not reported in these studies (2,9,10).

Hematologic

Significant depression of bactericidal activity of leukocytes and mitogen-induced lymphocyte transformation occurred after the administration of dl-tocopherol 300 mg/day for 3 weeks (11).

Reduced platelet adhesion to collagen has been described (12), and experimentally confirmed (13) and has been seen with doses of vitamin E from 400 mg/day (14).

Table 1 Adverse effects of high doses of vitamin E

Dosage (mg/day)	Symptoms or changes
	Clinical effects
>300	Gastrointestinal irritation, nausea, vomiting, headache, muscular weakness, dizziness, stomatitis, visual complaints
400	Thrombophlebitis, urticaria, vaginal bleeding
800	Faintness, fatigue, creatinuria
1200	Ecchymoses
1600	Deterioration of angina pectoris
Unknown	Deterioration of diabetes mellitus
Unknown	Transient hypertension
Unknown	Allergic contact dermatitis
Unknown	Gynecomastia, breast cancer
	Laboratory findings
300	Increased concentrations of lipids, cholesterol, carotenoids, and coagulation factors
>300	Reduced incorporation of thymidine into phytohemagglutinin-stimulated lymphocytes, reduced bactericidal activity of leukocytes, and reduced blood glucose concentrations
600	Decreased concentrations of triiodothyronine and thyroxine in serum
600	Increased concentrations of free cholesterol in LDL and VLVD fractions
800	Increased serum creatine kinase, creatinuria
1000	Increased excretion of steroids in the urine
1200	Increased warfarin action
Unknown	Increased dehydroepiandrosterone concentrations in blood
Unknown	Increased gonadotrophin concentrations

Skin

Although there is no proof of any beneficial effects of topical use of vitamin E, it continues to be popular. Allergic contact dermatitis has been reported rarely (15).

Susceptibility Factors

Age

Premature neonates are reported to have a relative deficiency of vitamin E at birth, which has been associated with hemolytic anemia (16). Since there was an increased incidence of necrotizing enterocolitis when oral tocopherol was given to such infants (7,8,17,18), parenteral tocopherol was for a while recommended for use in very ill neonates (19,20).

There were increasing numbers of commonly fatal cases of the so-called "E-Ferol syndrome" during the 1980s (SEDA-12, 329) (21), a condition characterized by progressive unexplained thrombocytopenia, renal dysfunction, cholestasis, and ascites (22). E-Ferol was an intravenous vitamin E formulation, but the syndrome was subsequently shown to be due to polysorbate 80, which was used as an emulsifier in the formulation (23–25).

Preterm infants receiving under 25 mg/kg/day of tocopherol acetate intravenously had highly variable serum tocopherol concentrations. High serum concentrations correlated with the occurrence of necrotizing enterocolitis (26).

An increased incidence of infection, even sepsis after intramuscular injection, as an adverse effect of megadose vitamin E therapy in very low birth weight infants was first reported in Japan in 1986 (SEDA-12, 330). In a review of the literature in 1992 it was concluded that pharmacological serum concentrations of vitamin E might predispose premature infants to infectious complications, possibly caused by an inhibitory effect of vitamin E on the formation of superoxide anion in leukocytes (27).

There was a statistically significant increase in the risk of retinal hemorrhage with parenteral vitamin E in premature infants (28). This has led some researchers to conclude that tocopherol should not be recommended for the prevention of retinopathy in prematurity (29), particularly in infants with birth weights of less than 1 kg.

Other features of the patient

An increased tendency towards gingival bleeding was noted in a recent 7-year prospective study of smokers who had been given alpha-tocopherol supplementation in comparison with non-receivers. Acetylsalicylic acid further increased the risk of bleeding.

Drug–Drug Interactions

Acetylsalicylic acid

Alpha-tocopherol supplementation may increase the risk of clinically significant bleeding, particularly when it is combined with acetylsalicylic acid (30). Although acetylsalicylic acid and its derivatives are widely used, reliable pharmacoepidemiological data about drug usage frequency in the population are sparse. Among reports of serious adverse effects resulting from acetylsalicylic acid and other salicylates (31–37), of special interest are potential adverse effects in those who concurrently take vitamin E formulations (38,39).

The first pharmacoepidemiological survey was published in 1995, covering data from 1984 to 1988 (40), and the population-based data collected in Germany from 1984 to 1999 have been analysed, including data from five epidemiological surveys, concerning total drug usage, physiological, clinical chemistry and hematological data, and information about the serum concentrations of active drugs and/or their metabolites (40). The data were analysed with regard to the usage of salicylates and drugs with potential interactions relevant to the highly sensitive balance between hemostasis and bleeding. Special attention was paid to serum concentrations of the various tocopherols, because of their potential activity in anticoagulation processes (39,41,42).

The data are representative of the resident population aged 25–69 years in the first four surveys and the age group 18–79 years in the last (1997–99), covering more than 20 000 study participants.

Patient drug usage data for the 7 days before the clinical examination were recorded using a standardized questionnaire in all the surveys (40). Measurements of salicylic acid and tocopherols were by HPLC with fluorescence detection or GC/MS (43).

In male users of salicylates and vitamin E the frequency of co-medication with lipid lowering drugs was 14%, with cardiovascular drugs 11%, and with analgesics 9%. Of female users of salicylates and vitamin E, 23% also took mineral products, 11% thyroid drugs, 10% estrogens, and 9% beta-blockers.

In all surveys salicylate use was higher in women (14%) than men (12%). Owing to massive advertising, vitamin E consumption has risen since the first survey, and was 5.6% in women and 3.6% in men in the German population aged 18–79 years (survey 1997–99). Co-medication with salicylates was observed in 17% of the vitamin E users (55% women, 45% men) and 90% of the reported concomitant use was in those over 50 years.

Mean salicylate concentrations in those who used acetylsalicylic acid as an analgesic were 8.3 µmol/l in 1985, and 16.5 µmol/l in 1988, 1991, and 1998, while salicylate concentrations in subjects who used acetylsalicylic acid as an antiplatelet drug fell from 9.8 µg/ml in 1985 to 7.8 µg/ml in 1988, 3.0 µg/ml in 1991, and 0.8 µg/ml in 1998. This fall in serum salicylate concentrations reflects changes in the usual dose of acetylsalicylic acid.

In contrast the mean concentrations of α-tocopherol in vitamin E users increased from 28 µmol/l in 1985 to 29 µmol/l in 1988, 35 µmol/l in 1991, and 56 µmol/l in 1998. Controls not taking any medications had much lower serum concentrations of α-tocopherol (7.5, 9.8, 11.8, and 18.3 µg/ml). Concentrations of β-tocopherol, γ- tocopherol, and δ-tocopherol in users of vitamin E were lower by up to 50% in users of vitamin E formulations. From these data the authors concluded that there is a considerable risk in the availability of over-the-counter drugs, especially those that can affect the balance between blood clotting and hemorrhage, such as salicylates and α-tocopherol. Since women over 40 in particular tend to use so-called dietary supplements, in the belief that such products might prevent illness, and because there is unrestricted advertising in the mass media, physicians should obtain a clear medication history from their patients.

The fact that blood concentrations of β-tocopherol, γ-tocopherol, and δ-tocopherol are lowered by α-tocopherol (42) should be taken into account in investigations on the clotting and bleeding balance and in cancer research.

Oral anticoagulants

Vitamin E therapy in vitamin K-deficient subjects and subjects taking anticoagulants reduces active plasma prothrombin concentrations (44).

There have been two cases of coagulation disorders with the herbal drug cucurbicin, each tablet of which contains vitamin E 10 mg (45). Cucurbicin is an approved herbal drug in Sweden, traditionally used for micturition difficulties. The active components are extracts from the fruit of *Serenoa repens* and the seed of *Cucurbita pepo*.

- A 73-year-old man with a common cold, who had been taking cucurbicin three tablets daily for more than 1 year, developed a coagulation disorder, with an international normalized ratio (INR) of 2.1, despite a normal albumin concentration and no anticoagulant treatment. His INR improved to 1.4 on treatment with vitamin K, but did not normalize until cucurbicin was withdrawn 1 week later.

- A 61-year-old man, who had taken warfarin and simvastatin for a long time and had an INR of 2.4, started to take cucurbicin five tablets daily for micturition difficulties. After 6 days his INR had increased to 3.4. After withdrawal of cucurbicin the INR returned to the previous value within 1 week.

No anticoagulant effect has been reported with either of the major components of cucurbicin. However, vitamin E antagonizes the effect of vitamin K and can cause an increased risk of bleeding, especially in patients taking oral anticoagulants. The amount of vitamin E in cucurbicin that these two patients consumed was 30–50 mg/day, corresponding to the recommended dose of 40–50 mg daily for vitamin E deficiency. The two cases suggest that caution should be exercised when cucurbicin is used concurrently with warfarin.

References

1. Schneider M, Verges B, Klein A, Miller ER, Deckert V, Desrumaux C, Masson D, Gambert P, Brun JM, Fruchart-Najib J, Blache D, Witztum JL, Lagrost L. Alterations in plasma vitamin E distribution in type 2 diabetic patients with elevated plasma phospholipid transfer protein activity. Diabetes 2004;53(10):2633–9.
2. Stephens NG, Parsons A, Schofield PM, Kelly F, Cheeseman K, Mitchinson MJ. Randomised controlled trial of vitamin E in patients with coronary disease: Cambridge Heart Antioxidant Study (CHAOS). Lancet 1996;347(9004):781–6.
3. Roberts HJ. Perspective on vitamin E as therapy. JAMA 1981;246(2):129–31.
4. Hale WE, Perkins LL, May FE, Marks RG, Stewart RB. Vitamin E effect on symptoms and laboratory values in the elderly. J Am Diet Assoc 1986;86(5):625–9.
5. Balistreri WF, Farrell MK, Bove KE. Lessons from the E-Ferol tragedy. Pediatrics 1986;78(3):503–6.
6. Meydani SN, Meydani M, Rall LC, Morrow F, Blumberg JB. Assessment of the safety of high-dose, short-term supplementation with vitamin E in healthy older adults. Am J Clin Nutr 1994;60(5):704–9.
7. Elmadfa IE. Nutzen und Gefahren hochdosierter Vitamin E-Präparate. Fette, Seifen, Anstrichmittel 1985;87:571.
8. Nako Y, Fukushima N, Tomomasa T, Nagashima K, Kuroume T. Hypervitaminosis D after prolonged feeding with a premature formula. Pediatrics 1993;92(6):862–4.
9. Stampfer MJ, Hennekens CH, Manson JE, Colditz GA, Rosner B, Willett WC. Vitamin E consumption and the

risk of coronary disease in women. N Engl J Med 1993;328(20):1444–9.

10. Rimm EB, Stampfer MJ, Ascherio A, Giovannucci E, Colditz GA, Willett WC. Vitamin E consumption and the risk of coronary heart disease in men. N Engl J Med 1993;328(20):1450–6.

11. Prasad JS. Effect of vitamin E supplementation on leukocyte function. Am J Clin Nutr 1980;33(3):606–8.

12. Steiner M. Effect of alpha-tocopherol administration on platelet function in man. Thromb Haemost 1983;49(2):73–7.

13. Jandok J, Steiner M. An effective inhibitor of platelet adhesion. Blood 1986;68:1153.

14. Srivastava KC. Vitamin E exerts antiaggregatory effects without inhibiting the enzymes of the arachidonic acid cascade in platelets. Prostaglandins Leukot Med 1986; 21(2):177–85.

15. Bazzano C, de Angeles S, Kleist G, Macedo N. Allergic contact dermatitis from topical vitamins A and E. Contact Dermatitis 1996;35(4):261–2.

16. Oski FA, Barness LA. Vitamin E deficiency: a previously unrecognized cause of hemolytic anemia in the premature infant. J Pediatr 1967;70(2):211–20.

17. Finer NN, Peters KL, Hayek Z, Merkel CL. Vitamin E and necrotizing enterocolitis. Pediatrics 1984;73(3):387–93.

18. Johnson L, Bowen P, Herman N. The relationship of prolonged elevation of serum vitamin E levels to neonatal bacterial sepsis (SEP) and necrotizing enterocolitis (NAC). Pediatr Res 1983;17:319A.

19. Pantoja A, Ukrainski C, Belendy D, et al. Vitamin E kinetics in children 1500 grams: intramusculair vs oral administration. Pediatr Res 1984;18:371A.

20. Phelps DL, Pool W, Bauernfeld JC, et al. Safety of intravascular tocopherol in a randomized double-blind trial in premature infants. Pediatr Res 1984;18:158A.

21. Jacobus CH, Holick MF, Shao Q, Chen TC, Holm IA, Kolodny JM, Fuleihan GE, Seely EW. Hypervitaminosis D associated with drinking milk. N Engl J Med 1992;326(18):1173–7.

22. Bove KE, Kosmetatos N, Wedig KE, Frank DJ, Whitlatch S, Saldivar V, Haas J, Bodenstein C, Balistreri WF. Vasculopathic hepatotoxicity associated with E-Ferol syndrome in low-birth-weight infants. JAMA 1985;254(17):2422–30.

23. Varma RK, Kaushal R, Junnarkar AY, Thomas GP, Naidu MU, Singh PP, Tripathi RM, Shridhar DR. Polysorbate 80: a pharmacological study. Arzneimittelforschung 1985;35(5):804–8.

24. Arrowsmith JB, Faich GA, Tomita DK, Kuritsky JN, Rosa FW. Morbidity and mortality among low birth weight infants exposed to an intravenous vitamin E product, E-Ferol. Pediatrics 1989;83(2):244–9.

25. Pesce AJ, McKean DL. Toxic susceptibilities in the newborn with special consideration of polysorbate toxicity. Ann Clin Lab Sci 1989;19(1):70–3.

26. Friedman CA, Wender DF, Temple DM, Parks BR, Rawson JE. Serum alpha-tocopherol concentrations in preterm infants receiving less than 25 mg/kg/day alpha-tocopherol acetate supplements. Dev Pharmacol Ther 1988;11(5):273–80.

27. Mino M. Clinical uses and abuses of vitamin E in children. Proc Soc Exp Biol Med 1992;200(2):266–70.

28. Rosenbaum AL, Phelps DL, Isenberg SJ, Leake RD, Dorey F. Retinal hemorrhage in retinopathy of prematurity associated with tocopherol treatment. Ophthalmology 1985;92(8):1012–14.

29. Phelps DL, Rosenbaum AL, Isenberg SJ, Leake RD, Dorey FJ. Tocopherol efficacy and safety for preventing retinopathy of prematurity: a randomized, controlled, double-masked trial. Pediatrics 1987;79(4):489–500.

30. Melchert HU, Knopf H, Pabel E, Braemer-Hauth M, Du Y. Co- and multimedication in users of ASA and vitamin E drugs in the Federal Republic of Germany. Results of the Federal Health Surveys 1984–1999. Int J Clin Pharmacol Ther 2001;39(11):488–91.

31. Derry S, Loke YK. Risk of gastrointestinal haemorrhage with long term use of aspirin: meta-analysis. BMJ 2000;321(7270):1183–7.

32. Jang AS. Severe reaction to lysine aspirin. Allergy 2000;55(11):1092–3.

33. Janssen T, Boege P, Oestreicher E, Arnold W. Tinnitus and 2f1-f2 distortion product otoacoustic emissions following salicylate overdose. J Acoust Soc Am 2000; 107(3):1790–2.

34. Karabulut AK, Ulger H, Pratten MK. Protection by free oxygen radical scavenging enzymes against salicylate-induced embryonic malformations in vitro. Toxicol In Vitro 2000;14(4):297–307.

35. Manfredini R, Ricci L, Giganti M, La Cecilia O, Kuwornu Afi H, Chierici F, Gallerani M. An uncommon case of fluid retention simulating a congestive heart failure after aspirin consumption. Am J Med Sci 2000; 320(1):72–4.

36. Tramer MR. Aspirin, like all other drugs, is a poison. BMJ 2000;321(7270):1170–1.

37. Wong KS, Mok V, Lam WW, Kay R, Tang A, Chan YL, Woo J. Aspirin-associated intracerebral hemorrhage: clinical and radiologic features. Neurology 2000; 54(12):2298–301.

38. Abate A, Yang G, Dennery PA, Oberle S, Schroder H. Synergistic inhibition of cyclooxygenase-2 expression by vitamin E and aspirin. Free Radic Biol Med 2000; 29(11):1135–42.

39. Liede KE, Haukka JK, Saxen LM, Heinonen OP. Increased tendency towards gingival bleeding caused by joint effect of alpha-tocopherol supplementation and acetylsalicylic acid. Ann Med 1998;30(6):542–6.

40. Melchert HU, Gorsch B, Hoffmeister H. Nicht-stationäre Arzneimittelanwendung und subjektive Arzneimittelverträglichkeit in der bundesdeutschen Wohnbevölkerung der 25–69-Jährigen—Ergebnisse der Erhebung des ersten nationalen Untersuchungs-Surveys 1984–1986. RKI-Schrift 195. Munchen: MMV Medizin-Verlag, 1995.

41. Melchert HU, Pabel E. Verbrauch acetylsalicylhaltiger Präparate im ersten und zweiten Durchgang des Nationalen Untersuchungs-Surveys. Tätigkeitsbericht 1991 des Bundesgesundheitsamtes. Munchen: MMV Medizin-Verlag, 1992:262–4.

42. Melchert HU, Pabel E. The tocopherol pattern in human serum is markedly influenced by intake of vitamin E drugs—Results of the German National Health Surveys. J Am Oil Chem Soc 1998;75:213–6.

43. Melchert HU, Pabel E. Quantitative determination of alpha-, beta-, gamma- and delta-tocopherols in human serum by high-performance liquid chromatography and gas chromatography-mass spectrometry as trimethylsilyl derivatives with a two-step sample preparation. J Chromatogr A 2000;896(1–2):209–15.

44. Helson L. The effect of intravenous vitamin E and menadiol sodium diphosphate on vitamin K dependent clotting factors. Thromb Res 1984;35(1):11–18.

45. Yue QY, Jansson K. Herbal drug curbicin and anticoagulant effect with and without warfarin: possibly related to the vitamin E component. J Am Geriatr Soc 2001; 49(6):838.

Vitamin K analogues

See also Vitamins

General Information

Vitamin K is the name of a group of compounds, all of which contain the 2-methyl-1,4-naphthoquinone moiety. Common nomenclature is:

- vitamin K_1 (phytomenadione; rINN)
- vitamin K_2 (phytonadione; rINN)
- vitamin K_3 (menadione; rINN).

Vitamin K is routinely administered in many countries to newborn babies in varying doses and by various routes, most commonly either orally or by intramuscular injection, to prevent hemorrhagic disease of the newborn (see Table 1).

Phytomenadione given intravenously is generally tolerated well. However, intravenous administration of small amounts (2–5 mg) can be followed by severe short-lasting cyanosis, dyspnea, tachycardia, and low blood pressure in patients with cardiac failure. Flushing and sweating can occur. Anaphylactoid reactions may be due to the excipient Cremophor EL. The most important adverse effects are jaundice and kernicterus, which can occur in small and premature babies, even after small doses, probably because of immature liver function.

Organs and Systems

Cardiovascular

Results of intravenous administration of 100 sequential doses of vitamin K in 45 patients (34 men, 11 women) have been retrospectively reviewed (1). Vitamin K_1 was administered as Aquamephyton. The dose averaged 9.7 (range 1–20) mg. The mean age was 44 (range 18–66) years. Many of the patients were seriously ill and had significant underlying surgical and medical problems, as evidenced by the fact that 16 died. However, none of the deaths was attributable to vitamin K. In the 11 instances in which the duration of administration was noted, the mean time was 49 (range 12.5–60) minutes. Only one patient had an episode of transient hypotension.

- A 37-year-old man with a history of ethanol abuse presented with hepatic failure and non-cardiogenic pulmonary edema after an overdose of paracetamol, codeine, ibuprofen, and diazepam. He received two doses of Aquamephyton (phytonadione) over 2 days and 10 minutes after the second dose his blood pressure fell to 79/40 mmHg.

In this study the incidence of adverse effects was 1%, contrasting with the impression that one obtains from reading the medical literature on vitamin K, which suggests an overall incidence of less than 1%.

Nervous system

Kernicterus can occur in small and premature babies, even after small doses of vitamin K, probably because of immature liver function. In its 1997 clinical practice guidelines, the Canadian Paediatric Society recommended that, in order to prevent haemorrhagic disease of the newborn, phytomenadione be given as a single intramuscular injection to all newborns within 6 hours of birth, in a dose of 1 mg for infants with a birth weight of more than 1500 g and half this dose for smaller infants. The dose is crucial, since overdosage carries a serious risk of kernicterus, especially in premature infants. There is only a remote possibility that this treatment might increase the risk of childhood cancer.

Cerebral vein thrombosis developed after the administration of 10 mg of phytomenadione in two patients with chronic intestinal inflammation assumed to be part of an autoimmune disease (2).

Hematologic

High doses of vitamin K can occasionally cause hemolytic anemia (3).

Severe hemolysis has been attributed to vitamin K in patients with glucose-6-phosphate dehydrogenase deficiency, particularly if infection is present (4,5).

In severe hepatocellular disease the prothrombin concentration can be further depressed by high doses of vitamin K (6,7).

Skin

Skin reactions have been observed after intramuscular injection of phytomenadione.

Presentation
The English-language literature on adverse skin reactions associated with intramuscular or subcutaneous phytomenadione has been reviewed (8). Vitamin K is generally well tolerated subcutaneously or intramuscularly. However, erythematous eczematous plaques have been well documented. Of 39 skin reactions due to

Table 1 Classification of hemorrhagic disease of the newborn

Syndrome	Time of presentation	Common bleeding sites	Comments
Early disease	0–24 hours	Cephalohematoma, intracranial, intrathoracic, intra-abdominal	Maternal drugs a frequent cause (for example warfarin, anticonvulsants)
Classic disease	1–7 days	Gastrointestinal, skin, nasal, circumcision	Mainly idiopathic, maternal drugs
Late disease	2–12 weeks	Intracranial, skin, gastrointestinal	Mainly idiopathic, can be the presenting feature of an underlying disease (for example cystic fibrosis, α_1-antitrypsin deficiency, biliary atresia; there is often some degree of cholestasis

phytomenadione, 32 were eczematous and 91% of the patients were women, average age 39 (range 9–64) years; in four cases there were small vesicles within the plaques (9–12).

As a rule, only a rash occurs, generally after high doses of the oil-soluble analogue. However, intramuscular injection of phytomenadione can also cause lumbar scleroderma around the injection site. The scleroderma is reported to develop in four stages; erythematous, erythematous pigmented, established scleroderma, and resolvent scleroderma. Localized pseudoscleroderma (Texier's syndrome) has also been reported (13). This particular adverse reaction has occurred mainly in patients with hepatic insufficiency (SEDA-12, 330), but skin reactions have also been seen in patients with a normal hepatic condition (14,15). Brown pigmentation in the trochanteric region has been reported in a patient with cirrhosis.

Localized eczema at the site of subcutaneous injection has been reported (8).

- A 50-year-old woman taking warfarin had an INR of 8 and was given phytomenadione 10 mg subcutaneously (Sabex, containing propylene glycol 2% and polyethylene glycol 10%) and 12 hours later another 5 mg. One week later she developed two red, pruritic, warm, indurated areas, measuring 2×4 and 8×10 cm, at the two separate injection sites. A skin biopsy showed minimal spongiosis of the epidermis and an edematous dermis with a dense perivascular lymphocytic infiltrate and numerous eosinophils.

A severe localized and subsequently generalized dermatitis occurred after intramuscular injection of phytomenadione (16).

- A 40-year-old woman with no pre-existing hepatic disease was given intramuscular phytomenadione (Konakion) 1 ml/day (10 mg/ml) on 4 days before open cholecystectomy for gallstones. She then noticed a pruritic erythematous patch on her anterior left thigh, and over the next 4 weeks four patches appeared on her thighs and became larger (maximum diameter 15 cm), vesicular, weeping, hot, indurated, and intensely itchy. Topical calamine lotion, 1% hydrocortisone cream, and Paxyl cream (lidocaine and benzalkonium chloride) and oral cefalexin had no effect. The eruption then spread to the operation wound site, the face, neck, and arms. Oral prednisolone resulted in gradual improvement over the next 4 weeks, but residual erythema persisted for nearly 6 months.

Other presentations include erythematous pruritic plaques associated with epidermal keratosis, focal spongiosis, and perivascular infiltrates of lymphocytes and eosinophils or scleroderma-like hypodermic indurations (17). In such cases, intradermal tests may be positive for phytonadione.

Timing

The lesions usually appear 4–16 days after intramuscular injection, and persist for up to 2 months (18,19), sometimes leaving a scar lasting for years (20). The median number of days between the administration of phytomenadione and the appearance of the eruption was 13 days, but eruptions have appeared as early as 30 minutes and as late as 4 weeks after injection. In 13 of 32 cases it took more than 2 months for the reaction to resolve.

Frequency

Skin reactions to vitamin K are rare, only about 40 cases having been reported.

Relation to dose

In some early reports it was postulated that a minimum dose was necessary to cause eruptions, but there have been later reports of adverse skin reactions after small doses (range 10–440 mg).

Histopathology

Histopathological examination typically shows epidermal changes, including spongiosis with or without intraepidermal vesicles. In the dermis there is a perivascular mononuclear cell infiltrate, which may also be interstitial, often containing eosinophils.

Mechanism

Various formulations of phytomenadione contain different inactive ingredients, including polysorbate 80, propylene glycol, sodium acetate, glacial acetic acid, polyethoxylated castor oil (Cremophor EL), dextrose, and benzyl alcohol. Based on negative results with these ingredients, it appears that phytomenadione itself is the antigen that leads to adverse skin reactions. Of 10 patients with liver disease and prior exposure to phytomenadione (Konakion), 4 had positive results to patch-testing with vitamin K (21). Intracutaneous tests have supported the generally accepted hypothesis that the phenomenon is due to type IV hypersensitivity.

Treatment

No particular therapy is effective. It is not known whether the minute quantities of phytomenadione that are present in some foods, such as parsley, kale, brussels sprouts, spinach, cucumber, soy bean oil, and green and black tea leaves, preclude effective dietary therapy. Since the mechanism of this reaction is thought to be delayed hypersensitivity, another potential therapeutic approach is topical application of tacrolimus (FK-506), a potent inhibitor of interleukin 2 and T cell activation. Tacrolimus up to now has only been shown to suppress allergic contact dermatitis to dinitrophenol.

Immunologic

Allergic reactions have been attributed to phytomenadione, menadione, and vitamin K_4. In mice, menadione caused marked hypodynamia and hypothermia. This effect was potentiated by riboflavin. Allergic reactions to the systemic administration of vitamin K are immunologically mediated, and generally arise in patients with coagulation or liver problems.

Intradermal tests with phytomenadione and menadione caused an allergic skin reaction 7–22 days after injection in 13 of 145 healthy subjects. The results suggested that the index of cutaneous sensitivity lies somewhere between 5.5 and 8.9%. On the other hand, the absence of adverse effects with oral phytomenadione is striking. Continuation of treatment orally can in some cases prevent dermatitis (10). No cross-sensitivity has been seen between phytomenadione and menadione (22). Anaphylactoid reactions, some fatal, to phytomenadione have been reported (SEDA-15, 416) mainly from intravenous use (23).

The recommendation that prolongation of the international normalized ratio (INR) to over 6.0 should be corrected with parenteral phytomenadione (24,25) is not accompanied by the caveat that the intravenous route entails the risk of life-threatening, non-IgE-mediated anaphylactic reactions and even death, due to the use of polyethoxylated castor oil (Cremophor EL) as a solvent (26). A severe reaction to intravenous phytomenadione has been reported (27).

- A 74-year-old woman, taking warfarin, presented with an INR of 6.2. She was given a slow intravenous injection of phytomenadione (Konakion, Roche Products Ltd) 0.25 ml (500 µg) over about 60 seconds, and soon after felt profoundly unwell and complained of severe backache. She was given chlorphenamine 10 mg by rapid intravenous injection and adrenaline 1 mg in 10 ml of water over 30 minutes, with a good result.

An unusual case of allergy to vitamin K, with a relapsing and remitting eczematous reaction, has been described after an intramuscular injection of vitamin K_1 (28).

- A 27-year-old woman with cystic fibrosis and pancreatic insufficiency was given intramuscular vitamin K_1 into her thigh. The next day transient erythema occurred over the injection site and 6 weeks later there was localized pain, erythema, and edema. She was given intravenous cefuroxime for presumed cellulitis, but over the next few days the features became more consistent with localized eczema; she was given oral prednisolone 30 mg/day, super-potent topical corticosteroids, corticosteroid injections, and corticosteroids under occlusion with Duoderm, all of which failed to result in improvement. She then also developed an eczematous reaction to the Duoderm dressing. Patch tests were positive to vitamin K_1 and cross-reacted with vitamin K_4. She was also positive to colophonium and ester gum rosin, the dressing adhesive. Recurrent angio-edema persisted for several months and 2 years later she still had symptoms at the injection sites.

In all reported cases, only the whole formulation of vitamin K_1 (in its vehicle) or vitamin K_1 alone elicited positive patch tests. When individual additives were tested the results were negative. No previous exposure to vitamin K_1 was required for the development of type IV hypersensitivity, and primary sensitization occurred within 1–2 weeks or after a longer time period, as in the patient described here.

Long-Term Effects

Tumorigenicity

The relation between neonatal vitamin K administration and childhood cancer has been investigated in three case-control studies.

In a retrospective study 685 children who developed cancer before their 15th birthday were compared with 3442 controls matched for date and hospital of birth (29). There was no association between the administration of vitamin K and the development of all childhood cancers (unadjusted odds ratio 0.89; 95% CI = 0.69, 1.15)

or of all cases of acute lymphoblastic leukemia (1.20; 0.75, 1.92), but there was a raised odds ratio for acute lymphoblastic leukemia 1–6 years after birth (1.79; 1.02, 3.15).

However, no such association was seen in a separate cohort-based study not dependent on case-note retrieval, in which the rates of acute lymphoblastic leukemia in children born in hospital units in which all babies received vitamin K were compared with those born in units in which less than a third received prophylaxis. It was concluded that on the basis of currently published evidence neonatal intramuscular vitamin K administration does not increase the risk of early childhood leukemia.

In another study children aged 0–14 years with leukemia ($n = 150$), lymphomas ($n = 46$), central nervous system tumors ($n = 79$), a range of other solid tumours ($n = 142$), and a subset of acute lymphoblastic leukemia ($n = 129$) were compared with 777 children matched for age and sex (30). Odds ratios showed no significant positive association for leukemias (1.30; 0.83, 2.03), acute lymphoblastic leukemia (1.21; 0.74, 1.97), lymphomas (1.06; 0.46, 2.42), central nervous system tumors (0.74; 0.40, 1.34), and other solid tumors (0.59; 0.37, 0.96). There was no association with acute lymphoblastic leukemia in children aged 1–6 years. The authors concluded that they had not confirmed the observation of an increased risk of childhood leukemia and cancer associated with intramuscular vitamin K.

In another study 597 cases and matched controls were compared. The association between cancer generally and intramuscular vitamin K was of borderline significance (odds ratio 1.44); the association was strongest for acute lymphoblastic leukemia (1.73) (31). However, there was also an effect of abnormal delivery. The authors suggested from the lack of consistency between the various studies so far published, including their own, and the low relative risks found in most of them, that the risk, if any, attributable to the use of vitamin K cannot be large, but that the possibility that there is some risk cannot be excluded. They recommended that prophylaxis using the commonly used intramuscular dose of 1 mg should be restricted to babies at particularly high risk of vitamin K deficiency; alternatively, a lower dose might be given to a larger proportion of those at risk.

Ecological studies of the relation between hospital policies on neonatal vitamin K administration and subsequent occurrences of childhood cancer have been analysed using data from selected large maternity units in Scotland, England, and Wales (32). The study covered 94 hospitals, with a total of 2.3 million births during periods when intramuscular vitamin K was routinely used and 1.4 million births when a selective policy was in operation. An increased risk was occasionally associated with vitamin K (highest odds ratio 1.25 for acute lymphoblastic leukemia in one hospital), but the overall results were not significant, and there was no evidence to support the previously suggested doubling of the risk of childhood cancer.

On the basis of all these results it is unlikely that there is a greatly increased risk of childhood cancer attributable to intramuscular vitamin K given to newborns, if indeed there is any risk at all.

Susceptibility Factors

High doses of vitamin K can cause relapses in patients with thrombosis and myocardial infarction treated with dicoumarol (33).

Drug Administration

Drug formulations

In a worldwide post-marketing surveillance program a conventional formulation of phytomenadione (Konakion), which contains Cremophor EL (polyethoxylated castor oil), was compared with a new mixed micellar formulation (Konakion MM) (34). During 1974–95 an estimated 635 million adults and 728 million children were given Konakion or Konakion MM. Of the 404 adverse events reported in 286 subjects (see Table 2) 387 (96%) were associated with Konakion, which had 95% of sales. Konakion MM accounted for 4% (n = 17) of the reported adverse effects and 5% of sales. Of the 17 adverse events 13 reported with Konakion MM were minor injection site reactions. Overall, 120 of the adverse events were serious, of which 117 (98%) were associated with Konakion. There were 85 probable anaphylactoid reactions (of which six were fatal) with conventional Konakion, compared with one non-fatal anaphylactoid reaction with Konakion MM. During the last 12 months of postmarketing surveillance, there were 14 serious adverse events reported in an estimated 21 million individuals treated with Konakion, but none in the 13 million who received Konakion MM. These results suggest that formulations of phytomenadione that are solubilized with Cremophor EL have a higher profile of adverse events, including anaphylactoid reactions, than the newer mixed micellar formulation Konakion MM.

Drug administration route

A case-control study in 1990 suggested a causal relation between intramuscular administration of vitamin K to neonates and the subsequent development of leukemia (35). Later studies have not been able to confirm this finding (30,36–38), although the results are not sufficiently conclusive to rule out the possibility that there is some risk (29,31).

Rapid intravenous administration of vitamin K can cause facial flushing, sweating, fever, a rise in blood pressure, a feeling of constriction in the chest, and cyanosis. Cases of cardiovascular collapse after intravenous injection of phytomenadione and phytonadione have been reported (39). Intravenous injection of phytomenadione is recommended to be performed slowly at a rate not exceeding 5 mg/minute.

The safety and efficacy of intravenously administered phytonadione have been retrospectively studied in patients taking long-term oral anticoagulants (40). Of 105 patients, 85 initially received intravenous phytonadione 0.5–1 mg,

Table 2 The distribution of 404 adverse events associated with phytomenadione in 286 patients, by system; the figures in parentheses refer to serious adverse events

System	Konakion (Cremophor EL)	Konakion (mixed micelles)	Total	% of total (n = 404)
General disorders	83 (37)	2 (1)	85 (38)	21.0
Cardiovascular				
Heart rate and rhythm disorders	31 (10)	1 (0)	32 (10)	7.9
Vascular	18 (11)		18 (11)	4.5
Extracardiac	8 (3)		8 (3)	2.0
Myocardial, endocardial, pericardial and valve disorders	1 (1)		1 (1)	0.2
Respiratory	31 (15)	1 (1)	32 (16)	7.9
Nervous system				
Central nervous and peripheral nervous systems	10 (4)		10 (4)	2.5
Autonomic nervous system	3 (0)		3 (0)	0.7
Sensory systems				
Hearing and vestibular disorders	2 (0)		2 (0)	0.5
Endocrine, metabolic, nutritional	1 (0)		1 (0)	0.2
Hematologic				
Erythrocyte disorders	3 (1)		3 (1)	0.7
Leukocyte and reticuloendothelial system disorders	2 (2)		2 (2)	0.5
Platelet, bleeding, and clotting disorders	5 (2)		5 (2)	1.2
Liver, biliary	14 (3)		14 (3)	3.4
Gastrointestinal	14 (2)		14 (2)	3.4
Urinary system	3 (3)		3 (3)	0.7
Skin	90 (9)	5 (0)	95 (9)	23.5
Musculoskeletal	2 (1)		2 (1)	0.5
Neonates and infants	13 (7)		13 (7)	3.2
Application site disorders	53 (6)	8 (1)	61 (7)	15.1
Total	387 (117)	17 (3)	404 (120)	100%

and 29 received a second dose. Only two of the 105 patients had suspected adverse reactions to phytonadione. Both were men with prior lung disease (one with an adenocarcinoma and one with chronic obstructive lung disease) and were to receive a 0.5 mg dose of phytonadione. During the phytonadione infusion both patients developed dyspnea and chest tightness, which resolved within 15 minutes of stopping the infusion; neither patient had hypotension.

Drug–Drug Interactions

Warfarin

An interaction of warfarin with a nutritional supplement containing vitamin K has been reported (41).

- A 72-year-old man taking warfarin (42.5 mg/week) to prevent thromboembolism related to atrial fibrillation/flutter wanted to take an over-the-counter nutritional supplement containing vitamin K (Nature's Life Greens, a blend of more than 20 herbs). He was instructed to withhold two doses of warfarin. Two weeks later he had an INR of 1.68; however, he had missed three doses of warfarin within the previous 10 days because of cataract surgery. Two weeks later his INR was 3.34. The warfarin dosage was reduced from 42.5 to 40.5 mg/week and the INR was in the target range 2 weeks later.

This report underlines the need for monitoring the use of nutritional and herbal products in patients taking warfarin.

Ubidecarenone (coenzyme Q10; ubiquinone-10) is chemically closely related to phytonadione. It is also widely available as a non-orthodox over-the-counter product, and several patients have been described in whom a reduced effect of warfarin was observed after the addition of non-orthodox ubidecarenone (42,43).

References

1. Bosse GM, Mallory MN, Malone GJ. The safety of intravenously administered vitamin K. Vet Hum Toxicol 2002;44(3):174–6.
2. Florholmen J, Waldum H, Nordoy A. Cerebral thrombosis in two patients with malabsorption syndrome treated with vitamin K. BMJ 1980;281(6239):541.
3. Jablonska A, Gadamska T. Niedokrwistosc hemolityczna u nowrodka po przedawkowaniu witaminy K. Med Wiejska 1973;1:79.
4. Ludin H. Blut- und Knochenmarkschädigungen durch Medikamente. [Blood and bone marrow damage caused by drugs.] Schweiz Med Wochenschr 1965;95(31):1027–32.
5. Garrett JV, Hallum J, Scott P. Urinary antiseptics causing haemolytic anaemia in pregnancy in a West Indian woman with red cell enzyme deficiency. J Obstet Gynaecol Br Commonw 1963;70:1073–5.
6. Roe DA. Nutrient toxicity with excessive intake. NY St J Med 1966;66:869.
7. Gupta KD, Banerji A. Paradoxical effect of vitamin K therapy in aggravating hypoprothrombinaemia. J Indian Med Assoc 1967;49(10):482–4.
8. Wilkins K, DeKoven J, Assaad D. Cutaneous reactions associated with vitamin K1. J Cutan Med Surg 2000;4(3):164–8.
9. Bruynzeel I, Hebeda CL, Folkers E, Bruynzeel DP. Cutaneous hypersensitivity reactions to vitamin K: 2 case reports and a review of the literature. Contact Dermatitis 1995;32(2):78–82.
10. Pigatto PD, Bigardi A, Fumagalli M, Altomare GF, Riboldi A. Allergic dermatitis from parenteral vitamin K. Contact Dermatitis 1990;22(5):307–8.
11. Joyce JP, Hood AF, Weiss MM. Persistent cutaneous reaction to intramuscular vitamin K injection. Arch Dermatol 1988;124(1):27–8.
12. Keough GC, English JC 3rd, Meffert JJ. Eczematous hypersensitivity from aqueous vitamin K injection. Cutis 1998;61(2):81–3.
13. Brunskill NJ, Berth-Jones J, Graham-Brown RA. Pseudosclerodermatous reaction to phytomenadione injection (Texier's syndrome). Clin Exp Dermatol 1988;13(4):276–8.
14. Sanders MN, Winkelmann RK. Cutaneous reactions to vitamin K. J Am Acad Dermatol 1988;19(4):699–704.
15. Moreau-Cabarrot A, Giordano-Labadie F, Bazex J. Hypersensibilité cutanée au point d'injection de vitamin K1. [Cutaneous hypersensitivity at the site of injection of vitamin K1.] Ann Dermatol Venereol 1996;123(3):177–9.
16. Wong DA, Freeman S. Cutaneous allergic reaction to intramuscular vitamin K1. Australas J Dermatol 1999;40(3):147–52.
17. Balato N, Cuccurullo FM, Patruno C, Ayala F. Adverse skin reactions to vitamin K1: report of 2 cases. Contact Dermatitis 1998;38(6):341–2.
18. Barnes HM, Sarkany I. Adverse skin reaction from vitamin K1. Br J Dermatol 1976;95(6):653–6.
19. Baer RL. Cutaneous skin changes probably due to pyridoxine abuse. J Am Acad Dermatol 1984;10(3):527–8.
20. Chung JY, Ramos-Caro FA, Beers B, Ford MJ, Flowers FP. Hypersensitivity reactions to parenteral vitamin K. Cutis 1999;63(1):33–4.
21. Bullen AW, Miller JP, Cunliffe WJ, Losowsky MS. Skin reactions caused by vitamin K in patients with liver disease. Br J Dermatol 1978;98(5):561–5.
22. Hwang SW, Kim YP, Chung BS, Kim HK. Vitamin K1 dermatitis. Korean J Dermatol 1983;21:91.
23. ADRAC Slow down on parenteral vitamin K. Aust Adverse Drug React Bull 1991;10:3.
24. Hirsh J, Dalen JE, Deykin D, Poller L, Bussey H. Oral anticoagulants. Mechanism of action, clinical effectiveness, and optimal therapeutic range. Chest 1995;108(Suppl 4):S231–46.
25. Routledge PA. Practical prescribing: warfarin. Prescr J 1997;37:173–9.
26. Martin JC. Anaphylactoid reactions and vitamin K. Med J Aust 1991;155(11–12):851.
27. Jolobe OM, Penny E. Severe reaction to i.v. vitamin K. Pharm J 1999;262:112.
28. Sommer S, Wilkinson SM, Peckham D, Wilson C. Type IV hypersensitivity to vitamin K. Contact Dermatitis 2002;46(2):94–6.
29. Parker L, Cole M, Craft AW, Hey EN. Neonatal vitamin K administration and childhood cancer in the north of England: retrospective case-control study. BMJ 1998;316(7126):189–93.
30. McKinney PA, Juszczak E, Findlay E, Smith K. Case-control study of childhood leukaemia and cancer in Scotland: findings for neonatal intramuscular vitamin K. BMJ 1998;316(7126):173–7.
31. Passmore SJ, Draper G, Brownbill P, Kroll M. Case-control studies of relation between childhood cancer and neonatal vitamin K administration. BMJ 1998;316(7126):178–84.
32. Passmore SJ, Draper G, Brownbill P, Kroll M. Ecological studies of relation between hospital policies on neonatal vitamin K administration and subsequent occurrence of childhood cancer. BMJ 1998;316(7126):184–9.
33. Reuter H. Vitamine, Chemie und Klinik. Stuttgart: Hippokrates Verlag, 1970.
34. Pereira SP, Williams R. Adverse events associated with vitamin K1: results of a worldwide postmarketing surveillance programme. Pharmacoepidemiol Drug Saf 1998;7(3):173–82.

35. Golding J, Paterson M, Kinlen LJ. Factors associated with childhood cancer in a national cohort study. Br J Cancer 1990;62(2):304–8.

36. Klebanoff MA, Read JS, Mills JL, Shiono PH. The risk of childhood cancer after neonatal exposure to vitamin K. N Engl J Med 1993;329(13):905–8.

37. Ekelund H, Finnstrom O, Gunnarskog J, Kallen B, Larsson Y. Administration of vitamin K to newborn infants and childhood cancer. BMJ 1993;307(6896):89–91.

38. McWhirter WR. Vitamin K and childhood cancer. Med J Aust 1993;159(8):499.

39. Pelletier G, Attali P, Ink O. Arrêt cardiorespiratoire après injection intraveineuse de vitamine K1. [Cardiopulmonary arrest after intravenous injection of vitamin K1.] Gastroenterol Clin Biol 1986;10(8–9):615.

40. Shields RC, McBane RD, Kuiper JD, Li H, Heit JA. Efficacy and safety of intravenous phytonadione (vitamin K1) in patients on long-term oral anticoagulant therapy. Mayo Clin Proc 2001;76(3):260–6.

41. Bransgrove LL. Interaction between warfarin and a vitamin K-containing nutritional supplement: a case report. J Herbal Pharmacother 2001;1:85–9.

42. Spigset O. Reduced effect of warfarin caused by ubidecarenone. Lancet 1994;344(8933):1372–3.

43. Anonymous. Coenzym Q10 (Qumin Q10 u.a.) stört orale Antikoagulation. Arznei-Telegramm 1994;12:120.

Vitamins

See also Individual agents

General Information

Vitamins are essential organic substances, usually obtained from food. They are required by humans in amounts ranging from micrograms to milligrams per day. The fat-soluble vitamins are:

- vitamin A (carotenoids)
- vitamin D (calciferols)
- vitamin E (tocopherols and tocotrienols)
- vitamin K

The water-soluble vitamins include:

- vitamin B_1 (thiamine, aneurin)
- vitamin B_2 (riboflavin)
- vitamin B_3 (niacin)
- vitamin B_5 (pantothenic acid)
- vitamin B_6 (pyridoxine)
- vitamin B_7 (folic acid)
- vitamin B_{10} (biotin)
- vitamin B_{12} (cobalamins)
- vitamin C (ascorbic acid)

The vitamins are chemically heterogeneous, but all are essential for normal growth, development, and maintenance of the human organism (1). They cannot be synthesized by the organism itself, with the exception of vitamin D, and have to be supplied externally. The main indications for vitamin supplementation are threatening or manifest deficiency states.

The word "vitamin" itself is a misnomer, created in 1911 by one of the early nutrition researchers, the Polish biochemist Casimir Funk (1884–1967). He knew that the substances he was trying to identify were not necessarily "amines," but felt that because of the great public health importance of these newly identified substances, a name was needed "that would sound well and serve as a 'catch word'" (2). His choice proved successful; the label "vitamin" has proved to have extraordinary appeal.

Vitamins are not infrequently used by medical workers as placebos against poorly defined general malaise, often without consideration of the patient's actual vitamin status (3). Self-medication with vitamin supplements is very common in most countries, and commonly the users are not objectively vitamin deficient (4). In general, physicians in an industrialized society can expect that about half of their adult patients will currently be taking vitamin supplements (5); among athletes 75% have been found to use supplements (6).

As micronutrient deficiencies more or less ceased to be a large public health problem in Western countries, the attention of scientists and manufacturers turned towards the many other functions that vitamins have in human metabolism. For the last several decades, pharmacological doses of most vitamins have been claimed to be of therapeutic value in a wide variety of conditions, which have only a superficial resemblance to the classic vitamin deficiency syndromes. The literature on which many of these claims are based unfortunately often consists of poorly conducted clinical trials or anecdotal reports. Properly designed studies are relatively few in number. No authoritative body has proposed quantitative recommendations or reference values for public health policy.

Reference values for vitamins

In the early 1990s European nutritionists, in the light of an increasing body of evidence, changed the nomenclature with regard to what used to be called the Recommended Dietary Allowance (RDA), Recommended Daily Intake (RDI), or Nutrient Reference Value (NRV) (7). When in 1993 the Scientific Committee for Food of the European Communities published a report entitled "Nutrient and Energy Intakes for the European Community" (8), a new approach was introduced, allowing for more flexibility in regard to quantitative values. Based on what is known about the Average Requirement (AR) for a nutrient in a population, and assuming a normal distribution of requirements, a value two standard deviations above the Average Requirement is called the Population Reference Intake, a dose at which deficiency of the micronutrient is probable in under 2.5% of any population. Similarly, a value two standard deviations below the Average Requirement, called the Lowest Threshold of Intake, denote a dose at which the probability of deficiency in a population is almost 97.5%. These values are given in Table 1. In the USA, the National Academy of Sciences has a different procedure and nomenclature (9). Each vitamin is treated separately and the reports of expert panels are published separately as they become available. US Dietary Reference Intakes commonly establishes four levels of reference values, including a Tolerable Upper Intake, which is the dose of greatest interest in the context of adverse effects. Values of Tolerable Upper Intake have also been recommended by

Table 1 Daily vitamin requirements for adults (men; women in parentheses if different)

Vitamin	Lowest Threshold of Intake	Average Requirement	Population Reference Intake	Tolerable Upper Intake
Vitamin A (carotenoids; micrograms RE)	300 (250)	500 (400)	700 (600)	3000
Vitamin B_1 (thiamine; micrograms/MJ)	50	72	100	–
Vitamin B_2 (riboflavin; micrograms)	0.6	1.3 (1.1)	1.6 (1.3)	–
Vitamin B_3 (niacin; mg/MJ)	1.0	1.3	1.6	8
Vitamin B_6 (pyridoxine; micrograms/g protein)	–	1.3	1.5	25
Vitamin B_7 (folic acid; micrograms)	160	230	300	1000
Vitamin B_{12} (cobalamins; micrograms)	0.6	1.0	1.4	–
Vitamin C (ascorbic acid; mg)	32	46	60	1000
Vitamin D (ergocalciferol; micrograms)	–	–	5–10	50

the European Commission's Scientific Committee on Food [http://europa.eu.int/comm/food/fs/sc/scf/out80_en.html].

Drug Administration

Drug overdose

The symptoms that are commonly reported in vitamin overdose are listed in Table 2.

Table 2 Notable symptoms reported with chronic and acute vitamin overdosage (SEDA-13, 345) (6,10)

Vitamin	Adverse effects
Vitamin A	Hypercarotenosis
	Increased intracranial pressure
	Headache
	Sleep disturbances
	Nausea, vomiting, diarrhea
	Chronic liver disease
	Dry skin, fissures, depigmentation, and pruritus
	Alopecia
	Bone tenderness
	Teratogenesis (renal and nervous system)
Vitamin B_3 (niacin)	Hypotension
	Dysrhythmias
	Headache
	Hyperglycemia
	Hyperuricemia, gout
	Peptic ulcer
	Hepatotoxicity
	Skin flushing
	Pruritus
	Alopecia
Vitamin B_6 (pyridoxine)	Peripheral sensory neuropathy
	Ataxia
Vitamin C	Impairment of work at high altitudes
	Gastrointestinal symptoms
	Oxalate stones in predisposed persons
	Possible teratogenesis and carcinogenesis in very high doses
Vitamin D	Hypertension
	Hypercalcemia
	Metastatic calcification
	Bone demineralization
	Renal calcinosis and kidney failure
Vitamin E	Increased action of warfarin
Vitamin K	Hemolytic anemia
	Neonatal jaundice

There is widespread and easy availability of high-dose single and multiple vitamin formulations, often presented as food supplements. This creates a potential for chronic or sporadic intake of high doses of vitamins and the occurrence of unanticipated adverse effects (11,12). The cases often involve children, who may be specially vulnerable to the effects of overdosage. The Canadian Paediatric Society's Nutrition Committee in 1990 issued a warning to physicians, based on an estimate that as many as 10% of healthy Canadian children were being exposed to vitamin polypharmacy and a substantial risk of accidental overdose (13).

According to some authors, the increased accessibility and use of high-dose vitamin formulations has been encouraged by the multi-million-dollar health food industry, increased emphasis placed by physicians on more "natural" approaches to disease treatment, a population of consumers interested in so-called "holistic medicine," and the marketing of these formulations in many countries without regulatory control. In therapeutic use, the physician has to keep in mind the benefit to harm balance of using high-dose vitamin supplements for disorders in which proof of efficacy is lacking (14).

Since vitamin overdose can produce unexpected, often vague, signs and symptoms, physicians should ask patients who present with inexplicable symptoms, including those listed in Table 2 (15), about their use of unusual or unapproved therapies, including vitamins in megadoses (10). It has been suggested that a medical history is not complete without vitamin/mineral supplement information (6).

Food fortification and "designer foods" specially formulated to prevent chronic diseases are enthusiastically advocated by the vitamin industry and its proponents (16). Unrestrained vitamin fortification added to unrestrained supplementation with these substances has now in some countries led to the potential for rather high cumulative amounts of intake in some populations. There is growing concern about the safety of chronically high doses of some of these, where the therapeutic margin between deficiency and toxicity may not be all that wide (15,17–19).

References

1. Council on Scientific Affairs. Vitamin preparations as dietary supplements and as therapeutic agents. JAMA 1987; 257(14):1929–36.

2. Combs GF. The Vitamins. Fundamental Aspects in Nutrition and Health. New York: Academic Press, 1992:22.

3. Schrijver J, Dukes MN, Helsing E, Bruce A. Use and Regulation of Vitamin and Mineral Supplements. A Study with Policy Recommendations. Groningen: Published for the WHO Regional Office for Europe by STYX Publications, 1993.

4. Koplan JP, Annest JL, Layde PM, Rubin GL. Nutrient intake and supplementation in the United States (NHANES II). Am J Public Health 1986;76(3):287–9.

5. Muncie HL Jr, Sobal J. The vitamin–mineral supplement history. J Fam Pract 1987;24(4):365–8.

6. Fike S. Vitamin preparations: recommendations for use. Natl Strength Condition Assoc J 1987;9:32.

7. Committee On Medical Aspects of Food Policy. Dietary Reference Values for Food Energy and Nutrients for the United Kingdom (1991). Report of the Panel on Dietary Reference Values. Report on Health and Social Subjects No. 41, Department of Health. London: Her Majesty's Stationery Office, 1991.

8. Scientific Committee for Food. Nutrient and energy intakes for the European Community. Directorate-General Industry. Luxembourg: Commission of the European Communities, 1993.

9. Levine M, Rumsey SC, Daruwala R, Park JB, Wang Y. Criteria and recommendations for vitamin C intake. JAMA 1999;281(15):1415–23.

10. Evans CD, Lacey JH. Toxicity of vitamins: complications of a health movement. BMJ (Clin Res Ed) 1986;292(6519):509–10.

11. Anonymous. Vitamin intoxication is new abuse. Am Pharm 1981;821:91.

12. Philen RM, Ortiz DI, Auerbach SB, Falk H. Survey of advertising for nutritional supplements in health and body-building magazines. JAMA 1992;268(8):1008–11.

13. Nutrition Committee, Canadian Paediatric Society. Megavitamin and megamineral therapy in childhood. CMAJ 1990;143(10):1009–13.

14. Ovesen L. Vitamin therapy in the absence of obvious deficiency. What is the evidence? Drugs 1984;27(2):148–70.

15. Positions of the American Dietetic Association: enrichment and fortification of foods and dietary supplements. J Am Diet Assoc 1994;94(6):661–3.

16. Gey KF, Stahelin HB, Eichholzer M. Poor plasma status of carotene and vitamin C is associated with higher mortality from ischemic heart disease and stroke: Basel Prospective Study. Clin Investig 1993;71(1):3–6.

17. Heiskanen K, Salmenpera L, Perheentupa J, Siimes MA. Infant vitamin B-6 status changes with age and with formula feeding. Am J Clin Nutr 1994;60(6):907–10.

18. Garewal HS, Diplock AT. How "safe" are antioxidant vitamins? Drug Saf 1995;13(1):8–14.

19. The Alpha-Tocopherol, Beta Carotene Cancer Prevention Study Group. The effect of vitamin E and beta carotene on the incidence of lung cancer and other cancers in male smokers. N Engl J Med 1994; 330(15):1029–35.

Voriconazole

See also Antifungal azoles

General Information

Voriconazole is a triazole that is structurally related to fluconazole. It has two interesting properties, activity against *Aspergillus* species and sufficient solubility in water to be administered parenterally. It is active against a wide spectrum of clinically important fungi, including *Candida* species, *Trichosporon beigelii*, *Cryptococcus neoformans*, *Aspergillus* species, *Fusarium* species, and other hyaline, dematiaceous, and dimorphic molds (1,2). It has demonstrated efficacy in various animal models of invasive fungal infections (1,2).

Pharmacokinetics

Voriconazole has a half-life of about 6 hours and undergoes complex hepatic metabolism. There is wide intersubject variability in the disposition of voriconazole, which is at least partly related to a CYP2C19 polymorphism. Voriconazole has the potential for drug–drug interactions mediated by CYP3A4, CYP2C9, and CYP2C19.

The kinetics of voriconazole are non-linear, as shown in 42 healthy men (3). Two groups of subjects participated. Group 1 ($n = 28$) took part in two study periods, each consisting of 14 days separated by a minimum 7-day washout period. During one of the periods, 14 subjects received intravenous voriconazole 6 mg/kg bd on day 1 followed by 3 mg/kg bd on days 2–7 and were then switched to 200 mg bd orally on days 8–14. During the other period, they received 6 mg/kg bd intravenously on day 1 followed by 5 mg/kg bd on days 2–7 and were then switched to 400 mg orally bd on days 8–14. The other 14 subjects in group 1 received a matching placebo throughout the study. In group 2 ($n = 14$), 7 subjects received 6 mg/kg intravenously bd on day 1 followed by 4 mg/kg bd on days 2–7 and were then switched to 300 mg bd orally on days 8–14. The other seven received a matching placebo. Voriconazole had non-linear pharmacokinetics, attributed to saturable metabolism. For intravenous dosing, a 1.7-fold increase in dose resulted in 2.4- and 3.1-fold increases in C_{max} and AUC respectively; a two-fold increase in oral dosing resulted in 2.8- and 3.9-fold increases in C_{max} and AUC respectively. The mean C_{max} after oral dosing was 63–90% of the intravenous C_{max}. After the switch from intravenous to oral dosing, most subjects achieved steady state by day 4. Voriconazole was well tolerated; the most commonly reported adverse events were mild to moderate headache, rash, and abnormal vision. Visual function tests conducted on all subjects detected no further abnormalities during voriconazole treatment and one abnormality (abnormal color vision test) during placebo treatment. All visual disturbances were mild to moderate in intensity, and all resolved spontaneously within 2 days of onset. No subject in any treatment group had a serious adverse event.

Observational studies

The efficacy of voriconazole has been demonstrated in non-comparative phase I/II studies in patients with oropharyngeal and esophageal candidiasis and acute and chronic invasive aspergillosis (4). In phase III clinical trials, it was superior to conventional amphotericin for first-line therapy of invasive aspergillosis and yielded comparable success rates but less proven and probable breakthrough infections compared with liposomal amphotericin as empirical antifungal therapy in patients with persistent neutropenia (5).

Voriconazole had excellent clinical efficacy in a non-comparative phase I/II studies in patients with oropharyngeal and esophageal candidiasis and acute and chronic invasive aspergillosis (6).

In an open, non-comparative, multicenter study in immunocompromised patients with proven or probable invasive aspergillosis, 116 patients were treated with intravenous voriconazole 6 mg/kg bd twice and then 3 mg/kg bd for 6–27 days, followed by 200 mg bd orally for up to 24 weeks; voriconazole was given as primary therapy in 60 (7). There were good responses in 56; 16 had a complete response and 40 a partial response; there was a stable response in 24 patients. There were adverse events in 91% of the patients who received at least one dose of voriconazole, but only 15% were attributed to the drug. The most common adverse events attributed to voriconazole were skin rash (8.7%), reversible visual disturbances (11%), and raised liver function tests (15%). There was evidence of a concentration-dependent incidence of adverse events: six of seven patients with voriconazole plasma concentrations over 10 µg/ml developed adverse events requiring drug withdrawal.

Comparative studies

Amphotericin

Voriconazole has been compared with liposomal amphotericin for empirical antifungal therapy in a randomized, international, multicenter trial in 837 patients (415 assigned to voriconazole, 4 mg/kg bd (6 mg/kg bd on day 1) and 422 to liposomal amphotericin, 3 mg/kg/day) (8). The overall success rates were similar (26% with voriconazole and 31% with liposomal amphotericin); however, there were significantly fewer documented breakthrough fungal infections in patients who received voriconazole (8 versus 21). Those who received voriconazole had fewer severe infusion-related reactions, less mild nephrotoxicity, as defined by increases in serum creatinine to over 1.5 times baseline, and less hypokalemia; however, there was no difference whatsoever in the proportion of patients with more profound renal compromise (increased serum creatinine to over 2.0 times baseline; 7.0 versus 7.6%). The incidence of hepatotoxicity, as measured by raised hepatic transaminases and alkaline phosphatase, was similar in the two groups; increased serum bilirubin to over 1.5 times baseline was more common in patients who took amphotericin. Patients who received voriconazole had more episodes of transient visual changes than those who received liposomal amphotericin (22 versus 1%) and more episodes of visual hallucinations (4.3 versus 0.5%). Parenteral voriconazole was changed to the oral formulation in 22%, with a reduction in the mean duration of hospitalization by 1 day in all patients but by 2 days in patients at high risk (with relapsed leukemia or after allogeneic bone marrow transplant). Toxicity or lack of efficacy caused 9.9% of those who received voriconazole and 6.6% of those who received amphotericin to withdraw.

In a comparative, randomized, unblinded trial for primary therapy of invasive aspergillosis, 144 patients received either intravenous voriconazole (6 mg/kg bd on day 1, then 4 mg/kg bd for at least 7 days) followed by 200 mg bd orally, and 133 received intravenous amphotericin deoxycholate (1–1.5 mg/kg/day); other licensed antifungal treatments were allowed if the initial therapy failed or if the patient had an intolerance to the first drug used (9). Most patients had allogeneic hemopoietic cell transplants, acute leukemia, or other hematological diseases. At week 12, 53% of the patients in the voriconazole group and 32% of those in the amphotericin group (difference = 21%; 95% CI = 10, 33%) had a successful outcome. The survival rate at 12 weeks was 71% in the voriconazole group and 58% in the amphotericin group (hazard ratio = 0.59; 95% CI = 0.40, 0.88). Transient visual disturbances were more common with voriconazole (45 versus 4.3%). The most frequent descriptions of such disturbances were blurred vision, altered visual perception, altered color perception, and photophobia. Of the patients who received voriconazole, 9% had hallucinations or confusion considered possibly related to the drug compared with 3.7% of those who received amphotericin. Infusion-related reactions (fever, chills, or both) were more common in those who received amphotericin (3.1 versus 25%), as were severe, potentially related adverse events (13 versus 24%); the most frequent events were renal impairment (14%) in those who received amphotericin and liver function abnormalities (4.8%) in those who received voriconazole.

Other antifungal azoles

In a multicenter, randomized, double-blind, double-dummy, parallel-group, dose-escalation comparison with fluconazole, the safety, tolerability, and pharmacokinetics of oral voriconazole were investigated in 24 subjects at high risk of fungal infections (with hematological malignancies, solid tumors, or autologous bone marrow transplants) (10). The subjects were randomized to receive voriconazole 200 mg bd ($n = 9$), voriconazole 300 mg bd ($n = 9$), or fluconazole 400 mg od ($n = 6$) for 14 days. There was an approximate five-fold accumulation of voriconazole during the dosing period and evidence of non-linear pharmacokinetics. Voriconazole was generally safe and well tolerated. Mild, reversible visual disturbances were the most commonly reported adverse events but they were not associated with treatment withdrawal. No patient developed a breakthrough fungal infection.

The efficacy, safety, and tolerability of voriconazole and fluconazole have been compared in 391 immunocompromised adults with esophageal candidiasis in a randomized, double-blind, multicenter trial (11). Most of the patients (94%) had AIDS. Following randomization, they took either voriconazole (200 mg bd) or fluconazole (400 mg on day 1 followed by 200 mg od) for a median of 14 or 15 days respectively. Treatment was continued for 7 days after the resolution of all signs and symptoms but was not allowed to exceed 42 days. The two drugs achieved comparable success rates (98% voriconazole, 95% fluconazole), as assessed by esophagoscopy in the primary efficacy analysis in 256 patients. More patients discontinued voriconazole because of laboratory test abnormalities (3.5 versus 1%) or treatment-related adverse events (2.5 versus 0.5%). The most frequent adverse event with voriconazole was transient visual disturbances (23 versus 8%); other clinical adverse events were similar in frequency. Increases of over three times the upper limit of the reference range in aspartate transaminase (20 versus 8%), alanine transaminase (11 versus 7%), and alkaline phosphatase (10 versus 8%) were more frequent with voriconazole.

Organs and Systems

Sensory systems

Visual adverse events, in particular enhanced brightness of light and color, are common with voriconazole (11). These visual adverse effects are transient and reversible. So far, comprehensive ophthalmological investigations have not shown any morphological correlates or long-term visual sequelae in any patient.

Liver

Liver function test abnormalities in patients taking voriconazole are not unexpected for an azole and can be explained by its extensive hepatic metabolic clearance (12).

Susceptibility Factors

Age

Although the disposition of voriconazole in children aged 12 years and over is similar to that in adults, children aged 2–11 years need larger dosages to achieve the same exposure that was effective in interventional trials in adults (13).

The safety and efficacy of voriconazole have been studied in 58 children (aged 9 months to 15 years; median 7 years) who were treated in the manufacturer's compassionate release program (14). They received voriconazole for an invasive fungal infection if they were refractory to or intolerant of conventional antifungal drugs. Voriconazole was given intravenously as a loading dose of 6 mg/kg every 12 hours on day 1 followed by 4 mg/kg every 12 hours thereafter. When feasible, the route of administration was changed from intravenous to oral (100 or 200 mg bd for patients weighing under or over 40 kg, respectively). At the end of therapy (mean 93 days, range 1–800), 26 patients had a complete or partial response, 4 had a stable response, 25 failed therapy, and 4 were withdrawn because of intolerance of voriconazole. Two had treatment-related serious adverse events (ulcerated lips with rash and raised hepatic transaminases or bilirubin). A total of 23 patients had voriconazole-related adverse events, three of which required withdrawal of voriconazole. The most commonly reported adverse events included raised hepatic transaminases or bilirubin ($n = 8$), skin rashes ($n = 8$), abnormal vision ($n = 3$), and a photosensitivity reaction ($n = 3$). The authors concluded that these data support the use of voriconazole for invasive fungal infections in children who are intolerant of or refractory to conventional antifungal drugs.

Drug–Drug Interactions

Ciclosporin

The interaction of voriconazole with ciclosporin has been investigated in a randomized, double-blind, placebo-controlled, crossover study in kidney transplant recipients with stable renal function (15). During the first study period (7.5 days), subjects taking ciclosporin 150 mg/day received either concomitant voriconazole (200 mg every 12 hours) or a matching placebo. After a washout period of at least 4 days, they were switched to the other treatment. In the seven subjects who completed both regimens, concomitant administration with voriconazole resulted in a 1.7-fold increase (90% CI = 1.47, 1.96) in mean ciclosporin AUC during a dosage interval. Ciclosporin C_{max} and t_{max} were not significantly affected, but C_{min} was increased by voriconazole by a mean of 2.48 (range 1.88–3.03) times. Seven subjects withdrew during voriconazole administration, six for reasons that were considered to be drug-related; most were attributable to increased ciclosporin concentrations. Although not serious, all causality-related adverse events were more frequent during voriconazole administration than during placebo administration. Thus, when voriconazole is initiated or withdrawn in patients who are already taking ciclosporin, blood ciclosporin concentrations should be carefully monitored and the dose of ciclosporin adjusted as necessary.

References

1. Hoffman HL, Ernst EJ, Klepser ME. Novel triazole antifungal agents. Expert Opin Investig Drugs 2000;9(3):593–605.
2. Chiou CC, Groll AH, Walsh TJ. New drugs and novel targets for treatment of invasive fungal infections in patients with cancer. Oncologist 2000;5(2):120–35.
3. Purkins L, Wood N, Ghahramani P, Greenhalgh K, Allen MJ, Kleinermans D. Pharmacokinetics and safety of voriconazole following intravenous- to oral-dose escalation regimens. Antimicrob Agents Chemother 2002;46(8):2546–53.
4. Marco F, Pfaller MA, Messer SA, Jones RN. Antifungal activity of a new triazole, voriconazole (UK-109,496), compared with three other antifungal agents tested against clinical isolates of filamentous fungi. Med Mycol 1998;36(6):433–6.
5. Groll AH, Gea-Banacloche JC, Glasmacher A, Just-Nuebling G, Maschmeyer G, Walsh TJ. Clinical pharmacology of antifungal compounds. Infect Dis Clin North Am 2003;17(1):159–91.
6. Groll AH, Walsh TJ. Antifungal chemotherapy: advances and perspectives. Swiss Med Wkly 2002;132(23–24):303–11.
7. Denning DW, Ribaud P, Milpied N, Caillot D, Herbrecht R, Thiel E, Haas A, Ruhnke M, Lode H. Efficacy and safety of voriconazole in the treatment of acute invasive aspergillosis. Clin Infect Dis 2002;34(5):563–71.
8. Walsh TJ, Pappas P, Winston DJ, Lazarus HM, Petersen F, Raffalli J, Yanovich S, Stiff P, Greenberg R, Donowitz G, Schuster M, Reboli A, Wingard J, Arndt C, Reinhardt J, Hadley S, Finberg R, Laverdiere M, Perfect J, Garber G, Fioritoni G, Anaissie E, Lee J; National Institute of Allergy and Infectious Diseases Mycoses Study Group. Voriconazole compared with liposomal amphotericin B for

empirical antifungal therapy in patients with neutropenia and persistent fever. N Engl J Med 2002;346(4):225–34.

9. Herbrecht R, Denning DW, Patterson TF, Bennett JE, Greene RE, Oestmann JW, Kern WV, Marr KA, Ribaud P, Lortholary O, Sylvester R, Rubin RH, Wingard JR, Stark P, Durand C, Caillot D, Thiel E, Chandrasekar PH, Hodges MR, Schlamm HT, Troke PF, de Pauw B; Invasive Fungal Infections Group of the European Organisation for Research and Treatment of Cancer and the Global Aspergillus Study Group. Voriconazole versus amphotericin B for primary therapy of invasive aspergillosis. N Engl J Med 2002;347(6):408–15.

10. Lazarus HM, Blumer JL, Yanovich S, Schlamm H, Romero A. Safety and pharmacokinetics of oral voriconazole in patients at risk of fungal infection: a dose escalation study. J Clin Pharmacol 2002;42(4):395–402.

11. Ally R, Schurmann D, Kreisel W, Carosi G, Aguirrebengoa K, Dupont B, Hodges M, Troke P, Romero AJ; Esophageal Candidiasis Study Group. A randomized, double-blind, double-dummy, multicenter trial of voriconazole and fluconazole in the treatment of esophageal candidiasis in immunocompromised patients. Clin Infect Dis 2001;33(9):1447–54.

12. Ullmann AJ. Review of the safety, tolerability, and drug interactions of the new antifungal agents caspofungin and voriconazole. Curr Med Res Opin 2003;19(4):263–71.

13. Walsh TJ, Karlsson MO, Driscoll T, Arguedas AG, Adamson P, Saez-Llorens X, Vora AJ, Arrieta AC, Blumer J, Lutsar I, Milligan P, Wood N. Pharmacokinetics and safety of intravenous voriconazole in children after single- or multiple-dose administration. Antimicrob Agents Chemother 2004;48(6):2166–72.

14. Walsh TJ, Lutsar I, Driscoll T, Dupont B, Roden M, Ghahramani P, Hodges M, Groll AH, Perfect JR. Voriconazole in the treatment of aspergillosis, scedosporiosis and other invasive fungal infections in children. Pediatr Infect Dis J 2002;21(3):240–8.

15. Romero AJ, Pogamp PL, Nilsson LG, Wood N. Effect of voriconazole on the pharmacokinetics of cyclosporine in renal transplant patients. Clin Pharmacol Ther 2002; 71(4):226–34.

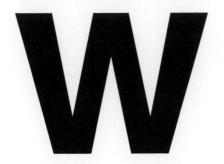

Wound dressings, substances used in

General Information

Substances that are used in wound dressings include hydrogels, hydrocolloids, alginates, and polyurethane foams. Medicaments that they contain include wool wax alcohols (amerchol, cetearyl alcohol, propylene glycol), plant resins/ethereal oils (balsam of Peru, colophony, fragrance mix, propolis), and topical antibiotics.

Organs and Systems

Immunologic

Patients with chronic venous insufficiency and venous leg ulcers are at risk of sensitization to topical medications. The frequency of sensitization in these patients is up to 67% (1). In a study using an expanded European standard series and 20 different wound dressings for patch-testing in 36 patients with chronic venous insufficiency, sensitization to modern wound dressings was found in 8.3% (three cases) and was caused by propylene glycol as an ingredient of hydrogels (2). However, it must be emphasized that positive patch test reactions to propylene glycol can indicate irritation rather than contact allergy. There were no cases of sensitization to hydrocolloids, alginates, or polyurethane foams. The rank order of allergens was headed by ointment bases (sensitization to wool wax alcohols in 33% of patients; amerchol 19%; cetearyl alcohol 14%; propylene glycol 8.3%), followed by plant resins/ethereal oils (balsam of Peru 22%; colophony 14%; fragrance mix 8.3%; propolis 5.6%), and topical antibiotics (neomycin sulfate 17%; chloramphenicol 14%) (3).

References

1. Wilson CL, Cameron J, Powell SM, Cherry G, Ryan TJ. High incidence of contact dermatitis in leg-ulcer patients—implications for management. Clin Exp Dermatol 1991;16(4):250–3.
2. Aberer W, Fuchs T, Peters K, PJ F. Propylenglykol: Kutane Nebenwirkungen und Testmethodik. Literaturübersicht und Ergebnisse einer Multicenterstudie der Deutschen Kontaktallergiegruppe (DKG). Dermatosen 1997;36:156–8.
3. Gallenkemper G, Rabe E, Bauer R. Contact sensitization in chronic venous insufficiency: modern wound dressings. Contact Dermatitis 1998;38(5):274–8.

WR-242511

General Information

WR-242511 is an 8-aminoquinoline that is being tested for activity against *Pneumocystis jiroveci* (1). In animals, it was more likely than primaquine to cause methemoglobinemia (SEDA-12, 703) (2).

References

1. Goheen MP, Bartlett MS, Shaw MM, Queener SF, Smith JW. Effects of 8-aminoquinolines on the ultrastructural morphology of *Pneumocystis carinii*. Int J Exp Pathol 1993;74(4):379–87.
2. Bartlett MS, Queener SF, Tidwell RR, Milhous WK, Berman JD, Ellis WY, Smith JW. 8-Aminoquinolines from Walter Reed Army Institute for Research for treatment and prophylaxis of *Pneumocystis* pneumonia in rat models. Antimicrob Agents Chemother 1991;35(2):277–82.

WR-243251

General Information

WR-243251 is a floxacrine analogue, a dihydroacridinedione. It is active in vitro against chloroquine-resistant, mefloquine-resistant, and pyrimethamine-resistant strains of malaria (1). By analogy to quinacrine and floxacrine, there is concern about possible dermatological, cardiac, and neuropsychiatric toxicity and vascular adverse effects.

Reference

1. Vennerstrom JL, Fu HN, Ellis WY, Ager AL Jr, Wood JK, Andersen SL, Gerena L, Milhous WK. Dispiro-1,2,4,5-tetraoxanes: a new class of antimalarial peroxides. J Med Chem 1992;35(16):3023–7.

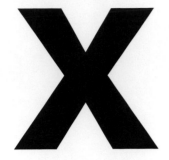

Xamoterol

See also Beta-adrenoceptor antagonists

General Information

Xamoterol is a beta-adrenoceptor antagonist/partial agonist that was developed for use in mild cases of cardiac failure and to treat atrial fibrillation (1). In more severe cases, however, it can actually worsen heart failure and increase mortality (2), because when sympathetic nervous system activity is high its beta-adrenoceptor antagonist properties predominate. It has therefore been withdrawn from the market (SEDA-18, 159).

References

1. Lawson-Matthew PJ, McLean KA, Dent M, Austin CA, Channer KS. Xamoterol improves the control of chronic atrial fibrillation in elderly patients. Age Ageing 1995;24(4):321–5.
2. Anonymous. New evidence on xamoterol. Lancet 1990;336(8706):24.

Xenon

See also General anesthetics

General Information

Xenon is a heavy gas (symbol Xe; atomic no 54) that is normally present in the atmosphere. It has been used as an anesthetic and as a diagnostic tool in functional neuroimaging (1).

Xenon has many characteristics of the ideal anesthetic (2). It has no effects on the cardiovascular system and has low solubility, enabling faster induction of and emergence from anesthesia. Although its high cost limits its use, the development of closed rebreathing systems has led to further interest. A European multicenter trial is under way.

Xenon-enhanced CT scanning in functional neuroimaging is based on the use of stable xenon gas, which is radiodense and lipid-soluble, as an inhaled contrast agent. The patient inhales a mixture of xenon, usually 26–33%, and oxygen for several minutes via a face mask. The inhaled xenon dissolves in the blood and passes into the brain parenchyma. CT scans can be acquired before, during, and after inhalation. Fast spiral CT has improved the capability of this technique.

General adverse reactions

Overall, about 10% of patients have unpleasant but usually transient adverse reactions. Xenon is a narcotic gas, more potent than nitrous oxide, and inhalation of 71% xenon is sufficient for anesthesia in 50% of patients. Lower concentrations of xenon are currently used, but some euphoric or dysphoric effects are still observed and can cause temporary exacerbation of neuropsychiatric symptoms. Mild nausea can also occur, and patients should have an empty stomach before the scan to reduce the risk of vomiting and possible aspiration. Very rarely, apnea can occur and can be reversed by instructing the patient to breathe. Like other narcotic gases, xenon causes mild cerebral vasodilatation.

Organs and Systems

Psychological, psychiatric

The subjective, psychomotor, and physiological properties of subanesthetic concentrations of xenon have been studied in 10 volunteers (3). Xenon sedation was well tolerated and was not associated with any adverse physiological effects. In particular, there was no nausea or vomiting. It was preferred to sedation with nitrous oxide and was subjectively dissimilar (xenon was more pleasant).

References

1. Taber KH, Zimmerman JG, Yonas H, Hart W, Hurley RA. Applications of xenon CT in clinical practice: detection of hidden lesions. J Neuropsychiatry Clin Neurosci 1999;11(4):423–5.
2. Leclerc J, Nieuviarts R, Tavernier B, Vallet B, Scherpereel P. Anesthésie an xénon: du mythe à la réalité. [Xenon anesthesia: from myth to reality.] Ann Fr Anesth Reanim 2001;20(1):70–6.
3. Bedi A, McCarroll C, Murray JM, Stevenson MA, Fee JP. The effects of subanaesthetic concentrations of xenon volunteers. Anaesthesia 2002;57(3):233–41.

Xipamide

See also Diuretics

General Information

Xipamide is a non-thiazide diuretic that acts mainly on the distal tubule (1). Its maximal diuretic effect is as great as that of furosemide, but its duration of action is longer and similar to that of the thiazides. Thus, like metolazone, it occupies an intermediate position between the two main groups of diuretics and can be used in renal insufficiency. However, xipamide does appear to present some risks, and it is not clear that these are outweighed by any advantages.

Organs and Systems

Metabolism

At equivalent therapeutic doses, the metabolic effects of xipamide are greater than those of the thiazides or furosemide (SED-11, 200).

Skin

A photoallergic skin reaction has been described in a patient taking xipamide (SEDA-16, 222).

Reference

1. Prichard BN, Brogden RN. Xipamide. A review of its pharmacodynamic and pharmaco kinetic properties and therapeutic efficacy. Drugs 1985;30(4):313–32.

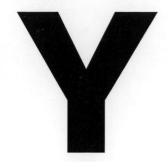

Yellow fever vaccine

See also Vaccines

General Information

Yellow fever vaccine contains the 17D virus strain grown in chick embryo tissue. The older (Dakar) yellow fever vaccine was prepared from more virulent material and often caused encephalitis, the risk in children being particularly high (SED-8, 712).

General adverse effects

The adverse effects of yellow fever vaccine have been documented by an expert group of the WHO (1).

Apart from minor postimmunization reactions the most common adverse effects are on the nervous system and allergic reactions.

On about the sixth day after immunization, under 5% of vaccinees develop fever, headache, and backache, lasting for 1–2 days.

Organs and Systems

Nervous system

About 20 cases of encephalitis have been recorded over a period of 40 years (SEDA-14, 1097). They all occurred in children: 12 in infants under 4 months old, two at 4 months, one at 6 months, one at 7 months, and one at 3 years of age. The last mentioned case was the only fatal one (17D virus was isolated from the brain), all the others recovered fully.

Encephalitis occurred after yellow fever immunization in a child older than 3 years of age and one over 9 months; a 13-year-old boy developed the disease 1 week after receipt of vaccine (2). The patient recovered after 1 month. There have been reports of encephalitis in a 29-year-old man and meningoencephalitis in two adults, suspected to be caused by the 17D yellow fever vaccine (3,4).

A case report of provocation of multiple sclerosis was published in 1967 (5), but this has not been confirmed.

Immunologic

Rash, erythema multiforme, urticaria, angioedema, and asthma occur infrequently, predominantly in people with a history of allergy, especially to eggs (1).

Severe immediate hypersensitivity reactions (type 1), sometimes accompanied by anaphylactic shock and circulatory collapse, have been described very rarely (1). Allergic reactions of the Arthus phenomenon type, characterized by local swelling and necrosis following less than 24 hours after immunization, have occurred in rare instances. Some of these cases have been fatal.

Two episodes have been reported from the Ivory Coast (1974) and Ghana (1982) (1). In the Ivory Coast, there were 39 cases of severe reactions with eight deaths following a mass campaign, in which 730 000 persons were immunized. The clinical features were uniform: a few hours after immunization the vaccinees developed signs of local inflammation. In severe cases, edema and inflammation were followed by cardiovascular collapse. Bacterial contamination could have been the cause: during the campaign, five-dose vaccine ampoules were pooled to prepare 50 and 100 doses for use in jet injectors. In Ghana, six vaccinees developed fulminant reactions 2–6 hours after immunization, including two deaths. The clinical features resembled those in the Ivory Coast episode. In 2001, during a mass vaccination campaign against yellow fever in Abidjan, the Ivory Coast, more than 2.6 million doses were administered and 87 adverse events were notified, of which 41 were considered to be vaccine-related. There was one case of anaphylaxis and 26 cases of urticaria, five of which were generalized (6).

People who are known to be suffering from allergy must be tested intradermally before immunization.

Multiorgan failure

There have been reports of seven cases of serious adverse events (including six deaths) after yellow fever immunization (7–11). The cases occurred from 1996 to 2001 in Australia ($n = 1$), Brazil ($n = 2$), and the USA ($n = 4$). The two people in Brazil were immunized with vaccine containing the live attenuated 17DD yellow fever strain and the others received vaccine containing the live attenuated 17D-204 strain; both strains are derived from the original 17D vaccine strain. All seven became ill within 2–5 days after immunization and required intensive care. Illness was characterized by fever, lymphocytopenia, thrombocytopenia, raised hepatocellular enzymes, hypotension, and respiratory failure. Most also had headache, vomiting, myalgia, hyperbilirubinemia, and renal insufficiency requiring hemodialysis. In some aspects the disease was similar to natural yellow fever. The causal association between multiorgan failure and the receipt of yellow fever vaccine is supported in most cases by isolation of the vaccine virus and histopathological changes; in cases with lack of specimens the temporal association and the similarity of the clinical presentations makes a causal association likely.

Susceptibility Factors

Age

Infants under 9 months old are not generally immunized, except if they live in rural areas with a history of yellow fever epidemics (immunization at 6 months) or in an active epidemic focus (immunization at 4 months) (1).

References

1. World Heath Organization. Prevention and Control of Yellow Fever in Africa. Geneva: WHO, 1986.
2. Schoub BD, Dommann CJ, Johnson S, Downie C, Patel PL. Encephalitis in a 13-year-old boy following 17D yellow fever vaccine. J Infect 1990;21(1):105–6.
3. Merlo C, Steffen R, Landis T, Tsai T, Karabatsos N. Possible association of encephalitis and 17D yellow fever

vaccination in a 29-year-old traveller. Vaccine 1993;11(6):691.

4. Drouet A, Chagnon A, Valance J, Carli P, Muzellec Y, Paris JF. Meningo-encephalite après vaccination anti-amanile par la souche 17 D: deux observations. [Meningoencephalitis after vaccination against yellow fever with the 17D strain: 2 cases.] Rev Med Interne 1993;14(4):257–9.

5. Miller H, Cendrowski W, Shapira K. Multiple sclerosis and vaccination. BMJ 1967;2(546):210–13.

6. Fitzner J, Coulibaly D, Kouadio DE, Yavo JC, Loukou YG, Koudou PO, Coulombier D. Safety of the yellow fever vaccine during the September 2001 mass vaccination campaign in Abidjan, Ivory Coast. Vaccine 2004;23(2):156–62.

7. Centers for Disease Control and Prevention (CDC). Fever, jaundice, and multiple organ system failure associated with 17D-derived yellow fever vaccination, 1996–2001. MMWR Morb Mortal Wkly Rep 2001;50(30):643–5.

8. Anonymous. Adverse events following yellow fever vaccination. Wkly Epidemiol Rec 2001;76(29):217–18.

9. Vasconcelos PF, Luna EJ, Galler R, Silva LJ, Coimbra TL, Barros VL, Monath TP, Rodigues SG, Laval C, Costa ZG, Vilela MF, Santos CL, Papaiordanou PM, Alves VA, Andrade LD, Sato HK, Rosa ES, Froguas GB, Lacava E, Almeida LM, Cruz AC, Rocco IM, Santos RT, Oliva OF; Brazilian Yellow Fever Vaccine Evaluation Group. Serious adverse events associated with yellow fever 17DD vaccine in Brazil: a report of two cases. Lancet 2001;358(9276):91–7.

10. Chan RC, Penney DJ, Little D, Carter IW, Roberts JA, Rawlinson WD. Hepatitis and death following vaccination with 17D-204 yellow fever vaccine. Lancet 2001;358(9276):121–2.

11. Martin M, Tsai TF, Cropp B, Chang GJ, Holmes DA, Tseng J, Shieh W, Zaki SR, Al-Sanouri I, Cutrona AF, Ray G, Weld LH, Cetron MS. Fever and multisystem organ failure associated with 17D-204 yellow fever vaccination: a report of four cases. Lancet 2001;358(9276):98–104.

Yohimbine

General Information

Yohimbine is a major carboline alkaloid in the bark of *Pausinystalia* species, such as *Pausinystalia yohimbe* (*Corynanthe yohimbe*), *Pausinystalia macrocerus*, *Pausinystalia paniculata*, and *Pausinystalia trillesi*. It is also found in *Pseudocinchona africana* and *Rauwolfia canescens*.

Yohimbine is an alpha$_2$-adrenoceptor antagonist and has been used in the treatment of erectile dysfunction. At high doses its most common effects are increased blood pressure, slight anxiety, and increased frequency of micturition (1). In a systematic review of randomized controlled trials (2), the following adverse events were noted: hypertension, allergic skin reactions, anxiety, dizziness, chills, headache, sweating, agitation, tachycardia, gastrointestinal symptoms, diarrhea, loss of energy, and increased urinary frequency.

Organs and Systems

Cardiovascular

In 25 unmedicated subjects with hypertension yohimbine 22 mg increased mean blood pressure by an average of 5 mm Hg, plasma noradrenaline by 66%, and plasma dihydroxyphenylglycol by 25% at 1 hour after administration (3). The magnitude of the pressor response was unrelated to baseline pressure but correlated positively with baseline noradrenaline concentration and with the yohimbine-induced increment in plasma noradrenaline.

In 25 healthy volunteers and 29 sex- and age-matched untreated hypertensive patients yohimbine 10 mg caused a significant increase in diastolic pressure only in the hypertensive patients (4).

In patients taking tricyclic antidepressants, hypertension can occur at a dose of 4 mg tds. The toxicity of yohimbine can be enhanced by other drugs, such as phenothiazines.

Angina pectoris has been attributed to yohimbine (5).

- A patient with CREST syndrome (calcinosis, Raynaud's phenomenon, esophageal dysfunction, sclerodactyly, and telangiectasia) paradoxically experienced worsening of Raynaud's phenomenon when using yohimbine for erectile dysfunction (6).

Respiratory

Bronchospasm has been attributed to yohimbine (7).

Nervous system

In a double-blind, placebo-controlled study in eight patients receiving methadone, yohimbine 4 mg/kg intravenously caused objective and subjective opioid withdrawal symptoms and increased craving for opioids (8). This was attributed to increased sensitivity of postsynaptic responses to noradrenaline.

Sensory systems

In a placebo-controlled, crossover study in seven healthy subjects oral yohimbine 0.4 mg/kg caused a significant but transient reduction in P50 auditory gating (9).

Psychological, psychiatric

Yohimbine commonly causes anxiety; in eight patients with panic disorder this effect was reduced by fluvoxamine (10).

Manic symptoms have been attributed to yohimbine (11).

In a placebo-controlled study in 18 combat veterans with post-traumatic stress disorder and 11 healthy controls, intravenous yohimbine 0.4 mg/kg significantly increased the amplitude, magnitude, and probability of the acoustic startle reflex (used as a model to investigate the neurochemical basis of anxiety and fear states) in the veterans with post-traumatic stress disorder but not in the controls (12).

Hematologic

Agranulocytosis has been attributed to yohimbine (13).

Immunologic

A lupus-like syndrome in conjunction with generalized erythroderma and progressive renal insufficiency has been attributed to yohimbine (14,15).

Drug Administration

Drug overdose

- In a 62-year-old man who took yohimbine 200 mg the only adverse effects were tachycardia, hypertension, and anxiety of brief duration (16).

This case suggests that yohimbine overdose is relatively benign.

- A 16-year-old girl who took yohimbine in the form of an alleged aphrodisiac known as "yo-yo" had an acute dissociative reaction accompanied by weakness, paresthesia, and incoordination, followed by anxiety, headache, nausea, palpitation, and chest pain; she also had hypertension, tachycardia, tachypnea, sweating, pallor, tremor, and an erythematous rash (17). Serum adrenaline and noradrenaline concentrations were raised. Her symptoms lasted about 36 hours and resolved spontaneously.

Drug–Drug Interactions

Phenytoin

Yohimbine can cause loss of the antiepileptic action of phenytoin (2).

Tricyclic antidepressants

Yohimbine has a sialogenic effect in depressed patients with a dry mouth due to tricyclic antidepressants or neuroleptic drugs (18).

However, there is an increased risk of hypertension when tricyclic antidepressants are combined with yohimbine (19).

References

1. Tam SW, Worcel M, Wyllie M. Yohimbine: a clinical review. Pharmacol Ther 2001;91(3):215–43.
2. Ernst E, Pittler MH. Yohimbine for erectile dysfunction: a systematic review and meta-analysis of randomized clinical trials. J Urol 1998;159(2):433–6.
3. Grossman E, Rosenthal T, Peleg E, Holmes C, Goldstein DS. Oral yohimbine increases blood pressure and sympathetic nervous outflow in hypertensive patients. J Cardiovasc Pharmacol 1993;22(1):22–6.
4. Musso NR, Vergassola C, Pende A, Lotti G. Yohimbine effects on blood pressure and plasma catecholamines in human hypertension. Am J Hypertens 1995;8(6):565–71.
5. Epelde Gonzalo F. Angor inducido por yohimbina. [Yohimbine-induced angina pectoris.] An Med Interna 1998;15(12):676.
6. Johnson S, Iazzetta J, Dewar C. Severe Raynaud's phenomenon with yohimbine therapy for erectile dysfunction. J Rheumatol 2003;30(11):2503–5.
7. Landis E, Shore E. Yohimbine-induced bronchospasm. Chest 1989;96(6):1424.
8. Stine SM, Southwick SM, Petrakis IL, Kosten TR, Charney DS, Krystal JH. Yohimbine-induced withdrawal and anxiety symptoms in opioid-dependent patients. Biol Psychiatry 2002;51(8):642–51.
9. Adler LE, Hoffer L, Nagamoto HT, Waldo MC, Kisley MA, Giffith JM. Yohimbine impairs P50 auditory sensory gating in normal subjects. Neuropsychopharmacology 1994;10(4):249–57.
10. Goddard AW, Woods SW, Sholomskas DE, Goodman WK, Charney DS, Heninger GR. Effects of the serotonin reuptake inhibitor fluvoxamine on yohimbine-induced anxiety in panic disorder. Psychiatry Res 1993;48(2):119–33.
11. Price LH, Charney DS, Heninger GR. Three cases of manic symptoms following yohimbine administration. Am J Psychiatry 1984;141(10):1267–8.
12. Morgan CA 3rd, Grillon C, Southwick SM, Nagy LM, Davis M, Krystal JH, Charney DS. Yohimbine facilitated acoustic startle in combat veterans with post-traumatic stress disorder. Psychopharmacology (Berl) 1995;117(4):466–71.
13. Siddiqui MA, More-O'Ferrall D, Hammod RS, Baime RV, Staddon AP. Agranulocytosis associated with yohimbine use. Arch Intern Med 1996;156(11):1235–8.
14. Sandler B, Aronson P. Yohimbine-induced cutaneous drug eruption, progressive renal failure, and lupus-like syndrome. Urology 1993;41(4):343–5.
15. De Smet PA, Smeets OS. Potential risks of health food products containing yohimbe extracts. BMJ 1994;309(6959):958.
16. Friesen K, Palatnick W, Tenenbein M. Benign course after massive ingestion of yohimbine. J Emerg Med 1993;11(3):287–8.
17. Linden CH, Vellman WP, Rumack B. Yohimbine: a new street drug. Ann Emerg Med 1985;14(10):1002–4.
18. Bagheri H, Schmitt L, Berlan M, Montastruc JL. A comparative study of the effects of yohimbine and anetholtrithione on salivary secretion in depressed patients treated with psychotropic drugs. Eur J Clin Pharmacol 1997;52(5):339–42.
19. Fugh-Berman A. Herb–drug interactions. Lancet 2000;355(9198):134–8.

Z

Zafirlukast

See also Leukotriene receptor antagonists

General Information

Zafirlukast is a leukotriene receptor antagonist, used in the treatment of asthma.

Organs and Systems

Liver

In the early clinical trials a range of doses of zafirlukast were used. With higher doses (80 mg bd) serum liver enzymes were occasionally raised. In subsequent clinical trials with 20 mg bd, a raised alanine transaminase activity was twice as common as in patients taking placebo [1].

Sporadic cases of severe hepatotoxicity [2–4], requiring orthotopic liver transplantation for subacute liver failure in two cases [5], prompted a revision of the "Adverse Events" section in the Physicians' Desk Reference [6].

Hepatitis has been attributed to zafirlukast in two cases.

- A 54-year-old asthmatic man developed subacute hepatitis and hepatic encephalopathy while taking zafirlukast 20 mg bd for 8 months and co-amoxiclav 2 g/day for a few days [3]. He also took antihistamines, inhaled glucocorticoids, and beta-blockers (not specified). A percutaneous liver biopsy showed severe hepatocellular necrosis and eosinophilic infiltrates without prominent cholestasis. Raised transaminases and total serum bilirubin normalized within 3 months after withdrawal of zafirlukast and co-amoxiclav and the use of intermittent, high-dose, parenteral glucocorticoids, followed by oral tapering.
- A 55-year-old asthmatic woman had subacute liver injury with severe hepatic necrosis and eosinophilic infiltrates while taking zafirlukast 20 mg bd and salbutamol sulfate nasal spray for 5 months [4]. There was no evidence of viral, metabolic, alcohol-related, or autoimmune hepatitis. Zafirlukast was withdrawn and liver function normalized within 2 months.

The authors concluded that subacute hepatitis in the second patient had been related to zafirlukast, but suggested that co-amoxiclav might also have been a precipitating factor. The long latency between the start of zafirlukast treatment and the onset of hepatotoxicity and the slow response to drug withdrawal and glucocorticoid treatment are reminiscent of previous cases of zafirlukast-related hepatotoxicity.

Drug–Drug Interactions

Aspirin

The plasma concentrations of zafirlukast rise when it is administered concurrently with aspirin [7].

Macrolide antibiotics

Zafirlukast 20 mg bd for 12 days did not interfere with the metabolism of azithromycin or clarithromycin [8]. However, the plasma concentrations of zafirlukast are reduced when it is administered concurrently with erythromycin [7].

Terfenadine

The plasma concentrations of zafirlukast are reduced when it is administered concurrently with terfenadine [7].

Theophylline

The plasma concentrations of zafirlukast are reduced when it is administered concurrently with theophylline [7]. Conversely, zafirlukast can increase serum theophylline concentrations.

- A 15-year-old girl with asthma, who had taken theophylline 300 mg bd for several years, with serum concentrations of about 61 μmol/l started to take zafirlukast [9]. Her serum theophylline concentration increased to 133 μmol/l. Rechallenge confirmed the effect.

The authors proposed that zafirlukast had inhibited CYP1A2, by which theophylline is metabolized.

Warfarin

Zafirlukast reduces the clearance of warfarin, resulting in a clinically significant prolongation of prothrombin time [10]. The mechanism for this interaction is thought to be inhibition of cytochrome P450 enzymes, such as CYP2C9.

References

1. Fish JE, Kemp JP, Lockey RF, Glass M, Hanby LA, Bonuccelli CM, Bronsky M, Condemi J, Golsdtein S, Norton J, et al. Zafirlukast for symptomatic mild-to-moderate asthma: a 13-week multicenter study. The Zafirlukast Trialists Group. Clin Ther 1997;19(4):675–90.
2. Danese S, De Vitis I, Gasbarrini A. Severe liver injury associated with zafirlukast. Ann Intern Med 2001;135(10):930.
3. Torres M, Reddy KR. Severe liver injury. Ann Intern Med 2001;135(7):550.
4. Physician's Desk Reference. Montvale. NJ: Medical Economics, 2001:611–3.
5. Bostanci I, Sarioglu A, Ergin H, Aksit A, Cinbis M, Akalin N. Neonatal goiter caused by expectorant usage. J Pediatr Endocrinol Metab 2001;14(8):1161–2.
6. Taylor J, Kotch A, Rice K, Ghafouri M, Kurland CL, Fagan NM, Witek TJ Jr; Ipratropium Bromide HFA Study Group. Ipratropium bromide hydrofluoroalkane inhalation aerosol is safe and effective in patients with COPD. Chest 2001;120(4):1253–61.
7. Dekhuijzen PN, Koopmans PP. Pharmacokinetic profile of zafirlukast. Clin Pharmacokinet 2002;41(2):105–14.
8. Garey KW, Peloquin CA, Godo PG, Nafziger AN, Amsden GW. Lack of effect of zafirlukast on the pharmacokinetics of azithromycin, clarithromycin, and 14-hydroxy-clarithromycin in healthy volunteers. Antimicrob Agents Chemother 1999;43(5):1152–5.
9. Katial RK, Stelzle RC, Bonner MW, Marino M, Cantilena LR, Smith LJ. A drug interaction between zafirlukast and theophylline. Arch Intern Med 1998;158(15):1713–15.
10. Kelloway JS. Zafirlukast: the first leukotriene-receptor antagonist approved for the treatment of asthma. Ann Pharmacother 1997;31(9):1012–21.

Zalcitabine

See also Nucleoside analogue reverse transcriptase inhibitors (NRTIs)

General Information

Zalcitabine is a nucleoside analogue reverse transcriptase inhibitor. Because of the high incidence of nervous system adverse effects and the availability of less toxic alternatives, zalcitabine is no longer used.

Comparative studies

Several large-scale studies of the efficacy of combined antiretroviral treatment with zalcitabine and zidovudine in HIV-infected patients (compared with zidovudine monotherapy or a combination of zidovudine and didanosine) have not shown unexpected adverse effects (1–4). The most common adverse effects in patients taking zalcitabine were peripheral neuropathy and aphthous mouth ulcers.

Organs and Systems

Nervous system

A peripheral neuropathy is often observed in patients treated with didanosine, stavudine, and zalcitabine (5,6). It usually occurs after prolonged treatment (more than 4 months), most often with zalcitabine, and often requires drug withdrawal, but it is sometimes not fully reversible. Mitochondrial alterations have been demonstrated in Schwann cells of peripheral nerves and dorsal root ganglia in rabbits treated with zalcitabine (7).

Hematologic

Thrombocytopenia has been observed in patients using zalcitabine and didanosine (8,9).

References

1. Delta Coordinating Committee. Delta: a randomised double-blind controlled trial comparing combinations of zidovudine plus didanosine or zalcitabine with zidovudine alone in HIV-infected individuals. Lancet 1996;348(9023):283–91.
2. Hammer SM, Katzenstein DA, Hughes MD, Gundacker H, Schooley RT, Haubrich RH, Henry WK, Lederman MM, Phair JP, Niu M, Hirsch MS, Merigan TC. A trial comparing nucleoside monotherapy with combination therapy in HIV-infected adults with CD4 cell counts from 200 to 500 per cubic millimeter. AIDS Clinical Trials Group Study 175 Study Team. N Engl J Med 1996;335(15):1081–90.
3. Schooley RT, Ramirez-Ronda C, Lange JM, Cooper DA, Lavelle J, Lefkowitz L, Moore M, Larder BA, St Clair M, Mulder JW, McKinnis R, Pennington KN, Harrigan PR, Kinghorn I, Steel H, Rooney JF. Virologic and immunologic benefits of initial combination therapy with zidovudine and zalcitabine or didanosine compared with zidovudine monotherapy. Wellcome Resistance Study Collaborative Group. J Infect Dis 1996;173(6):1354–66.
4. Saravolatz LD, Winslow DL, Collins G, Hodges JS, Pettinelli C, Stein DS, Markowitz N, Reves R, Loveless MO, Crane L, Thompson M, Abrams D.

Zidovudine alone or in combination with didanosine or zalcitabine in HIV-infected patients with the acquired immunodeficiency syndrome or fewer than 200 CD4 cells per cubic millimeter. Investigators for the Terry Beirn Community Programs for Clinical Research on AIDS. N Engl J Med 1996;335(15):1099–106.
5. Fichtenbaum CJ, Clifford DB, Powderly WG. Risk factors for dideoxynucleoside-induced toxic neuropathy in patients with the human immunodeficiency virus infection. J Acquir Immune Defic Syndr Hum Retrovirol 1995;10(2):169–74.
6. Simpson DM, Tagliati M. Nucleoside analogue-associated peripheral neuropathy in human immunodeficiency virus infection. J Acquir Immune Defic Syndr Hum Retrovirol 1995;9(2):153–61.
7. Feldman D, Anderson TD. Schwann cell mitochondrial alterations in peripheral nerves of rabbits treated with 2′,3′-dideoxycytidine. Acta Neuropathol (Berl) 1994;87(1):71–80.
8. Yarchoan R, Perno CF, Thomas RV, Klecker RW, Allain JP, Wills RJ, McAtee N, Fischl MA, Dubinsky R, McNeely MC, et al. Phase I studies of 2′,3′-dideoxycytidine in severe human immunodeficiency virus infection as a single agent and alternating with zidovudine (AZT). Lancet 1988;1(8577):76–81.
9. Dolin R, Lambert JS, Morse GD, Reichman RC, Plank CS, Reid J, Knupp C, McLaren C, Pettinelli C. 2′,3′-Dideoxyinosine in patients with AIDS or AIDS–related complex. Rev Infect Dis 1990;12(Suppl 5):S540–9.

Zaleplon

General Information

Zaleplon is a non-benzodiazepine that induces sleep comparable to other hypnotics but with significantly fewer residual effects (1), related at least in part to its short half-life. It is a pyrazolopyrimidine hypnotic that binds selectively to the $GABA_{A1A}$ receptor, previously known as the benzodiazepine type 1 (BDZ_1) receptor. Whereas such agonist selectivity was hoped to confer advantages in terms of the risk of adverse effects, in practice zaleplon is similar to the older non-selective benzodiazepines in terms of both efficacy and safety (2–4). The so-called "Z drugs," including zaleplon, are significantly more expensive than benzodiazepines and are therefore likely to be less cost-effective (5).

Pharmacokinetics

After oral administration zaleplon is well absorbed (71%) and peak concentrations are reached in about 60 minutes. However, it undergoes presystemic elimination and has a systemic availability of about 30%. Its adverse effects include anterograde amnesia, depression, paradoxical reactions (for example restlessness, agitation), dependence, and withdrawal symptoms (related to the dose and duration of treatment). Although the data are limited, it is thought to be relatively safe in overdose, unless it is combined with other CNS depressants.

The pharmacokinetics and absolute oral systemic availability of zaleplon have been assessed in a partially randomized, single-dose, crossover study in 23 healthy subjects, who received intravenous infusions of zaleplon 1 and 2.5 mg during the first and second periods and were then randomly assigned to receive an oral dose of 5 mg or an intravenous infusion of 5 mg in a crossover design (6). The oral and intravenous doses of zaleplon were well tolerated. Somnolence, abnormal vision, diplopia, and dizziness were the most commonly reported adverse events.

Pharmacological effects

Initial pharmacodynamic data suggested that sleep latency is improved by zaleplon and there is no significant next-day psychomotor impairment or memory impairment (7), and evaluations at zaleplon peak plasma concentrations show much less impairment than with other hypnotics, suggesting an improved benefit-to-harm balance for zaleplon compared with older agents. However, outcome data are mainly from industry-sponsored trials and are often difficult to compare. Differences between zaleplon and benzodiazepine hypnotics may have been exaggerated (3,4).

Zaleplon can be used to treat symptoms of insomnia with little next-day psychomotor or memory impairment. However, further research is needed.

Comparative studies

A review of published studies of zaleplon has shown that it has a quick onset of action and undergoes rapid elimination, which results in an arguably better safety profile than previously available agents (8). In addition, rebound insomnia and other withdrawal effects have not been demonstrated with zaleplon, and it is well tolerated in both young and older patients. These characteristics may be advantageous for patients who should not receive benzodiazepines.

Placebo-controlled studies

Three doses of zaleplon have been compared with placebo in outpatients with insomnia in a 4-week study (9). During week 1, sleep latency was significantly shorter with zaleplon 5, 10, and 20 mg than with placebo. The significant reduction in sleep latency persisted to week 3 with zaleplon 10 mg and to week 4 with zaleplon 20 mg. Compared with placebo, zaleplon 10 mg and 20 mg also had significant positive effects on sleep duration, number of awakenings, and sleep quality. Pharmacological tolerance did not develop with zaleplon and there were no indications of rebound insomnia or withdrawal symptoms after discontinuation. There was no significant difference in the frequency of adverse events with zaleplon compared with placebo. The authors concluded that zaleplon provides effective treatment of insomnia with a favorable safety profile.

Zaleplon versus triazolam

Zaleplon and triazolam have been compared in two concurrent multicenter, randomized, double-blind, placebo-controlled crossover studies in chronic insomniacs (10). Study 1 compared zaleplon (10 and 40 mg) with triazolam (0.25 mg) and placebo; study 2 compared zaleplon (20 and 60 mg) with triazolam (0.25 mg) and placebo. All doses of zaleplon produced significant reductions in sleep latency, and triazolam 0.25 mg reduced sleep latency comparable with zaleplon 10 mg. Only triazolam

and zaleplon 60 mg produced significant increases in total sleep time compared with placebo. Zaleplon 40 and 60 mg and triazolam also reduced the percentage of REM sleep compared with placebo. There was no evidence of residual daytime impairment with zaleplon, but triazolam produced significant impairment in performance on a digit copying test. There were more adverse events with zaleplon 60 mg compared with triazolam 0.25 mg and placebo. The most frequently reported adverse events with all treatments included headache, dizziness, and somnolence.

Zaleplon versus zolpidem

Zaleplon and zolpidem have been compared in two concurrent multicenter, randomized, double-blind, placebo-controlled crossover studies in chronic insomniacs (10). In study 1, zaleplon 10 mg, zolpidem 10 mg, or placebo were given double-blind to 36 healthy subjects under standardized conditions in a six-period, incomplete-block, crossover study (11). The subjects were gently awakened and given the medication at predetermined times, 5, 4, 3, or 2 hours before morning awakening, which occurred 8 hours after bedtime. When they awoke in the morning, subjective and objective assessments of residual effects of hypnotics were administered. There were no serious adverse experiences during the study; all adverse events were mild to moderate. The most commonly reported adverse events associated with zaleplon were weakness and somnolence. Weakness, depersonalization, dizziness, and somnolence were the most frequent nervous system adverse events associated with zolpidem.

Zaleplon has been compared with zolpidem 10 mg and placebo in 615 adult outpatients with insomnia (12). After a 7-night placebo (baseline) period, the patients were randomly assigned to receive one of five treatments in double-blind fashion for 28 nights (zaleplon 5, 10, or 20 mg; zolpidem 10 mg; or placebo), followed by placebo for 3 nights. Sleep latency, sleep maintenance, and sleep quality were determined from sleep questionnaires each morning. Rebound insomnia and withdrawal effects on withdrawal were also assessed. There was no evidence of rebound insomnia or withdrawal symptoms on withdrawal of zaleplon after 4 weeks. The frequency of adverse events in the active treatment groups did not differ significantly from that in the placebo group.

The pharmacokinetics and pharmacodynamics of zaleplon (10 or 20 mg) and zolpidem (10 or 20 mg) have been investigated in a randomized, double-blind, crossover, placebo-controlled study in 10 healthy volunteers with no history of sleep disorder (13). The half-life of zaleplon was significantly shorter than that of zolpidem. Zaleplon produced less sedation than zolpidem at the two doses studied, and the sedation scores in the zaleplon groups returned to baseline sooner than in the zolpidem groups. Zaleplon had no effect on recent or remote recall, whereas zolpidem had a significant effect on both measures.

Organs and Systems

Psychological, psychiatric

- A 25-year-old unmarried Asian woman with high intellectual functioning and psychiatric history developed illusions and hallucinations and a feeling of superior psychosocial adjustment, with no current or prior medical or depersonalization within several minutes of taking zaleplon 10 mg (14). The illusions and visual hallucinations resolved after 15 minutes, but she continued to have light-headedness and fatigue, which gradually resolved by the next day.

Drug–Drug Interactions

Alcohol

The addition of alcohol to the Z drugs, zaleplon, zolpidem, and zopiclone, produces additive sedative effects without altering their pharmacokinetics (15).

The effects of alcohol combined with either zaleplon or triazolam have been studied in 18 healthy volunteers (16). Triazolam, with and without ethanol, impaired digit symbol substitution, symbol copying, simple and complex reaction times, and divided attention performance compared with placebo. Zaleplon without ethanol impaired only digit symbol substitution and divided attention tracking, but when it was combined with ethanol all measures were impaired. However, zaleplon without ethanol was consistently better than triazolam alone. Zaleplon produced less performance impairment and a shorter period of ethanol potentiation than triazolam.

Cimetidine

Cimetidine increases plasma concentrations of the Z drugs and increases their sedative effects (15); this occurs to a lesser extent than the similar effect on benzodiazepines that are exclusively metabolized by CYP3A4.

Digoxin

The interaction of zaleplon with digoxin has been investigated in 20 subjects (17). There were one or more adverse effects in 18% of those who took digoxin alone and 35% of those who took digoxin plus zaleplon, but these were all mild and resolved quickly. Zaleplon had no significant effects on selected pharmacokinetic and pharmacodynamic properties of digoxin.

Erythromycin

Erythromycin increases plasma concentrations of the Z drugs and increases their sedative effects (15); this occurs to a lesser extent than the similar effect on benzodiazepines that are exclusively metabolized by CYP3A4.

Ibuprofen

The interaction of zaleplon with ibuprofen has been investigated in 17 subjects (18). Healthy adult volunteers were given zaleplon 10 mg alone, ibuprofen 600 mg alone, or zaleplon 10 mg plus ibuprofen 600 mg in an open, randomized, crossover study. The adverse effects were mild and resolved without intervention. The authors concluded that there was no evidence of a significant interaction between zaleplon and ibuprofen.

Ketoconazole

Ketoconazole increases plasma concentrations of the Z drugs and increases their sedative effects (15); this occurs to a lesser extent than the similar effect on benzodiazepines that are exclusively metabolized by CYP3A4.

Rifampicin

Rifampicin significantly induces the metabolism of zaleplon and reduces its sedative action (15), although the effect is less than the effect of rifampicin on triazolam or midazolam, probably because they are more exclusively metabolized by CYP3A4.

References

1. Mangano RM. Efficacy and safety of zaleplon at peak plasma levels. Int J Clin Pract Suppl 2001;116:9–13.
2. Landolt HP, Gillin JC. GABA(A1a) receptors: involvement in sleep regulation and potential of selective agonists in the treatment of insomnia. CNS Drugs 2000;13(3):185–99.
3. Anonymous. What's wrong with prescribing hypnotics? Drug Ther Bull 2004;42(12):89–93.
4. Holbrook AM. Treating insomnia. BMJ 2004; 329(7476):1198–9.
5. Dundar Y, Boland A, Strobl J, Dodd S, Haycox A, Bagust A, Bogg J, Dickson R, Walley T. Newer hypnotic drugs for the short-term management of insomnia: a systematic review and economic evaluation. Health Technol Assess 2004;8(24):iii–x, 1–125.
6. Rosen AS, Fournie P, Darwish M, Danjou P, Troy SM. Zaleplon pharmacokinetics and absolute bioavailability. Biopharm Drug Dispos 1999;20(3):171–5.
7. Anonymous. Does zaleplon help you sleep and wake refreshed? Drug Ther Perspect 1999;14:1–4.
8. Israel AG, Kramer JA. Safety of zaleplon in the treatment of insomnia. Ann Pharmacother 2002;36(5):852–9.
9. Fry J, Scharf M, Mangano R, Fujimori M. Zaleplon improves sleep without producing rebound effects in outpatients with insomnia. Zaleplon Clinical Study Group. Int Clin Psychopharmacol 2000;15(3):141–52.
10. Drake CL, Roehrs TA, Mangano RM, Roth T. Dose–response effects of zaleplon as compared with triazolam (0.25 mg) and placebo in chronic primary insomnia. Hum Psychopharmacol 2000;15(8):595–604.
11. Danjou P, Paty I, Fruncillo R, Worthington P, Unruh M, Cevallos W, Martin P. A comparison of the residual effects of zaleplon and zolpidem following administration 5 to 2 h before awakening. Br J Clin Pharmacol 1999;48(3):367–74.
12. Elie R, Ruther E, Farr I, Emilien G, Salinas E. Sleep latency is shortened during 4 weeks of treatment with zaleplon, a novel nonbenzodiazepine hypnotic. Zaleplon Clinical Study Group. J Clin Psychiatry 1999;60(8):536–44.
13. Drover D, Lemmens H, Naidu S, Cevallos W, Darwish M, Stanski D. Pharmacokinetics, pharmacodynamics, and relative pharmacokinetic/pharmacodynamic profiles of zaleplon and zolpidem. Clin Ther 2000;22(12):1443–61.
14. Bhatia SC, Arora M, Bhatia SK. Perceptual disturbances with zaleplon. Psychiatr Serv 2001;52(1):109–10.
15. Hesse LM, von Moltke LL, Greenblatt DJ. Clinically important drug interactions with zopiclone, zolpidem and zaleplon. CNS Drugs 2003;17(7):513–32.
16. Roehrs T, Rosenthal L, Koshorek G, Mangano RM, Roth T. Effects of zaleplon or triazolam with or without ethanol on human performance. Sleep Med 2001;2(4):323–32.

17. Sanchez Garcia P, Paty I, Leister CA, Guerra P, Frias J, Garcia Perez LE, Darwish M. Effect of zaleplon on digoxin pharmacokinetics and pharmacodynamics. Am J Health Syst Pharm 2000;57(24):2267–70.
18. Sanchez Garcia P, Carcas A, Zapater P, Rosendo J, Paty I, Leister CA, Troy SM. Absence of an interaction between ibuprofen and zaleplon. Am J Health Syst Pharm 2000;57(12):1137–41.

Zidometacin

See also Non-steroidal anti-inflammatory drugs

General Information

Zidometacin differs from indometacin in having an azido group in the *para*-position, where indometacin has a benzyl group. It appears to be less ulcerogenic in animals. However, epigastric pain, burning, and nausea have been experienced by patients taking zidometacin (1).

Reference

1. Friez L. Preliminary clinical experience with zidometacin. Acta Ther 1985;11:109.

Zidovudine

See also Nucleoside analogue reverse transcriptase inhibitors (NRTIs)

General Information

Zidovudine is a nucleoside analogue reverse transcriptase inhibitor. Its adverse effects include hematological complications, severe headache, insomnia, confusion, nausea, vomiting, abdominal discomfort, myalgia (myopathy), and nail pigmentation (1).

Observational studies

Oral zidovudine in a dosage of 200 mg every 4 hours for 42 days was used as prophylaxis in health-care workers after percutaneous exposure to blood or body fluids from HIV-infected patients. Adverse reactions occurred in 73%, the most frequent being nausea (47%), headache (35%), and fatigue (30%). Of selected hematological laboratory markers only platelet counts increased significantly over 4 weeks. Although adverse reactions were not very severe and none of the laboratory changes was considered clinically significant, treatment was poorly accepted and stopped prematurely by 30% (2). Current guidelines for postexposure prophylaxis recommend a much lower dosage (300 mg bd) with much better tolerance (3).

Comparative studies

The safety and efficacy of lamivudine (300–600 mg/day) in combination with zidovudine (600 mg/day) in the treatment of antiretroviral-naive and zidovudine-experienced HIV-infected persons has been compared with zidovudine monotherapy in two placebo-controlled studies of 129 and 223 patients (4,5). There were no significant differences in the incidence or severity of adverse effects between patients taking zidovudine alone or in combination with lamivudine. In both studies gastrointestinal symptoms, notably nausea, were the most commonly observed adverse reactions, occurring in 5–11% of zidovudine-experienced patients and 23–29% of antiretroviral drug-naive individuals. Although one antiretroviral drug-naive patient taking combined therapy had an asymptomatic rise in pancreatic amylase activity, acute pancreatitis was not observed in either study. Grade 1 peripheral neuropathy was reported in one zidovudine-experienced patient taking low-dosage lamivudine (150 mg bd) and zidovudine.

Several large-scale studies of the efficacy of combined antiretroviral treatment with zalcitabine and zidovudine in HIV-infected patients (compared with zidovudine monotherapy or a combination of zidovudine and didanosine) have not shown unexpected adverse effects (6–9). The most common adverse effects in patients taking zalcitabine were peripheral neuropathy and aphthous mouth ulcers.

Organs and Systems

Nervous system

Various nervous system adverse effects of zidovudine have been reported, which may or may not be directly related to the drug. These include seizures, confusion, and acute encephalopathy occurring after zidovudine dosage reduction (10).

Metabolism

Lipodystrophy is a common adverse effect of antiretroviral drugs, particularly the NRTIs and has been reported with zidovudine (11).

- A 42-year-old woman developed abdominal and dorsocervical fat enlargement after having taken zidovudine for over 10 years. Zidovudine was withdrawn and the lesions improved considerably over the next 26 months.

Hematologic

The main dose-limiting adverse reactions of zidovudine therapy in HIV-infected adults and children are hematological complications (12). When zidovudine was introduced it was given in about twice the dosage used today. Consequently, hematological adverse effects occur at a much lower frequency than previously reported (13,14).

Almost uniformly, zidovudine treatment results in a progressive increase in the erythrocyte mean cell volume, which cannot be prevented by supplementation with vitamin B_{12} and folinic acid (15). Zidovudine can cause anemia (16) and reversible pure red cell aplasia (17). While recombinant erythropoietin is useful in correcting zidovudine-induced anemia, some cases of anemia are associated with high serum erythropoietin concentrations and normocytic cells, indicating bone marrow unresponsiveness to erythropoietin (18). Measuring baseline serum erythropoietin concentrations may help to predict the response to this very costly hormone supplementation.

Zidovudine can cause neutropenia (16).

Thrombocytopenia has been observed in patients using zidovudine and didanosine (19,20).

Skin

Fatal toxic epidermolysis has been attributed to zidovudine (21) as has cutaneous hypersensitivity (22).

Zidovudine can occasionally cause unusual pigmentation, probably depending on the individual's pigmentary pattern (23).

Nails

The presenting sign of neutropenia in a neonate treated with prophylactic zidovudine for reduction of perinatal transmission was, unusually, severe paronychia of the large toes as a result of *Candida albicans* and *Escherichia coli* infection (24). The paronychia resolved after treatment with oral fluconazole and topical antiseptics. Paronychia of the large toes has also been observed when filgrastim (recombinant granulocyte colony stimulating factor) was used alongside chemotherapy in poor-risk patients with myelodysplastic syndrome (25), and there is some evidence that paronychia (even in the absence of blood disorders) can occur as an independent adverse reaction to various antiretroviral drugs, including indinavir and lamivudine (26).

Closely similar is the strong evidence from case-control studies that ingrowing toenails are associated with the use of indinavir (27) and possibly other similar compounds, but not lamivudine.

Musculoskeletal

Myopathy has been well described with long-term zidovudine and is reversible after withdrawal (28). Phosphorus magnetic resonance spectroscopy has been used to study the changes in phosphorylated metabolites (ATP, phosphocreatine, and inorganic phosphate) during exercise in 19 healthy volunteers, 6 untreated HIV-positive individuals, and 9 zidovudine-treated patients with biopsy-proven myopathy (29). Zidovudine altered the normal muscle energy metabolism in the patients with myopathy, suggesting that it reduces maximal work output, and thus the maximal rate of mitochondrial ATP synthesis, in human muscle. So far, the syndrome has not been associated with any other NRTI (30) and it has been suggested that other factors might contribute to the development of zidovudine-associated myopathy (31). Mitochondrial abnormalities have also been observed in biopsies from untreated patients infected with HIV-1, suggesting that the virus itself can also cause myopathy.

To assess the contribution of zidovudine to the mitochondrial damage, the effects of zidovudine on non-infected co-cultures of spinal ganglia, spinal cord, and skeletal muscle in fetal rats have been studied (32).

There were significant changes not only in the mitochondria but also in the nuclei of all cells tested. These changes depended less on the concentration of zidovudine than on the duration of exposure.

Multiorgan failure

A well-documented case has shown that zidovudine can cause type B lactic acidosis and acute respiratory and hepatic failure (33).

- A 34-year-old obese woman developed nausea, vomiting, and intermittent diarrhea. Her current medications included zidovudine. She had tachypnea and tender hepatomegaly, and a CT scan of the abdomen showed hepatomegaly with fatty infiltration. The serum bicarbonate concentration was low and the lactate concentration three times normal. The tachypnea and dyspnea worsened as the lactate concentration rapidly increased to 15 times normal, and she died in acute respiratory and hepatic failure with multiorgan dysfunction.

Second-Generation Effects

Pregnancy

Zidovudine during pregnancy and delivery, followed by treatment of the infant for 6 weeks, prevents maternofetal transmission of HIV, and is associated with minimal short-term toxicity to both mother and child and no increased incidence of neonatal structural abnormalities (SEDA-19, 279) (34).

Zidovudine is relatively well tolerated in pregnancy, with anemia, neutropenia, or thrombocytopenia occurring in 10% and abnormalities of serum electrolytes and liver function in 5% (34).

Teratogenicity

There has been a randomized cohort study in the USA of children from 122 pregnancies in which zidovudine was given and of children from 112 pregnancies in which only a placebo was used (35). The median age of the children at the last follow-up visit was 4.2 years. There were no significant differences between children exposed to zidovudine and those who received placebo in terms of sequential data on lymphocyte subsets, weight, height, head circumference, and cognitive/developmental function. There were no deaths or malignancies. Two children (both exposed to zidovudine) were still being followed for unexplained abnormal fundoscopy. One child exposed to zidovudine had a mild cardiomyopathy on echocardiography at the age of 48 months but was clinically asymptomatic.

Lactation

Since zidovudine seems to be relatively well tolerated both in pregnancy and in neonates, there is also much reason to consider its use during lactation in order to reduce vertical transmission of HIV. Indeed, many would regard it as highly preferable to abandoning breastfeeding by HIV-infected women. In a critical double-blind West African study the effects of a 6-month course of treatment in prenatal and lactating mothers were examined (36). Eligible participants were women aged 18 years or older who had confirmed HIV-1 infection, were 36–38 weeks pregnant, and gave written informed consent. Exclusion criteria were severe anemia, neutropenia, abnormal liver function, and sickle cell disease. They were randomly assigned to zidovudine ($n = 214$; 300 mg bd until labor, 600 mg at the start of labor, and 300 mg bd for 7 days) or to matching placebo ($n = 217$). The Kaplan-Meier probability of HIV infection in the infant at 6 months was 18% in the zidovudine group and 28% in the placebo group, a relative efficacy of 0.38. In current and follow-up observations over 6 months, no major adverse biological or clinical events were reported in excess among women or children in the zidovudine group. The authors concluded that a short course of oral zidovudine given during the peripartum period is well tolerated and provides significant reduction in early vertical transmission of HIV-1 infection despite breastfeeding.

A second related study showed similar results (37), and the two papers together provide impressive evidence that it is proper and defensible to use zidovudine in breast-feeding mothers.

Susceptibility Factors

Age

The only recognized toxic effect in infants is anemia within the first 6 weeks of life, which is not associated with premature delivery, duration of maternal treatment, degree of maternal immunosuppression, or maternal anemia. An 18-month follow-up of 342 children born to mothers who had taken zidovudine or placebo during pregnancy has recently been reported (38). There were no differences in growth parameters or immune function in uninfected children. In addition, no childhood neoplasias were reported in either group.

Drug–Drug Interactions

Atovaquone

Atovaquone can potentiate the activity of zidovudine by inhibiting its glucuronidation (39).

Clarithromycin

Clarithromycin has an unpredictable effect on the absorption of zidovudine; blood concentrations may rise or fall (40,41).

Cytotoxic drugs

In 13 HIV-infected patients with cancer, the mean pharmacokinetics of zidovudine (AUC, half-life, oral clearance, and oral apparent volume of distribution) were no different with or without chemotherapy (42). However, there was a 57% reduction in C_{max} and a 66% increase in t_{max} after chemotherapy. There were no differences in the urinary excretion of zidovudine or zidovudine glucuronide. The authors concluded that these minor changes did not warrant any change in the dosage of zidovudine during concurrent chemotherapy.

Oxazepam

There was a striking incidence of headache in a small series of patients when zidovudine was given with oxazepam (43).

Paracetamol (acetaminophen)

Paracetamol (acetaminophen) increased the clearance (and possibly reduced the effects) of zidovudine (44,45).

Probenecid

In two healthy volunteers, co-administration of probenecid 500 mg every 6 hours altered the pharmacokinetics of a single oral dose of zidovudine 200 mg (46). There was an increase in the average AUC, with a corresponding reduction in oral clearance, attributed to an inhibitory effect of probenecid on the glucuronidation and renal excretion of zidovudine.

Eight subjects took zidovudine for 3 days with and without probenecid 500 mg every 8 hours for 3 days, and then additional quinine sulfate 260 mg every 8 hours (47). Probenecid increased the AUC of zidovudine by 80%. Quinine prevented the probenecid effect but had no effect on zidovudine kinetics when it was taken without probenecid by four other subjects. All of the effects were secondary to changes in zidovudine metabolism, since neither probenecid nor quinine changed the renal elimination of zidovudine.

Rifamycins

Rifampicin, a well-known enzyme inducer, increased the metabolism of zidovudine, and the effect persisted for 2 weeks after rifampicin had been withdrawn (48).

References

1. Neuzil KM. Pharmacologic therapy for human immunodeficiency virus infection: a review. Am J Med Sci 1994;307(5):368–73.
2. Forseter G, Joline C, Wormser GP. Tolerability, safety, and acceptability of zidovudine prophylaxis in health care workers. Arch Intern Med 1994;154(23):2745–9.
3. Gerberding JL. Prophylaxis for occupational exposure to HIV. Ann Intern Med 1996;125(6):497–501.
4. Katlama C, Ingrand D, Loveday C, Clumeck N, Mallolas J, Staszewski S, Johnson M, Hill AM, Pearce G, McDade H. Safety and efficacy of lamivudine–zidovudine combination therapy in antiretroviral-naive patients. A randomized controlled comparison with zidovudine monotherapy. Lamivudine European HIV Working Group. JAMA 1996;276(2):118–25.
5. Staszewski S, Loveday C, Picazo JJ, Dellarnonica P, Skinhoj P, Johnson MA, Danner SA, Harrigan PR, Hill AM, Verity L, McDade H. Safety and efficacy of lamivudine–zidovudine combination therapy in zidovudine-experienced patients. A randomized controlled comparison with zidovudine monotherapy. Lamivudine European HIV Working Group. JAMA 1996;276(2):111–17.
6. Delta Coordinating Committee. Delta: a randomised double-blind controlled trial comparing combinations of zidovudine plus didanosine or zalcitabine with zidovudine alone in HIV-infected individuals. Lancet 1996;348(9023):283–91. Erratum in 1996;348:834.

7. Hammer SM, Katzenstein DA, Hughes MD, Gundacker H, Schooley RT, Haubrich RH, Henry WK, Lederman MM, Phair JP, Niu M, Hirsch MS, Merigan TC. A trial comparing nucleoside monotherapy with combination therapy in HIV-infected adults with CD4 cell counts from 200 to 500 per cubic millimeter. AIDS Clinical Trials Group Study 175 Study Team. N Engl J Med 1996;335(15):1081–90.

8. Schooley RT, Ramirez-Ronda C, Lange JM, Cooper DA, Lavelle J, Lefkowitz L, Moore M, Larder BA, St Clair M, Mulder JW, McKinnis R, Pennington KN, Harrigan PR, Kinghorn I, Steel H, Rooney JF. Virologic and immunologic benefits of initial combination therapy with zidovudine and zalcitabine or didanosine compared with zidovudine monotherapy. Wellcome Resistance Study Collaborative Group. J Infect Dis 1996;173(6):1354–66.

9. Saravolatz LD, Winslow DL, Collins G, Hodges JS, Pettinelli C, Stein DS, Markowitz N, Reves R, Loveless MO, Crane L, Thompson M, Abrams D. Zidovudine alone or in combination with didanosine or zalcitabine in HIV-infected patients with the acquired immunodeficiency syndrome or fewer than 200 CD4 cells per cubic millimeter. Investigators for the Terry Beirn Community Programs for Clinical Research on AIDS. N Engl J Med 1996;335(15):1099–106.

10. Langtry HD, Campoli-Richards DM. Zidovudine. A review of its pharmacodynamic and pharmacokinetic properties, and therapeutic efficacy. Drugs 1989;37:408–50.

11. Garcia-Benayas T, Blanco F, Gomez-Viera JM, Barrios A, Soriano V, Gonzalez-Lahoz J. Lipodystrophy body-shape changes in a patient undergoing zidovudine monotherapy. AIDS 2002;16(7):1087–9.

12. Pizzo PA, Wilfert C. Antiretroviral therapy for infection due to human immunodeficiency virus in children. Clin Infect Dis 1994;19(1):177–96.

13. Fischl MA, Parker CB, Pettinelli C, Wulfsohn M, Hirsch MS, Collier AC, Antoniskis D, Ho M, Richman DD, Fuchs E, et al. A randomized controlled trial of a reduced daily dose of zidovudine in patients with the acquired immunodeficiency syndrome. The AIDS Clinical Trials Group. N Engl J Med 1990;323(15):1009–14.

14. Collier AC, Bozzette S, Coombs RW, Causey DM, Schoenfeld DA, Spector SA, Pettinelli CB, Davies G, Richman DD, Leedom JM, et al. A pilot study of low-dose zidovudine in human immunodeficiency virus infection. N Engl J Med 1990;323(15):1015–21.

15. Falguera M, Perez-Mur J, Puig T, Cao G. Study of the role of vitamin B12 and folinic acid supplementation in preventing hematologic toxicity of zidovudine. Eur J Haematol 1995;55(2):97–102.

16. McLeod GX, Hammer SM. Zidovudine: five years later. Ann Intern Med 1992;117(6):487–501.

17. Blanche P, Silberman B, Barreto L, Gombert B, Sicard D. Reversible zidovudine-induced pure red cell aplasia. AIDS 1999;13(12):1586–7.

18. Kuehl AK, Noormohamed SE. Recombinant erythropoietin for zidovudine-induced anemia in AIDS. Ann Pharmacother 1995;29(7–8):778–9.

19. Yarchoan R, Perno CF, Thomas RV, Klecker RW, Allain JP, Wills RJ, McAtee N, Fischl MA, Dubinsky R, McNeely MC, et al. Phase I studies of 2′,3′-dideoxycytidine in severe human immunodeficiency virus infection as a single agent and alternating with zidovudine (AZT). Lancet 1988;1(8577):76–81.

20. Dolin R, Lambert JS, Morse GD, Reichman RC, Plank CS, Reid J, Knupp C, McLaren C, Pettinelli C. 2′,3′-Dideoxyinosine in patients with AIDS or AIDS-related complex. Rev Infect Dis 1990;12(Suppl 5):S540–9.

21. Murri R, Antinori A, Camilli G, Zannoni G, Patriarca G. Fatal toxic epidermolysis induced by zidovudine. Clin Infect Dis 1996;23(3):640–1.

22. Duque S, de la Puente J, Rodriguez F, Fernandez Pellon L, Maquiera E, Jerez J. Zidovudine-related erythroderma and successful desensitization: a case report. J Allergy Clin Immunol 1996;98(1):234–5.

23. Zazo-Hernanz V, Sanchez-Herreros C, Gonzalez-Beato-Merino MJ, Lazaro-Ochaita P. Zidovudine pigmentation. Med Oral 1999;4:441.

24. Russo F, Collantes C, Guerrero J. Severe paronychia due to zidovudine-induced neutropenia in a neonate. J Am Acad Dermatol 1999;40(2 Pt 2):322–4.

25. Kang-Birken SL, Prichard JG. Paronychia of the great toes associated with protease inhibitors. Am J Health Syst Pharm 1999;56(16):1674–5.

26. Tosti A, Piraccini BM, D'Antuono A, Marzaduri S, Bettoli V. Paronychia associated with antiretroviral therapy. Br J Dermatol 1999;140(6):1165–8.

27. Bourezane Y, Thalamy B, Viel JF, Bardonnet K, Drobacheff C, Gil H, Vuitton DA, Hoen B. Ingrown toenail and indinavir: case-control study demonstrates strong relationship. AIDS 1999;13(15):2181–2.

28. Peters BS, Winer J, Landon DN, Stotter A, Pinching AJ. Mitochondrial myopathy associated with chronic zidovudine therapy in AIDS. Q J Med 1993;86(1):5–15.

29. Sinnwell TM, Sivakumar K, Soueidan S, Jay C, Frank JA, McLaughlin AC, Dalakas MC. Metabolic abnormalities in skeletal muscle of patients receiving zidovudine therapy observed by 31P in vivo magnetic resonance spectroscopy. J Clin Invest 1995;96(1):126–31.

30. Pedrol E, Masanes F, Fernandez-Sola J, Cofan M, Casademont J, Grau JM, Urbano-Marquez A. Lack of muscle toxicity with didanosine (ddI). Clinical and experimental studies. J Neurol Sci 1996;138(1–2):42–8.

31. Benbrik E, Chariot P, Bonavaud S, Ammi-Said M, Frisdal E, Rey C, Gherardi R, Barlovatz-Meimon G. Cellular and mitochondrial toxicity of zidovudine (AZT), didanosine (ddI) and zalcitabine (ddC) on cultured human muscle cells. J Neurol Sci 1997;149(1):19–25.

32. Schroder JM, Kaldenbach T, Piroth W. Nuclear and mitochondrial changes of co-cultivated spinal cord, spinal ganglia and muscle fibers following treatment with various doses of zidovudine. Acta Neuropathol (Berl) 1996;92(2):138–49.

33. Acosta BS, Grimsley EW. Zidovudine-associated type B lactic acidosis and hepatic steatosis in an HIV-infected patient. South Med J 1999;92(4):421–3.

34. Connor EM, Sperling RS, Gelber R, Kiselev P, Scott G, O'Sullivan MJ, VanDyke R, Bey M, Shearer W, Jacobson RL, et al. Reduction of maternal-infant transmission of human immunodeficiency virus type 1 with zidovudine treatment. Pediatric AIDS Clinical Trials Group Protocol 076 Study Group. N Engl J Med 1994;331(18):1173–80.

35. Culnane M, Fowler M, Lee SS, McSherry G, Brady M, O'Donnell K, Mofenson L, Gortmaker SL, Shapiro DE, Scott G, Jimenez E, Moore EC, Diaz C, Flynn PM, Cunningham B, Oleske J. Lack of long-term effects of in utero exposure to zidovudine among uninfected children born to HIV-infected women. Pediatric AIDS Clinical Trials Group Protocol 219/076 Teams. JAMA 1999;281(2):151–7.

36. Dabis F, Msellati P, Meda N, Welffens-Ekra C, You B, Manigart O, Leroy V, Simonon A, Cartoux M, Combe P, Ouangre A, Ramon R, Ky-Zerbo O, Montcho C, Salamon R, Rouzioux C, Van de Perre P, Mandelbrot L. 6-month efficacy, tolerance, and acceptability of a short regimen of oral zidovudine to reduce vertical transmission

of HIV in breastfed children in Cote d'Ivoire and Burkina Faso: a double-blind placebo-controlled multicentre trial. DITRAME Study Group. DIminution de la Transmission Mere-Enfant. Lancet 1999;353(9155):786–92.

37. Wiktor SZ, Ekpini E, Karon JM, Nkengasong J, Maurice C, Severin ST, Roels TH, Kouassi MK, Lackritz EM, Coulibaly IM, Greenberg AE. Short-course oral zidovudine for prevention of mother-to-child transmission of HIV-1 in Abidjan, Côte d'Ivoire: a randomised trial. Lancet 1999;353(9155):781–5.

38. Sperling RS, Shapiro DE, McSherry GD, Britto P, Cunningham BE, Culnane M, Coombs RW, Scott G, Van Dyke RB, Shearer WT, Jimenez E, Diaz C, Harrison DD, Delfraissy JF. Safety of the maternal-infant zidovudine regimen utilized in the Pediatric AIDS Clinical Trial Group 076 Study. AIDS 1998;12(14):1805–13.

39. Lee BL, Tauber MG, Sadler B, Goldstein D, Chambers HF. Atovaquone inhibits the glucuronidation and increases the plasma concentrations of zidovudine. Clin Pharmacol Ther 1996;59(1):14–21.

40. Gustavson LE, Chu SY, Mackenthun A, Gupta MS, Craft JC. Drug interaction between clarithromycin and oral zidovudine in HIV-1 infected patients. Clin Pharmacol Ther 1993;53:163.

41. Vance E, Watson-Bitar M, Gustavson L, Kazanjian P. Pharmacokinetics of clarithromycin and zidovudine in patients with AIDS. Antimicrob Agents Chemother 1995;39(6):1355–60.

42. Toffoli G, Errante D, Corona G, Vaccher E, Bertola A, Robieux I, Aita P, Sorio R, Tirelli U, Boiocchi M. Interactions of antineoplastic chemotherapy with zidovudine pharmacokinetics in patients with HIV-related neoplasms. Chemotherapy 1999;45(6):418–28.

43. Mole L, Israelski D, Bubp J, O'Hanley P, Merigan T, Blaschke T. Pharmacokinetics of zidovudine alone and in combination with oxazepam in the HIV infected patient. J Acquir Immune Defic Syndr 1993;6(1):56–60.

44. Sattler FR, Ko R, Antoniskis D, Shields M, Cohen J, Nicoloff J, Leedom J, Koda R. Acetaminophen does not impair clearance of zidovudine. Ann Intern Med 1991;114(11):937–40.

45. Shriner K, Goetz MB. Severe hepatotoxicity in a patient receiving both acetaminophen and zidovudine. Am J Med 1992;93(1):94–6.

46. Hedaya MA, Elmquist WF, Sawchuk RJ. Probenecid inhibits the metabolic and renal clearances of zidovudine (AZT) in human volunteers. Pharm Res 1990;7(4):411–17.

47. Kornhauser DM, Petty BG, Hendrix CW, Woods AS, Nerhood LJ, Bartlett JG, Lietman PS. Probenecid and zidovudine metabolism. Lancet 1989;2(8661):473–5.

48. Gallicano KD, Sahai J, Shukla VK, Seguin I, Pakuts A, Kwok D, Foster BC, Cameron DW. Induction of zidovudine glucuronidation and amination pathways by rifampicin in HIV-infected patients. Br J Clin Pharmacol 1999;48(2):168–79.

Zileuton

General Information

Zileuton is an inhibitor of 5-lipoxygenase, the first step in the conversion of arachidonic acid to cysteinyl leukotrienes. It is starting to be used in the long-term control of asthma (1). It has also been used to treat acne (2), atopic dermatitis (3), and the Sjögren–Larsson syndrome (4).

Organs and Systems

Hematologic

In 10 patients with asthma, zileuton treatment for 2 weeks significantly increased thromboxane B2 concentrations and spontaneous platelet aggregation (5). These results suggest that zileuton may be associated with an increased risk of thrombosis.

Liver

In 2947 patients at 233 centers in the USA randomly assigned in a 5:1 ratio to zileuton plus usual asthma care or usual asthma care alone, the patients who took zileuton had significantly fewer corticosteroid rescues, required less emergency care, had fewer hospitalizations, and had greater increases in FEV_1 (6). They also had significantly greater improvements in asthma symptoms. There were increases in alanine transaminase activity to three times or more the upper limit of the reference range in 4.6% of patients taking zileuton and 1.1% of those receiving usual care; most of the increases occurred during the first 2–3 months. There were no cases of jaundice or chronic liver disease.

References

1. Dube LM, Swanson LJ, Awni W. Zileuton, a leukotriene synthesis inhibitor in the management of chronic asthma. Clinical pharmacokinetics and safety. Clin Rev Allergy Immunol 1999;17(1–2):213–21.

2. Zouboulis CC, Nestoris S, Adler YD, Orth M, Orfanos CE, Picardo M, Camera E, Cunliffe WJ. A new concept for acne therapy: a pilot study with zileuton, an oral 5-lipoxygenase inhibitor. Arch Dermatol 2003;139(5):668–70.

3. Taskapan MO. Zileuton and atopic dermatitis. Ann Allergy Asthma Immunol 2001;87(2):162–3.

4. Willemsen MA, Lutt MA, Steijlen PM, Cruysberg JR, van der Graaf M, Nijhuis-van der Sanden MW, Pasman JW, Mayatepek E, Rotteveel JJ. Clinical and biochemical effects of zileuton in patients with the Sjögren–Larsson syndrome. Eur J Pediatr 2001;160(12):711–17.

5. Wu X, Dev A, Leong AB. Zileuton, a 5-lipoxygenase inhibitor, increases production of thromboxane A2 and platelet aggregation in patients with asthma. Am J Hematol 2003;74(1):23–5.

6. Lazarus SC, Lee T, Kemp JP, Wenzel S, Dube LM, Ochs RF, Carpentier PJ, Lancaster JF. Safety and clinical efficacy of zileuton in patients with chronic asthma. Am J Manag Care 1998;4(6):841–8.

Zinc

General Information

Zinc is a bluish-white metallic element (symbol Zn; atomic no. 30) that is found in minerals such as franklinite, ghanite, goslarite, hemimorphite, smithsonite, sphalerite, willemite, and wurtzite. Sphalerite, which contains zinc sulfide, is the most abundant source.

Zinc deficiency and toxicity have been reviewed (1,2). Zinc supplementation reduces the incidence of infection and increases the survival rate after infections in elderly people (3). However, oral zinc sulfate has been overused in many fields of therapy, particularly in dermatology, despite the fact that some of the indications once claimed for it have been discredited and only a few disorders have been clearly shown to result from zinc deficiency. Dosages have often been high, for example the equivalent of 45 mg of metallic zinc three times a day. Zinc oxide is used topically as an astringent and protectant. Zinc chloride is used as an astringent and a desensitizer for dentine. Zinc sulfate is sometimes used as an ophthalmic astringent. Zinc oxide is used as an anti-infective agent. Zinc is also found in some freely available alternative remedies and in non-medicinal products such as shampoos.

Zinc acetate (Galzin, Gate Pharmaceutical Co), developed for the treatment of Wilson's disease (4), has been used in maintenance therapy of adult and pediatric disease, but it also has efficacy in the treatment of pregnant women and presymptomatic patients from the start. It also has value as adjunctive therapy for the initial treatment of symptomatic patients. Its mechanism of action involves induction of intestinal cell metallothionein, which blocks copper absorption from the intestinal tract. Negative copper balance is caused by blockade not only of absorption of food copper but by blockade of reabsorption of the considerable amount of endogenously secreted copper in saliva, gastric juice, and intestinal secretions. It is therefore effective in controlling copper concentrations and toxicity in Wilson's disease.

The main advantage of zinc over other anticopper agents is its extremely low toxicity. The only adverse effect is some degree of initial gastric irritation in about 10% of patients, which usually abates and becomes insignificant over time. As with all long-term therapies, compliance is a problem in some patients and dictates regular monitoring by measurement of 24-hour urine copper and zinc. As with all anticopper therapies, overtreatment can cause copper deficiency over a long period of time. This is to be avoided, particularly in children, because copper is required for growth.

Zinc can be beneficial in zinc deficiency. Severe depletion of zinc in two patients with advanced cancer and malnutrition was accompanied by cutaneous bleeding, a prolonged bleeding time, and abnormal platelet aggregation (5). Both had very low serum and urinary zinc concentrations. Oral zinc without any additional therapy was rapidly followed by control of bleeding and normalization of bleeding time and platelet aggregation. Discontinuation of zinc caused the return of the bleeding and abnormal laboratory findings.

Organs and Systems

Nervous system

Clioquinol (5-chloro-7-iodo-8-hydroxyquinoline) was used 30 years ago as an oral antiparasitic agent and to increase the intestinal absorption of zinc in patients with acrodermatitis enteropathica, a genetic disorder of zinc

absorption. However, the use of clioquinol was epidemiologically linked to subacute myelo-optic neuropathy (SMON), characterized by peripheral neuropathy and blindness, which affected 10 000 patients in Japan. Withdrawal of oral clioquinol led to the elimination of SMON, but the mechanism of how clioquinol induces neurotoxicity is unclear. There is now evidence that zinc may have been implicated.

The effect of clioquinol-metal chelates has been tested on neural crest-derived melanoma cells (6). The effect of clioquinol chelates on cells was further studied by electron microscopy and by a mitochondrial potential-sensitive fluorescent dye. Of the ions tested, only clioquinol-zinc chelate was cytotoxic. This cytotoxicity was extremely rapid, suggesting that its primary effect was on the mitochondria, and electron microscopic analysis showed that the chelate caused mitochondrial damage. This was further confirmed by the observation that the chelate reduced the mitochondrial membrane potential. The phenomenon of clioquinol-mediated toxicity appeared to be specific to zinc and was not seen with other metals tested. Since clioquinol causes increased systemic absorption of zinc, it is likely that clioquinol-zinc chelate was present in appreciable concentrations in patients with SMON and may have been the causative toxin.

Hematologic

The use of megadoses of vitamin and mineral supplements has become common, and adverse effects can occur.

- A 17-year-old man developed fatigue after taking large daily doses of zinc supplements for 6–7 months in an attempt to treat his acne (7). He initially took 50 mg/day, but because his acne did not improve he increased the dosage to 100 mg tds. He had anemia and neutropenia. His plasma zinc concentration was 1.95 (reference range 0.50–0.95) µg/ml 1 month after withdrawal and 1.69 µg/ml 1 month later. His plasma copper concentration was 0.12 (reference value 0.90–2.35) µg/ml. When his anemia and neutropenia had resolved 4 months later, the zinc and copper concentrations had returned to normal.

Zinc sulfate can cause copper deficiency by inducing the production of metallothionein in intestinal cells and thus lowering copper absorption; copper deficiency can lead in turn to sideroblastic anemia (8), neutropenia, and osteopenia (9).

- A 17-year-old man with anaemia, leukopenia, and neutropenia had been self-medicating with over-the-counter zinc formulations for acne for almost 2 years at doses of up to 300 mg/day (10). Serum copper and serum ceruloplasmin concentrations were less than 100 (reference range 70–155) ng/ml and 20 (23–49) µg/ml respectively. His serum zinc concentration was 2 (0.6–1.3) µg/ml. Within 1 month of withdrawal, and without copper supplementation, the ceruloplasmin concentration had risen to 90 µg/ml. By 2 months his complete blood count was normal.

It is not clear whether zinc itself also causes anemia directly, or whether the effect is exerted solely through this interaction with copper, but with the increasingly popular sale of zinc supplements this adverse effect merits attention as a possible cause of unexplained blood disorders (11).

Gastrointestinal

Zinc compounds that are soluble in water or in gastric fluid are poisonous. If zinc sulfate is given on an empty stomach, gastric acid can convert it to zinc chloride, which is a powerful caustic agent; it is therefore not surprising that gastric irritation, nausea, vomiting, hemorrhagic erosive gastritis, and diarrhea are common adverse reactions.

Bacitracin zinc has been used for giardiasis (12), in which it appears effective. In the doses used, adverse effects have been limited to nausea, abdominal discomfort, and diarrhea in a small number of patients. Similar effects have been noted when zinc gluconate lozenges were administered for the common cold (13).

- A 10-year-old girl accidentally ingested an acid soldering flux solution (pH 3.0; zinc chloride 30–60%) (14). Systemic effects after ingestion were unremarkable, except for lethargy. Thus, chelation therapy was not considered. Severe gastric corrosion was caused by local caustic action. An antral stricture of the stomach developed about 3 weeks later, and she had a modified Heineke–Mikulicz antropyloroplasty. Postoperatively, she made an uneventful recovery. However, although she was tolerating a normal diet, a barium meal showed that her stomach was totally aperistaltic.

In this case careful long-term follow-up was considered necessary, because of the potential risk of malignancy in the damaged stomach.

Liver

The use of zinc acetate in Wilson's disease has been reviewed and recommended rather than copper chelation, because of limited adverse effects. However, liver damage has been attributed to zinc in a patient with Wilson's disease (15).

- A 25-year-old woman with Wilson's disease took oral zinc acetate 50 mg tds and 21 days later developed right hypochondrial pain, nausea, vomiting, fever, arthralgia, and tender hepatomegaly. Her hemoglobin was at 10.5 g/dl, aspartate transaminase 393 U/l, and alanine transaminase 911 U/l. Oral zinc was withdrawn and oral D-penicillamine (250 mg qds) was prescribed. One week later she was asymptomatic, and her liver enzymes returned to normal within 4 months.

Skin

Lichen planus has been attributed to zinc in dental materials.

- A 74-year-old woman, who had extensive odontitis treated with root canal disinfection and dental metal restorations, developed painful erosion and erythema of the upper lip mucosa, white streaks on the buccal

mucosa, and white lesions on the gums (16). Histology showed lichen planus. Her 14 dental metal restorations contained 5.3% zinc, and patch-testing was positive with zinc chloride and negative with all the other metal components. The lichen planus resolved 3 months after removal of the metal restorations.

Zinc products are extensively used in shampoos and other non-medical items and severe reactions occasionally occur. In one instance a shampoo based on zinc pyrithione caused a serious relapse in a woman with stable psoriasis (SEDA-22, 251).

Reproductive system

The efficacy and safety of intravaginal zinc sulfate + usnic acid as adjuvant therapy for human papillomavirus genital infection has been studied before or after radiosurgical treatment in 100 patients (17). Papillomavirus lesions disappeared in 93% of the patients in the control group and in 100% of the others. Re-epithelialization after 1 month was complete in only 28% of the control group but in 65% of the treated patients; after 2 months it was complete in 76% of the controls and in 94% of the others. Treatment before radiosurgical treatment resulted in a reduction of the overall area of lesions in 88% of cases. Three months after radiosurgical treatment there was significantly less recurrence in those treated with usnic acid and zinc sulfate. Adverse effects were limited to local pain and irritation and were well tolerated.

Immunologic

Zinc can reportedly impair immune responses (18).

Drug Administration

Drug dosage regimens

When zinc is used therapeutically, the dosage of zinc often considerably exceeds the recommended daily allowance for healthy adults (15 mg of elemental zinc). In view of its adverse effects, it is advisable to limit the dosage to two or three times this amount. To reduce the unwanted gastrointestinal effects it may be helpful to use zinc acetate rather than zinc sulfate (19).

Drug overdose

- A very old woman accidentally ingested a formulation containing zinc and copper sulphate (20). At 90 minutes after ingestion, the peak plasma concentrations were 20 mg/ml for zinc and 2 µg/ml for copper. The major complications were gastric and bronchial inflammation, due to the corrosive properties of these compounds. There were also systemic manifestations, with cardiovascular failure and renal insufficiency, but the patient made a complete recovery.
- A schizophrenic patient died after ingesting 461 coins, the first reported case of a death associated with zinc intoxication (21). The patient presented with clinical manifestations consistent with the local corrosive as well as systemic effects of zinc intoxication and died 40 days after admission with multisystem organ failure. Many British post-1981 pennies, which contain mostly

zinc, were severely corroded through prolonged contact with gastric juice. Tissue samples of the kidneys, pancreas, and liver obtained at autopsy contained high concentrations of zinc and showed acute tubular necrosis, mild fibrosis, and acute massive necrosis respectively.

References

1. Barceloux DG. Zinc. J Toxicol Clin Toxicol 1999;37(2):279–92.
2. Abbasi A, Shetty K. Zink: Pathophysiologische Effekte, Mangelzustande und Wirkungen einer Supplementierung bei alteren Personen—ein Forschungsuberblick. [Zinc: pathophysiological effects, deficiency status and effects of supplementation in elderly persons—an overview of the research.] Z Gerontol Geriatr 1999;32(Suppl 1):I75–9.
3. Mocchegiani E, Muzzioli M, Giacconi R. Zinc and immunoresistance to infection in aging: new biological tools. Trends Pharmacol Sci 2000;21(6):205–8.
4. Brewer GJ. Zinc acetate for the treatment of Wilson's disease. Expert Opin Pharmacother 2001;2(9):1473–7.
5. Stefanini M. Cutaneous bleeding related to zinc deficiency in two cases of advanced cancer. Cancer 1999;86(5):866–70.
6. Arbiser JL, Kraeft SK, van Leeuwen R, Hurwitz SJ, Selig M, Dickersin GR, Flint A, Byers HR, Chen LB. Clioquinol–zinc chelate: a candidate causative agent of subacute myelo-optic neuropathy. Mol Med 1998;4(10):665–70.
7. Salzman MB, Smith EM, Koo C. Excessive oral zinc supplementation. J Pediatr Hematol Oncol 2002;24(7):582–4.
8. Fiske DN, McCoy HE 3rd, Kitchens CS. Zinc-induced sideroblastic anemia: report of a case, review of the literature, and description of the hematologic syndrome. Am J Hematol 1994;46(2):147–50.
9. Patterson WP, Winkelmann M, Perry MC. Zinc-induced copper deficiency: megamineral sideroblastic anemia. Ann Intern Med 1985;103(3):385–6.
10. Porea TJ, Belmont JW, Mahoney DH Jr. Zinc-induced anemia and neutropenia in an adolescent. J Pediatr 2000;136(5):688–90.
11. Singal DP, Green D, Reid B, Gladman DD, Buchanan WW. HLA-D region genes and rheumatoid arthritis (RA): importance of DR and DQ genes in conferring susceptibility to RA. Ann Rheum Dis 1992;51(1):23–8.
12. Andrews BJ, Panitescu D, Jipa GH, Vasile-Bugarin AC, Vasiliu RP, Ronnevig JR. Chemotherapy for giardiasis: randomized clinical trial of bacitracin, bacitracin zinc, and a combination of bacitracin zinc with neomycin. Am J Trop Med Hyg 1995;52(4):318–21.
13. Godfrey JC, Godfrey NJ, Novick SG. Zinc for treating the common cold: review of all clinical trials since 1984. Altern Ther Health Med 1996;2(6):63–72.
14. Yamataka A, Pringle KC, Wyeth J. A case of zinc chloride ingestion. J Pediatr Surg 1998;33(4):660–2.
15. Castilla-Higuero L, Romero-Gomez M, Suarez E, Castro M. Acute hepatitis after starting zinc therapy in a patient with presymptomatic Wilson's disease. Hepatology 2000;32(4 Pt 1):877.
16. Ido T, Kumakiri M, Kiyohara T, Sawai T, Hasegawa Y. Oral lichen planus due to zinc in dental restorations. Contact Dermatitis 2002;47(1):51.
17. Scirpa P, Scambia G, Masciullo V, Battaglia F, Foti E, Lopez R, Villa P, Malecore M, Mancuso S. Terapia adiuvante con un preparato a base di zinco solfato e acido usnico delle lesioni genitali da human papilloma virus (HPV) dopo trattamento chirurgico distruttivo. [A zinc sulfate and usnic acid preparation used as post-surgical adjuvant therapy in genital lesions by human papillomavirus.] Minerva Ginecol 1999;51(6):255–60.
18. Hunt JR. Position of the American Dietetic Association: vitamin and mineral supplementation. J Am Dietet Assoc 1996;96(1):73–7.
19. Mahajan SK, Abbasi AA, Prasad AS, Rabbani P, Briggs WA, McDonald FD. Effect of oral zinc therapy on gonadal function in hemodialysis patients. A double-blind study. Ann Intern Med 1982;97(3):357–61.
20. Hantson P, Lievens M, Mahieu P. Accidental ingestion of a zinc and copper sulfate preparation. J Toxicol Clin Toxicol 1996;34(6):725–30.
21. Bennett DR, Baird CJ, Chan KM, Crookes PF, Bremner CG, Gottlieb MM, Naritoku WY. Zinc toxicity following massive coin ingestion. Am J Forensic Med Pathol 1997;18(2):148–53.

Zingiberaceae

See also Herbal medicines

General Information

The genera in the family of Zingiberaceae (Table 1) include cardamom and ginger.

Zingiber officinale

Zingiber officinale (ginger) contains a variety of compounds, including diarylheptanoids and the phenol gingerol. It has been used to treat motion sickness and other forms of nausea and vomiting, and may have some efficacy (1).

Adverse effects
Skin
Of about 1000 patients with occupational skin diseases, five had occupational allergic contact dermatitis from spices (2). They were chefs, or workers in kitchens, coffee rooms, and restaurants. In all cases the dermatitis affected the hands. The causative spices were garlic, cinnamon, ginger, allspice, and clove. The same patients had positive patch test reactions to carrot, lettuce, and tomato.

Among 55 patients with suspected contact dermatitis, skin patch tests that were positive at concentrations of both 10% and 25% were most common with ginger ($n = 7$), nutmeg ($n = 5$), and oregano ($n = 4$); other spices produced no responses or one positive response (3). Positive

Table 1 The genera of Zingiberaceae

Aframomum (aframomum)
Alpinia (alpinia)
Amomum (cardamom)
Boesenbergia (boesenbergia)
Curcuma (curcuma)
Elettaria (elettaria)
Etlingera (waxflower)
Hedychium (garland-lily)
Hitchenia (hitchenia)
Kaempferia (kaempferia)
Renealmia (renealmia)
Zingiber (ginger)

reactions at only one concentration were more likely at 25%: nutmeg ($n = 5$), ginger and cayenne ($n = 4$), curry, cumin, and cinnamon ($n = 3$), turmeric, coriander, and sage ($n = 2$), oregano ($n = 1$), and basil and clove ($n = 0$).

Drug interactions

Ginger may potentiate the effects of oral anticoagulants (4).

- A 76-year-old white woman taking long-term phenprocoumon, with an INR in the target range, began using ginger products (5). Several weeks later, her INR rose to 10 and she had epistaxis. The INR returned to the target range after ginger was stopped and vitamin K1 was given.

References

1. Ernst E, Pittler MH. Efficacy of ginger for nausea and vomiting: a systematic review of randomized clinical trials. Br J Anaesth 2000;84(3):367–71.
2. Kanerva L, Estlander T, Jolanki R. Occupational allergic contact dermatitis from spices. Contact Dermatitis 1996;35(3):157–62.
3. Futrell JM, Rietschel RL. Spice allergy evaluated by results of patch tests. Cutis 1993;52(5):288–90.
4. Heck AM, DeWitt BA, Lukes AL. Potential interactions between alternative therapies and warfarin. Am J Health Syst Pharm 2000;57(13):1221–7.
5. Kruth P, Brosi E, Fux R, Morike K, Gleiter CH. Ginger-associated overanticoagulation by phenprocoumon. Ann Pharmacother 2004;38(2):257–60.

Zipeprol

General Information

Zipeprol is a centrally acting cough suppressant. Because it has hallucinogenic effects, it has been abused, particularly in Korea.

Long-Term Effects

Drug abuse

Abuse of zipeprol can be a problem (SEDA-17, 211), and has been associated with severe neurological symptoms.

Drug Administration

Drug overdose

A retrospective study of cases of eprazinone, eprozinol, and zipeprol intoxication collected at the Poison Control Center in Paris from 1975 to 1982 noted 199 cases of accidental or intentional acute poisoning. In seven cases, seizures were observed, all after ingestion of eight times the therapeutic dose. They resolved rapidly and without recurrence with symptomatic treatment (1).

In Korea, from 1991 to 1998, a total of 69 zipeprol-related deaths were reported (2). In 96% of cases involving zipeprol alone, the victims were in their teens and

twenties. The male/female ratio was 3.5:1. The blood concentration of zipeprol was 0.8–38 µg/ml when zipeprol was taken alone and 0.1–35 µg/ml zipeprol when it was taken with dextromethorphan.

References

1. Merigot P, Garnier R, Efthymiou ML. Les convulsions avec trois antitussifs dérivés substitués de la pipérazine (zipeprol, eprazinone, eprozinol). [Convulsions with 3 antitussive substituted derivatives of piperazine (zipeprol, eprazinone, eprozinol).] Ann Pediatr (Paris) 1985;32(6):504–6.
2. Chung HS, Choi HK, Kim EM, Park MJ, Chung KH, Yoo YC. Demographic characteristics of zipeprol-associated deaths in Korea. Arch Pharm Res 1998;21(3):286–90.

Ziprasidone

See also Neuroleptic drugs

General Information

Ziprasidone is a dibenzotheolylpiperazine compound with a receptor binding profile similar to that of other atypical antipsychotic drugs, and a high affinity for serotonin ($5\text{-}HT_{2A}$) receptors and a lower affinity for dopamine (D_2) receptors; it also has high affinities for $5\text{-}HT_{1A}$, $5\text{-}HT_{1D}$ and $5\text{-}HT_{2C}$ receptors and inhibits serotonin and noradrenaline reuptake. Two extensive reviews of the clinical pharmacology of ziprasidone have appeared (1,2).

On February 5, 2000, the FDA approved ziprasidone for the treatment of schizophrenia (www.fda.gov). However, the FDA has been concerned with the possibility that ziprasidone and a number of other drugs might increase the risk of the specific potentially fatal cardiac dysrhythmia, torsade de pointes. The FDA did not approve ziprasidone in 1998, because of evidence that it can cause prolongation of the QT interval, and they asked that specific safety data be gathered. The safety data were submitted in 1999. Although QT prolongation is still a theoretical concern, over 4000 patients have been treated in clinical trials without evidence of torsade de pointes. In addition, overall mortality in the trials was similar to that seen with placebo and other neuroleptic drugs. The FDA labelling does not include a so-called "black-box warning" and does not require an electrocardiogram before or during treatment. However, the labelling does warn physicians and patients about QT interval prolongation and the possible risk of sudden death. The labelling suggests that doctors use their best judgment, based on the health status of the individual, as to whether to use ziprasidone as first-line treatment or only after other available drugs have failed. There is no requirement that patients have regular heart check-ups while taking this drug.

Comparison with placebo

Ziprasidone has been used in 28 children and adolescents (aged 7–17 years) with Tourette's syndrome in an 8-week pilot study (3). They were randomly assigned to ziprasidone (5–40 mg/day; $n = 16$) or placebo ($n = 12$). Ziprasidone significantly reduced tic frequency. There was one case each of somnolence and akathisia, both with the highest dose of ziprasidone; these were considered to be severe but did not necessitate withdrawal.

Comparison with benzodiazepines

Ziprasidone 20 mg ($n = 30$) has been compared with diazepam 10 mg ($n = 30$) and placebo ($n = 30$) in a randomized, parallel-group, double-blind study in nonpsychotic subjects who were anxious before undergoing minor dental surgery (4). The peak anxiolytic effect of ziprasidone compared with placebo was similar to that of diazepam but had a later onset. However, at 3 hours after the dose, the anxiolytic effect of ziprasidone was significantly greater than that of placebo and somewhat greater than that of diazepam. The sedative effect of ziprasidone was never greater than that of placebo, whereas diazepam was significantly more sedative than placebo 1–1.5 hours after the dose. Ziprasidone was generally well tolerated; only one patient reported treatment-related adverse events (nausea and vomiting) and, unlike diazepam, ziprasidone did not reduce the blood pressure. Dystonia, extrapyramidal syndrome, akathisia, and postural hypotension were not seen with ziprasidone. Ziprasidone may therefore have anxiolytic effects in addition to its neuroleptic properties.

Organs and Systems

Cardiovascular

Three extensive reviews of ziprasidone have devoted particular attention to the possibility of QT interval prolongation (5–7). Ziprasidone up to 160 mg/day prolongs the QT_c interval on average 5.9–9.7 ms (data from 4571 patients); a QT_c interval of over 500 ms was seen in two of 2988 ziprasidone recipients and in one of 440 placebo recipients. In an open study in 31 patients with schizophrenia, ziprasidone given for 21–29 days prolonged the QT_c interval by 20 ms (95% CI = 14, 26).

- A 38-year-old woman with a psychosis who took 4020 mg of ziprasidone had borderline intraventricular conduction delay (QRS duration 111 ms); the QT_c interval was 445 ms (8). She oscillated between being drowsy and calm, and alert and agitated; her blood pressure fell from 129/81 to 99/34 mmHg 4 hours later. She also had diarrhea and urinary retention.

Nervous system

In a randomized, Phase III, double-blind study, ziprasidone 80 mg/day and 160 mg was more effective than placebo in patients with acute exacerbations of schizophrenia or schizoaffective disorders ($n = 302$) (9). After 6 weeks, somnolence (19%) and akathisia (13%) were more frequent with ziprasidone 160 mg than with placebo (5 and 7% each). Benzatropine was required at some time during the study by 20% of the patients taking ziprasidone

80 mg/day, 25% of those taking ziprasidone 160 mg/day, and 13% of those taking placebo. The long-term safety of ziprasidone is unknown.

Tardive dyskinesia has been associated with ziprasidone in a 49-year-old man with bipolar disorder (10).

Psychological, psychiatric

Three cases of hypomania in patients with depression have been reported (11).

Metabolism

Ziprasidone is said to be associated with less weight gain than the other atypical neuroleptic drugs and than most typical ones (1,2).

Musculoskeletal

Rhabdomyolysis with pancreatitis and hyperglycemia has been reported in a middle-aged woman with schizoaffective disorder (12).

Drug–Drug Interactions

Pfizer, the marketing authorization holder of ziprasidone, has promoted several pharmacokinetic studies. Oral contraceptives (ethinylestradiol 30 µg/day plus levonorgestrel 150 µg/day) (13), lithium 900 mg/day (14), ketoconazole 400 mg/day (15), and carbamazepine (100–400 mg/day) (16) had no effects on the pharmacokinetics of ziprasidone (40 mg/day).

References

1. Buckley PF. Ziprasidone: pharmacology, clinical progress and therapeutic promise. Drugs Today 2000;36:583–9.
2. Daniel DG, Copeland LF. Ziprasidone: comprehensive overview and clinical use of a novel antipsychotic. Expert Opin Investig Drugs 2000;9(4):819–28.
3. Sallee FR, Kurlan R, Goetz CG, Singer H, Scahill L, Law G, Dittman VM, Chappell PB. Ziprasidone treatment of children and adolescents with Tourette's syndrome: a pilot study. J Am Acad Child Adolesc Psychiatry 2000;39(3):292–9.
4. Wilner KD, Anziano RJ, Johnson AC, Miceli JJ, Fricke JR, Titus CK. The anxiolytic effect of the novel antipsychotic ziprasidone compared with diazepam in subjects anxious before dental surgery J Clin Psychopharmacol 2002;22(2):206–10.
5. Stimmel GL, Gutierrez MA, Lee V. Ziprasidone: an atypical antipsychotic drug for the treatment of schizophrenia. Clin Ther 2002;24(1):21–37.
6. Gunasekara NS, Spencer CM, Keating GM. Ziprasidone: a review of its use in schizophrenia and schizoaffective disorder. Drugs 2002;62(8):1217–51.
7. Caley CF, Cooper CK. Ziprasidone: the fifth atypical antipsychotic. Ann Pharmacother 2002;36(5):839–51.
8. House M. Overdose of ziprasidone. Am J Psychiatry 2002;159(6):1061–2.
9. Daniel DG, Zimbroff DL, Potkin SG, Reeves KR, Harrigan EP, Lakshminarayanan M. Ziprasidone 80 mg/day and 160 mg/day in the acute exacerbation of schizophrenia and schizoaffective disorder: a 6-week placebo-controlled trial. Neuropsychopharmacol 1999;20:491–505.

10. Rosenquist KJ, Walker SS, Ghaemi SN. Tardive dyskinesia and ziprasidone. Am J Psychiatry 2002;159(8):1436.

11. Davis R, Risch SC. Ziprasidone induction of hypomania in depression? Am J Psychiatry 2002;159(4):673–4.

12. Yang SH, McNeely MJ. Rhabdomyolysis, pancreatitis, and hyperglycemia with ziprasidone. Am J Psychiatry 2002;159(8):1435.

13. Muirhead GJ, Harness J, Holt PR, Oliver S, Anziano RJ. Ziprasidone and the pharmacokinetics of a combined oral contraceptive. Br J Clin Pharmacol 2000;49(Suppl. 1):S49–56.

14. Apseloff G, Mullet D, Wilner KD, Anziano RJ, Tensfeldt TG, Pelletier SM, Gerber N. The effects of ziprasidone on steady-state lithium levels and renal clearance of lithium. Br J Clin Pharmacol 2000;49(Suppl. 1):S61–64.

15. Miceli JJ, Smith M, Robarge L, Morse T, Laurent A. The effects of ketoconazole on ziprasidone pharmacokinetics—a placebo-controlled crossover study in healthy volunteers. Br J Clin Pharmacol 2000;49(Suppl. 1):71S–6S.

16. Miceli JJ, Anziano RJ, Robarge L, Hansen RA, Laurent A. The effect of carbamazepine on the steady-state pharmacokinetics of ziprasidone in healthy volunteers. Br J Clin Pharmacol 2000;49(Suppl. 1):65S–70S.

Zirconium

General Information

Zirconium is a metallic element (symbol Zr; atomic no. 40) that occurs in minerals such as baddeleyite and eudialyte.

Topical zirconium can cause hypersensitivity granulomas in sensitized persons, which has led to the removal of zirconium salts from antiperspirants (SEDA-22, 242). Complexes of zirconium and aluminum are non-sensitizing and are still commonly used as active ingredients in topical antiperspirants. However, a granulomatous reaction to this material has been reported (1).

Reference

1. Montemarano AD, Sau P, Johnson FB, James WD. Cutaneous granulomas caused by an aluminum–zirconium complex: an ingredient of antiperspirants. J Am Acad Dermatol 1997;37(3 Pt 1):496–8.

Zofenopril

See also Angiotensin converting enzyme inhibitors

General Information

Zofenopril is a prodrug that, once absorbed, undergoes rapid and complete hydrolysis to the sulfhydryl-containing active ACE inhibitor zofenoprilat. The use of zofenopril in hypertension and in acute myocardial infarction has been extensively reviewed (1).

Reference

1. Borghi C, Ambrosioni E. Zofenopril: a review of the evidence of its benefits in hypertension and acute myocardial infarction. Clin Drug Invest 2000;20:371–84.

Zolpidem

General Information

Zolpidem and alpidem are imidazopyridines, chemically distinct from the benzodiazepines and appear to bind selectively to a subset of benzodiazepine receptors (1). This property may account for their apparently milder withdrawal effects and, in the case of alpidem, a relative dominance of anxiolytic over sedative and cognitive effects (2). Zolpidem has hypnotic efficacy comparable to short- and medium-acting benzodiazepines, and has similar or possibly fewer adverse effects at therapeutic doses (3–5), except for gastrointestinal disturbances, which appear to be more common, and visual hallucinations, especially in women (SEDA-17, 46) (SEDA-18, 45) (SEDA-21, 40). On the other hand, zolpidem unexpectedly causes as much memory impairment as triazolam, if not more, at least in young healthy adults (SEDA-19, 33). Also surprising is the same author's later contention that zolpidem causes less memory impairment than do the benzodiazepine hypnotics (SEDA-21, 40), presumably including triazolam. Zolpidem may also be relatively toxic in overdose, owing to respiratory depression (6), but later observations have suggested that it may not be any more toxic than the benzodiazepines (SEDA-21, 40). At normal doses zolpidem is said to be at least as safe as standard benzodiazepines in patients with respiratory compromise (SEDA-21, 40). The effects of zolpidem are reversed by flumazenil (7).

Subjective responses to treatment with zolpidem were assessed in 16 944 outpatients with insomnia. Nausea, dizziness, malaise, nightmares, agitation, and headache were the most common adverse events reported. There was one serious adverse reaction in a 48-year-old woman, who developed paranoid symptoms during the documentation phase. There were no life-threatening adverse events (8).

The safety and tolerability of zolpidem have been investigated in two multicenter studies, in which 8.9% and 7.5% of the patients reported an adverse event (9). The most frequent events were related to the central nervous system (somnolence, headache, confusion, vertigo), but gastrointestinal and cutaneous symptoms were also frequently reported.

In a double-blind, placebo-controlled, crossover study, 10 patients with "probable progressive supranuclear palsy" took single oral doses of zolpidem (5 and 10 mg), co-careldopa (levodopa 250 mg plus carbidopa 25 mg), or placebo in four separate trials in random order (10). Zolpidem, unlike levodopa or placebo, reduced voluntary saccadic eye movements, and the 5 mg dose produced a statistically significant improvement in motor function. The adverse effects of zolpidem included drowsiness and increased postural instability and were more marked after a dose of 10 mg.

Zolpidem has been investigated in a multicenter, double-blind, placebo-controlled, parallel-group, randomized study in 138 adults, who were experienced air travelers (11). They were randomized to zolpidem 10 mg or placebo for three (or optionally four) consecutive nights, starting with the first night-time sleep after travel. Sleep was assessed with daily questionnaires. Compared with placebo, zolpidem was associated with significantly improved sleep, longer total sleep time, reduced numbers of awakenings, and improved sleep quality. It was not associated with improvement in sleep latency. No unexpected or serious adverse events were reported and the most common adverse event was headache in both groups.

Zolpidem 10 mg/day and zopiclone 7.5 mg/day, given at night, have been compared in a 14-day, double-blind study in 479 chronic primary insomniacs (12). With zolpidem 68% of the patients were rated at least "moderately improved," versus 62% with zopiclone. However, with zolpidem sleep-onset latency improved in significantly more patients (86 versus 78%). In addition, significantly fewer patients who took zolpidem had drug-related adverse events (31 versus 45%); bitter taste accounted for 5.8% of such complaints with zolpidem compared with 40% with zopiclone. In conclusion, zolpidem was at least as effective as zopiclone but showed significantly less rebound on withdrawal; overall it was better tolerated.

Improvement in social and occupational function has been attributed to zolpidem (13).

- A recovering 60-year-old alcoholic woman developed reduced cognitive function, including considerable memory loss, praxis disorders, and an inability to join in conversation. A CT scan showed non-specific cerebral atrophy. She was given zolpidem 10 mg for insomnia, which she took at first at 2200 hours, but then earlier, at 1900 hours. After starting to take it at the earlier time she talked more easily and could wash the dishes and do the housework, things that she had lost the ability to do. This beneficial effect was detectable 45–60 minutes after the dose of zolpidem, lasted for 3 hours after each administration, and then abated. The subjective improvement in cognitive function was confirmed several times by her general practitioner.

Three patients had improvements in dystonia and parkinsonism after taking zolpidem 10 mg (14). The improvement in dystonia began at 15–45 minutes and optimal benefits were observed after 1–2 hours. The mean duration of action was 4.5 hours initially, falling to 2–3 hours with chronic use. This is similar to that reported in patients with progressive supranuclear palsy, and corresponds to the drug's half-life (2.5 hours). Sleepiness was noted at doses over 10 mg bd.

Organs and Systems

Nervous system

Zolpidem 10 mg, temazepam 15 mg, and placebo have been compared in 630 healthy adults in a multicenter study (15). They were given 15 minutes before lights out, with polysomnographic monitoring for 7.5 hours. Subjective questionnaires and performance tests, including digit symbol substitution and symbol copying, were administered before and after sleep. Neither drug significantly reduced objective sleep latency, but zolpidem reduced awakenings compared with temazepam. Both improved sleep efficiency and most subjective sleep measures, and zolpidem was superior to temazepam in five of six subjective outcome measures. Symbol copying, morning sleepiness, and morning concentration were not altered. Zolpidem 10 mg provided greater subjective hypnotic efficacy than temazepam 15 mg in this model of transient insomnia, with reduced polysomnographic awakenings.

Zolpidem was identified in the blood of 29 subjects arrested for impaired driving (16). In those in whom zolpidem was present with other drugs and/or alcohol, the symptoms reported were generally those of nervous system depression and included slow movements and reactions, slow and slurred speech, poor coordination, lack of balance, flaccid muscle tone, and horizontal and vertical gaze nystagmus. In five subjects in whom zolpidem was the only drug detected, signs of impairment included slow and slurred speech, slow reflexes, disorientation, and lack of balance and coordination. Therapeutic doses of zolpidem can affect driving adversely, and concentrations above the target range further impair both driving ability and consciousness.

Psychological, psychiatric

Like the benzodiazepines, zolpidem can produce a variety of paradoxical effects, including disturbances of mood, perception, and behavior. In 192 surgical patients zolpidem 8 mg but not 16 mg caused such effects, particularly anxiety, 1 hour after administration (17).

The acute effects of zolpidem and triazolam have been compared in 10 non-drug-abusing subjects using a Digit-Enter-and-Recall task with varying delay intervals (9, 10, and 20 seconds) (18). Zolpidem and triazolam impaired performance as a function of dose after all intervals. However, zolpidem produced significantly less impairment than triazolam after the longest delay (20 seconds). Zolpidem and triazolam produced comparable dose-related impairment of the digit symbol substitution, circular lights, and picture recall/recognition tasks. The results suggested that zolpidem may have less potential than triazolam to impair recall, which may be due to differences between these compounds in terms of their benzodiazepine-receptor binding profiles.

Delirium has been attributed to zolpidem (19,20).

- A 26-year-old woman was treated at a psychiatric inpatient unit for psychotic depression. She had neither formal thought disorder nor perceptual disturbances and was cognitively intact. Ten days later she was stabilized on fluoxetine, risperidone, and benzatropine. She then developed flu-like symptoms, and 3 days later took zolpidem 10 mg to help her to sleep. After 30 minutes she was found agitated, confused, and rambling, and wanted to go to the beach. Her speech was disorganized and she had visual hallucinations. Her gait was ataxic. There were no signs of meningeal irritation. Her temperature was 37.3°C, her pulse 114/minute, and her blood pressure 116/78 mmHg. When she was evaluated the next morning, her delirium had cleared and she made a full recovery.

- An 86-year-old white woman with headaches and diplopia took zolpidem 5 mg and about 2 hours later became restless, disoriented, and physically agitated. She was given haloperidol and needed restraining for her own safety. Her symptoms resolved by day 5 and she had no recollection of the incident. Rechallenge was not attempted.

Liver

Liver damage has been attributed to zolpidem (21).

- A 53-year-old woman first took zolpidem for insomnia in July 1996. In September 1996 she again took zolpidem 20 mg/day and 2 days later had developed sudden epigastric pain associated with pale stools and dark urine but no fever; she stopped taking zolpidem and the abdominal pain resolved spontaneously within 12 hours. In April 1997, she had another episode of abdominal pain after taking zolpidem. Eleven days later her serum alanine transaminase and gamma-glutamyltranspeptidase activities were 50 IU/l and 89 IU/l respectively. In June 1997 ultrasound showed a normal biliary tract. Viral hepatitis and concurrent infections with Epstein-Barr virus and cytomegalovirus were excluded.

Long-Term Effects

Drug abuse

There has been a literature review of the abuse potential of zolpidem (22). There were 15 published cases of abuse or dependence. In six patients the abuse was secondary to other forms of abuse or dependence. The authors concluded that the abuse potential of zolpidem is much less than with other hypnotics and that it is also safer than conventional hypnotics. Patients with a history of other substance abuse may be considered as being at risk of later abuse of zolpidem.

However, there is a risk of abuse and dependence from chronic use of zolpidem in high doses (23).

- A 67-year-old Caucasian woman, who had previously been treated for depression, anxiety, and insomnia, as well as alcohol, barbiturate, and benzodiazepine dependence, was given zolpidem 10 mg at bedtime for insomnia. She increased the dose without the knowledge of her physicians, using up to 100 mg/day for 1.5 years, alternating it with various benzodiazepines obtained from multiple physicians when zolpidem was unobtainable. She developed severe generalized tremor, psychomotor agitation, facial flushing, and anxiety, despite taking chlordiazepoxide 300 mg in divided doses during the first 24 hours of detoxification. A tapering dose of zolpidem was initiated and the chlordiazepoxide was tapered. Her symptoms completely subsided within 30 minutes of a single dose of zolpidem 15 mg.

Drug dependence

Four cases of former drug or alcohol abusers with personality disorders have been described; all developed dependence while taking high doses of zolpidem (24).

Drug withdrawal

Zaleplon has been compared with zolpidem 10 mg and placebo in 615 adult outpatients with insomnia (25). After a 7-night placebo (baseline) period, the patients were randomly assigned to receive one of five treatments in double-blind fashion for 28 nights (zaleplon 5, 10, or 20 mg; zolpidem 10 mg; or placebo), followed by placebo for 3 nights. Sleep latency, sleep maintenance, and sleep quality were determined from sleep questionnaires each morning. Rebound insomnia and withdrawal effects on withdrawal were also assessed. After withdrawal of zolpidem, the incidence of withdrawal symptoms was significantly greater than after withdrawal of placebo, and there was suggestion of significant rebound insomnia in some patients who had taken zolpidem compared with placebo. The frequency of adverse events in the active treatment groups did not differ significantly from that in the placebo group.

Withdrawal-induced seizures have been described in a woman taking various benzodiazepines and zolpidem (26).

- A 43-year-old woman had had insomnia since she was a child. At the age of 15 benzodiazepine therapy improved her sleeping, but when she gradually stopped taking benzodiazepines the insomnia returned after a few days. At the age of 26 she was abusing several benzodiazepines, including diazepam and flunitrazepam. At the age of 30 she was taking high doses of bromazepam every evening before going to sleep. After 1 month, she abruptly stopped taking bromazepam and during withdrawal had an epileptic seizure. During the next few years, she had periods of relative well-being, but also two further periods of benzodiazepine abuse, both resulting in seizures after withdrawal. Finally, a physician prescribed zolpidem. Two months later she increased the dose to 450–600 mg/day. After another month of abuse, she was forced by an unexpected event to discontinue the zolpidem and 4 hours later had an epileptic seizure, similar to the previous ones. She started taking zolpidem again, the drug abuse continued, and her fits settled. Six months later she underwent a planned program of zolpidem withdrawal.

Susceptibility Factors

Hepatic disease

The adverse effects of zolpidem can be enhanced in hepatic cirrhosis (27).

- A 41-year-old white man developed postoperative complications 11 months after liver transplantation. His mental status began to deteriorate secondary to hepatic encephalopathy. One day before admission he was given zolpidem 5 mg for sleep and 1 hour later he awoke in a stupor and was not oriented to place or time. He became increasingly incoherent and verbally abusive.

Although this patient's worsening mental state could have been explained by the natural history of the encephalopathy, it is possible that zolpidem exacerbated his decline.

Drug Administration

Drug dosage regimens

A review of six studies in over 4000 patients has suggested that non-nightly administration of zolpidem is effective and does not appear to be associated with withdrawal symptoms or dose escalation (28). On the other hand, a case report has suggested that stopping and restarting zolpidem can trigger visual hallucinations; the same phenomenon was observed three times in a healthy 23-year-old Chinese woman (29).

Drug overdose

Two deaths due to acute intentional zolpidem overdose have been reported (30).

- A 36-year-old woman with a history of psychiatric illness, including paranoid disorder, depression with panic episodes, and stress disorder, was found dead in bed. Caffeine, risperidone, and zolpidem were found in her urine.
- A 58-year-old woman with a history of hypertension and mental illness (manic depression and schizophrenia) was found dead in bed, with white foam around her mouth. Zolpidem and carbamazepine were found in her urine.

The cause of death in both cases was thought to have been acute zolpidem overdose, but it is not clear how risperidone and carbamazepine could have been excluded as possible contributors.

- A 44-year-old white man, who had had major depression and anxiety disorder for 25 years, became drowsy after swallowing 20 tablets (10 mg) of zolpidem (31). He was not taking any other medications at the time. A few hours later he became unresponsive and comatose and developed respiratory depression with hypoxia and mild hypercapnia. He subsequently made a full recovery after appropriate medical support.

Drug–Drug Interactions

Antifungal imidazoles

Potential interactions of zolpidem with three commonly prescribed azole derivatives (ketoconazole, itraconazole, and fluconazole) have been evaluated in a controlled clinical study. Co-administration of zolpidem with ketoconazole impaired zolpidem clearance and enhanced its benzodiazepine-like agonist pharmacodynamic effects. Itraconazole and fluconazole had a small effect on zolpidem kinetics and dynamics. The findings were consistent

with in vitro studies of differentially impaired zolpidem metabolism by azole derivatives (32).

Similarly, itraconazole 200 mg did not alter the pharmacokinetics and pharmacodynamics of zolpidem 10 mg in 10 healthy volunteers (33). Therefore, unlike triazolam, zolpidem may be used in normal or nearly normal doses together with itraconazole.

Drugs that compete for hepatic oxidative pathways

Omeprazole, like cimetidine, can impair benzodiazepine metabolism and lead to adverse effects (SEDA-18, 43). Other drugs, including antibiotics (erythromycin, chloramphenicol, isoniazid), antifungal drugs (ketoconazole, itraconazole, and analogues), some SSRIs (fluoxetine, paroxetine), other antidepressants (nefazodone), protease inhibitors (saquinavir), opioids (fentanyl), calcium channel blockers (diltiazem, verapamil), and disulfiram also compete for hepatic oxidative pathways that metabolize most benzodiazepines, as well as zolpidem, zopiclone, and buspirone (SEDA-22, 39) (SEDA-22, 41).

Fluoxetine

The possible pharmacokinetic and pharmacodynamic interactions of repeated nightly zolpidem dosing with fluoxetine were evaluated in 29 healthy women. There were no clinically significant pharmacokinetic or pharmacodynamic interactions (34).

Rifampicin

Rifampicin, and presumably other CYP3A inducers, reduces concentrations of zolpidem (SEDA-22, 42).

Ritonavir

The inhibitory effect of ritonavir on the biotransformation of triazolam and zolpidem has been investigated (35). Short-term, low-dose ritonavir produced a large and significant impairment of triazolam clearance and enhancement of its clinical effects. In contrast, ritonavir produced small and clinically unimportant reductions in zolpidem clearance. The findings are consistent with the complete dependence of triazolam clearance on CYP3A activity, compared with the partial dependence of zolpidem clearance on CYP3A.

Sertraline

Interactions between zolpidem and sertraline have been studied in 28 healthy women, who took a single dose of zolpidem alone and five consecutive doses of zolpidem 10 mg while taking chronic doses of sertraline 50 mg (36). Co-administration of sertraline 50 mg and zolpidem 10 mg was safe but could result in a shortened onset of action and increased effect of zolpidem.

References

1. Lader M. Psychiatric disorders. In: Speight T, Holford N, editors. Avery's Drug Treatment. 4th ed. Auckland: ADIS International Press, 1997:1437.
2. Lader M. Clin pharmacology of anxiolytic drugs: Past, present and future. In: Biggio G, Sanna E, Costa E, editors.

GABA-A Receptors and Anxiety. From Neurobiology To Treatment. New York: Raven Press, 1995:135.

3. Langtry HD, Benfield P. Zolpidem. A review of its pharmacodynamic and pharmacokinetic properties and therapeutic potential. Drugs 1990;40(2):291–313.

4. Declerck AC. Is "poor sleep" too vague a concept for rational treatment? J Int Med Res 1994;22(1):1–16.

5. Rosenberg J, Ahlstrom F. Randomized, double blind trial of zolpidem 10 mg versus triazolam 0.25 mg for treatment of insomnia in general practice. Scand J Prim Health Care 1994;12(2):88–92.

6. Lheureux P, Debailleul G, De Witte O, Askenasi R. Zolpidem intoxication mimicking narcotic overdose: response to flumazenil. Hum Exp Toxicol 1990; 9(2):105–7.

7. Zivkovic B, Morel E, Joly D, Perrault G, Sanger DJ, Lloyd KG. Pharmacological and behavioral profile of alpidem as an anxiolytic. Pharmacopsychiatry 1990;23(Suppl. 3):108–13.

8. Hajak G, Bandelow B. Safety and tolerance of zolpidem in the treatment of disturbed sleep: a post-marketing surveillance of 16 944 cases. Int Clin Psychopharmacol 1998;13(4):157–67.

9. Ganzoni E, Gugger M. Sicherheitsprofil von zolpidem: zwei studien mit 3805 patienten bei schweizer praktikem. [Safety profile of zolpidem: two studies of 3805 patients by Swiss practitioners.] Schweiz Rundsch Med Prax 1999;88(25–26):1120–7.

10. Daniele A, Moro E, Bentivoglio AR. Zolpidem in progressive supranuclear palsy. N Engl J Med 1999;341(7):543–4.

11. Jamieson AO, Zammit GK, Rosenberg RS, Davis JR, Walsh JK. Zolpidem reduces the sleep disturbance of jet lag. Sleep Med 2001;2(5):423–30.

12. Tsutsui S. Zolipidem Study Group. A double-blind comparative study of zolpidem versus zopiclone in the treatment of chronic primary insomnia. J Int Med Res 2001;29(3):163–77.

13. Jarry C, Fontenas JP, Jonville-Bera AP, Autret-Leca E. Beneficial effect of zolpidem for dementia. Ann Pharmacother 2002;36(11):1808.

14. Evidente VG. Zolpidem improves dystonia in "Lubag" or X-linked dystonia–parkinsonism syndrome. Neurology 2002;58(4):662–3.

15. Erman MK, Erwin CW, Gengo FM, Jamieson AO, Lemmi H, Mahowald MW, Regestein QR, Roth T, Roth-Schechter B, Scharf MB, Vogel GW, Walsh JK, Ware JC. Comparative efficacy of zolpidem and temazepam in transient insomnia. Hum Psychopharmacol 2001;16(2):169–76.

16. Logan BK, Couper FJ. Zolpidem and driving impairment. J Forensic Sci 2001;46(1):105–10.

17. Uhlig T, Huppe M, Brand K, Heinze J, Schmucker P. Zolpidem and promethazine in pre-anaesthetic medication. A pharmacopsychological approach. Neuropsychobiology 2000;42(3):139–48.

18. Rush CR, Baker RW. Zolpidem and triazolam interact differentially with a delay interval on a digit-enter-and-recall task. Hum Psychopharmacol 2001;16(2):147–57.

19. Freudenreich O, Menza M. Zolpidem-related delirium: a case report. J Clin Psychiatry 2000;61(6):449–50.

20. Brodeur MR, Stirling AL. Delirium associated with zolpidem. Ann Pharmacother 2001;35(12):1562–4.

21. Karsenti D, Blanc P, Bacq Y, Metman EH. Hepatotoxicity associated with zolpidem treatment. BMJ 1999;318(7192):1179.

22. Soyka M, Bottlender R, Moller HJ. Epidemiological evidence for a low abuse potential of zolpidem. Pharmacopsychiatry 2000;33(4):138–41.

23. Madrak LN, Rosenberg M. Zolpidem abuse. Am J Psychiatry 2001;158(8):1330–1.

24. Vartzopoulos D, Bozikas V, Phocas C, Karavatos A, Kaprinis G. Dependence on zolpidem in high dose. Int Clin Psychopharmacol 2000;15(3):181–2.

25. Elie R, Ruther E, Farr I, Emilien G, Salinas E. Sleep latency is shortened during 4 weeks of treatment with zaleplon, a novel nonbenzodiazepine hypnotic. Zaleplon Clinical Study Group. J Clin Psychiatry 1999;60(8):536–44.

26. Aragona M. Abuse, dependence, and epileptic seizures after zolpidem withdrawal: review and case report. Clin Neuropharmacol 2000;23(5):281–3.

27. Clark A. Worsening hepatic encephalopathy secondary to zolpidem. J Pharm Technol 1999;15:139–41.

28. Hajak G, Cluydts R, Allain H, Estivill E, Parrino L, Terzano MG, Walsh JK. The challenge of chronic insomnia: is non-nightly hypnotic treatment a feasible alternative? Eur Psychiatry 2003;18(5):201–8.

29. Tsai MJ, Huang YB, Wu PC. A novel clinical pattern of visual hallucination after zolpidem use. J Toxicol Clin Toxicol 2003;41(6):869–72.

30. Gock SB, Wong SH, Nuwayhid N, Venuti SE, Kelley PD, Teggatz JR, Jentzen JM. Acute zolpidem overdose—report of two cases. J Anal Toxicol 1999;23(6):559–62.

31. Hamad A, Sharma N. Acute zolpidem overdose leading to coma and respiratory failure. Intensive Care Med 2001;27(7):1239.

32. Greenblatt DJ, von Moltke LL, Harmatz JS, Mertzanis P, Graf JA, Durol AL, Counihan M, Roth-Schechter B, Shader RI. Kinetic and dynamic interaction study of zolpidem with ketoconazole, itraconazole, and fluconazole. Clin Pharmacol Ther 1998;64(6):661–71.

33. Luurila H, Kivisto KT, Neuvonen PJ. Effect of itraconazole on the pharmacokinetics and pharmacodynamics of zolpidem. Eur J Clin Pharmacol 1998;54(2):163–6.

34. Allard S, Sainati S, Roth-Schechter B, MacIntyre J. Minimal interaction between fluoxetine and multiple-dose zolpidem in healthy women. Drug Metab Dispos 1998;26(7):617–22.

35. Greenblatt DJ, von Moltke LL, Harmatz JS, Durol AL, Daily JP, Graf JA, Mertzanis P, Hoffman JL, Shader RI. Differential impairment of triazolam and zolpidem clearance by ritonavir. J Acquir Immune Defic Syndr 2000;24(2):129–36.

36. Allard S, Sainati SM, Roth-Schechter BF. Coadministration of short-term zolpidem with sertraline in healthy women. J Clin Pharmacol 1999;39(2):184–91.

Zomepirac

See also Non-steroidal anti-inflammatory drugs

General Information

Although zomepirac is a pyrrole-acetic acid compound closely related to tolmetin, it was originally claimed to be a new type of analgesic drug. Its history is not unlike that of benoxaprofen. In 1982, because of the severity and frequency of hypersensitivity reactions, it was withdrawn voluntarily by the manufacturers worldwide on a temporary basis (1). It has not been relaunched.

The overall incidence of its adverse effects, according to numerous reviews (SEDA-7, 114), is similar to or somewhat higher than with other NSAIDs. After single oral doses 36% of 496 patients had some adverse effects. The percentage was even higher (43%; 458 of

1079 patients) during short-term therapy (2 weeks). Owing to adverse reactions, 3.5% of patients dropped out. When it was given over 2–3 weeks, 65–70% patients had adverse effects, but the discontinuation rate was similar to or lower than that of other NSAIDs (2,3). Only the most important adverse effects are presented here.

Organs and Systems

Gastrointestinal

Adverse effects of zomepirac on the gastrointestinal tract were the most frequent reason for interruption of treatment. They increase with duration of administration. Nausea, vomiting, dyspepsia, discomfort, abdominal pain, and diarrhea or constipation have been recorded, as have stomatitis and tongue pain (4). Zomepirac 300 mg/day increases fecal blood loss, but less than aspirin.

Urinary tract

In five patients with prior normal renal function, zomepirac caused acute renal insufficiency, with varying degrees of uremia, proteinuria, and oliguria (5). All recovered either after withdrawal or with prednisone therapy. In another case renal biopsy showed a tubulo-interstitial nephritis (6).

Immunologic

The manufacturers received 1100 reports of allergic reactions in the first 2 years after launch. Fatal anaphylactic and anaphylactoid reactions have been reported: 10% of all reports on anaphylactic reactions in the USA named zomepirac, making it second only to the much older drug tolmetin. Hypersensitivity reactions are characterized by hypotension, bronchospasm, and serious respiratory distress, with or without oropharyngeal edema. Type-III allergic reactions have also been described.

Long-Term Effects

Drug dependence

Suspicions based on cluster reports that zomepirac may be addictive have not been confirmed (7).

References

1. World Health Organization. Zomepirac (United States of America). PHA (DIA) 1983;83.3.8.
2. Ruoff GE, Andelman SY, Cannella JJ. Long-term safety of zomepirac: a double-blind comparison with aspirin in patients with osteoarthritis. J Clin Pharmacol 1980;20(5-6 Pt 2):377–84.
3. McMillen JI, Urbaniak JR, Boas R. Treatment of chronic orthopedic pain with zomepirac. J Clin Pharmacol 1980;20(5-6 Pt 2):385–91.
4. Bates LH, Triplett WC, Berry ER, Weddle RA. Stomatitis associated with zomepirac. JAMA 1982;247(4):461–2.
5. Miller FC, Schorr WJ, Lacher JW. Zomepirac-induced renal failure. Arch Intern Med 1983;143(6):1171–3.
6. McCarthy JT, Schwartz GL, Blair TJ, Pierides AM, Van den Berg CJ. Reversible nonoliguric acute renal failure associated with zomepirac therapy. Mayo Clin Proc 1982;57(6):351–4.
7. Mendelis PS. Abuse potential associated with nonsteroidal anti-inflammatory drugs. ADR Highlights 1982;82.

Zonisamide

See also Antiepileptic drugs

General Information

Original attempts to market zonisamide in the USA were halted by reports of nephrolithiasis, but successful marketing in Japan resulted in renewed interest elsewhere (1). Zonisamide has a broad spectrum of efficacy in the treatment of seizures, including infantile spasms and myoclonic seizures. It may also have neuroprotective and antimanic effects. Its mechanism of action is not known, but it blocks sodium channels and T-type calcium channels and scavenges free radicals.

In a large Japanese survey, adverse effects occurred in 51% of patients treated with zonisamide and led to drug withdrawal in 18%. The most common were drowsiness, ataxia, anorexia, mental slowing, and gastrointestinal symptoms (2). Other adverse effects include dizziness, nystagmus, dysarthria, diplopia, asterixis, tremor, confusion, anorexia, and weight loss. Some of these may be related to the rate of dosage escalation.

In a double-blind, placebo-controlled, add-on, randomized trial of zonisamide 400 mg/day in 203 patients over 14 years of age with refractory partial-onset seizures, the response rate was 42% (3). The most common treatment-emergent adverse events were somnolence, anorexia, rhinitis, dizziness, nausea or vomiting, ataxia, fatigue, and headache. With zonisamide, 22% of the patients lost over 2.3 kg compared with 10% on placebo.

In a Cochrane Collaboration meta-analysis of trials of zonisamide, levetiracetam, oxcarbazepine, and remacemide, there were no significant differences in efficacy among the four drugs (4). The relative risks for treatment withdrawal were also not significantly different.

Organs and Systems

Psychological, psychiatric

Behavioral problems and acute mania have been described (SEDA-16, 75) (SEDA-19, 76).

Of 74 epileptic patients who had taken zonisamide 14 had psychotic episodes, diagnosed retrospectively (5). The authors estimated that the incidence of psychotic episodes during zonisamide treatment was several times higher than the previously reported prevalence of epileptic psychosis, and that the risk was higher in young patients. In 13 patients, psychotic episodes occurred within a few years of starting zonisamide. In children, obsessive-compulsive symptoms were related to psychotic episodes.

A unique form of paramnesia has been attributed to zonisamide (6).

- After an episode of zonisamide-induced psychosis, a 28-year-old man with epilepsy consistently mistook people who were unknown to him, such as hospital staff, for people whom he had met long ago. However, he did not misidentify their names or other attributes, such as their occupations.

The authors could not fit this extraordinary form of misidentification into any known subcategory of misidentification syndromes, but rather thought that it fitted Kraepelin's description of "assoziierende Erinnerungsfälschungen".

Acid–base balance

Metabolic acidosis has been reported in patients taking zonisamide (7). Zonisamide inhibits carbonic anhydrase (8), which might have contributed, as has been suggested by another case of metabolic acidosis in a 7-year-old boy, in which the mechanism was renal tubular acidosis.

Ammonium chloride, bicarbonate, and furosemide loading tests in an epileptic man with metabolic acidosis and episodic hypokalemia taking zonisamide showed evidence of distal renal tubular acidosis (9). On re-examination 7 weeks after zonisamide had been replaced with phenytoin, the renal tubular acidosis had resolved.

Urinary tract

Zonisamide inhibits carbonic anhydrase, but the risk of nephrolithiasis seems to be lower than initially suspected (SEDA-21, 80). Further cases have been reported (10).

- A 13-year-old boy who had taken zonisamide and acetazolamide for 2 months developed abdominal pain due to left-sided hydronephrosis, which resolved after the passage of a stone. He had an alkaline urine, and acetazolamide was withdrawn. However, 2 months later he formed another stone. Zonisamide was withdrawn and he formed no more stones.
- A 7-year-old boy took zonisamide for 3 months and then formed a thick sludge of calcium phosphate in the bladder when dehydrated because of pneumonia.
- A 15-year-old girl, who had a history of recurrent urinary obstruction, formed a thick sludge of calcium oxalate in the bladder.

In all three patients the urine was alkaline and there was hypercalciuria.

Sweat glands

Zonisamide can cause lack of sweating (11).

- A 10-year-old boy who had taken zonisamide for about 9 months noticed that he had a dry skin and that he seldom sweated. His zonisamide blood concentration was very high. He discontinued zonisamide and became able to sweat.

The authors suggested that this effect was due to ion channel blockade.

In 16 patients taking zonisamide, acetylcholine stimulation testing after about 1 month was normal in four cases and reduced in 12 (12). There was reduced sweating in

four of the 12 who had a reduced test response, but not in the four with a normal response.

Children have a higher risk of zonisamide-associated oligohidrosis and hyperthermia (13). Elan Pharma issued a "Dear Doctor" letter reporting this adverse event in June 2002. During the zonisamide development program in Japan one case of oligohidrosis was reported among 403 children (an incidence of 1/285 patient-years of exposure). There were no cases reported in the US or European development programs, although under 100 children were included in those programs. In the first 11 years of marketing in Japan, 38 cases have been reported (about 1 per 10 000 patient-years). In the first year in the USA, two cases were reported (an estimated reporting rate of 12/10 000 patient-years). This rate might be an underestimate, owing to under-reporting.

There have been reports of heat stroke associated with reduced sweating in young patients.

- A 2-year-old mentally retarded boy with frontal lobe epilepsy developed hyperpyrexia with oligohidrosis and central neurological symptoms, including chorea-like involuntary movements, resting tremor, and cogwheel rigidity, while receiving zonisamide (14). A sweat test using pilocarpine iontophoresis showed a marked reduction in the sweat response, which suggested a postganglionic sweating dysfunction. A skin biopsy showed no morphological abnormality in the sweat glands. He regained the ability to sweat within 2 weeks of withdrawal.

Children receiving zonisamide should be monitored closely for evidence of reduced sweating and increased body temperature, especially in warm or hot weather and when taking other drugs that predispose to this (carbonic anhydrase inhibitors, anticholinergic drugs, topiramate).

Immunologic

Zonisamide-induced lupus erythematosus has been reported in a 5-year-old child taking zonisamide and ethosuximide (15). He had raised titers of antinuclear antibodies and anti-DNA antibodies and presented with fever, pericarditis, pleurisy, and arthralgia. Clinical recovery and a reduction in the anti-DNA-antibody titer promptly followed withdrawal. A lymphocyte transformation test against zonisamide was positive.

Second-Generation Effects

Lactation

Zonisamide concentrations in plasma and breast milk were measured, in order to investigate the transfer of zonisamide through the placenta and breast milk in two neonates (16). The transfer rates were 92% via the placenta and 41–57% via breast milk.

Drug–Drug Interactions

Carbamazepine

Evidence that zonisamide reduces serum carbamazepine concentrations is conflicting (SEDA-19, 61). Zonisamide can reduce carbamazepine-10,11-epoxide to carbamazepine ratios, possibly by reducing the rate of epoxidation.

CYP3A4 inhibitors

In vitro data suggest that the CYP3A4 inhibitors ketoconazole, ciclosporin, and miconazole reduce zonisamide clearance by 31%, 23%, and 17% respectively (SEDA-22, 93).

Enzyme-inducing anticonvulsants

Serum zonisamide concentrations are reduced by enzyme-inducing anticonvulsants (17).

Lamotrigine

Preliminary evidence suggests that serum zonisamide concentrations can be increased by lamotrigine (17).

Diagnosis of Adverse Drug Reactions

The recommended target plasma zonisamide concentration is 10–20 µg/ml.

References

1. Oommen KJ, Mathews S. Zonisamide: a new antiepileptic drug. Clin Neuropharmacol 1999;22(4):192–200.
2. Peters DH, Sorkin EM. Zonisamide. A review of its pharmacodynamic and pharmacokinetic properties, and therapeutic potential in epilepsy. Drugs 1993;45(5):760–87.
3. Faught E, Ayala R, Montouris GG, Leppik IE. Zonisamide 922 Trial Group. Randomized controlled trial of zonisamide for the treatment of refractory partial-onset seizures. Neurology 2001;57(10):1774–9.
4. Marson AG, Hutton JL, Leach JP, Castillo S, Schmidt D, White S, Chaisewikul R, Privitera M, Chadwick DW. Levetiracetam, oxcarbazepine, remacemide and zonisamide for drug resistant localization-related epilepsy: a systematic review. Epilepsy Res 2001;46(3):259–70.
5. Miyamoto T, Kohsaka M, Koyama T. Psychotic episodes during zonisamide treatment. Seizure 2000;9(1):65–70.
6. Murai T, Kubota Y, Sengoku A. Unknown people believed to be known: the "assoziierende Erinnerungs falschungen" by Kraepelin. Psychopathology 2000;33(1):52–4.
7. Imai K, Mano T, Shimono K, Ueda H, Okinaga T, Yanagihara K, Li Z, Okada S. [Three cases of hypoactivity and poor appetite with zonisamide-induced metabolic acidosis.] No To Hattatsu 2000;32(1):75–7.
8. Masuda Y, Karasawa T. Inhibitory effect of zonisamide on human carbonic anhydrase in vitro. Arzneimittelforschung 1993;43(4):416–18.
9. Inoue T, Kira R, Kaku Y, Ikeda K, Gondo K, Hara T. Renal tubular acidosis associated with zonisamide therapy. Epilepsia 2000;41(12):1642–4.
10. Kubota M, Nishi-Nagase M, Sakakihara Y, Noma S, Nakamoto M, Kawaguchi H, Yanagisawa M. Zonisamide-induced urinary lithiasis in patients with intractable epilepsy. Brain Dev 2000;22(4):230–3.
11. Matsuoka Y, Nakai N, Tada M, Nishigaki T, Onoe S. A case of hidropoietic disorder caused by zonisamide, antiepileptic drug. Skin Res 2000;42:58–62.
12. Okumura A, Ishihara N, Kato T, Hayakawa F, Kuno K, Watanabe K. Predictive value of acetylcholine stimulation testing for oligohidrosis caused by zonisamide. Pediatr Neurol 2000;23(1):59–61.
13. Glauser TA, Pellock JM. Zonisamide in pediatric epilepsy: review of the Japanese experience. J Child Neurol 2002;17(2):87–96.
14. Shimizu T, Yamashita Y, Satoi M, Togo A, Wada N, Matsuishi T, Ohnishi A, Kato H. Heat stroke-like episode in a child caused by zonisamide. Brain Dev 1997;19(5):366–8.
15. Mutoh K, Hidaka Y, Hirose Y, Kimura M. Possible induction of systemic lupus erythematosus by zonisamide. Pediatr Neurol 2001;25(4):340–3.
16. Kawada K, Itoh S, Kusaka T, Isobe K, Ishii M. Pharmacokinetics of zonisamide in perinatal period. Brain Dev 2002;24(2):95–7.
17. McJilton J, DeToledo J, DeCerce J, Huda S, Abubakr A, Ramsay R. Cotherapy of lamotrigine/lamictal results in significant elevation of zonisamide levels. Epilepsia 1996;37(Suppl. 5):173.

Zopiclone

General Information

Although it is chemically distinct to the benzodiazepines, zopiclone, a cyclopyrrolone, has similar pharmacology, binding close to the same site of the GABA receptor–chloride channel complex.

Zopiclone has been widely used as a hypnotic, comparable to estazolam (1), and appears to be relatively safe in overdose. It has no adverse effects that would not be expected from its pharmacological and pharmacokinetic properties, with three exceptions: bitter taste (in 3.6% of 20 513 patients) and, like zolpidem, increased risks of gastrointestinal disturbances and visual hallucinations (2,3). Subchronic zopiclone produces minimal changes in the sleep electroencephalogram (4), a potential advantage over benzodiazepines, and in direct comparisons was at least as effective as triazolam or flunitrazepam, with no rebound insomnia after 1 month (SEDA-19, 37). On the other hand, longer administration of zopiclone can cause physical dependence (5), emphasizing the importance of restricting treatment duration. Likewise, its potential for abuse and release of aggression (6) is similar to that of the benzodiazepines (SEDA-17, 47).

Organs and Systems

Nervous system

In a two-part, placebo-controlled, crossover comparison of the effects of zopiclone and zaleplon on car driving, memory, and psychomotor performance, zaleplon 10 mg had no residual effect on driving when taken at bedtime, 10 hours before driving (7). In contrast, zopiclone 7.5 mg caused marked residual impairment. Patients should be advised to avoid driving the morning after taking zopiclone.

Further concern that zolpidem can impair performance comes from a Chinese study (8). Zopiclone 7.5 mg, but not triazolam 2.5 mg, impaired simulated flight performance 2 hours and 3 hours after a dose at midday and sleeping for 1 hour; performance recovered after 4 hours.

Endocrine

The syndrome of inappropriate secretion of antidiuretic hormone has been attributed to zopiclone (9).

- A woman with a 2-week history of insomnia took zopiclone 7.5 mg nightly and over the next 9 days became confused, lethargic, and depressed, culminating in an overdose of six zopiclone tablets. Her previous medical history included hypertension and two episodes of diuretic-induced SIADH. Her serum sodium was 129 mmol/l and 4 days later fell to 113 mmol/l. Her serum osmolality was low (240 mmol/kg) and her urine sodium was 20 mmol/l. The serum sodium returned to normal 12 days after withdrawal of zopiclone.

The rapid resolution of symptoms and correction of the hyponatremia after withdrawal was consistent with an effect of zopiclone.

Long-Term Effects

Drug withdrawal

The acute polysomnographic effects of withdrawal of standard doses of zopiclone ($n = 11$), zolpidem ($n = 11$), triazolam ($n = 10$), and placebo ($n = 7$) have been studied in healthy men (10). They took zopiclone 7.5 mg, zolpidem 10 mg, triazolam 0.25 mg, or placebo for 4 weeks in double-blind, randomized order. Sleep EEG was performed. Total sleep time and sleep efficiency were lower in the first night after withdrawal of triazolam. After withdrawal from zopiclone or zolpidem there were slight but not significant rebound effects. Self-rating scales showed minimal rebound insomnia after withdrawal of all three hypnotics. In the placebo group there were no changes in sleep. These results suggest that the risks of tolerance and dependency are low after short-term zopiclone or zolpidem in the recommended doses.

Drug Administration

Drug overdose

- A 72-year-old with respiratory debilitation due to bronchogenic carcinoma died after taking zopiclone about 200–350 mg (11).

Drug–Drug Interactions

Nefazodone

An 86-year-old white woman taking nefazodone for depression started to take zopiclone for insomnia, but subsequently had morning drowsiness (12). The plasma concentration of zopiclone was measured 8 hours after administration on two occasions, during and after nefazodone therapy. After withdrawal of nefazodone, the plasma concentration of the S-enantiomer of zopiclone fell from 107 to 17 ng/ml, while the plasma concentration of the R-enantiomer fell from 21 to 1.5 ng/ml.

The substantial fall in plasma zopiclone concentration after withdrawal of nefazodone probably reflected a drug interaction due to inhibition of CYP3A4 by

nefazodone (13). Despite the normally short half-life of zopiclone, the residual sedation initially observed in this case suggests that the interaction had clinical significance.

References

1. Li S, Wang C. A comparative study of imovane and estazolam treatment on sleep disturbances. Chin Med Sci J 1995;10(1):56–8.
2. Goa KL, Heel RC. Zopiclone. A review of its pharmacodynamic and pharmacokinetic properties and therapeutic efficacy as an hypnotic. Drugs 1986;32(1):48–65.
3. Mahendran R, Chee KT, Peh LH, Wong KE, Lim L. A postmarketing surveillance study of zopiclone in insomnia. Singapore Med J 1994;35(4):390–3.
4. Roschke J, Mann K, Aldenhoff JB, Benkert O. Functional properties of the brain during sleep under subchronic zopiclone administration in man. Eur Neuropsychopharmacol 1994;4(1):21–30.
5. Jones IR, Sullivan G. Physical dependence on zopiclone: case reports. BMJ 1998;316(7125):117.
6. Shaw SC, Fletcher AP. Aggression as an adverse drug reaction. Adverse Drug React Toxicol Rev 2000;19(1):35–45.
7. Vermeeren A, Riedel WJ, van Boxtel MP, Darwish M, Paty I, Patat A. Differential residual effects of zaleplon and zopiclone on actual driving: a comparison with a low dose of alcohol. Sleep 2002;25(2):224–31.
8. Jing BS, Zhan H, Li YF, Zhou YJ, Guo H. [Effects of short-action hypnotics triazolam and zopiclone on simulated flight performance.] Space Med Med Eng (Beijing) 2003;16(5):329–31.
9. Cubbin SA, Ali IM. Inappropriate antidiuretic hormone secretion associated with zopiclone. Psychiatr Bull 1999;23:306–7.
10. Voderholzer U, Riemann D, Hornyak M, Backhaus J, Feige B, Berger M, Hohagen F. A double-blind, randomized and placebo-controlled study on the polysomnographic withdrawal effects of zopiclone, zolpidem and triazolam in healthy subjects. Eur Arch Psychiatry Clin Neurosci 2001;251(3):117–23.
11. Bramness JG, Arnestad M, Karinen R, Hilberg T. Fatal overdose of zopiclone in an elderly woman with bronchogenic carcinoma. J Forensic Sci 2001;46(5):1247–9.
12. Alderman CP, Gebauer MG, Gilbert AL, Condon JT. Possible interaction of zopiclone and nefazodone. Ann Pharmacother 2001;35(11):1378–80.
13. Nemeroff CB, DeVane CL, Pollock BG. Newer antidepressants and the cytochrome P450 system. Am J Psychiatry 1996;153(3):311–20.

Zotepine

See also Neuroleptic drugs

General Information

Zotepine is a dibenzothiepine neuroleptic drug, an antagonist at D_1 dopamine receptors and at 5-HT_1 and 5-HT_2 receptors (1). It rarely causes extrapyramidal disturbances, and when they do occur they are usually mild.

The efficacy and safety of zotepine have been explored in a 1-year open study in 253 patients with schizophrenia (mean age 38 years, range 18–65) who took zotepine 75–450 mg/day (2). The mean total BPRS score was reduced from 52 at baseline to 41. Since concomitant treatment was allowed, 173 patients reported 205 ongoing and 448 new neuroleptic medicaments during the study. A total of 826 adverse events were reported by 220 patients; 50 had serious adverse events and 5 died during the study, 2 taking zotepine; one death was a suicide and the other was due to a ventricular dysrhythmia. In all, 138 patients (55%) withdrew from the study; 60 withdrawals were due to adverse events. The most frequently reported adverse events were weight gain (28%; mean weight gain 4.3 kg), somnolence (15%), and weakness (13%). There were adverse events that could be related to extrapyramidal effects in 5%. In 14 patients with normal baseline electrocardiography there were abnormalities at the end of the study, most commonly sinus tachycardia; there were no reports of torsade de pointes. No clinically important hematological abnormalities have been reported to date.

References

1. Ackenheil M. Das biochemische Wirkprofil von Zotepin im Vergleich zu anderen Neuroleptika. [The biochemical effect profile of zotepine in comparison with other neuroleptics.] Fortschr Neurol Psychiatr 1991;59(Suppl. 1):2–9.
2. Palmgren K, Wighton A, Reynolds CW, Butler A, Tweed JA, Raniwalla J, Welch CP, Bratty JR. The safety and efficacy of zotepine in the treatment of schizophrenia: results of a one-year naturalistic clinical trial. Int J Psychiatry Clin Pract 2000;4:299–306.

Zuclopenthixol

See also Neuroleptic drugs

General Information

Zuclopenthixol is a thioxanthene neuroleptic drug.

Organs and Systems

Hematologic

Neutropenia has been associated with zuclopenthixol (1).

- A 66-year-old man with schizophrenia took zuclopenthixol 10 mg tds for 18 days and developed a mild leukopenia (2.9×10^9/l) and thrombocytopenia (109×10^9/l). He was asymptomatic, with no evidence of infection or a bleeding tendency. Zuclopenthixol was withdrawn, without any change in the rest of his drug therapy (glibenclamide 5 mg tds, biperiden 2 mg bd, oxazepam 10 mg tds, dipyridamole 75 mg tds, and ranitidine 150 mg/day). The leukocyte and platelet counts rose over the next 5 days.

Sexual function

Priapism, although infrequent, can occur during treatment with neuroleptic drugs and necessitates prompt urological consultation and sometimes even surgical intervention (SEDA-14, 149). A case has been associated with zuclopenthixol (2).

- A 31-year-old man developed priapism after taking zuclopenthixol 30 mg/day for 8 days, the dose having been increased to 75 mg the day before, while he was still taking oral carbamazepine 600 mg/day and clorazepate dipotassium 30 mg/day. He had a history of perinatal anoxic encephalopathy with severe motor sequelae and dyslalia, alcohol dependence, and a personality disorder. On the day before the priapism occurred, he had been physically restrained and given an extra dose of intramuscular clorazepate dipotassium 50 mg. When priapism occurred, all drugs except clorazepate were withdrawn and about 6 hours later the corpora cavernosa were washed and infused with noradrenaline in glucose (8 doses of 40 μg), after which the priapism resolved.

References

1. Coutinho E, Fenton M, Adams C, Campbell C. Zuclopenthixol acetate in psychiatric emergencies: looking for evidence from clinical trials Schizophr Res 2000;46(2–3):111–18.
2. Salado J, Blazquez A, Diaz-Simon R, Lopez-Munoz F, Alamo C, Rubio G. Priapism associated with zuclopenthixol. Ann Pharmacother 2002;36(6):1016–18.

Zygophyllaceae

See also Herbal medicines

General Information

The family of Zygophyllaceae (Table 1) contains nine genera.

Larrea tridentata

The major phenolic component of *Larrea tridentata* (chaparral, creosote bush) is a catechol lignan called nordihydroguaiaretic acid. It causes lymphatic and renal lesions when given chronically in high doses to rodents.

Table 1 The genera of Zygophyllaceae

Balanites (balanites)
Bulnesia (lignum vitae)
Fagonia (fagon bush)
Guajacum (lignum vitae)
Kallstroemia (caltrop)
Larrea (creosote bush)
Peganum (peganum)
Tribulus (punturevine)
Zygophyllum (bean caper)

Adverse effects

There have been several reports of hepatotoxicity attributed to herbal medicines containing *L. tridentata* leaves (1,2). Of 18 reports of illnesses associated with the ingestion of chaparral, there was evidence of hepatotoxicity in 13 cases (3). The presentation was characterized by jaundice with a marked increase in serum liver enzymes at 3–52 weeks after ingestion, and it resolved 1–17 weeks after withdrawal. The predominant pattern of liver damage was cholestatic; in four cases there was progression to cirrhosis and in two there was acute fulminant liver failure that required liver transplantation.

Chaparral-induced hepatotoxicity in 16 published cases has been summarized in the light of a further report (4).

- A 27-year-old Hispanic man presented with nausea and vomiting, diarrhea, and upper abdominal pain 12 months after starting to take chaparral capsules. A liver biopsy showed hepatocellular injury with necrosis and periportal inflammation. His liver function stabilized after withdrawal of chaparral.

However, in four patients who were given topical chaparral tincture there was no evidence of liver damage (5).

Contact dermatitis has been attributed to *L. tridentata* (6).

A cystic renal cell carcinoma and acquired renal cystic disease associated with consumption of chaparral tea has been reported (7).

References

1. Gordon DW, Rosenthal G, Hart J, Sirota R, Baker AL. Chaparral ingestion. The broadening spectrum of liver injury caused by herbal medications. JAMA 1995;273(6):489–90.
2. Batchelor WB, Heathcote J, Wanless IR. Chaparral-induced hepatic injury. Am J Gastroenterol 1995;90(5):831–3.
3. Sheikh NM, Philen RM, Love LA. Chaparral-associated hepatotoxicity. Arch Intern Med 1997;157(8):913–9.
4. Grant KL, Boyer LV, Erdman BE. Chaparral-induced hepatotoxicity. Integrative Med 1998;1:83–7.
5. Heron S, Yarnell E. The safety of low-dose *Larrea tridentata* (DC) Coville (creosote bush or chaparral): a retrospective clinical study J Altern Complement Med 2001; 7(2):175–85.
6. Shasky DR. Contact dermatitis from *Larrea tridentata* (creosote bush) J Am Acad Dermatol 1986;15(2 Pt 1):302.
7. Smith AY, Feddersen RM, Gardner KD Jr, Davis CJ Jr. Cystic renal cell carcinoma and acquired renal cystic disease associated with consumption of chaparral tea: a case report. J Urol 1994;152(6 Pt 1):2089–91.

APPENDIX

Appendix: List of miscellaneous compounds

General Information

Compound	Adverse effect(s)	References
Amaranth	Allergic reactions (asthma etc.)	(1)
Apnea monitors	Electrocution/burns	(SED-13, 1463)
Balsam of Peru	Dermatitis	(SEDA-21, 501)
Benzalkonium chloride	Exacerbation of rhinitis (nose-drops)	(2)
	Eye irritation or keratitis (eye-drops)	(3)
Benzyl alcohol	Gasping syndrome and infant deaths	(SEDA-19, 446)
Blue dye	Contact dermatitis	(4)
Butyl hydroxyanisole	Allergic contact dermatitis	(5)
Cementless hip arthroplasty	Failure	(SEDA-20, 435)
Cetyl-stearyl alcohol	Dermatitis	(SEDA-21, 501)
Chlorhexidine-impregnated devices	Hypersensitivity reactions	(SEDA-22, 525)
Cosmetics	Dermal reactions	(SEDA-19, 441)
Cinnamic aldehyde	Cutaneous vasodilatation	(6)
	Lichenoid skin eruptions, eczematous erythroderma	(7,8)
Dental amalgam fillings	Allergies	(SEDA-20, 440)
Dental materials	Allergic skin rash	(SED-13, 1456)
Detergents	Allergic contact dermatitis	(9)
Dimethylacetamide	Hallucinations, delusions, pulmonary edema	(10)
Dinitrochlorobenzene	Pruritic reaction	(SEDA-19, 446)
Electric heating pads	Burns, electric shocks	(SEDA-20, 435)
Enoxolone	Allergic contact dermatitis	(11)
Ethanolamine	Chest pain, dysphagia, strictures	(SEDA-20, 438)
Ethyl aminobenzoate	Allergic contact dermatitis	(SEDA-21, 497)
FD and C Blue No 1	Intense green hyperpigmentation	(12)
Food additives	Urticaria	(13)
Fructose	Hypoglycemia	(SEDA-21, 501)
Fructose-1,6-diphosphate	Nausea, local burning	(SEDA-19, 446)
Fumaric acid	Gastrointestinal disorders	(SEDA-21, 501)
Fumaric acid (alkyl ester)	Leukopenia, eosinophilia	(SEDA-20, 440)
Gamma-hydroxybutyric acid	Vomiting, dizziness, tremors, seizures	(SEDA-21, 501)
Gamolenic acid	Inadequate efficacy	(14)
	Hyperparathyroidism	(15)
Glycolic acid	Dermal wounding	(SEDA-19, 446)
Hair implants	Foreign body reactions, infections	(SEDA-20, 435)
Hemodiafiltration	Hypophosphatemia	(16)
Indigo carmine	Anaphylactoid reaction; cardiac arrest	(17)
	Allergic alveolitis	(18)
	Anaphylactoid reaction	(SEDA-19, 446)
K4-herbal product	Liver problems	(SEDA-21, 498)
Lactose	Skin eruptions	(19)
	Diarrhea, vomiting, hypoglycemia	
	Availability problem	(SEDA-19/21, 501)
Lanolin alcohol	Allergic contact eczema	(SEDA-21, 501)
Lecithin	Atopic dermatitis	(20)
Lipokinetix	Liver injury	(21)
Metabisulfite sodium	Allergic contact dermatitis	(22)
	Bronchospasm, anaphylaxis, contact dermatitis	(23)
	Nasal syndromes	(SEDA-19, 446)
Metered-dose inhalers	Bronchoconstriction	(SEDA-19, 446)
Methyl glucose dioleate	Erythematous dermatitis	(24)
Monofluorophosphate	Leg pain	(25)

Continued

Continued

Compound	Adverse effect(s)	References
Para-phenylenediamine	Contact allergies	(SEDA-20/21, 501)
Parabens	Allergic contact eczema	(SEDA-21, 501)
Parathion	Death	(26)
	Acute intoxication	(27)
Pharmaceutical excipients	Asthma, anaphylaxis, local irritation	(28)
Phenazone salicylate	Drug eruption	(SEDA-19, 446)
Phenol	Burns	(29)
Phosphate infusion	Calcified right atrial thrombus	(30)
Phosphate, sodium	Electrolyte disturbances	(SEDA-21/22, 526)
Polidocanol	Embolia cutis medicamentosa	(31)
	Allergic contact dermatitis	(32)
	Allergic reactions, thrombosis	(SEDA-20, 440)
Polyoxyethylene lauryl ether	Follicular contact dermatitis	(33)
	Contact dermatitis	(33)
Polyvinylpyrrolidone	Contact allergy (facial eczema)	(34)
	Allergic contact dermatitis	(35)
Potassium dichromate	Contact allergy	(SEDA-20, 440)
Potassium salts	Complex ventricular dysrhythmias	(36)
	Drug-induced esophagitis	(37)
Rasburicase	Skin rash, respiratory reaction, hemolysis	(38)
Royal jelly	Allergic reactions, death	(SEDA-22/21, 526)
"Slim 10"	Contamination with nicotinamide, fenfluramine, and thyroid gland components	(39)
Sodium picosulfate	Electrolyte disturbance, convulsions, syncope, metabolic alkalosis	(40)
Sodium prasterone sulfate	Anaphylactic reactions	(41)
Sorbic acid	Systemic contact dermatitis	(42)
Sorbitol	Adominal pain, diarrhea	(SEDA-21, 500)
Stearyl alcohol	Contact dermatitis	(43)
Sterile water	Hemolysis	(SEDA-22, 524)
Sulfan blue	Anaphylactic reactions	(44)
Synthetic food coloring	Hyperactivity, irritability children	(SED-13, 1462)
Tetraethylthiuram disulfide	Contact dermatitis	(45)
Thiuram mix	Contact allergy	(SEDA-20, 440)
Tiaprofenic acid	Cystitis	(SEDA-19, 446)
Tincture of orange	Nausea, vomiting, abdominal pain	(SEDA-19, 446)
Titanium alloy prosthesis	Cytogenetic damage	(46)
Trichloracetic acid	Dermal wounding	(SEDA-19, 446)
Visicol	Risk of seizures	(47)
Volume ventilators	Injuries and deaths	(SED-13, 1464)
Walnut oil	Foreign body reactions, tumors, pulmonary complications	(48)
White flower	Contact dermatitis	(49)
Yasmin	Venous thromboembolism	(50)

References

1. Bossert J, Wahl R. Amaranth: a new allergen in bakeries. Allergologie 2000;23:448–57.
2. Marple B, Roland P, Benninger M. Safety review of benzalkonium chloride used as a preservative in intranasal solutions: an overview of conflicting data and opinions. Otolaryngol Head Neck Surg 2004;130(1):131–41.
3. Noecker R. Effects of common ophthalmic preservatives on ocular health. Adv Ther 2001;18(5):205–15.
4. Guin JD. Seat-belt dermatitis from Disperse Blue dyes. Contact Dermatitis 2001;44(4):263.
5. Orton DI, Shaw S. Allergic contact dermatitis from pharmaceutical grade BHA in Timodine, with no patch test reaction to analytical grade BHA. Contact Dermatitis 2001;44(3):191–2.
6. VanderEnde DS, Morrow JD. Release of markedly increased quantities of prostaglandin D2 from the skin in vivo in humans after the application of cinnamic aldehyde. J Am Acad Dermatol 2001;45(1):62–7.
7. Aguilar A, Gallego MA, Pique E. Lichenoid drug eruption due to cyanamide. Int J Dermatol 1999;38(12):950–1.
8. Abajo P, Feal C, Sanz-Sanchez T, Sanchez-Perez J, Garcia-Diez A. Eczematous erythroderma induced by cyanamide. Contact Dermatitis 1999;40(3):160–1.
9. Belsito DV, Fransway AF, Fowler JF Jr, Sherertz EF, Maibach HI, Mark JG Jr, Mathias CG, Rietschel RL, Storrs FJ, Nethercott JR. Allergic contact dermatitis to detergents: a multicenter study to assess prevalence. J Am Acad Dermatol 2002;46(2):200–6.
10. Su TC, Lin PH, Chiu MJ, Chu TS, Chang MJ, Wang JD, Cheng TJ. Dimethylacetamide, ethylenediamine, and

diphenylmethane diisocyanate poisoning manifest as acute psychosis and pulmonary edema: treatment with hemoperfusion. J Toxicol Clin Toxicol 2000;38(4):429–33.

11. Tanaka S, Otsuki T, Matsumoto Y, Hayakawa R, Sugiura M. Allergic contact dermatitis from enoxolone. Contact Dermatitis 2001;44(3):192.

12. Czop M, Herr DL. Green skin discoloration associated with multiple organ failure. Crit Care Med 2002;30(3):598–601.

13. Kurek M, Grubska-Suchanek E. Challenge tests with food additives and aspirin in the diagnosis of chronic urticaria. J Allergy Clin Immunol 2001;41:463–9.

14. Anonymous. Gamolenic acid. Withdrawal of marketing authorizations. WHO Pharmaceuticals Newslett 2002;4:2.

15. Gupta SK, Khan TI, Gupta RC, Gupta AB, Gupta KC, Jain P, Gupta A. Compensatory hyperparathyroidism following high fluoride ingestion — a clinico – biochemical correlation. Indian Pediatr 2001;38(2):139–46.

16. Gatchalian RA, Popli A, Ejaz AA, Leehey DJ, Kjellstrand CM, Ing TS. Management of hypophosphatemia induced by high-flux hemodiafiltration for the treatment of vancomycin toxicity: intravenous phosphorus therapy versus use of a phosphorus-enriched dialysate. Am J Kidney Dis 2000;36(6):1262–6.

17. Gousse AE, Safir MH, Madjar S, Ziadlourad F, Raz S. Life-threatening anaphylactoid reaction associated with indigo carmine intravenous injection. Urology 2000; 56(3):508.

18. Steurich F, Feyerabend R. Campari-/Karmin-/Cochenille-Allergie. Farbstoffe in Lebensuitteln, Medikamenten und Kosmetika. Allergologie 2001;24:66–72.

19. Cox NH, Duffey P, Royle J. Fixed drug eruption caused by lactose in an injected botulinum toxin preparation. J Am Acad Dermatol 1999;40(2 Pt 1):263–4.

20. Palm M, Moneret-Vautrin DA, Kanny G, Denery-Papini S, Fremont S. Food allergy to egg and soy lecithins. Allergy 1999;54(10):1116–17.

21. Anonymous. Lipokinetix. Reports of liver injury. WHO Pharmaceuticals Newslett 2002;1:3.

22. Tucker SC, Yell JA, Beck MH. Allergic contact dermatitis from sodium metabisulfite in Trimovate cream. Contact Dermatitis 1999;40(3):164.

23. Harrison DA, Smith AG. Concomitant sensitivity to sodium metabisulfite and clobetasone butyrate in Trimovate cream. Contact Dermatitis 2002;46(5):310.

24. Corazza M, Levratti A, Virgili A. Allergic contact dermatitis due to methyl glucose dioleate. Contact Dermatitis 2001;45(5):308.

25. Ringe JD, Kipshoven C, Coster A, Umbach R. Therapy of established postmenopausal osteoporosis with monofluorophosphate plus calcium: dose-related effects on bone density and fracture rate. Osteoporos Int 1999;9(2):171–8.

26. Hamen J, Wennig R. Diagnostic d'une intoxicaiton aiguë au Parathion et consequences medico-legales. Acta Clin Belg 1999;54:54–8.

27. Marques EGP, Oliveira MM, Monsanto PV, Proenca P, Castanheira F, Vieira DN. Parathion and acute intoxication. The importance of toxicological analytic tests. Z Zagodnien Nauk Sadowych 2000;43:157–63.

28. Anonymous. Excipients-review of adverse reactions. WHO Newsletter 1998;11/12:5.

29. Sugden P, Levy M, Rao GS. Onychocryptosis-phenol burn fiasco. Burns 2001;27(3):289–92.

30. Spencer K, Weinert L, Pentz WH. Calcified right atrial mass in a woman receiving long-term intravenous phosphate therapy. J Am Soc Echocardiogr 1999; 12(3):215–17.

31. Geukens J, Rabe E, Bieber T. Embolia cutis medicamentosa of the foot after sclerotherapy. Eur J Dermatol 1999;9(2):132–3.

32. Gallo R, Basso M, Voltolini S, Guarrera M. Allergic contact dermatitis from laureth-9 and polyquaternium-7 in a skincare product. Contact Dermatitis 2001;45(6):356–7.

33. Kimura M, Kawada A. Follicular contact dermatitis due to polyoxyethylene laurylether. J Am Acad Dermatol 2000;42(5 Pt 2):879–80.

34. Smith HR, Armstrong K, Wakelin SH, White IR. Contact allergy to PVP/eicosene copolymer. Contact Dermatitis 1999;40(5):283.

35. Stone N, Varma S, Hughes TM, Stone NM. Allergic contact dermatitis from polyvinylpyrrolidone (PVP)/1-triacontene copolymer in a sunscreen. Contact Dermatitis 2002; 47(1):49.

36. Parisi A, Alabiso A, Sacchetti M, Di Salvo V, Di Luigi L, Pigozzi F. Complex ventricular arrhythmia induced by overuse of potassium supplementation in a young male football player. Case report. J Sports Med Phys Fitness 2002; 42(2):214–16.

37. O'Donnell J. Drug-induced esophagitis. J Pharm Pract 2000;13:290–6.

38. Easton J, Noble S, Jarvis B. Rasburicase. Paediatr Drugs 2001;3(6):433–7.

39. Anonymous. Slim 10. Withdrawal due to presence of undeclared substances. WHO Pharmaceuticals Newslett 2002;4:5,

40. Anonymous. Sodium picosulfate. Reports of severe electrolyte disturbances. WHO Pharmaceuticals Newslett 2002;2:9.

41. Anonymous. Sodium prasterone sulfate: anaphylactoid reactions. WHO Newslett 2000;2:6.

42. Raison-Peyron N, Meynadier JM, Meynadier J. Sorbic acid: an unusual cause of systemic contact dermatitis in an infant. Contact Dermatitis 2000;43(4):247–8.

43. Yesudian PD, King CM. Allergic contact dermatitis from stearyl alcohol in Efudix cream. Contact Dermatitis 2001;45(5):313–14.

44. Gimenez J, Botella-Estrada R, Hernandez D, Carbonell M, Martinez MA, Guillen C, Vazquez C. Anaphylaxis after peritumoral injection of sulphan blue 1% for identification of the sentinel node in lymphatic mapping of the breast. Eur J Surg 2001;167(12):921–3.

45. Gutgesell C, Fuchs T. Orally elicited allergic contact dermatitis to tetraethylthiuramdisulfide. Am J Contact Dermat 2001;12(4):235–6.

46. Stea S, Visentin M, Granchi D, Savarino L, Dallari D, Gualtieri G, Rollo G, Toni A, Pizzoferrato A, Montanaro L. Sister chromatid exchange in patients with joint prostheses. J Arthroplasty 2000;15(6):772–7.

47. Mackey AC, Shaffer D, Prizont R. Seizure associated with the use of visicol for colonoscopy. N Engl J Med 2002;346(26):2095.

48. Munch IC, Hvolris JJ. Bodybuilding ved hjaelp af intramuskulaer injektion af valnoddeolie. [Body building aided by intramuscular injections of walnut oil.] Ugeskr Laeger 2001;163(48):6758.

49. Saary MJ, Holness DL. Contact dermatitis from white flower embrocation. Contact Dermatitis 2001;44(2):100.

50. Anonymous. Yasmin and venous thromboembolism. WHO Pharmaceuticals Newslett 2002;1:14.

Index of drug names

Notes, *see also* classes and specific drugs. **Boldface** page numbers refer to main discussions

Index of adverse reactions

A

abdominal discomfort
aminosalicylates, 141
antimalarials, 771
antimalarials + mefloquine, 2236
biguanides, 511
carnidazole, 675
difetarsone, 1124
fenfluramine, 1333
furazolidone, 1454
ibuprofen, 1710
ion exchange resins, 1903
lactulose, 2011
local anesthetics, 2120
losartan, 2168
mefloquine, 2234
methylphenidate, 2310
osmotic laxatives, 2011
oxamniquine, 2642
pefloxacin, 2727
plasma products, 2848
praziquantel, 2911, 2912
proguanil, 2937
Rhamnus purshianus, 3036
rosiglitazone, 3385
stimulant laxatives, 2009
tosufloxacin, 3468
typhoid vaccine, 3539
zidovudine, 3713

abdominal distension
albendazole, 50
fluphenazine, 1424
gemtuzumab ozogamicin, 1489
gold and gold salts, 1523
indometacin, 1742
itraconazole + vinca alkaloids, 3638
magnesium salts, 2197
mebendazole + albendazole, 2224
mefenamic acid, 2230
neuroleptics, 2466

abdominal distress
anticholinergics, 266
cocaine, 859

abdominal disturbance
ivermectin, 1949

abdominal fullness
protease inhibitors, 2968

abdominal pain
abacavir, 3
acamprosate, 9
acecainide, 10
aciclovir, 29
albendazole, 48, 49, 50
allopurinol + meglumine antimoniate, 317
alpha-glucosidase inhibitors, 85, 86
aminosalicylates, 138, 143

anthracyclines, 250
anthracyclines–liposomal formulations, 256
anti-CD4 monoclonal antibodies, 264
antimalarials, 771
antimonials, 317
artemisinin derivatives, 343
artesunate + lumefantrine, 343
atorvastatin, 366
atovaquone, 368
azathioprine, 378
baclofen, 411
barium sulfate, 414, 415
bephenium, 445
beta-lactam antibiotics, 483
beta-lactamase inhibitors, 503
bile acids, 515
bisacodyl, 2010
bismuth, 520
calcitonin, 596
carbomers, 2831
carbon dioxide, 642
Cassia species, 1311
celecoxib, 686
cephalosporins, 692
cibenzoline, 741
cimetidine, 776
cisapride, 789
clioquinol, 1575
clofazimine, 808
clometacin, 810
clopidogrel, 821
clotiapine, 822
clozapine, 831, 832
cocaine, 860, 862, 870
codeine, 880
colchicine, 883
Coriariaceae, 905
Corynebacterium parvum, 983
COX-2 inhibitors, 1006
Crotalaria species, 1313
Cyamopsis tetragonoloba, 1313
cyclofenil, 1024
deferiprone, 1056
desmopressin, 1076
dextrans, 1086
dextropropoxyphene, 1092
diacerein, 1094
dichlorophen, 1109
diltiazem, 1126
dimethylsulfoxide, 1131
dirithromycin, 1144
Dysosma pleianthum, 448
eflornithine, 1208
enalapril, 1212
enprostil, 1219
entacapone, 1220

Ephedra, 1223
ergot derivatives, 1230
erythromycin, 1237, 1239
esomeprazole, 1252
estrogen + progestogens, 1640
estrogens, 1269
etacrynic acid, 1275
ethambutol, 1283
ethanol, 1286
felbamate, 1329
flubendazole, 2223
fluconazole, 1378, 1380
fluorouracil, 1411
fluphenazine, 1424
flutamide, 1427
fosamprenavir, 211
fosmidomycin, 1451
gadolinium, 1473
galactose, 3543
gemifloxacin, 1487
gemtuzumab ozogamicin, 1488
glucocorticoids, 920, 943
glycol, 1519
gold and gold salts, 1524
gonadotropins, 1530, 1532
hexachlorophene, 1626
hormonal contraceptives–oral, 1655, 1659
ibuprofen, 1710
infliximab, 1749
interferon alfa, 1807
interleukin-1, 1842
intravenous immunoglobulin, 1720
iodinated contrast media, 1850, 1879, 1884
iron salts, 1912
itraconazole, 1933, 1937
itraconazole + vinca alkaloids, 3638
ivermectin, 1947, 1949
ketorolac, 1978
lactulose, 2012
lansoprazole, 2001
Larrea tridentata, 3733
lead, 2014, 2015
leflunomide, 2019
levofloxacin, 2048
lithium, 2083
macrolide antibiotics, 2185
Mandragora species, 3159
manganese, 2201
MDMA, 2301
mefenamic acid, 2231
mefloquine, 2234
melarsoprol, 2244
meloxicam, 2248
meptazinol, 2257
metformin, 507

iloprost, 1717

infliximab, 1747, 1749

insulin + meglitinides, 2241

iodinated contrast media, 1883

iron salts, 1916, 1917

lidocaine, 2055

manganese, 2201

MDMA, 2294, 2298, 2299

MDMA + MDMA hydrochloride, 2295

meglitinides + thiazolidinediones, 2240, 3382

melatonin, 2245

mesalazine, 140

mesulergine, 2267

minocycline, 2352

monosodium glutamate, 2383

muromonab-CD3, 2397

parenteral nutrition, 2716

protirelin, 2972

radiopharmaceuticals, 3018

remacemide, 3029

respiratory anesthesia, 2146

risperidone, 3054

sclerosants, 3107

sibutramine, 3131

silicone, 3139

streptogramins, 3182

streptokinase, 3405

talc, 3293

tobramycin, 3437

topoisomerase inhibitors, 3458

triptans, 3526

urokinase, 3406

zolmitriptan, 3525

chest pressure

clozapine, 828

chest tightness

aluminium, 98

anthracyclines–liposomal formulations, 258

baxiliximab, 418

beta$_2$-adrenoceptor agonists, 451

fibrates, 1359

intravenous immunoglobulin, 1720

liposomal amphotericin, 195

megestrol, 2932

nedocromil, 2429

pentagastrin, 2772

platinum-containing cytostatic drugs, 2862

St. John's wort, 842

triptans, 3526

vitamin K analogues, 3687

chest wall rigidity

fentanyl, 1347

fentanyl + midazolam, 1353, 2340

opioid analgesics, 2626

remifentanil, 3032

sufentanil, 3212

chewing

haloperidol, 2457

methylphenidate, 2308

chewing difficulty

nicotine replacement therapy, 2510

Cheyne-Stokes respiration

diamorphine, 1098

lithium, 2078

Lobelia inflata, 612

topical salicylates, 3099

chills

aldesleukin, 58, 60

amphetamines, 187

amphotericin, 193, 197, 198, 200, 1378

amphotericin B colloidal dispersion, 193

amphotericin deoxycholate, 193

amphotericin lipid complex, 195

Anacardiaceae, 215

androgens and anabolic steroids, 220

anthracyclines–liposomal formulations, 258

anthrax vaccine, 260

anti-CD4 monoclonal antibodies, 263

antilymphocyte immunoglobulin, 1724

bleomycin, 529

bone marrow transplantation, 533

calcium channel blockers, 601

catheters, 680

chlorzoxazone, 736

Corynebacterium parvum, 983

diethylcarbamazine, 1115

etherified starches, 1287

ganciclovir, 1480

gentamicin, 1502

granulocyte-macrophage colony-stimulating factor, 1553

guanethidine, 2595

heparins, 1595

ibritumomab, 1709

immunoglobulin, 1724

infliximab, 1747

interferon, 1841

interferon alfa, 1794

interferon alfa + carmustine, 1818

interleukin-1, 1842

interleukin-3, 1843

intravenous immunoglobulin, 1720, 1725

iodinated contrast media, 1854, 1855

iron salts, 1912, 1917

ivermectin, 1947, 1949

lentinan, 2024

liposomal amphotericin, 194, 195

macrophage colony-stimulating factor (M-CSF), 2195

miconazole, 2336

misoprostol, 2357

monoclonal antibodies, 2381

muromonab-CD3, 2397

nitrofurantoin, 2542

pentoxifylline, 2780

phenytoin, 2815

PIXY321, 1844

propylhexedrine, 2954

prostaglandins, 2959

pyrimethamine + sulfadoxine, 2987

quinine, 3003, 3005

rifampicin, 3041

rituximab, 3070

rosiglitazone, 3385

smallpox vaccine, 3151

streptogramins, 3182

sulindac, 3243

suramin, 3252

teicoplanin, 3306, 3307

terconazole, 303

thrombolytic agents, 3405

tiabendazole, 3417

Ting kung teng, 1616

topoisomerase inhibitors, 3460

triclabendazole, 3489

vancomycin, 3594, 3596, 3599

yohimbine, 3704

Chinese herb nephropathy

Aristolochia species, 336

Chinese restaurant syndrome

monosodium glutamate, 2383

Chlamydia **infection**

hormonal contraceptives–oral, 1644

chloasma (melasma)

estrogens, 1257

hormonal contraceptives–oral, 1661

hormonal replacement therapy–estrogens, 1687

spironolactone, 3177

choanal atresia

thionamides, 3392

choking sensation

anthracyclines–liposomal formulations, 258

cholangiocarcinoma

thorotrast, 3401

cholangiolitis

kebuzone, 1964

cholangitis

carbamazepine, 631

MDMA, 2301

nicotinic acid and derivatives, 2513

penicillins, 2760

sulindac, 3243, 3245

cholecystitis

aldesleukin, 63

bismuth, 520

floxuridine, 1138

thiazide diuretics, 3377

choledochal sphincter spasm

morphine, 2388

cholelithiasis

ciclosporin, 749

hormonal contraceptives–oral, 1659

parenteral nutrition, 2709

somatostatin, 3161

cholera-like syndrome

eflornithine, 1208

melarsoprol, 2244

Eucalyptus species, 2411
pancuronium bromide, 2672
tubocurarine, 3533
hypovitaminosis C
aldesleukin, 62
hypovolemia
arsenic, 341
hypovolemic shock
azathioprine, 378
thiacetazone, 3371
hypoxemia
acrylic bone cement, 33
aldesleukin, 61
amphotericin lipid complex, 194
atracurium, 371
busulfan, 578
calcium channel blockers, 600
emetine, 1904
epidural anesthesia, 2128
epoprostenol, 1228
gonadorelin, 1532
interferon gamma, 1839
isoprenaline, 1920
lidocaine, 2055
melphalan, 2250
midazolam, 2338
naproxen, 2428
olanzapine, 2608
organic nitrates, 2531
phenytoin, 2814
pranlukast, 2909
retinoids, 3657
salbutamol, 3093
talc, 3293
vancomycin, 3601
hypoxia
alphaprodine, 90
amphotericin, 199
amphotericin B colloidal dispersion, 193
barium sulfate, 415
benzocaine, 428
beta$_2$-adrenoceptor agonists, 448
bone marrow transplantation, 533
brachial plexus anesthesia, 2122
dapsone, 1051
deferoxamine, 1059
diazepam + pethidine, 2791
diphenoxylate, 805, 1136
fenbufen, 1332
fentanyl, 1352
general anesthetics, 1496
granulocyte-macrophage colony-stimulating factor, 1553
itraconazole + vinca alkaloids, 3638
local anesthetics, 2118
MDMA, 2293, 2296, 2303
midazolam + opiates, 2338
mitomycin, 2361
opioid analgesics, 2622
parenteral nutrition, 2701
peribulbar anesthesia, 2143
retinoids, 3656
rituximab, 3069

thiamine, 3372
zanamivir, 2436
zolpidem, 3726
hysterical reactions to dreams
doxapram, 1187

I

ichthyosiform contact dermatitis
cetrimonium bromide, 704
ichthyosiform eruption
lovastatin, 2172
ichthyosis
clofazimine, 808
nicotinic acid and derivatives, 2514
ichtyosiform desquamation
maprotiline, 2205
icteric hepatitis
niflumic acid, 2523
icterus
see jaundice
idiopathic fetal loss
neuroleptics, 2468
idiopathic pneumonia syndrome
busulfan, 578
IgA deficiency
penicillamine, 2743
IgA depression
phenytoin, 2816
ileitis
glucocorticoids, 919
lamotrigine, 1996
ileum necrosis
retinoids, 3660
ileus
Cytisus scoparius, 1313
iodinated contrast media, 1866, 1880
ivermectin, 1952
mycophenolate mofetil, 2402
ileus, postoperative
dextrans, 1086
illusions
mescaline, 2266
zaleplon, 3711
imbalance
amphetamines, 182
gentamicin, 1501
haloperidol, 1579
immune complex disease
intravenous immunoglobulin, 1724
immune complex glomerulonephritis
sulfonylureas, 3235
immune complex vasculitis
cell therapy, 892
immunosuppression
cannabinoids, 620
parenteral nutrition, 2713
phenols, 2802
pyrimethamine + dapsone, 2987
imperforate anus
beta-lactam antibiotics, 491

thalidomide, 3351
thionamides, 3392
implant expulsion
hormonal contraceptives–progestogen implants, 1681
implant extrusion
androgens and anabolic steroids, 221
implant failure
cobalt, 848
impotence
aldosterone receptor antagonist, 1155
aminosalicylates, 143
antiepileptics, 279
beta-adrenoceptor agonists, 463, 467
bromocriptine, 560
carbonic anhydrase inhibitors, 643
Celastraceae, 683
cimetidine, 776
dextromethorphan, 1089
disopyramide, 1146
diuretics, 1161–1162
estrogens, 1268
fenfluramines, 1340
fibrates, 1360
flecainide, 1373
gonadorelin, 1530
histamine H$_2$ receptor agonists, 1630
hydroxyprogesterone caproate, 2931
indometacin, 1741
interferon alfa, 1812
interferon gamma, 1839
itraconazole, 1936
lidocaine, 2055
MAO inhibitors, 2372, 2374
medroxyprogesterone, 2227
methanthelinium, 2276
methotrexate, 2283
naproxen, 2428
nitrous oxide, 2551
phenoxybenzamine, 2803
propafenone, 2941
ranitidine hydrochloride, 3024
reboxetine, 3028
risperidone, 2446, 3052
statins, 1634
thiazide diuretics, 3377
thioridazine, 3398
impulsivity
cannabinoids, 621
inadvertent intra-arterial injection
temazepam, 3312
inarticulate vocalization
olanzapine, 2603
inattention
cannabinoids, 621
incoherence
valaciclovir, 3576
zolpidem, 3726
incontinence
acivicin, 32
amphotericin, 200

sulfasalazine, 140
topiramate, 3448
yohimbine, 3704
Raynaud's syndrome
amphotericin, 200
Aristolochia species, 337
bromocriptine, 559
stellate ganglion anesthesia, 2147
reaction time reduction
general anesthetics, 1494
reactive arthritis
hepatitis B vaccine, 1600, 1606
reading difficulty
remifentanil, 3032
rebound congestion
propylhexedrine, 2954
rectal bleeding
anti-CD4 monoclonal antibodies, 264
beta-lactam antibiotics, 483
celecoxib, 686
estrogens, 1256
gold and gold salts, 1524
ketoprofen, 1977
tenoxicam, 3314
rectal irritation
phenylbutazone, 2806
rectal necrosis
phosphates, 2821
rectal pain
ferristene, 1910
ibuproxam, 1713
rectal stenosis
ergot derivatives, 1232
rectal stricture
acetylsalicylic acid, 20
red cell aplasia
gonadorelin, 1531
oxazolidinones, 2645
red eye syndrome
leukodepleted blood products, 532
red man syndrome
rifampicin, 3043
teicoplanin, 3307
vancomycin, 3306, 3594, 3599, 3601
redness
see erythema
red reflex reduction
retrobulbar anesthesia, 2143
reflex sympathetic dystrophy
diamorphine, 1097
reflux
formaldehyde, 1440
reflux esophagitis
clozapine, 831
refractile opacity
tamoxifen, 3298
regenerative hyperplasia
see liver tumor
regional pain syndrome
glucocorticoids, 943
regurgitation
guar gum, 1562
suxamethonium, 3264

Reiter's syndrome
Bacille Calmette-Guérin vaccine, 397
hepatitis B vaccine, 1602
interferon alfa, 1810
REM sleep
nefazodone, 2430
renal
see also entries at kidney –; nephr–
renal adenocarcinoma
cyclophosphamide, 1028
renal artery stenosis
iodinated contrast media, 1868
renal artery thrombosis
iloprost, 1716
renal calcinosis
corticotrophins, 981
renal calculus
see kidney stone
renal cancer
acetylsalicylic acid, 23
diuretics, 1162–1163
Larrea tridentata, 3733
NSAIDs, 2572
paracetamol, 2684–2685
renal colic
benzbromarone, 423
indinavir, 1736, 1738
sulfonamides, 3220
renal cortical necrosis
tranexamic acid, 3477
renal dysfunction
aprotinin, 331
benzyl alcohol, 445
gabapentin, 1467
lamotrigine, 1996
melarsoprol, 2244
polysorbate 80, 3678
quinine, 3005
renal dysgenesis
indometacin, 1742
renal fibrosis
Aristolochia species, 337
renal function abnormality
indinavir, 1736
renal graft rejection
interferon alfa, 1809
renal impairment
ACE inhibitors, 228, 230, 232
ACE inhibitors + metformin, 1743
aciclovir, 30
chloroxylenol, 731
diclofenac + triamterene, 1111
formaldehyde, 1440
ganciclovir, 1480
lithium, 2087
MDMA + amphetamine, 2293
valaciclovir, 3577
renal infarction
cocaine, 861
renal injury
phenols, 2800
renal insufficiency
ACE inhibitors, 228

ACE inhibitors + furosemide, 1457
ACE inhibitors + spironolactone, 3178
acetylsalicylic acid, 21–22
Aesculus species, 1628
Aesculus species + aminoglycoside antibiotics, 1628
alemtuzumab, 71
allopurinol, 80
aloe, 84
aminocaproic acid, 115
aminoglycosides + cephalosporin, 128
aminoglycosides + gallium, 1478
aminoglycosides + ibuprofen, 1712
aminophenazone, 136
aminosalicylates, 143
amoxapine, 180
amphotericin, 193, 197, 1378
androgens and anabolic steroids, 220
antituberculars, 322
aprotinin, 332
Aristolochia species, 336, 337
azithromycin, 391
Bacille Calmette-Guérin vaccine, 397
baclofen, 410
benoxaprofen, 421
beta-adrenoceptor agonists, 456
bismuth, 520, 521
bone marrow transplantation, 533
Callilepis laureola, 363
captopril, 626
carbamazepine, 631
carboplatin, 2861
carp bile, 238
carvedilol, 677
Chelidonium majus, 2677
cholera vaccine, 736
chromium, 739
ciclosporin, 750–752, 756
cidofovir, 771
cimetidine, 775
ciprofibrate + ibuprofen, 1360
ciprofloxacin, 784, 785
clometacin, 810
clozapine, 832
cocaine, 860, 872
contrast media + metformin, 512
copper, 904
co-triamterzide + ketoprofen, 1978
coumarin anticoagulants, 985
COX-2 inhibitors, 1008
dapsone, 1051
deferiprone, 1055
deferoxamine, 1059, 1062
dextrans, 1083–1084
dextrans + radiocontrast media, 1087
diamorphine, 1097
diclofenac, 1110
diethylene glycol, 1517
dihydrocodeine, 1125
diltiazem, 1126
diuretics + tetracyclines, 3338
edetic acid, 1200
enalapril, 1212

3956 **Index of adverse reactions**

W